# TUMORS *and* TUMOROUS CONDITIONS *of the* BONES *and* JOINTS

By

Henry L. Jaffe, M.D.

*Director of Laboratories and Pathologist, Hospital for Joint Diseases, New York, N. Y., Consultant, Armed Forces Institute of Pathology, Washington, D. C.*

*701 Illustrations on 194 Figures*

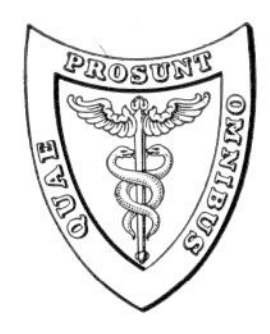


Lea & Febiger

Philadelphia

Reprinted
March, 1959
September, 1961
September, 1964
November, 1968

Library of Congress Catalogue Card Number: 58-7269

Printed in the United States of America

TO MY WIFE

CLARISSE K. JAFFE

WITH AFFECTION AND GRATITUDE

# Preface

THIS book is intended to present an integrated account of the tumors and tumorous conditions affecting the bones and joints. The clinical, roentgenographic, and pathologic findings pertaining to the various lesions are discussed and correlated. Facts about the clinical findings are given with attention to their value in narrowing down the diagnostic possibilities. The roentgenographic appearance presented by a particular lesion is explained as much as possible in terms of the actual gross anatomic changes. In addition, the microscopic findings will often be found coordinated with the gross findings and sometimes even with the roentgenographic reflections of the latter. On the other hand, in regard to the pathologic findings, an effort has been made to avoid distorting the account as a whole by an excess of histologic detail relating to the lesion. Altogether, the presentations have been guided by the idea that the problems of diagnosis and differential diagnosis raised by the skeletal tumors can best be met if, in the interpretation of a given lesion, its clinical, roentgenographic, and pathologic features are considered and evaluated together. In regard to treatment, attention is devoted mainly to the choice of procedure appropriate for each condition.

In the past, the author (alone or with colleagues) has contributed various articles to the periodical literature on the subject of the skeletal tumors. However, this book represents a fresh presentation, written in continuity. In the exposition of the various lesions, a great deal of reliance has been placed on the illustrative material. The illustrations have been arranged on full-page plates to permit the simultaneous display of a number of pictures for purposes of comparison. The accompanying legends give details about each illustration, and many of them embody sufficient information to constitute case histories. Indeed, though integrated with the text, the illustrations and their legends compose in themselves something like an atlas of the skeletal tumors.

In large measure, this book conveys the author's personal conceptions of the lesions discussed. Due cognizance has, of course, been taken of the work of others in the field, and many key articles have been mentioned. However, the pertinent literature is vast, and it has not been found practical to give detailed citations from it. In any event, it is hoped that pathologists, radiologists, and orthopedic surgeons will find the book useful in their work, and that it will also be of interest to other colleagues who are confronted from time to time by problems relating to skeletal tumors.

Throughout the composition of this book, I have had the unflagging assistance of Miss E. Marion Pilpel, who has worked closely with me for the past twenty-five years. The preparation of the manuscript for the press has received the meticulous and unstinting care of Miss Edith Ross. To both Miss Pilpel and Miss Ross I am also indebted for their aid in the correction of the proof and preparation of the index.

For the preparation of many of the gross specimens for photography and detailed study, my thanks are due to my associate, Dr. Golden Selin, who has shown special ingenuity in this connection. The tissue sections from which the photomicrographs were made represent the skilled work of Mrs. Rose Afford. Practically all of the illustrations were made by Mr. Julius Weber, who spared no effort in their production. I also wish to express my gratitude to the many colleagues in the Hospital for Joint Diseases and elsewhere who have so kindly permitted me to draw upon their experience and material relating to individual cases. Finally, it is a pleasure to acknowledge the patience and cooperation received from the publishers during the years in which this book was being planned and written.

Henry L. Jaffe

New York, N. Y.

# Contents


| CHAPTER | | PAGE |
|---|---|---|
| 1. | Introduction: Problems of Classification and Diagnosis | 9 |
| 2. | Giant-Cell Tumor | 18 |
| 3. | Benign Chondroblastoma | 44 |
| 4. | Aneurysmal Bone Cyst | 54 |
| 5. | Solitary Bone Cyst | 63 |
| 6. | Fibrous Cortical Defect and Non-ossifying Fibroma | 76 |
| 7. | Osteoid-Osteoma | 92 |
| 8. | Benign Osteoblastoma | 107 |
| 9. | Fibrous Dysplasia | 117 |
| 10. | Solitary and Multiple Osteocartilaginous Exostosis | 143 |
| 11. | Solitary Enchondroma and Multiple Enchondromatosis | 169 |
| 12. | Juxtacortical Chondroma | 196 |
| 13. | Chondromyxoid Fibroma | 203 |
| 14. | Adamantinoma of Limb Bones | 213 |
| 15. | Benign Vascular Tumors | 224 |
| 16. | Bone Lesions Associated with Neural Tumors | 240 |
| 17. | Osteogenic Sarcoma | 256 |
| 18. | Juxtacortical Osteogenic Sarcoma | 279 |
| 19. | Desmoplastic Fibroma and Fibrosarcoma | 298 |
| 20. | Chondrosarcoma | 314 |

Contents

CHAPTER PAGE

21. Malignant Vascular Tumors . . . . . . . . . . . . . . . . 341

22. Ewing's Sarcoma . . . . . . . . . . . . . . . . . . . 350

23. Myelomatosis (Multiple Myeloma) . . . . . . . . . . . . 369

24. Leukemia and Lymphoma . . . . . . . . . . . . . . . 396

25. Lesions Peculiar to the Jawbones . . . . . . . . . . . . 425

26. Chordoma . . . . . . . . . . . . . . . . . . . . . . 451

27. Tumors Developing at Sites of Pre-existing Bone Disease . . . . 463

28. Radiation Injury and Postradiation Sarcoma of Bones . . . . . . 479

29. Tumors Invading Bones from Overlying Soft Parts . . . . . . . 502

30. Pigmented Villonodular Synovitis, Bursitis and Tenosynovitis . . . 532

31. Synovial Chondromatosis and Other Benign Articular Tumors . . . 558

32. Synovial Sarcoma and Other Malignant Articular Tumors . . . . 576

33. Tumors Metastatic to the Skeleton . . . . . . . . . . . . 589

Chapter

# 1

# Introduction

In this chapter we shall consider questions relating to: the classification of the skeletal tumors; the matter of how their diagnosis should be approached; and the obtainment and interpretation of pertinent biopsy specimens.

## CLASSIFICATION

The tumors of the bones and joints make up a large and intriguing group of lesions. Their scope is indicated by the listing given below. This has been made on the basis of the different ways by which tumors (in the broadest sense of the term) may come to occur in the skeleton.

Tumors Developing as Primary Lesions in Bones
Tumors Developing at Sites of Pre-existing Bone Disease
Tumors Developing at Sites of Damage to Bone from Ionizing Radiation
Tumors Invading Bones from Overlying Soft Parts
Tumors Developing as Primary Lesions in Joints and Related Structures
Tumors Metastatic to the Skeleton

When the diagnostic problem relating to an individual skeletal tumor first presents itself, it is useful to keep such a comprehensive listing in mind. If one does this, one can often avoid the common error of concluding too hastily in a given case that the lesion in question is necessarily a primary bone tumor. However, the variety of the primary bone tumors (that is, the large number of different clinicopathologic entities composing the group) makes that group the one around which attention has largely centered. It also accounts for the fact that the schemata of classification in general use do not encompass the full scope of the skeletal tumors, but pertain mainly to the primary bone tumors.

The first systematic classification (at least in this country) of the tumors primary in bones was that proposed by the Registry of Bone Sarcoma of the American College of Surgeons. The Committee of the Registry (whose original members were Ewing, Codman, and Bloodgood) was formed to deal with the confusing nomenclature existing around 1920. If one studies the summarizing report of 1925 by Codman, one cannot fail to be impressed by the complexity of the Committee's task and by the advancement already represented by its original classification. Codman stressed the idea that the Committee's proposals would, of necessity, require modification as the understanding of skeletal tumors advanced. In 1939, Ewing published an official revision of the Registry's classification. This revision has undergone further modifications by others, but still constitutes the core of many of these later versions. For this reason, and also because it is of historic interest, the Registry's classification of 1939 is reproduced below.

REGISTRY'S REVISED CLASSIFICATION

| | *Malignant* | *Benign* |
|---|---|---|
| Osteogenic series | Osteogenic sarcoma<br>Medullary and subperiosteal<br>Telangiectatic<br>Sclerosing<br>Periosteal<br>Fibrosarcoma<br>(*a*) Medullary<br>(*b*) Periosteal<br>Parosteal, capsular | Exostosis<br>Osteoma |
| Chondroma series | Chondrosarcoma<br>Myxosarcoma | Chondroma |
| Giant cell tumor series | Malignant | Epiphyseal giant cell tumor |
| Angioma series | Angioendothelioma<br>Diffuse endothelioma | Cavernous angioma<br>Plexiform angioma |
| Myeloma series | Plasma cell<br>Myelocytoma<br>Erythroblastoma<br>Lymphocytoma | |
| Reticulum cell lymphosarcoma | | |
| Liposarcoma | | |

The modifications embodied in the classification proposed by Phemister in 1949 took cognizance of new concepts (many in line with the writer's published views) which had already evolved in the field of the bone tumors. These modifications included specifically: a stricter interpretation of what should be called a giant-cell tumor; the abolition of the many subtypes of osteogenic sarcoma; the transfer of fibrosarcoma from the osteogenic sarcoma category to an independent status; the reduction of the myeloma series to the so-called plasma cell myeloma alone; and formal recognition of the doubts that the Ewing sarcoma was a tumor derived from vascular endothelium, and classification of it as a tumor apparently derived from primitive mesenchymal cells instead.

PHEMISTER'S CLASSIFICATION

| *Tissue* | *Benign* | *Malignant* |
|---|---|---|
| Bone | Exostosis, osteoma | Osteogenic or osteosarcoma |
| Cartilage | Chondroma<br>hyaline<br>chondroblastoma | Chondrosarcoma |
| Fibroblast | Fibroma | Fibrosarcoma |
| Giant-cell | Benign giant-cell tumor | Giant-cell sarcoma |
| Vascular | Hemangioma<br>cavernous<br>organoid | Hemangioendothelioma<br>(Ewing's sarcoma?)<br>Cavernous angiosarcoma |
| Marrow | | Solitary myeloma and<br>multiple myelomas |
| Reticulo-endothelial | (?) | Reticulum-cell sarcoma |
| Lymphatic | (?) | Lymphosarcoma |
| Fatty | Lipoma (?) | Liposarcoma (?) |
| Undifferentiated-cell (mesenchyme) | (?) | Mesenchymal-cell sarcoma<br>(Ewing's sarcoma?) |

In both the Registry's and Phemister's classification (as in most of the more recent classifications founded upon them), the primary bone tumors are arranged in groups or series on the basis of the fundamental cell or tissue type, under the two general captions "Benign" and "Malignant." While the writer recognizes that classifying them in this manner has some value for general orientation, the practical utility of such classifications is open to question. Actually, the individual primary bone tumors are brought into sharper focus, and certain confusions about them are avoided, if one considers them outside of the framework of such classifications and views them simply as clinicopathologic entities. Toward the delimitation of these entities, the clinical findings, the roentgenographic picture, and the dominant histologic pattern all contribute.

For instance, if chondroma and chondrosarcoma are juxtaposed as the representatives of the cartilage series of tumors, one is merely contrasting the fundamentally benign with the malignant cartilage tumors. There is nothing in such an alignment to indicate that the essentially benign cartilage tumors include both solitary chondroma (enchondroma) and multiple enchondromatosis, which differ so importantly in regard to their clinical and roentgenographic aspects, as well as, incidentally, in regard to certain nuances in the histologic picture. Furthermore, in addition to the benign and malignant central cartilage tumors, there are benign and malignant cartilage tumors which develop in relation to the periosteum and which may be designated as juxtacortical chondroma and juxtacortical chondrosarcoma. Altogether, little is contributed to the understanding of the various cartilage tumors by considering them merely as members of a "cartilage series" of tumors. Furthermore, the restrictiveness of this type of classification invites the arbitrary placement of certain lesions in one category or another. Thus, in some of the more recent classifications based on tissue type, benign chondroblastoma and even chondromyxoid fibroma are forced into the category of the cartilage growths. Actually, as was brought out in the original descriptions of these lesions, they are not exactly cartilage tumors, despite the implication of "cartilage" in their names.

Let us now consider the conventional classification of lesions which have osseous tissue as an essential constituent. For example, one commonly finds exostosis and osteogenic sarcoma juxtaposed as the benign and malignant forms of the "bone" or "osteogenic" series of lesions. The alignment of these two lesions in this way implies a relationship which actually does not exist and obscures fundamental differences between them. An osteogenic sarcoma represents a bone-forming connective-tissue sarcoma. On the other hand, it is only in a superficial sense that a solitary exostosis (osteocartilaginous exostosis) is a tumor at all. Actually, it represents the expression of a developmental aberration of periosteal activity. Also, if one lists exostosis alone as the benign form in the "osteogenic" series of lesions, cognizance is not being taken of hereditary multiple exostosis. Though the latter bears a pathologic kinship to solitary exostosis, it reveals itself as a strikingly different disorder when viewed in its entirety as a clinicopathologic complex.

Still another illustration of difficulty which may arise from classification on the basis of fundamental tissue or cell type appears in connection with lesions containing multinuclear giant cells. The true giant-cell tumor of bone stands apart as a clinicopathologic complex from all the other lesions in which one may find multinuclear giant cells. It should not be classified even in the most general way with such other lesions containing giant cells as the fibrous cortical defect, the non-ossifying fibroma, and the giant-cell reparative granuloma. To avoid an alignment which invites confusion among the various lesions containing multinuclear giant cells is important both theoretically and practically.

These examples may suffice to indicate why a more dynamic approach to the primary bone tumors is attained if one turns away from the conventional classifications and considers each type of lesion as a clinicopathologic entity in its own right. The advantage of this approach is illustrated when one considers juxtacortical osteogenic sarcoma in relation to the common form of osteogenic sarcoma. It is now generally recognized that an osteogenic sarcoma which starts in the interior of a bone (the common form) represents a clinicopathologic entity entirely different from the so-called juxtacortical (or parosteal) osteogenic sarcoma. The latter, while a bone-forming sarcoma, is at first merely oriented to the regional bone in the sense of starting just beyond the confines of the cortex, though later the tumor may erode the cortex of the regional bone and even invade the marrow cavity. The juxtacortical osteogenic sarcoma and the common central osteogenic sarcoma also differ in respect to age incidence and clinical course. Indeed, the former has a much more favorable prognosis than the central osteogenic sarcoma, and even on this basis alone should be held apart from the latter.

Finally, let us consider fibrous dysplasia of bone. This is a lesion in which the basic tissue is a mixture of bone-forming connective tissue and osseous tissue in varying proportions. Should such a lesion be encompassed in the "osteogenic" series of lesions or placed among the "fibrous" lesions? Actually, it does not belong in either category. On the other hand, as a clinicopathologic entity it stands our as a condition which may occur in one, several, or many bones and which may to may not be associated with abnormal pigmentation and/or endocrine disorders.

## DIAGNOSTIC APPROACH

When one is viewing the primary tumors and tumor-like lesions of bone as clinicopathologic entities, the clinical findings are helpful in narrowing down the diagnostic possibilities in accordance with the age of the patient, the duration of the complaints, the particular bone or bone area affected, *etc.* The roentgenographic picture is more directly helpful. Indeed, one may well regard the latter as a sort of blueprint (sometimes sketchy and sometimes quite elaborate) of the gross pathology of the lesion. Specifically, the roentgenographic picture: (1) reveals where the lesion is located in relation to the bone as a whole; (2) shows what the lesional tissue has done to the original osseous tissue at the site of development of the tumor; (3) indicates any response which the lesion may be provoking in the perilesional bone area; and (4) often permits one to deduce a good deal of information about the gross character of the lesional tissue itself.

In regard to the original osseous tissue, the *x*-ray picture may show, for instance, "mottled" rarefaction indicating that that tissue is undergoing spotty dissolution. Or perhaps instead, one may find large individual foci of radiolucency reflecting mass dissolution of cortex and/or spongy trabeculæ. As to the perilesional response, this too varies with the nature of the provoking condition. The periphery of a lesion may be rather vague or, on the contrary, may reveal so-called "margination" indicating reactive densification of the perilesional osseous tissue. Then again, the roentgenograph may show that the presence of the lesion is associated with subperiosteal new bone deposition, while another lesion may give no evidence of such a reaction. In respect to the lesional tissue proper, the extent to which the *x*-ray picture shows radiopacity, for instance, represents the extent to which that tissue has undergone calcification and/or ossification.

The histologic tissue pattern remains, of course, the decisive factor in the diagnostic interpretation of any particular lesion. However, in evaluating the pattern in a given case, judgment should be based on the dominant histologic appearances, as determined by examination of tissue areas from various parts of the lesion. One should recognize the subordinate character of local variations in the total histologic pattern, and also the fact that, here and there in the lesion, tissue elements may be encountered which are not indigenous to it.

In illustration of these general histologic facts, let us consider a tissue section prepared from the actively growing peripheral portion of an osteogenic sarcoma of the common type. In such a section the tissue may be found to be composed largely of cartilage. If it is, and if undue diagnostic importance is attached to this finding, the lesion might be mistakenly interpreted as a chondrosarcoma instead of an osteogenic sarcoma. This mistaken impression may already be controverted by reference to the roentgenographic appearance of the lesion. Furthermore, the age of the patient is also an important consideration. If the subject is an older child or an adolescent, the great likelihood is that the lesion is an osteogenic sarcoma despite the impression created by the tissue section. Indeed, late childhood and adolescence is the period during which osteogenic sarcoma usually appears, except when it occurs as a complication of Paget's disease—a disorder rarely noted in persons under 40 years of age. Chondrosarcoma, in contrast to osteogenic sarcoma occurring *de novo,* appears mainly in persons of middle age, although occasionally it does occur in a young person. Of course, if the lesion is an osteogenic sarcoma, tissue sections taken from other parts of it will show the pattern which is characteristic of that tumor. That is, it will present the pattern of a sarcomatous connective-tissue growth in which the malignant stromal cells have osteogenic potentialities, as demonstrated by the presence of tumor osteoid and tumor bone.

To take another example, the value of correlating the impression gained from the histologic pattern with the clinical and *x*-ray findings stands out rather well in relation to the diagnosis of giant-cell tumor of bone. If one is dealing with a lesion thought to be a giant-cell tumor on the basis of the histologic findings, and if the clinical and *x*-ray findings deviate from those characteristic for that condition, the histologic findings should be re-evaluated in the light of these discrepancies. Consider, for example, a case in which the patient is a child or adolescent and in which the lesion, while in a long bone, is located in the shaft of the bone (somewhat eccentrically) and does not involve the epiphysial end of the bone. In such a case, even if the histologic tissue findings might lead one to conclude that the lesion was a giant-cell tumor, the great likelihood is that one is actually dealing with a non-ossifying fibroma. Indeed, a giant-cell tumor rarely occurs in persons under 20 years of age and nearly always involves the actual epiphysial end of the bone, along with some part of the adjacent metaphysis. Furthermore, the eccentrically located shaft lesion in question is likely to appear rather "loculated" and clearly marginated in the *x*-ray picture. When one once questions the histologic diagnosis in the light of these other findings and re-examines the tissue sections, certain details will now stand out which will turn one away from the diagnosis of giant-cell tumor toward that of non-ossifying fibroma. In particular, it will be noted that the multinuclear giant cells are small, sparse, and often concentrated about small areas of hemorrhage. Furthermore, the stromal cells will be found to differ from the stromal cells of a typical giant-cell tumor in that they are smaller, more drawn out, and often arranged in interlacing bundles.

These examples will probably suffice to make clear the necessity of bringing to the diagnosis of the bone tumors the light which can be shed jointly by the disciplines of radiology, pathology, and surgery. Moving forward in line with this approach, it appears to the writer, however, that, in evaluating a particular lesion, we should try to achieve something more than a collection of individual, compartmented opinions representing strictly each of these three disciplines. That is, we should strive for something more than a joint picture to which each person contributes from his point of view alone, as illustrated by the following diagram.

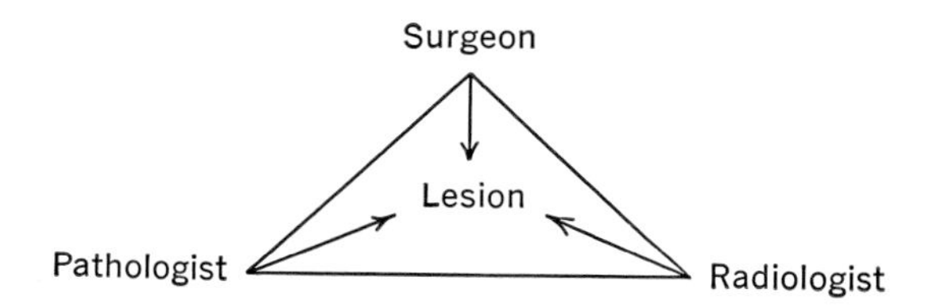


That type of cooperative approach, while valuable and creditable, is still not the one most likely to lead us out of diagnostic blind alleys. Let us suppose, for instance, that we are dealing with a benign chondroblastoma in the upper end of a humerus. The radiologist might have called it a Codman tumor—that is, a benign chondroblastoma. The surgeon, impressed by the gross appearance of the tissue encountered in the course of biopsy or curettage of the lesion, might think he was dealing with an ordinary cartilage tumor. The pathologist, struck particularly by the multinuclear giant cells in the tissue sections, might wish to designate the lesion as a giant-cell tumor. Unless such disparate opinions are integrated by being made to shed light on each other, the case will not have yielded its full meaning to any of the three persons concerned with it.

In fact, overemphasis on different individual aspects of a lesion may lead to entirely unnecessary confusion about the diagnosis. This is avoided when one sees each feature in its total setting, recognizing, for instance, that a benign chondroblastoma may show multinuclear giant cells (perhaps quite a few in some areas) and that, on the other hand, in tissue areas which have become calcified, the lesion may be quite gritty and suggest an ordinary cartilage tumor.

Accordingly, it seems to the writer that anyone concerned with the bone tumors should try to achieve what one may call a tridimensional view of them. This is possible only to the extent to which the surgeon, the radiologist or the pathologist, individually, is able to view the diagnostic problem not only from his angle, but from that of the other two. (See diagram below.)

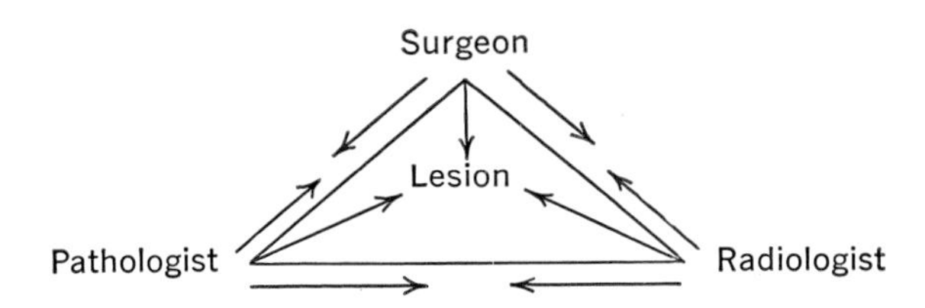


Thus, a pathologist attempting to interpret a particular bone tumor will be functioning best if his approach to its pathologic aspects is made in the light of a personal understanding of its roentgenographic and clinical setting. Conversely, the greater the extent to which the surgeon or the radiologist can interpret the clinical and *x*-ray findings presented by a given bone tumor against the background of bone tumor pathology, the better will he be equipped to avoid the pitfalls in bone tumor diagnosis. Even such an approach cannot abolish all diagnostic errors, but it can certainly make them fewer and less glaring.

## REMARKS ON THE BIOPSY

A biopsy should be regarded as a final diagnostic procedure and should not be lightly undertaken as a mere short cut to diagnosis. In any event, it should be preceded by a careful evaluation of the clinical history, a painstaking physical examination, analytic study of the pertinent *x*-ray pictures, and the consideration of any relevant hematologic and chemical laboratory data. If the information obtainable from the clinical, laboratory, and *x*-ray findings is thoughtfully correlated, this information suffices surprisingly often for the establishment of the diagnosis. Nevertheless, a biopsy is sometimes indicated to confirm the diagnosis reached on this basis. It usually permits a definitive diagnosis if the latter is not clear from these findings. It is certainly indicated in all cases in which an amputation or other radical surgery is contemplated, since under these circumstances one would naturally wish to avoid even the remote possibility that the clinical interpretation of the case may have been incorrect. Finally, a biopsy should be done (if at all possible) whenever radiation is to be the therapeutic procedure, to avoid the danger of radiating a lesion for which that form of treatment is contraindicated, or for which surgery would be more appropriate.

After a biopsy has been decided upon, the question of how the tissue should be obtained must likewise be considered with care. Shall an open (or surgical) biopsy be done, or shall there be a closed biopsy employing one of the several techniques for aspirating or coring out a small amount of tissue from the lesion? Such factors as the bone affected, the precise location of the lesion in relation to that bone, and the suspected nature of the lesion naturally enter into the decision. However, these factors are very often subordinated to the preferences cherished by the surgeon and/or the pathologist concerned in the case. Be that as it may, both methods of biopsy have their inherent virtues and deficiencies.

**Closed Biopsy.**—A lesion which is in an accessible site and which is not encased in a thick layer of cortical bone lends itself particularly well to a closed biopsy. Coley, who has had a wide experience with the closed biopsy, still employs simply a long 18-gauge needle fitted with a 20 cc. record syringe for this purpose. By using this equipment and being careful in the selection of cases and in the choice of the proper site for aspiration, he is very often able to obtain adequate material for histologic study. As a rule, the material aspirated from the lesion will include at least some minute fragments of tissue. These can be crushed between two slides and smeared and then stained and examined microscopically. Frequently one also obtains some plugs of tissue which are large enough to be imbedded in paraffin for sectioning and staining. Such tissue sections are, of course, likely to be more useful than the direct smears in supplying histologic information about the lesion. (For technical details on the procedures in question, see Coley.)

Certain special needles have also been devised for carrying out a closed biopsy on a bone tumor. However, for lesions in easily accessible sites, these needles seem not to present any general advantages over the 18-gauge needle attached to a record syringe, when the latter is skillfully employed. Altogether, needle biopsies carried out and interpreted by appropriately skilled surgeons and pathologists can be expected to permit correct and specific diagnoses on about 65 per cent of primary and metastatic bone tumors in favorable sites.

The obvious advantage of the needle biopsy is that it constitutes a limited intervention which disturbs the lesion only slightly and causes but little morbidity to the patient. However, even in the most experienced hands, it sometimes fails to yield sufficient material and may even yield none. Then again, the material yielded, though apparently adequate, may present problems of histologic interpretation to the pathologist. For instance, the tissue obtained may be largely or completely necrotic, so that even a pathologist experienced in reading needle biopsies may have difficulty in coming to a conclusion about the lesion. On the other hand, even if viable tissue has been obtained, the pathologist may be unable to make a definitive diagnosis as to the nature of the tumor, or perhaps even to decide whether the lesion is a tumor at all. Or the innate nature of the tissue obtained may raise problems in itself. For instance, if the lesion is a cartilage tumor, it may be very difficult to decide, on the basis of mere fragments of tissue, whether the growth in question is benign or malignant. These various difficulties relating to the obtainment and interpretation of needle biopsies from lesions in accessible sites make it evident that in some cases one has to resort to an open surgical biopsy even in respect to such sites.

Finally, in regard to closed biopsy, it should be noted that vertebral bodies have lately become approachable by this method. A technique for making an accurate needle approach to the vertebral bodies was suggested by Valls *et al.* This is now being largely supplanted by methods involving the coring out of a rather large biopsy specimen. Instruments and technical procedures for coring out biopsy specimens from vertebral bodies have been described by Siffert and Arkin, and by Craig, among others. A biopsy performed by these techniques presents obvious advantages when compared with open biopsy in relation to vertebral bodies. However, these procedures require rather special skill and experience and are not mere minor interventions in themselves. Therefore, when one is dealing with a vertebral lesion, every other possible avenue of diagnosis should be explored before the lesion is biopsied in this way.

**Open (Surgical) Biopsy.**—The decision to do a surgical biopsy in the case of a bone tumor should always be regarded as a major decision. A surgical biopsy should never be done without thorough previous evaluation of the clinical, roentgenographic, and laboratory data relating to the case. It may reasonably be undertaken because a needle biopsy has failed to yield, or is not likely to yield, satisfactory material for diagnosis. Furthermore, there are surgeons and pathologists who tend in general to prefer a surgical biopsy to a needle biopsy. Clearly, they wish their decision as to diagnosis and treatment to be based on examination of a frozen section (or if necessary a paraffin section) of a larger sample of tissue than is obtained by needle biopsy.

The open biopsy should be carried out in such a way that surgical trauma is kept to a minimum. For instance, in taking a biopsy specimen from a lesion which has broken out of a bone, a sliver of tumor tissue from the periphery of the extra-osseous tumor mass is very likely to constitute a satisfactory specimen. Instead, however, there is often the tendency to go much beyond this and to obtain tissue from the interior of the affected bone site. Under such circumstances, an excessive amount of material is usually obtained, and what is really deplorable is the fact that the lesion has been subjected to traumatic disruption. This is also not infrequently the case when the biopsy is done on a lesion which had not yet broken out of the bone. Thus, instead of merely taking an adequate specimen of lesional tissue for examination, the surgeon, in his eagerness to obtain material, actually does something like a curettage of the lesion. In addition, it should be noted that, if the tumor is a malignant one, an unduly traumatic biopsy may encourage its metastatic spread.

Finally, there is the matter of deciding: (1) whether the histologic diagnosis should be made on the basis of a frozen section of the biopsy specimen, so that additional surgery may be performed at once if this is indicated; or (2) whether the wound should be closed and the diagnosis and decision about further treatment postponed until after paraffin sections have been prepared. The answers to these questions depend largely on the kind of tissue yielded by the biopsy. If this tissue includes areas which are not calcified or ossified, properly prepared frozen sections from such soft areas will usually suffice for diagnostic purposes. In this connection, it is surprising to note how often it is the most ossified portions of the biopsy specimen that are actually taken for study, on the mistaken assumption that paraffin sections of decalcified tissue will be most likely to give the diagnostic information. On the other hand, if the biopsy specimen shows that the lesion is composed of cartilage, it is better to await the preparation of paraffin sections even if the cartilage tissue in question is not calcified and thus suitable for frozen sectioning. That is, paraffin sections offer a better basis than frozen sections for evaluating the details of a cartilage tumor in respect to benignity or malignity. In another case, a frozen section may show that the tumor is composed of round cells. In such a case the wound should be closed and paraffin sections prepared in addition. The tumor may be a Ewing sarcoma, a reticulum cell sarcoma, or a metastatic tumor (a neuroblastoma, for instance). Indeed, even after studying the paraffin sections one may still have difficulty in deciding exactly what the lesion is. Since these lesions are not treated surgically in any event, nothing will be lost through the delay. In general, the decisions relating to frozen sections *vs.* paraffin sections represent nice questions of judgment whose answers must often be adapted to the individual case.

## REFERENCES

CODMAN, E. A.: *Bone Sarcoma. An Interpretation of the Nomenclature Used by the Committee on the Registry of Bone Sarcoma of the American College of Surgeons,* New York, Paul B. Hoeber, Inc., 1925.

COLEY, B. L.: *Neoplasms of Bone,* New York, Paul B. Hoeber, Inc., 1949 (see p. 28).

CRAIG, F. S.: Vertebral-Body Biopsy, J. Bone & Joint Surg., *38-A,* 93, 1956.

EWING, J.: A Review of the Classification of Bone Tumors, Surg., Gynec. & Obst., *68,* 971, 1939.

——————:The Place of the Biopsy in Bone Sarcoma, Am. J. Surg., *27,* 26, 1935.

JAFFE, H. L.: *See* Discussion of paper by Hodges, P. C.: Pitfalls in the Roentgen Diagnosis of Bone Tumors, Radiations *vs.* Cancer, A Critical Evaluation, Proc. Am. Cancer Soc., 1952 (see p. 37).

——————:*See* Discussion of paper by Johnson, L. C.: A General Theory of Bone Tumors, Bull. New York Acad. Med., *29,* 164, 1953 (see p. 170).

JAFFE, H. L., and SELIN, G.: Tumors of Bones and Joints, Bull. New York Acad. Med., *27,* 165, 1951.

PHEMISTER, D.: Panel on Bone Tumors, Proc. First Nat. Cancer Conf., 1949 (see p. 217).

SIFFERT, R. S., and ARKIN, A. M.: Trephine Biopsy of Bone with Special Reference to the Lumbar Vertebral Bodies, J. Bone & Joint Surg., *31-A,* 146, 1949.

SNYDER, R. E., and COLEY, B. L.: Further Studies on the Diagnosis of Bone Tumors by Aspiration Biopsy, Surg., Gynec. & Obst., *80,* 517, 1945.

VALLS, J., OTTOLENGHI, C. E., and SCHAJOWICZ, F.: Aspiration Biopsy in Diagnosis of Lesions of Vertebral Bodies, J.A.M.A., *136,* 376, 1948.

Chapter

# 2

# Giant-Cell Tumor

THE *giant-cell tumor* of bone, in the strict sense in which the writer uses the term, presents a number of characteristic clinical and pathologic features. Grossly, the lesional tissue is soft and friable, and its color is predominantly reddish brown, though an individual lesion may show some areas which are yellowish or even grayish. Histologically, much of the tissue presents the pattern of a more or less vascularized network of plumpish or ovoid stromal cells, heavily interspersed with multinuclear giant cells. In the evaluation of a giant-cell tumor, detailed consideration should be given to the appearance of the stromal cells and to the quantity and grouping of the giant cells in relation to the stromal cells. It cannot be emphasized too strongly that the mere finding of some multinuclear giant cells in a bone lesion is not enough to justify designating it as a giant-cell tumor. It is this overemphasis on the mere presence of giant cells, without consideration of the histologic pattern of the lesional tissue as a whole, that has been responsible in the past for the loose inclusion of various other kinds of lesions under the heading of giant-cell tumor (see Jaffe, Lichtenstein, and Portis).

Clinically, it is to be noted in regard to giant-cell tumor that in the great majority of the cases the patients are between 20 and 40 years of age. In the great majority of the cases, also, the lesion is in an end of a long tubular bone. Roentgenographically, the affected bone part usually shows up as a rather large, more or less circumscribed area of striking radiolucency, with little if any suggestion of trabeculation. As to clinical behavior, giant-cell tumor of bone is a lesion which not infrequently recurs and which may even metastasize, so that the use of the term "benign" as part of its name is inappropriate.

**Nomenclature.**—While the designation of the lesion as "giant-cell tumor of bone" is now widely used, the term "osteoclastoma of bone" is also often employed. However, "giant-cell tumor" seems preferable, since it is a more neutral name than "osteoclastoma," which implies that the giant cells are osteoclasts and behave as such in the course of the lesion's evolution. Actually, they do not, and the lytic destruction of the bone at the site of the lesion is the result of growth of the tumor as a whole, rather than the result of selective osteoclastic action of the giant cells. Furthermore, just as the prefix "benign" should be discarded in connection with giant-cell tumor of bone, so, at the other extreme, should "giant-cell sarcoma" be rejected, as likewise not fitting the clinical facts in all cases. Some other names which have been applied to the lesion but which are no longer used are: "myeloid tumor," "tumeur à myéloplaxes," "myeloid sarcoma," and "hemorrhagic osteomyelitis."

## CLINICAL CONSIDERATIONS

**Incidence.**—The giant-cell tumor, in the strict sense of the term, is not a very common lesion. Notably, it is very much less common than the non-ossifying fibroma (p. 83), the lesion with which it is most likely to be confused on a histologic basis.

As to the age incidence of giant-cell tumor, some further details are worth noting. The lesion is observed only infrequently in persons under 20 years of age, and only very rarely in a person under 10. We did observe a giant-cell tumor in the lower end of a femur of a child of 10, but in general, in such a young subject, the age is strongly against the probability that a tumor suspected of being a giant-cell tumor really is one. The great bulk of the cases (about 75 per cent) fall into the age group 20 to 40 years, the age group 30 to 40 years perhaps being slightly predilected. For the patient to be between 40 and 50 years old is not unusual. It is only rarely, however, that the patient is over 50, though we did also observe 1 case of a giant-cell tumor in the upper end of a tibia in a woman of 58. In further analyzing the age incidence in our own series of 60 cases (collected to 1953), we found that the median age of the patients was 32 and the average age 33 years.

In general, as to age incidence, we have come to view with skepticism any conclusions about giant-cell tumor drawn from reports heavily weighted with cases in the age group below 20. This is not to deny, as noted, the occasional occurrence of giant-cell tumor of bone in the young. However, what one encounters much more frequently in the young are lesions which merely mimic giant-cell tumor in one respect or another, and which, on critical evaluation, are found not to justify the diagnosis of giant-cell tumor of bone.

As to sex incidence, females predominate slightly in our own series of cases, but not sufficiently to controvert the general finding that males and females are affected in about equal numbers.

**Localization.**—That in the vast majority of cases the tumor is in an end of some long tubular bone has already been pointed out. At the initial examination, the lesion in a given long bone is usually already found implicating some part of the epiphysial end of the bone, and the adjacent metaphysis. Part of the end may be affected, either toward one side or centrally, or the lesion may involve practically the entire bone end. The lower end of the femur, the upper end of the tibia, and the lower end of the radius are the three most common sites for the lesion. Together they account for about 60 to 70 per cent of the localizations in any representative series of cases, and the lower end of the femur and upper end of the tibia together may account for as much as 50 per cent. The only other fairly common site of involvement so far as long bone ends are concerned is the upper end of the femur. Such sites as the upper end of the humerus and the upper end of the fibula are occasionally found affected, and, even less frequently, some other long bone end, not yet mentioned, may be involved.

Very exceptionally, a giant-cell tumor is found limited to a nonepiphysial part of a long bone, and the writer has seen one such case. In that case, the lesion was in the upper part of the shaft of a tibia, its upper limit being several centimeters below the epiphysial bone end.

It is estimated that instances of localization of giant-cell tumor of bone elsewhere than in a long tubular bone make up only about 15 to 20 per cent of the cases. Of the limb bones other than long bones, the patella is an occasional site for the tumor, as are the astragalus and the calcaneus, while it is only rarely that the lesion appears in a carpal bone. A phalanx is sometimes the site of the tumor, and so, though less often, is a metacarpal or metatarsal bone. In these short tubular bones, too, the tumor tends to begin in the epiphysial end of the bone and generally comes to involve much of the shaft.

The frequency with which one encounters reports of giant-cell tumor in some bone of the skull would lead one to think that it is not rare in these bones, but actually it is uncommon there. Undoubtedly, the older statistics on giant-cell tumor in jawbones mistakenly include many instances in which the lesion was not a giant-cell tumor but merely one of the "brown tumors" in a case of hyperparathyroidism.

Also, probably, some of the reported instances of giant-cell tumor of jawbones represent lesions of the nature of giant-cell organizational reaction to intramedullary hemorrhage, such as those which the writer denotes as "giant-cell reparative granuloma of jawbones." Furthermore, there are a few reported instances of giant-cell tumor of the calvarium, but most of these, too, are unacceptable as cases of primary giant-cell tumor. With one exception, the only instances of giant-cell tumor of the calvarium which the writer has seen were cases in which the lesion was present as a complication of Paget's disease in that location. (See Differential Diagnosis, p. 32.)

As to the trunk bones, the vertebral column, too, is supposed to be a not unusual site for giant-cell tumor. However, in many of the reported supposed instances, the unavailability of pertinent pathologic material leaves the diagnosis doubtful. The writer has encountered personally only two instances of giant-cell tumor primary in the vertebral column. In one case, the lesion was in a vertebral body, and

***Figure 1***

*A*, Roentgenograph of a giant-cell tumor in the lower end of a femur. The lesional area appears radiolucent and not trabeculated. The bone cortex in that area is thin, but the contour of the bone is not expanded. The patient was a woman 39 years of age, and her complaints on admission to the hospital were of 2 months' standing. Her chief complaint was of pain in the knee, exacerbated by walking and relieved by rest. The lesional area was curetted and packed with bone chips. It has healed in, and the patient has remained free of recurrence for 3½ years.

*B*, Roentgenograph of a giant-cell tumor in the upper end of a femur. The lesional area as a whole is strikingly radiolucent, and the cortex of a substantial part of the femoral neck has been destroyed by the tumor. The patient was a man 33 years of age whose complaint was of pain in the right hip for 10 months. The treatment consisted of excision of the femoral head and neck, and there has been no local recurrence. Of great interest in connection with this case is the fact that, 2½ years after resection of the femoral lesion, the patient developed a tumor in the prepuce of the penis. This penile tumor was removed, and on histologic examination it, too, showed the pattern of a giant-cell tumor. One can only speculate on the route by which the metastasis to the penis took place. In any event, the patient was alive and well 5 years after excision of the penile tumor and 7½ years after resection of the femoral giant-cell tumor.

*C*, Roentgenograph of a giant-cell tumor in the upper end of a tibia. Characteristically, this tumor, too, involves the epiphysial end and part of the adjacent shaft of the bone. There is a very slight suggestion of trabeculation. The patient was a woman 45 years of age who gave a history of increasing pain in the knee for 3 months. The initial surgical intervention was curettage. The curettings showed the pattern of a giant-cell tumor in which the stromal cells were very prominent and plump, and more than an occasional one was in mitotic division. On the basis of these findings, the tumor was interpreted as a giant-cell tumor of grade II presenting changes in the direction of malignancy. Within 4 months there was a recurrence and even local extension of the tumor. An amputation was done, and histologic examination of the recurrent tumor tissue showed that the lesion was now clearly a malignant growth. Death occured 7 months later from widespread metastases.

*D*, Roentgenograph of a giant-cell tumor in the lower end of a radius. The cortex in the lesional area is thinned, and the area is characteristically radiolucent, the lesion extending to the articular cartilage. The patient was a man 44 years of age. His complaints were of only a few months' standing when this picture was taken. The lesion was treated by curettage, and this was followed by radiation therapy, 2,500 r of $x$-radiation being given. One year later there was not only a recurrence, but a local extension of the tumor. The second intervention consisted of resection of the lower end of the radius, well beyond the region of tumorous involvement, removal of the first row of carpal bones, and the introduction of a large fibular graft to fill the gap. Follow-up 4 years later showed that the patient had remained free of recurrence and was gainfully employed in spite of a stiff wrist.

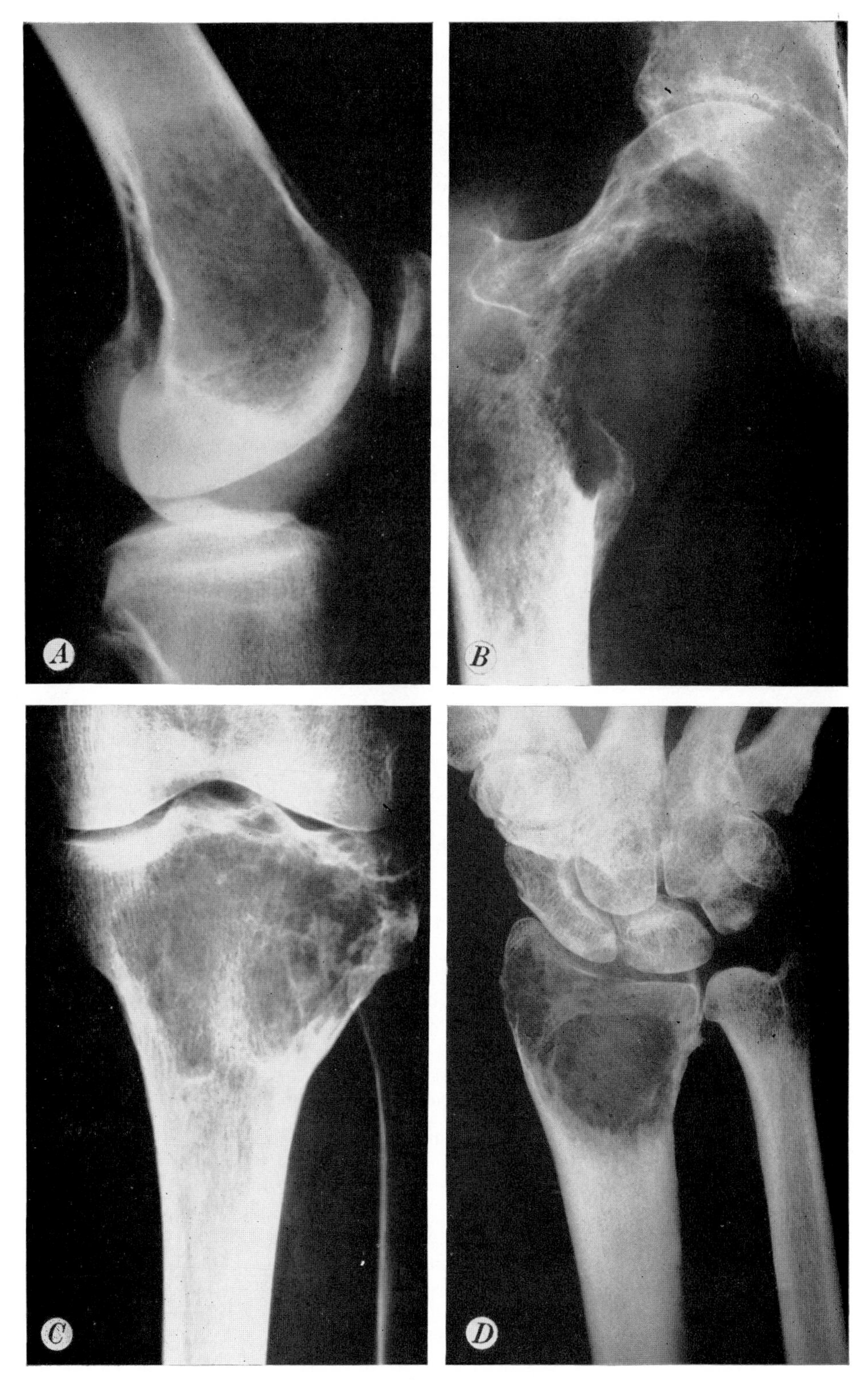


*Figure 1*

in the other in the sacrum. In most instances, however, cases reported as giant-cell tumor of vertebræ actually represent, in his opinion, so-called aneurysmal bone cyst (p. 54). Some instances of giant-cell tumor of a rib, clavicle, or sternum have been reported, but in regard to some of these, also, one cannot be at all certain that they actually represented giant-cell tumor of bone. A giant-cell tumor involving some portion of an innominate bone is sometimes encountered. The writer has seen it once involving practically an entire ilium and once involving the entire superior ramus of a pubic bone.

The presence of more than one giant-cell tumor of bone in the same person (*i.e.*, the appearance of the tumor otherwise than as a solitary lesion) is so unusual that one accepts only with great hesitancy an apparent instance of this. Cases of this kind must be carefully scrutinized for the presence of hyperparathyroidism. A case apparently showing two independent giant-cell tumors (one in an astragalus and the other in the adjacent scaphoid) is cited by Konjetzny. Coley and Higinbotham mention having observed a case in which, at different times, the lesion developed in both femora. The writer observed a case of giant-cell tumor involving the lower end of an ulna, the fifth metacarpal, the proximal phalanx of a fourth finger, and perhaps the upper end of a humerus. In this case, the possibility of hyperparathyroidism was definitely excluded, and the giant-cell tumor character of three of the lesions was established by histologic examination of tissue removed from them.

**Clinical Complaints and Findings.**—The tumor is likely to be well developed before the clinical difficulties appear. In its usual site, a long bone, dull, aching pain (often intermittent) is generally the earliest complaint, but pain may fail to appear until an infraction or incomplete pathologic fracture has occurred. In this connection, the subject may state that, some weeks before medical attention was sought, the region had been slightly traumatized, for instance by a blow, fall or twist. In fact, the difficulties may be dated from this trauma. Soon, motion of the adjacent joint becomes more or less restricted and painful. Furthermore, enlargement of the affected bone region may now become visible or at least palpable. As this increases, local tenderness is likely to appear, and the skin over the affected region may feel warm and even show reddish mottling. If, as rarely happens now, the tumor has become very large, "parchment crackling" may be elicitable and the veins in the skin be found engorged. When the lesion appears elsewhere than in a long bone, this general picture is modified by the special conditions imposed by the individual location.

In regard to the role of *trauma*, it is undoubtedly true that many of the patients give no history of possibly relevant trauma. On the other hand, when one does obtain a history of a traumatic incident antecedent to the discovery of the lesion, one can frequently conclude from the clinical and roentgenographic data that the lesion was present before the trauma, and that the latter merely directed attention to it by causing an infraction of the undermined bone cortex.

There are no clinical laboratory tests which are helpful in making the diagnosis. The serum calcium and inorganic phosphate values are normal, as is the serum alkaline phosphatase activity. An elevated serum calcium value in a case suspected of being one of giant-cell tumor points rather to hyperparathyroidism or multiple myeloma. Though the roentgenographic picture is exceedingly helpful in arriving at a diagnosis, it is nevertheless true that examination of a biopsy specimen is often necessary before one can be certain of it.

**Roentgenographic Findings.**—It is usually on the basis of the roentgenographic findings that the diagnosis of giant-cell tumor is first attempted. The roentgenographic picture is largely determined by the following facts: that the tumor develops rather rapidly; that the tumor tissue causes rapid lytic destruction of the osseous tissue at the site of its growth; that the tumor tissue itself possesses no osteogenic capacity; and that, even peripherally, as long as the tumor is in a dynamic phase, there is very little, if any, perilesional new bone formation.

In relation to the lesion in its typical location (the end of a long bone), these facts are reflected roentgenographically in the following picture: The epiphysial end of the bone, sometimes alone but most often with part of the adjacent metaphysis, shows a large and somewhat eccentric area of striking radiolucency, with little if any suggestion of trabeculation. The involvement may extend to the articular cartilage, and occasionally an intra-articular fracture line is visible. The bone cortex in the affected region is found thinned and expanded, and may even show fracture. Despite this, there is likely to be very little periosteal new bone formation over the thinned and expanded cortex. (See Fig. 1.)

It is to be noted that, in this general picture of the *x*-ray findings, no stress has been laid upon trabeculation and the resultant multilocular cyst-like effect as being important in the roentgenographic pattern of the lesion. The diagnostic value of this multilocular appearance has, we believe, been overemphasized, and one may easily be led astray if the presence of this appearance is necessarily expected. As a matter of fact, it is really rather unusual (at least in its full efflorescence) with giant-cell tumor.

Far more important, diagnostically, than trabeculation are the location of the area of rarefaction in the end of the bone and the thinning and expansion of the cortex, particularly on one side. Likewise a significant point is the practical absence of periosteal new bone formation over the thinned and expanded cortex, not infrequently even where the latter has undergone pathologic fracture. However, in this connection, it should not be forgotten that a fibrosarcoma, for instance, which has started in an end of a long bone may produce a roentgenographic picture completely simulating that of a giant-cell tumor. We have also seen a few cases in which a myeloma did so, too.

On the whole, however, when a giant-cell tumor is in a long tubular bone, one can often surmise the correct diagnosis on the basis of the *x*-ray picture. This is often not the case when, as occasionally happens, the giant-cell tumor involves a bone other than a long tubular bone. In relation to these other locations, the difficulties are perhaps smallest when the giant-cell tumor is in a phalanx. In a phalanx, a giant-cell tumor involves, in characteristic fashion, the epiphysial end and a variable part of the adjacent shaft. In the differential diagnosis, one would have to consider the possibilities that the phalangeal lesion is an enchondroma or a bone cyst. The enchondroma is the most common tumor of phalanges. However, an enchondroma is usually, though not always, limited to the shaft of the bone. A solitary bone cyst can be ruled out because that lesion rarely (if ever) involves a phalanx, and, even if it should appear in a phalanx, would characteristically spare the end of the bone.

## PATHOLOGY AND PATHOGENESIS

**Gross Pathology.**—The older descriptions of giant-cell tumor usually relate to lesions of long standing which had attained large size, associated with pronounced secondary changes. Consequently, these descriptions, with their emphasis on extensive necrosis, hemorrhage, cystic softening, and the formation of large blood spaces, though accurate so far as very advanced lesions are concerned, do not, on the whole, fit the gross picture of giant-cell tumor as we see it, now that it is being treated more promptly.

In bygone days, when the lesion had a chance to run its natural course, the tumor often also came to disrupt the periosteal cuff and perhaps grow along intermuscular septa. It may even have advanced into a neighboring bone, either by transgressing into the joint space or by extending through an interosseous membrane. These various consequences used also to be seen in connection with postsurgical recurrences of the tumor, or in the wake of malignant transformation of a recurrent tumor. They were especially likely to be found in cases in which renewed attempts at surgical treatment of a recurrent tumor had been undertaken after a course of radiation therapy, and in which an infection had supervened. Under the latter circumstances, the tumor often even fungated through a wound in the skin.

If one now obtains a giant-cell tumor intact in its setting (for instance, in the end of a long bone) and sections it in its long axis, it will be found that, where the original cortex has been destroyed and the contour of the bone has been expanded, the lesion is nevertheless contained by a thin shell of subperiosteal new bone which may even not have been apparent roentgenographically. Also, if one runs a finger over the lesional area, one will find that the cancellous bone which had been present at the site is largely or entirely lacking, so that, altogether, the tumor area is nonosseous. Though the tumor tissue usually extends to the articular cartilage in one place or another, the cartilage is not likely to be found perforated. Shaftward—*i.e.*, in the direction of the major marrow cavity—the tumor is delimited by a thin wall of fibrous tissue or bone. (See Fig. 2.)

As to the tumor tissue itself, its gross appearance naturally depends, to a considerable extent, on the degree to which it has already undergone secondary changes.

***Figure 2***

*A*, Photograph showing a giant-cell tumor in the upper end of a tibia. Note that the tumor occupies the epiphysial end of the bone and part of the adjacent shaft, and that in some places it reaches the articular cartilage. The patient was a man 48 years of age. For 8 months prior to the surgical intervention, he had complaints of pain and swelling relating to the left knee. The clinical diagnosis was confirmed by biopsy, and the treatment consisted of resection of the proximal 4 inches of the tibia, filling the gap with an autogenous bone graft, and arthrodesis of the knee joint. There was no local recurrence after this procedure, and the patient was thus cured of his giant-cell tumor.

*B*, Photograph of a recurrent giant-cell tumor in the lower end of a radius. The tumor tissue extends to the articular cartilage. The contour of the bone is very much expanded. The original tumor was a relatively small one and was treated by curettage and chemical cauterization of the tumor bed. The patient, a man, was 37 years of age at the time when he was first admitted for treatment. Within 8 months after the curettage there was evidence of a recurrence, and the recurrent lesion was subjected to *x*-radiation. However, it was not contained by this treatment, and it was then decided to resect the lower end of the radius and fill the gap with a fibular bone graft. The patient died at our hospital about 12 years after this second intervention, but his death was not connected with the lesion in question.

*C*, Photograph of a giant-cell tumor in the upper end of a fibula. In the lesional area, the bone contour is much distended in consequence of complete destruction of the regional cortex. The tumor tissue extends to the deep surface of the articular cartilage and is confined by the expanded periosteum. The patient was a woman 27 years of age. She complained of progressive pain of about 6 months' standing at the lateral aspect of the left knee, and had become aware of swelling of the area about 1 month before admission. The treatment consisted of resection of the upper end of the fibula, and the patient was cured of her giant-cell tumor.

*D*, Photograph of a giant-cell tumor in the upper end of a radius. The lesion, though relatively small, again involves both the actual end of the bone and part of the adjacent shaft. It has not yet completely destroyed the local shaft cortex, and the bone contour is therefore not much modified. The patient was a man 32 years of age whose complaints were of 6 months' standing and consisted of pain connected with functional use of the elbow joint. The treatment consisted of resection of the upper end of the radius and was successful in eliminating further morbidity relating to the giant-cell tumor.

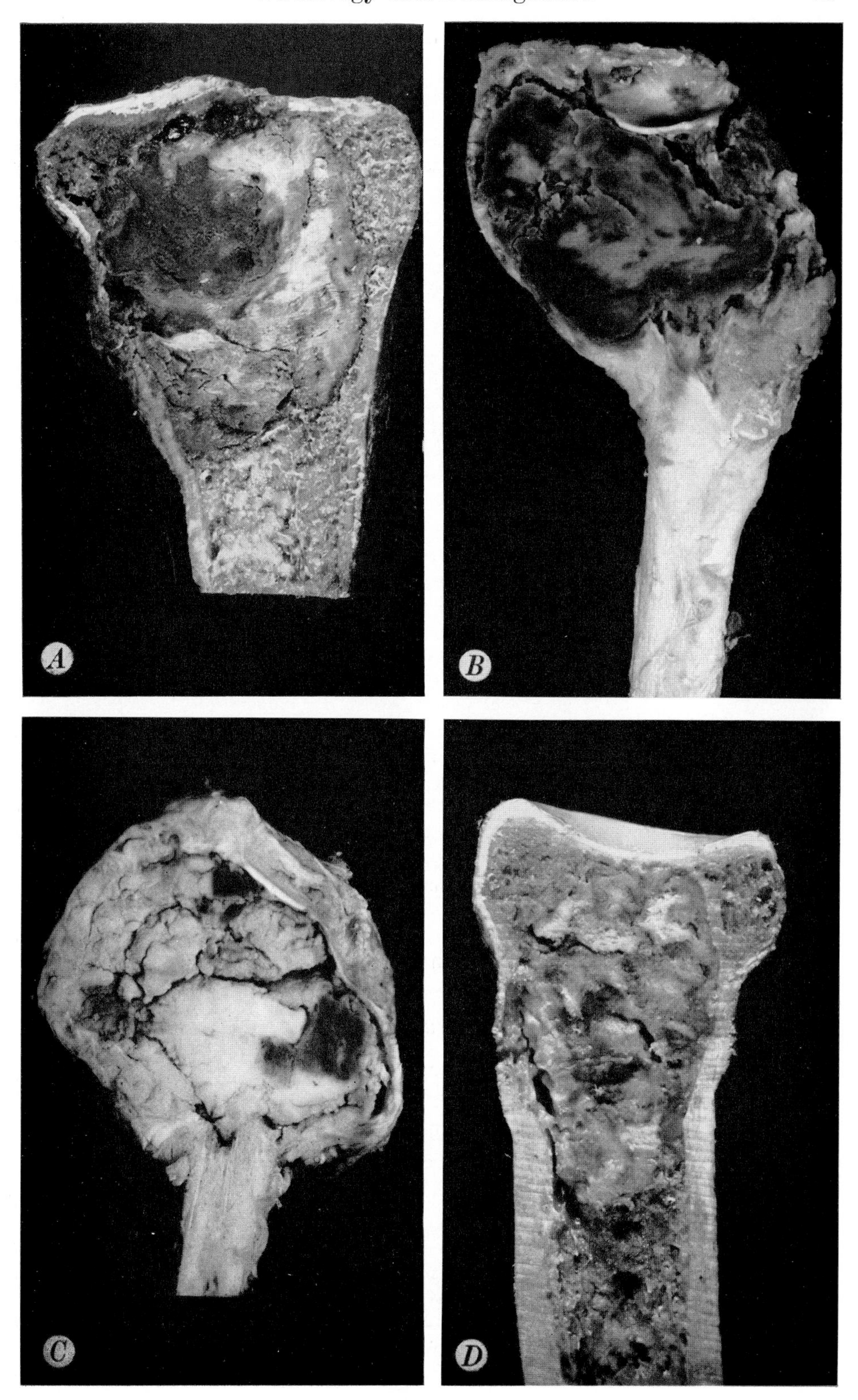


*Figure 2*

Tumor tissue which has undergone but little modification is likely to be of a rather uniform reddish or reddish brown color and of a fleshy consistency, though friable. In fact, practically the entire lesion may present this appearance, especially if it is still small. In most specimens, however, the color and consistency are found altered by secondary changes which have occurred here and there throughout the tumor. Some firmer, gray-yellow areas may be encountered where the tumor tissue has undergone fibrosis and collagenization. The presence of hemorrhage is evidenced in spots or blotches of bright red or blackish red and in greater softness of the tissues. Necrotic areas appear yellowish, amber, or orange, and may be found partly liquefied. In the wake of necrosis and hemorrhage, some cystification of the tumor tissue may occur, the cystic areas containing serous, serosanguineous, or frankly hemorrhagic fluid.

**Microscopic Pathology.**—It is, of course, the viable and not otherwise modified tumor areas that show to best advantage the relational pattern of giant cells and stromal cells which is characteristic of the lesion cytologically. The following brief sketch of this pattern represents what one may call a typical or average picture. The stromal cells are mononuclear, plumpish cells, spindle-shaped or ovoid in varying proportions. Correspondingly, the nucleus, which occupies much of the cell body, is longish or roundish. Occasional stromal cells may present evidence of mitotic division. The multinuclear giant cells are found distributed between the stromal cells. The giant-cell nuclei tend to be agglomerated toward the middle of the cell, and some cells have several dozen nuclei. On the whole, the nuclei of the giant cells are not much different from those of the stromal cells, and they may even be indistinguishable from them. An occasional giant cell may show pyknosis of its nuclei, apparently reflecting degeneration of the cell. The cytoplasm of the giant cells is usually considerable in amount, frequently granular, and sometimes vacuolated. The giant cells of giant-cell tumors contain a considerable amount of acid phosphatase. However, acid phosphatase is found also in normal bone osteoclasts, foreign-body giant cells, and the Langhans giant cells of tuberculous tubercles.

In evaluating a giant-cell tumor, if, in all the viable areas under observation, the stromal cells are numerous and are crowding the giant cells, the likelihood of recurrence of the tumor in question is stronger than it would be if the stromal cells were less abundant and proliferating less actively. In any case, in a lesion representing a recurrence of a giant-cell tumor, one can often note that the stromal cells are more crowded and plumper than they were in the original lesion. Still, this does not signify that the recurrent lesion will necessarily metastasize or take on locally the features of a frankly malignant giant-cell tumor. (See Fig. 3.)

***Figure 3***

*A*, Photomicrograph (× 150) showing the tissue pattern which is characteristic of a giant-cell tumor. In this lesion, the ovoid stromal cells are not particularly crowding the giant cells. A lesion presenting this pattern may or may not recur. Actually, in this case the lesion, which was in the lower end of a radius, did recur. In its recurrence it showed an increase both in the amount of the stromal cells and in their plumpness, so that the histologic pattern of the recurrent lesion clearly represented a giant-cell tumor of grade II.

*B*, Photomicrograph (× 150) showing the histologic pattern of a giant-cell tumor in which there are a considerable number of spindle-shaped stromal cells crowding the giant cells. A giant-cell tumor presenting this pattern is rather prone to recurrence, though the latter is not inevitable. The pattern is not to be regarded as that of a malignant giant-cell tumor. (See Fig. 4-*C*.) The patient in this case was a man 44 years of age, and the tumor was in the lower end of a femur. The treatment was curettage, but some months later there was a recurrence. Since the recurrent tumor was growing rapidly, the limb was ablated. The histologic pattern of the recurrent tumor tissue remained that of grade II.

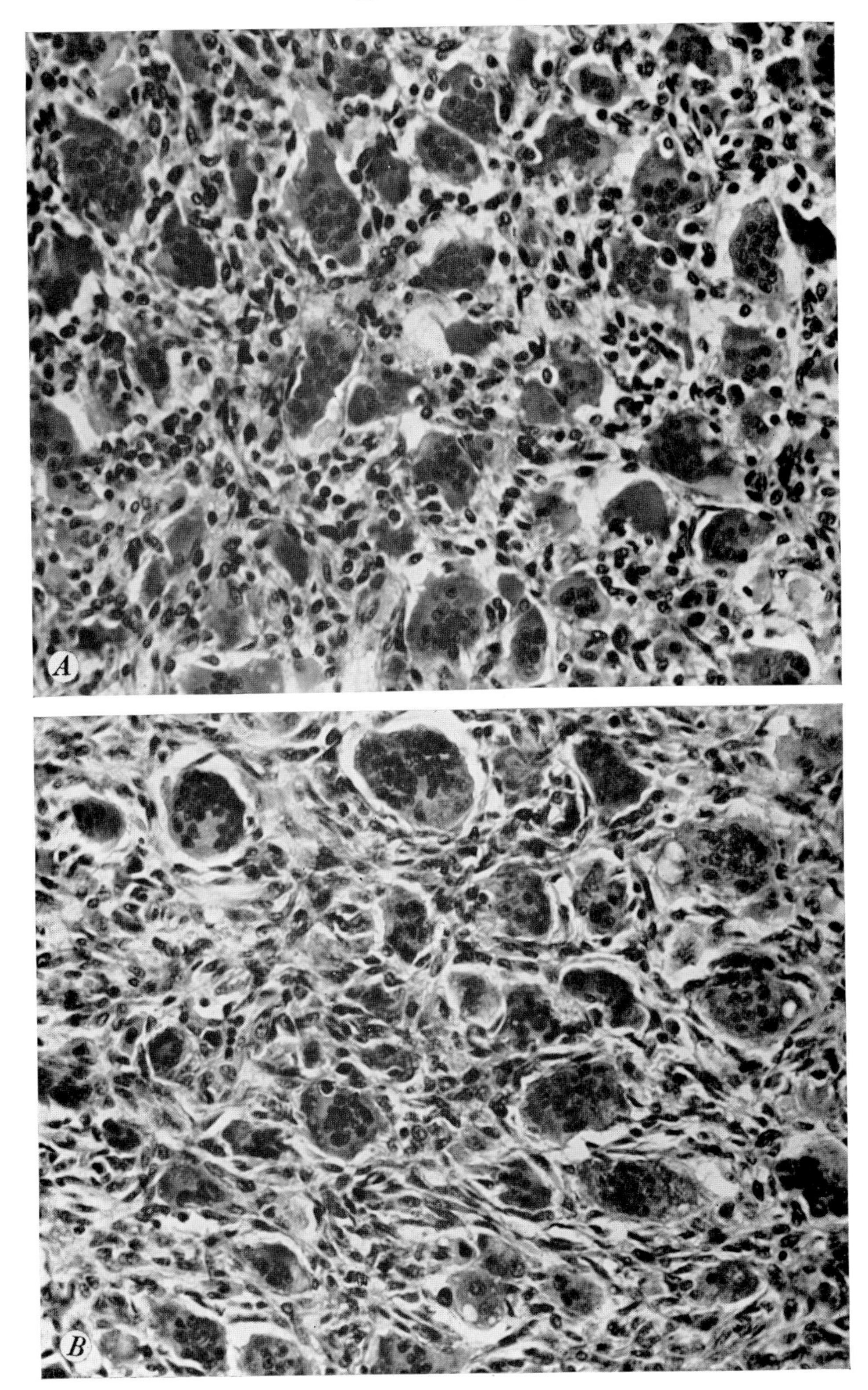


*Figure 3*

If a substantial amount of tissue from a particular giant-cell tumor is examined, it will be found that, in addition to areas showing the characteristic cytologic pattern, there are some areas which show spindling and whorling of the stromal cells, the presence of abundant intercellular collagenous material, sparsity of the giant cells, and the presence of lipid-bearing (cholesterol-bearing) foam cells. Such appearances apparently reflect spontaneous regression and healing occurring in the tumor. In an occasional giant-cell tumor, tissue showing this healing reaction even predominates over the characteristic tissue. Whether the pattern of a giant-cell tumor ever comes to be totally of this scarifying-healing type we do not know. At any rate, the conspicuous presence of this scarifying-healing reaction is a favorable finding when one is evaluating a particular giant-cell tumor, and the response to treatment in such a case can be expected to be good. (See Figs. 4-*A* and *B*.)

Occasionally, one encounters a giant-cell tumor which is already frankly sarcomatous when tissue is first taken from it for study. In these rare cases, the stromal cells of the lesional tissue have an indubitable sarcomatous aura, and metastasis is to be expected. It is held by some that these "malignant giant-cell tumors" are not actually giant-cell tumors but instead represent so-called "osteolytic osteogenic sarcoma" which has been misdiagnosed. There can be no doubt that in an osteolytic osteogenic sarcoma one may see numerous giant cells of the type observed in giant-cell tumor. However, if, in these cases, one is not misled by the presence of such giant cells and is guided by the total histologic pattern of giant-cell tumor, one will not fall into the error of misclassifying such osteogenic sarcomas as malignant giant-cell tumors. What the writer has in mind when he refers to a malignant giant-cell tumor is a tumor which, if a substantial amount of viable tumor tissue is examined, shows consistently the characteristic pattern of giant cells and stromal cells, but in which the appearance of the stromal cells is such as to give the tissue a sarcomatous cast. (See Fig. 4-*C*.)

**Nature and Genesis.**—The idea that the giant-cell tumor is a neoplasm seems to have been taken for granted until the early part of the present century. This idea is now again the prevailing one among American and British students of the subject, and is shared by the present writer. Furthermore, as will be brought out presently, the giant-cell tumor can metastasize and still maintain the conventional seemingly "benign" giant-cell tumor pattern in its metastases. Or it can change its character and appear as a fibrosarcoma in its metastases. Occasionally, also, a

***Figure 4***

*A*, Photomicrograph (× 100) showing lipid-bearing (cholesterol-bearing) foam cells adjacent to an area presenting the conventional histologic pattern of giant-cell tumor. (See *B*.)

*B*, Photomicrograph (× 100) showing sparsity of giant cells, spindling and whorling of the stromal cells, and the presence of abundant intercellular collagenous material. Tissue fields presenting such a histologic pattern and the pattern of lipoidification shown in *A* represent the alterations associated with the scarifying and healing which often take place spontaneously in some (or even many) areas of a giant-cell tumor.

*C*, Photomicrograph (× 150) showing the histologic pattern of a malignant giant-cell tumor. While the general interrelational pattern of giant cells and stromal cells is still present, the stroma is given a sarcomatous aura by the largeness and abundance of the stromal cells. Note also that the multinuclear giant cells tend to be smaller than in a giant-cell tumor which is as yet not malignant. The patient was a woman 23 years of age. This grade III giant-cell tumor involved the right 11th rib, and the treatment was resection of the affected rib. The patient died about 6 months after this, and the lungs showed metastatic foci of giant-cell tumor, but there was no recurrence at the site of the rib resection. (I am indebted to Dr. Ephraim Woll for kindly supplying the material and history in this case.)

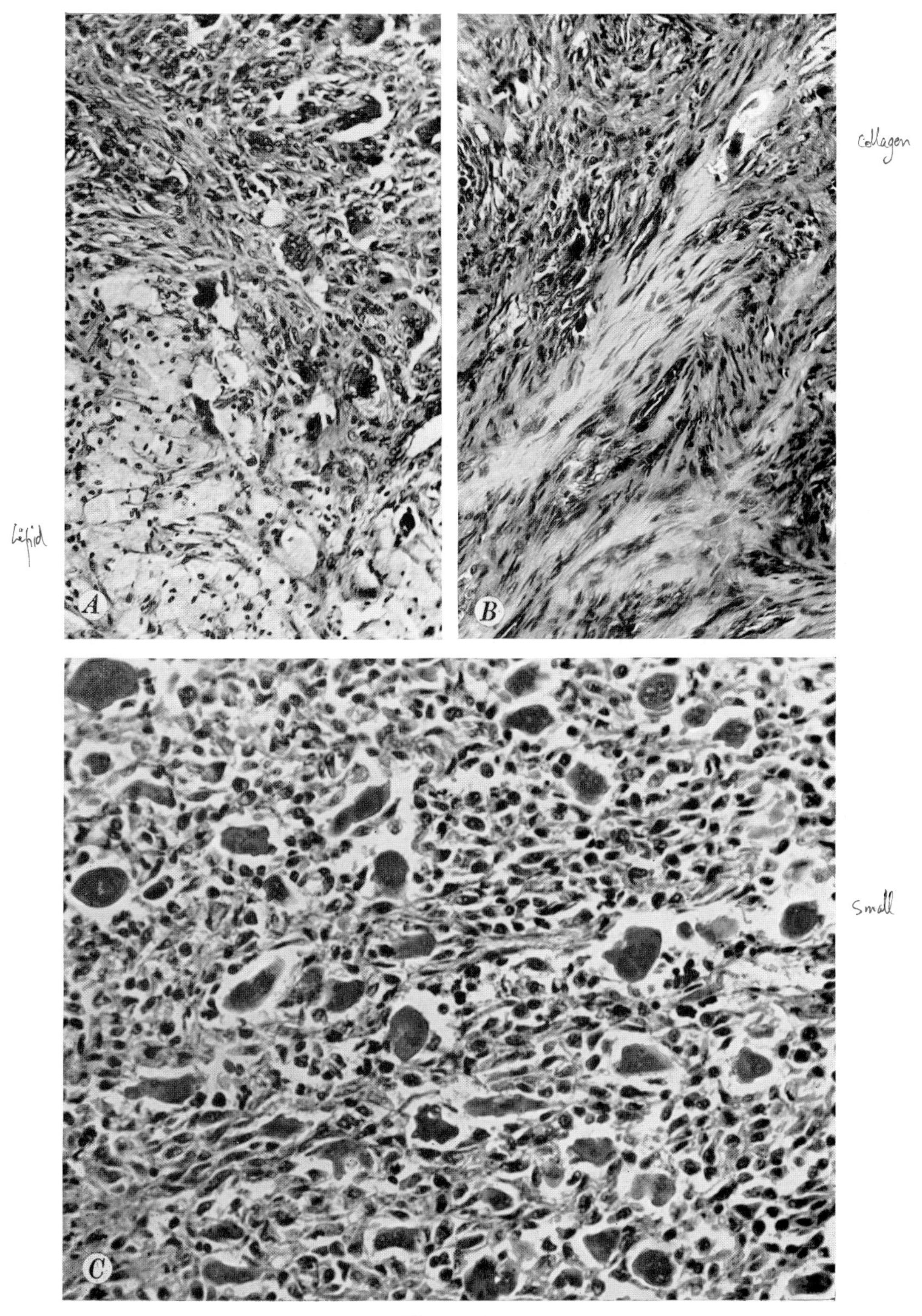


*Figure 4*

giant-cell tumor is encountered which, from the very beginning, is to be interpreted as a malignant giant-cell tumor.

As a neoplasm, the giant-cell tumor seems best interpretable as a connective-tissue growth, and more specifically as developing out of the mesenchyme-like supporting connective tissue of the bone marrow. The stromal cells of the tumor seem most plausibly explainable as arising through proliferation of this tissue. As to the origin of the giant cells, there is difference of opinion even among those who agree in holding that the lesion is a neoplasm. We, like Aegerter, for instance, believe that the giant cells are derived from the stromal cells. In any case, the giant cells ought not to be given the primal position in the genesis of the growth that has been assigned to them by many writers. An extreme expression of overemphasis upon the giant cells is represented by the idea of Geschickter and Copeland that the lesion is the result of an abnormal hyperplasia of osteoclasts left at a site of endochondral ossification.

In contrast to the neoplastic conception of the lesion is the idea that it represents a non-neoplastic reactive process. This opinion is the prevailing one among continental European (and especially German) students of the subject, enjoying the support of Lubarsch (see Gaugele), and Konjetzny, for instance. The exponents of this view hold that giant-cell tumors represent an abnormal healing process, expressed in the exuberant formation of granulation tissue. In accordance with this conception, the lesion has sometimes been described as a "granuloma," "granulation tumor," "inflammatory-resorptive tissue growth," and even "resorptive-regenerative malformation and exuberance."

The idea that a giant-cell tumor develops on the basis of an abnormal healing process necessarily presupposes antecedent local tissue damage. The latter is generally held to be an intramedullary hemorrhage. It has sometimes been postulated that a significant local intramedullary hemorrhage may appear without previous trauma, but this idea is purely speculative. It is true that many cases of giant-cell tumor give no history of trauma such as could plausibly lead to an intramedullary hemorrhage. On the other hand, when one does obtain a history of an acute trauma antecedent to the discovery of the lesion, one can frequently conclude that the lesion was present before the trauma and that the latter merely directed attention to it by causing an infraction of the bone cortex. Furthermore, it is well known that giant-cell tumors do not develop at the site of fracture (and incidental hemorrhage) through an epiphysial bone end. Finally, it has not been found possible to induce a lesion resembling a giant-cell tumor by causing intramedullary hemorrhage experimentally in any of several ways. Thus, the weight of the evidence is against the lesion being anything but a neoplasm.

## HISTOLOGIC PATTERN IN RELATION TO CLINICAL BEHAVIOR

Many writers, both early and contemporary, speak simply of "typical benign giant-cell tumor." Actually, however, the study of a series of giant-cell tumors will reveal certain cytologic variations which may be of value in grading them. Indeed, Goforth, and Stewart, Coley, and Farrow already sensed this, and Ewing laid down certain presumptive criteria for this purpose. We, too, feel that, in addition to making a diagnosis of giant-cell tumor of bone in a given case, one should attempt to grade the lesion. Our system of grading is based on variations relating mainly to the stromal cells. On this basis, we think, giant-cell tumor of bone can be subclassified into three grades—I, II, and III—showing, respectively, no appreciable, moderate, and pronounced atypism of the stromal cells, the giant-cell tumors of grade III presenting a sarcomatous stroma and being already frankly malignant. (See Figs. 3 and 4-*C*.)

In connection with grading, the details of the stromal cells should be closely scrutinized, and one should judge the tumor by its most ominous-looking areas. It follows from this that, for a relatively safe judgment, more material is usually needed than is obtained in a needle or punch biopsy specimen. In fact, when a mass of curettings is available, one should submit a considerable portion of it to cytologic study, using particularly the areas least modified by spontaneous secondary changes. Previous irradiation of the growth, too, is likely to be a confusing factor in the grading, since it may have induced fibrosis, hyalinization, and calcification, as well as distortion of the stromal cells. Even though it has not been irradiated, a recurrent tumor which has become infected may also be somewhat difficult to grade, as it tends, on the whole, to look somewhat more ominous than it really is.

As to clinical behavior, one must, of course, expect an unfavorable outcome in the case of a giant-cell tumor whose stroma has a sarcomatous cast, unless an amputation has been promptly done. However, in the vast majority of cases, as already noted, the stroma of the virginal lesion is clearly not sarcomatous. Nevertheless, even among these cases there will be a good many in which the tumor will recur after surgical intervention (perhaps more than once) and even some in which, sooner or later, it will metastasize to the lungs. Unfortunately, one really cannot predict from the histologic pattern which cases these will be. However, as already mentioned, those giant-cell tumors presenting evidence of considerable scarification and healing reaction are the ones least likely to recur. On the other hand, in a lesion representing a recurrence of a giant-cell tumor, one is likely to note that the stromal cells are more crowded and plumper than they were in the original lesion. Still, this does not signify that the recurrent lesion will necessarily metastasize or take on locally the histologic features of a frankly malignant giant-cell tumor.

The writer's experience indicates that the incidence of *recurrence* after treatment by curettage averages about 55 per cent among cases of giant-cell tumor classified as belonging to grades I and II on the basis of histologic examination of the originally curetted tissue. For grade I considered separately, the average incidence of recurrence is about 40 per cent, and for grade II about 60 per cent. Only a small percentage of giant-cell tumors present, in the originally curetted tissue, a pattern placing them in grade III. Almost all of these tumors could be expected to recur. However, when the lesion is in a limb bone, as it usually is in these cases, the part is usually ablated before recurrence has had a chance to take place. The over-all incidence of metastasis in any representative series of cases of primary giant-cell tumor is about 15 per cent. These statistical data are in accord with those reported by Thomson and Turner-Warwick.

In connection with the question of *metastasis*, it is clear that one can often find giant-cell tumor plugs in venous channels at the periphery of the tumorously involved bone site. There can also be no doubt that some of these tumor plugs become detached and reach the lungs as emboli. Undoubtedly, the story usually ends there, the tumor emboli being destroyed, but sometimes the emboli do become established as metastatic tumor foci, and grow in the cytologic pattern of the original giant-cell tumor.

Indeed, we have seen 4 cases in point. In none of these cases did either the metastatic tumor tissue or the tumor tissue at the original site acquire a frankly malignant giant-cell tumor pattern. In one of these instances the patient was a man 27 years of age who had a giant-cell tumor in the lower end of a femur. Interestingly enough, even before his femoral lesion was biopsied and curetted, a small, abnormal shadow was visualized in the middle lobe of the right lung. At that time, the pulmonary lesion was not believed to be related to the femoral lesion, and the latter was curetted and filled with bone chips. In the course of a number of months, the pulmonary lesion enlarged somewhat, and subsequently the femoral lesion recurred. About a year after the original curettement, a midthigh amputation was done, and the solitary tumor nodule in the right lung was resected. The pattern of the pulmonary lesion was that of a conventional giant-cell tumor, not differing from the pattern of the tissue originally curetted from the femur or that found in the femoral recurrence. (See Fig. 5.)

In another instance of giant-cell tumor metastasizing to the lungs and retaining its "innocent-looking" tissue pattern, the pulmonary metastases nevertheless grew to massive size, and led to the patient's death. In this case, the patient was a man 22 years of age, and the primary lesion was in the proximal phalanx of a finger. At the time of the original local intervention, difficulty was encountered in resecting the affected phalanx, and therefore the entire digit and part of the related metacarpal bone were amputated. A local recurrence appeared fairly promptly, and more of the hand was amputated about a year after the original intervention. Locally, there was never any difficulty after this, and it was complaints from the pulmonary metastases that led to further hospitalization and to the patient's death three years after the original surgical intervention. Autopsy failed to disclose any other metastases than those in the lungs.

However, there are also cases in which a giant-cell tumor undergoes progressive cytologic changes in the direction of frank malignancy locally and, in its metastases, even fails to show the histologic pattern characteristic of a giant-cell tumor at all. In a case in point—that of a woman 35 years of age—the site of the giant-cell tumor was the ascending ramus of a pubic bone. The cytology of the tissue removed at biopsy in this case was that of a conventional giant-cell tumor with a rather succulent but not frankly malignant stroma. Subsequently, the tumor showed widespread local extension, and also metastasized widely. In the metastatic foci, the tumor tissue had completely lost its giant-cell tumor pattern and presented the pattern of a spindle cell sarcoma. (See Fig. 6.)

## DIFFERENTIAL DIAGNOSIS

The problem of diagnosis and differential diagnosis of giant-cell tumor is not that it is difficult to identify the lesion when one is actually dealing with it. Indeed, under these circumstances, the correct diagnosis is easy to make. The problem, as already noted, resides in the tendency to place in the category of giant-cell tumor one lesion or another which is not really a giant-cell tumor. However, it is increasingly being recognized that a bone lesion should not necessarily be designated

***Figure 5***

*A*, Roentgenograph of a giant-cell tumor in the lower end of a femur of a man 27 years of age. Before the femoral lesion was curetted, there was already a focus of metastasis in the middle lobe of the right lung. *X*-ray examination of the lungs 4 months after the curettage showed that the pulmonary nodule, which had been very small, was increasing in size. About 1 year after curettage of the femoral lesion, the limb was amputated because of a recurrence of the giant-cell tumor. About 1 month after the amputation, the tumor nodule in the middle lobe of the right lung was resected (see *C*).

*B*, Photomicrograph (× 100) of the giant-cell tumor tissue curetted from the lesion shown in *A*. The tissue pattern is that of a giant-cell tumor of grade II.

*C*, Photomicrograph (× 100) showing the pattern of the pulmonary metastasis excised from the patient mentioned in connection with *A*. About a year after excision of this metastatic pulmonary focus, other pulmonary metastases appeared which again showed the pattern conventional for giant-cell tumor. Of great interest in connection with this case is the fact that the patient was still surviving with pulmonary metastases 6 years after the first pulmonary metastases had appeared.

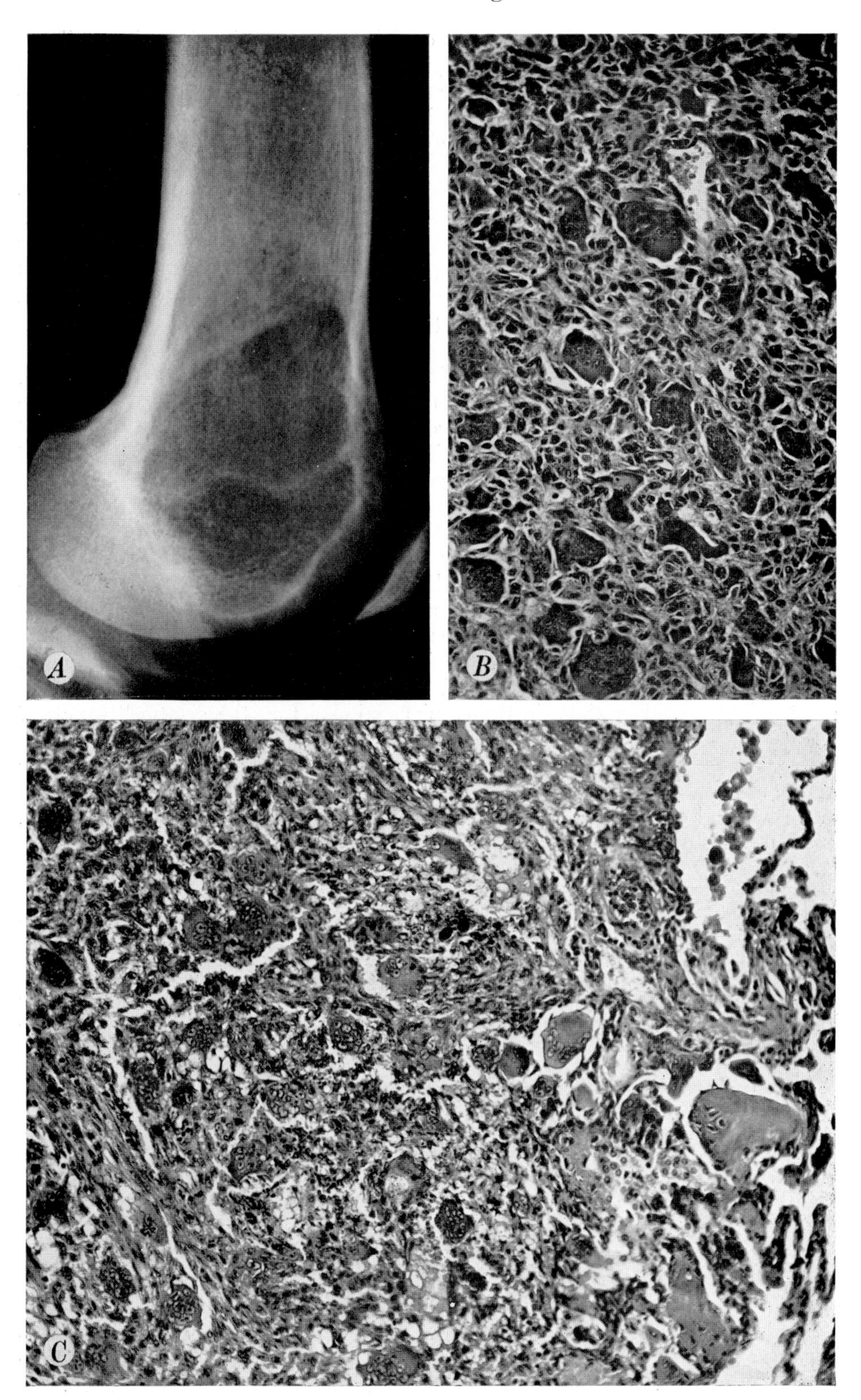


***Figure 5***

as a giant-cell tumor merely because it contains some multinuclear giant cells, to the neglect of the lesion's total histologic picture. Also, in connection with the diagnosis of giant-cell tumor, there are, as noted, significant clinical and roentgenographic features which are helpful in piecing together the total picture.

The diagnostic clinicopathologic highlights can be briefly resummarized as follows: In the great majority of the cases, the patient is between 20 and 40 years of age. In the great majority of the cases, the lesion is in an end of a long tubular bone. Roentgenographically, the affected bone part usually shows up as a rather large, more or less circumscribed area of striking radiolucency, with little if any suggestion of so-called "trabeculation." Cytologically, the pattern of the lesional tissue in characteristic areas is that of a vascularized network of plumpish, spindle-shaped or ovoid stromal cells, heavily intermingled with multinuclear giant cells.

A bone lesion presenting the cytologic pattern outlined would, of course, have to be denoted as a giant-cell tumor even if it was uncharacteristic in all other respects. However, we have not encountered a bone lesion conventional for giant-cell tumor in its cytologic pattern and aberrant in respect to all the other features of the total general picture. Indeed, the greater the extent to which a supposed giant-cell tumor is uncharacteristic in these other particulars, the greater the need for caution in interpreting the tissue sections as representing giant-cell tumor of bone.

**"Brown Tumor" Focus of Hyperparathyroidism.**—There can be no doubt that a "brown tumor" focus of hyperparathyroidism is likely to be miscalled a giant-cell tumor. It is likely that the relatively high incidence of giant-cell tumor of jawbones reported in the older literature can be explained largely on the basis of this error. Actually, in the writer's experience, conventional giant-cell tumor as we know it in relation to long tubular bones is rare in jawbones. Thus, on the basis of location alone, one should already hesitate in designating a jawbone lesion as a giant-cell tumor. Elsewhere in the craniofacial skeleton, the giant-cell tumor of bone seems likewise to be rare.

In the tissue of a "brown tumor" focus (whether in a jawbone or in some other bone), the size and distribution of the multinuclear giant cells, and the character of the stromal cells, help to distinguish this lesion from genuine giant-cell tumor. Specifically, the giant cells are small and often clumped or bunched (sometimes in nodular arrangement), especially about areas of hemorrhage; the stromal cells are delicate; and there is often evidence of osseous metaplasia of the stroma. What such a "brown tumor" focus apparently represents is a reparative scarring reaction associated with the presence of giant cells in an area heavily damaged by the local effects of hyperparathyroidism. (See Figs. 7 and 8-*A*.)

The age of the patient and the roentgenographic appearance of the jawbone lesion are not likely to be helpful in the differential diagnosis. Of course, in a case

***Figure 6***

*A*, Roentgenograph of a giant-cell tumor involving the right pubic bone in a woman 35 years of age. The history was one of pain, which had been present for 6 months at the time when this *x*-ray picture was taken. Tissue removed from the lesion established the latter as a giant-cell tumor of grade II (see *B*). The tumor underwent rapid local extension and the patient died 2 years after the onset of her complaints, with widespread metastases, especially to the lungs. The metastatic tumor tissue presented the histologic pattern of an anaplastic fibrosarcoma (see *C*).

*B*, Photomicrograph (× 150) of the tumor tissue curetted from the lesion shown in *A*. The histologic pattern is that of a conventional giant-cell tumor.

*C*, Photomicrograph (× 150) showing the tissue pattern of a focus of pulmonary metastasis in the case mentioned in connection with *A*. The histologic pattern of the metastatic focus is that of an undifferentiated sarcoma, the giant-cell tumor pattern having disappeared.

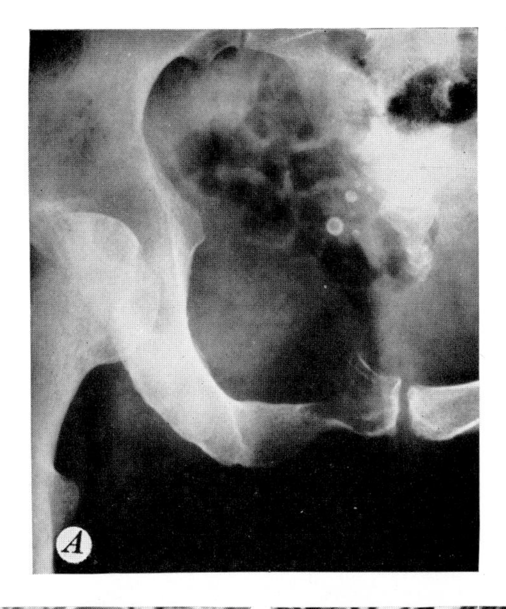

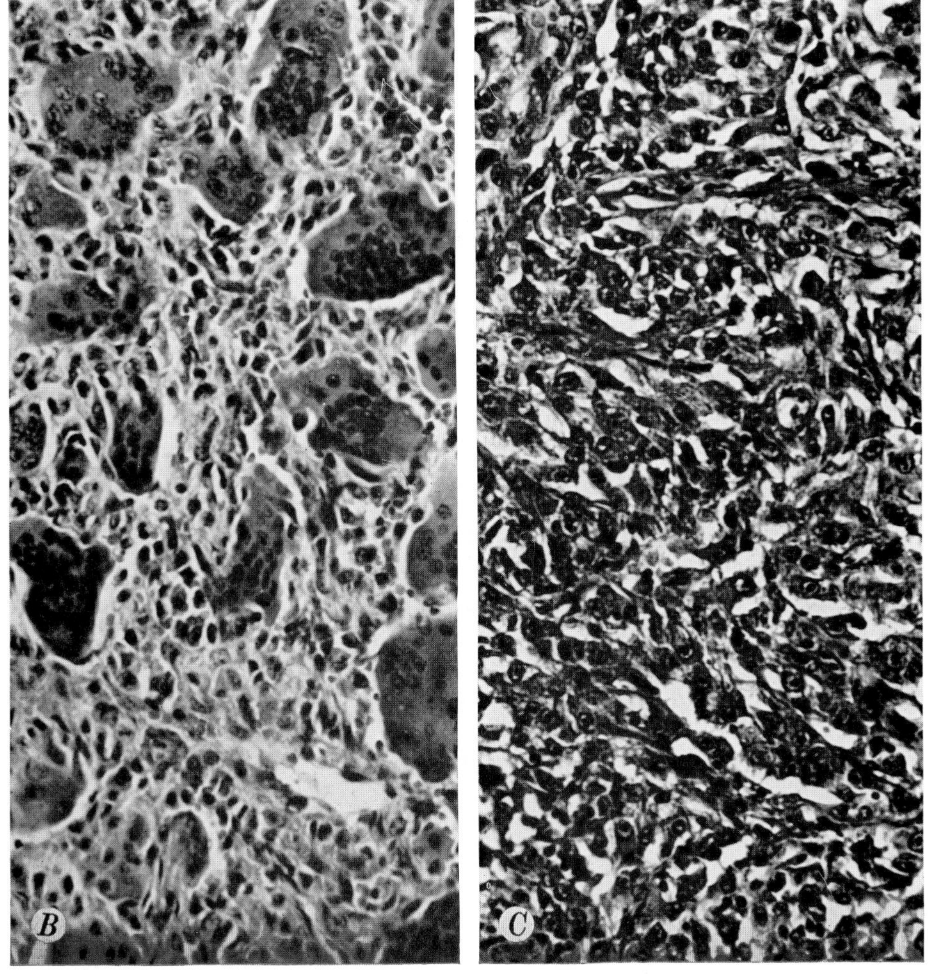

*Figure 6*

in which hyperparathyroidism is suspected, it is advisable that the entire skeleton be roentgenographed in a search for porosity of the bones and the possible presence of other circumscribed lytic lesions. However, one does encounter cases of hyperparathyroidism in which roentgenographic survey of the skeleton fails to reveal significant porosity of the bones in general, and/or the presence of more than a single localized lytic lesion. When there is only a single localized lytic lesion in a case of hyperparathyroidism, it is most likely to be in a jawbone.

To reinforce a histologic diagnosis of "brown tumor," biochemical determinations are of primary importance. The decisive determination is the serum calcium value. Provided that one can be certain of the accuracy of the determination, a serum calcium value of 11.0 mg. per 100 cc. should already make one suspect that hyperparathyroidism may be present, and a value of 11.5 mg. or more is of definite diagnostic significance in favor of hyperparathyroidism. The only other common condition which leads to an elevation of the serum calcium value is multiple myeloma, and, in relation to that condition, the biopsy findings eliminate all danger of confusion. In a case of hyperparathyroidism, the serum alkaline phosphatase value is likely to be at least somewhat above normal, though it is not necessarily so. Calcium balance studies are too complex in proportion to their practical value in arriving at a diagnosis, and the Sulkowitch test often yields equivocal results.

**Giant-cell Reparative Granuloma of Jawbones.**—Independently of hyperparathyroidism, one also occasionally encounters a jawbone lesion which, though commonly interpreted as a giant-cell tumor, likewise seems not to warrant this designation. The cytologic peculiarities of this jaw lesion make the name of "giant-cell reparative granuloma of jawbones" seem appropriate for it. Specifically, this name seems to have the advantage of conveying the idea that the lesion is not a neoplasm in the true sense, but, instead, a local reparative reaction.

It is difficult to reconstruct mentally, on the basis of the mature lesion, the successive stages of the reparative granulomatous process which has taken place. However, it seems clear that the giant cells observed in the lesional tissue bear a relation to the occurrence of hemorrhage, and are not elements in a tumorous proliferation, as they are in a bona fide giant-cell tumor of bone.

Giant-cell reparative granuloma of jawbones is not a common lesion. It occurs more often in the mandible than in the maxilla. Most often, the patients are between 10 and 25 years of age.

Roentgenographically, the lesion appears as a roundish or oval area of increased radiolucency, which is sometimes faintly trabeculated. It thins and expands, but does not perforate, the cortex of the affected jawbone. In general, the roentgenographic appearance of the lesion is thus rather nondescript, and not such as, in itself, to permit a definitive preoperative diagnosis.

***Figure 7***

*A*, Roentgenograph of the mandible in a case of hyperparathyroidism in a woman 53 years of age. Complaints relating to the mandibular lesion were the presenting complaints in this case. The area of rarefaction to be observed represents the presence of a "brown tumor" of hyperparathyroidism. Roentgenographic examination of the rest of the skeleton revealed no other lesions. Examination of a blood specimen taken after the lesion was biopsied (see *B*) showed the serum calcium to be 13.1 mg. per 100 cc. Subsequently, a parathyroid adenoma weighing about 1 gm. was removed.

*B*, Photomicrograph (× 100) showing the histologic tissue pattern in some fields of the "brown tumor" shown in *A*. Note the sparsity and bunching of the giant cells.

*C*, Photomicrograph (× 100) showing the histologic pattern in other fields of the "brown tumor" shown in *A*. Note that some osseous trabeculæ are being formed in the organizing spindle cell stroma.

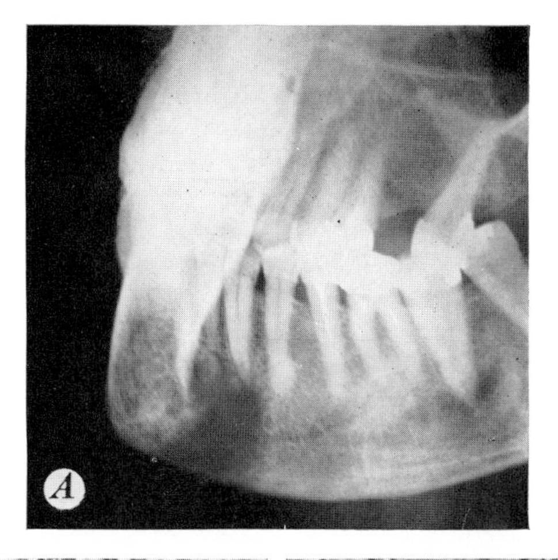


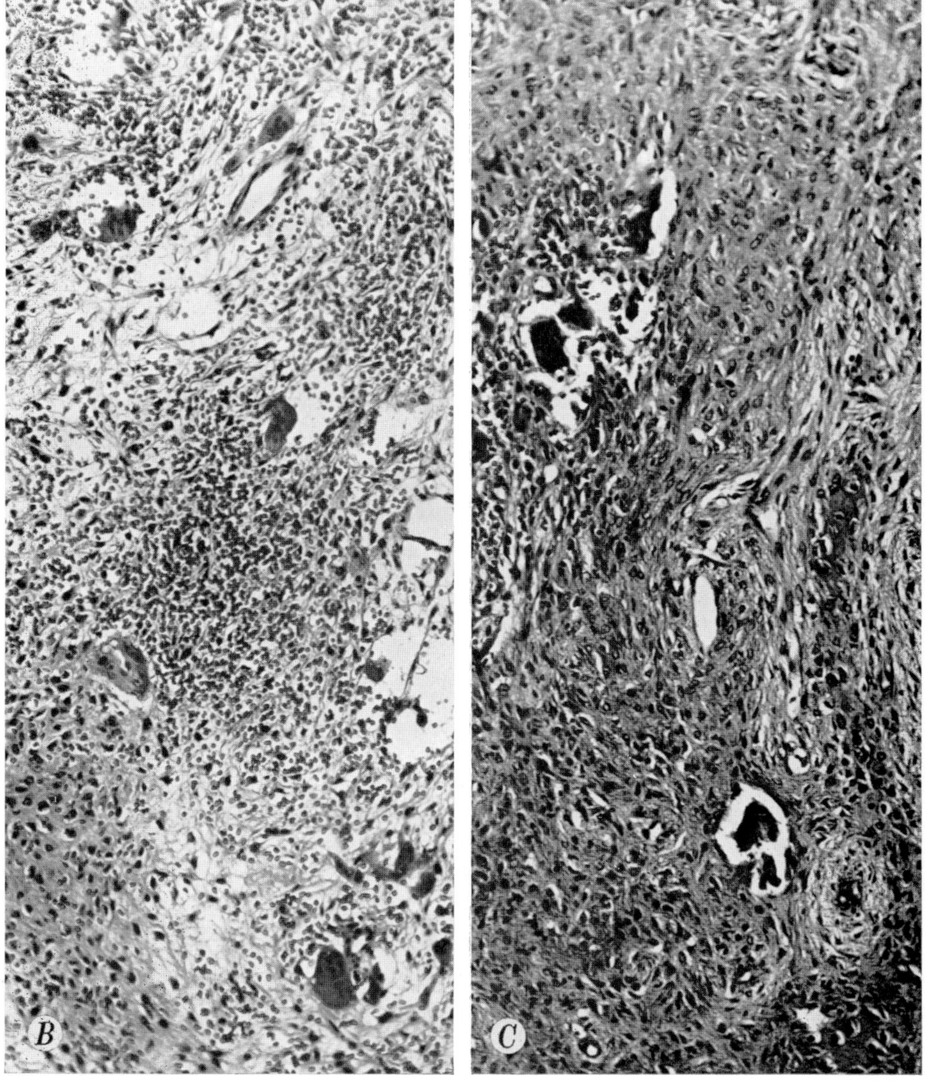


***Figure 7***

When the lesional area is entered, one finds that it contains a variable amount of soft, spongy, reddish, friable tissue. The histologic pattern presented by the lesional tissue is a rather distinctive one. In a fairly loose vascular stroma composed of small spindle-shaped cells, one notes a good deal of hemorrhagic extravasation. The multinuclear giant cells present are sparse, small, and unevenly distributed, and often clumped in areas of hemorrhage. One will note also some microscopic fields of edema and even cystification. Between microscopic lobules of such lesional tissue, one may see, here and there, some newly formed osteoid and bone. (See Fig. 8.)

When one encounters a giant-cell reparative granuloma in a jawbone, one should make sure (through chemical study of the blood and roentgenographic survey of the bones) that the patient is not suffering from hyperparathyroidism. Indeed, cytologically, it is difficult and sometimes impossible to distinguish between tissue from a jaw lesion representing a so-called "brown tumor" of hyperparathyroidism (see above) and tissue from a giant-cell reparative granuloma lesion which has developed in a jaw as a solitary lesion unrelated to hyperparathyroidism.

Giant-cell reparative granuloma of jawbones yields readily to therapy. The therapeutic procedure of choice is curettage, after which the lesion usually heals in. Occasionally, the curettage has to be repeated subsequently, but if a lesion which was thought to represent a giant-cell reparative granuloma has recurred, one must make doubly sure that the patient is not suffering from hyperparathyroidism and that the jaw lesion in question does not represent an expression of that disease. Cases of giant-cell reparative granuloma established by biopsy have also been found to yield to radiation therapy. However, the results obtained through curettage of the lesion are usually so satisfactory that, in view of the benignity, it seems unnecessary to run such risks as radiation therapy, even in small doses, may entail.

**Other Lesions in Which the Presence of Some Giant Cells May Create Confusion with Giant-cell Tumor.**—There is an expansile lesion which one not infrequently sees in relation to vertebræ and which undoubtedly accounts for many reported supposed instances of giant-cell tumor of vertebræ. This lesion (which

***Figure 8***

*A*, Roentgenograph of a giant-cell reparative granuloma in the upper jaw of a girl 10 years of age. The history was that the patient had fallen about 1 year prior to the time when this *x*-ray picture was taken, striking and loosening her upper left central and lateral incisors. A roentgenograph taken shortly after this traumatic incident showed no changes in the maxilla, and clinical examination revealed merely the loosening of the teeth. The girl came under definitive care because of the eventual appearance of a local swelling of the maxilla. Note that the roots of the teeth project into the area of the rarefaction, and that they show evidence of erosion. (I am indebted to Dr. Adolph Berger for the data in this case and the one illustrated in *B*.)

*B*, Roentgenograph of a giant-cell reparative granuloma in the lower jaw of a girl 15 years of age. The lesional area, extending from the second premolar nearly to the midline, appears radiolucent. For 3 months before this picture was taken, the patient had complained of periodic pain in the left side of the lower jaw and moderate sensitiveness of the bicuspid teeth to thermal changes. The onset of the complaints was preceded by a traumatic incident connected with skating.

*C*, Photomicrograph (× 100) of a tissue field from a giant-cell reparative granuloma. Note that the giant cells are sparse, small, and unevenly distributed in an edematous stroma. There is often a good deal of similarity in the cytologic pattern between tissue removed from a giant-cell reparative granuloma and a "brown tumor" of hyperparathyroidism. (Compare with 7–*B*.)

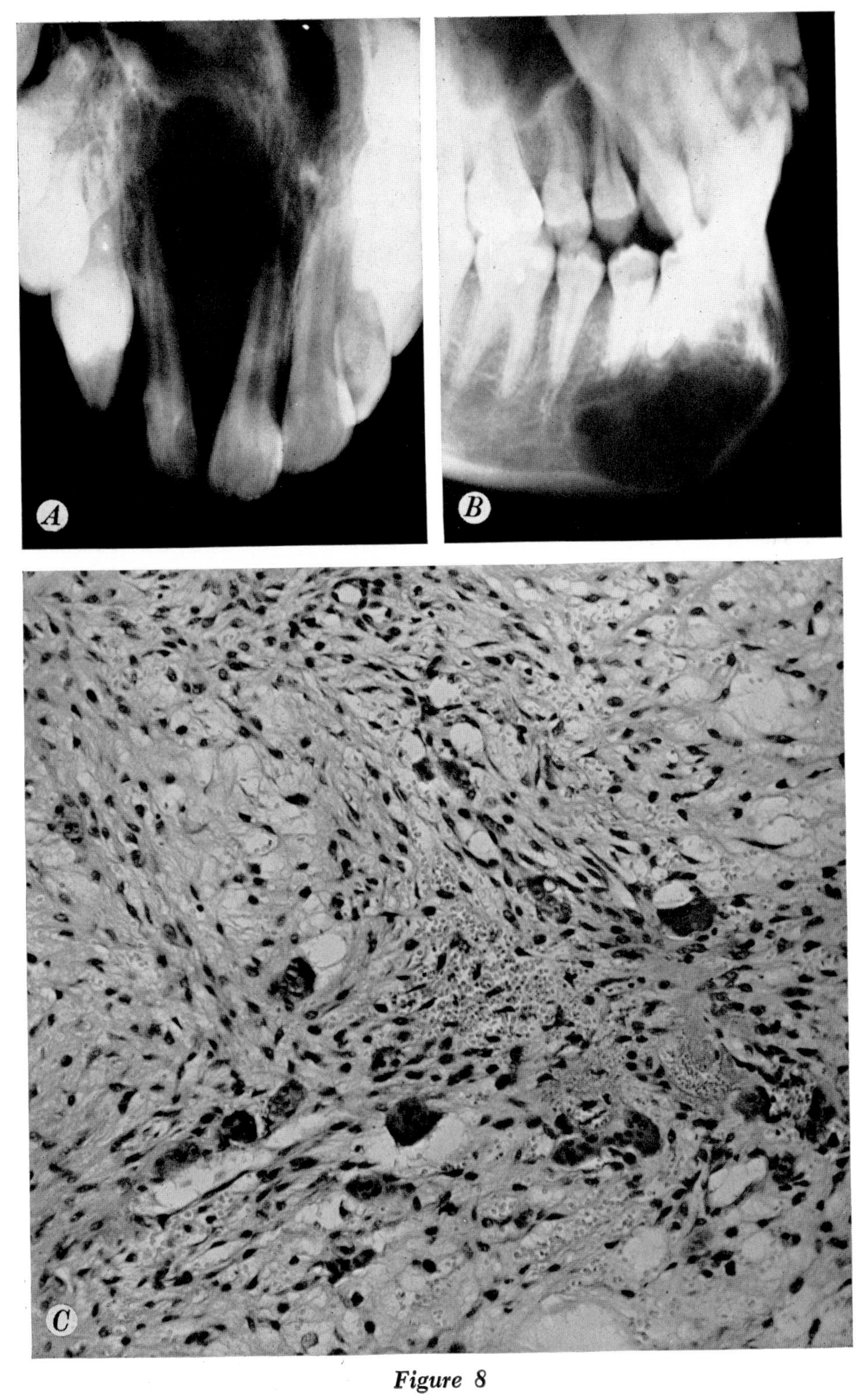


*Figure 8*

occurs in long bones also) may be encountered in any of the segments of the column. Its subjects are mainly older children and adolescents. We denote it as the "aneurysmal bone cyst," and consider it more fully elsewhere (p. 54). The term "aneurysmal" in the name relates to a sort of "blowout" distention of part of the contour of the affected bone area, creating the striking roentgenographic picture so often presented by the lesion. The term "bone cyst" in the name relates to the fact that what one finds when the lesion is entered through the thin shell of the bulged area is so largely a blood-filled cavity. The tissue on its wall is usually meager, and what there is of it is rather meshy and honeycombed by vascular spaces, and one certainly does not see any substantial tissue areas presenting the cytologic pattern of unequivocal giant-cell tumor. The burden of proof is upon those who would maintain that the cystic lesion in question is merely an "atypical" or a "subperiosteal" giant-cell tumor—terms often applied to this lesion when its appears in relation to long bones.

The writer has also occasionally seen cases in which the finding of some multinuclear giant cells in the curettings from the wall of a "solitary bone cyst" (p. 63) has led to the misinterpretation of this lesion, too, as a giant-cell tumor. The solitary bone cyst ordinarily appears as a nonloculated, fluid-filled cavity in a bone, lined by a thin fibrous membrane. In relation to a long bone, which is nearly always its site, it starts its development in one end of the shaft but rarely if ever comes to involve the corresponding epiphysial end of the bone, as a giant-cell tumor nearly always does. The findings in regard to age and location are likewise not in harmony with what one usually notes in connection with giant-cell tumor. Actually, in at least 50 per cent of the cases, the cyst is in the proximal portion of a humeral shaft, and about 80 per cent of the patients are between 3 and 14 years of age when the condition is discovered clinically. Altogether, then, there is nothing about solitary bone cyst, clinically, roentgenographically, or pathologically, which should make one regard it (as some still do) as the healing or cystic variant of giant-cell tumor.

Another lesion which should be, and is more and more frequently being, detached from the giant-cell tumor category is the "Codman tumor," or, as we prefer to call it, "benign chondroblastoma of bone" (p. 44). This lesion used commonly to be interpreted as the calcifying or chondromatous variant of giant-cell tumor. When occurring in a long bone, the benign chondroblastoma resembles giant-cell tumor in that it involves the epiphysial end of the bone. However, its roentgenographic picture is not likely to present the clear-cut radiolucency of the latter tumor. In any case, the benign chondroblastoma does not have the stroma or the general histologic pattern of a giant-cell tumor as described in this chapter, and, furthermore, it presents the highly characteristic feature resulting from the presence of focal areas of calcification. Though the lesion is now generally accepted as an entity independent of giant-cell tumor, one still encounters reports in which it is linked to giant-cell tumor.

In relation to the shafts of long bones of children and adolescents, the "non-ossifying fibroma" (p. 83) is not infrequently encountered. This lesion, which, on the basis of its histology, has often been held to represent the "xanthic" variant of giant-cell tumor, has a mere sprinkling of giant cells in a stroma of attenuated spindle cells, often containing hemosiderin-bearing phagocytes and sometimes showing areas having groups of lipophages. The non-ossifying fibroma not only appears in youthful subjects, but, in further contrast to giant-cell tumor, spares the end of the affected bone when, as is usually the case, a long bone is involved. Within the bone shaft, the lesion is ordinarily located eccentrically in the metaphysial area. Furthermore, roentgenographically, the lesional area tends to appear trabeculated. Altogether, then, though the histologic picture of non-ossifying fibroma does vaguely mimic that of giant-cell tumor of bone, its clinical and roentgenographic features are entirely different from those of giant-cell tumor.

## TREATMENT

The treatment of giant-cell tumor should be guided by the idea that the lesion (considered independently of its supposed variants or other lesions with which it may be confused) is a rather serious one. In the writer's opinion, the most practical approach to its treatment is the surgical approach, provided, of course, that the lesion is in a surgically accessible site. For a giant-cell tumor in a surgically inaccessible site, *x*-ray therapy is the only practical treatment.

In connection with surgery, resection of the tumor intact in its setting is the procedure of choice, whenever feasible. This procedure is certainly appropriate when the bone part affected is one which can be dispensed with altogether—for instance, a patella or the upper end of a fibula. Resection of the tumor-bearing portion of the bone may also be reasonable for a lesion in the lower end of a radius or possibly even the upper end of a humerus, or in any other site where the affected bone part can be replaced by a bone graft without serious mutilation or functional loss. The writer recognizes that this procedure might be held to be too radical in such cases, but it seems to him to be worth a great deal to have a chance of ridding the patient of his lesion once and for all. At any rate, for a lesion in the lower end of a radius, the functional end result from resection and grafting could at least not be worse than it has been in some cases in which the lesion in this site has been treated by curettage or *x*-ray therapy alone.

For a giant-cell tumor in the lower end of the femur or upper end of the tibia (or any analogous site), surgeons generally practice curettage and filling of the cavity with bone chips, while radiotherapists are strong in their advocacy of *x*-ray therapy. There can be no doubt that either procedure gives good results in a certain percentage of the cases. Nevertheless, in other cases, curettage fails to prevent recurrence, necessitating further surgical intervention. Though the baleful results of a supervening infection are no longer as much to be feared as they used to be in these cases, one is likely to get a prolonged morbidity, and ultimately a stiff joint. As to *x*-ray therapy, even in those cases of giant-cell tumor (about the knee, for instance) in which this is employed with relative success, one has to anticipate a morbidity of a year or even 2 years. Generally, a tumor dose of 2,000 to 3,000 roentgens is delivered over a period of 3 or 4 weeks. A second series may have to be given after 3 to 6 months, and even a third series may be necessary a year later. One must also recognize that after the initiation of *x*-ray therapy one may at first note clinical and roentgenographic exacerbation of the lesion. Though eventually the tumor diminishes in size and the cortex becomes sclerotic, the affected area never becomes completely reconstructed. Altogether, the writer wonders, even in connection with lesions in the knee joint area, whether resection of the tumor-bearing part of the bone and fusion of the knee is not to be preferred over either curettage or radiation therapy.

The question of whether one should use some *x*-ray therapy first and follow it by curettage is by no means settled. This combined procedure is still practiced by some, the precaution being taken to give no more than about 1,000 to 1,500 roentgens before curettage. The underlying belief is that, under these circumstances, the conditions for doing a curettage 2 or 3 months later are rendered more favorable because the vascularity of the tumor has been reduced and the curettage can be more thorough. The question of whether one should give supplementary irradiation therapy after curettage is also a debated one. While formerly widely practiced, such combined treatment is no longer in strong favor, the consensus of opinion being that better results are achieved by pursuing either curettage or *x*-radiation therapy consistently.

In any event, in a small percentage of giant-cell tumor cases, amputation may finally have to be done because of failure of previous therapy (either irradiation or surgery) to produce a cure. Also, in an occasional case, amputation may have to be resorted to because of malignancy of the lesion. Even if amputation is done, the ultimate prognosis is grave in these latter cases, since the likelihood is that pulmonary metastases will ensue nevertheless. It should be remembered, too, that a giant-cell tumor may undergo malignant degeneration no matter what method of treatment has previously been used. Finally, we come to the matter of malignancy appearing at the site of an irradiated giant-cell tumor.

**Postirradiation Sarcoma.**—That this may develop is no longer open to question, and the occurrence is probably not even rare. The interval between the irradiation and the appearance of the sarcoma in the original giant-cell tumor site is usually 5 to 8 years, but may be shorter or much longer. The sarcoma formation in such cases is to be interpreted as a noxious effect of the irradiation upon the bone area as a whole, rather than upon any residual giant-cell tumor tissue *per se*. The sarcoma developing under these conditions often has the histologic characteristics of a mixed mesodermal sarcoma, and may include fields of osteogenic sarcoma, fibrosarcoma, and even giant-cell tumor.

In a particularly illuminating case studied by the writer, the patient was a man 28 years of age who was treated in 1928 by curettage and irradiation for a giant-cell tumor in the upper end of a tibia. He was free from complaints for the following 23 years, during which time he went about his duties as a police officer. In 1951, he developed pain in the upper part of the leg, and a sarcoma was found to have evolved in the upper part of the tibia, in the area where the giant-cell tumor had been present. An amputation was done, and the malignant tumor was found to be an osteogenic sarcoma of a rather complex pattern. Some evidences of residual radiation osteitis could still be noted. The patient succumbed to metastases about a year after the amputation. For further details relating to this case, see page 496.

## REFERENCES

AEGERTER, E. E.: Giant Cell Tumor of Bone, Am. J. Path., *23*, 283, 1947.

ANDERSON, W.: Giant Cell Tumor of Bone, Am. J. M. Sc., *234*, 334, 1957.

BRAILSFORD, J. F.: Treatment of Osteoclastoma, Lancet, *1*, 776, 1943.

CAHAN, W. G., WOODARD, H. Q., HIGINBOTHAM, N. L., STEWART, F. W., and COLEY, B. L.: Sarcoma Arising in Irradiated Bone, Cancer, *1*, 3, 1948.

COLEY, B. L., and HIGINBOTHAM, N. L.: Giant-cell Tumor of Bone, J. Bone & Joint Surg., *20*, 870, 1938.

COMPERE, E. L.: The Diagnosis and Treatment of Giant-cell Tumors of Bone, J. Bone & Joint Surg., *35*-A, 822, 1953.

DALAND, E. M., and HAINES, C.R.: Giant-cell Tumors of Bone, New England J. Med., *254*, 587, 1956.

EWING, J.: A Review of the Classification of Bone Tumors, Surg., Gynec. & Obst., *68*, 971, 1939. (*See* Giant Cell Tumors, p. 974.)

GAUGELE, K.: Zur Frage der Knochencysten und der Ostitis fibrosa von Recklinghausen's, Arch. f. klin. Chir., *83*, 953, 1907.

GESCHICKTER, C. F., and COPELAND, M. M.: *Tumors of Bone*, 3rd ed., Philadelphia, J. B. Lippincott Co. 1949. (*See* Chapter on Giant-cell Tumor.)

GOFORTH, J. L.: Giant Cell Tumor of Bone, Arch. Surg., *13*, 846, 1926.

GROSS, S. W.: Sarcoma of the Long Bones, Am. J. M. Sc., *78*, 17, 1879.

HAAS, A., and RITTER, S. A.: "Benign" Giant-cell Tumor of Femur with Embolic Metastasis in Prepuce of Penis, Am. J. Surg., *89*, 573, 1955.

HAGGART, G. E., and HARE, H. F.: Combined Roentgen Radiation and Surgical Treatment of Large Benign Giant Cell Tumors of Bone, Ann. Surg., *124*, 228, 1946.

HATCHER, C. H.: The Development of Sarcoma in Bone Subjected to Roentgen or Radium Irradiation, J. Bone & Joint Surg., *27*, 179, 1945.

JAFFE, H. L.: Giant-cell Tumour (Osteoclastoma) of Bone: Its Pathologic Delimitation and the Inherent Clinical Implications, Ann. Roy. Coll. Surgeons England, *13*, 343, 1953.

——————: Giant-cell Reparative Granuloma, Traumatic Bone Cyst, and Fibrous (Fibro-osseous) Dysplasia of the Jawbones, Oral Surg., *6*, 159, 1953.

——————: Giant Cell Tumor of Bone: Problems of Differential Diagnosis, Bull. Hosp. Joint Dis., *5*, 84, 1944.

JAFFE, H. L., LICHTENSTEIN, L., and PORTIS, R. B.: Giant Cell Tumor of Bone: Its Pathologic Appearance, Grading, Supposed Variants and Treatment, Arch. Path., *30*, 993, 1940.

KIRKLIN, B. R., and MOORE, C.: Roentgenologic Manifestations of Giant-cell Tumor, Am. J. Roentgenol., *28*, 145, 1932.

KONJETZNY, G. E.: Zur Beurteilung der gutartigen Riesenzellengeschwülste der Knochen, Chirurg, *9*, 245, 1937.

LEUCUTIA, T., and COOK, J. C.: Malignant Degeneration of Benign Giant Cell Tumor of Bone, Am. J. Roentgenol., *62*, 685, 1949.

MÖNCKEBERG: Ueber Cystenbildung bei Ostitis fibrosa, Verhandl. d. deutsch. path. Gesellsch., *7*, 232, 1904.

MORTON, J. J.: Giant-Cell Tumor of Bone, Cancer, *9*, 1012, 1956.

MOULONGUET, P.: Tumeurs à myéloplaxes des os, Mém. Acad. de chir., *76*, 733, 1950.

MURPHY, W. R., and ACKERMAN, L. V.: Benign and Malignant Giant-Cell Tumors of Bone, Cancer, *9*, 317, 1956.

NÉLATON, E.: *D'une nouvelle espèce de tumeurs bénignes des os, ou tumeurs à myéloplaxes*, Paris, A. Delahaye, 1860.

PAGET, J.: *Lectures on Surgical Pathology*, Philadelphia, Lindsay & Blakiston, 1854, p. 446.

PLATT, H.: Osteoclastoma or Giant-Cell Tumour of Bone, J. Bone & Joint Surg., *31-B*, 157, 1949.

PROSSOR, T. M.: Treatment of Giant-cell Tumours of Bone, J. Bone & Joint Surg., *31*-B, 241, 1949.

SCHAJOWICZ, F., and MONDOLFO, S.: Tumores de células gigantes de los huesos, Rev. ortop. y traumatol., *21*, 3, 1951.

SLADDEN, R. A.: Intravascular Osteoclasts, J. Bone & Joint Surg., *39-B*, 346, 1957.

STEWART, F. W., COLEY, B. L., and FARROW, J. H.: Malignant Giant Cell Tumor of Bone, Am. J. Path., *14*, 515, 1938.

STONE, W. S., and EWING, J.: An Unusual Alteration in the Natural History of a Giant Cell Tumor of Bone, Arch. Surg., *7*, 280, 1923.

THOMPSON, P. C.: Subperiosteal Giant-cell Tumor: Ossifying Subperiosteal Hematoma – Aneurysmal Bone Cyst, J. Bone & Joint Surg., *36*-A, 281, 1954.

THOMSON, A. D., and TURNER-WARWICK, R. T.: Skeletal Sarcomata and Giant-cell Tumour, J. Bone & Joint Surg., *37-B*, 266, 1955.

WILLIAMS, R. R., DAHLIN, D. C., and GHORMLEY, R. K.: Giant-cell Tumor of Bone, Cancer, *7*, 764, 1954.

WILLIS, R. A.: The Pathology of Osteoclastoma or Giant-cell Tumour of Bone, J. Bone & Joint Surg., *31*-B, 236, 1949.

WINDEYER, B. W., and WOODYATT, P. B.: Osteoclastoma, J. Bone & Joint Surg., *31*-B, 252, 1949.

Chapter

# 3

# Benign Chondroblastoma

THE *benign chondroblastoma* is the lesion which was denoted in the past as the "calcifying giant cell tumor" (see Ewing) and as the "epiphyseal chondromatous giant cell tumor" (see Codman). However, though linking it to giant-cell tumor, both of these workers already recognized that the lesion differed in a number of ways from the ordinary giant-cell tumor. The present writer has gone further, holding that the lesion should be completely dissociated from giant-cell tumor and regarded as an independent entity (see Jaffe and Lichtenstein). This opinion has gained general acceptance, and the name "benign chondroblastoma" suggested for the lesion is now widely used (see Hatcher and Campbell, and Kunkel *et al.*).

The lesional tissue of a benign chondroblastoma presents a striking cytologic pattern, distinguished not only by the appearance of the basic polyhedral tumor cells, but also by the presence of areas of focal necrosis and calcification scattered through the tumor tissue. The name "benign chondroblastoma" implies that the lesion develops from cartilage germ cells, and it is true that the cytologic appearance of the unmodified tumor cells suggests that they might be chondroblasts. However, this idea should perhaps not be taken too rigidly, and certainly the lesion should be held apart from the tumors whose cartilaginous nature is beyond question.

## CLINICAL CONSIDERATIONS

**Incidence.**—Benign chondroblastoma is one of the less common primary tumors of bone. The writer's experience with the lesion now covers about 30 cases. As to sex incidence, the striking predilection for males seems well worth mentioning. As to age distribution, the rather strong tendency of the cases to fall into the teen-age group is likewise of clinical interest. Indeed, in all but a few of the cases studied by the writer, the patients were from 10 to 17 years of age. The ages in Codman's 9 cases ranged between 12 and 24 years. Certainly, a case in which the patient is less than 10 or more than 25 years of age is uncommon.

**Localization.**—In connection with localization, it is to be noted that, in all of the cases reported by Codman, the lesion was in the upper end of a humerus. It should be pointed out, however, that when Codman was culling his cases from the Registry of Bone Sarcoma, he was concentrating his attention upon the shoulder region, in accordance with his special interest. Nevertheless, such references to the lesion as exist in textbooks and articles sometimes include the statement that there is predilection for this region and, perhaps, even that the lesion is found there alone. Codman himself did not think it necessarily had such a restricted localization, but he did think that that localization was characteristic for it. Our experience does not confirm this idea.

In the cases studied by the writer, the sites affected, in descending order of frequency, were the following: lower end of the femur; upper end of the tibia; upper end of the humerus; lower end of the tibia; upper end of the femur; calcaneus; astragalus; ilium; ischium. Together, involvement of the lower end of the femur and upper end of the tibia accounted for more than half of the cases. Accumulating experience may shift this order of frequency and also add new sites. However, it seems clear that the humerus is not the predominant site that it was at first thought to be.

In connection with involvement of long bones, the lesion may be found limited to part of an epiphysis or involving the epiphysis and part of the adjacent metaphysis. It may be surmised that the tumor originates in the epiphysis, and that any involvement of the metaphysis is secondary. In several cases in which the patients were observed over many months, the growth of the lesion could be followed roentgenographically as it spread from the epiphysis into the adjacent metaphysis.

In connection with involvement of the upper end of the humerus, it should be noted that the lesion tends to begin its development in the greater tubercle. It is significant in this connection that this tubercle nearly always develops from an ossification center separate from that for the head proper. The lesion then spreads from the tubercle into the adjacent portion of the metaphysis, sometimes sparing the capital humeral epiphysis altogether. This pattern of involvement is also observed in connection with the upper end of the femur. Here, the lesion is likely to take its departure from the greater trochanter—again a bone part which develops from a separate center of ossification. In the cases observed by the writer in which the lesion was in the os calcis, it was once in the anterior part and the other time in the superior-posterior part of that bone. In the case in which it involved the ilium, it was located in the acetabular region.

**Clinical Complaints.**—Complaints are usually mild, so that they may be of many months' standing before medical aid is sought. Some patients give a history of an injury—usually a fall or twist—which they connect with the condition in some way, while others give no history of any possibly relevant injury. The complaints are nearly always referred to the joint closest to the lesion. This joint is generally painful, more or less swollen, and somewhat limited in its motion. Examination usually also reveals some increase of local heat, a point of tenderness, limping when a lower extremity is concerned, and even some flexion deformity, in association with local muscle atrophy. Slight hydrarthrosis, too, is to be discovered in some cases.

## ROENTGENOGRAPHIC FINDINGS

In a benign chondroblastoma the lesional area usually appears oval or round. It is rather small, ordinarily being between 3 and 6 cm. in its greatest diameter. In a long bone, as noted, the lesion is confined to part of an epiphysis or also implicates part of the adjacent metaphysis. Furthermore, the lesion is usually eccentrically located within the affected portion of the bone, so that when *x*-ray pictures taken from various angles are available, distention of the regional cortex can often be noted.

In most cases, the lesional area appears as a fuzzily rarefied and even mottled focus. That is, in most cases, the rarefied area as a whole is not strikingly radiolucent, though, in one lesion or another, parts of it may be more so than others. In one instance or another, the lesional area may appear trabeculated in addition. The fuzzy, mottled appearance of the tumor area reflects the calcification which is going on unevenly within it. In a heavily calcified lesion, the mottling will be correspondingly pronounced. Beyond the limits of the tumor, but not necessarily evenly around the lesion, a smaller or larger area of the bone may appear densified. When the tumor has bulged the regional cortex, it is not unusual to find some periosteal new bone deposition on the cortex beyond the lesional area in the metaphysis. (See Fig. 9.)

In relation to the upper end of the humerus, the lesion has become somewhat familiar and is often correctly diagnosed on a clinicoroentgenographic basis alone. When the correct diagnosis is not surmised on this basis, the lesion may be misconstrued roentgenographically as a malignant tumor and, more specifically, as a chondrosarcoma or an osteogenic sarcoma. When the lesion is small and is located in the knee region, it might be thought to represent an infectious process, such as tuberculosis. On the other hand, if the lesion is larger and the roentgenographic appearance suggests a neoplastic process, there is the possibility of miscalling it a giant-cell tumor. Undoubtedly also, on account of the mottled, spotty radiopacity which the benign chondroblastoma shows in its *x*-ray picture in some cases, the lesion may sometimes be misinterpreted as an enchondroma of bone. When, as happens only occasionally, the lesion is located elsewhere than the end of a long tubular bone, the correct diagnosis is not likely to suggest itself at all except on the basis of tissue examination.

## PATHOLOGIC FINDINGS

**Gross Pathology.**—To have the opportunity of examining a benign chondroblastoma intact in its setting is exceptional, the pathologist usually receiving only bits of curetted tumor tissue. This tissue is likely to appear in part reddish gray, rather cellular and quite vascular or even hemorrhagic, and in part more grayish and gritty and flecked with yellowish calcific material. While in one case the curetted material may show the full variety of these appearances, in another case it may be predominantly reddish gray, cellular, and vascular, and in still another mainly gritty and yellowish.

### *Figure 9*

*A*, Roentgenograph of a benign chondroblastoma in the upper end of a humerus. In this location, the lesion usually first involves the greater tubercle, but eventually may come to involve the neck and head of the bone, also, as it does in this case. The lesional area appears somewhat multiloculated, and its relative radiolucency is attributable to the fact that the lesional tissue is not much calcified. The patient was a boy 14 years of age who had had complaints referable to the right shoulder joint for about 9 months. The shoulder was painful on motion and tender to touch, and the area had become obviously enlarged by the time the boy was admitted to the hospital. The lesional area was curetted and filled with bone chips. One year after the surgical intervention, the boy was discharged from the outpatient department as cured, since he no longer presented any complaints clinically and there was satisfactory ossification at the site of the lesion roentgenographically.

*B*, Roentgenograph of a benign chondroblastoma in the upper end of a tibia. The lesional area involves the epiphysis and part of the adjacent metaphysis. A lateral view showed the tumor to be eccentrically located and to lie mainly in the posterior part of the bone, where it bulged the cortex considerably. The patient was a girl 15 years of age, and her complaints relating to the left knee were of 9 months' standing. The lesion was treated by curettage, and in the course of the subsequent 9 months, the lesional area had undergone substantial healing. Re-examination of the patient 3 years later showed her to be cured of the benign chondroblastoma.

*C*, Roentgenograph of a benign chondroblastoma involving the greater trochanter of a femur, an area which develops from an independent center of ossification. The writer has seen a lesion of analogous appearance involving the epiphysis of the femoral head alone, and several others involving only the epiphysis of the lower end of the femur or upper end of the tibia.

*D*, Roentgenograph of a benign chondroblastoma involving the acetabular area of an ilium. There is a good deal of radiopacity in the lesional area, reflecting the calcification of the lesional tissue. The patient was a boy 16 years of age who had complained of pain in the hip for about 2 months. The lesion was treated by curettage and healed in rather promptly.

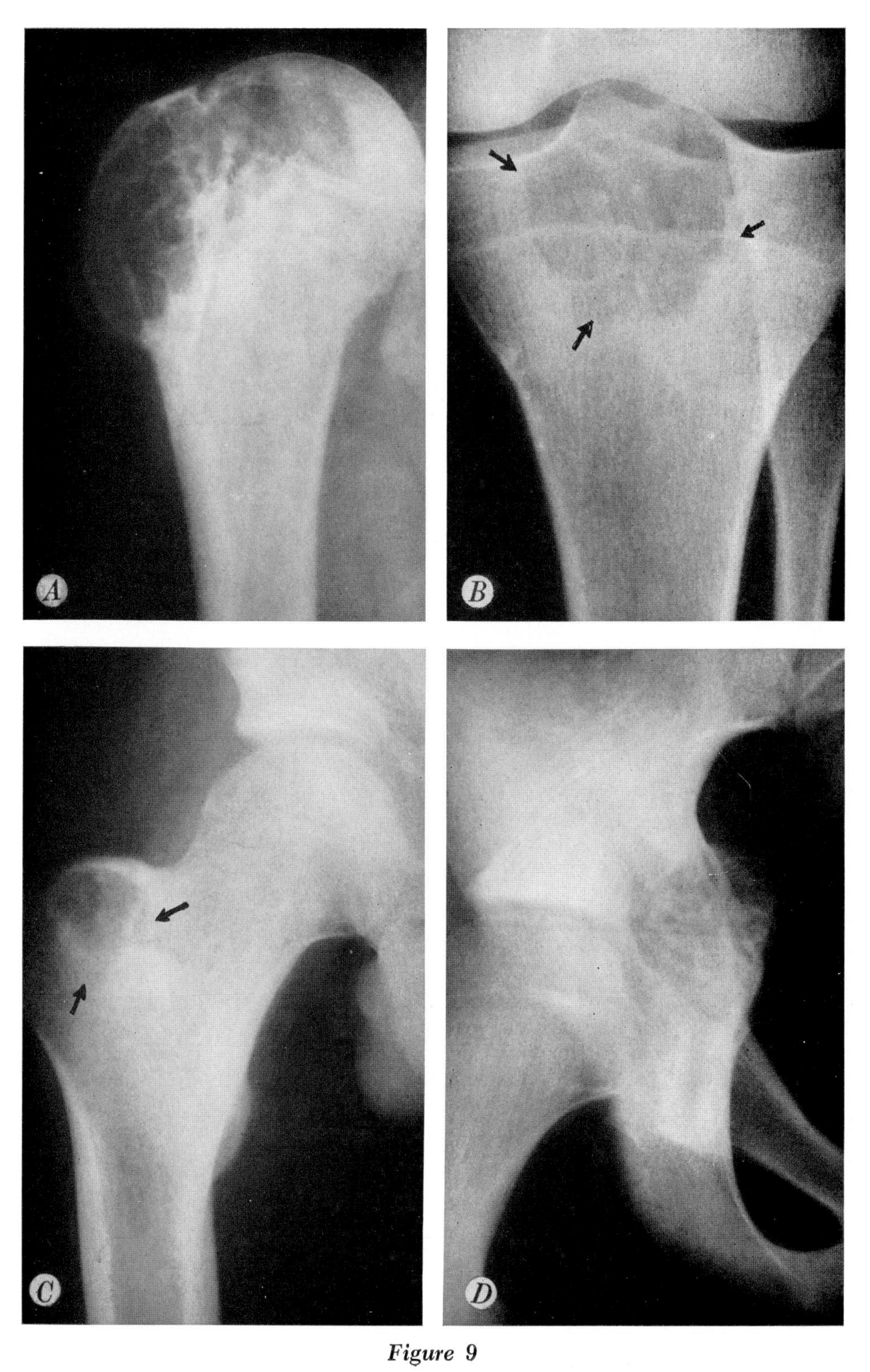


*Figure 9*

In a lesion which had been resected intact in its setting from the upper end of a humerus, the gross findings were as follows: The tumor involved the tubercles, metaphysis, and an adjacent bit of the capital epiphysis. In the cut section, it measured 6 cm. in its long axis and 4 cm. across. The tumor tissue was sharply delimited from the neighboring uninvolved bone, and the delimiting margin was convexly lobulated. Such tumor tissue as was not cystic or hemorrhagic (as it was in fully two-thirds of the lesion) was soft but rather firm and in some places even gritty, and of a gray-yellow or gray-brown color. Within the tumor, and quite enclosed by tumor tissue, one could note residual islands of epiphysial cartilage plate which had been displaced from their original position. The cystic and hemorrhagic areas were disposed mainly about the periphery. The cysts were 1 cm. or less in diameter and were outlined by a thin wall of connective tissue. Some of the hemorrhagic areas showed cystic softening and were apparently in the process of resolution into well-defined cysts. The appearance of the tumor in this case was in harmony with that of the resected humeral specimen studied by Phemister, in which the tumor proper was a soft mass of mottled brown, blue, and gray tissue.

**Microscopic Pathology.**—If one wishes to observe the full range of the histologic picture which is characteristic of benign chondroblastoma, one should make certain that at least some of the lesional tissue is processed without decalcification. The histopathology of the lesion can be outlined as follows: The basic cells are polyhedral cells of moderate size which may be closely compacted or somewhat separated by a small amount of interstitial ground substance. But, as already noted, what is striking and specific about the histologic picture is, in the first place, the presence of focal areas of calcification and the fact that, where the cells and ground substance have become heavily incrusted with calcium, the tissue is necrotic. These aspects are best visualized in sections prepared from lesional tissue which has not been decalcified. Furthermore, in the necrotic areas, one sees evidence of collagenization, resorption of the necrotic calcified debris, and replacement of the latter by hyaline chondroid tissue. This tissue itself may come to show patchy calcification and, in some places, even direct metaplasia into osseous tissue. The multinuclear giant cells to be found, either singly or in small collections, here and there in the lesions and especially about areas of hemorrhage and necrosis, are not part of the primary cytologic pattern of the tumor, but secondary to the occurrence of hemorrhage and necrosis.

As to detail, it will be noted that the polyhedral or roundish basic tumor cell has a relatively large nucleus, which is more or less centrally placed. Mitotic division figures ordinarily have to be searched for, but in some areas they are more numerous. The cytoplasm and the delimiting membrane of the tumor cells fail to stand out prominently in some places, though in others they are quite evident. As to the spotty calcification, in some low power fields two or three spots of calcification can be seen, some barely perceptible and others quite large and obvious. The calcium granules are not only deposited between the cells, but are also found in the cytoplasm of the cells, especially where the focal deposition of calcium is relatively intense. The calcium deposition in such areas is associated with swelling of the tumor cells. (See Fig. 10.)

***Figure 10***

*A*, Photomicrograph (× 420) showing the cytologic pattern of a relatively unmodified tissue area of a benign chondroblastoma. The stippling toward the right of the picture represents beginning calcification between some of the tumor cells. Toward the center of the picture, there is beginning swelling of the tumor cells, and a small multinuclear giant cell.

*B*, Photomicrograph (× 420) showing the cytologic pattern in a tumor field in which the deposition of calcium is further advanced than in *A*.

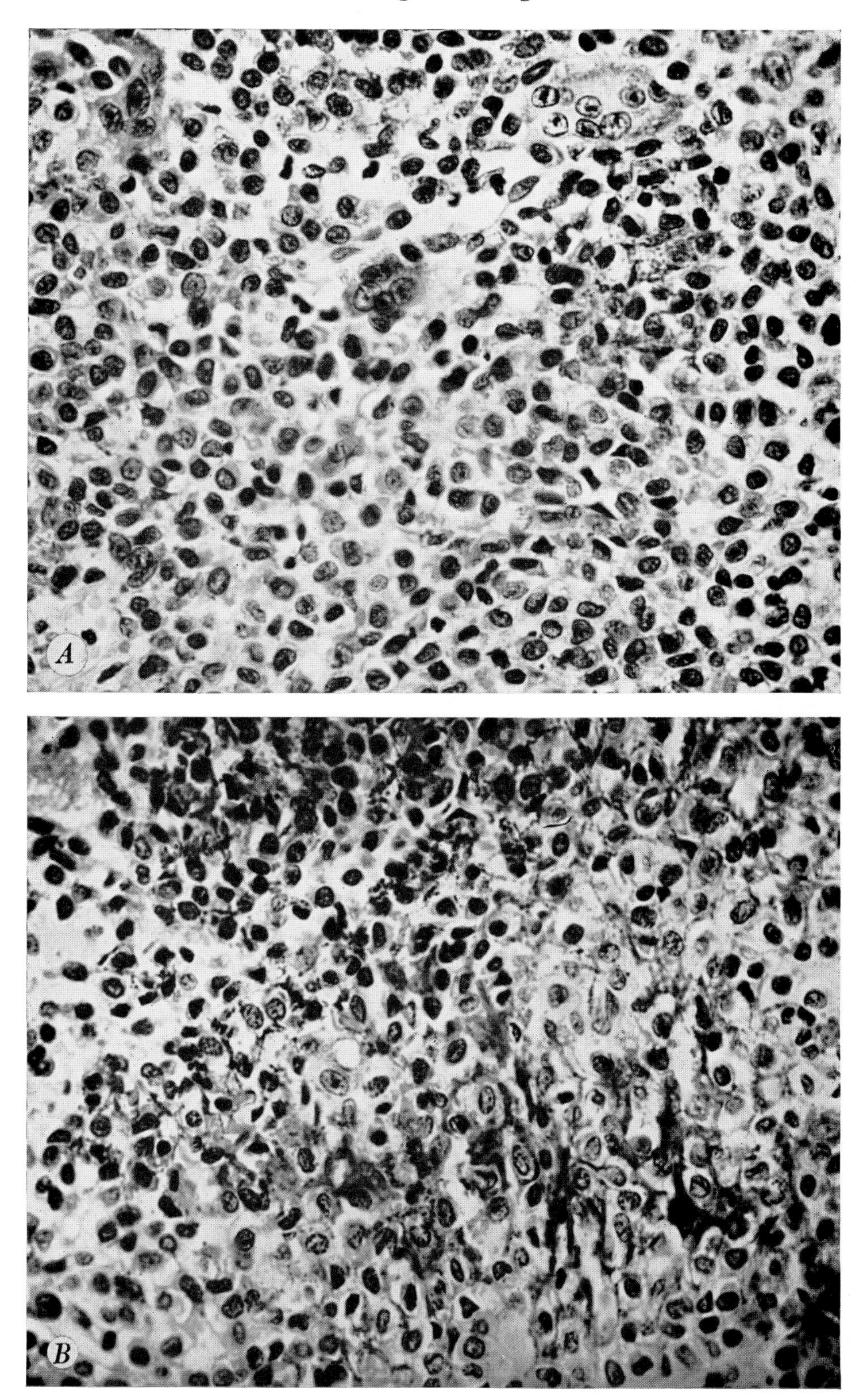


*Figure 10*

In surveying different fields of the tumor, one can thus see clumps or nodules of tumor cells with large, pale nuclei and purple-staining granules in their cytoplasm, surrounded by varying amounts of calcareous intercellular ground substance. In some fields, also, the focal calcium incrustation results in the appearance of calcareous blotches. When such an area is examined under high magnification, it becomes evident that most of the cell nuclei within it are either disintegrating or have already disappeared, and the cellular architecture is sometimes found represented merely by the faint outlines of the former cell walls. Thus, where the calcification has become more intense, focal areas of necrosis appear in the tumor tissue. Neighboring areas of focal calcification and necrosis may spread and fuse, leaving little if any intervening viable tumor tissue. Such areas represent the yellowish calcareous bits of gross material which can be found among the curettings from a benign chondroblastoma. Altogether, when one traces the evolution of the focal calcification, one cannot doubt that the necrosis of the tumor cells is secondary to the calcification and does not provoke it.

Let us consider now the fate of the calcified and necrotic areas. About the periphery of these areas, one sees evidence of collagenization and the appearance of what seems to be hyalinized connective tissue. This collagenized connective tissue progressively encroaches upon and replaces the necrotic and calcified debris. In the course of this encroachment, the calcified material becomes confined more and more closely to the center of the area undergoing replacement, and steadily diminishes in amount. Finally, large patches of collagenous hyaline or chondroid tissue come to replace the necrotic tissue. (See Fig. 11.)

In the description of the gross appearance of the tumor, it was noted that the latter may present areas of gross hemorrhage, softening, and small cysts resulting from the organization of hemorrhage. Microscopically, it can be seen that, about the periphery of necrotic areas undergoing hyaline and chondroid metaplasia, and especially in the vicinity of large vascular sinuses and areas of free hemorrhage, there are large multinuclear giant cells, often in aggregates or clumps. As already noted, it is because of the presence of such clumps of giant cells in areas of necrosis that benign chondroblastoma has been interpreted, especially in the past, as a form of giant-cell tumor of bone. These giant cells undoubtedly represent multinuclear macrophages such as are commonly found in any skeletal lesion in the vicinity of local hemorrhage, organization, fibrosis, chondrification, or ossification. At any rate, as already indicated, they do not form part of the basic cytology of the lesion.

Because of overlapping histologic patterns occasionally encountered, it has been suggested that benign chondroblastoma and chondromyxoid fibroma are closely related lesions (see Kunkel *et al.*). It should be pointed out, however, that histologic diagnosis of any bone tumor should be based on the predominating tissue pattern.

### *Figure 11*

*A*, Photomicrograph (× 450) showing a field in which the calcification is rather considerable. Where this is the case, the tumor cells are undergoing necrosis.

*B*, Photomicrograph (× 100) showing intermingled viable and necrotic (and previously heavily calcified) tumor tissue also presenting areas of microcystic softening. The tissue from which this slide was prepared had been decalcified with nitric acid.

*C*, Photomicrograph (× 230) showing an area in which the calcification had originally been intense. The tissue had been decalcified with nitric acid before imbedding. Pale shadows of necrotic tumor cells may be seen where the calcification had been particularly intense.

*D*, Photomicrograph (× 70) showing chondroid areas intermingled with cellular areas. Here and there in the chondroid tissue, secondary calcification is apparent. In some lesions, the calcified chondroid material may undergo spotty osseous metaplasia.

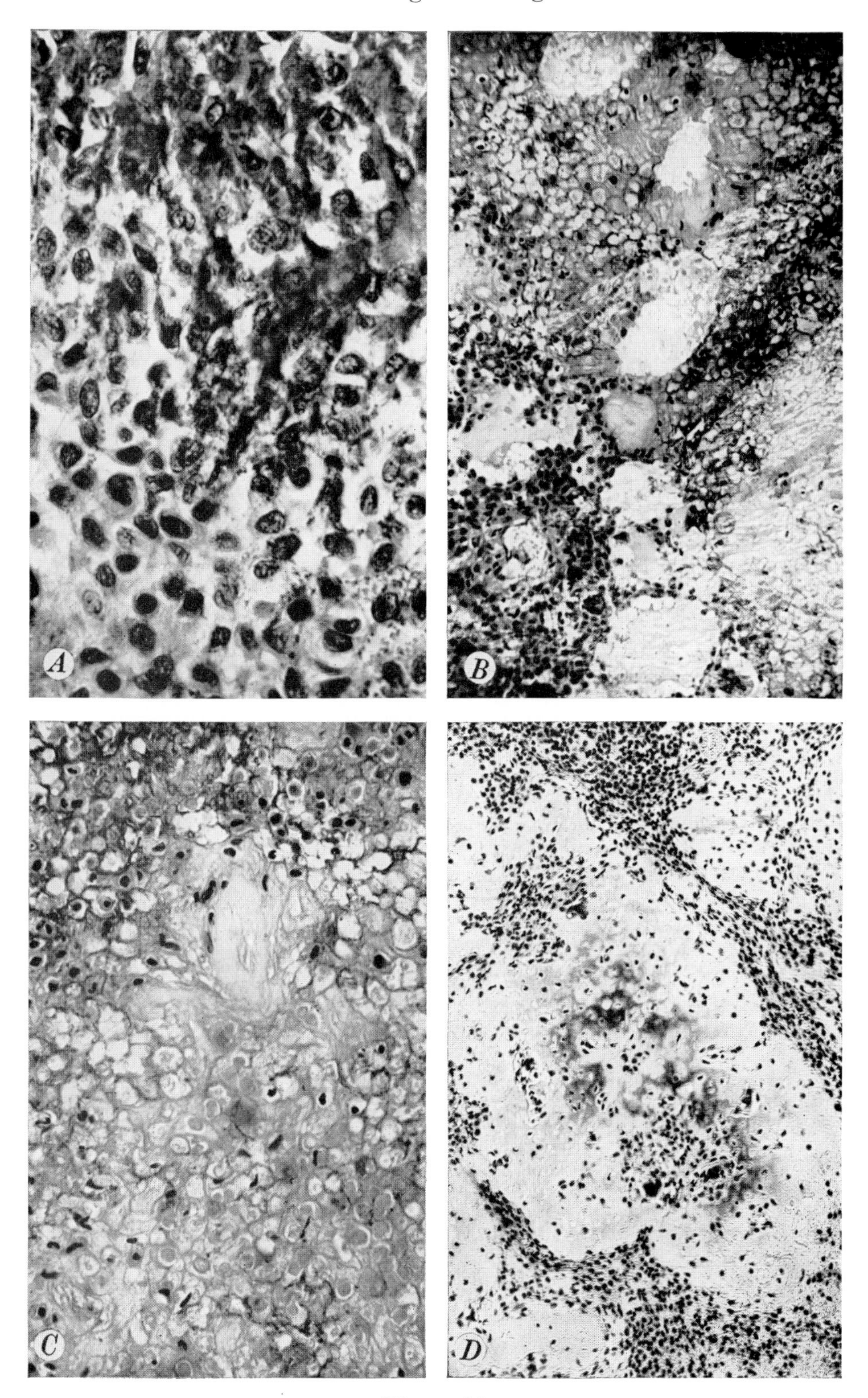


*Figure 11*

In any event, the writer believes that these two lesions should be held apart as distinct clinicopathologic entities. The question of the suggested cytologic interrelationship between them is discussed in connection with the microscopic pathology of chondromyxoid fibroma (see p. 210).

## DIFFERENTIAL DIAGNOSIS

There can be no doubt that cases of benign chondroblastoma are still being misinterpreted in various ways. Designation of the lesion as a giant-cell tumor (albeit as a variant) probably still represents the most common confusion. The interpretation of it as a chondrosarcoma or chondroblastic sarcoma is also not rare. Now and then, too, a lesion which is probably a benign chondroblastoma is regarded as an enchondroma (central chondroma)—that is, as a benign tumor of mature cartilage. Search of the literature even reveals an occasional case in which the lesion has been widely misinterpreted as a myeloma, endothelioma, or even fibrosarcoma, or, in a paradoxical way, as a "benign" osteogenic sarcoma.

**Giant-cell Tumor.**—It is true that, like the benign chondroblastoma, the giant-cell tumor predilects the ends of long tubular bones. In cases of giant-cell tumor, however, the patients are usually between 20 and 40 years of age, instead of in their teens or slightly younger, as in cases of benign chondroblastoma. In the *x*-ray picture, the giant-cell tumor shows up, on the average, as a larger and more radiolucent lesion. As to histology, the stromal cells of a giant-cell tumor are spindle-shaped or ovoid, rather than polyhedral, and one does not observe the spotty calcification and necrosis characteristic of the lesional tissue of the benign chondroblastoma. In viable and not otherwise modified tissue areas of a giant-cell tumor, the giant cells are numerous and freely interspersed between the stromal cells. In viable and relatively unmodified areas of a benign chondroblastoma, on the other hand, multinuclear giant cells are sparse and do not constitute an essential element of the histologic pattern. Indeed, in a benign chondroblastoma, one is not likely to find more than a sprinkling of giant cells, except in areas in which there has been a considerable amount of necrosis and hemorrhage, or around those areas showing chondroid organization. Altogether, in respect to the differential histologic diagnosis between the two lesions, one must keep in mind that, in the benign chondroblastoma: The basic tumor cell is polyhedral; the lesional tissue shows patchy calcification and necrosis; the necrotic areas undergo chondroid organization; and multinuclear giant cells are sparse except in areas undergoing secondary change.

**Chondrosarcoma.**—The possibility of confusion between benign chondroblastoma and chondrosarcoma arises only in connection with central chondrosarcoma (p. 315). On the clinical side, while an occasional chondrosarcoma is found in a youthful subject, most instances of it are observed in young or middle-aged adults. As to histology, one can be guided by the fact that the tissue of a chondrosarcoma is clearly cartilage tissue. Specifically, its constituent cells are usually surrounded by lacunæ and set in a considerable amount of clearly defined intercellular matrix. Furthermore, a central chondrosarcoma shows at least numerous binuclear cartilage cells with plump nuclei. In addition, it may show a number of large or giant cartilage cells with large single or multiple nuclei, and, if its malignancy is full blown, many of the tumor cells will be seen in mitotic division. Particularly if the chondrosarcoma has developed in a child or adolescent, these cytologic stigmata of malignancy are usually very pronounced.

It is true that some benign chondroblastomas show tissue fields suggesting cartilage because of the development of a sort of hyaline chondroid material which has replaced the calcified and necrotic tumor tissue. Nevertheless, if the chondroid areas are considered in their total setting, it will be clear that the cells in relatively unmodified fields of a benign chondroblastoma do not present the appearance of mature cartilage cells or the nuclear aberrations shown by the cells of a chondrosarcoma.

**Enchondroma.**—Less likely to happen than confusion with chondrosarcoma is the possibility of misinterpreting a benign chondroblastoma as an enchondroma (solitary central chondroma). This possibility is most likely to arise on the basis of the roentgenographic appearance, in connection with a rather heavily calcified and otherwise modified benign chondroblastoma in an epiphysial end of a long bone. It should be remembered, however, that, though a solitary enchondroma (p. 169) is sometimes found involving the epiphysial end of the bone, it is usually located in the bone shaft only. Phalanges and metacarpal and metatarsal bones are common sites for the solitary enchondroma, and exceptional ones for benign chondroblastoma. Also, a patient affected with a solitary enchondroma is much more likely to be an adult than an adolescent.

As to pathology, in a solitary enchondroma the lesional tissue as a whole is indubitable mature cartilage tissue. Furthermore, this tissue is less cellular than that of a benign chondroblastoma. The individual cartilage cell nuclei are relatively small and show no atypism. Altogether, then, even if one sets the clinical guideposts aside, the histologic distinctions are sufficiently clear-cut to prevent confusion between the two lesions.

## TREATMENT

As indicated in its name, the benign chondroblastoma is a benign lesion. It is a question whether the tumor ever undergoes spontaneous malignant transformation, and the writer himself has seen no case in which it did so.

The treatment of choice is thorough curettement of the lesion, and the writer has not observed recurrence after such treatment alone. Radiation therapy (alone or supplemental to curettage) has been employed in some cases, but hardly seems advisable in view of the amenability of the lesion to curettage. Hatcher and Campbell report a case of benign chondroblastoma in the upper end of a humerus which was treated by curettage supplemented by 3,600 r of radiation. Three and a half years after treatment, a chondrosarcoma developed in the lesional area, and they interpreted this as having been induced by the radiation therapy.

## REFERENCES

Bergstrand, H.: A Note on Chondroblastic Sarcoma, Am. J. Cancer, *27*, 326, 1936.

Codman, E. A.: Epiphyseal Chondromatous Giant Cell Tumors of the Upper End of the Humerus, Surg., Gynec. & Obst., *52*, 543, 1931.

Coley, B. L., and Santoro, A. J.: Benign Central Cartilaginous Tumors of Bone, Surgery, *22*, 411, 1947.

Ewing, J.: The Classification and Treatment of Bone Sarcoma, Report Internat. Conf. on Cancer, London, John Wright and Sons, Ltd., Bristol, 1928. (*See* Calcifying Giant Cell Tumor, p. 370.) *and* A Review of the Classification of Bone Tumors, Surg., Gynec. & Obst., *68*, 971, 1939. (*See* Giant Cell Tumors, p. 974.)

France, W. G.: Benign Chondroblastoma of Bone, Brit. J. Surg., *39*, 357, 1952.

Hammarström, S.: Ein Fall von Chondroblastischem Sarkom, Acta radiol., *15*, 668, 1934.

Hatcher, C. H., and Campbell, J. C.: Benign Chondroblastoma of Bone: Its Histologic Variations and a Report of Late Sarcoma in the Site of One, Bull. Hosp. Joint Dis., *12*, 411, 1951.

Jaffe, H. L., and Lichtenstein, L.: Benign Chondroblastoma of Bone: A Reinterpretation of the So-called Calcifying or Chondromatous Giant Cell Tumor, Am. J. Path., *18*, 969, 1942.

King, E. S. J.: An Example of Benign Osteogenic Sarcoma, Brit. J. Surg., *19*, 330, 1931–32.

Kunkel, M. G., Dahlin, D. C., and Young, H. H.: Benign Chondroblastoma, J. Bone & Joint Surg., *38-A*, 817, 1956.

Phemister, D. B.: Chondrosarcoma of Bone, Surg., Gynec. & Obst., *50*, 216, 1930. (*See* p. 223.)

Treasure, E. R.: Benign Chondroblastoma of Bone, J. Bone & Joint Surg., *37*-B, 462, 1955.

Valls, J., Ottolenghi, C. E., and Schajowicz, F.: Condroblastoma epifisario, Rev. ortop. y traumatol., *19*, 17, 1949. (*Also* J. Bone & Joint Surg., *33-A*, 997, 1951.)

Chapter

# 4

# Aneurysmal Bone Cyst

ONE occasionally encounters a rather arresting benign bone lesion for which the writer has formulated the name *aneurysmal bone cyst* as being descriptive in a general way. The term "aneurysmal" in the name relates to a sort of "blowout" distention of part of the contour of the affected bone area, creating the striking roentgenographic picture so often presented by the lesion. The term "bone cyst" in the name relates to the fact that, when the lesion is entered through the thin shell of the bulged area, what one finds is mainly a blood-filled cavity. The tissue on its wall is usually meager, and what there is of it is rather meshy and honeycombed by vascular spaces. The lesion usually affects some long bone shaft or some part of the vertebral column, but has been encountered in various other bone sites also. The lesion has no relation to the familiar solitary bone cyst (p. 63).

**Nomenclature.**—Examples of the "aneurysmal bone cyst" are to be found most often among cases classified as "atypical" or "subperiosteal" giant-cell tumor. Some of the cases recorded in the older literature as instances of "benign bone aneurysm" probably likewise represent it. Furthermore, especially when located in the vertebral column, the lesion has sometimes been denoted as a "hemangioma of bone," albeit of a peculiar character. The name "hemangiomatous bone cyst" has also been suggested for the lesion in question. However, that name might lead to the misinterpretation that the latter has its basis in a hemangioma. More importantly, it sacrifices the feature of "blowout" distention which is so conspicuous in the $x$-ray picture of the lesion and which is all that the term "aneurysmal" was intended to convey.

***Figure 12***

√ *A*, Roentgenograph of an aneurysmal bone cyst in a femur. Note the ballooned-out distention outlined by the arrows, and also the fact that the lesion is eccentric and the regional cortex is disintegrated. The patient was a man 22 years of age whose difficulties relating to the left hip were of about 6 months' standing. His chief complaint was pain, which he dated back to a fall sustained during jujitsu practice. The pain became progressively worse, and, on the basis of this $x$-ray picture, the lesion was misinterpreted at first as an osteogenic sarcoma. On biopsy of the lesion, however, a large, blood-filled cavity was encountered, and the specimen removed from the periphery of the lesion showed the characteristic pattern of an aneurysmal bone cyst (see 14-*A*).

*B*, Roentgenograph of an aneurysmal cyst in the upper end of a tibia of a boy 15 years of age. Note again the ballooned-out appearance of the lesional area.

*C*, Roentgenograph of an aneurysmal bone cyst in the clavicle. Note the "blowout" distention in the lesional area. The patient was a woman 35 years of age, and her chief complaint was of pain in the right shoulder region. She had been aware of the pain for about 1 month, and stated that it was present only when the arm was moved. Shortly after the onset of her local difficulties, she noted a swelling of the outer part of the clavicle. Treatment consisted of excision of the blister-like cystic area and curettement of its base. The defect in the clavicle healed in within a few months.

*D*, Roentgenograph of an aneurysmal bone cyst involving the 5th lumbar vertebra. The patient was a child 8 years of age. Note the ballooned-out distention present in relation to the collapsed vertebral body.

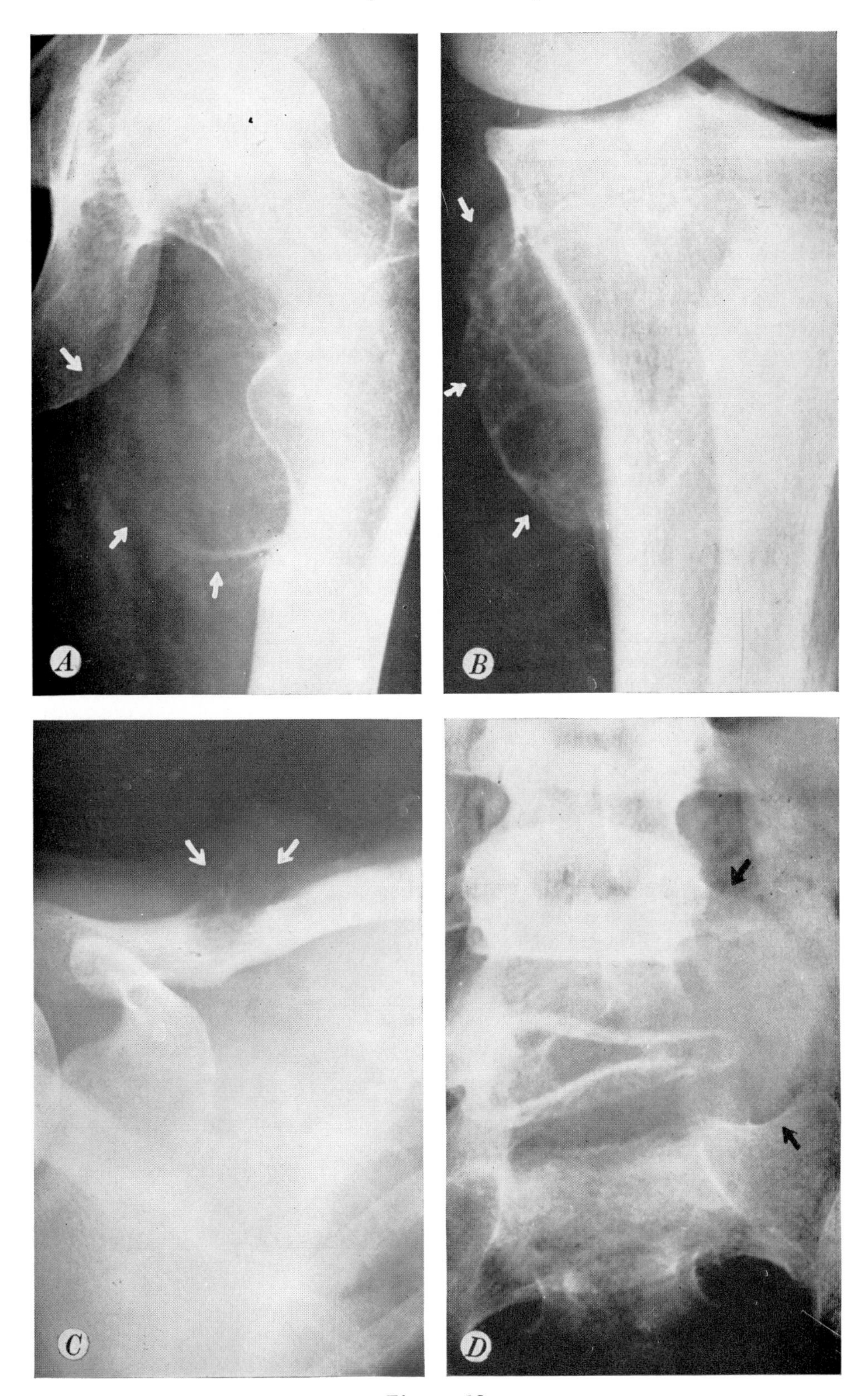


***Figure 12***

## CLINICAL CONSIDERATIONS

**Incidence.**—Almost all of the patients are older children, adolescents, or young adults. In our series of about 35 cases, females definitely predominated over males, but it is not certain that this finding is statistically reliable.

**Localization.**—As noted, a relatively common location of the lesion is in some long bone—most often a femur. In relation to a long bone, the lesion is usually somewhere near one end of the shaft, generally sparing the actual epiphysial end of the bone. However, it may be found somewhere near the middle of the shaft. In either case, the lesion is likely to be located eccentrically—that is, to involve only one side of the bone shaft.

Involvement of some part of the vertebral column is about as common as involvement of a long bone. However, the lesion shows no particular predilection for any one segment of the column. The writer has seen it in the cervical, dorsal, lumbar, and even sacral part of the column. The lesion may be practically confined to the vertebral body, extending only very slightly beyond it, or it may be mainly in the arch and processes, affecting the body only slightly if at all. On the other hand, it may be found to involve the body, arch, and even processes. In such cases, when thoracic vertebræ are affected, neighboring ribs on one side or another and even an adjacent vertebra may come to show pressure erosion.

In a representative series of cases, the likelihood is that localization to the long bones and vertebral column will account for about three-quarters of the cases. Other locations in which the writer has observed the aneurysmal bone cyst include an os calcis, the superior ramus of a pubic bone, and the shaft of a clavicle, of a metacarpal bone, and of a phalanx.

**Clinical Complaints.**—Not infrequently, the patients give a history of local trauma antedating the onset of the complaints by a relatively short interval. It is doubtful, however, that trauma instigates the lesion. Probably it usually only calls attention to the lesion by exacerbating it locally.

In connection with involvement of a long bone, for instance, the history is usually one of pain, not severe, and at most of a few months' standing. There may also be an awareness of a gradually increasing swelling. Lesions which approach the joint end of the bone are likely to be associated also with some pain on motion. When the lesion is in some part of the vertebral column, pain and stiffness relating to the affected segment of the column are the initial complaints. As the lesion progresses, there are usually also associated neural complaints. In connection with a lesion in the thoracic region, for instance, there may be girdle pains or progressive weakness of the lower limbs, associated even with numbness. With a lesion in the lumbar part of the column, there may even be loss of bladder and bowel control. In any

### *Figure 13*

*A*, Roentgenograph of an aneurysmal cyst in a lower femoral metaphysis of a girl 12 years of age. Note the disintegration of the cortex in the region of the "blowout" distention indicated by the arrows. The patient gave a history of local pain and tenderness dating back only 3 weeks. The lesional area was excised *in toto* (see *B*), and the patient had no further difficulty relating to the lesion.

*B*, Photograph of the specimen removed in the case illustrated in *A*. One is looking into the interior of the cyst. Below it, there is a small margin of the epiphysial end of the bone. Note the meager meshy tissue within the cystic area (see *C*).

*C*, Photomicrograph (× 5) illustrating the appearance of the ballooned area. From above down, one notes the periosteum, the thin subperiosteal shell of new bone, and the large, sinuous spaces, which were filled with blood.

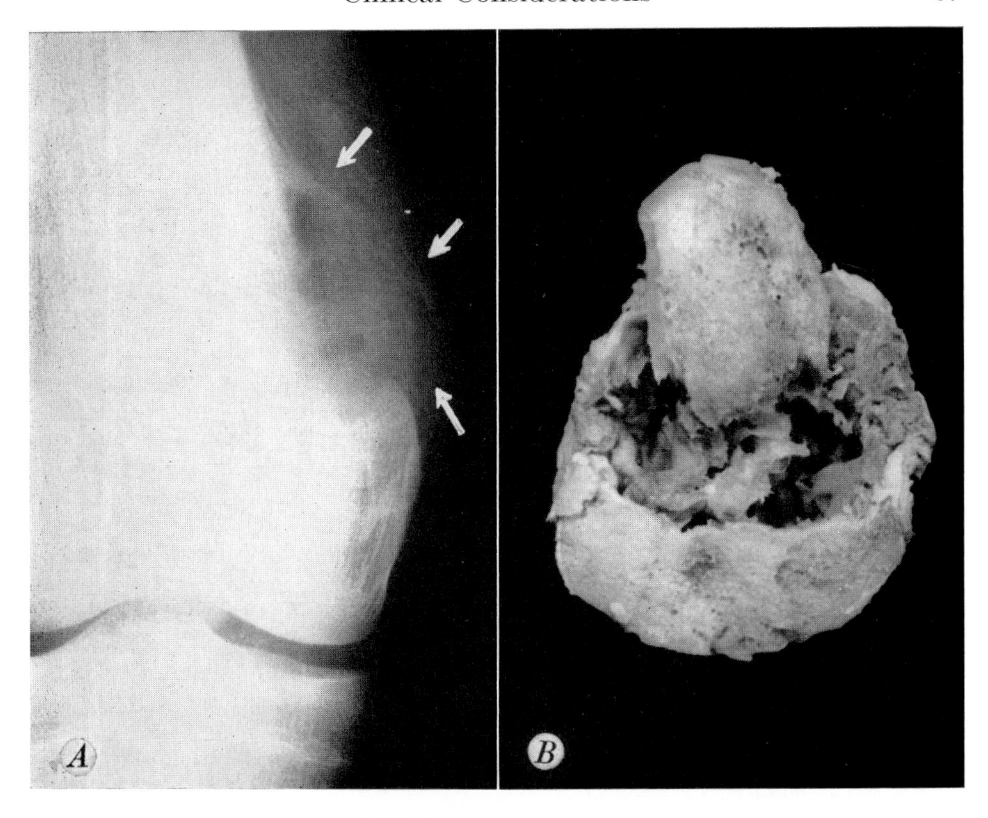


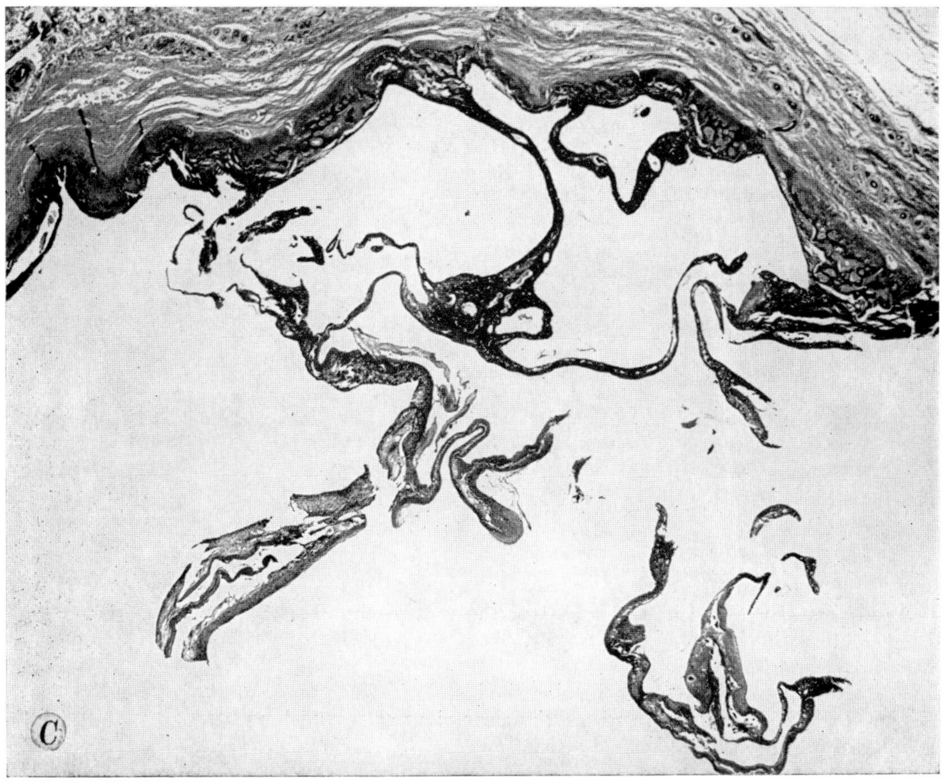


***Figure 13***

case, all complaints connected with a lesion in some part of the vertebral column become accentuated if the integrity of the affected vertebral body becomes undermined so that it partially collapses.

## ROENTGENOGRAPHIC FINDINGS

It is usually the *x*-ray picture that directs attention to the possibility that one is dealing with an aneurysmal bone cyst. In fact, the lesion came to light because its roentgenographic picture stood out from that observed in the course of a survey of cases representing the ordinary solitary bone cyst (see Jaffe and Lichtenstein). Further experience with the lesion has led the writer to re-emphasize its striking *x*-ray picture (see Jaffe). It is also stressed in the growing literature on the subject (see Lichtenstein, Dahlin *et al.*, Taylor, Barnes, and Cruz and Coley).

In general, what characterizes the lesion roentgenographically is a ballooned-out distention of the periosteum, usually outlined by a paper-thin subperiosteal bone shell. The ballooned-out area is often found overlying a region of disintegration of the cortex. The bulged area and the rest of the affected part of the bone may present faintly a coarse "soap bubble" pattern. The impression created by this picture is that of a subperiosteal "blowout," most plausibly interpretable on the basis of a massive hemorrhage in the affected area. It is when the lesion is in a long bone that its "blowout" character is most strikingly demonstrated in the *x*-ray picture. It may also be striking when the lesion is in the vertebral column, but if the lesion is largely confined to the vertebral body and this has collapsed, this feature may not be so clear-cut or may actually be lacking. (See Fig. 12.)

As noted, in affected long bones, the position of the lesion in relation to the shaft is eccentric. That is, the lesion does not traverse the entire diameter of the bone. Furthermore, it does not tend to extend into the actual epiphysial end of the bone. Generally, in relation to a long bone, the bulged-out area is rather large. It may measure as much as 5 to 8 cm. in its greatest dimension, which is generally in the long axis of the bone. Lesions involving some segment of the vertebral column sometimes also attain large size, particularly if not only a vertebral body but also its arch and processes are affected. In fact, one of the largest aneurysmal bone cysts which the writer has seen (about 10 cm. in diameter) involved the sacrum. He also saw a very large lesion implicating the superior ramus of the pubis. This caused such pronounced distention of the bone (especially inward and backward) that an expansion of the pelvic wall as big as a large orange could be felt through the rectum.

## PATHOLOGIC FINDINGS

When exposing the lesion and opening into its thin wall, the surgeon is confronted by a hole containing fluid blood. Blood continues to exude from the inner wall of the cyst, though without spurting. The bulged shell of the lesion is covered by periosteum. Beneath the latter there is a variable amount of new bone which has been laid down by the periosteum. (See Fig. 13.)

***Figure 14***

*A*, Photomicrograph (× 20) of part of the wall of the distended area shown in Figure 12–*A*. Note again the abundant vascular spaces, some of which are supported by filamentous trabeculæ of connective-tissue bone.

*B*, Photomicrograph (× 100) showing the histologic detail of the wall of one of the spaces shown in *A*. Note the scattered multinuclear giant cells, which are present mainly in the vicinity of collections of red blood cells.

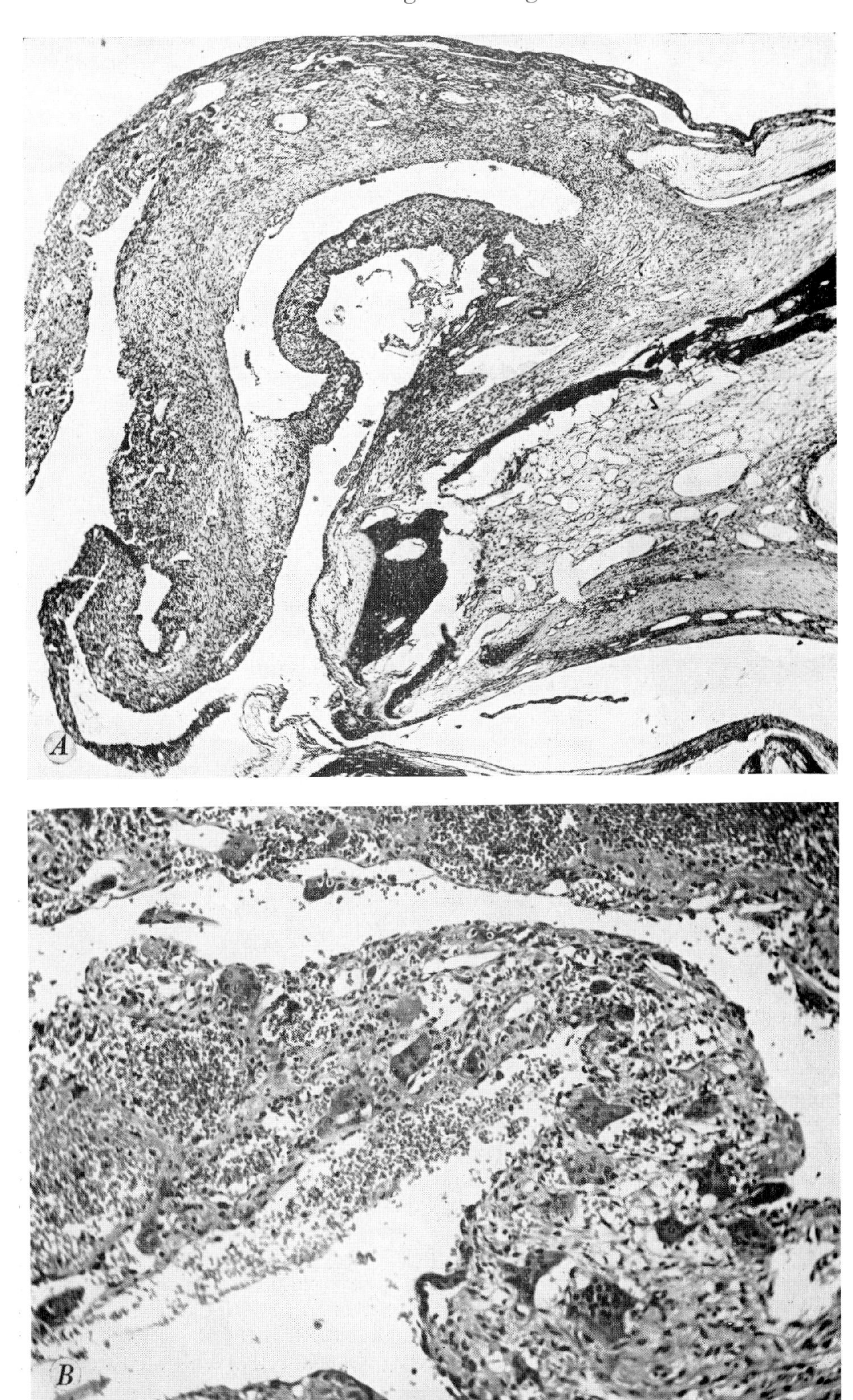


*Figure 14*

The lesional area contains only a meager amount of tissue, and what there is of it is stringy, meshy and honeycombed by spaces. Small amounts of reddish brown soft tissue may also be present between and on the walls of the spaces. In general, the tissue of the cystic area is heavily permeated with delicate blood-filled capillaries and large distended or distorted thin-walled blood spaces. In some places, there is much free hemorrhage between these blood channels, which, incidentally, have no muscular coats, and in these areas hemosiderin-bearing phagocytes and multinuclear giant cells are sometimes numerous. In fact, some of the larger blood spaces, though lined by endothelial-like cells, are also collared by small, multinuclear giant cells in variable numbers. Further, between the vascular spaces and sometimes even around the larger ones, there are filamentous trabeculæ of connective-tissue bone. The soft reddish tissue which may also sometimes be curetted from the cyst wall in small amounts usually contains large collections of multinuclear giant cells. These giant cells (rather small ones) are usually disposed about areas of hemorrhage and probably appear in the wake of organization of hemorrhage.

The numerous and intercommunicating vascular channels are apparently the source of bleeding into the cyst proper. The absence of blood clot on the cyst wall and in the vascular spaces indicates that the blood is not stagnant and that the lesion as a whole represents, from the dynamic point of view, a large blood pool being steadily drained and freshly supplied. (See Fig. 14.)

As already emphasized, the aneurysmal bone cyst is characterized by a "blowout" distention of part of the bone contour, associated with the presence of a largely blood-filled cavity in the underlying area. The question of the origin and basic nature of the lesion still has to be left open. Specifically, it is by no means clear whether: (1) The hemorrhagic "blowout" occurs in a previously normal bone area or (2) is engrafted upon a pre-existing lesion (possibly not always the same) in the course of which the identity of that lesion is lost. However, in none of the cases studied by the writer has examination revealed anything in the tissue sections which would favor the latter hypothesis. There is no clinical or anatomic evidence that aneurysmal bone cyst results even from modification of the usual solitary bone cyst (p. 63). This is already clear from the fact that the solitary bone cyst predilects the upper end of the humerus—a site certainly uncommon for aneurysmal bone cyst. At any rate, whether it actually develops as a primary or as a secondary lesion, the aneurysmal bone cyst stands out quite adequately as a clinicopathologic complex.

## DIFFERENTIAL DIAGNOSIS

If one keeps the "blowout" character of the roentgenographic appearance in mind, the lesion in a classic case can often already be diagnosed on the basis of its *x*-ray picture. On the other hand, to one not familiar with it, this picture may look ominous. In relation to a long bone, it may create the impression that one is dealing with a so-called osteolytic osteogenic sarcoma or with some other form of malignant bone tumor. Actually, the *x*-ray picture of an osteogenic sarcoma rarely raises the problem of differential diagnosis from aneurysmal bone cyst. Indeed, on only one occasion has the writer observed an osteogenic sarcoma presenting, in the *x*-ray picture, a "blowout" distention which raised this question. The lesion in that case was in the lower end of a femur. However, even in that instance, there was a focus of dense radiopacity in the interior of the bone in the lesional area which pointed correctly in the direction of osteogenic sarcoma. Thus, the "blowout" distention also seen in the *x*-ray picture in that case was to be interpreted as representing merely the consequence of massive hemorrhage in connection with the sarcoma in the femur.

Another problem of differential diagnosis relates to the question of giant-cell tumor—the lesion with which the aneurysmal bone cyst is most often confused. Occasionally, one encounters a giant-cell tumor which pulsates. Ewing referred to the pulsating giant-cell tumor as the "aneurysmal giant-cell tumor." He conceived it as a giant-cell tumor which grows to large size, pulsates, and occasionally yields a bruit, apparently because it is freely fed by communicating arterioles and large arteries. Shallow and Wagner have collected a number of such cases and have added one of their own. Undoubtedly, some instances of aneurysmal bone cyst may be included among these cases of so-called "pulsating giant-cell tumor." However, several important differences can be pointed out. The aneurysmal cyst does not pulsate. In relation to long bones it is often strictly limited to the end of the shaft and does not involve the epiphysial bone end. Usually, the patients are below 20 years of age (that is, in an age group in which giant-cell tumor is rarely found). Above all, the tissue pattern of aneurysmal bone cyst as a whole is not really that of giant-cell tumor.

On the other hand, there can be no doubt that certain of the cases which have been described as instances of "atypical" or "subperiosteal" giant-cell tumor in the shafts of long bones actually represent the aneurysmal bone cyst. Cases of what the writer would call aneurysmal bone cyst are discussed by Coley in his textbook under the heading of "atypical (subperiosteal) giant-cell tumor." He recognized, nevertheless, that these cases deserved special classification as representing a rather distinctive group. He thought, like the writer, that one of the factors in the evolution of these lesions was subperiosteal hemorrhage, and he was also impressed by their benignity. Coley has now come all the way over to the idea that the lesion should be held completely distinct from giant-cell tumor, and he, too, now refers to it as the "aneurysmal bone cyst." (See Cruz and Coley.)

An aneurysmal bone cyst involving some part of the vertebral column is very likely to raise difficulties of diagnosis and differential diagnosis on clinical and roentgenographic grounds. In the first place, the lesion can rather easily be misinterpreted as a malignant bone tumor. This is especially true when the presence of the lesion is associated with collapse of the affected vertebral body. On the other hand, in other cases of involvement of the vertebral column, the lesion may be interpreted as representing an expansile hemangioma. Although the *x*-ray picture may suggest this diagnosis, the findings from tissue examination will, of course, not support it.

## TREATMENT

The aneurysmal bone cyst in a benign lesion. In principle, the treatment is thorough curettage of the wall and packing of the cavity with autogenous bone chips. Naturally, in certain sites, such as the vertebral column, this is not always feasible. There, evacuation of the cyst may be all that is possible. Even this may be associated with so much hemorrhage that the intervention has to be quickly concluded, and fusion, which would otherwise be desirable, has to be postponed. However, even incomplete curettage of the cystic area is likely to be followed by healing.

## REFERENCES

Barnes, R.: Aneurysmal Bone Cyst, J. Bone & Joint Surg., *38-B*, 301, 1956.
Booher, R. J.: Aneurysmal Bone Cyst of a Metatarsal, J. Bone & Joint Surg., *39-A*, 435, 1957.
Coley, B. L.: *Neoplasms of Bone*, New York, Paul B. Hoeber, Inc., 1949. (*See* p. 168.)
Cruz, M., and Coley, B. L.: Aneurysmal Bone Cyst, Surgery, *103*, 67, 1956.
Dahlin, D. C., Besse, B. E., Jr., Pugh, D. G., and Ghormley, R. K.: Aneurysmal Bone Cysts, Radiology, *64*, 56, 1955.

DAWSON, G. R., JR.: Giant-Cell Tumor of the Pelvis at the Acetabulum, Ilium, Ischium, and Pubis, J. Bone & Joint Surg., *37-A*, 1278, 1955.
EWING, J.: *Neoplastic Diseases*, 4th ed., Philadelphia, W. B. Saunders Co., 1940.
GURI, J. P.: Tumors of the Vertebral Column, Surg., Gynec. & Obst., *87*, 583, 1948.
JAFFE, H. L., and LICHTENSTEIN, L.: Solitary Unicameral Bone Cyst, with Emphasis on the Roentgen Picture, the Pathologic Appearance and the Pathogenesis, Arch. Surg., *44*, 1004, 1942. (*See* Aneurysmal Cyst, p. 1021.)
JAFFE, H. L.: Aneurysmal Bone Cyst, Bull. Hosp. Joint Dis., *11*, 3, 1950.
LICHTENSTEIN, L.: Aneurysmal Bone Cyst, Cancer, *3*, 279, 1950.
MAYER, L., and KESTLER, O. C.: Aneurysmal Bone Cyst of Spine, Bull. Hosp. Joint Dis., *5*, 16, 1944.
SHALLOW, T. A., and WAGNER, F. B. JR.: Pulsating Benign Giant Cell Tumors of Bone, Arch. Surg., *52*, 661, 1946.
TAYLOR, F. W.: Aneurysmal Bone Cyst, J. Bone & Joint Surg., *38-B*, 293, 1956.
THOMPSON, P. C.: Subperiosteal Giant-cell Tumor: Ossifying Subperiosteal Hematoma—Aneurysmal Bone Cyst, J. Bone & Joint Surg., *36*-A, 281, 1954.

Chapter

# 5

# Solitary Bone Cyst

THOUGH the *solitary bone cyst* is not a tumor in the strict sense, it is ordinarily included among the tumors in discussions of bone lesions. The lesion is nearly always located in the shaft of some long tubular bone. Its site of predilection is the humerus, and specifically the upper part of the humeral shaft. Unless there has been a recent fracture through the bone cyst, the fluid which it usually contains is straw-colored. Under these conditions, the cavity is unicameral and lined by a thin membrane from which relatively little material can be curetted when the cyst is entered. A cyst which is examined in the wake of one or more fractures through it may not show this "unicameral" character. Indeed, in consequence of hemorrhage into the cyst, and organization of the blood clot, the cavity may be found subdivided by fibrous partitions, though never by bony ones.

## CLINICAL CONSIDERATIONS

**Incidence.**—The solitary bone cyst is not an uncommon lesion, and the writer's experience with it covers about 75 cases. There seems to be a definite preponderance of males among the patients, in the proportion of about 2 to 1.

In regard to age incidence, it is in the period between early childhood and adolescence that the great majority of the cases first come under observation. In any fairly large series of cases, it will probably be found that about 80 per cent of the patients were between 3 and 14 years of age when the condition began to give them trouble. It is only rarely that the patient is younger than 3 years, though the writer has observed a case in an infant two months old. As to the patients over 14 years of age, most of them will be found to be between 15 and 20. In fact, a solitary bone cyst rarely becomes clinically manifest for the first time in a mature adult. Once in a great while, the lesion is discovered incidentally on roentgenographic examination in an adult who had never had any complaints relating to it at all.

**Localization.**—As already noted, the site of the lesion is nearly always some long tubular bone, and the humerus is strongly predilected. It is probably safe to say that in somewhat more than half of the cases in any large series the cyst will be located in the proximal portion of the humeral shaft. In respect to relative frequency of involvement of the other long tubular bones, there is likely to be variation from series to series. However, it is clear that the upper and lower ends of the femoral and tibial shafts and the upper end of the fibular shaft together account for most of these localizations.

As to still other localizations, the writer has seen only a single instance in which the cyst was in a metacarpal and one in which it was in a metatarsal bone. In these short tubular bones, the cyst was again located in the juxta-epiphysial part of the shaft, and both patients were adolescents. In still other bone sites, the cyst seems to be of even rarer occurrence. The writer has observed it once in the calcaneus, twice in a rib, and twice in the ilium. In both cases of iliac involvement, the cyst was only a few centimeters in diameter; was located just below the epiphysis for the crest; contained yellowish serous fluid; and was lined by a delicate fibrous membrane. Occasional instances of these rarer localizations of the cyst have also been reported by others.

**Clinical Complaints.**—It is often not until some trauma (direct or indirect) to the affected bone has been followed by the occurrence of an infraction or fracture through the cyst that the presence of the latter is discovered. Often, the muscle pull connected with throwing a ball, or a casual stumble or jolt during play, is sufficient to instigate the fracture. In other cases, the history may even reveal that, some time in the past, there had been some disability relating to the area where a cyst was later discovered, but that the complaints were mi'd and passed off by themselves, and no *x*-ray picture was taken. In these cases, there is reason to believe that a cortical infraction had occurred which, because it was not associated with tearing of the periosteum, caused but little discomfort and healed rapidly. In general, though inquiry may reveal that a fracture had actually been preceded by slight recurrent local pain and some stiffness of the neighboring joint, it is remarkable how little difficulty there usually is before the fracture occurs. This often applies even when the lesion is in a lower limb bone, but some cases—particularly those in which the lesion is in the upper portion of a femoral shaft—may have attention drawn to them by a limp.

## ROENTGENOGRAPHIC FINDINGS

It is when the cyst is in the upper metaphysis of a humerus that the roentgenographic findings are most likely to guide one to the correct diagnosis, because of the well-known predilection of the lesion for this location. In relation to other long bones, the roentgenographic picture is usually just as characteristic, but failure to take the possibility of bone cyst into consideration is more likely to lead to misinterpretation of the picture. When the cyst is in one of its rarer locations, one is even less secure in attempting a diagnosis on the basis of the *x*-ray findings alone.

Though located in the shaft of the long tubular bone, the lesion is frequently found lying near or relatively near an epiphysial plate, but is sometimes already

### *Figure 15*

*A*, Roentgenograph of a solitary bone cyst in the upper part of the shaft of a humerus of a boy 7 years of age. The existence of the cyst had been known for 2 years, and there had been two previous fractures. Note the vaguely trabeculated appearance of the lesional area, and the thinning of the cortex. Note also that, despite the previous fractures, the cyst is still near the epiphysial cartilage plate.

*B*, Roentgenograph of a solitary bone cyst in the upper part of a humerus of a boy 13 years of age. Five years previously, the presence of the cyst, which was then near the epiphysial cartilage plate, was discovered through the occurrence of a fracture. In the interim, the cyst moved down the shaft. A recent slight trauma induced a comminuted fracture in the cyst. A cyst such as this, which has definitely moved away from the plate area, may be designated as a latent cyst.

*C*, Roentgenograph of a solitary bone cyst in the lower part of a femoral shaft of a boy 5 years of age. The cyst abuts on the epiphysial cartilage plate, and the thinned and somewhat expanded cortex is the site of a fracture. A cyst abutting on an epiphysial plate may be designated as an active cyst.

*D*, Roentgenograph of an active solitary bone cyst in the upper part of the shaft of a fibula of a boy 7 years of age. Attention had been only recently drawn to this cyst by the occurrence of a fracture through it. (See also Figs. 16-*A* and *B*.)

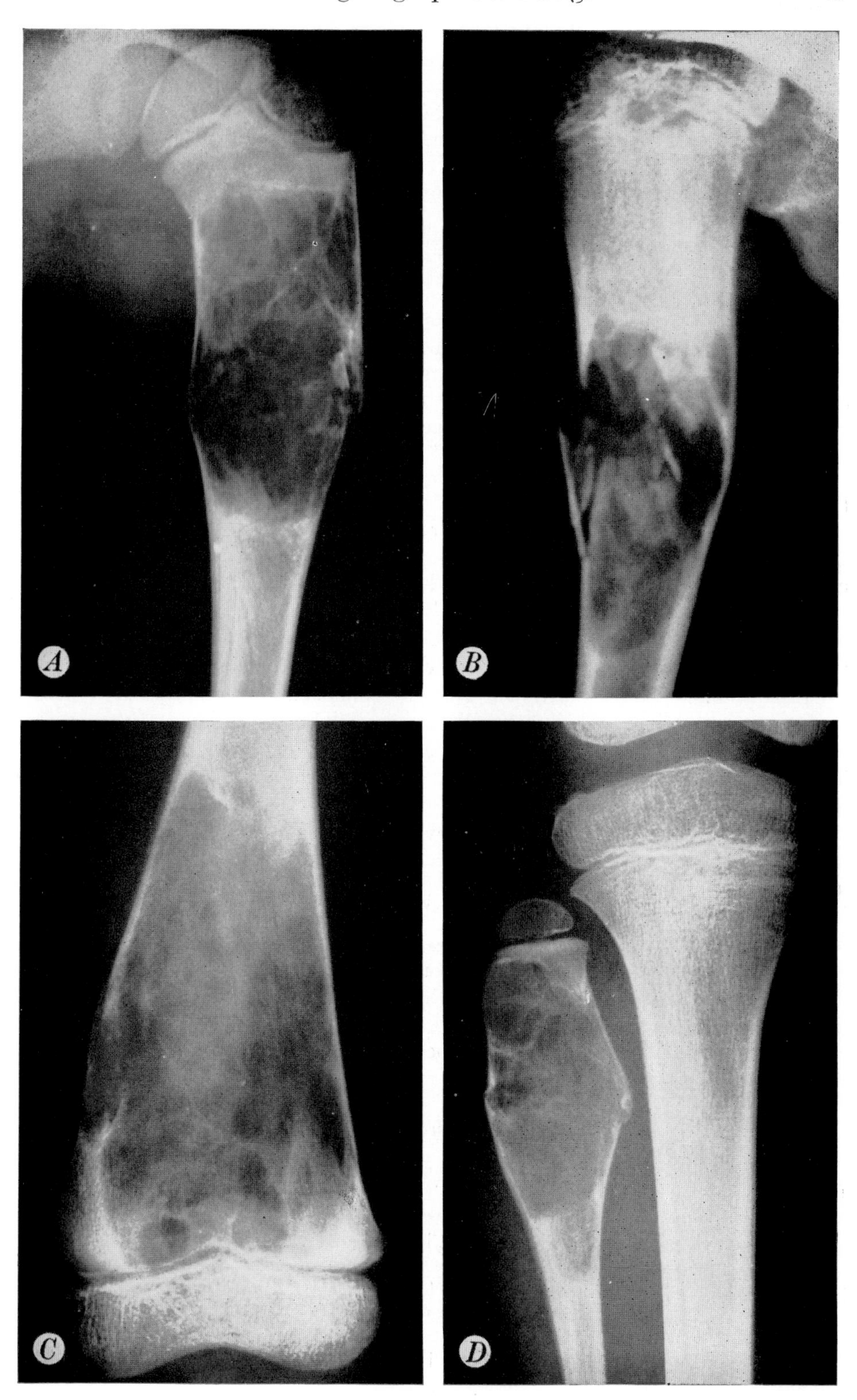


*Figure 15*

several inches away from the plate. In any event, a solitary bone cyst rarely if ever violates the plate so as to implicate also the actual epiphysial end of the bone of a youthful subject. As to roentgenographic detail, a cyst in the upper portion of the humeral shaft, for instance, if seen directly or shortly after an initial infraction or fracture, is commonly found to extend from the immediate vicinity of the epiphysial cartilage plate downward for several inches. The diameter of the humeral shaft in the affected region may be found slightly expanded over a limited area or uniformly. The regional cortex appears attenuated. The thinning can be seen to have taken place from the medullary surface, which may even appear somewhat scalloped. The periosteal surface of the cortex is generally smooth and presents no obvious evidence of new bone apposition, except in the immediate vicinity of the infraction or fracture if the latter is in process of healing. Furthermore, on account of the disappearance of spongiosa markings, the affected shaft area appears rarefied to a greater or lesser degree. In some cases the rarefied area may appear irregularly "trabeculated" here and there. The loculated appearance reflects the presence of ridges on the medullary surface of the modified cortex rather than bony partitions traversing and dividing the cyst. (See Fig. 15.)

The initial cortical infraction or fracture line is usually in the proximal half of the cystic area. The line may be transverse or oblique, but in any case, even if there is complete severance of continuity, this is not likely to be associated with significant displacement at the site of the fracture, since the periosteum is usually not torn through. The fracture tends to heal very rapidly, and, within a month or so, continuity has usually been completely re-established and only a ridge in the cortex may mark the site of the previous fracture line. Sometimes within two or three months after the first fracture one can note that the cystic area proximal to the fracture line is largely filled in with spongy bone, so that the upper limit of the cyst is now as much as an inch below the epiphysial cartilage plate. If this process has not taken place after an initial fracture, it is common, though not inevitable, for it to follow after a second fracture has occurred, most often some months after the first.

Thus, within a year after the first, or even less after the second fracture, an inch or more of reconstructed metaphysis may be present between the plate and the upper end of the cyst. At the same time, the longitudinal axis of the cyst may be found reduced but is not necessarily so, since the cyst may have progressed somewhat at its distal end. In time, in consequence of growth of the bone and reconstruction of the metaphysis between the upper end of the cyst and the plate, the cyst may move a considerable distance down the shaft. Should there be no such filling in of the metaphysis after a succession of fractures, the cyst usually shows additional progression and may come to occupy a substantial portion of the shaft.

### *Figure 16*

*A*, Photograph of the longitudinally sectioned upper end of the fibula shown in Figure 15-*D*. The upper part of the cyst area contains coagula of blood. The membranous lining of the cyst is apparent only in the lower portion of the lesional area.

*B*, Roentgenograph of the specimen shown in Figure *A*.

*C*, Photograph showing a longitudinal section of another active bone cyst in the upper part of the shaft of a fibula. The affected part of the fibula was resected because, during the previous 2 years, two vain attempts had been made to obliterate the cyst. Note the thin lining of the cyst, and the partitioning fibrous membrane.

*D*, Roentgenograph of the specimen shown in Figure *C*. The shadows of compacted bone chips can be seen in the lower part of the picture.

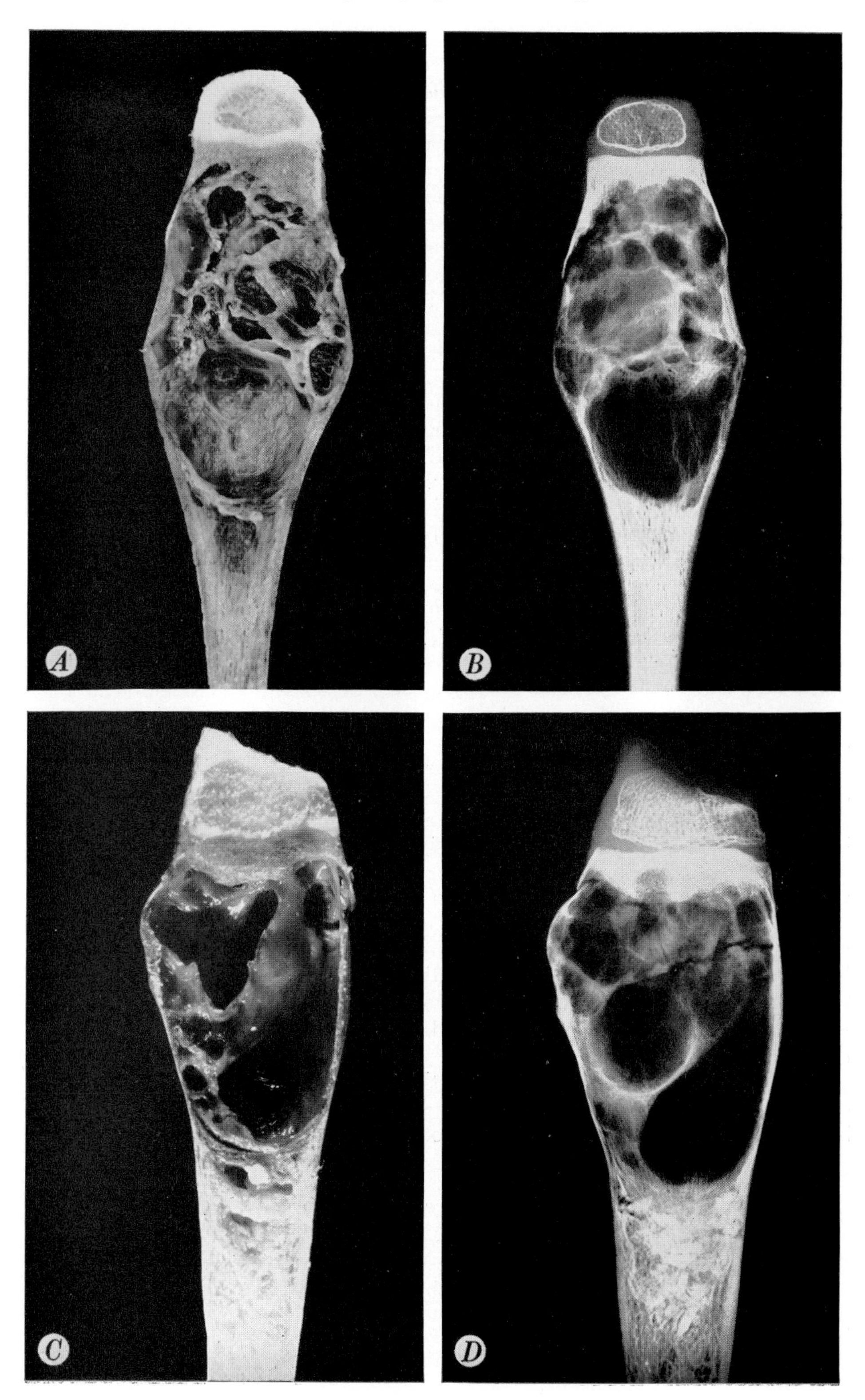


*Figure 16*

## PATHOLOGIC FINDINGS

In the course of exposing the cyst, the surgeon finds the muscles overlying it unaltered unless there has been a recent fracture. In the latter case they are likely to be discolored from hemorrhage. When the muscles are retracted, the cortical wall of the cyst may present a bluish sheen, apparent even through the periosteum. This is accounted for by the thinness of the cortex and its consequent translucency to the fluid in the cyst. Indeed, in some places the cyst wall may be of almost eggshell thinness. On stripping off the periosteum, it may be found that where the cortex is especially attenuated, parts of the latter may even show tiny defects. The fluid which is evacuated when the cortex is opened may be clear and yellowish, or else serosanguineous. If there has been a recent fracture through the cyst, the fluid may even be heavily discolored by blood, and the cyst may even contain coagula of it. (See Fig. 16.)

On evacuating the fluid and exploring the cavity, it is found that the latter is not divided off into compartments. However, the inner wall of the cortex may show some meager bony ridging, and in an occasional case a few projections may be found jutting quite prominently into the cavity. Further exploration commonly shows that the inner surface of the cortex is lined by a connective-tissue membrane which, most often, is smooth and very thin. If the fluid content was not frankly sanguineous, the basic color of the membrane will be gray-white, though patches of it may show rust-brown discoloration. If one curets the inner wall of a cyst, it is striking to find how little tissue can usually be obtained from it, unless there has been a relatively recent hemorrhage into it. Indeed, a cyst several inches in length may yield only 2 or 3 curet spoonfuls of material. If there has been hemorrhage into the cyst and the blood clot is substantially organized, a considerable amount of yellowish and brownish material, obviously containing a good deal of lipid, can be curetted from a few places on the cyst wall.

On microscopic examination, the thin cortical wall of the cyst is found composed of rather loose-meshed osseous tissue. This represents a new cortex which has slowly been laid down by the periosteum as the old cortex was being resorbed. It is only at sites of infraction that obvious signs of active periosteal new bone apposition are present. The fairly large vascular spaces of the cortical shell usually show many dilated and thin-walled vessels. On the walls of these spaces, a scattering of osteoclasts may be seen, and some osteoclasts may be present also between the periosteum and the outer surface of the cortical shell on the one hand and between its inner surface and lining membrane on the other. Any spongiosa that may have been removed from beyond the immediate limits of the cyst is likely to show remodeled trabeculæ, while the intertrabecular marrow appears mucoid or fibrous and contains thin and dilated blood vessels.

As noted, the lining membrane is very thin in most places, consisting in these of only a few superposed layers of connective-tissue cells. In other places, the membrane may be slightly thicker and be composed essentially of a rather vascular

***Figure 17***

*A*, Photomicrograph (× 6) showing a survey view of a cyst in the upper end of a fibula. From above down, one notes: the epiphysis; the epiphysial cartilage plate; and the thin membrane which is adherent to the spongy trabeculæ immediately under the plate area.

*B*, Photomicrograph (× 25) showing in somewhat greater detail than *A* how the membrane adheres to the osseous trabeculæ being formed in the plate area.

*C*, Photomicrograph (× 25) of a portion of the modified cortex of a bone cyst, lined on its inner surface by a thin membrane.

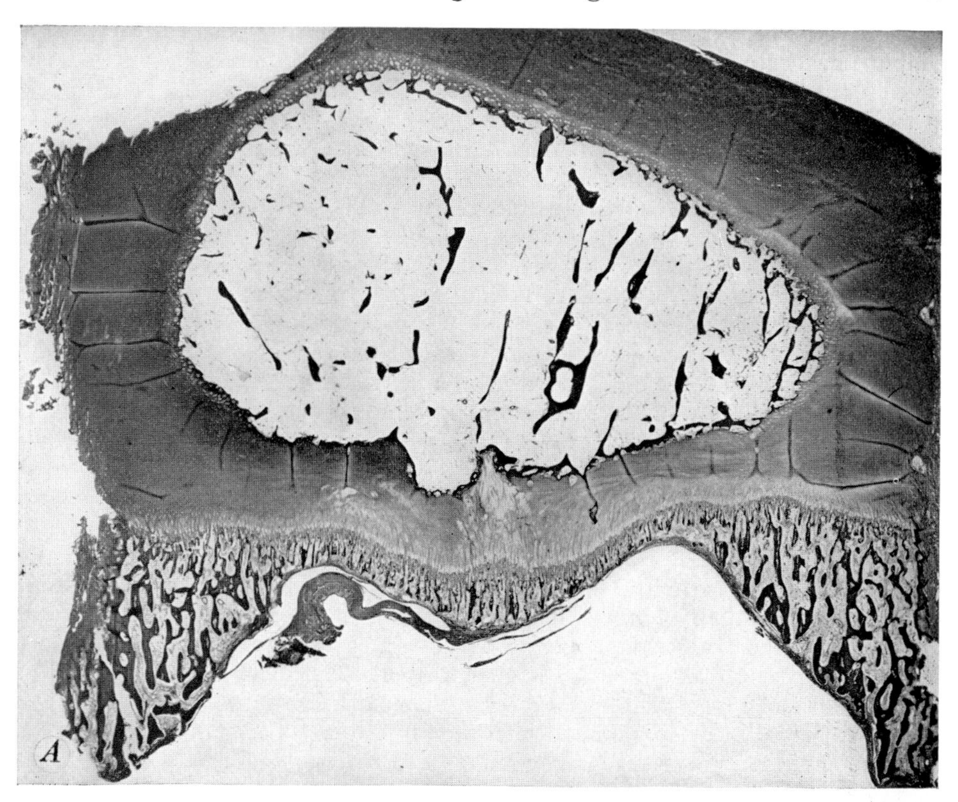


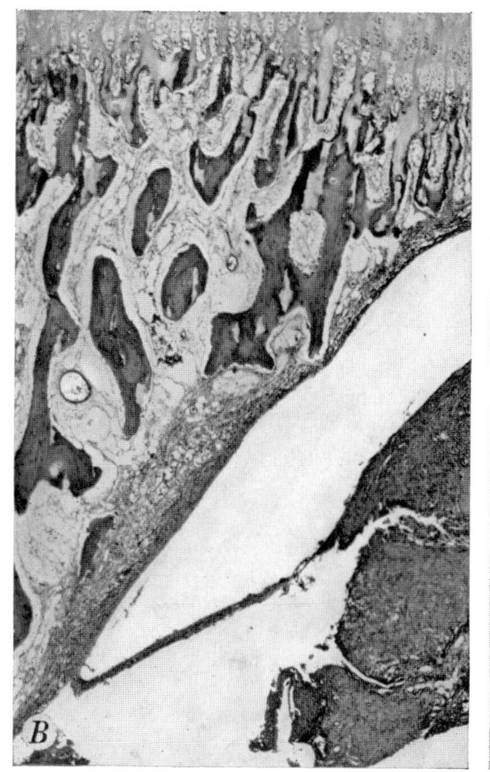


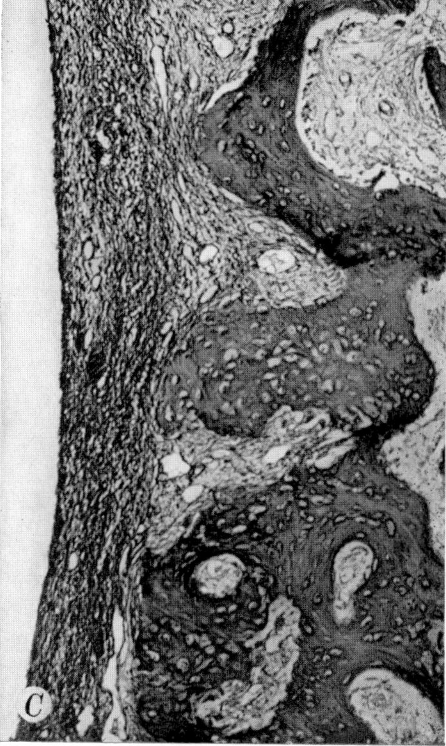


*Figure 17*

connective tissue. It may also show a scattering of blood pigment, either free or within phagocytes. Here and there in the lining membrane, some osteoid and osseous trabeculæ may be seen to have formed through metaplasia. The bits of tissue which are usually found adherent to the lining of the cyst will appear, on microscopic examination, to be mainly fibrin clots often containing some red blood cells and undergoing organization and even calcification and ossification. In the occasional instance in which a generous amount of brownish material can be curetted from some places on the cyst wall, the fibrin mass has imbedded in it cholesterol crystals and/or lipid- and hemosiderin-bearing phagocytes and small multinuclear giant cells. (See Figs. 17 and 18-*A*, *B*.)

**Pathogenesis.**—Mönckeberg suggested the idea (favored and elaborated by Konjetzny and by Geschickter and Copeland) that the bone cyst represented a "healing form of giant-cell tumor or osteitis fibrosa." The term "osteitis fibrosa" as used in the older literature had widely varying connotations. Some authors used it to mean (or at least to include) Paget's disease of bone, and others used it to signify the skeletal changes of hyperparathyroidism. Others, again, employed it to cover what we now call fibrous dysplasia of bone.

Certainly the lesion being discussed in this chapter as "solitary bone cyst" is in no way related to any of these conditions. Nor does it develop through cystic softening of a fibro-osseous disease focus, of the kind formerly denoted as "localized osteitis fibrosa" or "localized fibrocystic disease." Furthermore, it has no clinical, roentgenographic, or anatomic characteristics which would support the idea that it might represent a healing or cystic form of giant-cell tumor.

On the positive side, as to pathogenesis, Pommer held that a solitary bone cyst results from the encapsulation and alteration of a focus of intramedullary hemorrhage. This theory is confronted with the contradictory fact that cysts do not develop at the site of an ordinary traumatic fracture. To meet this objection, the proponents of the Pommer theory (see, for instance, Lang) reason that, when such a fracture occurs, the periosteum is torn, so that the possibility of development of a closed hemorrhagic pressure cyst is removed. Hence, they postulate that it is only after mild trauma, without fracture but with intramedullary hemorrhage, that a solitary bone cyst can develop. However, it is debatable whether intramedullary hemorrhage ever follows upon a mild trauma without fracture. Also, the most common site of the cyst is the upper part of the humeral shaft—a site less subject to nonfractural traumatic damage than the bones entering into the knee and ankle.

***Figure 18***

*A*, Photomicrograph (× 150) showing some multinuclear giant cells, such as are often found in the curettings from the wall of a solitary bone cyst.

*B*, Photomicrograph (× 115) showing the histologic pattern of the bits of organizing and calcifying fibrin and blood clot such as are likewise not infrequently curetted from the wall of a solitary bone cyst.

*C*, Roentgenograph of a multiloculated lesion in the shaft of a radius. One could not be certain from this *x*-ray picture just what one would encounter on entering the lesion. Actually, the lesional area contained only a small amount of loose, edematous, gritty tissue. The lesion might well be an old and static solitary bone cyst. The patient was a boy 17 years of age. The history was that in the course of the previous 3½ years he had sustained 3 other fractures through the affected shaft of the radius. Furthermore, on each of these occasions the fracture had healed rather promptly, as usually happens in connection with a bone cyst.

*D*, Photomicrograph (× 150) representative of the material removed from the lesion shown in *C*. This tissue has apparently been formed as a reparative response to the repeated fractures.

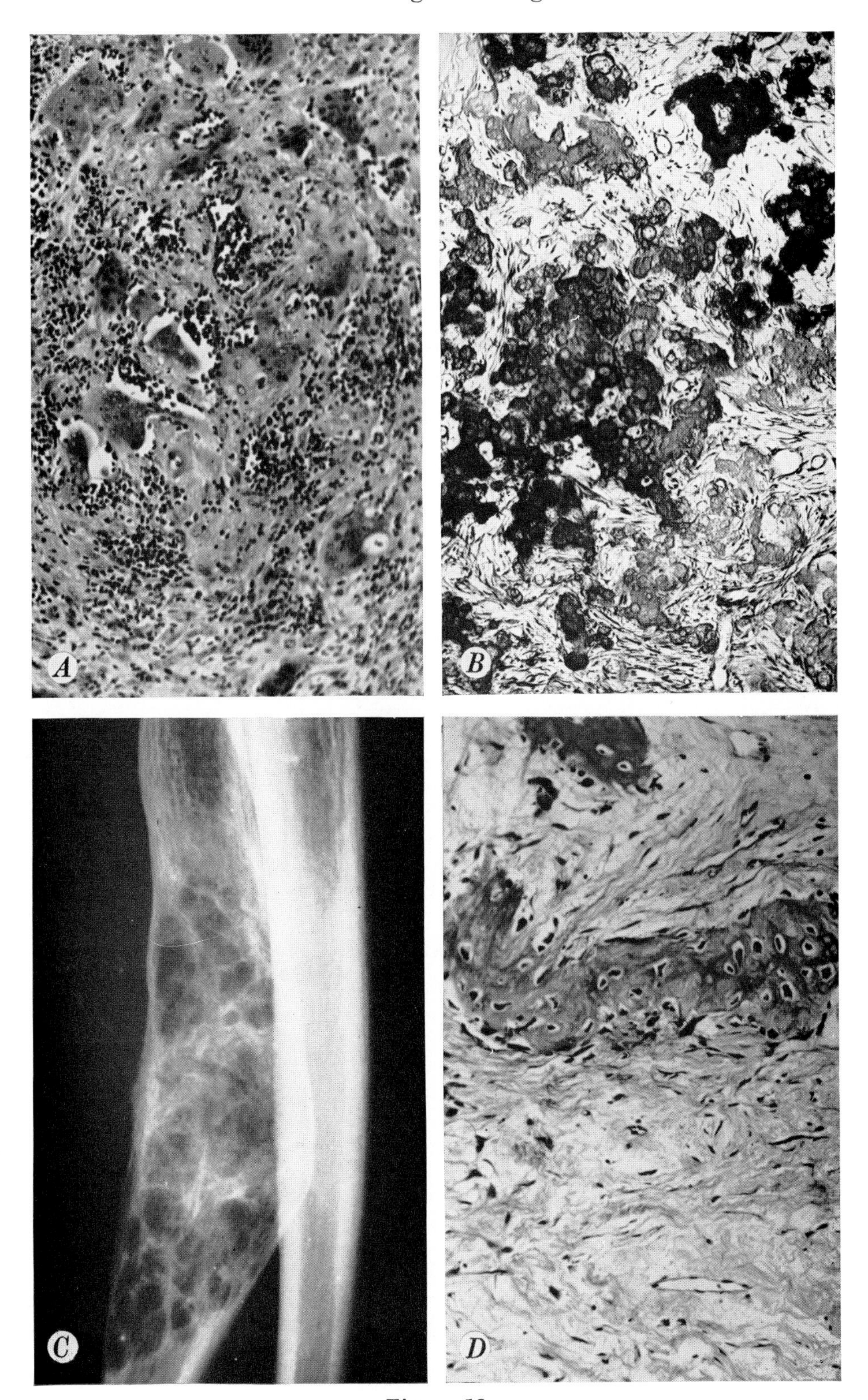


*Figure 18*

Whatever it may be that instigates the formation of the cyst, it is important to realize that the abnormality underlying its development and growth is confined to the spongy part of the affected shaft region. Indeed, there is no interference with periosteal bone formation at the end of the shaft, and the periosteal cortical cuff therefore continues to grow. Hence, longitudinal growth of the bone is uninterrupted, even though the cystic cavity continues to abut upon the plate area. Also, as long as the lining of the cyst is contiguous with the spongy trabeculæ being newly formed at the plate area, and there is pressure from the fluid against that area, the cyst will not move away from the end of the shaft.

**Natural Course of the Cyst.**—The writer divides the solitary bone cysts into two groups—the *active* and the *latent*. A cyst which extends to the immediate vicinity of, or abuts upon, the epiphysial cartilage plate is to be regarded as one still possessing potentialities for growth, and hence as an active cyst. On the other hand, a cyst which has definitely moved away from the plate, so that there is now a reconstructed area of shaft between it and the plate, has entered into the latent stage of its life cycle, since its growth activity has ceased. The lesion may now be regarded as a mere static defect in the bone, though this defect may maintain itself for years and even be the basis for subsequent refractures.

The question of whether a solitary bone cyst ever undergoes spontaneous healing is a natural one. Adams reports an instance of complete disappearance of a cyst without surgical intervention. Such a course is certainly exceptional. As a rule, unless the cystic defect is obliterated by surgery, it persists indefinitely. Indeed, the writer has seen 1 case in which a cyst endured for almost 25 years and then had to be obliterated by surgical intervention.

A persistent latent cyst will continue to be visible in the *x*-ray picture as a loculated defect in the shaft of the bone. In several such cases seen by the writer, it was found, when the lesional area was finally entered, that it contained some loose, edematous, and somewhat gritty tissue, interspersed with cystic spaces. Histologic examination of the tissue removed showed that it was a loose-meshed, vascular granulation tissue containing some trabeculæ of new bone. The inference to be drawn from the total picture in these cases is that cysts of long standing may come to be partly filled in through a process of reparative osteofibrosis, though the likelihood that the area ever undergoes complete spontaneous reconstruction so as to present a normal roentgenographic appearance is certainly small. (See Figs. 18-*C* and *D*.)

## DIFFERENTIAL DIAGNOSIS

The clinical findings in a case of solitary bone cyst, and the roentgenographic appearance of the lesional area, are often already sufficient to make it clear that that is the lesion in question. Specifically, the diagnosis of solitary bone cyst has a firm foundation if (to review the facts briefly): the patient is a child or adolescent; the lesion is at or near the end of a long bone shaft; complaints are absent or relatively mild, at least until a fracture occurs; and the *x*-ray picture shows a relatively large centrally located radiolucent area in the affected part of the shaft, associated with thinning of the cortex and relatively slight expansion of the bone contour.

As to the pathologic findings, if the lesion is entered while the condition is no longer complicated by a fracture, there will be very little curettable material on the wall of the cyst. Essentially, this material consists of fibrin intermingled with small numbers of multinuclear giant cells and perhaps even some loose trabeculæ of new bone. If the cyst has been curetted not long after the occurrence of a fracture through it, much of the cyst may be occupied by blood clot in the process of organization. Under these circumstances, the organizing blood clot may be permeated by blood-filled spaces lined by flattened cells and even collared in many places by multinuclear giant cells, and there may also be evidence of new bone formation in the tissue walls between the spaces.

Although the differentiation of solitary bone cyst from other lesions is usually not difficult, problems of differential diagnosis do occasionally arise, especially if only the clinical history and *x*-ray picture are available. In particular, under these conditions, the question of differentiation between a bone cyst and an eosinophilic granuloma, an enchondroma, or a solitary focus of fibrous dysplasia may sometimes come up. If undue significance is attached to the giant cells present in the curettings from a solitary cyst, the problem of differential diagnosis from aneurysmal bone cyst or giant-cell tumor of bone might also present itself.

**Eosinophilic Granuloma.**—It is, of course, only when a solitary focus of eosinophilic granuloma is located in the shaft of a long bone that the question of its clinical differentiation from a bone cyst may arise. In this connection, it is useful to remember that, though an eosinophilic granuloma may be located at or near the end of the shaft, it is more likely to lie toward the middle. Also, an eosinophilic granuloma, when first seen, is not usually as large a lesion as a solitary bone cyst, but, on the other hand, is definitely more likely to be painful. In contrast to a bone cyst, an eosinophilic granuloma in a long bone shaft almost invariably provokes a good deal of subperiosteal new bone deposition, which often extends for a considerable distance beyond the radiolucent defect.

On the anatomic side, it is to be noted that an eosinophilic granuloma, when entered, may show relatively little tissue in the lesional area, just as a bone cyst often does. However, whatever tissue is curetted from an eosinophilic granuloma does show numerous eosinophilic leukocytes and also histiocytes in the tissue sections—findings which are characteristic for that lesion.

**Enchondroma.**—The ordinary site of an enchondroma (that is, a solitary, benign cartilaginous tumor) is the shaft of a tubular bone. However, its most common location is in the shaft of a short tubular bone such as a metacarpal or metatarsal bone, or a phalanx. These are precisely the rarest locations for solitary bone cyst. Thus, a radiolucent defect in the shaft of a short tubular bone is, *a priori,* not likely to represent a solitary bone cyst. If the lesional area shows punctate radiopacities, one can be quite sure that it is not a bone cyst, since these would indicate calcification and/or ossification taking place within a cartilaginous tumor. In relation to the shaft of a long tubular bone, one may occasionally see a radiolucent area without punctate radiopacities which actually represents an enchondroma which might be interpreted as a bone cyst on the basis of the *x*-ray picture. In these exceptional cases, the pathologic findings are decisive, since the material removed from the lesional area is clearly cartilage.

**Solitary Focus of Fibrous Dysplasia.**—In these cases, too, when the lesion is in a long bone, it is likely to be confined to some part of the shaft. The tissue in the lesional area is fibro-osseous in general, but in some lesions it is more fibrous than osseous, in others more osseous than fibrous, and in still others perhaps cystic in part. Thus, on a pathologico-anatomic basis, there is no likelihood of confusing a focus of fibrous dysplasia with a solitary bone cyst. Roentgenographically, however, a focus of fibrous dysplasia which is predominantly fibrous and perhaps cystic in part might conceivably be misinterpreted as a solitary bone cyst. This is so because the lesional tissue, being predominantly fibrous and in part cystic, would cast a rather radiolucent shadow, suggestive of a cyst. On the other hand, a focus of fibrous dysplasia whose lesional tissue is rather on the osseous side of the fibro-osseous complex often casts a "ground glass" shadow quite inconsistent with that from a solitary bone cyst.

**Giant-cell Tumor.**—If one keeps in mind the clinical and roentgenographic features which characterize giant-cell tumor, there is very little likelihood that a solitary bone cyst will be mistaken for a giant-cell tumor. In the great majority of cases of giant-cell tumor, the patients are adults, while in the great majority of cases of solitary bone cyst they are children or adolescents. With rare exceptions, a giant-cell tumor affecting a long bone involves the actual epiphysial end of the bone, while in regard to a bone cyst it is a question whether the lesion ever violates the plate and extends into the epiphysial end of the bone. As to its anatomic features, the lesional area in the giant-cell tumor is usually filled with tissue much of which presents the histologic pattern of plumpish spindle-shaped or ovoid stromal cells heavily intermingled with multinuclear giant cells. In the curettings from a bone cyst, some multinuclear giant cells may be seen, but these are small, rather sparse, irregularly distributed, and not set in the type of stroma which one sees in connection with giant-cell tumor.

**Aneurysmal Bone Cyst.**—As has been stated in the chapter devoted to aneurysmal bone cyst (p. 54), there is apparently no connection between that lesion and the solitary bone cyst. Still, if a solitary bone cyst has become filled with an organizing blood clot in consequence of a fracture, the histologic appearance of the tissue removed from it might make one think that one was dealing with an aneurysmal bone cyst. This possibility of confusion is created by the fact that in the tissue removed from such a solitary bone cyst there will be large blood-filled spaces reminiscent of what is characteristic of an aneurysmal bone cyst. For differential diagnosis under these conditions, the roentgenographic appearance of the lesional area is of crucial importance. Specifically, if, in the *x*-ray picture, the lesion is central and not eccentric, and if one does not observe a "blowout" distention of part of the contour of the bone, the possibility of aneurysmal bone cyst can safely be rejected.

## TREATMENT

In describing the *x*-ray picture of bone cyst, it was pointed out that some months after an initial fracture, but more often after the second or third fracture, it will be observed that an area of reconstructed metaphysis is now present between the cyst and its neighboring epiphysial cartilage plate. In the discussion of the natural course of the cyst, it was emphasized that, if it has moved away from the neighboring plate, the growth activity of the cyst has ceased, the latter having changed from an active to a latent cyst. It is in this latent and static stage that the cyst responds best to surgical intervention (see Jaffe and Lichtenstein).

The treatment of choice (whether or not the lesion has moved away from the plate) is to expose the cyst, curet its wall, fill it with autogenous bone chips, collapse the cyst wall, and close the wound tightly. As much as possible of the lining membrane should be removed in any case. If the cyst is in its active stage, it seems imperative to remove at least that part of the membrane which abuts upon the metaphysial spongiosa near the plate, since otherwise the likelihood of recurrence is considerable.

In the past, the over-all recurrence rate was about 40 to 50 per cent. As indicated, the recurrence rate is higher for those cases (in any large series) in which the cyst was near the plate at the time of the original surgical intervention. Cysts which recur are nearly always cured by a second intervention with renewed curettage and refilling with bone chips. It is only very rarely indeed that a third intervention is needed.

In no case has the writer found that any benefit resulted from radiation therapy to the cyst. Indeed, when given before or after surgical intervention, there is at least the theoretical possibility that radiation may even delay the healing. Furthermore, the writer has seen a case in which a cyst in the shaft of a humerus was given a course of heavy radiation therapy with baleful consequences. In this case, $6\frac{1}{2}$

years after the radiation treatment, a fibrosarcoma developed at the site of the bone cyst (*see* p. 496).

## REFERENCES


Adams, A. W.: Report of a Case of Solitary Fibrocystic Disease of the Humerus Exhibiting Spontaneous Resolution, Brit. J. Surg., *13*, 734, 1926.

Garceau, G. J., and Gregory, C. F.: Solitary Unicameral Bone Cyst, J. Bone & Joint Surg., *36*-A, 267, 1954.

Geschickter, C. F., and Copeland, M. M.: *Tumors of Bone*, 3rd ed., Philadelphia, J. B. Lippincott Co., 1949, p. 245.

Gieseking, H.: Das familiäre Auftreten von "jugendlichen Knochencysten," Chirurg, *21*, 670, 1950.

Graham, J. J.: Solitary Unicameral Bone Cyst, Bull. Hosp. Joint Dis., *13*, 106, 1952.

Heublein, G. W., and Baird, C. L.: Solitary Unicameral Bone Cyst of Right Ilium, Am. J. Roentgenol., *59*, 699, 1948.

Jaffe, H. L.: Giant-Cell Tumor of Bone: Problems of Differential Diagnosis, Bull. Hosp. Joint Dis., *5*, 84, 1944.

Jaffe, H. L., and Lichtenstein, L.: Solitary Unicameral Bone Cyst, with Emphasis on the Roentgen Picture, the Pathologic Appearance and the Pathogenesis, Arch. Surg. *44*, 1004, 1942.

Konjetzny, G. E.: Die sogenannte "lokalisierte Ostitis fibrosa," Arch. f. klin. Chir., *121*, 567, 1922.

Lang, F. J.: Beiträge zu den mikroskopischen Befunden bei Knochenzysten, Deutsche Ztschr. f. Chir., *172*, 193, 1922.

Lasthaus, M.: Jugendliche Knochencyste und Unfall, Chirurg, *21*, 672, 1950.

von Mikulicz, J.: Über cystische Degeneration der Knochen, Verhandl. d. Gesellsch. Deutscher Naturforsch. u. Ärzte, 76th meeting, 2nd Half, Pt. II, p. 107, 1905.

Mönckeberg.: Ueber Cystenbildung bei Ostitis fibrosa, Verhandl. d. deutsch. path. Gesellsch., *7*, 232, 1904.

Platt, H.: Cysts of the Long Bones of the Hand and Foot, Brit. J. Surg., *18*, 20, 1930.

Pommer, G.: Zur Kenntnis der progressiven Hämatom- und Phlegmasieveränderungen der Röhrenknochen, Arch. f. orthop. u. Unfall-Chir., *17*, 17, 1920.

Stewart, M. J., and Hamel, H. A.: Solitary Bone Cyst, South. M. J., *43*, 927, 1950.

Verstandig, C. C.: Solitary Unicameral Cyst of the Os Calcis, New England J. Med., *237*, 21, 1947.

Chapter

# 6

# Fibrous Cortical Defect and Non-ossifying Fibroma

THE so-called *fibrous cortical defect* is a very common lesion. Knowledge of it has been gathered mainly through roentgenographic study of the growing skeleton in normal young children. The lesional tissue consists essentially of a small focus of connective tissue often containing some multinuclear giant cells. The lesion is usually located in the metaphysial cortex of a long bone—most often the distal metaphysis of a femur—and the lesional tissue erodes the cortex at its site. In itself, the fibrous cortical defect has but little clinical importance and hardly merits the designation of tumor. Indeed, it only rarely gives rise to clinical manifestations, and it usually disappears spontaneously. Even when it does persist, it usually remains rather small and clinically silent.

Once in a while, a fibrous cortical defect not only persists but undergoes proliferative activity, perhaps attaining a fairly large size. Occasionally, it even penetrates into, and continues to grow in, the medullary cavity. When it does this, the lesion ceases to be a mere *fibrous cortical defect* and becomes what we call a *non-ossifying fibroma of bone.* Clinically, the ultimate larger lesion, with its invasion of the marrow cavity, is certainly more than a mere fibrous cortical defect. What

***Figure 19***

*A*, Roentgenograph of a fibrous cortical defect (shown in profile view) in the cortex of the lower end of a femoral shaft. Note that the defect is small and shallow. The patient was a boy 8 years of age. The lesion was discovered incidentally when the left knee area was roentgenographed because the boy had suffered a soft tissue laceration of the upper part of the leg. Serial *x*-rays taken during the subsequent 9 months revealed what appeared to be a slight increase in size of the lesional area. Because of this, the lesion was excised. In the area of the defect, the bone cortex was found to have been eroded by a focus of rather collagenous connective tissue which was continuous with the deep layer of the overlying periosteum.

*B*, Roentgenograph giving a frontal view of the fibrous defect pictured in *A*. In this view, its orientation to the cortex is less evident. Note that the periphery of the defect is outlined by a narrow ring of sclerosis.

*C*, Roentgenograph of a fibrous defect in the cortex on the medial aspect of the upper end of a tibial shaft. The patient was a girl 10 years of age. She complained of pain relating to the upper medial aspect of the tibia in question (the right), and also had pain at the corresponding site of the left tibia, where another defect was discovered. This case illustrates the common finding of bilateral and symmetrical cortical defects. It is unusual, however, for such small defects to give rise to clinical complaints.

*D*, Roentgenograph of a rather large fibrous cortical defect in a femur. Note the loculated appearance and considerable longitudinal extent of the lesional area. A lesion of this size suggests the beginnings of a non-ossifying fibroma. The patient was a boy 10 years of age. The lesion was discovered incidentally when the knee area was roentgenographed after the boy had bruised his thigh in a fall from a bicycle. Thus, despite its size, the cortical defect in this case had not given rise to any complaints.

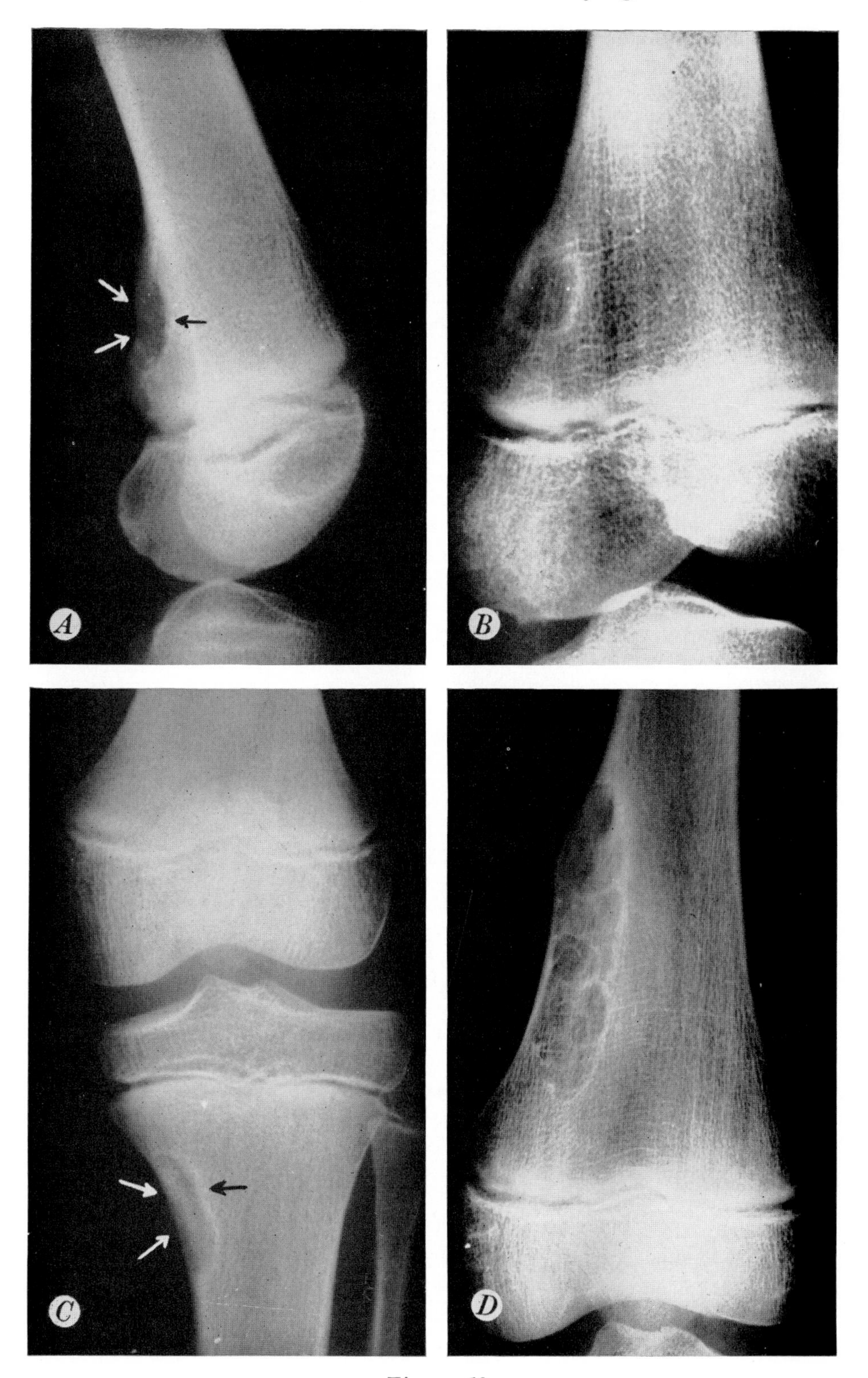


*Figure 19*

the non-ossifying fibroma thus seems to represent is a tumorous evolutionary form occasionally attained by the fibrous cortical defect. In harmony with this conception, its subjects are mainly older children and adolescents, rather than young children as in most cases of fibrous cortical defect. Furthermore, a non-ossifying fibroma may become large enough to provoke such clinical complaints as pain and swelling, and occasionally a pathologic fracture occurs at its site. It is to be noted that, though the writer now prefers the term "non-ossifying fibroma" for the lesion, the latter was originally designated as the *non-osteogenic fibroma* of bone (see Jaffe and Lichtenstein). Subsequently, Hatcher referred to the lesion as representing a *metaphysial fibrous defect*. Indeed, these various designations have since been used more or less interchangeably (see Maudsley and Stansfeld, Campbell and Harkess, and Compere and Coleman).

## FIBROUS CORTICAL DEFECT

As already noted, the so-called fibrous cortical defect is a very common but small, innocent, and usually ephemeral lesion. Recognition of it dates from an article by Sontag and Pyle published in 1941. That article, which was essentially a roentgenographic and statistical study, was entitled: "The Appearance and Nature of Cyst-like Areas in Distal Femoral Metaphyses of Children." As to the nature of the condition, those authors held speculatively that the "cyst-like" rarefactions reflected the presence of rests of cartilage which had presumably migrated to the metaphysis from the epiphysial plate area. However, studies of the pathology of these "cyst-like" lesions by the present writer and also by Hatcher have shown that the abnormal tissue is not cartilage but fibrous tissue. Furthermore, it has become clear that this fibrous tissue develops out of the local periosteum and invades the underlying cortex to create the roentgenographic picture characterizing the fibrous cortical defect. The more recent large-scale roentgenographic study by Caffey has confirmed and extensively supplemented previous findings in connection with the lesion.

### CLINICAL CONSIDERATIONS

**Incidence.**—From the roentgenographic surveys already made, it is clear that a large percentage of children (about 30 to 40 per cent) develop one or more fibrous cortical defects. The defect is rarely found in a child under 2 years of age; is most commonly encountered between the ages of 4 and 8; and rarely appears for the first time after the age of 14. Whenever it appears, it is likely to persist for about 2 years, but it may persist much longer. The lesion is encountered more frequently in males than in females, in the proportion of about 2 to 1.

**Localization.**—An individual subject may present the condition in solitary or in multiple form. In the latter case, the lesions may be bilateral and even symmetrical, or they may involve several different bones.

***Figure 20***

*A*, Photomicrograph (× 20) showing the histologic pattern of a small fibrous cortical defect which is eroding the cortical bone seen on the left. The spindle cell character of the stroma of the lesion is evident even under this low magnification.

*B*, Photomicrograph (× 175) showing in histologic detail an area from the tissue pictured in *A*. Note the whorling of the spindle-shaped stromal cells and the occasional small multinuclear giant cell.

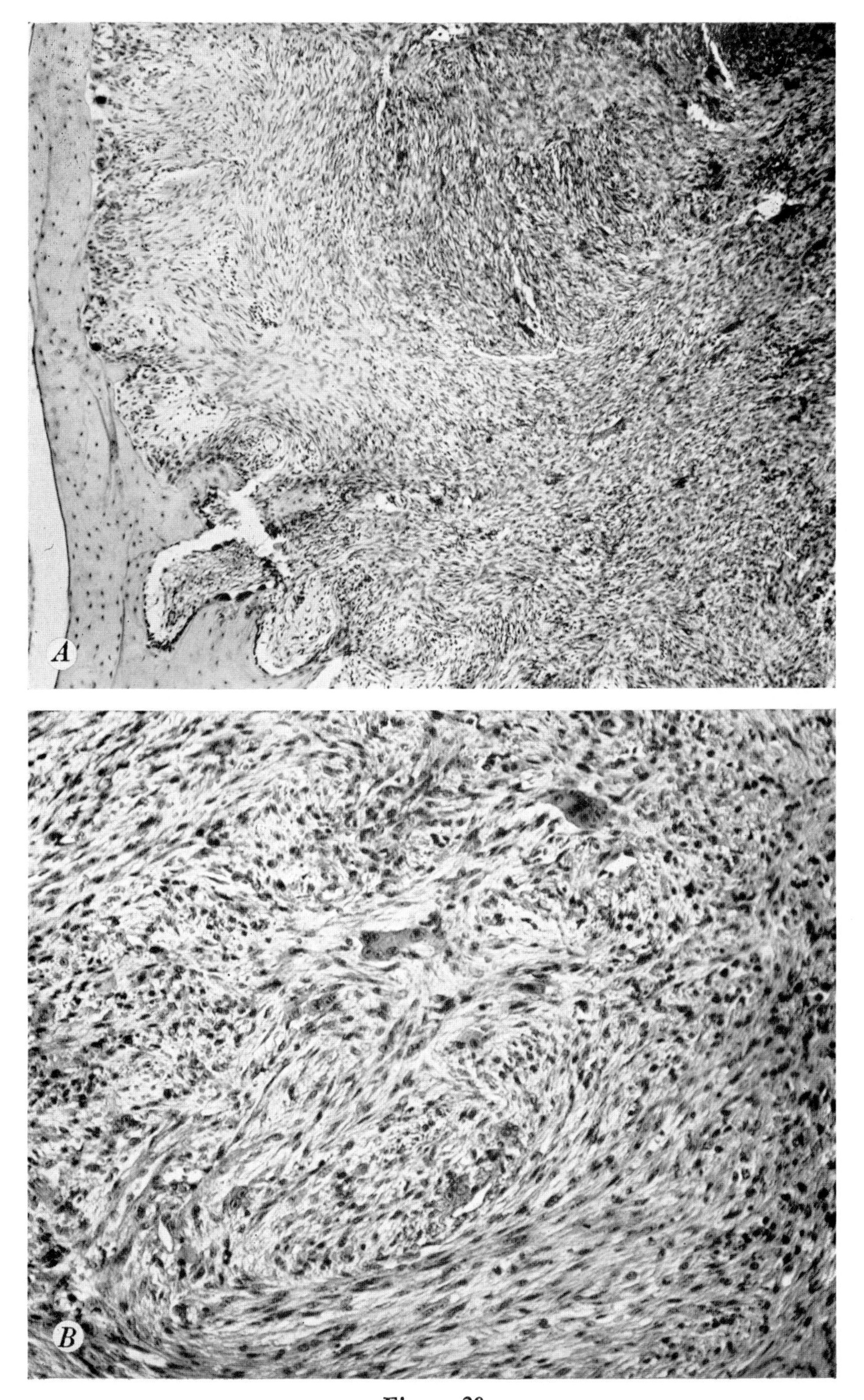


*Figure 20*

By far the most common site of the lesion is the lower part of the femoral shaft, close to, or at most a few inches from, the epiphysial cartilage plate. The lesion is more often in the right femur than in the left. Furthermore, in relation to the lower part of the femoral shaft, the defect is most often oriented to the posteromedial part of the cortex. Next in order of frequency of involvement, though far behind the femur, is the upper part of the tibial shaft. Localization in the upper or lower part of a fibular shaft ranks third in order of frequency, but far behind the tibial shaft. Occasionally, a fibrous cortical defect is found in the upper end of a femoral or lower end of a tibial shaft. Even more rarely, it appears in the shaft of a humerus, radius, or ulna, or in the shaft of some short tubular bone.

While many of the defects do not move away from the place where they were first noticed, some do. While some disappear whether or not they have moved away, others persist for years. Also, persisting defects may enlarge, and occasionally, as already indicated, an enlarging defect penetrates into the medullary cavity and acquires the character of the so-called *non-ossifying fibroma of bone*. (See Fig. 19.)

**Clinical Complaints.**—Ordinarily, a fibrous cortical defect does not give rise to any clinical manifestations. Indeed, except when attention is especially directed toward it in skeletal research surveys, it usually represents an incidental finding in the course of roentgenographic examination of a skeletal area (especially the knee area) in some other connection. For instance, a child may have suffered some trauma to a knee area, and roentgenographic examination might disclose the presence of the defect. If one is not familiar with the lesion, or not cognizant of its high incidence, one might associate its presence with the trauma in question or think one had discovered some serious lesion in an early stage. Again, a child might have some serious lesion developing in the hip area and be complaining of pain referred to the knee. In such a case, a fibrous defect which happened to be present in the femur, for instance, might be misinterpreted as the basis for the complaints. Thus, the main need for understanding the fibrous cortical defect lies not in any clinical importance attaching to the lesion in itself, but in the hazard that it presents as a possible source of confusion. (See Differential Diagnosis, p. 88.)

## ROENTGENOGRAPHIC AND PATHOLOGIC FINDINGS

As already noted, the location of a fibrous cortical defect is always at or fairly near one end of the affected bone shaft. Specifically, it may be found in the cortex

### *Figure 21*

*A*, Roentgenograph of a rather small fibrous defect in the lower part of a tibial shaft, showing substantial obliteration of the defect through sclerotization. The patient was a boy 8 years of age. He had no complaints referable to the lesion, which was discovered incidentally on *x*-ray examination because he suffered an injury to the foot.

*B*, Roentgenograph of a larger defect in the lower part of the tibial shaft, again in process of obliteration through sclerotization. The patient was a man 22 years of age. The lesion was discovered on *x*-ray examination of the lower part of the leg on account of pain.

*C*, Roentgenograph of a fibrous cortical defect in the lower part of a femoral shaft. There were no clinical complaints at the time when this roentgenograph was taken. The patient, a girl, was $9\frac{1}{2}$ years of age at that time. The cortical defect in question was an incidental finding, noted when the part was roentgenographed in connection with an injury to the kneecap (see *D*).

*D*, Roentgenograph, taken $3\frac{1}{2}$ years later, of the lesion shown in *C*. The lesion has grown considerably, and had given rise to clinical complaints. On surgical intervention, the lesional tissue was found to have extended into the medullary cavity. Thus, the lesion had made the transition from a fibrous cortical defect into a non-ossifying fibroma.

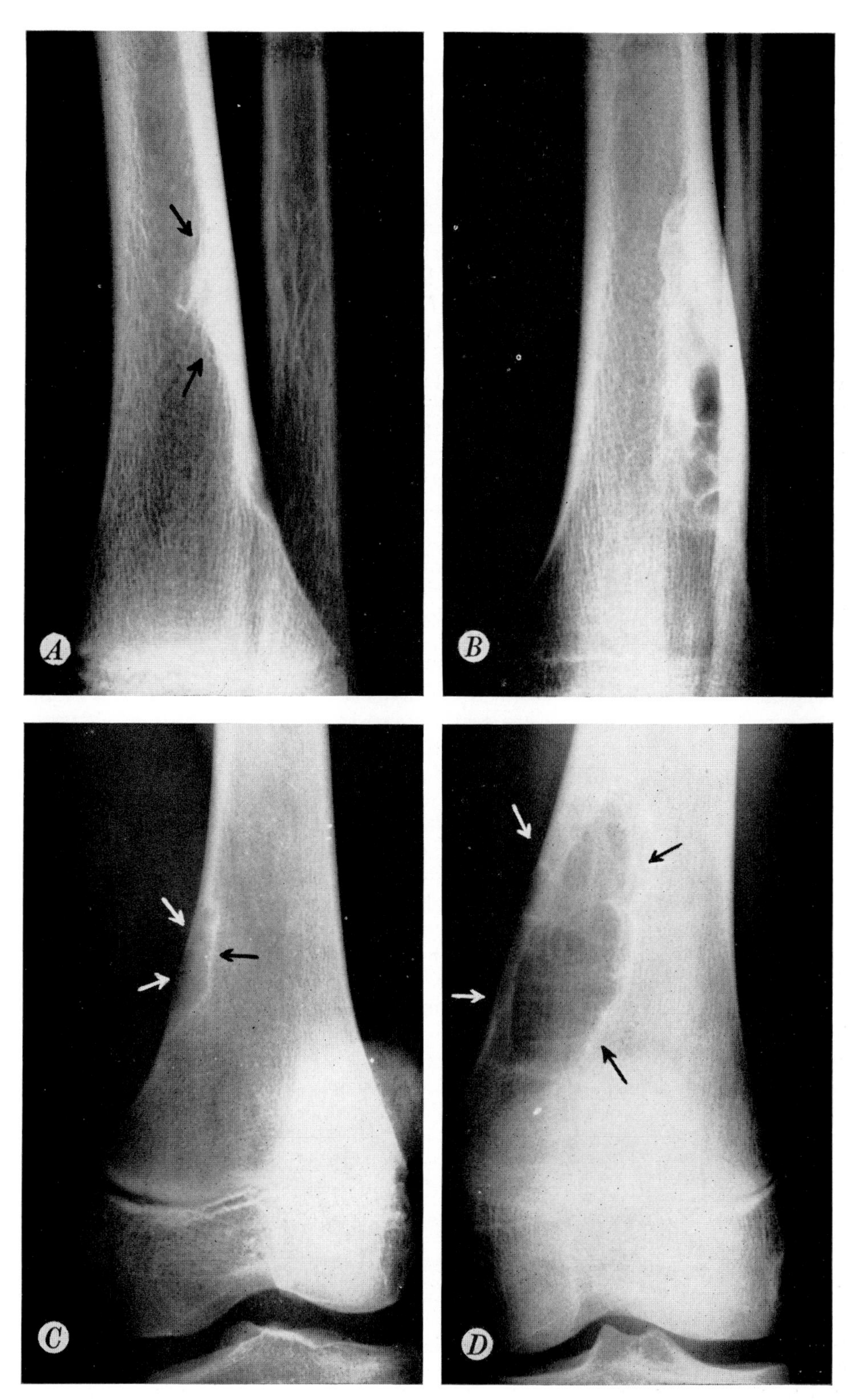


*Figure 21*

close to the epiphysial cartilage plate or several or more centimeters away from the plate. The lesional area may be roundish but is usually oval, in which case its long axis tends to parallel the long axis of the shaft. The greatest length of the defect ranges from about 1 cm. to 3 or even 4 cm. When observed in profile view, the defect is found to be superficial and shallow and located in the cortical wall. When it is seen in frontal view, its orientation to the cortex is likely to be obscure, so that the lesion may mistakenly be thought to lie in the interior of the bone. Around the periphery of the defect, there may be a radiopaque sclerotic border, which may be smooth or scalloped. On the other hand, some defects (especially larger ones) may appear divided off into loculæ by abutting zones of sclerosis.

The writer has had the opportunity of examining several small fibrous cortical defects intact in their setting. These have shown unmistakably that, at the site of a defect, the local cortex comes to be invaded by fibrous tissue which has developed out of the periosteum. This fibrous periosteal scar tissue may be composed, in part or throughout, of intertwining bundles of rather collagenous connective tissue which is continuous with the periosteum. A fibrous cortical defect in which collagenized connective tissue is conspicuous corresponds to the cortical defect due to periosteal desmoid which has been discussed by Kimmelstiel and Rapp.

More often, the lesional tissue is rather cellular connective tissue. When this is the case, the constituent connective-tissue cells may even have a sprinkling of small, multinuclear giant cells among them. The lesional tissue of a fibrous cortical defect which is surrounded and/or subdivided by densely sclerotic osseous tissue is likely to show a good deal of lipid. The lipid is cholesterol, which is present in nests of foam cells scattered among the spindle-shaped stromal cells. Where such cells are present, multinuclear giant cells are likely to be sparse. (See Fig. 20.)

It is not possible to speak with any confidence about the pathogenesis of the fibrous cortical defect. Caffey has carefully considered the various etiologic possibilities, including traumatic injury to the periosteum, directly or through the agency of muscle pull. He found none of these explanations completely satisfactory, but concluded that, on the whole, the most reasonable tentative hypothesis was that the defect represents a local developmental aberration. Hatcher, too, thought that the defect might be explained on such a basis. Specifically, he conceived the lesion as a mass of fibrous tissue appearing in consequence of a flaw in the ossification process in the juxta-epiphysial region, and postulated that the reason for the flaw was a local vascular derangement.

At any rate, we do know that, in the great majority of cases, the fibrous cortical defect undergoes spontaneous regression. Indeed, usually it disappears altogether, and the normal architecture of the region becomes completely reconstituted. Or, in regressing, the lesion may become substantially but not completely obliterated and persist for years as a small focus of radiopacity, within which there are one or more radiolucent loculæ. Occasionally, the lesional area is ultimately marked merely by a uniformly dense patch of radiopacity representing the result of intense sclerotization of the cortex in the area where the lesional tissue of the fibrous defect had been present and been slowly squeezed out of existence. It is interesting to note that the sclerotization occurring in connection with obliteration of the lesion usually begins in the part of the lesion most remote from the epiphysial end, and advances toward that end.

Be that all as it may, an occasional fibrous cortical defect fails to disappear and does not even become sclerotized and static. These cases, as already indicated, are the ones in which the lesional tissue takes on proliferative activity and undergoes transition into the more tumor-like lesion we have come to call non-ossifying fibroma of bone (see below). That the two lesions represent the same basic condition is shown by the fact that the histologic appearance of the lesional tissue is essentially the same whether it has been removed from a fibrous cortical defect or from a non-ossifying fibroma. Also, the present writer has actually been able to follow a few cases in which the course of transition of a fibrous cortical defect into a non-ossifying fibroma could be traced in successive roentgenographs. (See Fig. 21.)

### TREATMENT

Small, asymptomatic fibrous cortical defects, of course, require no treatment. Larger dormant lesions which are likewise picked up incidentally in the course of roentgenographic examination made in some other connection again do not require treatment. In the occasional instance in which the lesion, though small, appears to be the cause of some clinical difficulty, the condition is best treated by curettage, in accordance with the surgical indications. However, in view of the fact that a fibrous cortical defect is nearly always clinically silent, one must try to make quite certain, before undertaking any surgical intervention, that it is not some other condition, entirely unrelated, that is responsible for the complaints.

## NON-OSSIFYING FIBROMA

As already indicated, the non-ossifying fibroma apparently represents an occasional sequela of the fibrous cortical defect. The interrelation between these two forms of what appears to be the same basic lesion was already suggested by Hatcher in 1945, but has only recently come to be better understood. Actually, the concept of non-ossifying (or non-osteogenic) fibroma was first formulated in 1942, in a different connection. It was developed by the writer and his colleagues to make a place for a lesion supposedly representing one of the so-called "variant forms" of giant-cell tumor which we felt should be completely detached from the category of giant-cell tumor. Specifically, the name *non-ossifying fibroma* was evolved to designate cases previously held to represent the "xanthic variant" or the "fibrous" or "healing" variant of giant-cell tumor. When not considered a variant form of giant-cell tumor, the lesion in question was sometimes designated as a "xanthoma" or "xanthogranuloma" of bone.

In the formulation of the name for the lesion, we were governed by the following considerations: 1) That the dominant cellular element of the lesion was the fibroblast; 2) that the basic fibrous tissue did not undergo osseous metaplasia; 3) that the foam cells present resulted from the imbibition of lipid by the fibroblasts, and 4) that the age distribution, localization, and clinical behavior of the lesion were not in line with that of indubitable giant-cell tumor of bone.

### CLINICAL CONSIDERATIONS

**Incidence.**—Since it is only occasionally that a fibrous cortical defect undergoes tumorous evolution into a non-ossifying fibroma, the latter lesion is, of course, much less common than the former. Also, the great majority of the patients are older children or adolescents at the time when the presence of the lesion is first recognized. The patient is not often under 8 or over 20 years of age when the condition is first observed. As to sex, if there is any significant difference in incidence, it is males that are slightly predilected.

**Localization.**—In harmony with the findings relating to the fibrous cortical defect, the non-ossifying fibroma strongly predilects the long bones of the lower limbs. Occasionally, however, the lesion is observed in a long bone of an upper limb. Within a particular long bone so affected, it nearly always lies toward the end of the shaft. However, there is usually an inch or two, though seldom much more, of unaffected shaft between the lesion and the adjacent cartilage plate. In this typical location, the lesion may or may not extend all the way across the shaft. In connection with localization, it seems worth pointing out also that one may encounter a non-ossifying fibroma in one long bone and one or more fibrous cortical defects in other long bones. Thus, in one case observed by the writer, there was a non-ossifying fibroma in the lower part of the shaft of one femur and a fibrous cortical defect in the upper end of each tibia. Also, in a unique case studied by the writer, large tumorous lesions of the nature of non-ossifying fibroma developed in the upper and lower ends of both femora and both tibiæ.

**Clinical Findings.**—Altogether, there is nothing distinctive or characteristic about the clinical findings in cases of non-ossifying fibroma. The lesion is one which progresses very inconspicuously and may lie dormant, sometimes for years, before attention is drawn to it. A patient presenting the lesion in the shaft of a long bone usually indicates that the complaints were of only a few weeks' or months' standing before admission to the hospital. However, from what is known in general about the evolutionary course, it is likely that the condition had been present much longer in asymptomatic form.

In some cases, the patients report their difficulty as beginning with some trauma, of moderate severity, to the general region in which the bone lesion was subsequently discovered. In some of these cases, palpation reveals a point of bone tenderness and sometimes even of bone swelling, and when an *x*-ray picture is taken the lesion (not caused, though perhaps aggravated, by the trauma) is discovered. In other cases, the trauma may even have induced a pathologic fracture through the lesional area. Other patients, while giving no history of trauma, likewise have pain and local swelling, not of long standing, as their central complaint. Not infrequently, also, a lesion in a long bone is discovered by chance during the roentgenographic examination of the part in some other connection, the patient still being free of clinical complaints relating to the lesion.

## ROENTGENOGRAPHIC FINDINGS

When a non-ossifying fibroma of bone has its characteristic location in the shaft of a long bone, the *x*-ray picture is usually so distinctive that one can make

### *Figure 22*

*A*, Roentgenograph of a non-ossifying fibroma in the lower part of a fibular shaft. As shown by the resection specimen, the lesional tissue occupied the medullary canal. It consisted of several adjacent but more or less discrete foci of firm tissue, brownish and yellowish in color and having a fibrous character. The patient was a girl 10 years of age who had had pain in the lower part of the leg for about 4 months and dated her difficulty from the time of a kick to that area. On the basis of the roentgenograph, one might have thought that the lesion was a solitary bone cyst, but actually the lesional area was completely filled by the tissue already described.

*B*, Roentgenograph of a non-ossifying fibroma in the lower part of the shaft of a tibia. Note the fracture, which was a pathologic one having followed upon a slight twist of the ankle.

*C*, Roentgenograph of a large non-ossifying fibroma in the upper part of a tibial shaft. The case was an unusual one in that similar large lesions were present in the upper end of the opposite tibia, the lower ends of both femora, and the lower ends of both tibiæ. Tissue was removed from four of these lesions. The biopsies showed consistently the histologic pattern of whorled bundles of spindle-shaped cells interspersed with small multinuclear giant cells, and some of the tissue areas also contained foam cells.

*D*, Roentgenograph representing a profile view of the lesion shown in *C*. (Details relating to this case are to be found in the paper by Adams and Goldner.)

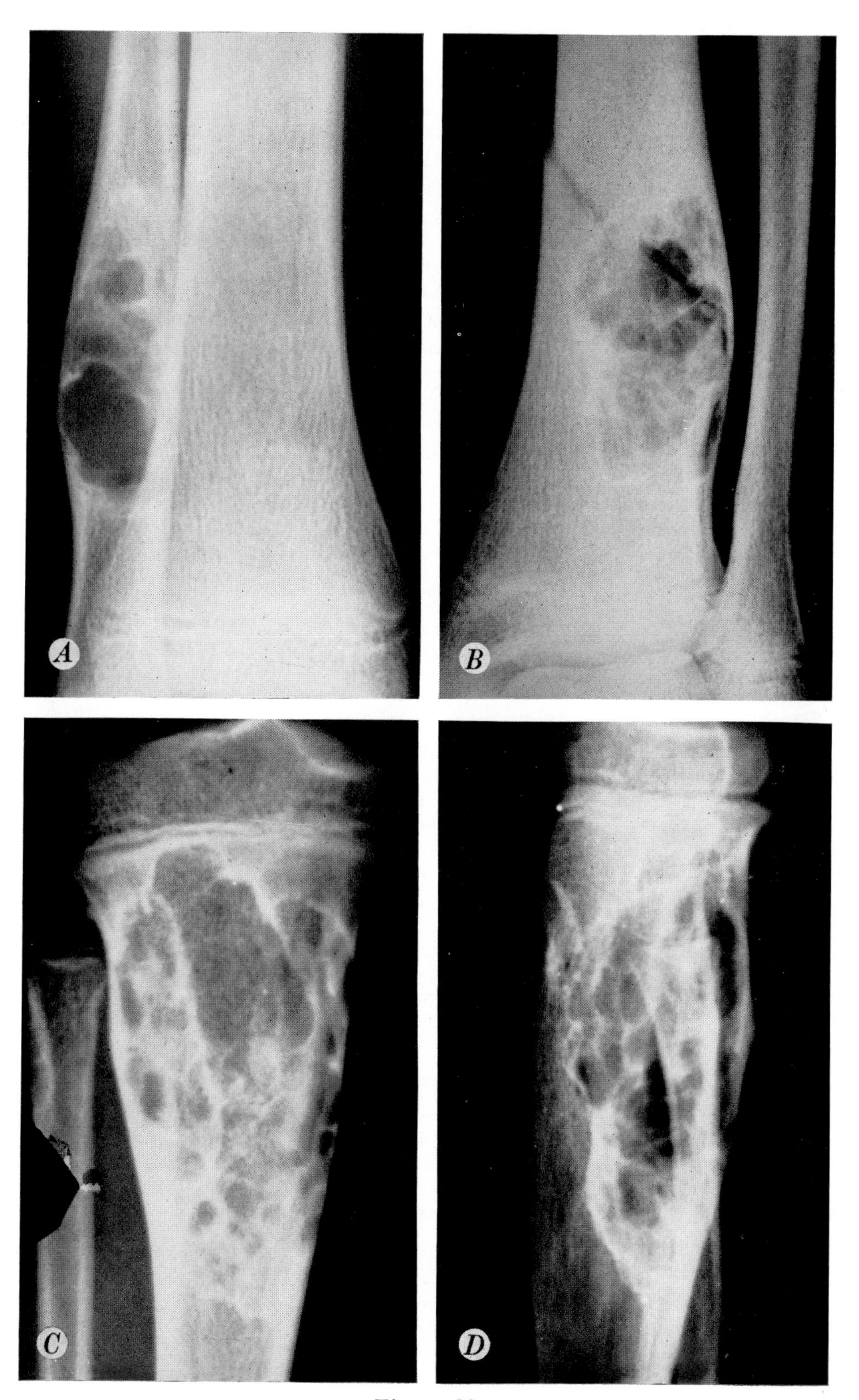


*Figure 22*

the diagnosis from this alone with a high degree of assurance. Although when first seen in a long bone shaft the lesion is almost always at some distance from the epiphysial cartilage plate, it actually usually starts its development close to the plate and moves shaftward in the course of growth of the bone. In a few cases, we have been able to demonstrate this from roentgenographs of the same lesion taken at different times during several years. Furthermore, as noted, the lesion is frequently oriented to one side of the shaft—*i.e.*, eccentric. It is less likely to be found extending all the way across the shaft in thick long bones (*e.g.*, tibia) than in thin ones (*e.g.*, fibula).

In a tibia or femur, for instance, an eccentrically located lesion is likely to be represented by a somewhat loculated rarefaction shadow, usually longer than it is wide, and commonly somewhere between 4 and 7 cm. in its greatest dimension. Where it abuts upon the cortex, the latter may be thinned and in part bulged, or, on the other hand, densified and sclerosed. Toward the interior, these eccentric lesions are outlined by an encapsulating and often scalloped sclerotic shell. The loculated roentgenographic appearance of the lesion is produced by one or more "partitioning" shadows which traverse the lesion irregularly. In a fibula, for instance, while the lesion may be eccentrically located, it is more likely to extend across the entire diameter of the shaft. In such a bone, too, the lesion is longer than it is wide, and is ordinarily about 3 to 4 cm. in length. The area of rarefaction representing the lesion may or may not appear loculated. The cortex in the area of the lesion tends to be thinned and slightly expanded. If there is an infraction through the lesion, the cortex toward the side of the infraction may be found thickened by periosteal new bone apposition. (See Fig. 22.)

## PATHOLOGIC FINDINGS

When a typical lesion which has been removed intact in its setting is cut in the long plane, the cut surface usually presents several more or less discrete but adjacent foci of tough tissue having a fibrous consistency. The color of this tissue is brownish or yellowish. Some lesions may be more or less uniform in color throughout. Others present a mottled appearance, created by a mixture of yellowish and brownish foci. The shaft cortex neighboring upon the brown-yellow tissue of the lesion is usually found eroded and thinned in some places, but may be abnormally thickened in others. Each focus may be outlined in part by a thin shell of sclerotic bone. Some of the individual foci may also be separated from each other by sclerotic spongiosa. In larger lesions, the tumoral tissue has essentially the same gross appearance, but is less likely to be found divided into clear-cut foci surrounded by encapsulating walls of bone. (See Fig. 23.)

### *Figure 23*

*A*, Roentgenograph of a relatively small non-ossifying fibroma in the shaft of a fibula. Note that the lesional area appears loculated and is surrounded by a narrow zone of radiopacity. The patient was a girl 6 years of age. She had been complaining of pain in both knees and both ankles for about 9 days, but these complaints were certainly not related to the lesion shown in the *x*-ray picture. The lesion was resected on the mistaken assumption that it represented a cyst (see *B*).

*B*, Photograph (somewhat enlarged) of the sectioned fibula presenting the lesional area shown in *A*. Note that the lesional tissue is within the medullary cavity of the bone.

*C*, Photomicrograph (× 8) showing the general histologic pattern of the lesion shown in *B*. A whorled arrangement of the stromal cells is apparent. The scattered larger dots represent the multinuclear giant cells. There is complete absence of osseous trabeculæ within the lesional tissue.

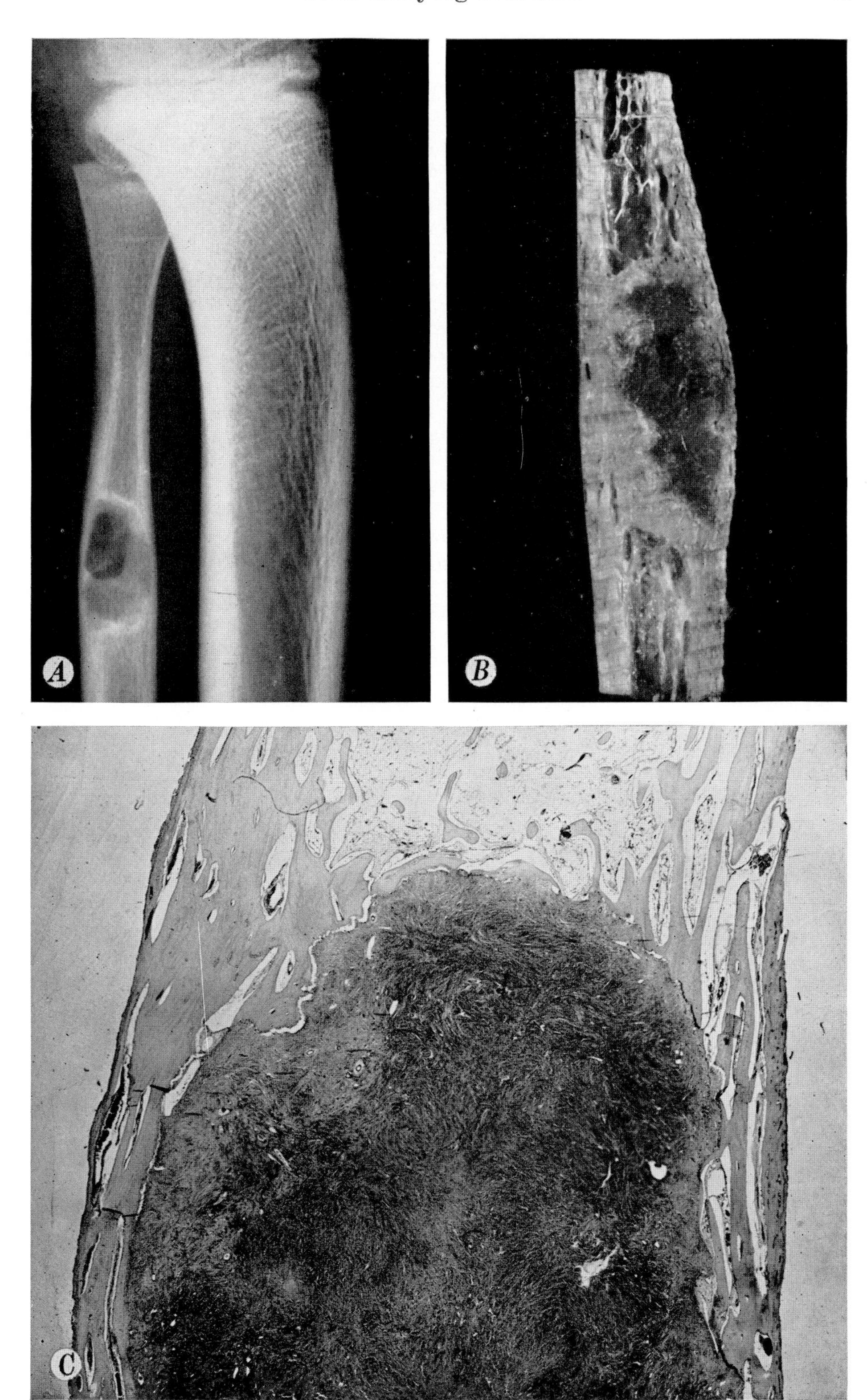


*Figure 23*

On microscopic examination, it appears that the general cytologic pattern of the stroma of the lesion is whorled bundles of spindle-shaped connective-tissue cells. However, the cellularity of the stroma varies from one lesion to another and from one focus to another within the same lesion. In a distinctly brownish lesion or focus, the stromal connective-tissue cells are spindle-shaped and closely compacted, being interspersed with but little collagenous intercellular material. Many of the stromal cells are likely to contain granules of hemosiderin in their cytoplasm. It is this that mainly accounts for the brownish color of the lesion or focus, though some scattered capillary hemorrhages may also contribute to it. Irregularly dispersed among the stromal cells are small, often elongated multinuclear giant cells. These cells are sparse on the whole. However, they may be more numerous and clustered together in some fields, and especially about areas of recent capillary hemorrhage. The giant cells seem to be formed through fusion of the spindle-shaped stromal cells. Like the latter, many of them also contain granules of hemosiderin in their cytoplasm. It is the presence of the giant cells, especially if they are found in clumps in areas of hemorrhage, that may lead to misdesignation of the lesion as a giant-cell tumor, albeit a healing one.

In a distinctly yellowish lesion or focus, one finds large and small nests of foam cells. In such areas, the stromal tissue is likely to be composed of rather collagenous spindle-shaped connective-tissue cells in winding thick strands or whorled bundles. It can be shown that the interspersed foam cells arise through conversion of the spindle cells into lipophages. The lipid contained within the latter is, to a large extent, of the nature of cholesterol esters. On the whole, the more yellow the lesion or focus, the more lipophages does it contain and the more collagenous does the intervening stromal tissue appear. Furthermore, the less does it show of hemosiderin pigment in the stromal cells, or of multinuclear giant cells among them. Lipid deposition apparently represents merely a regressive change, associated with walling off and an attempt at spontaneous healing of the lesion. The presence of the foam cells, in greater or lesser numbers, is the factor which has influenced some observers in the direction of designating the lesion as a xanthic variant of giant-cell tumor, as a xanthogranuloma, or possibly as a healed, lipidized focus of eosinophilic granuloma.

The absence of bone formation within the lesional stromal tissue is consistent and striking. It is true that individual foci may be walled off or delimited at their periphery by a narrow zone of bone. Also, abutting upon the cortex of the shaft, the lesion may even provoke the former to thickening in some places, just as, in other places, it may erode it. However, in either case, such bone formation represents a response of the neighboring tissue to the lesion, and not a feature of the lesion itself. (See Fig. 24.)

## DIFFERENTIAL DIAGNOSIS

The problems of differential diagnosis are somewhat different in regard to a lesion which is still a mere fibrous cortical defect from what they are in regard to a

**Figure 24**

*A*, Photomicrograph (× 125) showing the cytologic pattern usually presented by most of the tissue in an actively proliferating non-ossifying fibroma. Note the whorled spindle-shaped stromal cells and the small and sparse multinuclear giant cells.

*B*, Photomicrograph (× 100) showing foam cells resulting from the imbibition of lipid by the spindle-shaped stromal cells.

*C*, Photomicrograph (× 200) showing the hemosiderin pigment (the black granules) sometimes to be found in and between the stromal cells.

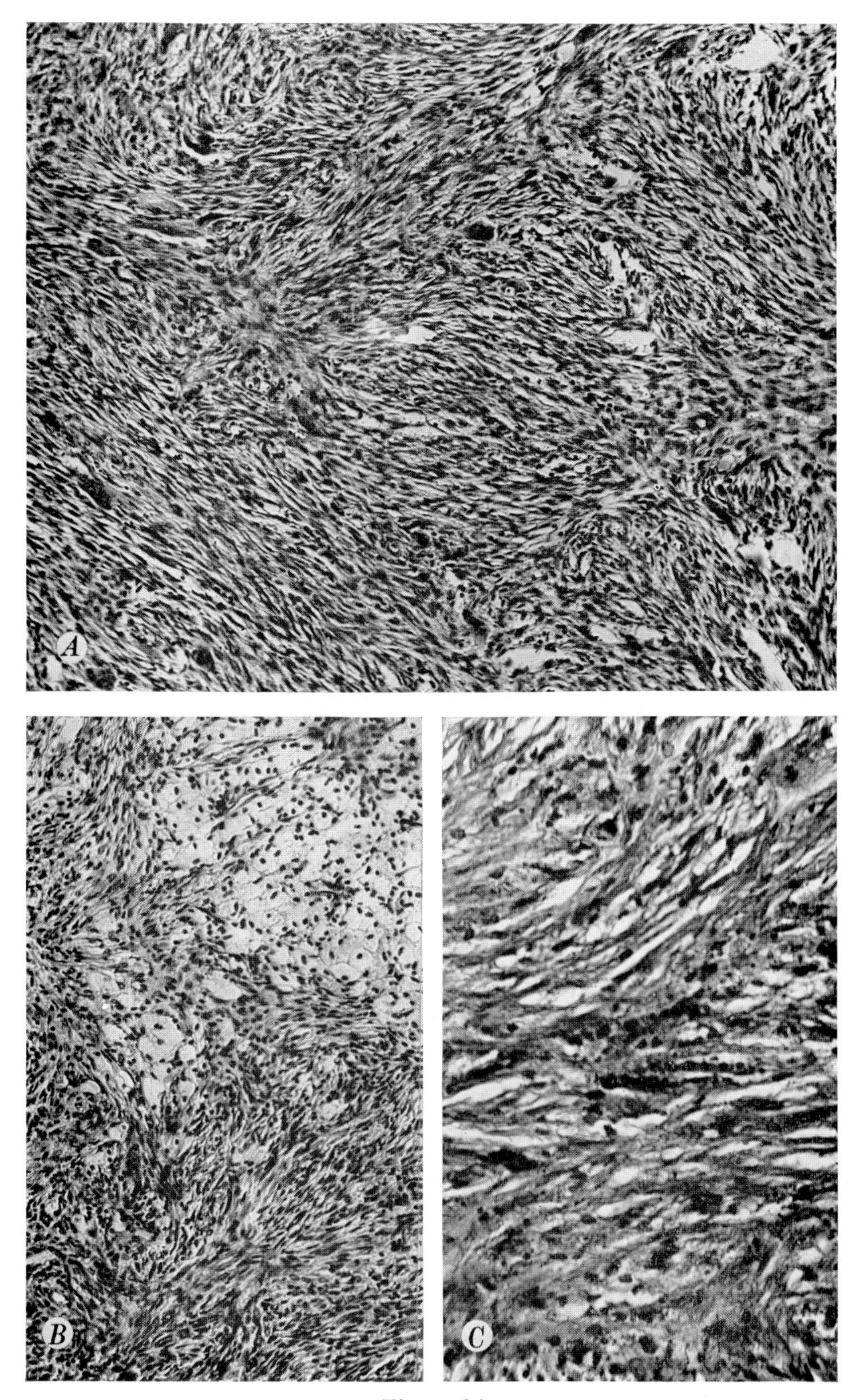


*Figure 24*

full-fledged non-ossifying fibroma. In connection with a fibrous cortical defect, these problems relate mainly to osteoid-osteoma and intracortical bone abscess. In connection with non-ossifying fibroma, the problems are largely those of differentiation from giant-cell tumor and xanthogranuloma (healed focus of eosinophilic granuloma).

**Osteoid-osteoma.**—In contrast to a fibrous cortical defect, an osteoid-osteoma is a painful lesion. In fact, it is not unusual for an osteoid-osteoma to manifest its presence by pain, months before it can be distinguished in the roentgenographic picture. Whether intracortical or medullary, the osteoid-osteoma nidus in itself is rather small—usually not more than 1 cm. in its greatest dimension. Furthermore, particularly when the nidus is oriented to the cortex, its presence is usually associated with considerable thickening of the cortex, not only in the vicinity of the nidus but along the shaft for several inches. Altogether, then, it should not usually be difficult to distinguish clinically between a fibrous cortical defect and an osteoid-osteoma oriented to the cortex.

**Intracortical Bone Abscess.**—A localized cortical abscess is of rare occurrence. Its site in the cortex is usually somewhere in the midportion of the shaft, rather than toward an end of the shaft, where the fibrous cortical defect is usually located. Roentgenographically, the abscess in the cortex appears as a minute area of radiolucency lying in a zone of thickened cortex. In contrast to the fibrous cortical defect, it is painful, though the pain may be only intermittent and periodic. Actually, there is greater likelihood of confusing an intracortical bone abscess clinically with an osteoid-osteoma than with a fibrous cortical defect. Histologically, the lesional area of the cortical abscess is clearly characterized by a minute cavity lined by a thick pyogenic membrane.

**Giant-cell Tumor.**—Misinterpretation of a non-ossifying fibroma (or a rather large fibrous cortical defect) as a giant-cell tumor is still common. The confusion is usually due to misreading of the histologic picture presented by the tissue removed from the lesion. It is true that the lesional tissue is likely to present the pattern of spindle-shaped cells interspersed with some multinuclear giant cells and thus to mimic the pattern of giant-cell tumor. However, the stromal cells of a non-ossifying fibroma are smaller, and the giant cells are smaller and much more sparse than those of a giant-cell tumor. On the clinical side, in any case, there are many facts which delimit the non-ossifying fibroma from the giant-cell tumor. These are: 1) Its subjects, with only occasional exceptions, are under 20 years of age; 2) the lesion is located in the bone shaft, almost always sparing the actual epiphysial end of the bone; and 3) the lesion is completely innocuous, tending to heal spontaneously and, in any event, not recurring after surgical intervention.

**Xanthogranuloma.**—In the healing phases of a fibrous cortical defect or a non-ossifying fibroma, many of the stromal cells in certain of the tissue fields may, as noted, become lipidized and converted into foam cells. On this account, one finds occasional instances in which the lesion in question has been described as a solitary xanthoma, xanthofibroma, or xanthogranuloma, often with the specific implication that the lesion represents a healed, lipidized focus of eosinophilic granuloma. The writer, however, has yet to encounter an indubitable solitary focus of eosinophilic granuloma which, even in part, has become so lipidized as to present the pattern of the lipidized tissue fields sometimes seen in a non-ossifying fibroma. In fact, his experience is to the effect that, if a solitary focus of eosinophilic granuloma is undergoing spontaneous healing, it heals by resolution and not by being converted into a xanthogranuloma.

## TREATMENT

The differences in indications for treatment between the non-ossifying fibroma and the fibrous cortical defect are, of course, dictated by the greater size and the likelihood of fracture in connection with the former lesion. In large lesions, curettage may leave defects so great that they have to be filled in with bone chips. Large lesions in favorable locations, such as a fibula, can also be removed by block resection. Postoperative radiation therapy is not necessary. Whether the lesion would be amenable to radiation therapy alone (that is, without surgical intervention) we cannot say.

## REFERENCES


Adams, J. P., and Goldner, J. L.: Fibrous Lesions of Bone, South. M. J., *46*, 529, 1953.

Bahls, G.: Über ein solitäres Xanthom im Knochen, Zentralbl. f. Chir., *63*, 1041, 1936.

Caffey, J.: On Fibrous Defects in Cortical Walls of Growing Tubular Bones, Advances Pediat., *7*, 13, 1955.

Campbell, C. J., and Harkess, J.: Fibrous Metaphyseal Defect of Bone, Surg., Gynec. & Obst., *104*, 329, 1957.

Compere, C. L., and Coleman, S. S.: Nonosteogenic Fibroma of Bone, Surg., Gynec. & Obst., *105*, 588, 1957.

Devlin, J. A., Bowman, H. E., and Mitchell, C. L.: Non-Osteogenic Fibroma of Bone, J. Bone & Joint Surg., *37-A*, 472, 1955.

Fenton, R. L., and Hoffman, B. P.: Osteoid Osteoma and Non-Ossifying Fibromas Co-existing in One Femur, Bull. Hosp. Joint Dis., *14*, 217, 1953.

Geschickter, C. F., and Copeland, M. M.: *Tumors of Bone*, 3rd ed., Philadelphia, J. B. Lippincott Co., 1949. (See p. 246.)

Hatcher, C. H.: The Pathogenesis of Localized Fibrous Lesions in the Metaphyses of Long Bones, Ann. Surg., *122*, 1016, 1945.

Jaffe, H. L., and Lichtenstein, L.: Non-Osteogenic Fibroma of Bone, Am. J. Path., *18*, 205, 1942.

Kimmelstiel, P., and Rapp, I.: Cortical Defect Due to Periosteal Desmoids, Bull Hosp. Joint Dis., *12*, 286, 1951.

Kolodny, A.: Bone Sarcoma: the Primary Malignant Tumors of Bone and the Giant Cell Tumor, Surg., Gynec. & Obst., *44*, (suppl. 1), 1-214, 1927. (*See* Fig. 83, p. 186.)

Maudsley, R. H., and Stansfeld, A. G.: Non-osteogenic Fibroma of Bone (Fibrous Metaphysial Defect), J. Bone & Joint Surg., *38-B*, 714, 1956.

Phélip, J-A.: Ostéite kystique vacuolaire juvénile xanthomateuse de l'extrémité inférieure du fémur, Mém. Acad. de chir., *61*, 443, 1935.

Phemister, D. B., and Grimson, K. S.: Fibrous Osteoma of the Jaws, Ann. Surg., *105*, 564, 1937.

Ravelli, A.: Röntgenbild und Deutung bestimmter Knochenherde in den Metaphysen von Tibia und Femur, Arch. f. klin. Chir., *280*, 205, 1955.

Schlumberger, H. G.: Fibrous Dysplasia of Single Bones (Monostotic Fibrous Dysplasia), Mil. Surgeon, *99*, 504, 1946.

Schröder, F.: Ein zentraler xanthomatöser Riesenzellentumor der Fibula. Gleichzeitig ein Beitrag zur Kenntnis der xanthomatösen Gewebsneubildungen, Arch. f. klin. Chir., *168*, 118, 1931–32.

Sontag, L. W., and Pyle, S. I.: The Appearance and Nature of Cyst-like Areas in the Distal Femoral Metaphyses of Children, Am. J. Roentgenol., *46*, 185, 1941.

Chapter

# 7

# Osteoid-Osteoma

THE *osteoid-osteoma* is a small but painful bone lesion, and it is its small size and consistent painfulness that strikingly characterize it clinically. Indeed, it often gives rise to pain for months before its presence is even demonstrable in the *x*-ray picture at all, and sometimes longer before the *x*-ray picture is reasonably clear-cut. The patients are predominantly children and young adults. While the lesion may appear in almost any bone, the femur and tibia are by far the most common locations for it.

Anatomically, the essential components of the osteoid-osteoma lesion are: a small core or nidus of osteoid and/or osseous tissue (the osteoid-osteoma proper) and a zone of bone sclerosis or thickening (the perifocal reactive zone). The lesion is also peculiar in that, even when it has been present for several years, the osteoid-osteoma nidus tends not to exceed 1 cm. in its greatest diameter.

In a particular case, the osteoid-osteoma nidus may lie within the spongiosa of the affected bone, perhaps close to an articular surface. On the other hand, the nidus may be oriented to the cortex, in which case it may lie against the inner surface of the cortex, within it, or even, though rarely, between the cortex and the periosteum. The reactive perifocal zone is much more likely to be striking when the osteoid-osteoma is oriented to the cortex than when it is oriented to the spongiosa. In the latter case, one may find merely a zone of thickened, condensed, and otherwise altered spongiosa surrounding the nidus as a ring or band of variable extent. When the nidus is oriented to the cortex, the latter may be found thickened over a considerable part of its circumference. This is true particularly when the lesion is in a long bone, in which case, furthermore, the cortical thickening may even extend for a number of inches in the longitudinal direction.

**Delimitation of the Concept.**—The concept of osteoid-osteoma as a clinicopathologic entity was proposed by the writer in 1935. The concept was rather

***Figure 25***

*A*, Roentgenograph of an osteoid-osteoma in the lower end of a humerus. The nidus appears as a round focus of relative radiolucency set in an area of cortical thickening. The patient, a boy 19 years of age, had suffered for 2 years from increasing and persistent pain in the right elbow region.

*B*, Roentgenograph of an osteoid-osteoma in the neck of a femur. The lesion appears as an oval area of relative radiolucency surrounded by a zone of radiopacity. The perifocal reactive bone thickening is most conspicuous, however, in the cortex below the neck.

*C*, Roentgenograph of an osteoid-osteoma involving the pedicle and the adjacent part of the lamina of the 4th dorsal vertebra, on the left side. The patient was a boy 15 years of age who complained of pain in the upper part of the back for over a year before the nidus was clearly visualized.

*D*, Roentgenograph of an osteoid-osteoma in a proximal phalanx. Note the considerable perinidal reactive bone thickening. The patient stated that there had been intermittent pain in the finger for 5 years. For a number of years before the lesion was diagnosed and removed, it was thought that the affected phalanx was the site of a "low-grade osteitis."

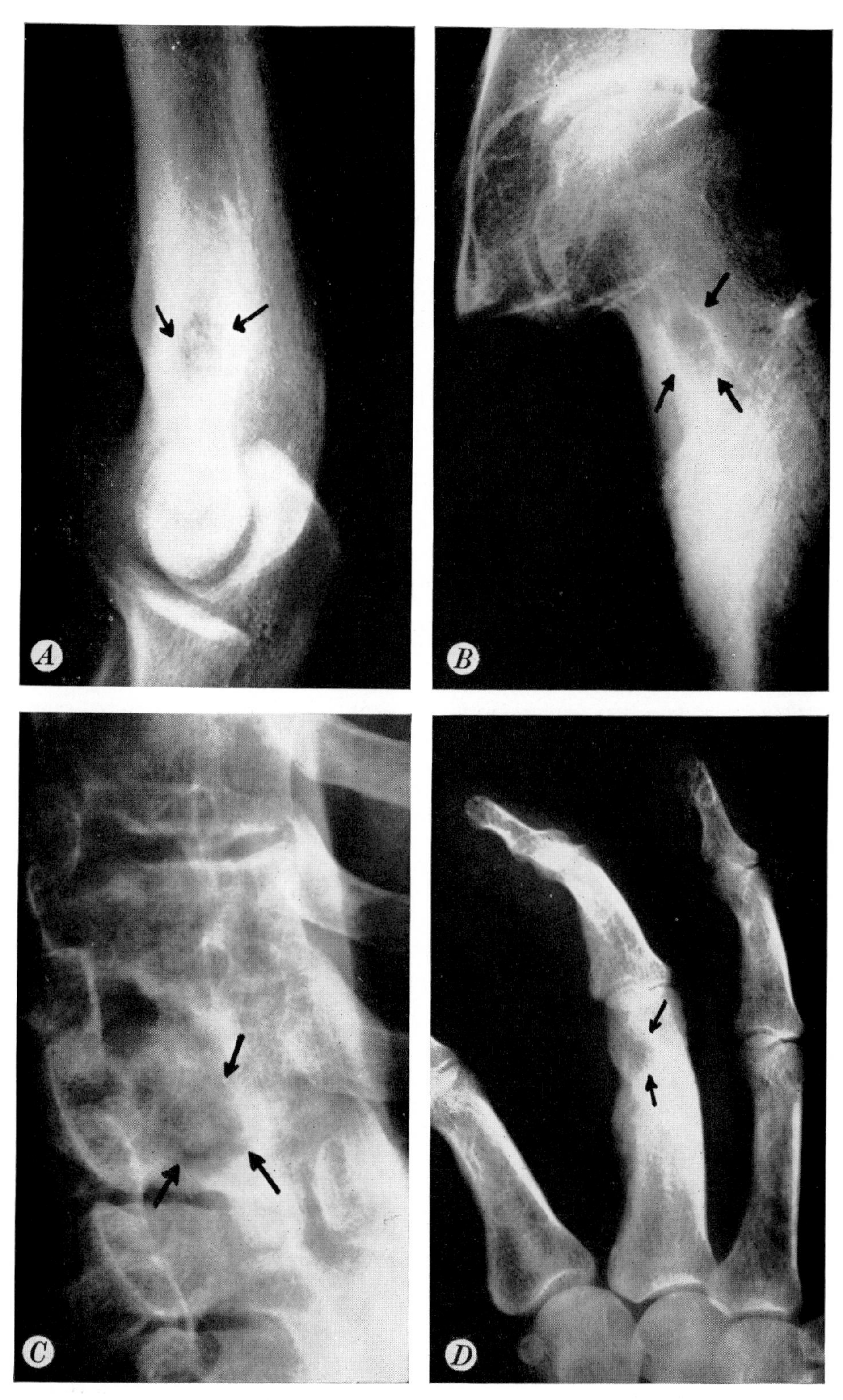


*Figure* 25

slow in gaining acceptance, but is now generally accepted and well sustained by reports on groups of collected cases from various clinics. Whatever may still be debatable about the nature of the lesion, it seems plain that it does not develop on the basis of an infection. However, in the older literature, many examples of the lesion can be found among the cases reported as instances of: "osteomyelitis with annular sequestrum," "cortical bone abscess," "localized bone abscess," "sclerosing nonsuppurative osteomyelitis" ("osteomyelitis of Garré"), "osteomyelitis chronic from the beginning," "fibrous osteomyelitis," etc. With the acceptance of osteoid-osteoma as an entity, the incidence of case reports under these other headings has radically declined. It is not to be denied, however, that when the distinction from osteoid-osteoma is made, there still remains a category of cases properly classified as localized chronic bone infection, though these cases are becoming increasingly rare.

Recently, the term "giant osteoid-osteoma" has been introduced to designate a lesion which should likewise be held apart from the osteoid-osteoma lesion as we conceive it. In its histologic appearance, the so-called "giant osteoid-osteoma" does mimic the genuine osteoid-osteoma. However, it is not only a larger lesion, but does not provoke the characteristic pain suffered by patients affected with osteoid-osteoma. Furthermore, the "giant osteoid-osteoma" usually becomes heavily calcified under treatment by irradiation. That the lesion which has been called "giant osteoid-osteoma" is an entity, there can be no doubt. In the writer's opinion, however, it is probably better characterized by the name of *benign osteoblastoma* (p. 107).

## CLINICAL CONSIDERATIONS

**Incidence.**—The osteoid-osteoma is not a rare lesion. On the average, the writer sees 6 or 7 cases per year, and his total experience with it covers about 150 cases. As to age incidence, fully 75 per cent of the cases are distributed rather evenly through the age group 10 to 25 years. Among the patients under 10, only an occasional one is under 2 years of age, and among those over 25 it is rare to find one over 50. As to sex incidence, it appears that the lesion is at least twice as common in males as in females.

**Localization.**—The lesion strongly predilects the femur and tibia. In any large series of cases, the femur will be found affected in about 25 per cent and the tibia in about 25 per cent. The distribution of the cases among the other bones will naturally vary from series to series. In our material, the fibula, humerus, vertebra (arch or process), astragalus and calcaneus together accounted for about 35 per cent of the locations. A large variety of other bone sites made up the remaining 15 per cent. In one or another of these miscellaneous cases, the lesion was observed in a rib, iliac bone, patella, or some hand or foot bone not already mentioned. The writer has not yet observed the lesion in a calvarium. As to jawbones, an indubitable instance of osteoid-osteoma has been described in relation to the mandible. In regard to other cases reported as instances of osteoid-osteoma of jawbones, there can be no doubt that most of them represent a nidus of osteocementum about one or another tooth, and not the lesion in question. (See Fig. 25.)

**Clinical Complaints and Findings.**—The duration of complaints at the time of admission to the hospital for removal of the lesion ordinarily ranges between a few months and a few years. Histories of less than 6 months are the exception; of 6 months to 2 years, the rule; and of over 2 years not common. In 2 cases seen by the writer, the difficulties dated back 5 and 10 years respectively. Probably the main reason for the common delay of about 6 months in the clinical identification is that, during the early stages of the clinical course of the case, it may be difficult to demonstrate the osteoid-osteoma roentgenographically, even under favorable technical conditions. Another reason undoubtedly is that the general medical practitioner—the one most likely to see the patient during the early part of the clinical course—is not likely to think of the possibility of an osteoid-osteoma.

Clinically, as already noted, the principal complaint is of pain, and it is this that consistently leads the patient to seek medical attention. Occasional and mild at first, the pain usually increases in persistence and severity and often becomes bad enough to interfere with sleep. Fortunately, most of the patients learn quickly that an adequate dose of *aspirin* almost invariably relieves the pain for several hours at a stretch.

The principal clinical finding is local tenderness—often exquisite "point" tenderness. Sooner or later, and particularly if the lesion is in a bone site not very thickly covered by soft tissue, a slight local swelling may become apparent. Limping is complained of by a considerable number of patients in whom a lower limb bone is involved. Stiffness and weakness of the part are observed in some cases—notably those in which the lesion is near a joint. In connection with the pain, it may be worth while to point out that, ordinarily, immobilization of the part does not relieve it. In some cases, on account of the fact that the part has been spared in use, there may also be a slight amount of muscle atrophy. Only rarely does one note even slight local heat and redness, and even when these are observed there is no history of febrile episodes in connection with the lesion.

In a case in which the lesion is in a vertebra or a rib, the patient may present a scoliotic deformity. Furthermore, a lesion located under the articular cartilage of a large joint or not far from it may incite a "sympathetic" synovitis, and ultimately even lead, as Sherman points out, to secondary degenerative hypertrophic arthritis. Exceptionally, also, a case is seen in which the clinical complaints have a neurologic coloring. Thus, in a case in which the lesion was in the upper part of the shaft of a humerus there was not only local pain and extensive muscle atrophy but also excessive perspiration of the related hand, which also was abnormally cold to touch. In another case, in which the lesion was in the upper end of a femur, the neurologic complaints simulated those of the sciatic syndrome. The reflex relation of the neurologic phenomena in any particular case to the lesion is shown by the fact that they disappear when the lesion is removed.

**The Question of Antecedent Trauma.**—A definite majority of the patients (about 70 per cent) do not relate the onset of their complaints to an antecedent local trauma. Some of those who do so relate it state that the trauma preceded the onset of symptoms by weeks, months, or even years. The others date the onset of the complaints directly from the injury. Since, however, only about 30 per cent of the patients bring up the factor of trauma at all, and it is in only about half of these cases that the alleged injury is directly inculpated, the writer is inclined to regard trauma as irrelevant to the causation of the lesion.

## ROENTGENOGRAPHIC FINDINGS

It is the roentgenographic picture that constitutes the most valuable single diagnostic guide to the lesion. As noted, the nidus itself is usually roundish or oval and is not more than 1 cm. in its greatest diameter. The clarity with which it shows up in the *x*-ray picture is affected by such variants as: the position of the nidus in the affected bone; the radiodensity of the nidus itself; the extent and radiodensity of the perinidal zone of reaction; and the attention given to techniques such as taking the picture from various angles, "coning down," overexposure, etc.

Characteristically, the nidus appears as a relatively radiolucent or (less frequently) radiopaque focus in the affected bone part. It is usually, though not always, surrounded by a shadow reflecting a reactively thickened or altered zone of neighboring bone. The area of perilesional radiopacity may be only a narrow ring or it may spread out for some distance from the lesion, even if the latter is in the spongiosa. Especially if the lesion develops in relation to the cortex of a long bone, the region of reactive thickening and densification may extend for several inches beyond the site of the osteoid-osteoma proper. In cases in which roentgenographic pictures such as these are supported by the clinical findings and history characteristic of osteoid-osteoma, one can already feel quite confident that one is dealing with that lesion. However, as previously noted, in cases in which the complaints are of only recent date, it may be difficult at first to demonstrate the osteoid-osteoma nidus roentgenographically. Thus, in a case in which the history is suggestive of osteoid-osteoma but in which the lesion has not yet evolved sufficiently to show up in the *x*-ray picture, re-examination at intervals of a few months may be necessary for the ultimate confirmation of the diagnosis. (See Fig. 26.)

Even if the complaints are already of long standing when the patient is first seen, the roentgenographic demonstration of the osteoid-osteoma nidus still presents certain difficulties in some cases. This may happen for instance in a case in which the lesion is in relation to the cortex of a long bone and the surrounding bone area is already much thickened and sclerosed. Under ordinary conditions of roentgenographic exposure, one may note only diffuse thickening and densification of the affected bone part. However, the osteoid-osteoma nidus can usually be made to stand out clearly in the thickened area if the field is "coned down" upon, increased kilovoltage is used for the *x*-ray pictures, and these are taken in various planes. In relation to dorsal vertebræ, the nidus is very likely to be extremely difficult to visualize in the *x*-ray picture unless such techniques are used.

There are also certain pitfalls in the roentgenographic diagnosis of osteoid-osteoma. For instance, the writer has seen several cases in which the condition was misdiagnosed as osteochondritis dissecans because the nidus was radiopaque and located at the articular end of a long bone. Again, a solitary enostosis ("bone fleck") may be confused with an osteoid-osteoma roentgenographically, though

***Figure 26***

*A*, Roentgenograph of an osteoid-osteoma oriented to the cortex of the upper part of a femoral shaft. The lesion presents as an area of faint radiolucency. The patient was a girl 16 years of age who had complained for 16 months of pain referred mainly to the knee area. (See also 26-*C*.)

*B*, Roentgenograph of an osteoid-osteoma oriented to the cortex of the upper part of a tibial shaft. The location of the nidus is indicated by the arrows, but the nidus does not stand out clearly in the view shown; nor did it stand out clearly in the lateral view. The reason for this is that the cortex about the nidus is very much thickened and the nidus itself is radiopaque, so that there is a lack of contrast between it and the cortex. (See also 26-*D*.)

*C*, Roentgenograph (enlarged) of a slice of the resection specimen from the case illustrated in 26-*A*. The relatively radiolucent osteoid-osteoma nidus is shown intact in its setting of thickened cortex.

*D*, Roentgenograph (enlarged) of a slice of the resection specimen from the case illustrated in 26-*B*. The relatively radiopaque osteoid-osteoma nidus is shown intact in its setting of thickened cortex.

*E*, Roentgenograph of an osteoid-osteoma located in a femoral condyle, beneath the articular cartilage. The patient, a woman 49 years of age, had pain in the knee for 2 years, and the condition remained undiagnosed for most of that time. An osteoid-osteoma in this location might be misinterpreted as representing an osteochondritis dissecans body.

*F*, Roentgenograph of an osteoid-osteoma in a terminal phalanx. The nidus is radiopaque and might be misinterpreted as an "annular sequestrum." The patient was a boy 10 years of age. He gave a history of pain in the affected phalanx of 3 months' standing.

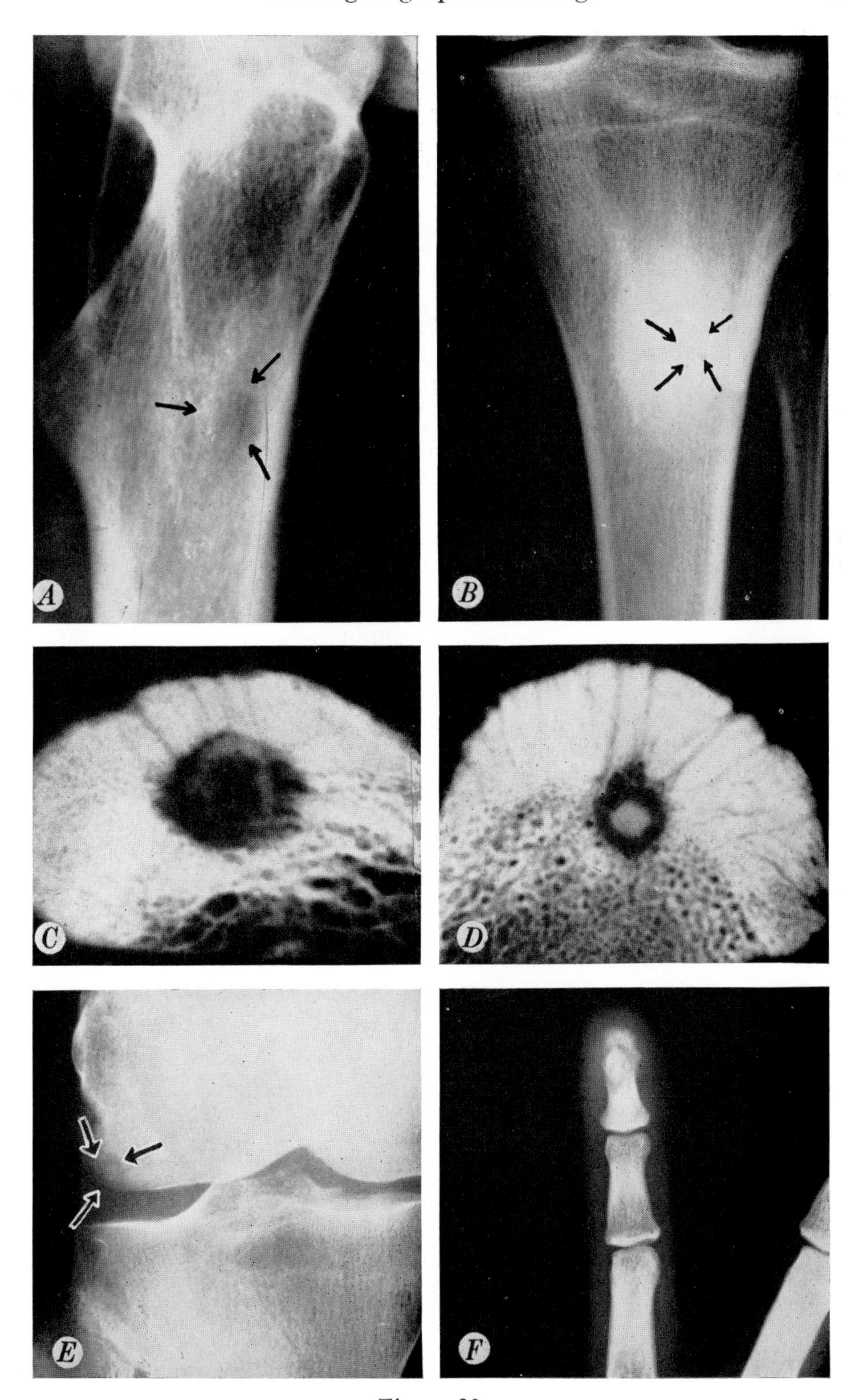


*Figure 26*

clinically the former lesion is asymptomatic. In this connection, the writer has even seen a case, probably unique, in which an osteoid-osteoma was developing within an enostosis, but in that case the clinical complaints were those appropriate to osteoid-osteoma. Furthermore, a solitary bone abscess occasionally raises the problem of differential diagnosis between it and osteoid-osteoma. For further details on these problems, see Differential Diagnosis, page 104.

## PATHOLOGIC FINDINGS

That an osteoid-osteoma may be located completely within the cortex, abut on the inner surface of the cortex, or even lie in the spongiosa at some distance from the cortex has already been indicated. In its greatest diameter, the nidus is usually between 0.5 and 2.0 cm., and, as noted, is most likely to be about 1.0 cm. It is very often more or less oval in shape if within the cortex, and globular if in the spongiosa or straddling the spongiosa and cortex. When observed intact in its setting, it stands out clearly as a sharply delimited core from the surrounding tissue, even though the latter is also modified. Its color and consistency vary from case to case and apparently reflect the stage of evolution of the lesion. As a rule, the core-like nidus is of a granular, gritty consistency, and reddish brown throughout, or reddish brown with whitish or yellowish mottling. The roentgenographic shadow cast by a nidus of this character is usually radiolucent. On the other hand, especially if located in the cortex, the nidus sometimes appears as a rather reddish white, firm or even compact osseous core delimited from the neighboring bone by a narrow, congested ring-like zone. Such a nidus usually shows up roentgenographically as a relatively radiopaque core.

On microscopic examination, a granular, gritty osteoid-osteoma nidus is found to consist, in varying proportions, of osteoid tissue and trabeculæ of newly formed osseous tissue, set in a substratum of highly vascularized osteogenic connective tissue. An individual lesion or part of a lesion may show the osteoid tissue in broad sheets, or in the form of trabeculæ undergoing calcification and consequently osseous transformation. Or, instead, one may note that delicate trabeculæ of newly formed osseous tissue pervade the lesion and predominate over the osteoid. The stromal tissue is, as noted, highly vascular. In accord with the active osteogenesis that is going on in the lesion, some osteoclasts are to be observed. In areas where hemorrhage has occurred, these may even be present as small clumps of rather small multinuclear giant cells. (See Fig. 27.)

***Figure 27***

*A*, Photograph of an osteoid-osteoma nidus in its bed. The lesion was removed from a tibia of a boy 18 years of age, and the nidus stood out as a relatively radiolucent area in a setting of thickened cortex and spongiosa. Grossly, the nidus appeared as a brownish globule of friable but gritty tissue. The histologic pattern is shown in *C* and *E*.

*B*, Photomicrograph of an osteoid-osteoma nidus, part of which is still imbedded in thickened cortex. The lesion was removed from the femur of a boy 12 years of age, and grossly the nidus appeared as a dark red, gritty, friable tissue mass.

C, Photomicrograph (× 10) showing the general histologic pattern of part of the osteoid-osteoma nidus of *A* in its setting of cortex.

*D*, Photomicrograph (× 10) showing the general histologic pattern of part of the osteoid-osteoma nidus of *B* in its setting of cortex.

*E*, Photomicrograph (× 250) made from the nidus shown in *C*. Note the evidence of active osteogenesis. A nidus such as this, removed from its setting and considered apart from the clinical and roentgenographic aspects of the case, might present a diagnostic problem.

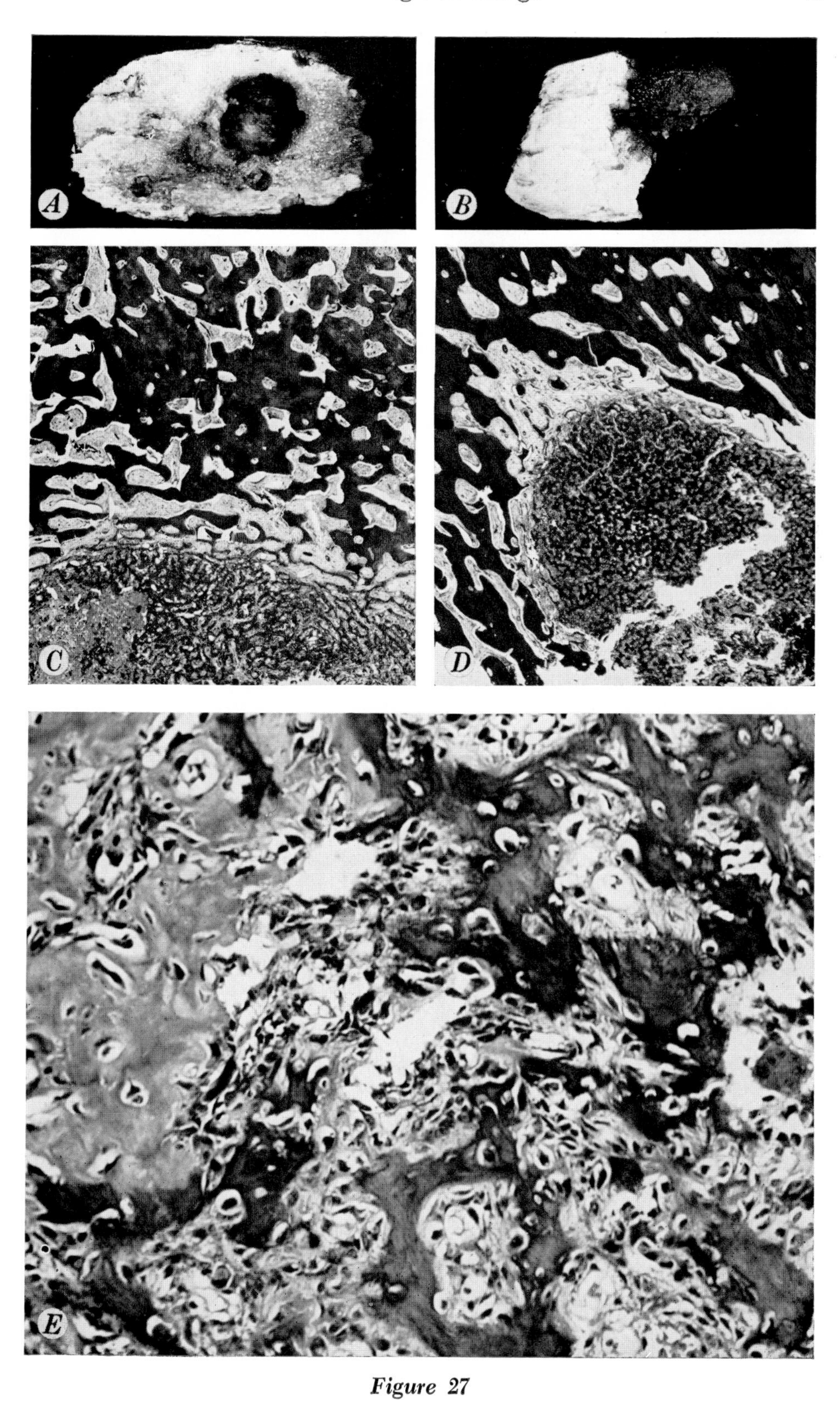


*Figure 27*

One familiar with the histopathology of an osteoid-osteoma nidus such as has been described above is not likely to mistake the lesion for anything else. This is true particularly if the nidus is examined intact in its setting—that is, if it and some of the surrounding bone bed are studied in the same section. However, one unfamiliar with the histopathology of the condition may have difficulties in arriving at the correct diagnosis. These difficulties are enhanced if the nidus has been removed from its setting, so that one can no longer be aided by its relation to the surrounding bone. Indeed, under these circumstances, and because of the presence of active osteogenesis and swollen osteoblasts, one may occasionally be led into the error of mistaking the tissue composing such an osteoid-osteoma nidus for tissue coming from an osteogenic sarcoma. The likelihood of this error is, of course, reduced when one considers the histopathologic picture in question in the light of the total (clinical and roentgenographic) picture of the case.

On the other hand, the histopathology of an osteoid-osteoma nidus appearing as a firm osseous core is not likely to be misconstrued as representing an osteogenic sarcoma. Such a nidus is usually composed of closely set trabeculæ of highly atypical new bone on residual fragments of the original bone. The intertrabecular spaces in such a core contain numerous dilated blood channels. The walls of the trabeculæ are likely to be lined by osteoblasts. Some osteoclasts in Howship's lacunæ may also be seen, reflecting the reconstruction which is going on during the evolution of the lesion.

Between a nidus which is firm and rather compact, and one which is gritty and granular, there are nidi representing various intermediary appearances. However, it must be pointed out that the histologic details of individual osteoid-osteoma nidi cannot be rigidly correlated with the clinical duration of the complaints. Nevertheless, there does seem to be some parallelism in the sense that the more granular and friable nidi tend to be those from cases of longer clinical standing. (See Fig. 28.)

In any case, the osteoid-osteoma nidus comes to be clearly set off from the surrounding bone. In the junctional area, in favorable sections, one may note many prominent arterioles. These may even sometimes be found clumped in one area, as though that point constituted a hilus for the entrance of the blood supply into the nidus. Quite possibly, it is the rather large blood supply confined to a small area contained within a rigid wall that accounts for the pain which is so conspicuous a feature of osteoid-osteoma. One often thinks of this pain, disproportionate to the size of the lesion, as reminiscent of that associated with a glomus tumor. However, histologic studies have failed to reveal any abnormal neurogenic tissue or glomus cell hypertrophies about the blood vessels as a possible explanation for the pain.

***Figure 28***

*A*, Photograph of a slice from a resected specimen in which the nidus presented grossly as a firm, compact core. The nidus is situated on the inner side of the cortex. The patient was a girl 10 years of age, and the lesion was in a tibia. The nidus could not be visualized roentgenographically because there was not enough contrast between it and the overlying thickened cortex. (See *B*.)

*B*, Roentgenograph (enlarged) of the specimen slice pictured in *A*. Note the radiopaque shadow cast by the nidus.

*C*, Photomicrograph (× 10) showing the topographic pattern of the compact nidus standing out clearly in contrast to the surrounding cortical bone.

*D*, Photomicrograph (× 250) showing the cytologic details of the nidus pictured in *C*. Note the closely set trabeculæ of atypical new bone on residual fragments of original bone.

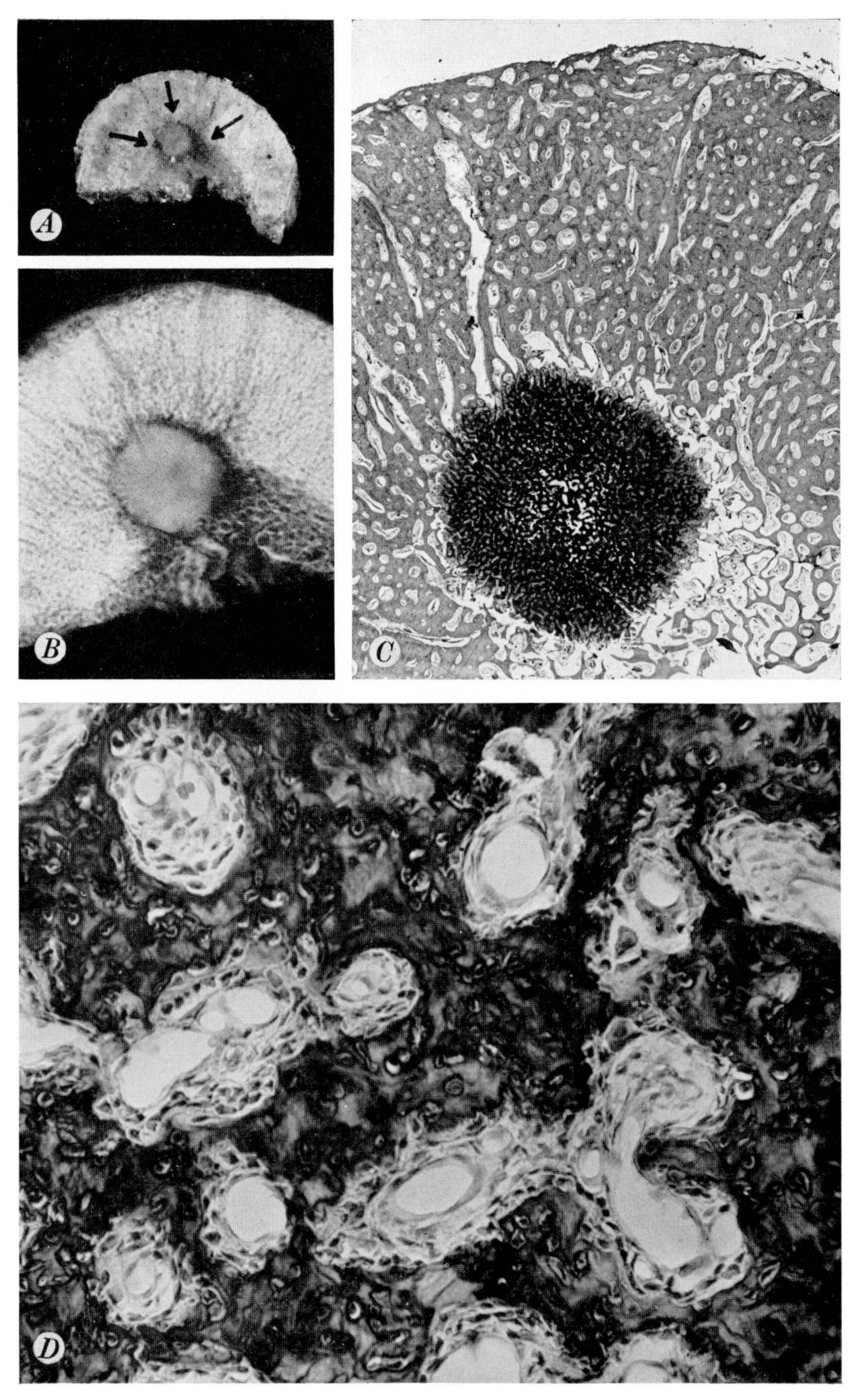

***Figure 28***

In regard to the area of perinidal reactive response, it is to be noted that, if the nidus has developed in the spongiosa, the sclerotic osseous tissue surrounding it is composed of thick and irregular bony trabeculæ, interspersed with a rather fibrillar marrow. If the nidus has developed in relation to the cortex, the thickened cortical area is usually found to be composed of two layers. These are a layer of more or less transformed original cortex, and, on the surface of the latter, a layer of compacted, newly apposed periosteal bone.

**Nature and Genesis.**—It is now generally accepted that osteoid-osteoma of bone is a lesion *sui generis*. That the lesion does not have an inflammatory basis is now also generally acknowledged; nor can it be held that the lesion represents a peculiar healing or reparative form of some familiar lesion, or that it originates from an embryonic rest. Altogether, then, the writer has been led, both by the processes of elimination and by consideration of the anatomic characteristics of the lesion itself, to the conclusion that it should be interpreted as a neoformation, and specifically as a peculiar benign tumor-like lesion of bone.

However, while interpreting the lesion as a neoformation, the writer appreciates that it has certain features which may be held to be inconsistent with this interpretation. First among these are the small size of the nidus and its seemingly self-limited nature, irrespective of its duration. Then there is the fact that it tends to incite the formation of a perifocal zone of bone sclerosis or thickening, sometimes of considerable magnitude, especially when the nidus has developed in relation to the shaft cortex of a long bone. The fact, however, that microscopically the osteoid-osteoma nidus, when well evolved, does have the characteristics of a neoformation seems to outweigh in importance these apparently inconsistent or controverting features. The latter are frankly puzzling and require explanation, but they only emphasize the peculiarity of the condition as a whole.

Very puzzling, also, are certain features of the pathology of the lesion itself, and especially the problem of interpreting the evolutionary sequence of the pathologic patterns seen in the various specimens. The writer feels that this problem is by no means settled as yet, and what is being said about it must be regarded as tentative. The genesis of the nidus is, of course, the same whether the lesion is developing in relation to a spongy bone area or in relation to bone cortex. However, it is much easier to line up what seems to be a series of developmental stages for lesions oriented to cortex.

At a site where an osteoid-osteoma nidus has started to evolve, the osseous tissue comes to stand out from the surrounding bone. The contrast is created by the

***Figure 29***

*A*, Roentgenograph of a fibula of a girl 21 years of age, showing a small area of radiolucency in the cortex, representing an intracortical abscess. Though the roentgenograph might suggest that one was dealing with an osteoid-osteoma, neither the clinical history nor the clinical findings could support this diagnosis.

*B*, Photomicrograph (× 10) showing, in the cortex of the fibula, the abscess which is extending to the surface of the bone and which is lined by a thick connective-tissue membrane found to be heavily infiltrated by leukocytes.

*C*, Roentgenograph of the tibia of a woman 42 years of age, who suffered from an intracortical bone abscess. From the *x*-ray picture and from the clinical findings, one might have suspected an osteoid-osteoma, but the clinical history was not that characteristic of the latter lesion.

*D*, Photomicrograph (× 8) showing a full cross section of the tibial abscess, which is located in the interior of the original cortex. The thickening of the cortex is due to periosteal new bone apposition.

*E*, Photomicrograph (× 250) showing the abscess wall of *D*, which is heavily infiltrated with polymorphonuclear leukocytes.

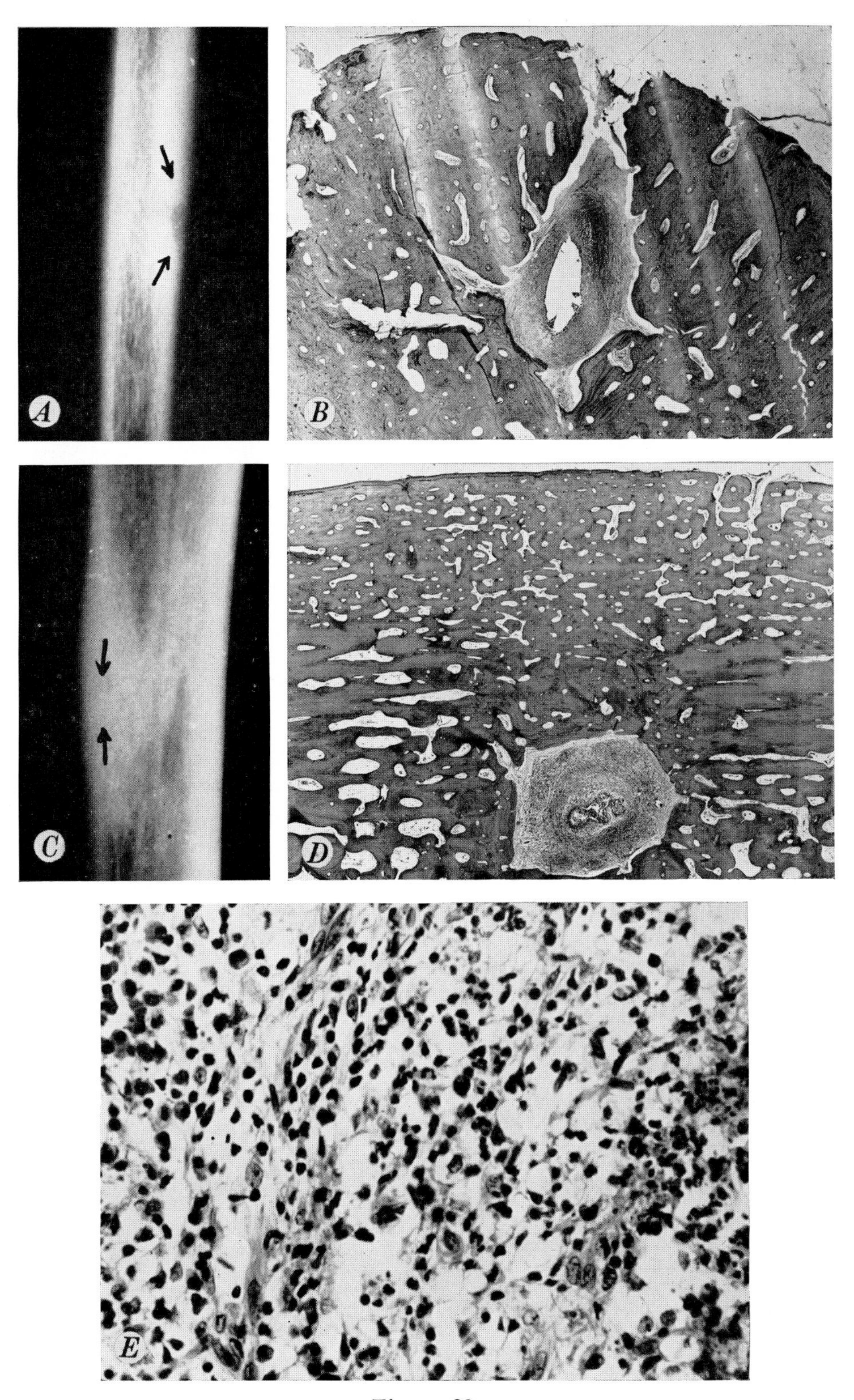


*Figure* 29

effects of increased vascularization and active reconstruction at the site. In consequence of this, the original osseous tissue in the area comes to be resorbed and simultaneously replaced by new bone laid down in a process of creeping replacement. The new bone presents a rather atypical histologic pattern, and its deposition is most striking around blood vessels. Sooner or later, the periosteum overlying the area where the nidus is forming becomes stimulated to deposit new bone on the outer surface of the cortex.

Eventually, the area under reconstruction becomes completely converted into a nidus of closely compacted trabeculæ of highly atypical osseous tissue. Between these trabeculæ there are numerous thin-walled blood channels set in a sparse stroma of osteogenic connective tissue.

From comparative study of many lesions, one gathers that if an osteoid-osteoma nidus presenting such a histologic pattern is not removed and thus has a chance to evolve further, the nidal area continues to undergo reconstruction. Its trabeculæ of highly atypical bone are reworked and resorbed, and a much more productive nidus comes into being. In the foreground of such a nidus, we now have a substratum of very vascular osteogenic connective tissue in which osteoid and osseous tissue in varying proportions are being laid down.

In fact, if one took an osteoid-osteoma nidus in this advanced stage of evolution out of its setting, it might, as already noted, quite reasonably be misinterpreted, in some cases, as a tumor field from an osteogenic sarcoma. The neoplastic aura is given it by the evidence of active osteogenesis within it. In fact, it is this aura of neoformation that the writer had in mind when he gave the lesion the name of "osteoid-osteoma" in spite of its consistent smallness and apparently self-limited nature.

## DIFFERENTIAL DIAGNOSIS

**Solitary Enostosis.**—Occasionally, a solitary enostosis (also called "bone fleck" or "medullary osteoma") may raise the problem of differential diagnosis from osteoid-osteoma. For instance, a patient may have pain localized to some bone or joint area in which roentgenographic examination reveals a roundish focus of radiopacity. The question to be resolved then is whether the radiopacity observed represents a radiopaque osteoid-osteoma nidus or a solitary enostosis. In the latter case, the patient's clinical complaints are not to be related to the roentgenographic findings at all, since a solitary enostosis is asymptomatic. The absence of sclerosis or thickening of the bone about the radiopaque focus favors its representing an enostosis rather than an osteoid-osteoma. The absence of point tenderness over the lesional area also favors the diagnosis of enostosis. Anatomically, an enostosis consists of a nest of compacted trabeculæ of mature lamellar bone, thus bearing no resemblance to an osteoid-osteoma nidus.

This problem of differential diagnosis comes up most often in relation to the hip joint area. It is rather common to encounter a solitary enostosis in the neck of a femur. It is also very common to have patients complain of persistent pain in the hip area for which no plausible explanation is readily available. When one is dealing with so crucial an area as the hip, if one has the least suspicion that the lesion might be merely an enostosis, the evidence in favor of osteoid-osteoma should be overwhelming before surgical intervention is undertaken against it.

**Bone Abscess.**—A small bone abscess, particularly an intracortical bone abscess, may raise the problem of differential diagnosis between that lesion and osteoid-osteoma. The problem arises mainly on a roentgenographic basis. Specifically, in such a case, a part of the bone cortex is found thickened, and there may be a small focus of radiolucency within the thickened area. Clinically, however, most examples of cortical bone abscess bear little resemblance to osteoid-osteoma. On the clinical side, however, it should be noted, in the first place, that the pain pattern is different from that of osteoid-osteoma. Also, the past history may indicate that there was some local heat and swelling. Indeed, the clinical features of the case, alone, can nearly always solve the diagnostic problem. If tissue becomes available from the lesional area, it is soon evident that there is no anatomic resemblance whatever between an intracortical bone abscess and an intracortical osteoid-osteoma. The radiolucent area observed in the *x*-ray picture in a case of cortical bone abscess is found to represent a tiny cavity in the cortex, lined by an inflammatory membrane, heavily permeated by leukocytes and/or lymphocytes. (See Fig. 29.)

## TREATMENT

Surgical removal of the lesion brings dramatically prompt and also lasting relief from the complaints. The nidus and some of the neighboring bone may be removed by curettement, but unless this is thorough the complaints will reappear. If the lesion is resected intact in its setting of surrounding bone, this danger will be avoided. In any case, especially if the lesion is in a site difficult to approach surgically, experience has shown that it is best to conduct the intervention under *x*-ray control.

Since an osteoid-osteoma is always a small lesion of limited growth propensity, one may ask what would ultimately happen to the lesion if no surgical intervention were done. We know at least that it persists and continues to cause clinical complaints for years if left to itself. Nevertheless, it is conceivable that, after many years, an osteoid-osteoma might undergo spontaneous clinical arrest or even anatomic involution. However, in view of the persistence and increasingly annoying character of the clinical complaints, and the ready accessibility of the lesion, in most cases, for surgical removal, it is not likely that much information will be collected on this point.

Radiation therapy has not often been tried for osteoid-osteoma. What little experience there is has indicated that this treatment is not effective in destroying the disease focus and permanently relieving the patient of the clinical complaints.

The question of the possibility of recurrence of an osteoid-osteoma occasionally arises. As already noted, if the lesion is not completely eradicated in the course of surgical intervention against it, the clinical complaints are either not relieved or relieved only temporarily. In the latter case, the interval before they return may be as long as a year or so. This sequence of events does not, of course, represent an actual recurrence, but rather a mere recrudescence of the lesion. The writer has, however, been able to follow one case which does seem to present a true recurrence. In that case, an osteoid-osteoma was removed from the tibia of a girl of 3 who then remained free of complaints for 13 years. After this long interval, she developed another osteoid-osteoma in precisely the same location in the tibia, and the recurrent lesion was likewise removed, with the usual prompt relief from pain.

## REFERENCES


Bado, J. L., and Larghero Ybarz, P.: A propósito del osteoma-osteoide de Jaffe; comentario de dos observaciones personales, Rev. brasil. de orthop. e traumatol., *2*, 139, 1941.

Barnes, R.: Osteoid Osteoma, J. Roy. Coll. Surgeons, Edinburgh, *2*, 144, 1956.

Dockerty, M. B., Ghormley, R. K., and Jackson, A. E.: Osteoid Osteoma, Ann. Surg., *133*, 77, 1951.

Domenici, A.: Sull'osteoma-osteoide, Tumori, *37*, 539, 1951.

Foss, E. L., Dockerty, M. B., and Good, C. A.: Osteoid Osteoma of the Mandible, Cancer, *8*, 592, 1955.

Goidanich, I. F., and Zanasi, R.: Osteoma osteoide ed osteomielite sclerosante: due entità cliniche definite e distinte, Chir. d. org. di movimento, *43*, 427, 1956.

Goldenberg, R. R.: Osteoid-Osteoma, J. M. Soc. New Jersey, *45*, 104, 1948.

Golding, J. S. R.: The Natural History of Osteoid Osteoma, J. Bone & Joint Surg., *36*-B, 218, 1954.
Gomes, M. de A.: Osteoma ostéoide, Gaz. méd. port., *2*, 511, 1949.
Gschnitzer, F., and De Gennaro, P. F.: Das Osteoid-Osteom. Klinik, Pathomorphologie und Gedanken zur Ätiologie, Ztschr. f. Orthop., *86*, 1, 1955.
Hamilton, J. F.: Osteoid Osteoma, Surg., Gynec. & Obst., *81*, 465, 1945.
Jaffe, H. L., and Lichtenstein, L.: Osteoid-Osteoma: Further Experience with this Benign Tumor of Bone, J. Bone & Joint Surg., *22*, 645, 1940.
Jaffe, H. L.: Osteoid-Osteoma of Bone, Radiology, *45*, 319, 1945.
———: Osteoid-Osteoma, Proc. Roy. Soc. Med., *46*, 1007, 1953. (Section of Orthopaedics, p. 29.)
———: "Osteoid-Osteoma": A Benign Osteoblastic Tumor Composed of Osteoid and Atypical Bone, Arch. Surg., *31*, 709, 1935.
Kleinberg, S.: Osteoid-Osteoma, New York State J. Med., *43*, 332, 1943.
Lewis, R. W.: Osteoid-Osteoma, Am. J. Roentgenol., *52*, 70, 1944.
Löfgren, L.: "Osteoid-Osteoma," Acta chir. scandinav., *104*, 383, 1953.
Mayer, L.: The Surgery of Osteoid-Osteoma, Bull. Hosp. Joint Dis., *12*, 174, 1951.
Ponseti, I., and Barta, C. K.: Osteoid Osteoma, J. Bone & Joint Surg., *29*, 767, 1947.
Pritchard, J. E., and McKay, J. W.: Osteoid Osteoma, Canad. M. A. J., *58*, 567, 1948.
Sabanas, A. O., Bickel, W. H., and Moe, J. H.: Natural History of Osteoid Osteoma of the Spine, Am. J. Surg., *91*, 880, 1956.
Schmidt, S.: Ostéome-ostéoide, Rev. orthop., *35*, 427, 1949.
Sherman, M. S.: Osteoid Osteoma, J. Bone & Joint Surg., *29*, 918, 1947.

Chapter

# 8

# Benign Osteoblastoma

THE name *benign osteoblastoma* is being used here for a peculiar, rather vascular, osteoid-and-bone forming benign tumor of bone, characterized cytologically by the abundant presence of osteoblasts. The benign osteoblastoma is a rather uncommon lesion. While it does affect limb bones, it seems to predilect the vertebral column.

Though osteoblasts are consistently prominent in the lesional tissue, there may be a good deal of variety in cytologic detail in other respects. Specifically, there may be a good deal of variety in the amount of osteoid and primitive osseous tissue which has been laid down, and in the intensity of calcification of this tissue. These facts have been a source of difficulty in defining and naming the lesion, and sometimes cause difficulty in distinguishing it from other lesions.

The writer's interest in this tumor dates from 1932, when he and Mayer discussed an instance of it, under the descriptive title of "An Osteoblastic Osteoid Tissue-forming Tumor of a Metacarpal Bone." That report already indicated that the lesion is one which raises problems of nomenclature and differential diagnosis, and altogether is not a simple one to interpret histologically. In respect to histologic differential diagnosis, the benign osteoblastoma may have to be distinguished, in one case or another, from osteoid-osteoma on the one hand and osteogenic sarcoma on the other.

**Nomenclature.**—The literature dealing with the lesion in question is sparse. In recent years, several reports discussing it have appeared under the heading of "osteogenic fibroma of bone." (See Golding and Sissons, and Kirkpatrick and Murray.) However, this name, to which the writer was once resigned, no longer strikes him as the best choice in relation to the lesion. In the first place, the lesion is too poor in well-differentiated fibroblastic connective tissue to justify the use of "fibroma" as part of its name. In the second place, the term "osteogenic fibroma" is likely to introduce confusion with the so-called "ossifying fibroma." The latter name has been used mainly for a lesion which, in most instances, represents fibrous dysplasia localized to a jawbone or some other facial bone (p. 136). Under whatever name, that lesion is clearly different from the one being described in this chapter.

Another name which has been used for the lesion is "giant osteoid-osteoma." (See Dahlin and Johnson.) They chose this name because of the lesion's mimicry of the histologic pattern of osteoid-osteoma, though they recognized that, clinically and roentgenographically, the "giant osteoid-osteoma" was different from the conventional osteoid-osteoma. Certainly it seems undesirable to blur the well-established clinicopathologic entity of osteoid-osteoma by use of the term "giant osteoid-osteoma" for a lesion which, in many aspects, is so different from it.

In advocating the name "benign osteoblastoma" for the lesion in question, the writer has been guided by several considerations. One is that the lesion is a benign one, though histologically, in one case or another, it may be mistaken for an osteogenic sarcoma. At the same time, the name gives appropriate emphasis precisely to the proliferating osteoblasts which are so conspicuous a feature of the lesion's histologic pattern. Finally, the name "benign osteoblastoma" seems not to have been used previously for any already established bone tumor entity.

## CLINICAL CONSIDERATIONS

**Incidence.**—As already indicated, the benign osteoblastoma is not a common lesion. The writer's total experience with it covers 10 cases from his own institution and about the same number from outside sources. As to sex incidence, there is some indication that females may be somewhat predilected. As to age incidence, most of the patients are between 10 and 25 years old, but an occasional one is a young child or a middle-aged adult.

**Localization.**—The most common location is somewhere in the vertebral column, where the lesion may involve part or much of the arch and/or body of a vertebra. On 3 occasions, the writer has observed the lesion in the sacral part of the column, and in one of these cases the tumor was found to be about 7 cm. in its greatest diameter. Next to the vertebral column, the most common location is a short tubular bone of a hand or foot. Occasionally, the lesion is observed in some other bone site, as, for instance, a long tubular bone, a rib, a scapula, or an innominate bone.

**Clinical Complaints and Findings.**—In detail, these vary, of course, with the location of the lesion. When the latter is in some part of the vertebral column, the complaints (usually of some months' standing) of pain or aching somewhere in the back usually become overshadowed by neurological difficulties. Specifically, a lesion localized to some part of a thoracic vertebra is very likely to give rise to weakness of the lower limbs, paresthesias, or even paraplegia, due to pressure upon the spinal cord. Complaints from a lesion in some part of a lumbar vertebra are

***Figure 30***

*A*, Roentgenograph showing a benign osteoblastoma in the spinous process of the third cervical vertebra of a boy 16 years of age. The affected bone part is very much expanded, appears somewhat trabeculated, and presents also some mottled radiopacity. When the lesional area was entered surgically, it was found completely filled with deep red, friable and somewhat gritty tissue.

*B*, Roentgenograph of a benign osteoblastoma which has caused extensive lytic destruction and expansion of the sacrum of a boy 15 years of age. After a biopsy done to establish the nature of the lesion, *x*-ray therapy was given. In the course of about 6 months, the lesional area became heavily calcified (see Fig. 33-*B*), and the clinical complaints subsided.

*C*, Roentgenograph showing a benign osteoblastoma in the second metacarpal bone of a girl 12 years of age. The lesional area shows a good deal of radiopacity. This is the result of spontaneous heavy calcification of the tumor osteoid (see Fig. 33-*A*), and not a response to radiation therapy. In the course of about $2\frac{1}{2}$ years, the lesion in this case developed into a very large tumor mass and destroyed practically the entire metacarpal bone. Despite the ominous clinical and gross pathologic appearance of the lesion (which suggested an osteogenic sarcoma), there was no evidence of recurrence in the course of a 10-year follow-up after mere resection of the tumorously involved metacarpal bone. (The details relating to this case can be found in the paper by Jaffe and Mayer.)

*D*, Roentgenograph of a benign osteoblastoma involving the fourth metacarpal bone in the case of a man 48 years of age. The lesional area is expanded, somewhat trabeculated and, on the whole, radiolucent. The resected metacarpal bone showed that the affected area was occupied by a dark red, friable, and somewhat granular tissue which, on histologic examination, was found to be composed practically throughout of poorly calcified osteoid, set in a very vascular substratum.

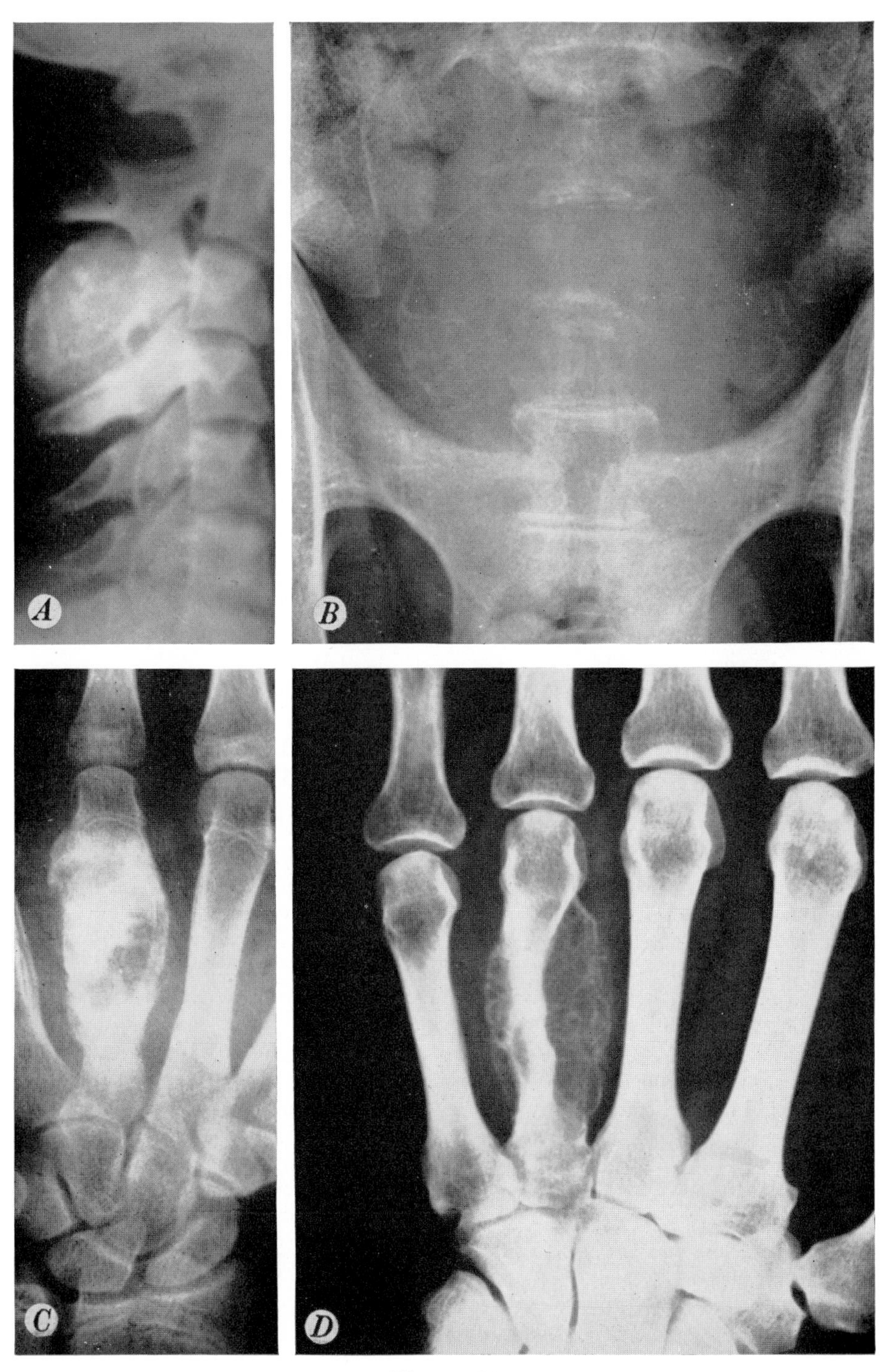


*Figure 30*

likely to be dominated eventually by pains radiating down the legs, associated with a good deal of spasm of the lumbar part of the column. Complaints from a lesion in the sacrum, too, are likely to become dominated by the effects of pressure on the local nerves.

Complaints from a lesion in a long or short tubular bone, which likewise are usually of only a few months' standing, consist mainly of some dull, aching pain. Usually, the affected bone part becomes visibly enlarged through the presence of a palpable tumor mass. Local tenderness is usually not severe. If the bone affected is involved in weight bearing, the patient may limp.

## ROENTGENOGRAPHIC AND PATHOLOGIC FINDINGS

**Roentgenographic Findings.**—There is nothing distinctive about the roentgenographic picture of a benign osteoblastoma. The picture may vary from case to case, in accordance not only with the size of the lesion but with the extent to which the lesional tissue is calcified. A small lesion may be no more than 2 cm. in its greatest dimension, while a large one may measure as much as 7 to 10 cm. A lesion in which the tumor tissue is highly vascular and relatively poorly calcified tends on the whole to cast a relatively radiolucent shadow. A lesion in which some parts of the tumor tissue are heavily calcified will show radiopacity of the corresponding areas. In any case, the contour of the bone in the affected area is likely to be expanded. In connection with involvement of tubular bones, the bone abutting on the lesion sometimes shows reactive thickening. In one case studied by the writer, the lesion was in the upper end of a tibia, and a pathologic fracture developed at its site. (See Fig. 30.)

**Gross Pathology.**—The writer has had the opportunity of examining 5 benign osteoblastomas intact in their settings. None of these lesions came from the vertebral column, since, from that area, it is usually only curettings that are obtainable. One of the resection specimens was from a fibula, another from a rib, and still another from a scapula, and the two other specimens were affected metacarpal bones. The smallest of the 5 lesions was the one in the fibula, and this lesion measured 2 × 1.5 × 1.4 cm. From its gross appearance and location, it might have passed as an osteoid-osteoma. However, it was much larger than an osteoid-osteoma usually is. Furthermore, it had perforated the cortex at one point, which an osteoid-osteoma starting in the medullary cavity of a bone would almost certainly not have done. The largest of the completely resected lesions studied was in a metacarpal bone, it being the one previously reported by the writer and Mayer. This lesion, which had practically destroyed the entire bone, was a tumor mass measuring 10 × 6.5 × 6 cm., and its gross appearance strongly suggested a malignant tumor, and specifically an osteogenic sarcoma.

The lesional tissue has, on the whole, a gritty consistency. Here and there, one or another area may have a firmer, sclerotic texture, in accordance with heavy

***Figure 31***

*A*, Photograph of part of a resected scapula showing a benign osteoblastoma intact in its setting. The lesional area measured about 4 cm. in length and 3 cm. across. The patient was a girl 10 years of age who had been complaining, for about 3 months, of pain and swelling in the region of the scapula. The roentgenograph revealed the lesional area as a circumscribed focus of lytic destruction.

*B*, Photomicrograph (× 125) showing the histologic pattern presented by many of the tissue areas of the lesion shown in *A*. Note the numerous osteoblasts, agglomerated into nests and sheets and interspersed with intercellular matrix,

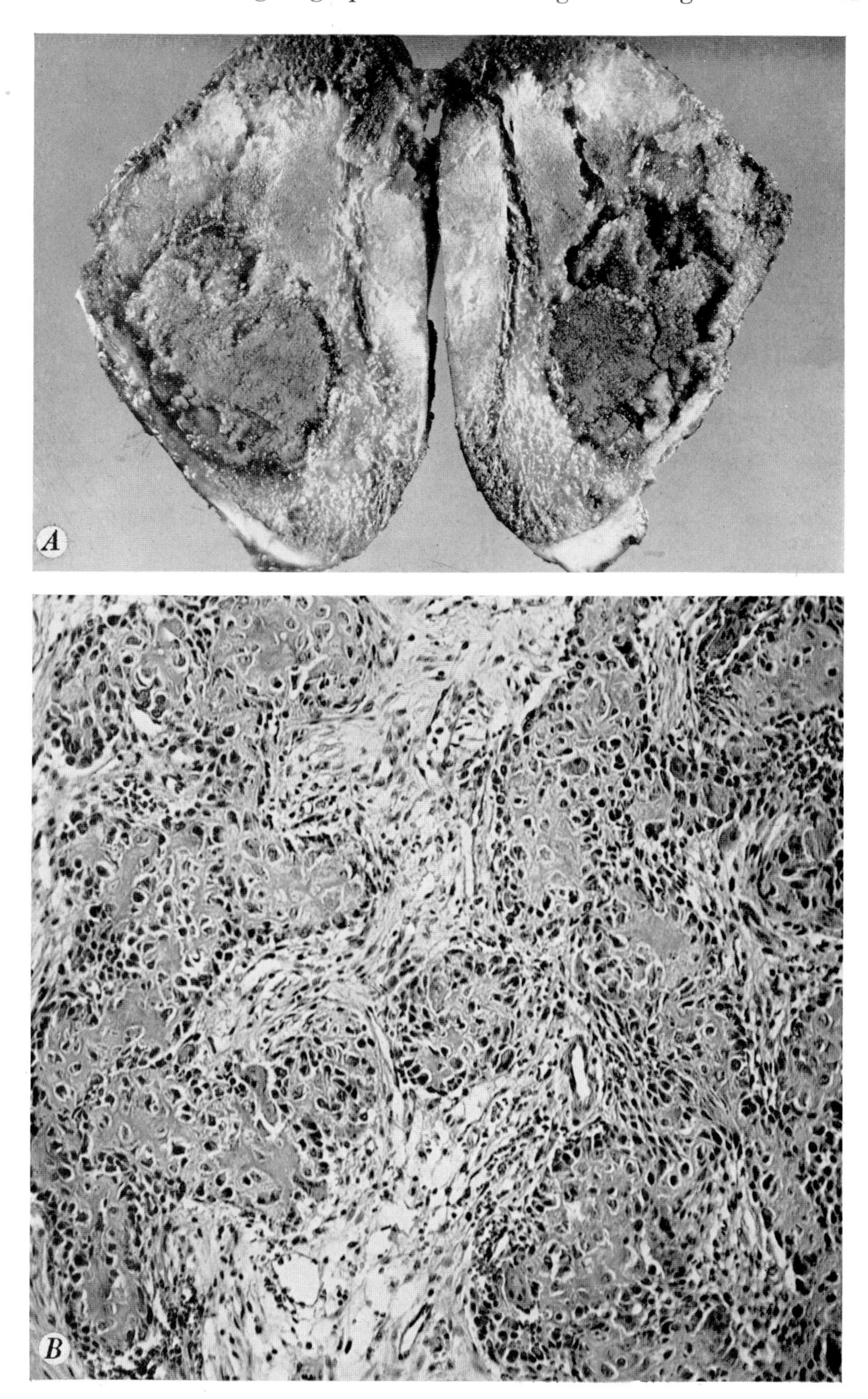


*Figure 31*

calcification of the lesional tissue in that area. The color of the tumor tissue is likely to be purplish red or reddish brown or even pinkish, reflecting its great vascularity. A lesion which has attained a large size may also show some small areas of softening and cystification. (See Fig. 31-*A*.)

**Microscopic Pathology.**—The variations in histologic detail between one lesion and another and between various parts of the same lesion reflect variations in the evolutionary sequences within the lesion. Always, the basic tissue consists of a loosely fibrillar and highly vascular matrix or substratum rich in osteoblasts.

As to the variations, in some lesions or parts of lesions, agglomerated nests, cords, or sheets of osteoblasts are a very conspicuous feature of the tissue pattern. In other areas of the same lesion, one can note that intercellular material has appeared between these proliferated masses of osteoblasts, so that osteoid trabeculæ have become delineated. About the peripheries of these trabeculæ, a fair number of small osteoclasts are also to be seen. In an area showing further progression of the histologic changes, one can note that the osteoid trabeculæ, having become calcified, have been transformed into trabeculæ of primitive osseous tissue. In many places, one may also note that this tissue has been undergoing osteoclastic resorption in the process of reconstruction into somewhat more mature osseous tissue. Nevertheless, one can still note, everywhere, numerous osteoblasts bordering upon the thin-walled blood vessels and apposed upon the osseous trabeculæ in the process of reconstruction.

In other lesions or lesional areas, the osteoblasts in the vascular osteoblastogenic substratum proceed to lay down trabeculæ of osteoid without first becoming hypertrophied and agglomerated into nests or cords. These osteoid trabeculæ are lined by osteoblasts, but also show, here and there, osteoclasts, which are subjecting them to resorption. In still other lesions or lesional areas, these osteoid trabeculæ can be seen to have fused into wide sheets which often appear heavily calcified. The heavily calcified sheets and plaques of osteoid are rather poor in cells. However, they form a matrix which, in some areas, may eventually show conversion into relatively mature osseous tissue.

In any event, what is characteristic of the benign osteoblastoma histologically is the fact that the lesional tissue is exceedingly rich in osteoblasts. Through the mediacy of the osteoblasts, large amounts of osteoid tissue are formed, and this tissue eventually becomes converted into primitive bone, and/or becomes heavily calcified in some places. (See Figs. 31-*A*, 32 and 33-*A*.)

## DIFFERENTIAL DIAGNOSIS

**Osteoid-osteoma.**—There can be no doubt that the histologic tissue pattern of the benign osteoblastoma bears a certain similarity to that of the osteoid-osteoma.

### *Figure 32*

*A*, Photomicrograph (× 125) showing the histologic pattern presented by still other tissue fields of the lesion shown in Figure 31-*A*. Note, on the left, the collections of hypertrophied osteoblasts, and, on the right, the trabeculæ of primitive osseous tissue which have been formed in consequence of the development and calcification of intercellular matrix between the osteoblasts.

*B*, Photomicrograph (× 125) from another benign osteoblastoma presenting a histologic pattern somewhat different from the one illustrated in *A*. Note the irregular, delicate trabeculæ of osteoid which, in some places, are being calcified. A number of small multinuclear cells (osteoclasts) are to be observed. Note again the absence of mature fibroblastic stroma in the lesional tissue. A lesion in which this histologic pattern is the dominant one is likely to appear quite radiolucent in the *x*-ray picture.

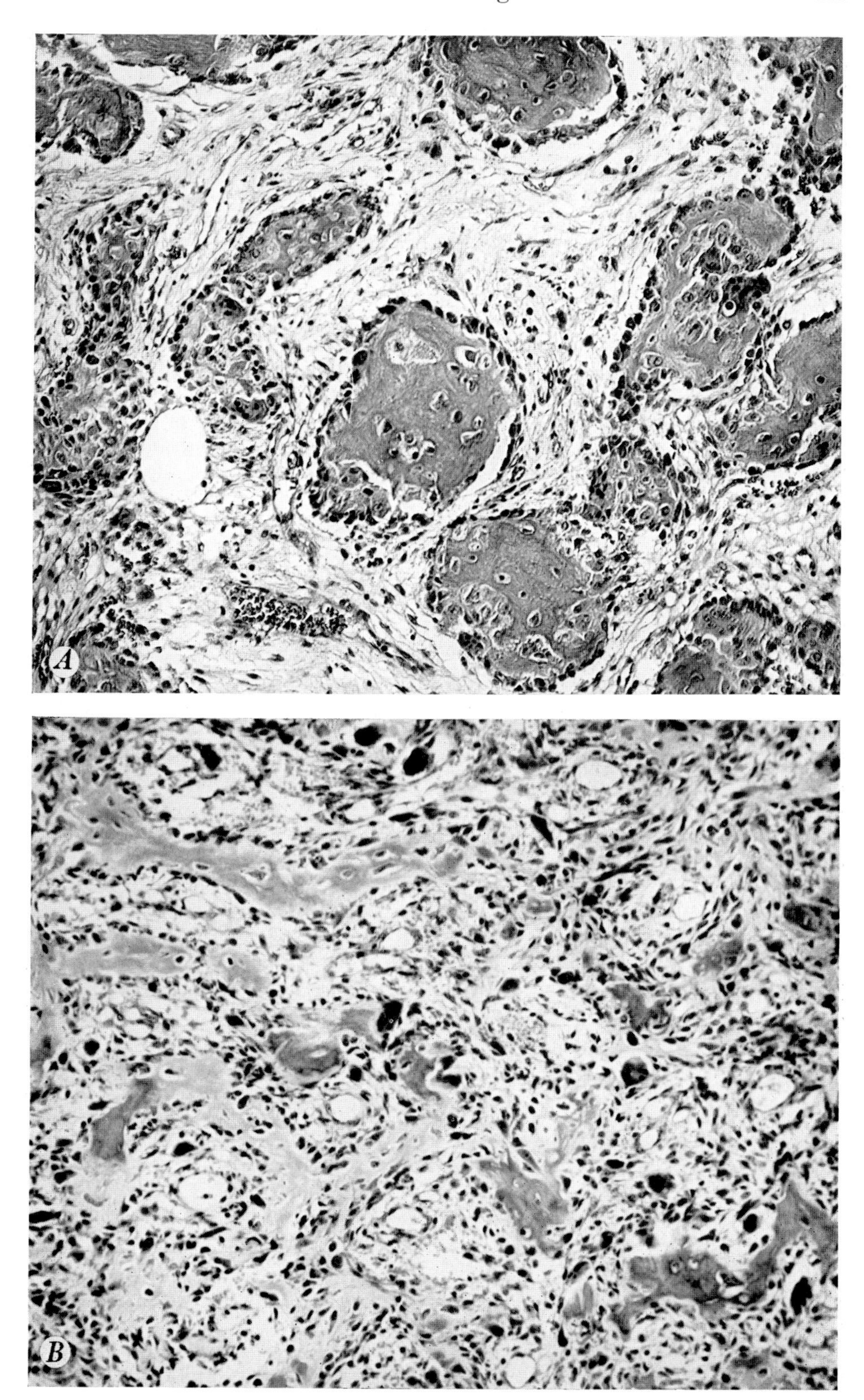


*Figure 32*

Indeed, it is solely on this histologic basis that Dahlin and Johnson decided to designate as "giant osteoid-osteoma" the lesion denoted in the present chapter as "benign osteoblastoma." However, they stressed the idea that the so-called "giant osteoid-osteoma" should be kept apart from the clinical entity represented by the *conventional* osteoid-osteoma. Nevertheless, it appears to the writer that, to prevent any possible confusion, the name of "giant osteoid-osteoma" had better be avoided altogether. (See Nomenclature, p. 107.)

Though the histologic tissue patterns of benign osteoblastoma and conventional osteoid-osteoma mimic each other in a general way, the number of osteoblasts is much greater in the former. On the clinical side, the benign osteoblastoma does not tend to produce the pain pattern so characteristic of osteoid-osteoma. Also, the benign osteoblastoma is consistently a larger lesion than the osteoid-osteoma. Indeed, the latter does not tend to exceed 1 cm. in its greatest diameter, no matter how long it may have been present. On the other hand, the benign osteoblastoma is a lesion which characteristically increases in size, sometimes quite rapidly, and may become a relatively large lesion within a period of several months. Furthermore, unlike the conventional osteoid-osteoma, which merely provokes the regional bone to reactive thickening, the enlarging benign osteoblastoma causes a good deal of local bone destruction and may even bulge out the contour of the affected bone part.

Nevertheless, one might contend, on the basis of certain similarities in the histologic appearance of the lesional tissue, that the benign osteoblastoma represents merely a conventional osteoid-osteoma which has, as it were, "run amuck." To sustain this conception, however, one would have to find cases in which, for 6 months or a year or so, the clinical history and roentgenographic appearance of the lesion had conformed to those of an osteoid-osteoma. However, this has not happened in any of the cases of benign osteoblastoma which we have studied, or in any relevant cases reported in the literature. This problem of differential diagnosis between benign osteoblastoma and osteoid-osteoma brings out again the importance of conceiving the individual bone tumors as clinicopathologic entities. In the delineation of these entities, the clinical facts and the roentgenographic findings are indeed often very important in the diagnostic evaluation of the lesion, and must be considered along with the histologic findings.

**Osteogenic Sarcoma.**—Another diagnostic pitfall in connection with the benign osteoblastoma is the possibility of histologic confusion with osteogenic sarcoma. This may arise in part because of the presence of the great numbers of osteoblasts in the osteoblastic substratum of the lesional tissue. To a greater extent, however, it may be due to the fact that, in some tissue fields, osteogenesis has been proceeding rapidly and large sheets of osteoid have been laid down. However, careful scrutiny of the tissue sections will make it plain that: The stromal cells are not large, plump, sarcomatous connective-tissue cells; mitoses are rare; sarcoma giant cells are absent; tumor cartilage is not being formed anywhere; and the cells enmeshed in the osteoid matrix are all relatively small.

***Figure 33***

*A*, Photomicrograph (× 125) showing the tissue pattern of a benign osteoblastoma in which, on the whole, the osteoid is heavily calcified. Note, on the left, the numerous osteoblasts and individual small, still sparsely calcified trabeculæ of osteoid. Note, on the right, that many of the osteoid trabeculæ have fused into large sheets and are heavily calcified. Lesions or lesional areas in which this histologic pattern dominates cast a radiopaque shadow in the *x*-ray picture.

*B*, Roentgenograph of a benign osteoblastoma in the sacrum (compare with Fig. 30-*B*) which has ossified and become radiopaque within 6 months after *x*-ray treatment.

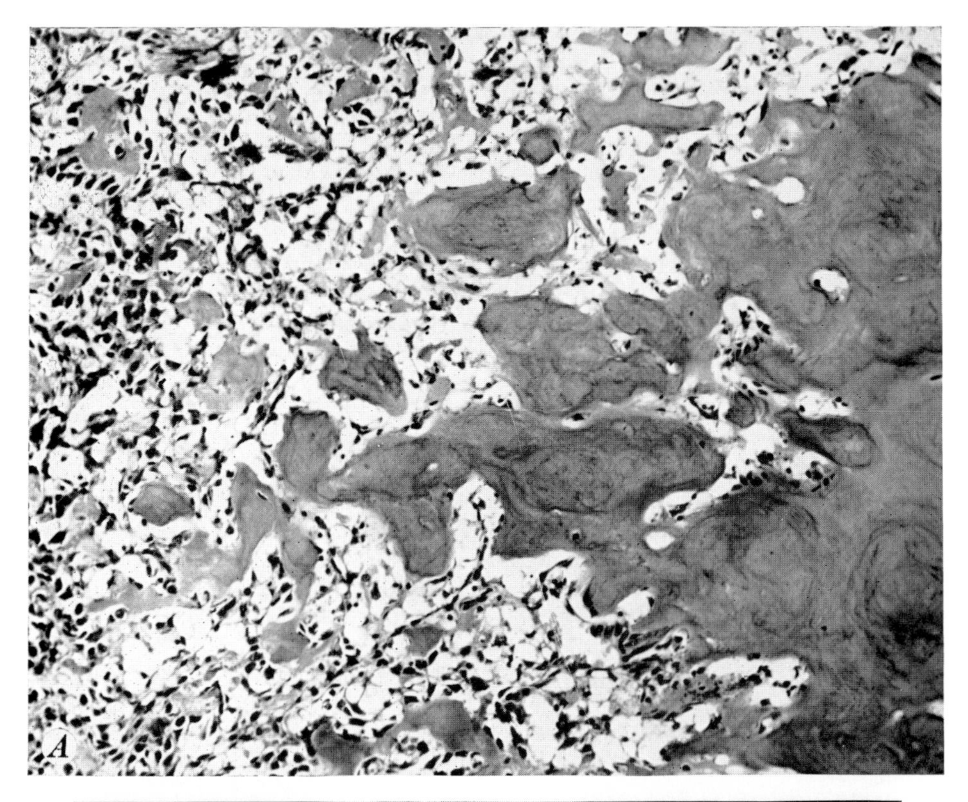


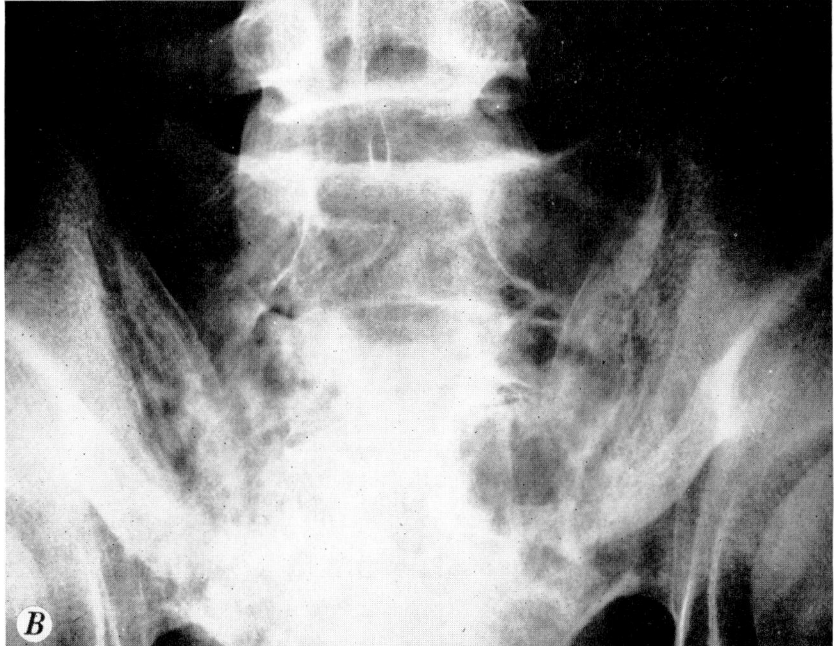


*Figure 33*

Fortunately, in several reported pertinent cases first misjudged as instances of osteogenic sarcoma, the lesion was in the vertebral column, and therefore no radical surgery was carried out. After irradiation undertaken as a palliative measure in these cases, the clinical improvement led to revision of the diagnosis.

**Giant-cell Tumor.**—In view of the clearer understanding of giant-cell tumor (and especially of its histologic appearance) which has been reached in recent years, the likelihood of misinterpretation of a benign osteoblastoma as a giant-cell tumor is no longer great. When it does happen, it occurs because undue diagnostic emphasis is placed on the scattered multinuclear giant cells (osteoclasts) which are regularly present in the benign osteoblastoma. Still, if one goes back to the older literature (see Geschickter and Copeland), one can note that this error was formerly not uncommon. Specifically, one finds references to cases of the so-called "spindle cell variant" of giant-cell tumor, which, to judge from the case histories and histologic descriptions, seem to represent benign osteoblastoma.

## TREATMENT

The treatment of choice for the benign osteoblastoma is excision of the lesional area. This is not technically feasible in all cases, of course, and especially not if the lesion is located in some part of the vertebral column. Even if the lesional area is only partly curetted, however, the lesion can be made to ossify and heal in through the use of moderate doses of *x*-ray therapy (see Fig. 33-*B*).

### REFERENCES

Dahlin, D. C., and Johnson, E. W., Jr.: Giant Osteoid Osteoma, J. Bone & Joint Surg., *36-A*, 559, 1954.

Geschickter, C. F., and Copeland, M. M.: *Tumors of Bone,* 3rd ed., Philadelphia, J. B. Lippincott Co., 1949. (See p. 326 and Fig. 237.)

Golding, J. S. R., and Sissons, H. A.: Osteogenic Fibroma of Bone, J. Bone & Joint Surg., *36-B*, 428, 1954.

Jaffe, H. L.: Benign Osteoblastoma, Bull. Hosp. Joint Dis., *17*, 141, 1956.

Jaffe, H. L., and Mayer, L.: An Osteoblastic Osteoid Tissue-Forming Tumor of a Metacarpal Bone, Arch. Surg., *24*, 550, 1932.

Kirkpatrick, H. J. R., and Murray, R. C.: Osteogenic Fibroma of Bone, J. Bone & Joint Surg., *37-B*, 606, 1955.

Chapter

# 9

# Fibrous Dysplasia

*Fibrous* (or *fibro-osseous*) *dysplasia* of bone is a disorder in which skeletal involvement is the central feature, but in which extraskeletal abnormalities not infrequently form part of the total disease complex. As to the skeleton, one, several, or many bones may be involved in any particular case. The involvement is characterized by the presence of fibro-osseous tissue in the interior of the affected part or parts of the bone. The proportion of fibrous to osseous elements in the lesional tissue may vary considerably, sometimes even from area to area in the same involved bone. Furthermore, some affected bone areas may show islands of cartilage and/or cysts within the basic lesional fibro-osseous tissue.

In some cases, the skeletal aberration constitutes the entire disorder, so far as one can tell. In other cases, the disorder is expressed as an association of the skeletal aberration with the presence of one or more nonelevated light yellow or yellow-brown areas of cutaneous pigmentation. Indeed, the vast majority of the cases of fibrous dysplasia show either the dysplastic fibro-osseous skeletal changes alone (in one, several, or many bones) or only such skeletal changes and some abnormal cutaneous pigmentation. In fact, such cases constituted the basis for the formulation of the concept of fibrous dysplasia as a disease entity by the writer and his associate.

On the other hand, there are cases in which the patient not only presents the skeletal changes (usually together with some abnormal pigmentation) but also shows, or has shown, premature skeletal maturation and precocious puberty, sometimes along with hyperthyroidism and even some other abnormalities. It is these full-blown cases that are commonly denoted as instances of Albright's disease. The identity of the skeletal lesions in so-called Albright's disease with those in cases in which fibrodysplastic skeletal changes are present alone, or at most in association with cutaneous pigmentation, has been confirmed by many workers. As Falconer, Cope, and Robb-Smith have succinctly put it: "Albright's disease must be regarded as an association of cutaneous pigmentation and endocrine disturbances—of which the most striking is precocious puberty in girls—with a characteristic skeletal disorder [fibrous dysplasia] which may occur by itself."

It is the writer's estimate that for every case of the florid (Albright) type there are about 30 or 40 cases of the type in which the fibrodysplastic involvement of the skeleton is limited to one bone or at most a small number of bones and is not associated with any striking cutaneous pigmentation, apparently not with any skeletal precocity, and certainly not with sexual precocity. In spite of their small number, these florid cases bulk large in the literature, because their spectacular qualities make them attractive subjects for reporting.

**Nature and Genesis.**—We know nothing of the etiology of the condition. The complexity of the more advanced cases, and particularly the fact that in these cases the skeletal involvement tends to be exclusively or predominantly on one side of the body, suggests that the disease may have its basis in some deep-rooted developmental defect. However, the disease does not show any familial or hereditary factor. There seems to be no reason for assuming, as some have done, that the skeletal aspect of the disorder has its basis in endocrine dysfunction. The individual bone lesions are malformations which, in a sense, are tumor-like. However, they are tumor-like only in the way that the skeletal lesions of enchondromatosis (p. 184) and hereditary multiple exostosis (p. 150) are so.

**Nomenclature.**—The number of different titles under which cases representing the disorder in different degrees of severity have been discussed in the past is bewildering. They do fall into certain groups, however. Specifically, most of these titles represent variations on the theme of "osteitis fibrosa," sometimes qualified by such terms as "focal," "unilateral," or "disseminated" and often also supplemented by references to some of the extraskeletal abnormalities. Most of the rest of the titles ring the changes on "fibrocystic disease of bone," or on "a form of Recklinghausen's disease of bone." These names are often likewise qualified by such terms as "regional" and "unilateral" and sometimes likewise supplemented by references to associated extraskeletal changes. In relation to fibrous dysplasia of skull bones and particularly of jawbones, such terms as "fibrous osteoma" or "ossifying fibroma" have most often been employed (p. 136).

Though actually denoting only the dysplastic skeletal changes common to all cases, the term "fibrous (or fibro-osseous) dysplasia of bone" as applied to the disease complex as a whole has the advantage that it emphasizes the central and constant feature of the disease complex and can be qualified in accordance with the special features of individual cases. Thus, if only one bone is affected, one can speak of *monostotic fibrous dysplasia.* If several or many bones are affected but there are no associated endocrine abnormalities, the case might be denoted as one of *polyostotic fibrous dysplasia.* When the skeletal involvement is polyostotic and the case has also endocrine aspects, it could be designated as an instance of fibrous dysplasia with endocrine manifestations, or of *Albright's disease.*

## CLINICAL CONSIDERATIONS

**Incidence.**—Fibrous dysplasia of bone is by no means a rare disorder. The type of case most commonly encountered is one in which several bones are involved. Cases presenting only monostotic involvement are also fairly common. In the past, many of the cases of monostotic involvement have undoubtedly been interpreted as instances of "bone cyst," or relegated to the vague general category of "fibrocystic disease." On the other hand, if it is not recognized that the florid cases, in which the skeleton is extensively involved, represent merely an extreme expression of the disorder as a whole, one may gain the impression that fibrous dysplasia is rather rare. As to sex incidence, fibrous dysplasia is definitely more common in females than in males, in the proportion of 2 or 3 to 1. As to age incidence, irrespective of when a case becomes manifest clinically, there can be no doubt that the bone lesions have their inception in childhood, and indeed they may have a congenital basis. However, most of the cases come to light clinically during childhood or adolescence.

**Distribution of the Skeletal Involvement.**—In a case in which only one bone is involved, the writer has found that this is most often a femur, a tibia, a rib, or a facial bone (particularly a jawbone), but it may be almost any bone. Others, too, have found that the monostotic lesions tend to predilect the bones mentioned. When a number of bones are involved, these are quite likely to be bones of one limb—especially a lower one. Typically, then, in these cases of polyostotic involvement, one finds the femur, tibia, and fibula affected, and perhaps also some bones of the foot and part of the innominate bone on the same side. When bones of an upper limb are involved, it is not unusual to find one or another of the skull bones also implicated. On the other hand, there are cases in which, though only a limited number of bones are involved, these are exclusively trunk bones—for instance, several ribs (not necessarily on one side), alone or with several vertebræ.

These cases in which a limited number of bones are affected merge without sharp delimitation into those cases in which the skeletal involvement can be said to be moderately or frankly severe. Thus one sees cases in which, while the lesions are located particularly in bones of the upper and lower limb on one side of the body, there are also at least some in limb bones on the other side, along with lesions of some skull bones, ribs, and pelvic bones, especially on the side on which the limb bones are more extensively affected.

Altogether, segmental distribution of the lesions in the polyostotic cases represents an important clinical and roentgenographic hallmark of the disease. Specifically, there is a definite tendency toward restriction of the lesions to the bones of one limb, or at least more extensive involvement of the bones on one side of the body when the skeleton as a whole is severely implicated. It is to be noted also that segmental distribution of lesions is likewise characteristic of skeletal enchondromatosis (p. 184)—a condition from which fibrous dysplasia may have to be differentiated in a given case.

**Clinical Complaints.**—When only one bone is affected, the clinical complaints tend to be rather mild. They depend more on what bone is affected than on the extent of the involvement. Thus, if it is a rib that is involved, the condition may be entirely asymptomatic. On the other hand, if the upper end of a femur is involved, there is usually a history of a limp and intermittent pain, due to deformity. Especially when a bone of very superficial location, such as a maxilla, a clavicle, or a rib is involved, a local swelling can often be palpated, irrespective of whether or not the condition is creating clinical difficulties.

In regard to the cases in which several bones of a single limb, or several bones irrespective of their relation to a limb, are affected, it is to be noted that the earlier in life the skeletal lesions become pronounced, the more likely it is that they will give rise to clinical complaints. Thus, a child or an adolescent in whom some bones of a lower limb are affected may have pain in the hip, a limp, or even bowing deformity. Also there may be a history of pathologic fractures, perhaps dating back some years. On the other hand, in some cases with involvement limited to one limb or to a few scattered bones, the condition may be present for years and even well into adult life before it is discovered. The discovery may come about through the ultimate appearance of some clinical complaint, or, less often, incidentally in the course of a general physical examination.

In the severest form of the disease, the condition usually manifests itself early in life—that is, in childhood or even in infancy. Moreover, the skeletal involvement often leads to serious deformities and crippling disability. Affected limb bones are frequently found considerably expanded, bowed, shortened, and otherwise deformed. Furthermore, such limb bones are rendered susceptible to repeated spontaneous fractures. As the result of the implication of the lower limbs, disturbance in gait is likely to appear because of coxa vara and bowing of the femora. Indeed, waddling may be observed early in childhood as one of the first signs of the disorder. Extensive involvement of the innominate bones may be followed by deformity of the pelvic girdle. Substantially involved vertebral bodies may become partially collapsed and angulated, so that various degrees of kyphoscoliosis develop. Lesions of ribs may present as localized tumor-like expansions, and such areas, too, are prone to pathologic fracture. In the calvarium, a focus of fibrous dysplasia may bring about a localized expansion of the outer table, which may become quite prominent clinically. In addition to calvarial changes and deformity of facial bones, skull roentgenographs in such cases often reveal striking thickening and radiopacity of the bones comprising the base of the skull, especially around the pituitary fossa.

**Abnormal Cutaneous Pigmentation.**—Of the nonskeletal manifestations of fibrous dysplasia, the most common is abnormal cutaneous pigmentation. A pigmented skin area is not elevated, has the same texture as the rest of the skin, and is yellowish or yellowish brown. It may appear as a small uniform patch, a patch of clustered freckles, or a large blotch or very extensive field with a rather irregular border. When the pigmentation is not extensive and the pigmented area or areas are light yellow, it may easily be overlooked in the clinical examination. (See Fig. 34.)

As already indicated, abnormal skin pigmentation is not a necessary accompaniment of the fibrodysplastic skeletal changes. Indeed, the writer has seen some patients in whom the skeletal involvement was fairly severe but in whom careful search, including examination of the scalp and buttocks, failed to reveal a single patch or blotch. In such cases, one may, it is true, find scattered individual freckles on the upper part of the back, or an occasional pigmented or vascular nevus. However, the commonness of these in the general population, even at the younger age levels, is well recognized, and one cannot attach to them the same significance that belongs to a patch or blotch or to an area of pigmentation constituted by freckles gathered in a cluster. On the other hand, one occasionally observes a case in which the skeletal involvement appears to be limited to a single bone and the patient nevertheless presents a number of abnormally pigmented skin areas. Furthermore, in cases destined to represent fibrous dysplasia in severe form, large patches of abnormal skin pigmentation are sometimes already present at birth as the first clinical manifestation of the disorder.

Sometimes, the site of the abnormal pigmentation corresponds to that of severe skeletal involvement. However, the cutaneous pigmentation may be in a region where the bones are not affected. Thus, in one of our cases, in which the only focus of fibrous dysplasia was in the upper portion of the shaft of a femur, a patch of cutaneous pigmentation several inches in diameter was present on the dorsum of the foot on that side. In another case, in which the fibrodysplastic changes were in bones of the right lower limb, a single patch of cutaneous pigmentation was found on the skin of the middle of the left leg.

The discoloration is caused by the presence of an abnormal amount of melanin pigment, particularly in the basal cells of the epidermis. Some of the cells of the granulosa layer may also show pigment granules, and an occasional pigment-bearing cell may likewise be seen in the corium. Otherwise, a pigmented skin area

***Figure 34***

*A*, Photograph of a very large blotch of pigmentation on the right side of the face of a young boy affected with fibrous dysplasia. The skeletal involvement in this case was most striking in the bones of the left lower limb. (See *B*.)

*B*, Photograph of the boy referred to in *A*. Note the deformity of the left thigh. This is due to curvature of the femur in general, and coxa vara deformity of the femoral neck.

*C*, Photograph showing extensive pigmentation on the right side of the back and the left buttock and thigh of a young woman. The pigmentation also extended somewhat on to the front of the body. The patient gave a history of precocious menstruation. However, despite this and the abnormal pigmentation, only a few of the bones were affected with fibrous dysplasia.

*D*, Photograph showing, in another young woman, pigmentation most striking on the right buttock but also extending down the back of the right thigh. In this case, there was no history of precocious menstruation. However, the skeletal involvement was quite generalized.

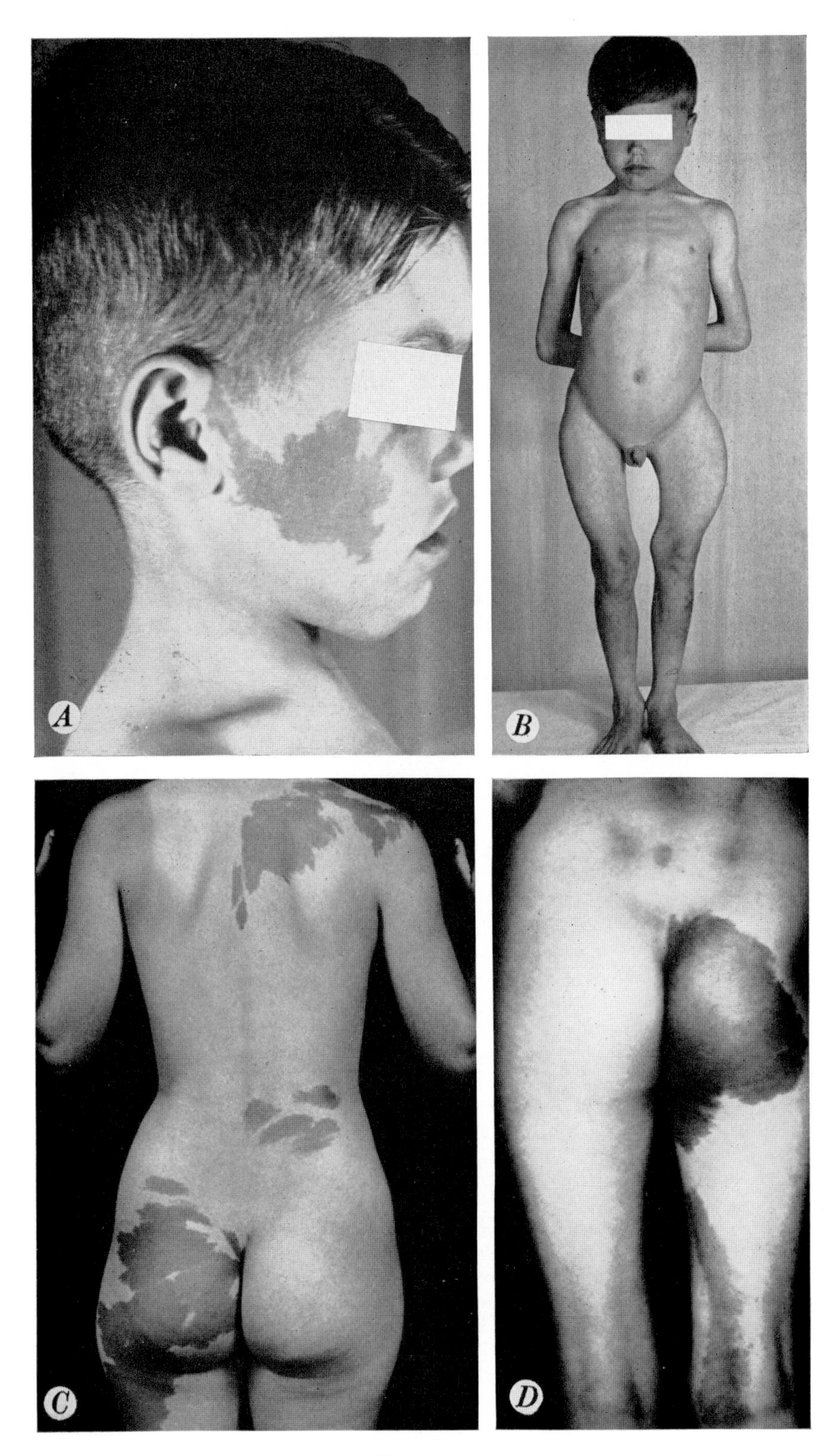


*Figure 34*

does not differ histologically from the unaffected adjacent skin. We do not know, as yet, the explanation for the pigmentation.

**Precocity in Growth.**—In some of the florid cases of fibrous dysplasia, both skeletal growth and skeletal maturation (that is, the ossification and fusion of epiphyses) are accelerated. These two effects work at cross purposes. Thus, for a time during childhood, the patient may be excessively tall for his or her age and show a skeletal age several years in advance of the chronological age. However, because there is premature epiphysial fusion, and consequent premature cessation of growth, the ultimate height of the patient is usually below the average. This ultimate shortness is usually accentuated by curvature of the vertebral column and deformity of the lower limb bones, especially the femora.

Skeletal precocity has been observed mainly in cases in which the widespread fibrodysplastic skeletal lesions were associated with sexual precocity. However, it appears that skeletal precocity may be present even in the absence of sexual precocity. Whether it ever occurs in the milder cases—for instance, those in which the bones of one limb alone are involved—is difficult to say, for often these cases do not come to light until near the end of the growth period. In any event, the basis for the skeletal precocity is apparently some endocrine imbalance.

**Sexual Precocity.**—Sexual precocity is found in only a small proportion of cases of fibrous dysplasia, and, as noted, especially in those in which the skeletal lesions are pronounced and extensive. This precocity was at first thought to occur exclusively among the female patients, but several instances of its occurrence in male patients also have now been reported. In the female, it is manifested in catamenia at an abnormally early age (exceptionally even at 1 or 2 years of age), enlargement of the external genitals, and the premature appearance of secondary sex characteristics, notably the development of large breasts showing prominent areolæ, and the growth of pubic and axillary hair. The onset of precocious menstruation often coincides, more or less, with the genital hypertrophy and the premature appearance of the secondary sex characteristics. In the male, of course, the sexual precocity follows the male pattern.

***Figure 35***

*A*, Photograph of the cut surface of the right tibia of a boy 14 years of age in whom the bones of the trunk and all 4 extremities were heavily involved by fibrous dysplasia. Despite this extensive skeletal involvement, he did not show any clear-cut skin pigmentation. Note the lesional tissue (largely whitish) in the interior of the shaft of the tibia. The roundish, more translucent areas represent foci of cartilage. Also, note, near the bottom of the picture, the large cyst, which was filled with blood clot.

*B*, Roentgenograph of the specimen shown in *A*. Where the lesional tissue is rather on the osseous side of the fibro-osseous complex, the shadow cast is radiopaque. The small, roundish radiolucencies represent the foci of cartilage in the lesional tissue.

*C*, Roentgenograph of the specimen shown in *D*. The trabeculated appearance was shown to be due to the presence of osseous ridges on the inner surface of the expanded new cortex of the affected rib area. Because the lesional tissue was more fibrous than osseous, the roentgenographic shadow which it cast tended toward radiolucency.

*D*, Photograph of the cut surface of the affected left 7th rib of a woman in whom a number of other ribs and several vertebræ, but no skeletal parts elsewhere, were involved. The lesional area is expanded and filled with tissue which was more or less uniformly, but only slightly, gritty. The tissue was also hemorrhagically discolored in some places. The patient was 36 years of age at the time when this chondral end of the rib was resected. She had been aware for 8 years of a local swelling. Roentgenographic examination revealed that the left 7th rib was involved also at its posterior end and that the 7th and 8th ribs on the right side were also extensively altered, as were several dorsal vertebrae. The patient did not present any patches or blotches of skin pigmentation, though she did show a number of small, scattered, elevated pigmented nevi and some vascular nevi. (See also 36-*A*.)

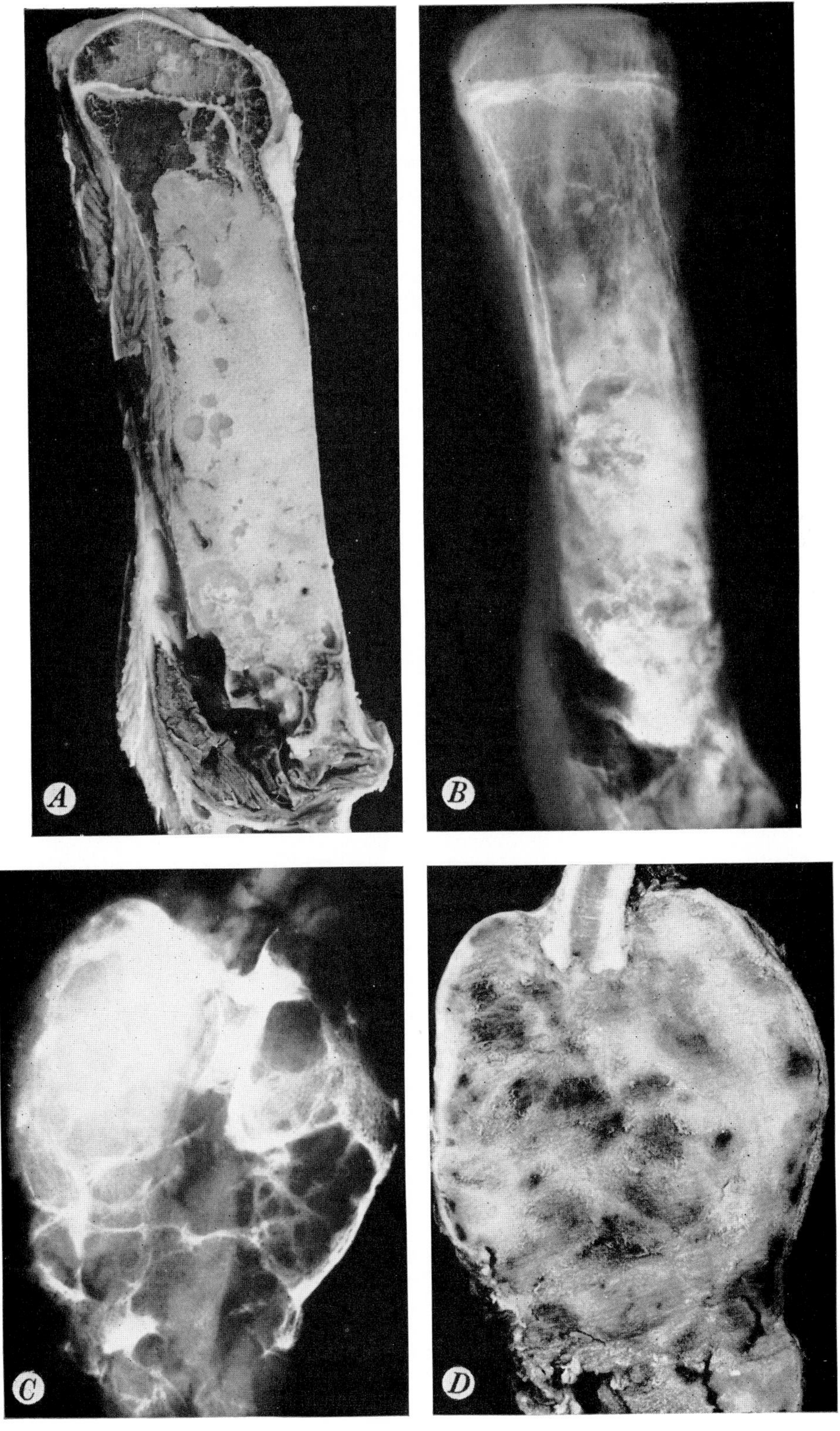


*Figure 35*

All the studies which have been undertaken in regard to the gonadotropic, follicle-stimulating, or estrogenic hormone content of the urine of these subjects have failed to yield any abnormal findings. Nor do the sex glands themselves show anything abnormal. Possibly there is, in these cases, an abnormality or lesion in the hypothalamus, conditioned by fibrodysplastic changes in the base of the skull, which is indeed often thickened in these cases. Finally, it is of interest in connection with the sexual precocity that there are a few recorded instances in which female patients who showed it have later gone successfully through pregnancies and given birth to children who showed no signs of the disease.

**Other Aberrations Occasionally Observed.**—In an occasional instance of fibrous dysplasia, there have also been observed such diverse phenomena as: hyperthyroidism, diabetes mellitus, congenital arteriovenous aneurysm, rudimentary kidney and coarctation of the aorta, and visual disturbances from pressure atrophy of the optic nerve. In rare instances, too, multiple fibrous or fibromyxomatous soft-tissue tumors, quite independent of the bone lesions, have been found.

**Biochemical Findings.**—In cases of fibrous dysplasia, the only aberration which one may find in the blood by clinical biochemical analysis is an elevation of the serum alkaline phosphatase activity value. Though in some cases, in spite of the fact that many bones are involved, this value is hardly above normal, in other cases we have found it around 20 Bodansky units. On the other hand, the serum calcium value and the serum inorganic phosphate values are within normal limits. In cases in which mineral balance studies (calcium and phosphorus) have been done, these have always yielded values within the normal range.

## PATHOLOGIC FINDINGS

**Gross.**—Often an affected bone or bone area is found distended, at least in part (see Fig. 35). The distention is due to erosion of the original cortical bone by the growing lesional tissue in the medullary cavity, and the yielding of the newly formed subperiosteal cortical bone to pressure from this expanding tissue. Whether the affected bone area is distended or not, the outer surface is usually smooth, but the inner surface can sometimes be shown to be more or less ridged. The lesional tissue occupying the interior of the affected bone area (usually part of the shaft when a tubular bone is involved) is mainly rather firm and whitish, but some areas may appear reddishly speckled on account of exceptional vascularity. The tissue may vary from lesion to lesion, and even from area to area, in respect to grittiness, also.

### *Figure 36*

*A*, Photograph of the sectioned, tumorously expanded right 8th rib of a woman 40 years of age who also presented fibrous dysplasia in other bones of the thorax. The upper part of the specimen is occupied by a number of large cysts. Some of these were found filled with blood clot and others with serous fluid. On the right, there is a ball-like mass of whitish tissue. This tissue was highly collagenous, having, indeed, practically no osseous elements in it. To the left of it there is an essentially solid lesional area. This area was rather uniformly fibro-osseous throughout. The specimen shown in Figure 35-*C* came from the same patient, and represents another rib lesion, which had been removed 4 years earlier.

*B*, Photograph showing fibrodysplastic involvement of a metatarsal bone and a phalanx. The tissue in the interior of these bones was more osseous than fibrous—that is, it was on the osseous side of the fibro-osseous complex. Note that the contour of these affected bones is not modified.

*C*, Photograph of other foot bones from the case illustrated in *B*. There are foci of fibrous dysplasia in various bone areas, but the bone contours are again not modified. The lesional areas in these bones, too, were much more osseous than fibrous.

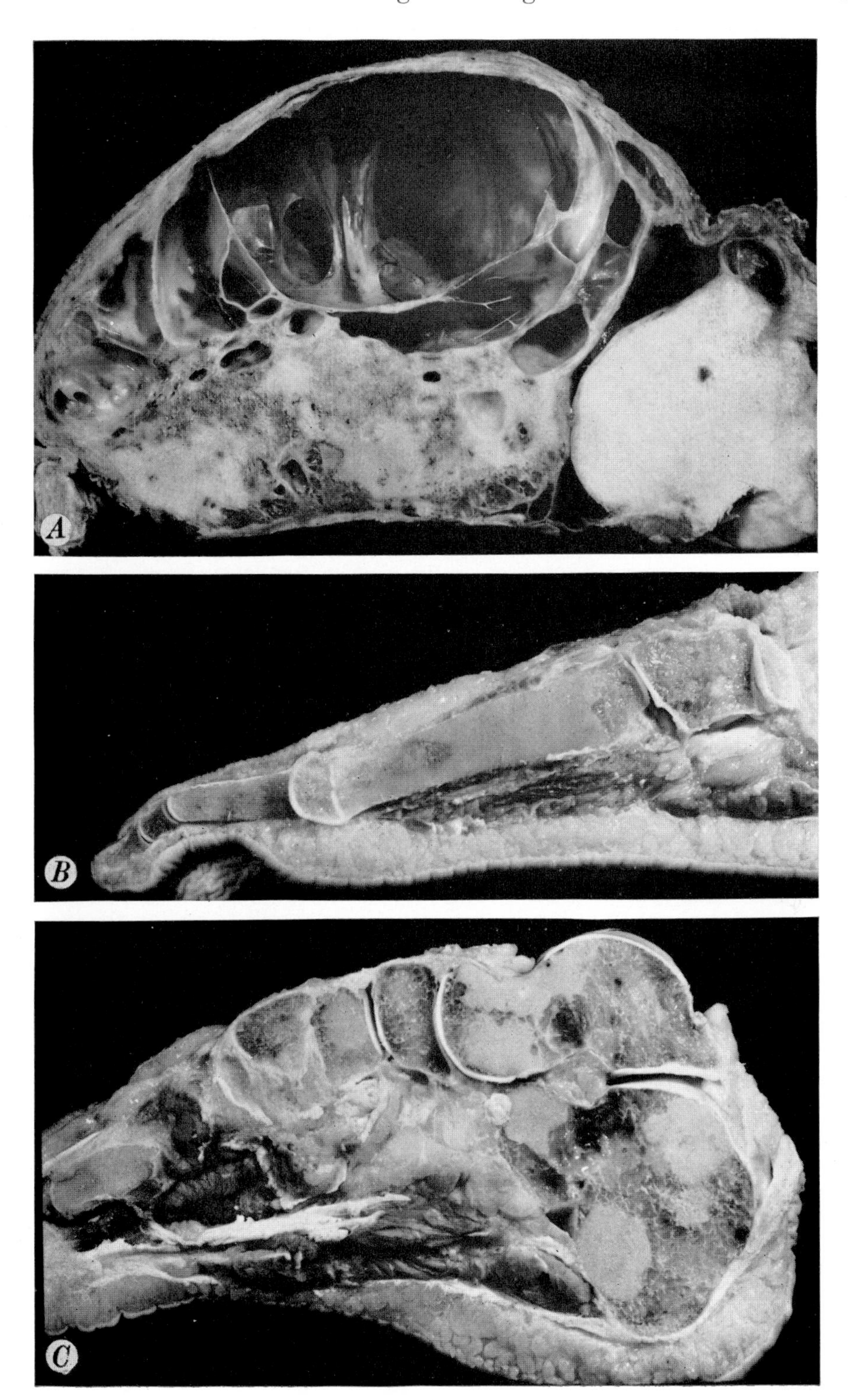


*Figure 36*

In some lesions, it is slightly but fairly uniformly gritty throughout, in accordance with a more or less even intermingling of the basic fibrous tissue with delicate osseous trabeculæ. In other areas or other lesions, the grittiness is less conspicuous, the lesional tissue being predominantly fibrous and collagenous. On the other hand, in still other areas or lesions, the lesional tissue has a definitely sclerotic character because so much osseous tissue is present in the connective-tissue substratum that the latter sinks into the background.

In some lesions, the pathologic replacement tissue may contain islands of hyaline cartilage. If cartilage foci are present, and if the subject is still growing, one may be able to show that they are derived from the epiphysial cartilage plate. Specifically, if an affected bone containing cartilage is cut open in its long axis, it will be found that the cartilage is most abundant in the metaphysial regions, at or near the epiphysial cartilage plates, and some cartilage foci may even be seen budding off from the plates. The cartilage foci are generally rather small, most of them being considerably less than a centimeter in diameter. In some instances, however, they are larger and fairly numerous and may even constitute a striking feature of the lesional tissue as a whole. They tend to become calcified peripherally. Eventually, many of them undoubtedly disappear.

Small cysts arising through edematous degeneration or hemorrhagic softening of the lesional tissue are sometimes observed. Further, we need only note that occasionally even large cysts (some centimeters in diameter) filled either with blood or with serous fluid may be encountered. The cysts filled with serous fluid have delicate, smooth, shiny lining membranes. (See Fig. 36.)

**Microscopic.**—If one examines an area in which the lesional tissue is only slightly but more or less uniformly gritty, it is seen to be composed of slender spindle cells in rather loose or whorled arrangement, interspersed with trabeculæ of newly formed bone, of variable size and shape. It can be observed further that the bone trabeculæ have been formed through osseous metaplasia of the connective tissue in which they are imbedded. If a rather fibrous and essentially nongritty tissue area is studied microscopically, the constituent tissue is likely to be found rather poor in cells and even heavily collagenized. (See Fig. 37.)

It is especially in the collagenized and poorly osseous tissue areas that one is likely to observe microscopic foci of edematous degeneration and cystic softening. The cysts large enough to be observed grossly apparently arise through fusion of such microcysts and/or hemorrhagic softening, which may occur here and there in a lesional area. Particularly within an area undergoing cystification, one may encounter tissue fields containing numerous multinuclear giant cells. Occasionally, a lesion may show some nests of foam cells within the fibrous connective-tissue substratum. These appear mainly in connection with hemorrhage or focal degeneration, and hardly represent a noteworthy feature of the pathology, except insofar as they may lead to a mistaken diagnosis of lipid granulomatosis. (See Differential Diagnosis, p. 134.)

***Figure 37***

*A*, Photomicrograph (× 10) showing a rib altered by fibrous dysplasia. In this survey view, one can see that the cortex of the rib is thinned and otherwise modified. Also, it is apparent that the fibro-osseous tissue in the interior of the bone is rather poor in osseous trabeculæ.

*B*, Photomicrograph (× 20) showing an island of cartilage bordered by fibro-osseous tissue. In this lesion, the pathologic tissue shows more osseous trabeculæ than it does in *A*. The cartilage is more or less calcified at its periphery.

*C*, Photomicrograph (× 15) of a focus of fibrous dysplasia in which the fibro-osseous tissue is more on the osseous side of the fibro-osseous complex, containing numerous thick, irregular osseous trabeculæ.

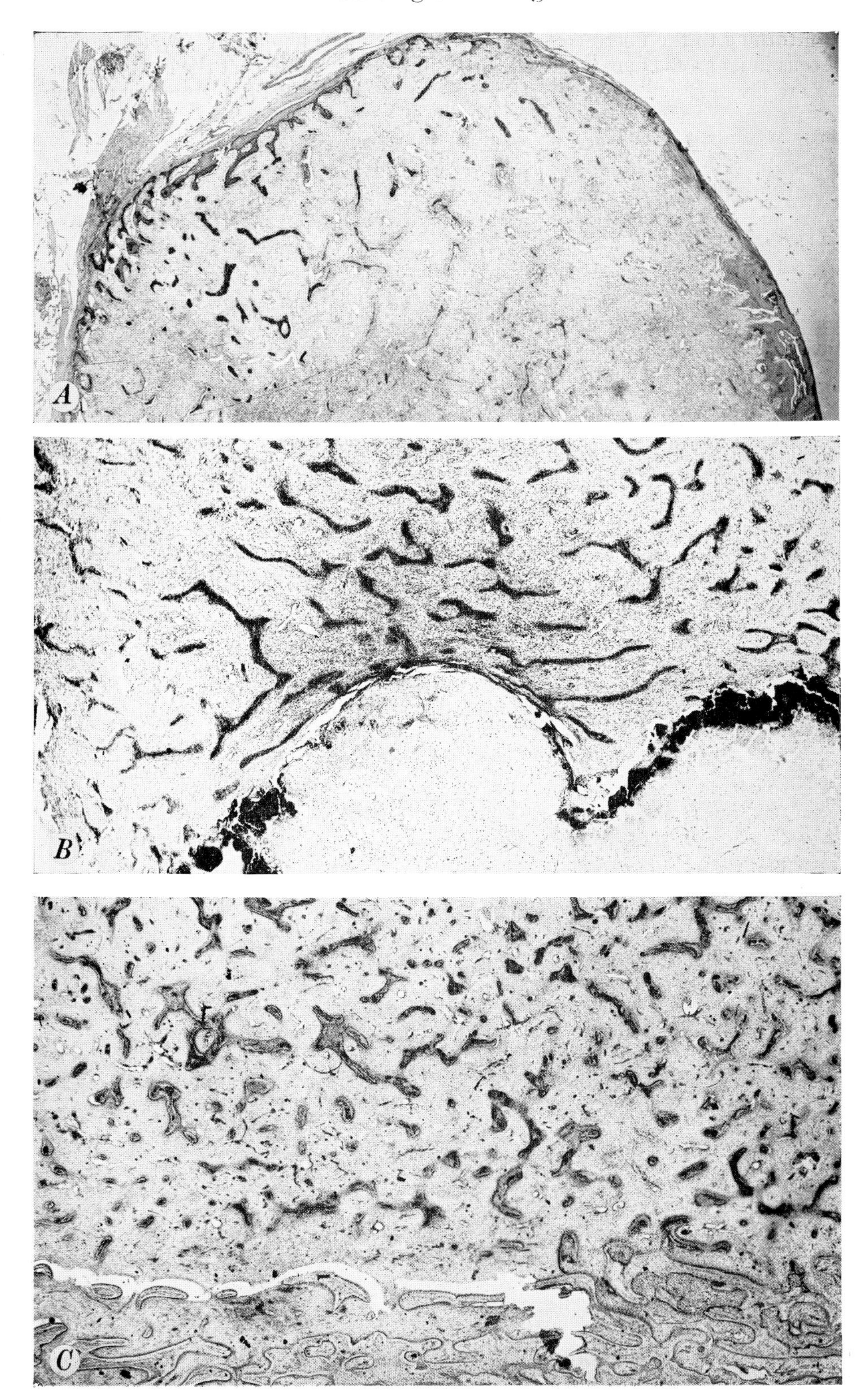


*Figure 37*

In turning to the microscopic pattern of a lesion or lesional area which is rather osseous in its gross appearance, one finds, in the first place, that the osseous trabeculæ are thick, irregularly contoured, and set in relatively little supporting connective tissue. Furthermore, the thick trabeculæ may show large numbers of cement lines. This picture may remind one vaguely of the cytologic pattern presented by the osseous tissue of Paget's disease, but nothing else in connection with the case is likely to suggest that disease. However, it should be remembered that while an individual lesion may be highly osseous throughout, another may be so only in part. In a lesion of the latter type, some parts will be definitely fibro-osseous and some even rather collagenous. Furthermore, in a case presenting multiple lesions, one lesion may be substantially or completely on the osseous side of the fibro-osseous complex, while another may be highly fibrous and only slightly osseous. (See Fig. 38.)

## ROENTGENOGRAPHIC FINDINGS

The roentgenographic picture presented by an affected bone or bone area is determined in its essentials by the character of the replacement tissue in the bone interior and by the effects of this tissue on the neighboring cortical bone. Thus this picture varies from one affected bone or bone area to another in accordance with the degree to which the bone contour has been expanded by erosion of the cortex, ridges have developed upon the inner aspect of the newly formed cortex, osseous tissue has been formed in the connective-tissue substratum, or cysts have appeared.

In lesions or parts of lesions in which the replacement tissue in the interior of the bone is not highly osseous or is cystic in part, it will tend to cast a rather radiolucent shadow. On the other hand, in lesions or parts of lesions (especially of long bones) in which the replacement tissue has undergone extensive ossification, it will tend to cast a shadow resembling ground glass. In relation to involvement of the facial bones (especially the maxilla and the sphenoid and ethmoid) the lesions are generally quite sclerotized and their shadows hence quite radiopaque. If much cartilage is interspersed through the replacement tissue, the *x*-ray shadow may even suggest clouds of smoke. If the replacement tissue has eroded the original cortical bone and distended the newly formed cortex, and if the latter has bony ridges on its inner surface, the affected area may present a "multilocular" appearance, although, as tissue examination has repeatedly shown, the area in question may actually be solidly filled by the basic fibro-osseous tissue. (See Fig. 39.)

***Figure 38***

*A*, Photomicrograph (× 50) showing in some detail the histologic pattern presented by an area of fibrous dysplasia in which the tissue is uniformly, though only moderately, gritty. The connective-tissue substratum is composed of whorled bundles of spindle cells, and osseous tissue is being formed in it by metaplasia.

*B*, Photomicrograph (× 50) showing the histologic pattern presented by an area of fibrous dysplasia in which, grossly, the tissue was rather osseous and sclerotic. Note the thick, irregular trabeculæ of well calcified osseous tissue imbedded in the spindle cell connective-tissue substratum.

*C*, Photomicrograph (× 125) showing the histologic pattern presented by an area of fibrous dysplasia in which, grossly, the tissue was highly collagenous. Osseous metaplasia is manifest in some places. This histologic section represents the tissue from the ball-like mass visible on the right in Figure 36-*A*.

*D*, Photomicrograph (× 65) showing the histologic pattern presented by an area of fibrous dysplasia containing a number of small microcysts resulting from edema and cystic degeneration. Some multinuclear giant cells are also to be seen.

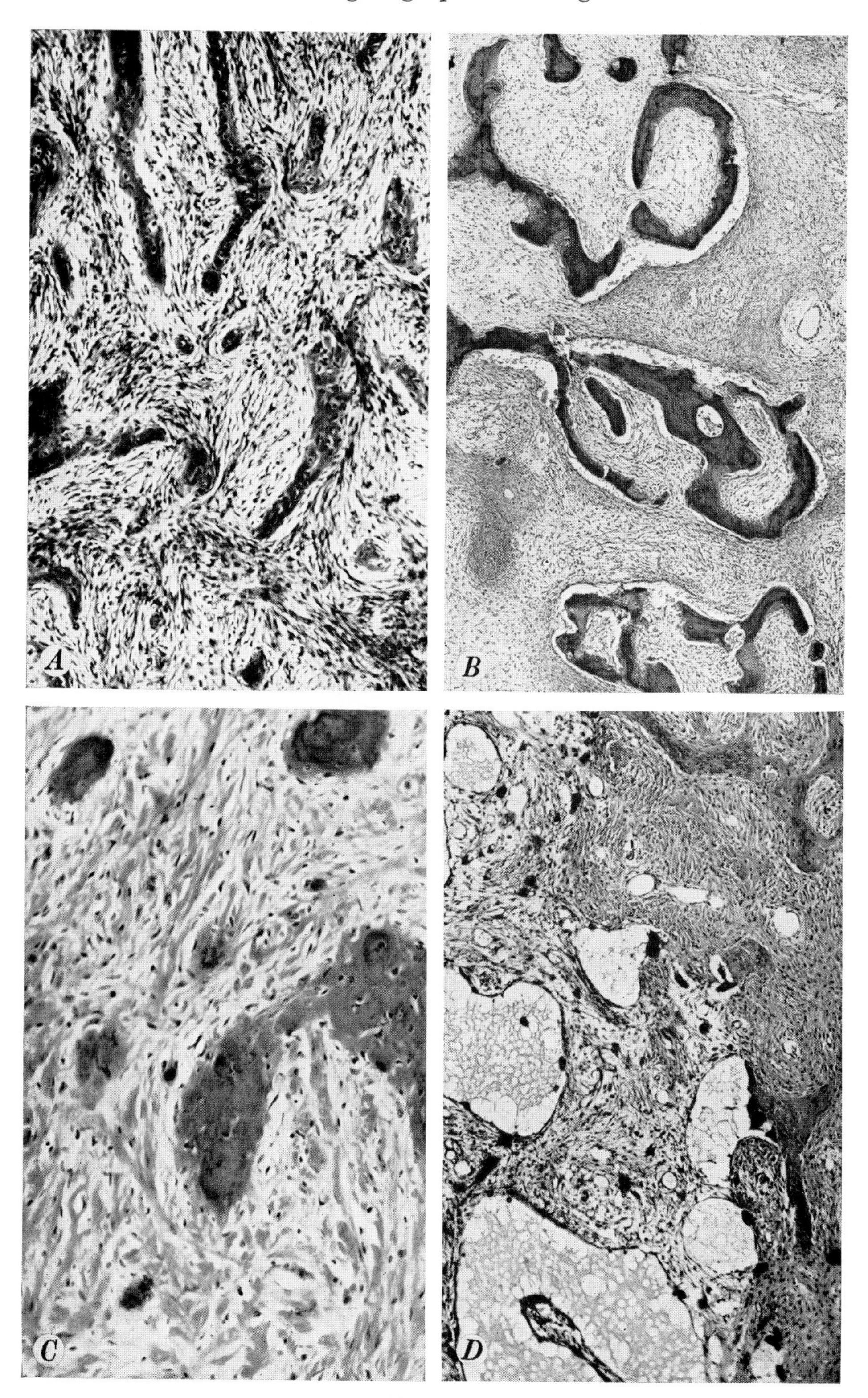


*Figure 38*

In regard to the solitary fibro-osseous lesions, the point of special interest is that the roentgenopathologic pattern is basically the same and may show the same variations from case to case that one encounters in the lesions of cases presenting polyostotic involvement. Thus, in a femur, for instance, one may demonstrate a solitary focus of fibrous dysplasia in which the lesional tissue appears relatively radiolucent and trabeculated roentgenographically. In such a lesion, the replacement tissue will be found to be rather heavily on the fibrous side and may even be cystified in part. Again, an affected femur may show a solitary focus which casts a "ground glass" shadow roentgenographically. In such a case, the lesional tissue is rather heavily on the osseous side of the fibro-osseous complex. Or a solitary femoral focus may cast a cloud-like puffy shadow, and in such a case the lesional replacement tissue is likely to include a good deal of cartilage.

When only one bone or part of one bone is involved, tissue examination may be necessary to support the roentgenographic diagnosis of fibrous dysplasia. This is so because the differentiation between a solitary focus of fibrous dysplasia and a solitary bone cyst or an enchondroma or even a large non-ossifying fibroma of bone cannot always be made on a roentgenographic basis. On the other hand, in cases in which a number of trunk or limb bones are involved, the diagnosis is usually fairly easy to make on a roentgenographic basis. This is particularly so when the involvement is predominantly on one side of the body. Under these circumstances (and, even then, only in the absence of skull lesions), the only condition which can sometimes raise the problem of differential diagnosis on a roentgenographic basis is skeletal enchondromatosis of the Ollier type. (See Fig. 40.)

## COURSE OF THE DISEASE IN THE SKELETON

**Tendency Toward Stabilization.**—Experience indicates that the period of active progression of the skeletal involvement tends to end when adult life is reached, in the sense that bones which were not involved by this time do not begin to become so now. Thus, even when fibrous dysplasia of bone is first uncovered in adult life, the skeletal lesions apparently date back to childhood. It is true that in a case

### *Figure 39*

*A*, Roentgenograph of an ilium in the case of a woman 20 years of age affected with fibrous dysplasia involving that bone and the bones of the lower limb on the same side. The ilium is enlarged and expanded and appears loculated. Actually, as tissue examination showed, the affected ilium was solidly filled with fibro-osseous tissue. The latter was more fibrous than osseous, and the appearance of loculated trabeculation was created by ridging on the inner surface of the new cortex in the affected area.

*B*, Roentgenograph showing the 7th and 8th ribs, affected by fibrous dysplasia, in the case of a woman 40 years of age. The ribs are expanded and again appear loculated. One can gather that the lesional tissue within them is more fibrous than osseous and may also be cystified.

*C*, Roentgenograph of part of a humerus, radius, and ulna of an adolescent boy affected with fibrous dysplasia involving numerous other bones also. The shadow cast by the replacement tissue in the interior of the bones shown is, on the whole, a "ground glass" shadow. One can gather from the shadow cast that the lesional tissue within these bones is more on the osseous than on the fibrous side of the fibro-osseous complex.

*D*, Roentgenograph of the upper part of the femur from the case illustrated in *C*. The femur presents the "shepherd's crook" deformity not infrequently encountered in florid cases of fibrous dysplasia when the upper end of a femur is severely affected. The roundish areas of relative radiolucency undoubtedly represent foci of cartilage within the fibro-osseous replacement tissue.

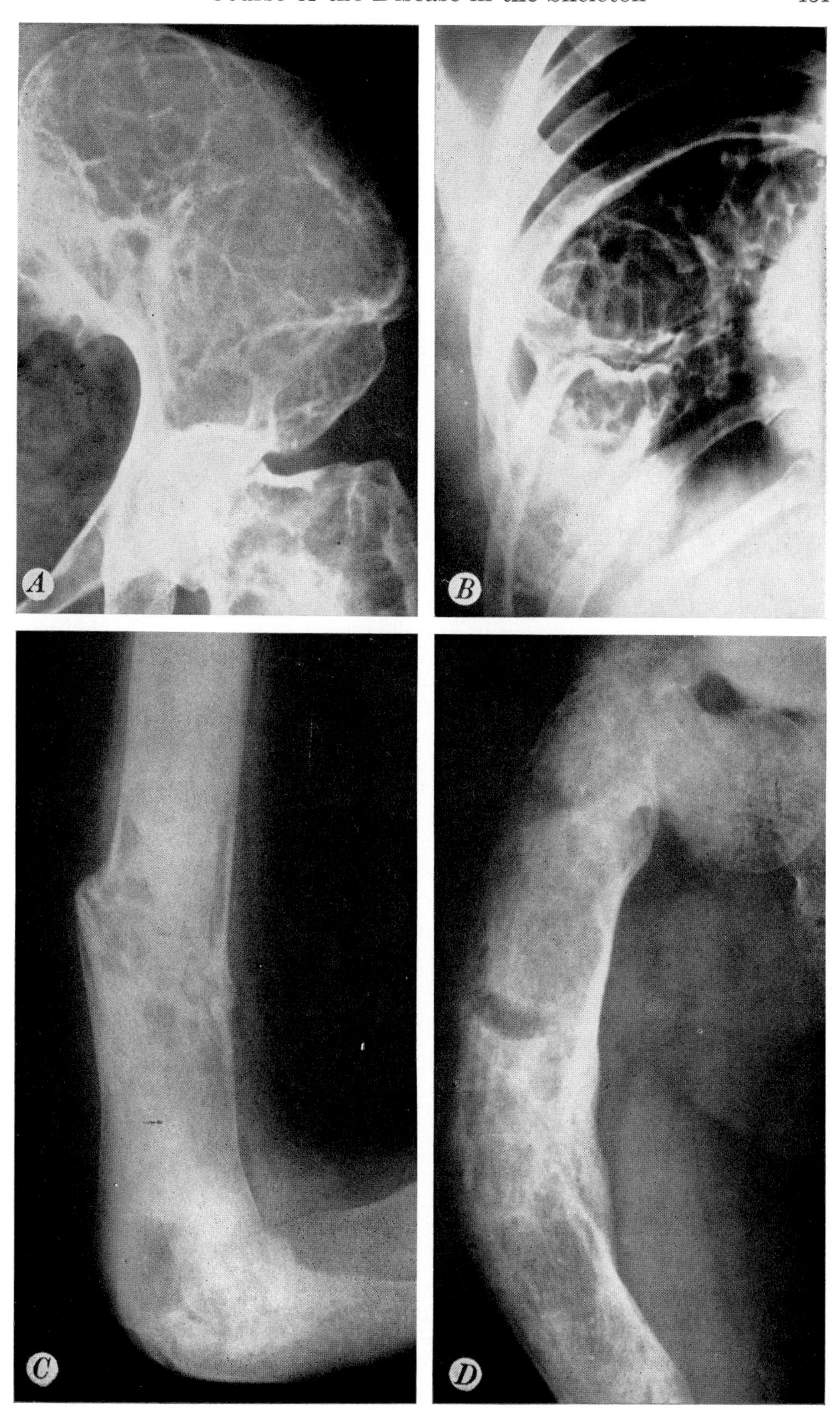


***Figure 39***

showing extensive skeletal involvement already in childhood, one or more of the severely affected bones may show progressive deformity later on. However, this is due to weakening of the bone, and is not inconsistent with the appearance of increasing ossification of the fibrodysplastic tissue as another aspect of the process of stabilization. In fact, in some cases, sclerotization of the fibrodysplastic tissue in some or many of the affected bones may become very pronounced. On the other hand, it is well known that fibrodysplastic lesions which may have been stabilized for years can subsequently take on some growth activity. Thus a patient may come in even during middle life because of complaints of only recent origin, due to a spurt of growth (perhaps quite slight) in a lesion which has clearly been present for decades.

Infrequently, rather rapid enlargement of one or more fibrodysplastic lesions may occur in a given case. The writer has seen, for instance, a case of polyostotic involvement in which one of the affected ribs, which had not undergone any significant change over a period of years, suddenly underwent tremendous enlargement in the course of a few months. Clinically, it was then suspected that this rib lesion, which attained approximately the size of a standard football, had undergone malignant transformation. When the rib was extirpated and sectioned in its long axis, the exposed cut surface showed that fully half of the mass was represented by a huge multilocular cystic area in which some of the cysts were filled with clotted blood and others with yellow-green fluid. The rest of the mass was made up of one large oblong area, composed of quite gritty fibrous tissue, and one ball-like area of highly collagenous tissue with little if any grit in it. The gross appearance of the lesion was already against the idea of its being a sarcoma, and the results of histologic examination were also against it. Furthermore, the subsequent clinical course in this case was a favorable one. Evidently, the huge distention of the rib had been due largely to the secondary changes of hemorrhage and cystification. (See Fig. 36-*A*.)

The writer has seen an analogous clinical picture developing in connection with hemorrhage and cystification of an affected tibia in a case of extensive fibrous dysplasia in a young boy. Clinically in this case, too, the fibrodysplastic bone had been held to have undergone sarcomatous transformation. However, study of the amputation specimen proved that the apparently ominous changes observed clin-

***Figure 40***

*A*, Roentgenograph showing a dense, radiopaque shadow cast by a maxilla affected with fibrous dysplasia. The patient was a man 20 years of age who had long presented a local swelling of the face in that area. The bones of the upper limb on the same side were also involved, and *C* shows the appearance of the changes in the affected hand in this case.

*B*, Photomicrograph (× 25) showing the histologic pattern of tissue removed from the maxillary lesion shown in *A*. The pattern is that of fibro-osseous tissue representing the result of metaplastic ossification in a spindle cell connective-tissue stroma. The histologic appearance of the tissue removed from the maxilla in this case was identical with that of the tissue removed from the fibrodysplastically affected humerus.

*C*, Roentgenograph of the hand in the case illustrated in *A*. Many of the bones are affected. Some cast a uniform "ground glass" shadow. Others, in which the fibro-osseous tissue is more osseous, cast an even more radiopaque shadow. The roundish areas of relative radiolucency in some of the metacarpal and phalangeal bones undoubtedly represent small foci of cartilage imbedded in the replacement tissue.

*D*, Roentgenograph of a solitary focus of fibrous dysplasia in the upper end of a femur. Much of the lesional area casts a radiopaque shadow. This is due to the fact that, in this lesion also, the fibro-osseous tissue removed from the lesion was rather on the osseous side of the fibro-osseous complex.

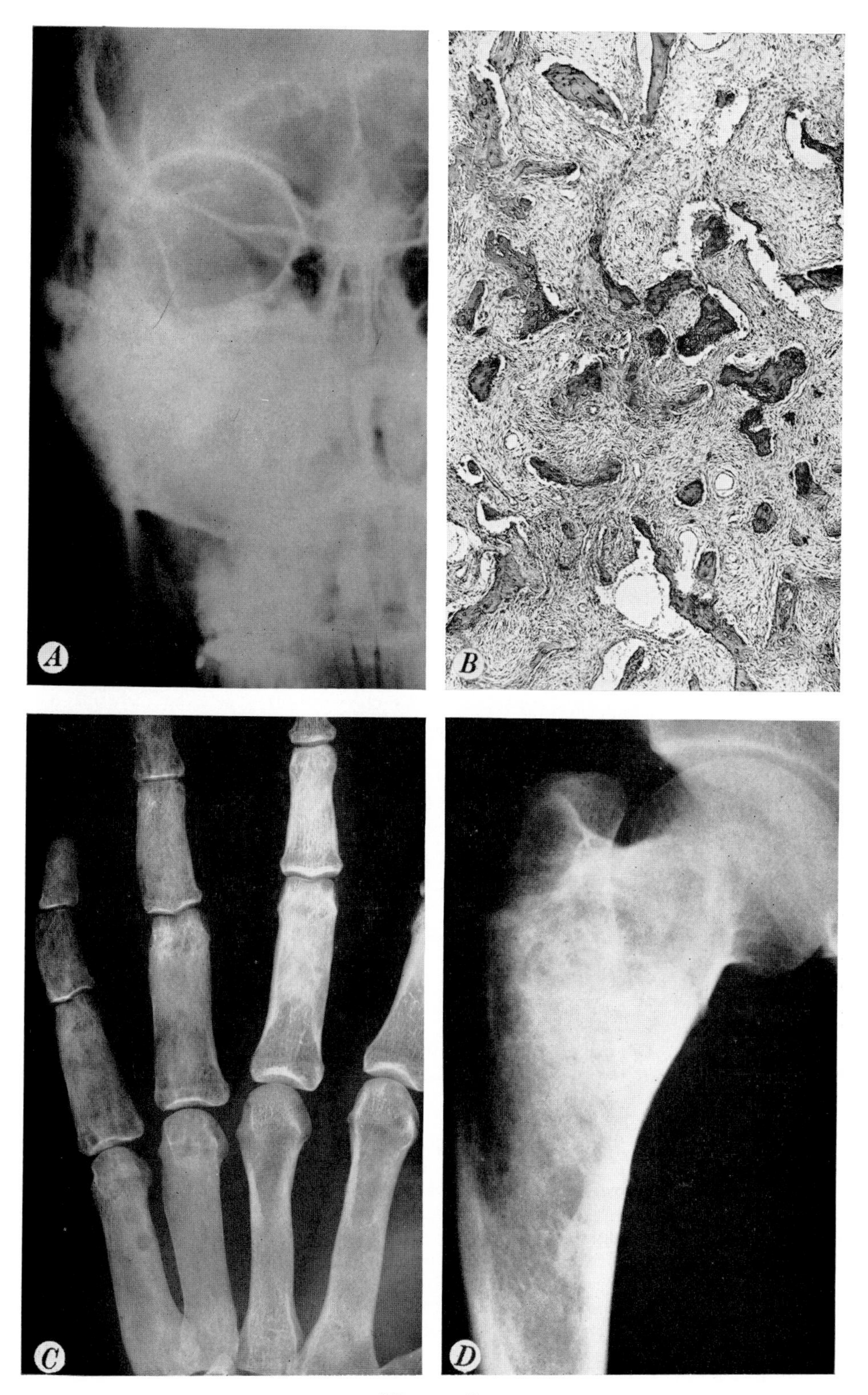


*Figure 40*

ically and roentgenographically did not have a sarcomatous basis and represented merely extensive local cystification. (See Figs. 35-*A* and *B*.)

**Sarcoma Complicating Fibrous Dysplasia.**—It is only occasionally that a bone affected with fibrous dysplasia comes to show sarcomatous transformation. This may happen in one or another of the affected bones in a case of polyostotic involvement, and occasionally even when the fibrous dysplasia is limited to a single bone. In each of the two cases reported by Coley and Stewart, the sarcoma appeared in a single fibrodysplastic bone site, though the fibrous dysplasia was polyostotic, as was confirmed by biopsy. In these two cases, the patients survived for 4 and 11 years respectively, death being due presumably to metastases. The course run by the sarcoma in both these cases was also unusual in that small doses of radiation therapy apparently held the sarcoma in check for years. Ordinarily, sarcomas developing in fibrous dysplasia are more rapidly fatal, especially if they are frank osteogenic sarcomas instead of fibrosarcomas (that is, non-bone-forming sarcomas) as they apparently were in these two cases. A number of other case reports relating to this complication of fibrous dysplasia have also appeared in the literature.

The writer himself has studied several cases of sarcoma complicating fibrous dysplasia. In one case (reported in detail by Sutro), the patient was a man 25 years of age whose first difficulty relating to his skeleton was of only a few months' standing and consisted of some pain in the right leg and the appearance of a slowly enlarging swelling in the middle of the tibia. Roentgenographic examination revealed the presence, in this limb, of fibrous dysplasia, of which, as noted, the patient was entirely unaware. The disorder involved the right femur, tibia, and fibula, and there was a bone-forming sarcoma more or less in the middle of the shaft of the tibia. Both grossly and histologically, the sarcoma proved to be an osteogenic sarcoma. Below the sarcomatous area, the marrow cavity of the tibia contained nonsarcomatous fibro-osseous tissue such as one sees in sclerotized fibrous dysplasia lesions. Similar tissue was observed in the marrow cavity of the femur and fibula.

In still another case—that of a girl 20 years of age—the fibrous dysplasia was limited to the upper part of the left femur but was known to have been present since the age of 7. The lesional area became the site of a chondrosarcoma. Eventually, the latter substantially replaced the fibrodysplastic tissue whose presence had been established by biopsy years before. In accordance with the better prognosis of chondrosarcoma, a segmental resection was carried out, and a 5-year follow-up showed neither local recurrence nor metastasis. (See Fig. 41.)

## DIFFERENTIAL DIAGNOSIS

**Solitary Bone Cyst.**—Occasionally, one encounters a long bone lesion whose roentgenographic appearance suggests a focus of fibrous dysplasia but whose

### *Figure 41*

*A*, Roentgenograph showing a pathologic fracture of a humerus, conditioned by an osteogenic sarcoma complicating fibrous dysplasia. Note the "ground glass" radiopacity below the fracture area in the humerus, and also in the radius. Examination of the amputation specimen established the presence of fibrous dysplasia in these sites.

*B*, Roentgenograph of the resected upper end of a femur in which a chondrosarcoma became engrafted upon fibrous dysplasia. The numerous radiopacities represent calcification and ossification going on in and about the cartilaginous tumor.

*C*, Photograph of the sectioned specimen shown in *B*. Residual areas of fibrous dysplasia can be noted in the head and neck of the bone, and at the lower end of the lesional area.

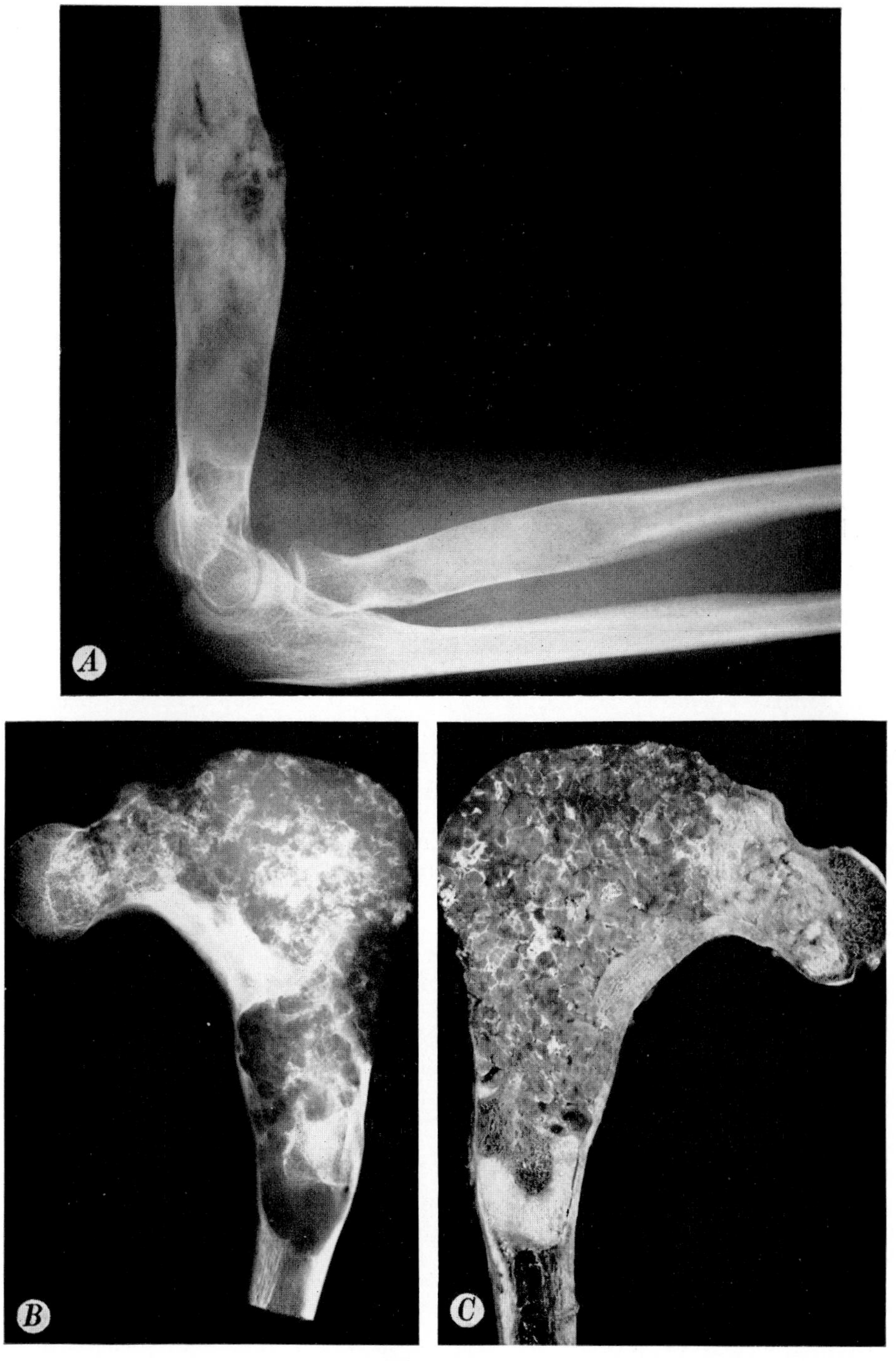


*Figure 41*

anatomic features do not confirm that diagnosis. Specifically, when one enters the lesional area, one finds some loose, edematous, and somewhat gritty tissue in the interior of the bone, interspersed with cystic spaces. Histologic examination of the tissue shows that it is a loose-meshed, vascular granulation tissue containing some trabeculæ of new bone. Thus there is nothing in the tissue removed from such a lesion to sustain a diagnosis of fibrous dysplasia, even in the form of an extensively cystified focus of fibrous dysplasia. Such lesions may well represent old solitary bone cysts which have become partly filled in through a process of reparative osteofibrosis. (See Figs. 18-*C* and 18-*D*, p. 71.)

**Solitary Enchondroma.**—Once in a while, one encounters a solitary focus of fibrous dysplasia which, because it contains a good deal of cartilage, might suggest roentgenographically that one was dealing with a solitary enchondroma instead. Specifically, it is the presence of punctate radiopacities in the *x*-ray picture that creates this impression. The differential diagnosis in such a case has to rest on tissue examination. When one is dealing with a focus of fibrous dysplasia containing cartilage, histologic examination will show that the islands of cartilage are imbedded in tissue which is essentially fibrous or fibro-osseous. An enchondroma (p. 179), on the other hand, never shows fibrous or fibro-osseous tissue within its constituent cartilage.

**Non-ossifying Fibroma.**—A large non-ossifying fibroma (see Fig. 22-*B*, p. 85) may, because of its "trabeculated" appearance in the *x*-ray picture, suggest a focus of fibrous dysplasia. However, tissue removed from such a lesion does not show the fibro-osseous pattern characteristic of a focus of fibrous dysplasia. Nevertheless, one can find, in the literature dealing with solitary foci of fibrous dysplasia, an occasional case of non-ossifying fibroma misdiagnosed as fibrous dysplasia.

**"Fibrous Osteoma" or "Ossifying Fibroma" of Jawbones vs. Fibrous Dysplasia of Jawbones.**—Phemister and Grimson, reporting some years ago on a group of solitary fibro-osseous lesions of jawbones, referred to them as "fibrous osteomas of the jaws." These jawbone lesions have often also been denoted by variants of this name, such as "ossifying fibroma" and "osteofibroma." They are composed of intermingled fibrous connective tissue and osseous tissue in various proportions. Usually, the osseous element is rather prominent in them, so that the lesional tissue tends to be quite firm and gritty. Roentgenographically, those lesions in which the osseous element is dominant consequently show considerable "ground glass" or even more intense radiopacity.

As to the jawbone affected, it appears that the maxilla is slightly predilected over the mandible. The condition is definitely more common in females than in males. As to the time of clinical emergence of the condition, it appears that a swelling of the affected maxilla or mandible is often already noted by the time the patient has reached adolescence. On the other hand, it is only infrequently that the cases come to clinical light in this way after the patient has reached the age of 30 or 35.

### *Figure 42*

*A*, Roentgenograph of a solitary focus of fibrous dysplasia in the maxilla of a girl 12 years of age. Note the "ground glass" radiopacity. There was a history of swelling of the cheek, of only a few months' standing.

*B*, Photomicrograph (× 25) showing the histologic pattern of the tissue removed from the lesion shown in *A*. Note the presence of fibro-osseous tissue, and the fact that the osseous trabeculæ are numerous and thick.

*C*, Roentgenograph of a solitary focus of fibrous dysplasia in the mandible. The patient was a girl 17 years of age who had not been aware of any abnormality relating to the jaw until a few weeks before this *x*-ray picture was taken. The tissue removed from this lesion had essentially the same pattern as the tissue shown in *B*.

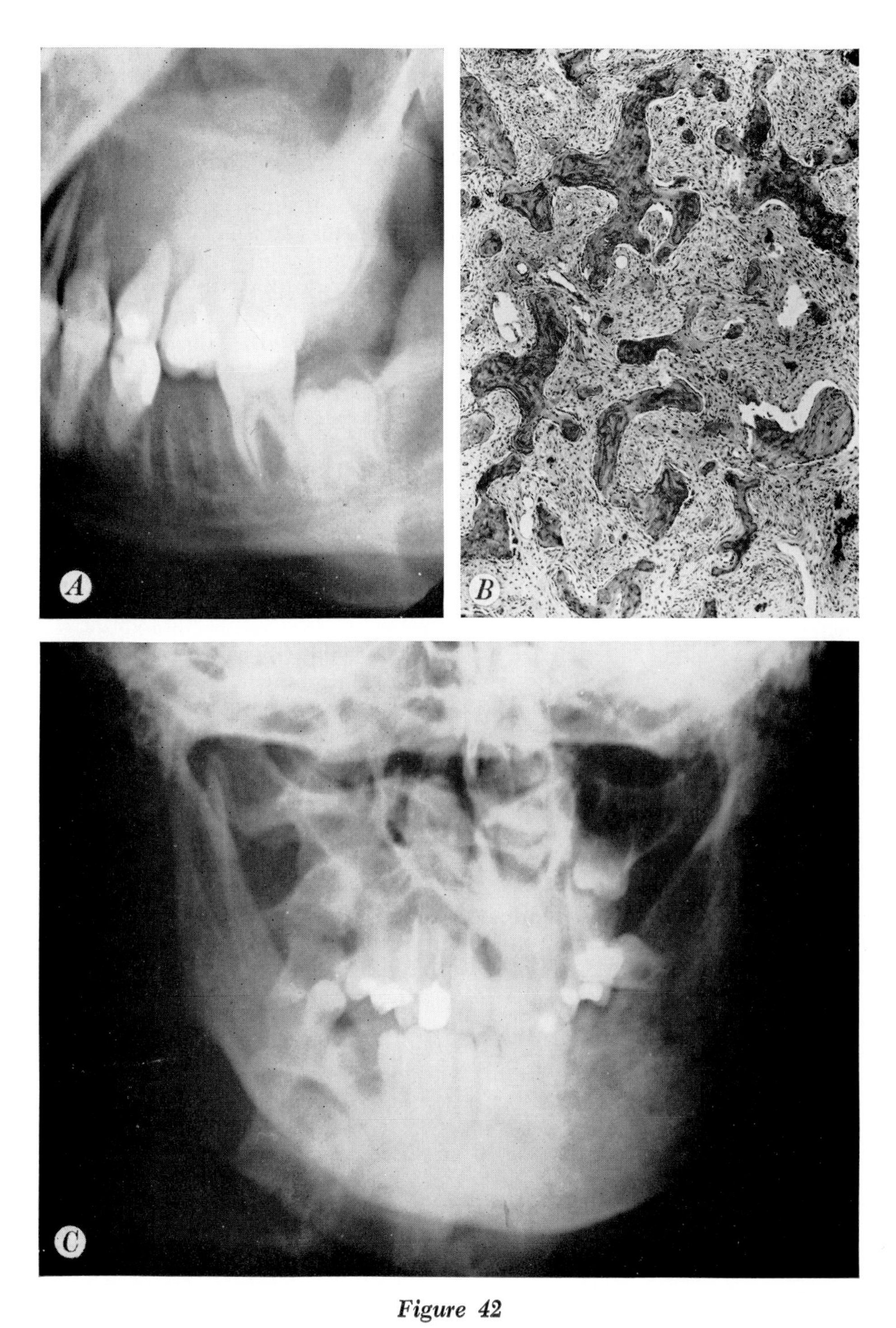

*Figure 42*

In any event, whatever the age when the patient comes under treatment for the condition, inquiry reveals that the swelling is of long standing, sometimes having been present for years. It is nearly always merely the swelling that first draws attention to the condition, for the lesion itself is seldom painful. Occasionally, the facial asymmetry is so slight that it has gone unnoticed by the patient altogether until dental care sought in some other connection has led to discovery of the abnormality in the jaw. Furthermore, when discovered and observed over a period of time, the swelling may seem to be stationary, or at least be found to be increasing very slowly. In only a very occasional case does one get a history of rapid enlargement of the affected jawbone. In a case in which a maxilla is involved, one sometimes finds deformity of the orbit and ocular proptosis. Occasionally, also, the progressive growth of the lesion may cause pressure upon one or another of the local nerves.

Now, what is the relation of these so-called fibrous osteomas of jawbones to the entity of fibrous dysplasia of bone? It should be noted in this connection that, in 1937, when Phemister designated these lesions as fibrous osteomas of jawbones, the concept of fibrous dysplasia of bone was just evolving. It soon came to be recognized that some patients presenting a so-called fibrous osteoma of a maxilla or mandible had analogous fibro-osseous lesions in extracranial parts of the skeleton. That in such cases the jaw lesion is to be correlated into a total picture of fibrous dysplasia seems clear. (See Figs. 40-*A*, *B*, and *C*.)

The difficult question is whether the solitary fibro-osseous lesions of jawbones should likewise be interpreted as representing fibrous dysplasia. There can be no doubt that, in many of these cases, the histologic tissue pattern of the jawbone lesion is indistinguishable from that of a rather heavily ossified fibrodysplastic lesion in an extracranial skeletal location. Thus, the tendency of the solitary fibro-osseous jawbone lesions to be on the osseous side of the fibro-osseous complex does not militate against classifying them as lesions of fibrous dysplasia. (See Fig. 42.)

Whether the completely osseous or eburnated solitary lesions of jawbones and other facial bones (often denoted as osteomas) should likewise be regarded as solitary expressions of fibrous dysplasia is still an open question. If one could prove that they represent the terminal stage of a lesion which, in an earlier stage, was fibro-osseous, the answer would be "yes." If, on the contrary, these lesions are highly eburnated from the beginning, they may represent a different condition, for which the name "osteoma" would indeed be warranted. At any rate, the writer is inclined, on the whole, to draw even rather highly ossified solitary lesions of jawbones into the category of fibrous dysplasia because of the exceptionally strong tendency of primary fibro-osseous lesions toward sclerotization when they occur in jawbones.

**Leontiasis Ossea and Unilateral Cranial Hyperostosis vs. Fibrous Dysplasia.**— As originally used by Virchow, "leontiasis ossea" was a descriptive term. Specifically, it was applied to leonine disfigurement of the head, resulting from more or less symmetrical hyperostotic thickening of the bones of the craniofacial skeleton. Such cases (that is, genuine cases of leontiasis ossea) are rare. There can be no doubt that, in an occasional instance, the leontiasis ossea has an inflammatory basis and is the result of a protracted and creeping osteoperiostitis. In the other instances, the widespread thickening is the result of a process of fibro-osseous replacement and thickening of the cranium. Certainly, leontiasis ossea on an inflammatory basis has nothing in common with fibrous dysplasia, and it is to be doubted that the other cases of leontiasis ossea are to be related to fibrous dysplasia either.

However, the term "leontiasis ossea" has come to be applied also to cases of "unilateral cranial hyperostosis" and "hemihypertrophy of the cranium." In these various types of cases, tissue examination usually shows that the bone thickening results from a process of fibro-osseous replacement and overgrowth which does simulate, to some extent, what one finds in fibrous dysplasia. The question still to be answered is whether, in such cases, the cranial lesions are to be interpreted (in analogy with the solitary jawbone lesions already discussed) merely as localized forms of fibrous dysplasia.

The writer still has an open mind on this point. On the one hand, he has yet to see a case in which such widespread cranial alterations were associated with extensive changes clearly representing fibrous dysplasia elsewhere in the skeleton. On the other hand, in cases of fibrous dysplasia in which many trunk and limb bones are affected, though one almost always finds one or more foci of cranial involvement, the latter does not, in the writer's experience, reach the magnitude of "unilateral cranial hyperostosis" or "hemihypertrophy of the cranium." Thus the noting of cases in which the presence of such cranial involvement is associated with extensive fibro-osseous changes elsewhere in the skeleton would be very welcome in support of the conception that such cranial lesions, too, represent an expression of fibrous dysplasia of bone.

**Hyperparathyroidism.**—Before the concept of fibrous dysplasia had become well delineated it was not unusual for cases in which the skeletal involvement was extensive to be misdiagnosed as cases of hyperparathyroidism. The confusion of such cases of fibrous dysplasia with hyperparathyroidism usually arose on the basis of misinterpretation of the *x*-ray findings. To avoid the error, however, one has only to bear in mind that the only aberration at all likely to be shown by the blood in cases of fibrous dysplasia is an elevation of the serum alkaline phosphatase activity value. Although in some cases of fibrous dysplasia this value is hardly above normal in spite of the fact that many bones are involved, there are other cases in which we have found the value as high as 17 or even 20 Bodansky units. On the other hand, in contrast to what one finds in hyperparathyroidism, the serum calcium value is never elevated in cases of fibrous dysplasia. Also, in cases of fibrous dysplasia in which mineral balance studies (calcium and phosphorus) have been done, these have always yielded values within the normal range, which is again not what is encountered in hyperparathyroidism.

**Skeletal Enchondromatosis.**—In the writer's experience, the only condition which is at all likely to raise the problem of differential diagnosis from fibrous dysplasia on a clinical basis is skeletal enchondromatosis of the Ollier type—that is, enchondromatosis limited to some bones of one limb, or involving predominantly the bones on one side of the body. However, in cases of this type, if hand or foot bones are involved, the punched-out rarefactions in the shafts of the phalanges and metacarpal bones, and the bulging of the contours of some of them, as seen roentgenographically, are almost sufficient in themselves to show that the condition is enchondromatosis (p. 184) and not fibrous dysplasia. Anatomically, of course, in enchondromatosis, the abnormal tissue occupying the interior of the affected bones is primarily and essentially cartilage, so that, on this basis, there is no likelihood of confusion with the abnormal tissue in the interior of bones affected with fibrous dysplasia.

**Lipid Granulomatosis.**—It has been maintained (notably by Snapper) that fibrous dysplasia does not represent a disease entity at all, and that it represents instead an atypical clinical expression of Hand-Schüller-Christian disease (lipid granulomatosis). This idea is already partly controverted by the fact that the lesions of lipid granulomatosis tend to be irregularly distributed over the skeleton, while the lesions of fibrous dysplasia in multiple foci are often limited even strictly to some bones of one limb. Furthermore, though "foam cells" are sometimes found in the lesional tissue of fibrous dysplasia, they are found only occasionally and are not numerous. In lipid granulomatosis, they are found regularly and in striking numbers. Again, one sometimes sees, in the lesions of fibrous dysplasia, larger or smaller foci of hyaline cartilage imbedded in the connective-tissue substratum. This finding is not a feature of the pathology of the bone lesions in Schüller-Christian disease. Also, in cases of the latter disease (including cases showing the Christian triad) yellow-brown melanin pigmentation of the skin, in the form of plaques, patches or spots does not occur. In pronounced cases of fibrous dysplasia, it is commonly seen and is indeed part of the disease syndrome as a whole. Furthermore, sexual precocity, especially in females, does not appear in connection with lipid granulomatosis, while it is sometimes a feature in pronounced cases of fibrous dysplasia.

**Neurofibromatosis.**—It has been contended (see Thannhauser) that fibrous dysplasia of bone (or, as he preferred to call it, "osteitis fibrosa cystica localisata et disseminata") is not an independent entity. He related it by its clinical and histological features to neurofibromatosis of Recklinghausen. Specifically, he connected these two conditions on the basis of supposedly similar skeletal lesions, abnormalities in pigmentation, and endocrine abnormalities (especially precocious puberty). This idea distorts the essential nature of both neurofibromatosis and fibrous dysplasia. It does so especially by overemphasizing the skin pigmentation and underemphasizing the specific character of the skeletal lesions in fibrous dysplasia. The idea of the unity of the two disorders also neglects the genetic difference between them. This difference is indicated by the recognized hereditary and familial character of neurofibromatosis in contrast to fibrous dysplasia. (For further details relating to the skeletal changes of neurofibromatosis, *see* Chapter 16.)

## TREATMENT

As to the skeletal lesions in a given case of fibrous dysplasia, the mere fact of their presence is not in itself an indication for treatment. Only those lesions should be treated which are causing pain or predisposing the bone to fracture or which (notably in facial bones) have created disfiguring swellings. For lesions in the maxilla, mandible, or other facial bones, resections have commonly been done in the past. Actually, however, such radical surgical treatment is contraindicated for them. Surgery can safely be held to the minimum which will be effective in reducing the size of the lesion sufficiently for cosmetic purposes, or for relieving pressure on adjacent structures.

For a long bone lesion which is small but is causing clinical difficulty, thorough curettage and filling of the resultant cavity with bone chips is indicated. On the other hand, for a symptomatic lesion in a rib, resection is preferable to curettement. If an individual lesion is large and the area affected is one subjected to heavy loading (notably the upper end of a femoral shaft) it is advisable to supplement curettage by the insertion of a massive autogenous bone graft. In fact, such a graft may have to be used subsequently in a case in which curettement and the introduction of autogenous or homogenous bone chips was the treatment used, since such chips may be resorbed and the lesion recur. A severe deformity of a long bone may make it necessary to support the area with a metal prosthesis.

Apparently nothing can be done for the abnormal skin pigmentation. Probably nothing should be done for the pubertas praecox, which, as noted, sometimes ceases to cause difficulty as the patient grows up.

The outlook as a whole need not be too pessimistic, even in the cases of severest disease. It is true that life expectancy is short in some of these—particularly the ones in which the associated extraskeletal (and especially glandular) abnormalities are already present in early childhood. However, the patients presenting only limited or moderate expressions of the disorder (the vast majority) seem to have a normal life expectancy, and those in whom only one bone is affected certainly do. The danger that a bone which is the site of fibrous dysplasia will undergo malignant transformation is certainly slight, but, as noted, does exist.

## REFERENCES


ALBRIGHT, F.: Polyostotic Fibrous Dysplasia: A Defense of the Entity, J. Clin. Endocrinol., *7*, 307, 1947.

ALBRIGHT, F., BUTLER, A. M., HAMPTON, A. O., and SMITH, P.: Syndrome Characterized by Osteitis Fibrosa Disseminata, Areas of Pigmentation and Endocrine Dysfunction, with Precocious Puberty in Females, New England J. Med., *216*, 727, 1937.

ARNESEN, H. C., and NITTER, L.: Polyostotisk fibrøs dysplasi (Albright's syndrom) med multiple bløtdelstumores, Nord. med., *45*, 735, 1951.

BERGER, A., and JAFFE, H. L.: Fibrous (Fibro-Osseous) Dysplasia of Jawbones, J. Oral Surg., *11*, 3, 1953.

COLEMAN, M.: Osteitis Fibrosa Disseminata, Brit. J. Surg., *26*, 705, 1939.

COLEY, B. L., and STEWART, F. W.: Bone Sarcoma in Polyostotic Fibrous Dysplasia, Ann. Surg., *121*, 872, 1945.

DOCKERTY, M. B., GHORMLEY, R. K., KENNEDY, R. L. J., and PUGH, D. G.: Albright's Syndrome (Polyostotic Fibrous Dysplasia with Cutaneous Pigmentation in Both Sexes and Gonadal Dysfunction in Females), Arch. Int. Med., *75*, 357, 1945.

DUSTIN, P., JR., and LEY, R. A.: Contribution à l'étude des dysplasies osseuses: description anatomo-clinique d'un cas d'ostéosarcome polymorphe chez un enfant atteint de fibro-xanthomatose osseuse avec prématuration sexuelle, Rev. belge path. et méd. expér., *20*, 52, 1950.

FALCONER, M. A., COPE, C. L., and ROBB-SMITH, A. H. T.: Fibrous Dysplasia of Bone with Endocrine Disorders and Cutaneous Pigmentation (Albright's Disease), Quart. J. Med., *11*, 121, 1942.

FERRERO, C.: La Maladie de Jaffe-Lichtenstein: Ostéofibromatose kystique, Presse méd. 55, 142, 1947.

JAFFE, H. L.: Fibrous Dysplasia of Bone: A Disease Entity and Specifically not an Expression of Neurofibromatosis, J. Mt. Sinai Hosp., *12*, 364, 1945.

————: Fibrous Dysplasia of Bone, Bull. New York Acad. Med., *22*, 588, 1946.

————: Lesioni solitarie osteofibrose delle ossa in rapporto alla displasia fibrosa (osteofibrosa) delle ossa in generale, Arch. "Putti," *4*, 33, 1954.

LICHTENSTEIN, L.: Polyostotic Fibrous Dysplasia, Arch. Surg., *36*, 874, 1938.

LICHTENSTEIN, L., and JAFFE, H. L.: Fibrous Dysplasia of Bone: A Condition Affecting One, Several or Many Bones, the Graver Cases of Which May Present Abnormal Pigmentation of Skin, Premature Sexual Development, Hyperthyroidism or Still Other Extraskeletal Abnormalities, Arch. Path., *33*, 777, 1942.

LUNDBAEK, K., and OLSEN, T.: Dysplasia fibrosa ossium, Ugesk. f. laeger, *113*, 455, 1951.

MCCUNE, D. J., and BRUCH, H.: Osteodystrophia Fibrosa: Report of a Case in Which the Condition was Combined with Precocious Puberty, Pathologic Pigmentation of the Skin and Hyperthyroidism, Am. J. Dis. Child., *54*, 806, 1937.

PECK, F. B., and SAGE, C. V.: Diabetes Mellitus Associated with Albright's Syndrome (Osteitis Fibrosa Disseminata, Areas of Skin Pigmentation, and Endocrine Dysfunction with Precocious Puberty in Females), Am. J. M. Sc., *208*, 35, 1944.

PHEMISTER, D. B., and GRIMSON, K. S.: Fibrous Osteoma of the Jaws, Ann. Surg., *105*, 564, 1937.

PUGH, D. G.: Fibrous Dysplasia of the Skull: A Probable Explanation for Leontiasis Ossea, Radiology, *44*, 548, 1945.

RUSHTON, M. A.: Regional Osteitis Fibrosa Affecting the Facial Bones, Proc. Roy. Soc. Med London, *40*, 316, 1947.

SCHLUMBERGER, H. G.: Fibrous Dysplasia of Single Bones (Monostotic Fibrous Dysplasid), Mil. Surgeon, *99*, 504, 1946; *and* Fibrous Dysplasia (Ossifying Fibroma) of the Maxillaaan Mandible, Am. J. Orthodontics, *32*, 579, 1946.

SHERMAN, R. S., and STERNBERGH, W. C. A.: The Roentgen Appearance of Ossifying Fibroma of Bone, Radiology, *50*, 595, 1948.

SMITH, A. G., and ZAVALETA, A.: Osteoma, Ossifying Fibroma, and Fibrous Dysplasia of Facial and Cranial Bones, Arch. Path., *54*, 507, 1952.

SNAPPER, I.: *Medical Clinics on Bone Diseases*, Interscience Publishers, Inc., New York, 1943 (pp. 157–171).

STAUFFER, H. M., ARBUCKLE, R. K., and AEGERTER, E. E.: Polyostotic Fibrous Dysplasia with Cutaneous Pigmentation and Congenital Arteriovenous Aneurysms, J. Bone & Joint Surg., *23*, 323, 1941.

STERNBERG, W. H., and JOSEPH, V.: Osteodystrophia Fibrosa Combined with Precocious Puberty and Exophthalmic Goiter, Am. J. Dis. Child., *63*, 748, 1942.

STRASSBURGER, P., GARBER, C. Z., and HALLOCK, H.: Fibrous Dysplasia of Bone, J. Bone & Joint Surg., *33-A*, 407, 1951.

SUTRO, C. J.: Osteogenic Sarcoma of the Tibia in a Limb Affected with Fibrous Dysplasia, Bull. Hosp. Joint Dis., *12*, 217, 1951.

THANNHAUSER, S. J.: Neurofibromatosis (von Recklinghausen) and Osteitis Fibrosa Cystica Localisata et Disseminata (von Recklinghausen), Medicine, *23*, 105, 1944.

UEHLINGER, E.: Osteofibrosis deformans juvenilis: (Polyostotische fibröse Dysplasie Jaffe-Lichtenstein), Virchows Arch. f. path. Anat., *306*, 255, 1940.

VINES, R. H.: Polyostotic Fibrous Dysplasia, Arch. Dis. in Childhood, *27*, 351, 1952.

WINDHOLZ, F.: Cranial Manifestations of Fibrous Dysplasia of Bone, Am. J. Roentgenol., *58*, 51, 1947.

ZIMMER, J. F., DAHLIN, D. C., PUGH, D. G., and CLAGETT, O. T.: Fibrous Dysplasia of Bone: An Analysis of 15 Cases of Surgically Verified Costal Fibrous Dysplasia, J. Thoracic Surg., *31*, 488, 1956.

Chapter

# 10

# Solitary and Multiple Osteocartilaginous Exostosis

Both solitary and multiple osteocartilaginous exostosis are characterized by the presence of sessile and/or stalked cartilage-capped protrusions from the affected bone part or parts. In cases of *solitary exostosis,* only a single skeletal part is affected—most often a juxta-epiphysial area of a long bone shaft. In cases of *multiple exostosis* the lesions are usually widely distributed over the skeleton, though most prominent in the juxta-epiphysial areas of the long bones. The two conditions tend to differ also in that the extent of involvement of an individual affected bone area is greater in cases of multiple than in cases of solitary exostosis. For instance, at the lower end of an affected femoral shaft in a case of multiple exostosis the entire circumference of the shaft is likely to be modified, while in a case of solitary exostosis involving the area in question only a small part of the shaft circumference is altered. The clinical implications of the two conditions are also different, since multiple exostosis is a hereditary disorder while solitary exostosis apparently is not.

## SOLITARY OSTEOCARTILAGINOUS EXOSTOSIS

The condition of solitary osteocartilaginous exostosis is often also denoted as *solitary osteochondroma* or simply *osteochondroma.* It is one of the most common of the primary tumorous skeletal affections. As already indicated, an osteocartilaginous exostosis represents a more or less cartilage-capped osseous projection from a bone. It appears only in relation to bones preformed in cartilage, and is most likely to be found in a juxta-epiphysial area of the shaft of a long tubular bone.

In relation to the terminal phalanges, and particularly the terminal phalanx of the great toe, one occasionally encounters the *subungual exostosis.* This outgrowth, too, is cartilage-capped. However, it develops at the distal end of the bone—that is, in an area not adjacent to an epiphysis. Hence, the subungual exostosis, though suggesting an osteocartilaginous exostosis, is probably not precisely the same type of lesion.

In relation to skull bones, one occasionally encounters a so-called *ivory exostosis.* This is a bump on the affected bone area, but one which is not capped by cartilage. Its usual site is a calvarial bone, in accordance with the fact that an ivory exostosis ordinarily develops in relation to a bone preformed in membrane and not one preformed in cartilage.

### CLINICAL CONSIDERATIONS

**Incidence.**—There appears to be no significant sex difference in the incidence of the condition, to judge from personal experience with several hundred cases. As to age, one finds that an appreciable number of the patients are young children at the time when the lesion is discovered. However, the great majority of the patients are between 10 and 20 years of age when they are admitted to a hospital for treatment. In regard to these patients, the presence of a bony bump or lump may already have been known for some years.

**Localization.**—As noted, cartilage-capped exostoses develop only in relation to bones preformed in cartilage. The juxta-epiphysial localization of solitary osteocartilaginous exostosis has likewise already been mentioned. Specifically, in relation to an affected bone, the lesion lies away, but not far away, from the nearest growth zone. By far the most common locations of the lesion are the lower metaphysis of the femur and the upper metaphysis of the tibia. Indeed, these sites together will be found to account for about half of the locations in any large series of cases. The other metaphysial long bone areas together account for a large proportion of the remaining half of the localizations. Among these, the ones predilected are the upper end of the humerus, the lower end of the radius, the lower end of the tibia, and the upper and lower ends of the fibula. An osteocartilaginous exostosis may also appear at any other juxta-epiphysial site. However, the more common of these less frequent localizations are a juxta-epiphysial area of the metacarpal or metatarsal bone, an iliac bone, or a scapula. (See Fig. 43.)

Though the bones of the wrist and midtarsus are preformed in cartilage, they are only exceptionally the site of a solitary cartilaginous exostosis. These bones develop like the epiphysis of the tubular bones, from a centrifugally expanding center of ossification. Hence, the sparing of these bones would seem to have the same basis as the fact that even in predilected bones the exostosis develops not on the epiphysis, but on the shaft, juxta-epiphysially. The occurrence of a cartilage-capped exostosis on one or another of the skull bones preformed in cartilage is also rare. If one does appear there, it is usually a relatively small lesion.

**Clinical Complaints.**—Ordinarily, the exostosis creates no clinical difficulties of any consequence. It is usually discovered merely through the palpation of a lump on the affected bone, being painless in most instances. Even when an exostosis does become painful, the pain is seldom severe. It may result from irritation of the lesion in the course of function, or from pressure on the overlying soft parts and

***Figure 43***

*A*, Roentgenograph showing a hook-like solitary exostosis projecting from the lower lateral aspect of a femoral shaft. The patient was a man 20 years of age. He had first become aware of the presence of a bump in this area 4 years previously, after being struck there by a baseball. The resected specimen showed only a thin layer of residual cartilage at the extreme tip of the outgrowth.

*B*, Roentgenograph showing a stalked solitary exostosis springing from the medial part of a femoral shaft. The end of the exostosis flares out and is rather knobby. The patient was a girl 16 years of age who had been aware of a bump in the region in question for about a year, but who had no other complaints. When removed, the exostosis was found covered with cartilage only at its flared end. Just beneath this cartilage there were some calcific areas extending for only a slight distance below the surface. The ring of radiopacity to be seen at the end of the exostosis represents the presence of the calcific material near the end of the lesion.

*C*, Roentgenograph showing a flat, sessile exostosis on the anteromedial aspect of a tibia of a girl 13 years of age. There were no clinical complaints, although the patient had been aware of a local prominence for about 2 years. In conformity with the *x*-ray picture, the specimen showed merely a cartilage-capped protrusion, beneath which endochondral ossification was proceeding in an orderly fashion, as shown in Figure 44-*E*.

*D*, Roentgenograph of a large, essentially sessile, exostotic outgrowth from the posterior surface of the upper part of a tibial shaft in a girl 17 years of age. The considerable radiopacity of the lesion reflects the presence of large amounts of calcified cartilage and calcium detritus extending into the interior of the lesion from the surface, as shown in Figure 45-*D*.

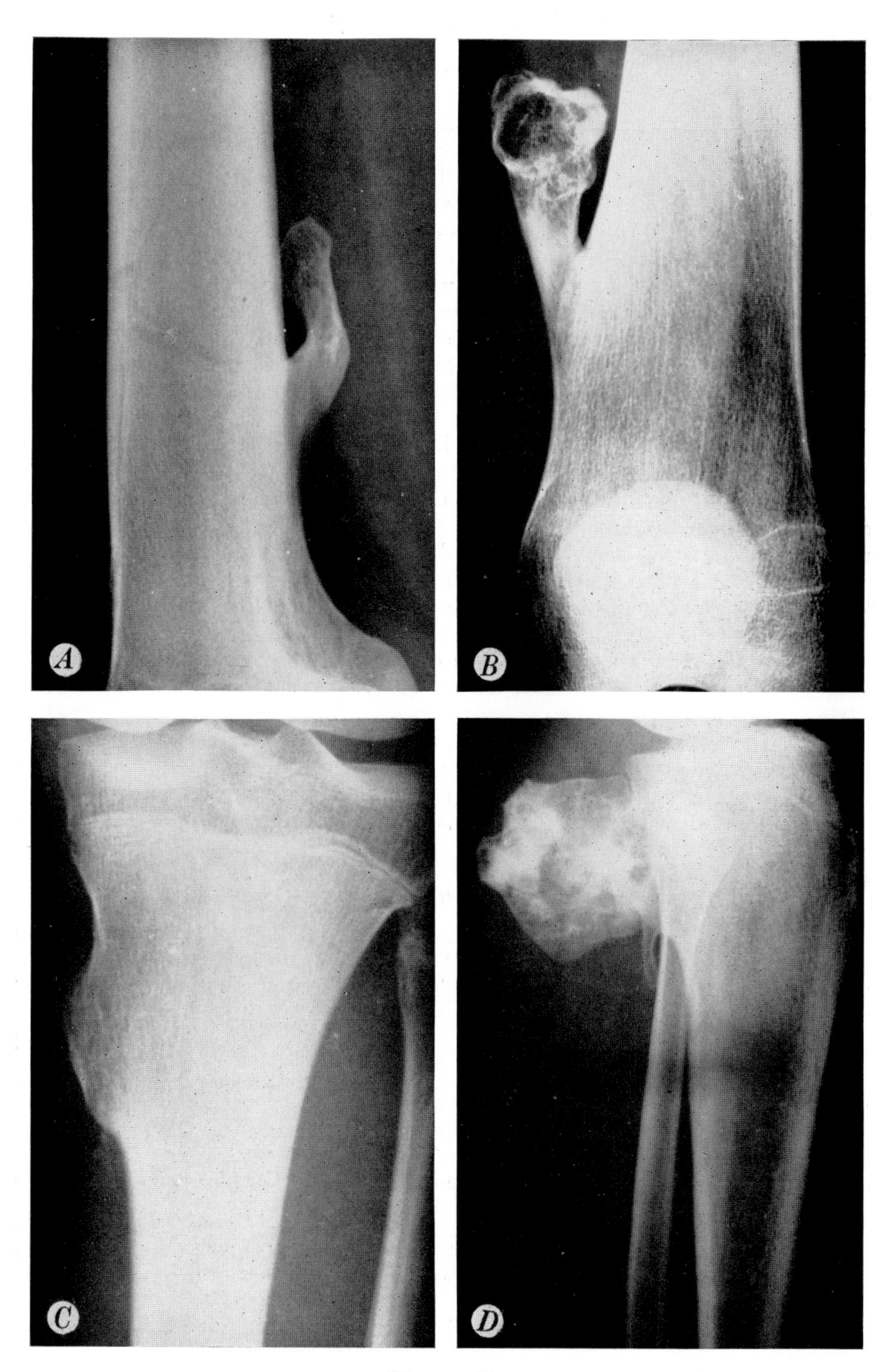


*Figure 43*

especially from impingement on a nerve. Or the pain may have been induced by a trauma to the lesion. Also, a hitherto painless exostosis sometimes becomes painful after a trauma which had actually induced a fracture through the base or stalk of the lesion.

## PATHOLOGIC AND ROENTGENOGRAPHIC FINDINGS

**Pathology.**—In general, an osteocartilaginous exostosis takes the form of a sessile or stalked protuberance jutting from the affected bone and merging at its base into the cortex. In one case or another, the exostosis may be no more than 1 or 2 cm. in its largest diameter, while in still other cases it may measure 10 cm. or more. The contour of a sessile lesion may be plateau-like or roundish, and its surface may be rather smooth or quite knobby. A stalked lesion may have a short stem, and its end may be rather flat or even mushroom-like, or rounded and perhaps knobby. On the other hand, a stalked lesion may appear elongated and mainly tubular or conical in shape and present a pronged end which may even be spiked or hooked.

In any case, the exostosis is covered by periosteum, which is continuous with that covering the adjacent cortex. This periosteum adheres closely to any knobs or depressions on the surface of the lesion. It is composed of poorly vascularized collagenous connective tissue. This may be thin and delicate, but, more often, it is rather thick and strips away with difficulty. On stripping the periosteum from a sessile lesion, one finds that part or much of its surface is covered by a cap of hyaline cartilage. If the lesion is a stalked one, cartilage is found merely toward its end, the rest of the stalk surface being osseous.

To study the gross architecture of an osteochondroma more fully, it is best to section the lesion at right angles to its convexity. When a lesion is so cut, the cartilage may be found continuous over the entire surface or covering only its central part. In general, the younger the patient, the greater the proportion of surface that is covered by cartilage and the thicker the layer. In any case, the thickness of the cartilage is not uniform and ordinarily measures only a few millimeters at most. Wherever the surface is not cartilaginous, it consists of a thin plate of osseous tissue.

***Figure 44***

*A*, Photograph of a sessile, cauliflower-shaped exostosis springing from a scapula. The surface of the outgrowth has been denuded of its periosteal covering. Note that the cortex of the scapula is continuous with the cortex of the exostotic protrusion. Note also that the cap of the outgrowth is covered with cartilage.

*B*, Photograph of specimen shown in *A*, after sectioning at right angles to the surface. Note the thickness of the cartilage in the cap region. Note also that most of the interior of the lesion consists of loose-meshed spongy bone. The picture also shows very well the continuity of the cortex of the scapula with that of the exostosis.

*C*, Photograph of a stalked exostosis terminating in a globular knob. The lesion had been removed from the lower metaphysial area of a femur of a boy 10 years of age. Note that the surface of the knob is covered with cartilage and that its interior consists of rather loose-meshed spongy bone.

*D*, Roentgenograph of a femur presenting a stalked solitary exostotic lesion like the one shown in *C*. Note the absence of radiopacities in the lesional area. This absence is due to the fact that the lesion does not contain any calcified cartilage and/or calcific detritus below the surface of the knob.

*E*, Photomicrograph (× 5) showing the histologic pattern of an osteocartilaginous exostosis which is covered by a proliferating cap of cartilage. At the cartilage-bone junction, endochondral ossification is proceeding in an orderly fashion, essentially as it takes place in a growing epiphysial cartilage plate.

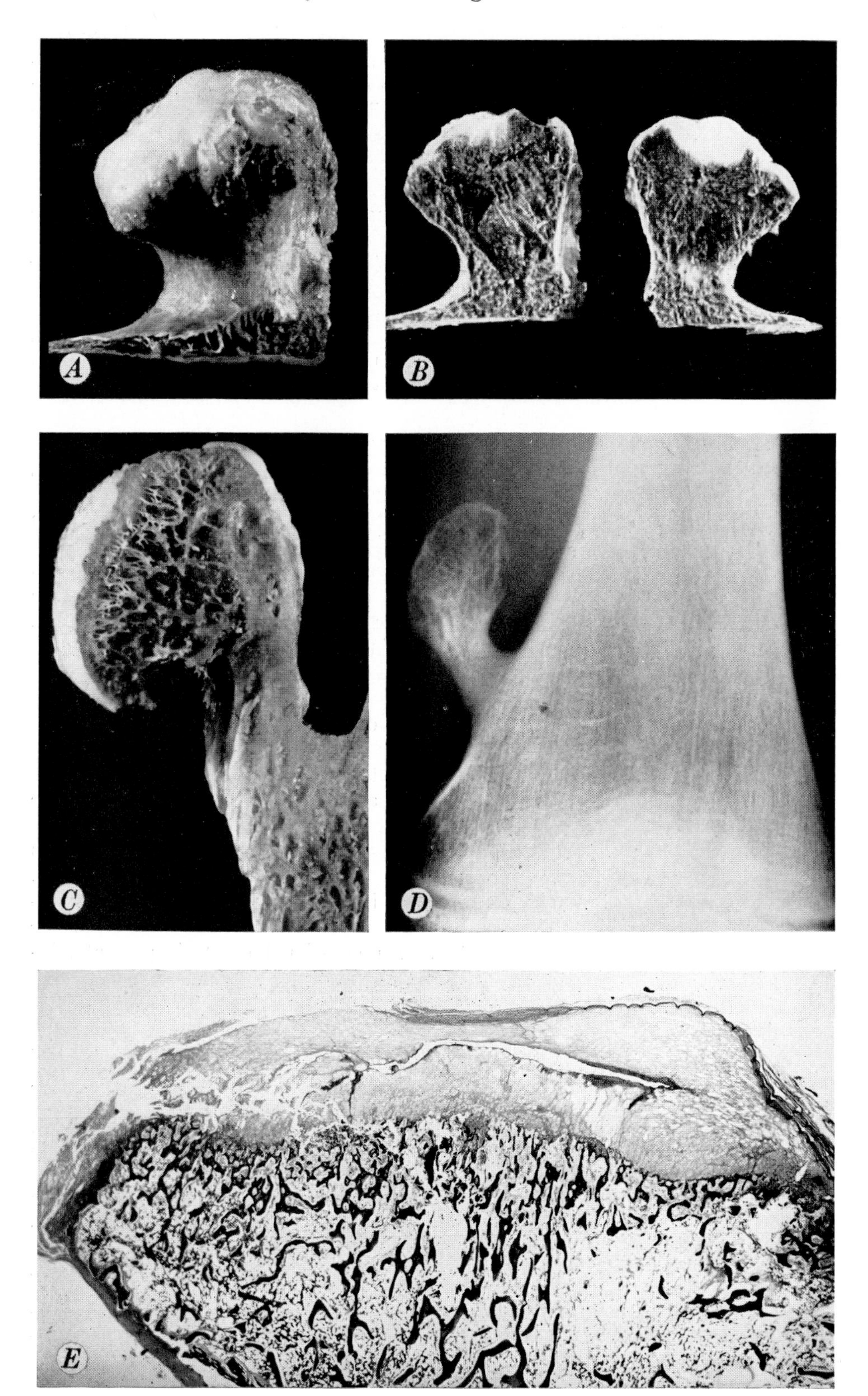


*Figure 44*

Internally, the lesion is composed of spongy bone, and indeed spongy bone constitutes the bulk of an exostosis. The marrow between the bony trabeculæ is predominantly fatty. Occasionally, one or more smaller or larger irregular, yellow gritty foc i may be observed beneath the cartilage cap. These are made up, as histologic examination shows, of a complex mosaic of highly calcified cartilage and bone and calcium detritus. Apparently, they result from the piling up of cartilage matrix in the interior of the exostosis, in connection with disordered endochondral growth of the lesion, possibly due to interference with the local blood supply (see Fig. 44 and also Fig. 45).

An osteocartilaginous exostosis grows by endochondral ossification on the inner surface of the cartilage cap, after the manner of growth of an epiphysial cartilage plate. Thus, in a lesion removed from a child or adolescent, microscopic examination will usually still reveal evidences of growth activity on the inner surface of the cap. As a rule, the cartilage has ceased to proliferate by the time the patient has reached the end of his growth. The quiescent cartilage becomes closed off by a thin plate of bone, and the residual cartilage itself may undergo regressive changes. It should be noted that, in connection with an occasional lesion, the cartilage ceases to proliferate even though the patient is still a child or adolescent. In any event, remnants of quiescent cartilage can still be found in the cap, far into adult life.

Not infrequently, a bursa (exostosis bursata) appears in connection with an osteocartilaginous exostosis. This is so particularly when the exostosis is large and presses upon overlying soft parts. The bursal sac is generally attached around the base of the exostosis. The bursal wall may be quite thin, but the writer has seen several instances in which the bursal wall came to reach about 1 cm. in thickness. In one instance or another, the inner surface of the bursa is lined by a layer of cells resembling synovial lining cells. In other instances, especially when there has been considerable local traumatic irritation of the bursa, the bursal wall is found to be quite vascularized and may even show deposits of fibrin on the surface. The bursal sac contains mucinous fluid, often fibrinoid rice bodies, and occasionally also fairly large calcified cartilage bodies, entirely like joint mice. Indeed, in one of the cases personally studied, the bursa contained about a dozen flat, calcified bodies of the shape of lima beans.

**Roentgenographic Appearances.**—The osteocartilaginous exostosis is an obvious lesion roentgenographically. In fact, it can hardly be mistaken for anything else. It is to be noted that the exostosis, whatever its shape, is usually directed shaftward—that is, away from the epiphysial end of the bone. The contour of the exostosis is usually sharply demarcated. An occasional exostosis presents, in-

***Figure 45***

*A*, Roentgenograph of a large solitary exostosis which springs from the juxta-epiphysial region of the crest of an ilium. The patient was a man 28 years of age who, for many years, had been aware of the presence of a mass in the left side. His only complaint was of slight local discomfort. Note that there is considerable radiopacity, especially in the upper half of the lesional area. This reflects the presence of calcified cartilage and calcific detritus in the interior of the lesion (see *D*).

*B*, Photograph of the cut surface of part of an osteochondroma which likewise sprang from an ilium. Note, in the upper left-hand part of the picture, the white, tonguelike projection, which is composed of calcified cartilage and calcareous detritus.

*C*, Roentgenograph of the area shown in *B*. Note the area of radiopacity corresponding to the tonguelike projection shown in *B*.

*D*, Photomicrograph (× 5) showing the histologic pattern presented by the radiopaque area shown in *A*. Note the considerable calcified cartilage matrix and detritus below the cartilage cap of the exostosis.

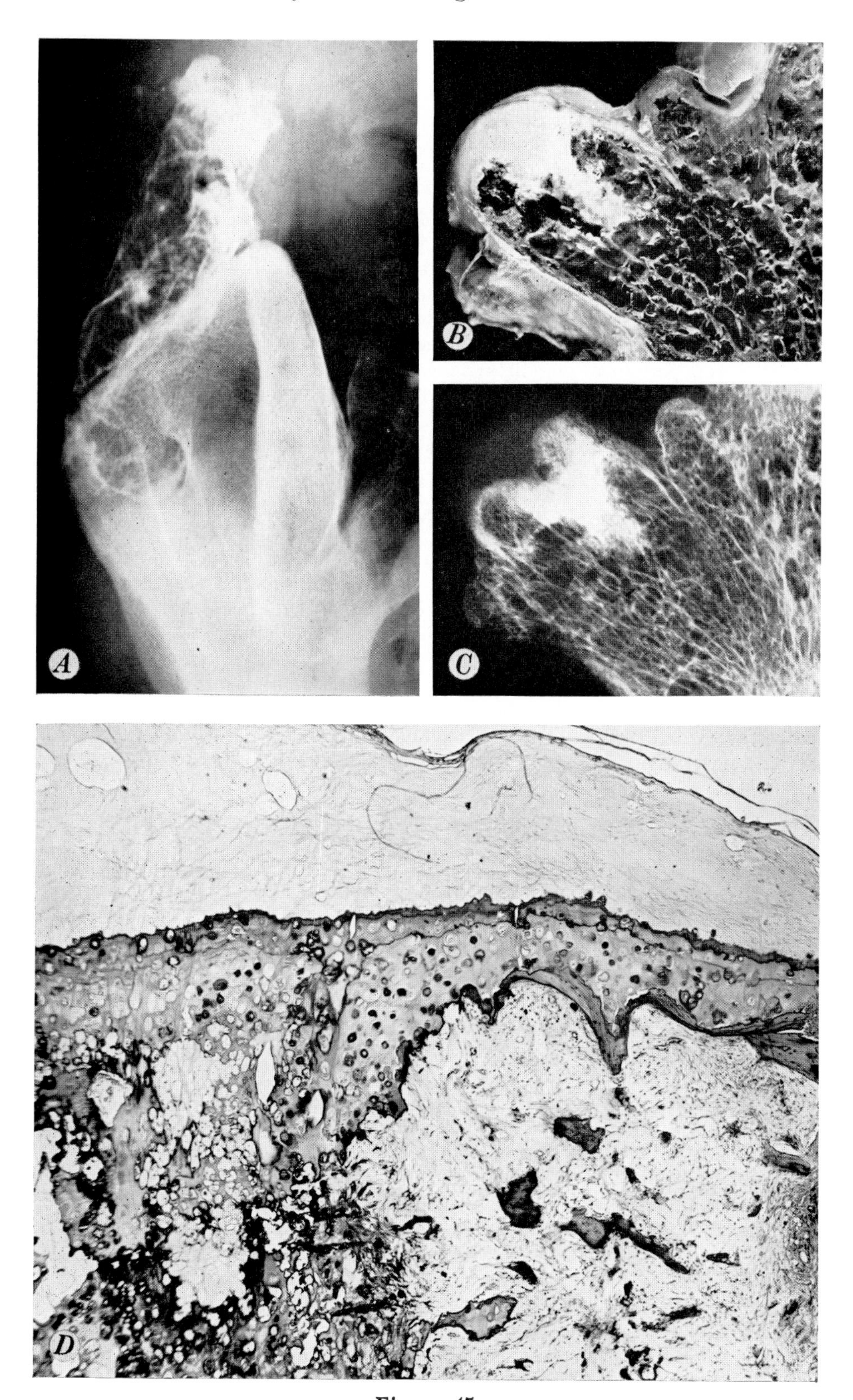


*Figure 45*

teriorly to its delimiting wall, smaller or larger blotches of radiopacity. These represent the piled-up masses of calcified cartilage matrix noted above in connection with the pathology of the lesion. When the blotchy radiopacity is very pronounced, one may make the erroneous deduction that the osteochondroma is undergoing malignant change. However, this idea can be rejected if the outline of the exostosis is uninterrupted and there is no soft-tissue mass outside of it showing streaky radiopacity (see Fig. 45).

**Chondrosarcoma as a Complication.**—Chondrosarcomatous transformation of a *solitary* osteocartilaginous exostosis occurs in only about 1 per cent of the cases, at most. Also, the complication tends not to appear before adulthood, and even not until rather late in life. If an osteochondroma takes on rapid growth activity in adult life, one should suspect that it is undergoing malignant transformation. The chondrosarcoma which develops out of an osteocartilaginous exostosis is often designated as a peripheral chondrosarcoma. Peripheral chondrosarcomas usually grow slowly. Even when incompletely extirpated, they tend to recur only locally and do not metastasize for a long time. Thus, this complication is one which can often be completely controlled by surgery. For further details on peripheral chondrosarcoma, see page 332.

### TREATMENT

The mere presence of a solitary exostosis is not in itself a valid reason for its removal. This is indicated, however, if the lesion creates any clinical difficulties or any disfigurement. Obviously an osteochondroma which, after having been quiescent, takes on a sudden spurt of growth should be removed, and, specifically, should be widely resected. In general, when a solitary exostosis is being removed, its periosteal covering should also be removed (rather than merely stripped back), since, at least theoretically, this covering may be a source for recurrence. Actually, however, this usually does not take place unless one is dealing with one of the rare cases in which the cartilage cap is undergoing malignant transformation.

## HEREDITARY MULTIPLE EXOSTOSIS

Hereditary multiple exostosis (multiple exostosis) represents an anomaly of skeletal development whose characteristic feature is the presence of bony protrusions (of widely different sizes) on the skeleton. The disorder is one which has long been known to have a hereditary background, about half of the offspring of an affected subject coming to manifest the condition.

When the disorder is present in severe form, practically all the bones preformed in cartilage may show the abnormality, at least to some extent. In any case, however, the exostotic protrusions are likely to be most conspicuous on the long bones, and especially in the vicinity of the knees and ankles. Furthermore, the exostoses tend, in general, to have a bilateral and symmetrical distribution. Clinically, multiple exostosis often comes to light in early childhood, through the discovery of one or more painless lumps on bone parts close to the surface of the body. Not infrequently, the subject also presents, even before adolescence, a bowing deformity of one or both forearms, often in association with ulnar deviation of the hand.

**Nomenclature.**—Hereditary multiple exostosis has also been denoted by various other names. These include "diaphysial aclasis" and "hereditary deforming chondrodysplasia." The term "diaphysial aclasis" (commonly used in the British literature), while valuable in pointing out that the modeling of the entire affected bone area is abnormal, emphasizes pathogenesis to the exclusion of concrete appearances, which "multiple exostosis" brings out so well. "Hereditary deforming chondrodysplasia" (a name formerly common in the American literature) is vague and again creates no mental picture of the disorder or its individual lesions. One frequently also encounters descriptions of the condition under the heading of "dyschondroplasia." This name introduces a confusion, since it was coined by Ollier, and is frequently used for cases of predominantly unilateral enchondromatosis (p. 184). Finally, notice must be taken of the name "osteogenic disease," which was formerly often used for the condition in the French and Italian literature. The term was coined to fit the conception of the existence of a basic disorder expressing itself in: multiple exostosis alone, multiple enchondromatosis alone, or these two conditions together. However, the idea of kinship between, and/or coexistence of, these two disorders is not sustained by the actual anatomic findings in the two conditions (p. 166). Hence, the comprehensive name "osteogenic disease" had better be avoided altogether.

## CLINICAL CONSIDERATIONS

**Incidence.**—Though not exactly common, multiple exostosis is by no means rare. Indeed, it is the most common of the systematized anomalies of skeletal development encountered clinically. This is understandable in the light of the absence, in connection with it, of an inherent lethal factor such as is present, for instance, in achondroplasia, osteogenesis imperfecta, and osteopetrosis. Specifically, multiple exostosis does not constitute, as these other disorders commonly do, a hindrance to maturation or birth of the stigmatized fetus. Furthermore, the postnatal skeletal abnormalities characterizing multiple exostosis seldom offer any threat to continued existence before adult life is reached. Later on, it is true, life may be endangered, in one case or another, by the evolution of a chondrosarcoma. However, since the development of a chondrosarcoma is usually a relatively late and only slowly progressive complication, it is not likely to have much effect on the hereditary transfer of the disorder to the next generation.

Males predominate among the affected persons. This is likely to be much more evident if the sex incidence is calculated on the basis of cases in groups of family trees than if one considers merely collected individual cases or groups of individual cases. As calculated on the former basis, the ratio of males to females affected is about 7 to 3.

**Emergence and Clinical Features of the Disorder.**—Apparently, the stigmatized infant only rarely presents any outward manifestations of the disorder at birth. Whether, in a family in which the disorder is known to be present, it would be possible to pick out regularly, by roentgenography, those newborn infants in whom it will subsequently become grossly manifest, one cannot say on the basis of our present knowledge. Most cases of the disorder come to light during childhood. There can be no doubt, however, that some cases (especially mild ones) are never identified clinically at all.

In the clinical cases, one or more bumps on the skeleton have usually been discovered accidentally by the patient or a relative. The writer's own experience is in harmony with the idea that it is only exceptionally that a case comes to light in this way before the patient is 2 years of age. However, from then on until puberty, but more particularly during the earlier years of childhood, the large bulk of the clinical cases is thus brought to medical attention. The discovery of a bump on some bone is followed in the course of time by the appearance and recognition of similar lesions on other bones. As our case records also show, there may be an interval of months or years between the time when lesions are first noted and the time when medical advice is first sought in regard to them. In a general way, this lag is a consequence of the absence of clinical complaints from the condition in young children. In addition, it may result from the fact that a similar condition is present and has proved harmless in one or more adult members of the family. After adolescence, growth of the exostoses slows down, and during adult life new ones apparently do not form.

The presenting protuberance is not infrequently on a scapula (particularly along its vertebral margin). More commonly, however, the bump is to be felt on the metaphysis of some long bone, and especially in the region of the knee, ankle, or shoulder. As more and more exostoses appear, the tendency of the condition to involve the long bones heavily becomes increasingly apparent. In the course of childhood, a subject may come to show a considerable number of obvious prominences on many of the bones, presenting, indeed, a knobby appearance so striking that the condition can be diagnosed by mere inspection of the subject.

In addition to presenting a knobby appearance, the more severely affected subjects may show definite shortness of the limbs in relation to the trunk. Consequently, the superficial appearance may resemble that of mild achondroplasia, but the patients do not present other stigmata of that disease. The shortness of the long bones is due, in the main, not to direct interference with longitudinal growth at the epiphysial cartilage plates (as is the case in achondroplasia), but to dissipation of the longitudinal growth force in a lateral direction at the metaphyses. Through the supplementary agency of curvature and deformity of the forearm, one or both upper limbs are likely to be even more strikingly shortened than the lower (see Fig. 46).

In the early stages of the evolution of the disorder, there are rarely any sub jective complaints—even of discomfort or inconvenience—relating to it. However, sooner or later, most of the subjects experience at least some minor difficulty. For instance, a large exostosis may cause discomfort from direct pressure on the neighboring tissues, though this is often mitigated by the development of a bursa between the growth and the overlying soft parts. Prominent exostoses around the ankle, knee, or hip may not only cause pressure pain but may hinder full normal articular function or gradually disturb the stance and gait. Some subjects present curvature of the tibia and fibula. Disproportionate shortening of the lower limbs may result in some degree of scoliosis.

**Figure 46**

*A*, Photograph of the lower limbs of a boy 15 years of age affected with multiple exostosis Note the knobby swellings and protuberances, especially prominent in the knee region Bumps on many bones had been known to be present at least since the boy was 10 years of age. There were no clinical complaints, however, up to a few months before admission, when he began to experience pain referred to the inner aspect of the right ankle. The boy was of short stature for his age. His parents and his sister seem to be clinically free of exostoses, but nothing is known of the status of other relatives.

*B*, Photograph showing knobby prominences in the ankle regions of another boy 15 years of age affected with multiple exostosis. This boy's younger brother (see *C*) and father likewise showed the disorder, and an uncle, grandfather, and granduncle (all on the paternal side) were reported as also showing it.

*C*, Photograph of the back of a boy 9 years of age (brother of *B*) showing protuberances on the left humerus and right scapula. The bump on the scapula was the presenting lesion in this case.

*D*, Photograph showing typical forearm deformity in the case of a man 21 years of age affected with hereditary multiple exostosis. Both forearms are abnormally short—the right more so than the left. There is ulnar deviation of the right hand, and the head of the radius has been dislocated (see Fig. 48-*C*).

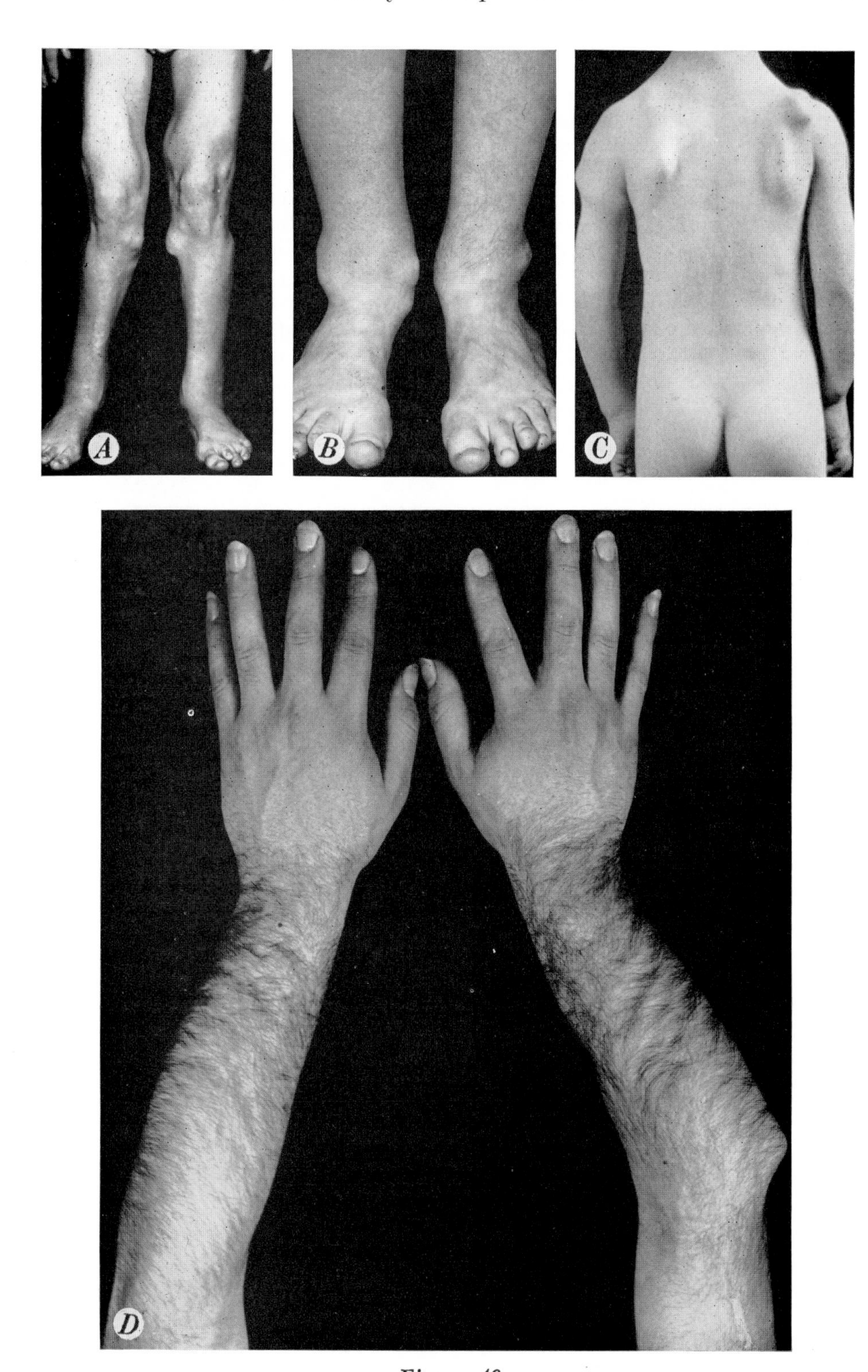


*Figure 46*

Deformity of the forearm, which Hagen was one of the first to discuss in detail, is another common and obvious manifestation of the disorder. The severity of the deformity may be approximately equal in the two forearms, but is usually not so. Indeed, in some cases, one forearm shows no clinical deformity at all, while the other does show it. A deformity of one or both of the forearms may already begin to be noted fairly early in childhood. It is to be found in practically all cases presenting pronounced skeletal involvement by multiple exostoses, and in about one-third of the cases in general. Furthermore, exostotic involvement of the forearm and consequent deformity of it is seen even in some cases in which the rest of the skeleton is relatively lightly affected.

Characteristically, in connection with this deformity one finds that: The ulna is strikingly shortened and its exostotically deformed distal end more or less thimble-shaped or conical; the radius, much less shortened than the ulna, is bowed outward, and the head of the radius may be found more or less dislocated outward and posteriorly. The factors operating in the causation of this deformity are striking retardation of growth at the lower end of the exostotically affected ulna (where about three-quarters of the longitudinal growth of this bone normally occurs) associated with a much lesser degree of retardation of growth of the corresponding end of the less severely affected radius (where only about one-fifth of the total longitudinal growth of this bone takes place).

The outward bowing of the radius represents an attempt at adaptation to the shortening of the ulna, and when the proximal end of the radius has become completely dislocated, the bowing of this bone is likely to be found less pronounced. When the shortened and deformed lower end of the ulna no longer articulates properly with the bones of the wrist, the hand comes to deviate toward the ulnar side. In consequence of the exostotic changes immediately above the wrist in the radius and ulna, blocking interference with supination and pronation of the forearm may even develop. There are variations of this typical pattern of the forearm deformity, referable mainly to relatively greater severity of involvement of the radius as compared with that of the ulna.

**Inheritance.**—As already noted, it may be expected that about half of the offspring in families in which one parent has multiple exostosis will show the condition. The recognition of an inheritance factor in the occurrence of the disorder dates clearly from the description by Stanley, in 1849, of a family manifesting it in three generations. Between that time and the present, numerous observers have collected and recorded pedigrees of persons presenting the condition, to emphasize this aspect of it. Quite the fullest and most comprehensive presentation of the hereditary features of the disorder is the one by Stocks and Barrington. They analyzed 1,124 recorded cases of multiple exostosis. The deep-rootedness of the hereditary factor is clearly revealed in the finding that 727 of these cases came from 163 family trees. Thus in 64 per cent of the 1,124 cases, the disorder was definitely not limited to one member of a family tree, but occurred also in one or more antecedents or relatives. In the remaining 36 per cent (the other 397 cases) it was found that either the relevant information about the family tree was vague or missing, or else the records definitely stated that no other member of the subject's family was known to be affected. In the latter group of cases—that is, those with a definitely negative family history—the possibility must be considered that the disorder represents a mutation in the affected subject. However, this postulate is safe only if one can be certain that the disorder was absent not only in the immediate family of the affected subject, but also for at least two generations back.

As to the clearly inherited cases, Stocks and Barrington found that in somewhat more than half (about 60 per cent) the condition could be traced directly from an affected parent to an affected child. The parent in question was the father in 73 per cent and the mother in only 27 per cent of these directly inherited cases. It should be noted, however, because of its practical significance, that an unaffected male in a family tree in which the disorder is prevalent apparently does not transmit it to the children. On the other hand, an unaffected female in such a family tree may do so, for it appears that in the female the disorder may be latent or suppressed. Indeed, this latency seems to be not uncommon, apparently existing in about 1 of every 4 females who transmit the disorder to their children, as indicated by the presence of the disorder on the mother's side of the family. Furthermore, the proportion of children affected is just as great when the condition is transmitted through an unaffected (though tainted) mother as when it comes through an affected mother.

As to position in the family, the earlier-born members of exostotic stock are more likely to be affected than the younger children. As to sex distribution, the disorder shows, as already noted, a definite predilection for males, for, when large numbers of cases are considered, about 70 per cent are found to be in males and only about 30 per cent in females. One reason for this preponderance of males among the subjects is that, altogether, deviations from the norm tend to be more common in males than in females. In addition, however, as already pointed out, a considerable proportion of unaffected females in families showing the disorder are yet able to transmit the disease. It is the fact that these latent cases do not, of course, show up to be counted as instances of the disorder that is mainly responsible for the relatively low incidence in females as compared with males.

Certain observations on inheritance have been made also in regard to the number and distribution of the exostoses themselves. All in all, the offspring of subjects with relatively few exostoses tend to have relatively few, while the offspring of subjects with numerous exostoses tend to have large numbers. However, in any given affected family tree, the exostoses tend to become more numerous from generation to generation.

## PATHOLOGIC AND ROENTGENOGRAPHIC FINDINGS

**Gross Pathology and Roentgenographic Picture.**—As has long been recognized, the lesions of multiple exostosis develop particularly, though not solely, in relation to sites of bone growth at epiphysial cartilage plates. They appear mainly as outgrowths on the body of the bones, in the general vicinity of the plates. Furthermore, one can note that there is a general positive relation between the severity of involvement of a particular juxta-epiphysial part and the rate of growth normal for that part. Thus, it is not surprising that it is the long tubular bones, and especially those of the lower limbs, that show the most exuberant involvement.

In the lower limbs (in contrast to the upper) both ends of the long bones will usually be found rather severely affected, although the involvement is likely to be heaviest in the knee regions. Because of the impingement of large exostotic outgrowths upon each other at both the upper and lower ends of the shafts of the tibia and fibula, these bones may be found interlocked or even synostotic over several inches at these ends. In the humeri, though the upper juxta-epiphysial ends of the shafts are likely to be considerably altered, the lower ends are usually but slightly affected, if at all. On the other hand, the upper ends of the shafts of the radii and ulnæ are likely to be found less affected than the lower ends. (See Fig. 47.)

Even in a case in which the skeletal lesions are widespread and well developed, the skull bones are likely to be found exempt from involvement. However, the cartilage-preformed base of the skull is sometimes found affected. Specifically, in an occasional case, one or more tiny or even pea-sized excrescences, usually composed entirely of cartilage (ecchondroses), are to be noted. These have been found particularly on the clivus or along the synchondrosis between the sphenoid and occipital bones. In connection with parts of the skull preformed in membrane, exostoses apparently do not form. The carpal and tarsal bones are, on the whole, also spared, with the exception of the os calcis. The latter, since it develops a secondary center of ossification posteriorly, may show a few small exostoses on the main body of the bone.

On the other hand, the bodies of the ribs are likely to show little wreaths of small pointed or warty cartilage-covered exostoses. These are located especially at the chondral end, but also, though to a lesser extent, posteriorly, particularly where the head of the rib articulates with the neck. Also, there are often some small, flat, broad-based exostoses further along the rib body, both anteriorly and posteriorly. Furthermore, certain rib bodies may show, in addition, one or two relatively large sessile or stalked exostoses. These are sometimes situated even as far out as the midaxillary region, projecting either externally or into the pleural cavity. Not far from the costochondral junctions, the costal cartilages themselves may show a number of pinhead-sized or even much larger bits of cartilage under the perichondrium (ecchondroses). However, the sternal ends of the costal cartilages are generally free of ecchondroses. It is not at all likely that the sternum itself or the clavicles will show many exostoses. If the clavicles do show any, they are at the sternal end of the body and are few and very small.

The scapulæ are likely to be quite definitely affected. There may be a more or less continuous row of flat, knobby exostoses protruding from the body, both anteriorly and posteriorly along the line of attachment of the epiphyses for the vertebral border and the inferior angle. Not infrequently, also, along this line on the body, there are one or more exostoses so large and prominent that they have often been the ones which had first directed clinical attention to the condition. Still on the body of the scapula, along the line of attachment of the epiphyses for the acromion and coracoid process, one may also note some small warty exostoses. The innominate bones, like the scapulæ, generally show rows of flat or knobby, cartilage-covered excrescences located peripherally along the attachments of the secondary centers of ossification (the epiphyses) to the main bodies of the constituent bones. In regard to these bones, the exostoses are, on the whole, most prominent and numerous on the anterior and posterior surfaces of the ilium, along the line of attachment of the epiphysis for the crest.

Such few exostoses as are present on the vertebral column obey the general rule in being located close to secondary centers of ossification (epiphyses). These

***Figure 47***

*A*, Roentgenograph of the lower part of the shaft of a femur in a case of multiple exostosis. The entire circumference of the shaft is somewhat expanded, and a number of small protrusions are to be noted.

*B*, Roentgenograph of the lower part of the shaft of a femur in a case of multiple exostosis showing changes more pronounced than those apparent in *A*. Note the large, hooked projection present posteriorly.

*C*, Roentgenograph of the lower part of the shaft of a femur in a case of multiple exostosis showing still more pronounced changes. Note the large, sessile projection and the smaller additional protuberances.

*D*, Roentgenograph of the lower part of the shaft of a femur in a case of multiple exostosis showing, in addition to general widening of the shaft, a very large exostotic outgrowth which is blotchily radiopaque. Tissue examination showed that the radiopacity was due to the presence, beneath the surface of the exostosis, of a considerable amount of calcified cartilage matrix and calcareous detritus.

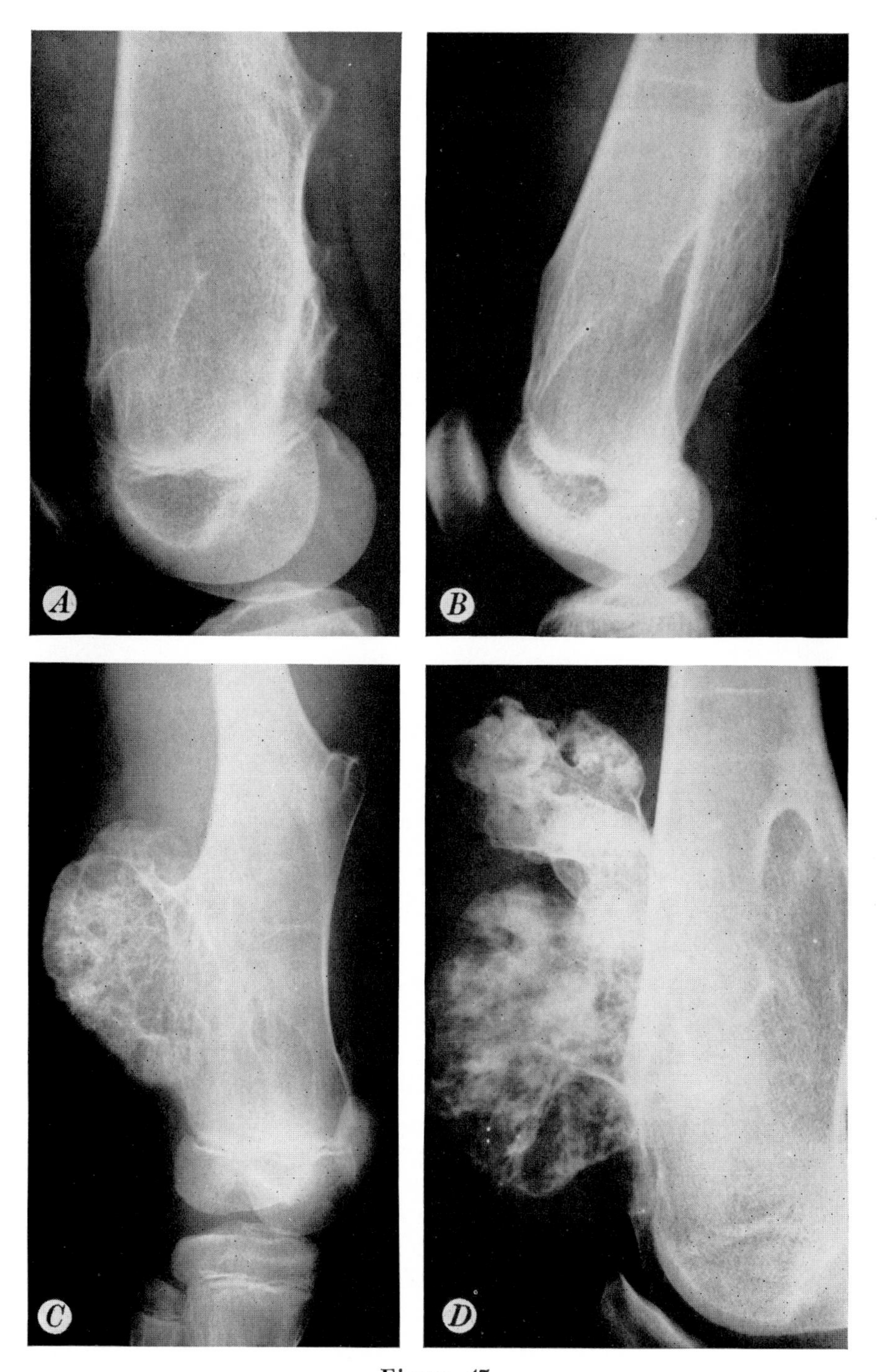


*Figure 47*

exostoses are small, on the whole, and are located most commonly near the tips of spinous processes. When the disorder is severe, the phalanges and the metacarpal and metatarsal bones may also show some exostotic outgrowths on their shafts.

From this sketch of the topographic anatomy of the involvement in multiple exostosis it is clear: that the long tubular bones, and especially those of the lower limbs, are the ones most strikingly involved; that the bones of the trunk show less florid involvement than the long bones; and that the vertebræ are the least affected of the trunk bones. If a rather strikingly affected bone is examined, it will be found that, over a considerable distance away from each epiphysial end, the shaft is wider and blunter than it would normally be. In fact, instead of tapering toward the middle of the diaphysis, the juxta-epiphysial shaft regions appear more or less cylindrical or even ballooned out. Also, instead of being smooth, the surface is knobby and bumpy over at least a large part of the circumference of these regions. This abnormality of the bone outline may be accentuated by the presence of one or more pedicled knobby protuberances, or of tubular projections ending bluntly or in a hook or point. It is worth noting that, on the whole, the nodosities and projections tend to curve away from, rather than to envelop, the epiphysial ends of the bone. It is true that, especially in connection with the upper end of the fibula and the lower end of the ulna, the modified juxta-epiphysial region may so expand as partly to encuff and even deform the epiphysis. Nevertheless, even then, the epiphysial end remains distinct from the encuffing metaphysial outgrowths. (See Fig. 48.)

Long bone areas modified by the presence of large exostoses, especially if the latter have displaced and pressed upon overlying muscle masses, may be found covered by bursæ. Specifically, a more or less vascularized connective-tissue membrane, even several millimeters thick, may come to be formed between the modified bone area and the overlying muscle. The membrane is attached all around the base of the modified bone area, forming a sort of encasing bag, and, in the latter, fluid (sometimes containing fibrin) may accumulate so that the muscle is more or less cushioned from the outgrowth. Occasionally, in such an "exostosis bursata," the bursal lining becomes villously modified and the sac may even come to contain a number of calcified bodies such as one sees in certain arthritic joints.

If one starts stripping the periosteum from the shaft of an affected long bone, working in the direction of an exostotically modified juxta-epiphysial area, it is

***Figure 48***

*A*, Photograph of the lower end of a femur and upper end of a tibia from the case of a man 41 years of age affected with multiple exostosis. Note the general bulging of the contour of the lower part of the femoral and upper part of the tibial shaft, and, in addition, the hooked and knobby protrusions present.

*B*, Photograph of the opposite surface of the femur and tibia shown in *A*.

*C*, Roentgenograph showing the characteristic deformity of the forearm in a case of multiple exostosis. Note the shortened ulna and the generally altered shape of its exostotically deformed distal third. Note also that the radius is disproportionately long in relation to the ulna, that it is bowed, and that its head is dislocated. Pronation and supination of the forearm were considerably restricted, and motion of the elbow was also somewhat impaired. The patient was a woman 26 years of age who stated that she had been aware of an abnormality of the forearm since early childhood.

*D*, Roentgenograph showing deformity of the forearm bones in the case of a child affected with multiple exostosis. In this case, the deformity presents a pattern somewhat different from the characteristic one shown in *C*.

*E*, Roentgenograph of a hand of a child affected with multiple exostosis. Note the numerous small exostotic outgrowths on the shafts of the phalanges and metacarpal bones.

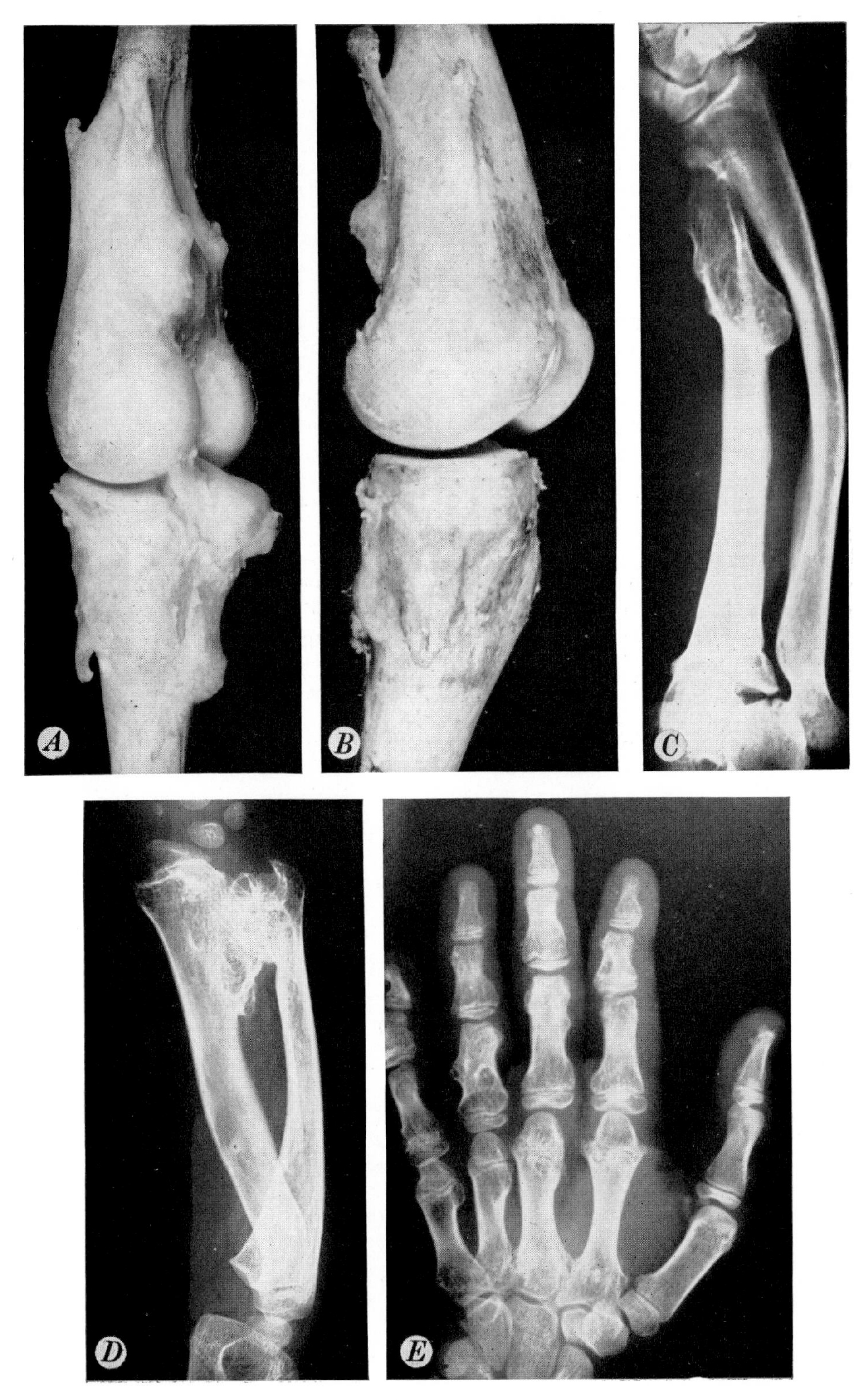


*Figure 48*

found that the periosteum of the unaffected part of the shaft continues over the exostotic area. It is considerably thicker there, and merges with the wall of the bursa if one is present. If no bursa is present, the periosteum is more closely adherent over the exostotic area than elsewhere on the bone, dipping in and out in such a way as to cover snugly the various prominences and depressions, also tending to fill in the latter. After it is removed, one can see clearly that the knobby surface of the affected region is cartilage-capped in some places and osseous in others, and that even the tubular projections are cartilage-capped at least at the tips, though the surfaces of their stems may be entirely osseous. One should note that, in general, the younger the subject, the greater the proportion of the affected area that is likely still to be covered by cartilage, and that in a mature subject this area may show only tiny sparse islands of cartilage, if any at all.

When the bone is sectioned, it will be seen that the outline of the surface in the affected area coincides with the periphery of the bone. That is, the exostotic area is not superposed upon a delimiting cortex, but instead the outline of the exostotic area represents an irregularly outpouched cortex. In the places where this cortex is still capped by cartilage, the latter may vary in thickness between about 2 and about 5 mm., even from place to place in the same exostotic area. Where the outpouched cortex is solely osseous, it is represented by a very thin plate of bone. Beneath the cortical surface, the bulged out modified area is composed of spongy bone whose trabeculæ are interspersed with considerable marrow, which on the whole is mainly fatty marrow. Within the substance of the exostosis, but generally near its surface, one may find smaller or larger yellow-white, gritty, compacted areas. These may be continuous with the covering cartilage. As described in connection with the microscopic pathology, they are composed of calcified cartilage and calcareous material. When abundant, they impart a good deal of radiopacity to the roentgenographic picture of the exostotic area.

If the exostotic long bone studied comes from a young subject, it can be noted that the centers of ossification for its epiphyses have apparently been growing normally and that the epiphyses themselves are fairly normal in shape. The epiphysial cartilage plates *per se* tend to show no abnormalities. Also, the chronology of fusion of the epiphyses with the shafts seems to be fairly normal. So also is the chronology of ossification and of fusion of the epiphyses elsewhere than in the long bones.

**Microscopic Pathology.**—In those parts of the exostotic area where there is a cartilaginous surface, it can be seen that the cartilage is hyaline. It may be rela-

***Figure 49***

*A*, Roentgenograph showing striking, though not unusual, alterations of the upper end of a fibula in a case of multiple exostosis. Outgrowths from the abutting portion of the tibia, interlocking with those from the fibula, had resulted in a synostosis, so that when the upper end of the fibula was resected a part of the adjacent portion of the tibia had to be removed also. As was shown by anatomic study of the resected specimen (see *B*, *C*, and *D*), the radiopaque patch in the left upper corner of the picture represents a focus of highly calcareous cartilage and cartilage matrix. Though it penetrates deeply into the interior of the affected area, the calcareous focus is still continuous with the cartilage capping the exostotic area in that region.

*B*, Photograph showing, in the upper left part of the picture, the calcareous focus which cast the radiopaque shadow shown in *A*. The relation of this focus (appearing as a white patch) to the surface of the lesion is clear.

*C*, Roentgenograph of the sectioned specimen shown in *B*.

*D*, Photomicrograph (× 35) showing cartilage of the cap on the right and, beyond it, the calcareous material which cast the radiopaque shadow in the fibular lesion illustrated.

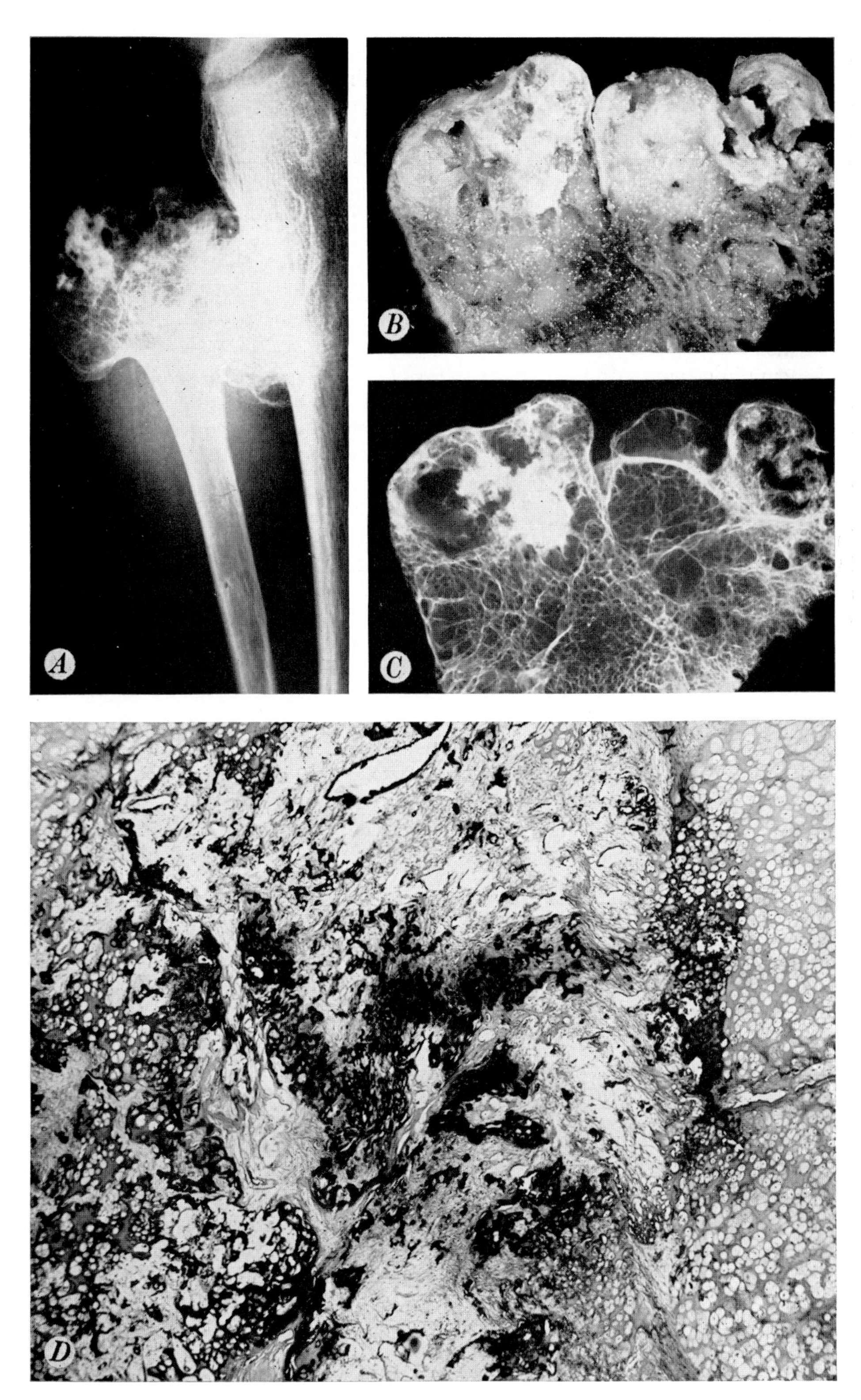


*Figure 49*

tively thick and may show, on its inner surface, considerable growth activity in the form of active endochondral ossification. If it does, the deeper-lying cartilage cells will be found lined up in columns and in general going through the gamut of changes associated with such ossification. In these areas, the subchondral spongiosa is rather likely to show congested marrow spaces and some myeloid marrow. Where the cartilage is not proliferating, columnar arrangement of its deeper cells is usually not apparent and the cartilage will be seen resting on a thin plate of bone which is continuous with the plate of bone outlining the surface of the exostotic area where this surface is devoid of cartilage.

As already noted, the periosteum covering the surface of the affected area is continuous with the periosteum over the unaffected areas. Where it runs over prominent cartilaginous surfaces it appears as a thin, rather poorly cellular, highly collagenous connective-tissue layer corresponding to the outer fibrous coat of periosteum in general. In areas not capped by cartilage, there is also a relatively thick inner cellular zone which corresponds to the cambium layer of periosteum in general, but this layer is remarkable on account of its thickness. If one searches different microscopic fields, one can find evidence of focal cartilaginous metaplasia occurring in this cellular, cambium-like layer of the periosteum.

One additional point should be noted. Occasionally one sees, below the surface in an exostotic area, a smaller or larger focus of gritty calcareous material. Histologically, this consists, in the main, of calcified (largely necrotic) cartilage, calcified acellular cartilage matrix, and calcium detritus. The presence of such a focus probably results from some local disturbance of the normal course of endochondral ossification associated with the growth of the exostotic area, so that calcified cartilage matrix which should have been destroyed and replaced by bone has accumulated under the proliferating cartilage. The finding of such a focus should not, however, be regarded as evidence that, in the exostotic area in question, an enchondroma is present along with the osteocartilaginous exostosis. Indeed such gritty calcified foci originate not from the interior of the bone, but from the surface of the lesions and are related to the proliferating cartilage on that surface. As already noted, a lesional area containing considerable calcified cartilage and calcium detritus is represented in the *x*-ray picture by a focus of radiopacity. Occasionally, even a large portion of an exostotic outgrowth may appear radiopaque on this account (see Fig. 49).

***Figure 50***

*A*, Roentgenograph of a large, calcifying chondrosarcoma which has sprung from the sacrum and has grown in the area of the hip joint in a case of multiple exostosis. The patient was a man 37 years of age. The tumor was treated by wide resection rather than by hindquarter amputation. In the course of 10 years from the time of the original surgical intervention, there were 3 local recurrences, each of which was likewise treated by resection. This case history points up the fact that chondrosarcomas complicating multiple exostosis are frequently, though not always, tumors which do not readily metastasize, though they tend to recur again and again.

*B*, Roentgenograph of the resected tumor. The radiopacities represent calcification and ossification going on in the tumor cartilage.

*C*, Photograph of the tumor resected at the original intervention. The area of bone to be seen in the lower part of the picture represents part of the sacrum, from whose outer surface the tumor developed.

*D*, Photomicrograph (× 250) showing the pattern of the tumor cartilage in the most ominous areas. Note the large, bizarre cartilage cells with multiple nuclei.

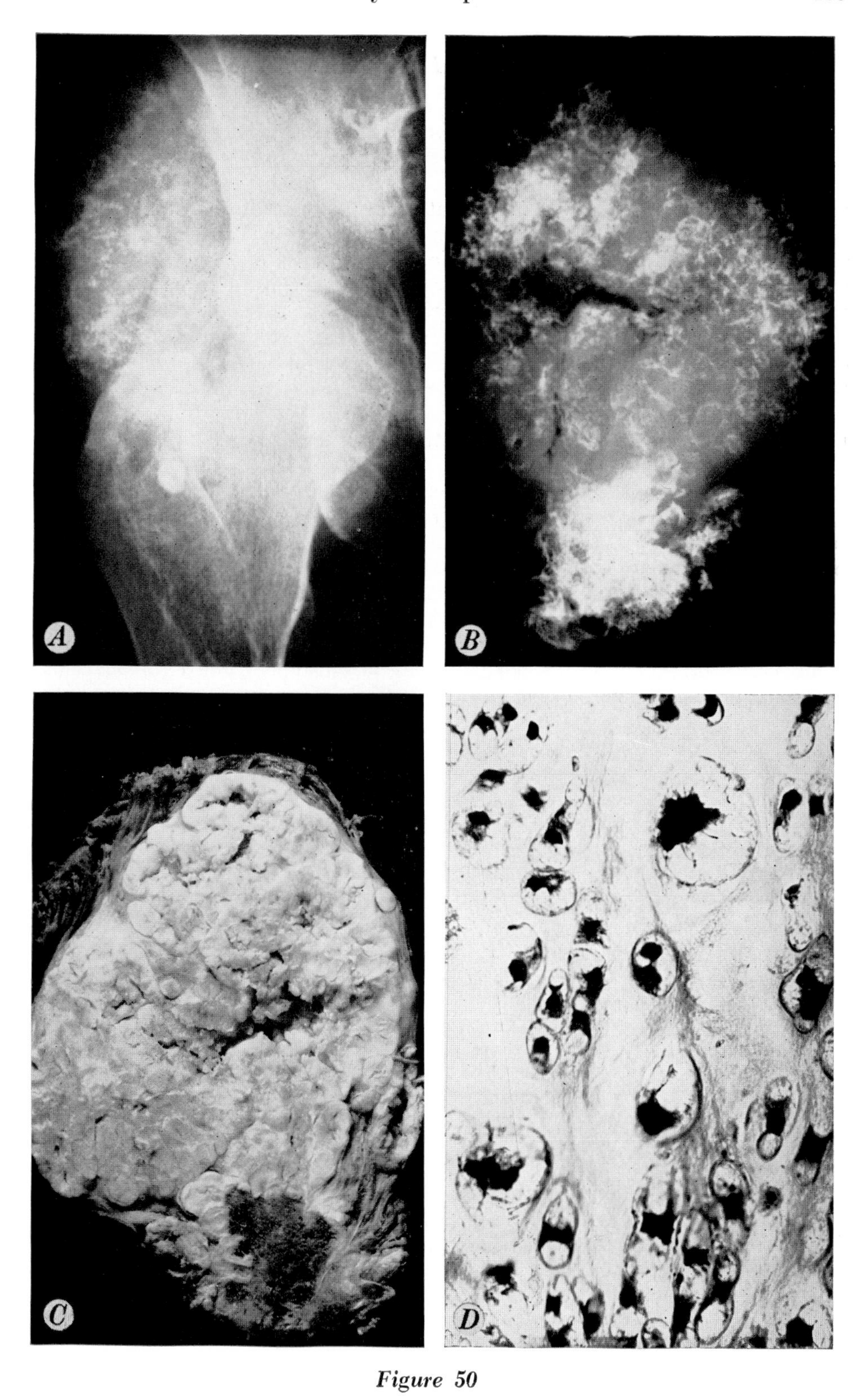


*Figure 50*

## CHONDROSARCOMA AS A COMPLICATION

That in a case of multiple exostosis a chondrosarcoma may develop in one or another of the affected bone areas has been known for a long time. Numerous accounts can be found scattered through the relevant literature, and most of these take the form of individual case reports. By far the most common location is the general area of the hip joint. The patients are usually adults, and often not even young adults, when the chondrosarcoma appears, yet children and adolescents sometimes likewise show this complication. In a series of 28 cases of multiple exostosis reported by the writer, 3 (nearly 11 per cent) showed it. Since the great majority of the patients in this series were still children or adolescents, one must allow for the possibility that, later in life, some of these, too, might develop chondrosarcoma. Thus, the full returns on the incidence of this complication in this reported series will not be in for a long time (theoretically not until all the subjects have died) and will almost certainly be higher than 11 per cent. In fact, in a comparable series of new cases seen subsequently, the writer already found the incidence to be nearer 20 than 11 per cent.

It appears that the chondrosarcoma may evolve out of the cartilaginous cap of one or another of the exostoses, or out of the residuum of this cap. It may conceivably also evolve out of a mere cartilage rest which had been lying between the periosteum and the cortex of the affected bone area before the tumor appeared. The latter may grow very rapidly to large size, soon break into regional venous channels, reach the heart and lungs by intravascular growth, and even give rise to parenchymal metastases, at least in the lungs. Death may ensue in the course of 5 or 6 months after appearance of the malignancy in such instances, but so rapid a course is exceptional. A course leading to death within a few years is more common. Furthermore, a very torpid course, of 10 years or more, is not at all unusual. In the cases of slower evolution, the malignant tumor may remain only locally invasive for years, without spreading distantly through the venous channels, and indeed death may take place from some cause only accidentally connected with the tumor, without its having spread distantly at all. (See Fig. 50.)

In the literature, the malignant tumor which develops in association with lesions of multiple exostosis is by no means uniformly referred to as a chondrosarcoma or even as a malignant chondroma. Indeed, it is often denoted with unfortunate vagueness as a chondroma or enchondroma, albeit a large, recurrent, or otherwise peculiar one. Again, it may be found referred to as an osteochondrosarcoma (chondro-osteosarcoma) or even, altogether incorrectly, as an osteogenic sarcoma. For details on the pathology of chondrosarcoma developing in connection with multiple exostosis, the reader is referred to the chapter on chondrosarcoma (p. 333).

## PATHOGENESIS

There are several different interpretations which have been proposed to explain the processes by which the lesions of multiple exostosis develop. For a long time, the dominant conception was the one given prestige by Virchow. He derived cartilage-covered exostoses on bones (as well as cartilage islands within bones—*i.e.*, enchondromata) from epiphysial cartilage plates or their analogues. Specifically, in regard to exostoses, he held that bits of cartilage become snared off from the lateral margins of the plates, and, moving on to the body of the bone, constitute the beginnings of the lesions.

Another conception of the pathogenesis is that the lesions have their beginnings in cartilage derived from the periosteum. This, too, is an old conception, but it is one which has been revived and which is gaining ground. Müller surveyed the literature relating to both the epiphysial plate theory and the periosteal theory. He weighed them against each other, and, adding evidence from the autopsy findings in a case of his own, gave impetus to the contemporary trend in favor of the periosteal mode of origin. From the findings in his case, he concluded that cartilage-covered exostoses on the bones have their beginnings in small nests of cartilage formed by the osteogenic layer (cambium layer) of the periosteum. As to the small cartilaginous nodules (ecchondroses) found on the costal cartilages and sometimes on the cartilage-preformed base of the skull, he concluded that they originate from the perichondrium. Furthermore, he held that, in multiple exostosis, there was an abnormal capacity of the periosteum and perichondrium to form cartilage during the entire growth period and even beyond it. This capacity, he held, represented a perverted activity of these tissues under the influence of some constitutional aberration.

We now come to the conception expounded by Keith. It is based on the well-established fact that normally at growth zones (epiphysial cartilage plates and their analogues) a core of bone formed by endochondral ossification becomes encased in a sheath of bone formed by the ring of periosteum surrounding the growth zone. On this foundation, he maintains that the primary basis of the pathogenesis of multiple exostosis is defectiveness of this periosteal ring. Thus he holds that on account of the deficiency or absence of deposition of bone by the periosteal ring, the cartilage-preformed bone at the growth zone is free to expand in abnormal directions, so that the normal confining and modeling at that zone fails to take place. Consequently, in his opinion, the new bone formed at the growth zone, not being restrained and subjected to active remodeling, "spills out," as it were, onto the outer surface of the body of the bone, producing the cartilage-covered excrescences. The latter, according to Keith, are thus merely the secondary results of the primary disorder of bone growth and especially bone modeling which he denotes in the name "diaphysial aclasis."

Material ideally suited for establishing the facts on the pathogenesis of multiple exostosis would be represented by whole affected bones with evolving lesions from children (especially very young ones). Strategic studies of such material have apparently not been reported even yet. Though not ideal, the material available to the present writer does seem to permit conclusions on the pathogenesis, since it included widely excised lesions from affected bones of children.

In a number of the specimens, the appearances were such as to favor one part of Keith's hypothesis—namely, the part which maintains that, where the exostotic outgrowths appear in juxta-epiphysial regions, there has been a lack of cortical bone formation by the periosteal ring, such as normally occurs in these regions and guides the normal shaping or modeling of the part. While favoring this part of Keith's theory, the findings from these specimens permitted one to hold at the same time that perverted activity of the periosteum is also a factor in the pathogenesis of the lesions. This idea, which is in line with Müller's, would mean that precisely in the juxta-epiphysial regions, periosteal activity is disordered or perverted on a deeply-rooted hereditary basis, and specifically that the periosteum is forming cartilage instead of bone.

In many of the other specimens examined by the present writer, evidence that the periosteal covering of the lesions does possess the capacity to form islands of cartilage in this disorder could be demonstrated. Furthermore, the inculpation of the coverings of bones and cartilages would explain the presence of nests of cartilage in the perichondrium (ecchondroses) such as one often observes on the costal cartilages in these cases. It would likewise account for the occasional occurrence of an excrescence on one or another of the bones at the base of the skull, which are preformed entirely in cartilage. Also, it would harmonize with the occasional finding of a large cartilage-covered exostosis on the body of a rib near the midaxillary line when the shaft of the rib near the costochondral junction is relatively well modeled, showing perhaps only a wreath of tiny, nodular excrescences.

Altogether, on the basis of histologic study of material such as could shed some light on the question, the present writer holds that the theory of defective modeling and that of perverted periosteal and perichondral activity are not only mutually compatible but reinforce each other in explaining the pathogenesis of the disorder as a whole.

## DIFFERENTIAL DIAGNOSIS

**Skeletal Enchondromatosis.**—As indicated under "Nomenclature," it was formerly thought by many that multiple exostosis and enchondromatosis represent manifestations of a general "osteogenic disease" which: (1) may express itself in either multiple exostoses or multiple enchondromata (even in different subjects of the same family tree), and (2) is also commonly manifested in the appearance of both disorders in the same person.

In the cases which have come under the writer's observation, there was no evidence of enchondromatosis in the family of the persons affected with multiple exostosis. Instead, when any other member of the family was known to have any sort of possibly similar skeletal disorder, it was always skeletal exostosis. Conversely, among the cases, far fewer, of skeletal enchondromatosis studied by the writer (p. 184), there were no instances of multiple exostosis in the family of the patient, nor was there even skeletal enchondromatosis in other members of the family. That is, skeletal enchondromatosis did not follow the pattern of a hereditary disease at all. Also, in our own material, we found no anatomic basis, either, directly linking the two disorders.

Nevertheless, it is not difficult to discover, by a survey of the literature, some of the sources of the confusion between cases of enchondromatosis and multiple exostosis. Such a survey will show, for instance, that a great many authors loosely refer to the peripheral cartilaginous caps of the cancellous exostoses as "enchondromata," in spite of the fact that etymologically the word "enchondroma" should be limited to a cartilage mass definitely involving the interior of a bone. As to the focus of calcified cartilage sometimes seen under the cap of an exostotic area, it has already been pointed out that such a focus does not represent anything akin to an enchondroma. Instead, as noted, it represents merely an area of calcified cartilage which has accumulated in consequence of a localized disturbance of endochondral ossification of the cartilage cap in an exostotic area. Nowhere does one find, in the exostotic lesions, frank masses of cartilage spreading out from the interior of the bone and distending its surface. In contrast, the lesions of skeletal enchondromatosis are composed essentially of such masses, which, especially in the bones of the hands and feet, may widely distend the cortex and make its contour irregularly bumpy by bulging from within. Again, a chondrosarcoma developing out of the cartilaginous cap of one of the cartilage-covered exostoses is sometimes loosely denoted as a malignant chondroma or even enchondroma.

Finally, some confusion has also resulted from incorrect interpretation of roentgenographic appearances. Often, if the affected bone area is roentgenographed in one plane only, an exostosis will not show up as a projection from the bone cortex. Instead, it will cast a shadow revealing only the outline of its margin where it extends out from the cortex, and the outlined area may thus appear as though framed within the bone and be misinterpreted as an enchondroma.

Altogether, it seems clear that multiple exostosis and skeletal enchondromatosis should be regarded as clinically and anatomically independent disorders.

## TREATMENT

The mere presence of multiple exostosis in a subject is not in itself a reason for intervention against the lesions. However, the removal of one or another of the bony prominences may be sought, for cosmetic reasons or on account of local pain. It may also be indicated when the lesions have resulted in interference with movement of joints, or given rise, directly or indirectly, to some gross skeletal deformity. The choice of procedure is, of course, a matter for the surgeon and will be governed by the aim to be accomplished in a given case. In general, when exostotic areas are excised, the periosteum should be removed with them, and not stripped back. That is, the excision should not be subperiosteal, since remaining periosteum may invite recurrence.

The management of an affected bone area which has undergone chondrosarcomatous transformation is likely to try surgical judgment. In general, the surgical decision should lean toward the radical side. Fortunately, chondrosarcoma (at least in easily accessible areas such as limbs) does not offer the gloomy prognosis of osteogenic sarcoma, provided that amputation is done well beyond the level of the lesion. In sites such as the pelvis, in which thorough eradication of the affected area is surgically difficult and may even be unfeasible, one may have to be content with resection, though the results of this are very likely to be unsatisfactory in the long run. In regard to the value of irradiation for chondrosarcoma, it has become clear that this has no therapeutic effect upon the course of these growths.

Finally, there are two additional points which seem worth mentioning. In exostotic women, it appears advisable to roentgenograph the pelvis in case there should be a large exostosis which might act as an obstruction during childbirth. Also, an exostotic adult should, of course, be informed that the condition would be likely to reappear in about half of his or her offspring.

## REFERENCES


Bennett, G. E., and Berkheimer, G. A.: Malignant Degeneration in a Case of Benign Exostoses Surgery, *10*, 781, 1941.

Cappellin, M.: Evoluzione tipica e atipica delle esostosi di crescenza. Esostosi condroblastomatosa, Chir. d. org. di movimento, *39*, 44, 1953.

Chiari, H.: Zur Lehre von den multiplen Exostosen, Prag. med. Wchnschr., *17*, 403, 1892.

Cohnheim, J.: Ein Fall von multiplen Exostosen, Virchows Arch. f. path. Anat., *38*, 561, 1867.

Ehrenfried, A.: Hereditary Deforming Chondrodysplasia—Multiple Cartilaginous Exostoses, J. A. M. A., *68*, 502, 1917.

Ellis, V. H., and Taylor, J. G.: Diaphysial Aclasis, J. Bone & Joint Surg., *33-B*, 100, 1951.

Fairbank, H. A. T.: Diaphysial Aclasis, J. Bone & Joint Surg., *31-B*, 105, 1949.

Hagen, F. B.: Ueber Knochen- und Gelenkanomalieen, insbesondere bei partiellem Riesenwuchs und bei multiplen cartilaginären Exostosen, Arch. f. klin. Chir., *41*, 749, 1891.

Henking, F.: Ein neuer Fall von multipler Exostosis cartilaginea, Virchows Arch. f. path. Anat., *77*, 364, 1879.

Huber, K.: Ein seltenerer Fall von "multiplen cartilaginären Exostosen," Virchows Arch. f. path. Anat., *88*, 256, 1882.

Jaffe, H. L.: Hereditary Multiple Exostosis, Arch. Path., *36*, 335, 1943.

Keith, A.: Studies on the Anatomical Changes which Accompany Certain Growth-Disorders of the Human Body, J. Anat., *54*, 101, 1920.

Müller, E.: Über hereditäre multiple cartilaginäre Exostosen und Ecchondrosen, Beitr. z. path. Anat. u. z. allg. Path., *57*, 232, 1913–14.

Ollier, L.: Exostoses ostéogéniques multiples, Lyon méd., *88*, 484, 1898, and: De la Dyschondroplasie, Bull. Soc. de chir. de Lyon, *3*, 22, 1900.

von Recklinghausen, F.: Ein Fall von multiplen Exostosen, Virchows Arch. f. path. Anat., *35*, 203, 1866.

Scherer, E.: Exostosen, Enchondrome und ihre Beziehung zum Periost, Frankfurt. Ztschr. f. Path., *36*, 587, 1928.

Sjövall, H.: Über solitäre Exostosen, Chirurg, *15*, 737, 1943.

Stark, J. D., Adler, N. N., and Robinson, W. H.: Hereditary Multiple Exostoses, Radiology, *59*, 212, 1952.

Stocks, P., and Barrington, A.: Hereditary Disorders of Bone Development, Eugenics Lab. Memoirs, 1925, No. 22, London (Cambridge U. Press).

Virchow, R.: Ueber multiple Exostosen, mit Vorlegung von Präparaten, Berl. klin. Wchnschr., *28*, 1082, 1891.

Weber, O.: Zur Geschichte des Enchondroms namentlich in Bezug auf dessen hereditäres Vorkommen und secundäre Verbreitung in inneren Organen durch Embolie, Virchows Arch. f. path. Anat., *35*, 501, 1866.

Chapter

# 11

# Solitary Enchondroma and Multiple Enchondromatosis

SOLITARY enchondroma and multiple enchondromatosis apparently occur only in bones preformed in cartilage. The term *solitary enchondroma* refers to a benign cartilage growth which starts its development in the medullary cavity of a bone and involves only a single bone in a given affected person. In cases of *multiple enchondromatosis*, on the other hand, at least several bones are involved. However, the extent of the involvement in these cases runs a very wide gamut. In some of them, only a few bones are affected, while at the other extreme there are cases in which practically every bone preformed in cartilage is involved. Furthermore, in multiple enchondromatosis, though much of the lesional cartilage originates in the interior of the affected bones, there can be no doubt that some of the cartilage is formed by the periosteum and comes to penetrate into the bones.

## SOLITARY ENCHONDROMA

The solitary enchondroma is a fairly common lesion. It is encountered mainly in the long and short tubular bones of the limbs. As it grows, the lesional tissue in the bone interior may distend the affected bone area, at least in part, by thinning and bulging the local cortex. This is especially true if the enchondroma is in a phalanx, metacarpal or metatarsal bone. However, a solitary enchondroma may be present without causing any distention of the contour of the affected bone. That a solitary enchondroma may undergo malignant transformation into a chondrosarcoma is well known. This is by no means a rare occurrence when the enchondroma is in a long tubular bone, but is very unusual when it involves one of the short tubular bones.

### CLINICAL CONSIDERATIONS

**Age and Sex Incidence.**—The disorder does not strikingly predilect any one age group. However, the patients are usually not under 10 or over 50 years of age at the time when the condition first comes under treatment. As to sex incidence, there seems to be no predilection of one sex over the other.

**Localization.**—As already noted, solitary benign enchondroma predilects limb bones. Specifically, in the writer's experience, the limb bones most commonly implicated are, in descending order of frequency: finger phalanges, metacarpal bones, humerus, femur, toe phalanges, metatarsal bones, tibia, fibula, ulna. In other series, the precise order will probably be somewhat different. In any event, however, it is clear that solitary enchondroma predilects finger phalanges and metacarpal bones in particular, and our findings on this point are in harmony with those of Mason. As to localization in long tubular bones, the writer's experience is also in accord with the literature in suggesting that, among these, the femur and humerus are the most likely to be affected.

A solitary enchondroma of a short or long tubular bone usually (though not always) begins its development in a metaphysial region. An enchondroma beginning within a metaphysis may eventually involve a large portion of the shaft and even extend into the corresponding epiphysial end of the affected bone. It by no means necessarily grows into the adjacent epiphysis, however, and apparently does not do so in any case until the epiphysis has fused with the shaft. That is, it does not tend to violate the epiphysial cartilage plate.

One only infrequently encounters a solitary enchondroma in a bone other than a limb bone. Among the rarer localizations, those in a rib or the sternum are probably the least exceptional. Localization in a pelvic bone or a vertebra has also been described. The writer, too, has encountered a few cases of solitary enchondroma involving one or another part of an innominate bone. As to the skull bones, of course, only those preformed in cartilage can possibly be the site of an enchondroma. In any event, the condition is rare in these bones. Furthermore, as Menne

***Figure 51***

*A*, Roentgenograph showing a solitary enchondroma in the shaft of a phalanx of a girl 16 years of age. Note that the lesion has bulged the bone contour. Note also that the lesional area shows no radiopacities such as would represent calcification of the lesional cartilage. Despite this fact, experience shows that a lesion of this location and roentgenographic appearance is almost certainly an enchondroma.

*B*, Roentgenograph showing a solitary enchondroma in a metacarpal bone of a girl 18 years of age. She complained of pain and a slowly progressive swelling in the area in question. In this lesion, too, there are no radiopacities to help establish the diagnosis of enchondroma roentgenographically. On a statistical basis alone, however, a lesion in this location in a metacarpal bone is very likely to be an enchondroma.

*C*, Roentgenograph of a calcifying enchondroma in a metacarpal bone of a girl 20 years of age. About a year earlier, she had sustained a fracture through this bone, and the existence of the metacarpal tumor was discovered at that time. The fracture healed, but pain persisted. The calcification and ossification going on in the tumor cartilage are represented by the roundish radiopacities, which help to establish the diagnosis.

*D*, Roentgenograph of an enchondroma in the shaft of a metacarpal bone of a man 34 years of age. There were no complaints referable to the area until 4 months before the picture was taken, when he suffered a traumatic injury to the part. At the time of the injury, an *x*-ray picture disclosed the presence of the lesion. Note the distention of the contour of the affected part of the bone shaft, and the radiopacities in the lesional area.

*E*, Roentgenograph of an enchondroma in the shaft of an ulna of a woman 42 years of age. About 25 years previously, she had suffered a fracture through the shaft of the bone. The picture taken at that time already disclosed the enchondroma. The latter has apparently increased only slightly in size in the interim, but recently there has been increasing pain referable to the area. Note the telltale radiopacities which help establish the nature of the lesion.

*F*, Roentgenograph of an enchondroma in the midshaft of a humerus of a boy 8 years of age. The lesional area is radiolucent and shows an infraction through its upper end. Because of the absence of radiopacities in the lesional area, the definitive diagnosis had to await tissue examination.

*G*, Roentgenograph of an enchondroma in the lower part of the shaft of a femur of a woman 41 years of age. She complained of local pain of 6 months' standing, and also limped. The lesion is entirely central and has not bulged the contour of the bone. The stippled radiopacities help establish the diagnosis. (Fig. 53-*A* is a photomicrograph of tissue curetted from this lesion.)

*H*, Roentgenograph of a rather extensive enchondroma in a humerus of a girl 14 years of age who complained of mild pain in the arm for about a year. Because of the "trabeculated" appearance of the lesional area, and the absence of clear-cut radiopacity, the definitive diagnosis of the lesion as an enchondroma had to await tissue examination.

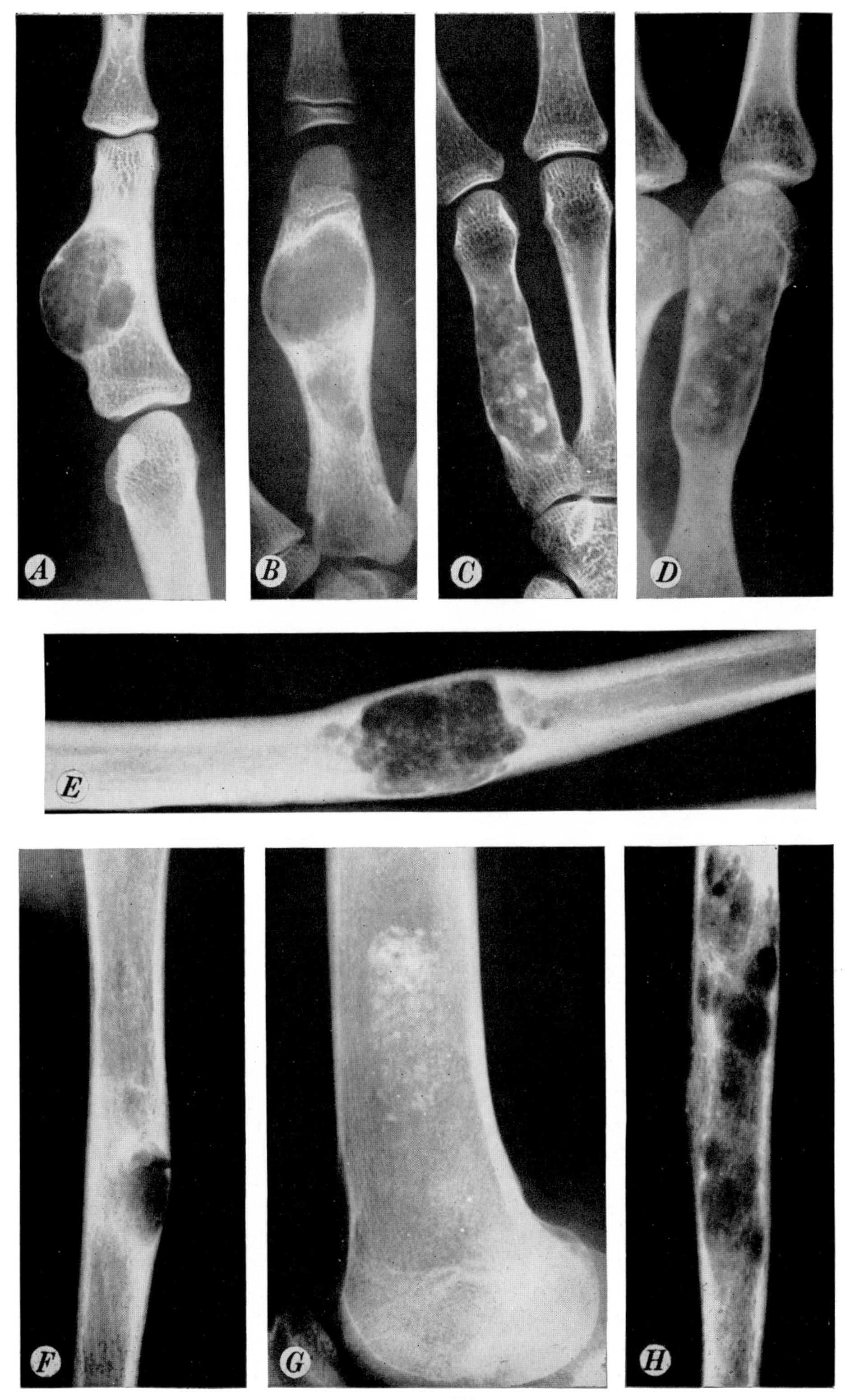


*Figure 51*

and Frank point out, one is often uncertain of the origin and real nature of reported instances of skull bone enchondromas.

**Clinical Complaints and Findings.**—A common history in the cases of phalangeal involvement is that the patient was not aware of anything wrong until a local trauma was followed by some pain and swelling, and a roentgenograph revealed an altered phalanx with a pathologic fracture. On the other hand, other patients give a history of spontaneous swelling of the region of the affected phalanx, dating back perhaps several years. This swelling may have been painless or only slightly and intermittently painful. It may be complained of only because it was recently exacerbated by a local trauma, which may have given rise to an infraction or fracture. On palpation, the enlarged region of the phalanx is likely to be rather firm, and if there has been a recent fracture through the area there may be considerable local tenderness and even some heat.

The history patterns in the cases of metacarpal and metatarsal bone involvement are essentially the same as in those of phalangeal involvement. These patients, also, usually present a local swelling of the affected bone. When there is pain (apparently from a fracture) after trauma, the pain subsequently subsides, though the swelling persists.

In the cases in which long tubular bones are affected, the clinical complaints are usually of rather recent date when the patient appears for definitive treatment. Nevertheless, it seems probable that in these cases, too, the lesion had been present for years, though latent, before the onset of the current complaints. Thus, in one case in point, a patient whose femoral enchondroma showed by its heavy calcification that it must have been in existence for many years presented herself only because of local pain, of 6 months' duration, aggravated by walking. In another case, the lesion (again in a femur) was discovered by chance 17 years before it began to cause any trouble. Still another patient, presenting an extensive enchondroma in a humerus, was admitted because of pain, tenderness, and disability attributable to a pathologic fracture 10 days previously. She stated, however, that, a year before, there had been a fracture through the same area, which had healed promptly, but the nature of the underlying lesion had apparently not been recognized. In another case in point, in which the enchondroma was in the shaft of an ulna, the patient stated that 25 years previously there had been a fracture through the ulna. The fracture was a pathologic one through a lesion which was clearly an enchondroma. The fracture healed promptly, and the patient remained free of complaints until her recent admission for treatment of the ulnar enchondroma. This enchondroma had thus apparently remained clinically latent for a quarter of a century after a pathologic fracture through it had healed.

## ROENTGENOGRAPHIC FINDINGS

In a phalanx, a solitary enchondroma appears as a more or less oval rarefaction shadow, usually limited to the shaft—that is, sparing the epiphysial end of the bone. The lesion may be situated centrally within the affected bone shaft, and may even fail to cause distention of the neighboring cortex. More often, however, it is situated off to one side (eccentrically), and it may even cause a pronounced bulging distention and thinning of the overlying cortex. Those enchondromas which are situated eccentrically usually show a delicate, radiopaque line where they abut upon the uninvolved portion of the phalanx. The rarefaction shadow as a whole usually looks more or less cloudy. It may present a vaguely trabeculated appearance or even several pinhead- to matchhead-sized densifications. The latter reflect foci of calcification and ossification in the lesional cartilage and constitute telltale indications of an enchondroma. Frequently, one can note evidence of a still unhealed fracture. Also, as already suggested, so long as the epiphysis has not fused with the shaft, the former is not involved. Even after fusion, as already noted, the epiphysis is not necessarily invaded (see Fig. 51-*A*).

Solitary benign enchondroma is by far the most common and indeed the principal solitary lesion affecting phalanges. In fact, any lesion situated in a middle or proximal phalanx of a finger and presenting anything like the roentgenographic picture described and illustrated is almost certainly a benign enchondroma. Nevertheless, a phalangeal enchondroma is not infrequently misinterpreted roentgenographically as a cyst, a giant-cell tumor, or an osteochondroma. Actually, a solitary bone cyst of the type common in long tubular bones is very unusual in phalanges. As to giant-cell tumor, that lesion, too, is definitely uncommon in phalanges, though not so uncommon there as cysts are. At any rate, a giant-cell tumor of a phalanx regularly involves the epiphysial end of the bone, and the bulk of the lesion is in the bone end. This is not true of phalangeal enchondromas, even when it does happen that they extend into the end of the bone. A phalangeal enchondroma which has conspicuously distended part of the cortex may also be misinterpreted as an osteochondroma, if attention is concentrated upon the bulge to the neglect of the appearance of the bone's interior. On the other hand, a squamous epithelium-lined inclusion cyst of a phalanx, though of rare occurrence, may strongly suggest an enchondroma in the *x*-ray picture. However, the epithelium-lined cyst, when involving a phalanx, seems to occur exclusively in terminal phalanges of fingers and indeed nearly always in the terminal half of such a phalanx—a location which would be exceptional for an enchondroma.

In regard to metacarpal and metatarsal bones, the roentgenographic findings are essentially similar to what they are in regard to phalanges. It is to be noted, however, that in metacarpal or metatarsal bones the enchondroma tends to be more or less in the distal instead of the proximal part of the shaft, though it is thus still oriented toward the epiphysis of the bone. The remarks on the differential diagnosis insofar as they pertain to solitary unicameral cyst, giant-cell tumor, and osteochondroma apply as closely to metacarpal or metatarsal as to phalangeal enchondroma. The epithelium-lined inclusion cyst apparently does not occur in metacarpal or metatarsal bones. However, a solitary focus of fibrous dysplasia (p. 117) occasionally does occur in a metacarpal or metatarsal bone. Roentgenographically, such a lesion in a metacarpal bone could simulate an enchondroma quite closely. Merely on the basis of statistical probability, however, the likelihood is that one would be dealing with an enchondroma rather than a focus of fibrous dysplasia. This is so because enchondroma is the more common lesion in the bones in question. Should the lesion under consideration present stippled foci of densification, one would have strong roentgenographic evidence of its actually being an enchondroma (see Figs. 51-*B*, *C*, and *D*).

In regard to long tubular bones, much of what has been said about the *x*-ray picture of enchondromas of phalanges and metacarpal bones is still applicable. A considerable part of the shaft may be involved, and the lesion is likely to be more strictly central. If the cortex does bulge, it is probable that the bulge will be slight and limited to a relatively small area. The presence of spotty or blotchy radiopacity points rather definitely in the direction of an enchondroma. Indeed, even a few scattered pinhead- to matchhead-sized spots of densification would point in that direction. On the other hand, when the presence of radiopaque spots is doubtful or when they are absent entirely, the *x*-ray diagnosis of enchondroma cannot be made with any confidence. Especially if the lesion (of course solitary) should also appear somewhat expanded and trabeculated, the strongest likelihood is that it represents a solitary focus of fibrous dysplasia, and another, though weaker, possibility is that it represents a solitary unicameral bone cyst, rather than an enchondroma.

In relation to long bones, furthermore, one sometimes encounters a highly calcified and ossified enchondroma more or less completely occupying an end of the bone. These enchondromata probably start their development in the epiphysis rather than in the shaft of the bone. In filling out the end, these enchondromata extend to the articular cartilage, but in the opposite direction they generally do not extend very far along the shaft (see Figs. 51-*E*, *F*, *G*, and *H*, and Figs. 52-*A* and *B*).

## PATHOGENESIS AND PATHOLOGIC FINDINGS

**Pathogenesis.**—The traditional conception of the origin of solitary enchondroma is that it arises from a misplaced cartilage rest. The source of such a rest is generally stated to be cartilage snared from an epiphysial cartilage plate. The principal basis for this conception is represented by autopsy findings dating from the time when rickets was a common disease and many severely rachitic children came to autopsy. Specifically, in such cases one often used to find, in the metaphyses of

***Figure 52***

*A*, Roentgenograph of an enchondroma in the superior ramus of an innominate bone of a woman 33 years of age. The patient had complained of mild pain in the hip region for about 5 months, after a fall. However, the presence of the lesion in the pubic bone was discovered only incidentally, in connection with *x*-ray examination of the pelvic organs. The pubic ramus is expanded, and the small radiopacities to be seen in the *x*-ray picture are consistent with the diagnosis of a cartilage tumor, but the location is rather atypical for it.

*B*, Roentgenograph of an enchondroma in the head and neck of a femur of a woman 42 years of age. At the time when this picture was taken, the patient had been complaining of pain in the hip for only 10 days. There can be no doubt that the lesion was present prior to the onset of this complaint. The stippled radiopacities in the lesional area suggest a cartilage tumor. However, in the clinical diagnosis, one would have to consider not only benign enchondroma but also benign chondroblastoma. The latter possibility is made tenuous by the age of the patient, since benign chondroblastomas are seen mainly in adolescents and very young adults.

*C*, Photograph of a small cartilage rest in the lower part of the shaft of a fibula of a man 54 years of age. This rest was an incidental finding in connection with amputation of the limb on account of a sarcoma in the lower end of the femur. The cartilage rest in the fibula was discovered during routine gross sectioning of the various bones of the amputated limb. Since the focus of cartilage was not calcified, it did not show up in the roentgenographic picture of this fibular specimen.

*D*, Photograph (enlarged) of an enchondroma in the upper end of a fibula of a man 21 years of age, whose complaints were of only a few months' standing. The lesional tissue is pearly white hyaline cartilage.

*E*, Roentgenograph of the fibular lesion illustrated in *D*. Since the lesional cartilage is neither calcified nor ossified, this clinical roentgenograph shows no radiopacities in the lesional area. On this account, it was difficult to make the diagnosis of enchondroma from the roentgenographic picture in this case.

*F*, Photograph (enlarged) of another enchondroma in the upper end of a fibula. The lesional tissue in this case showed a good deal of grittiness due to calcification and ossification going on in it.

*G*, Roentgenograph of the specimen illustrated in *F*. The calcification and ossification in the lesional tissue is represented by the radiopacities.

*H*, Roentgenograph of the calcifying and ossifying enchondroma illustrated in *F* and *G*. The numerous agglomerated radiopacities and the clear-cut circumscription of the lesional area justify the clinical diagnosis of enchondroma from this picture.

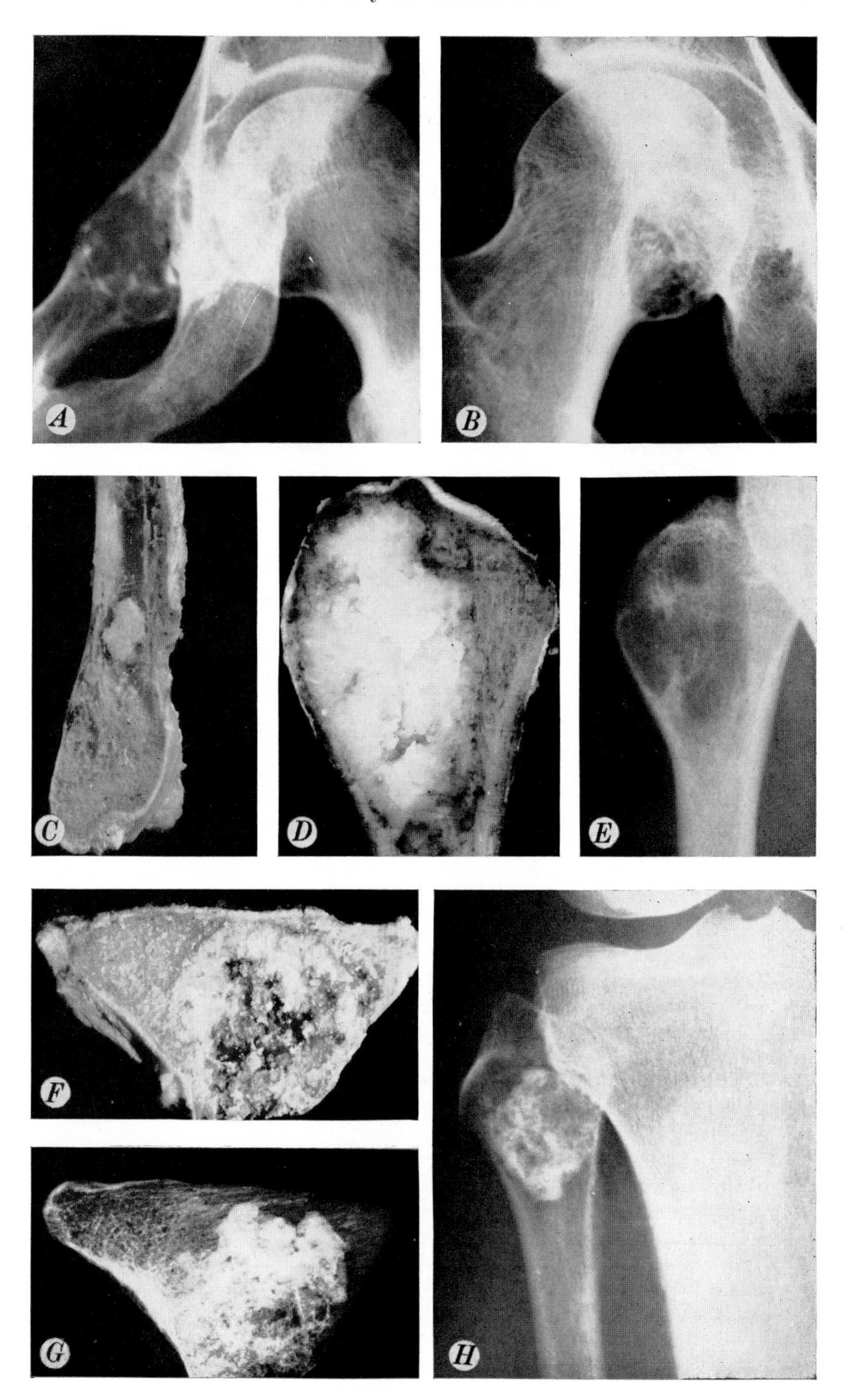


*Figure 52*

long bones, smaller or larger cartilage foci apparently derived from the cartilage plates. To what extent these findings relating to rickets are really applicable to the genesis of solitary enchondroma is a moot question and one which is now, of course, no longer subject to systematic investigation.

However, we do know that even in persons who have not had rickets, cartilage apparently derived from the plates may be found persisting in the metaphyses, even into old age. Scherer looked for such rests in the right femur, routinely removed at autopsy. He found them in 20 out of 1,125 femora (1.7 per cent) in subjects over 25 years of age. The rests were of lentil to cherry-pit size and were located in one or the other metaphysis of the femur, at most a few centimeters from where the epiphysial cartilage plate had been. They usually showed considerable evidence of regressive change, the cartilage having undergone a good deal of calcification and cystification in some cases, and even heavy ossification in others. Such rests are encountered occasionally in autopsy material from other bones, also. Unless a small rest is heavily calcified, it may not even show up in a clinical roentgenograph. If heavily calcified, it will show up as a roundish or oval, more or less stippled focus of radiopacity. Furthermore, after undergoing involutionary calcification, a small cartilage rest may even eventually disappear (see Fig. 52-*C*).

Quite apart from such findings, it may very well be that solitary enchondroma can develop *de novo*—that is, without dependence on a pre-existing cartilage rest. On the other hand, it may well be that an enchondroma might develop from a cartilage rest which has failed to become calcified. At any rate, we do know that a persisting cartilage rest may slowly increase in size, and even while increasing, undergo progressive calcification. Such an enlarging calcified cartilage focus (which may already be said to represent an enchondroma) may even attain a diameter of 2 or 3 cm. or more, and still be completely asymptomatic. Under these conditions, its presence may only be discovered incidentally, during roentgenographic examination of the bone part in some other connection. Or instead, a relatively large, heavily calcified, and essentially static cartilage focus may take on a spurt of growth, causing some pain. The latter may lead to roentgenographic examination of the affected area, and in that way to discovery of the lesion.

**Gross Pathology.**—Ordinarily, the gross material available from an enchondroma consists merely of fragments of cortex from the site of surgical entry and curettings from the interior of the affected bone area. It can be said in general that the fragments of cortical bone will be found thin and even shell-like if they come from an affected area where the cortex has been bulged out, as is commonly the case when the lesion is in a phalanx or a metacarpal or metatarsal bone. On the other hand, the cortical fragments may show but little thinning or none if they come from a lesion which has failed to bulge the cortex—a state of affairs not uncommon when a long tubular bone is affected. The medullary surface of the cortical fragments, whether they are only slightly or very much thinned, usually shows some erosive ridging and grooving. The periosteal surface is ordinarily found smooth and without evidence of apposition of new bone unless the cortical fragments have come from a site of recent infraction.

The tissue obtained by curettement from the interior of the lesion consists in some cases almost entirely of faceted bits of bluish white, firm or even somewhat myxomatous hyaline cartilage. However, such lesions may also yield some bits of dull white cartilage and yellowish, definitely gritty tissue representing heavily calcified and even ossified cartilage. On the other hand, the curettings from still other lesions may consist mainly of obviously calcified and ossified cartilage and may be only meagerly interspersed with islands of hyaline cartilage. In our cases, calcification and ossification of the lesional cartilage was more pronounced, on the whole, in the enchondromas involving long bones, especially of adults. It was also moderately pronounced in some of the phalangeal and metacarpal bone lesions, especially of the middle-aged adults.

The writer has also studied several specimens showing a solitary enchondroma intact in its setting. In one of these cases, the lesion was in the upper end of a fibula of a man 21 years of age. The major portion of the enchondroma was situated in the metaphysis, but part of it was also in the actual epiphysial end of the bone. Because the lesional tissue was neither calcified nor ossified, the lesional area appeared as a focus of relative radiolucency in the clinical roentgenograph. On the basis of the age of the patient, the location of the lesion, and the absence of radiopacity in the lesional area, it was held clinically that one was dealing with a giant-cell tumor. On this account, the upper end of the fibula was resected. When the specimen was cut in its long axis, the lesional area was found occupied by pearly white hyaline cartilage showing no evidence of calcification or ossification. The regional cortex on one side was thinned and also expanded (see Figs. 52-*D* and *E*).

Another instance of an enchondroma intact in its setting in the upper end of a fibula was also studied. The patient in this case was a woman 54 years of age. Since the lesional area showed numerous roundish radiopacities in the *x*-ray picture, the nature of the lesion as a calcifying and ossifying enchondroma was correctly surmised. When the resected specimen was sectioned in its long axis, the lesional area was found to be composed of highly calcified cartilage which, in places, was still clearly hyaline. The lesional tissue extended to beneath the articular cartilage, but the contour of the bone in the affected area was not expanded (see Figs. 52-*F*, *G*, and *H*).

An extirpated affected metacarpal bone showed general bulging of the contour of its shaft anteriorly, exaggerated on the distal half by two distinct hemispherical bulges—a smaller and a larger one. Sectioning of the bone in both the longitudinal and transverse axes revealed that the marrow cavity of the shaft was substantially filled by cartilage which, in general, was bluish white and faceted. Where the contour of the bone was distended, it could be seen that tumor cartilage was bulging forward under an attenuated cortex. In the region of the two humps, the cortex had been reduced to paper thinness. Finally, in a fourth case, the resected involved lower end of a femur showed, when sawed sagittally, an eccentrically situated tumor mass the size of a large walnut. The tumor hugged the cortex on one side but did not distend the latter. Also, it was so located that about half of the tumor mass was situated in the lower end of the metaphysis and half extended into the epiphysial end of the bone. The tumor was so highly calcified and ossified that it appeared, on the whole, yellowish and gritty, though islands of tissue clearly recognizable as cartilage were still in evidence.

**Microscopic Pathology.**—If one surveys the lesional tissue of a number of enchondromas with a scanning lens, the tendency of the cartilage to be divided off into fields or lobules will be apparent, though it will be more so in some lesions or lesional areas than in others. Frequently, the lobules of cartilage are separated by clefts, and it is not difficult to deduce, from comparison of different fields, the course of evolution of these spaces. They are formed at sites of swelling and fusion of cartilage cell lacunæ, associated with disintegration of the cells within. Eventually, many of the spaces thus created are invaded by blood vessels. If the cartilage immediately bordering upon the spaces becomes calcified or ossified, these may even come to contain some fatty and myeloid marrow.

The individual benign enchondromas vary in respect to cellularity. Some are richer in cells than others, and in still other lesions relatively cellular areas are found intermingled with areas poor in cells. In any event, a benign central cartilage tumor is never so cellular as a central chondrosarcoma (p. 315). Furthermore, the lesional tissue of a benign *solitary* enchondroma is, on the whole, much less cellular than tissue from a lesional area in a case of *multiple* enchondromatosis.

In part or throughout, the intercellular substance of the lesional tissue from a solitary enchondroma may be hyaline. When it is, the cells usually lie in lacunæ, many of which may be quite large, and a lacuna does not usually contain more than one cell, though some lacunæ show two and an occasional one may show even a nest of cells. In some areas, the intercellular substance may appear edematous or even mucoid, and where it does, the cartilage cells tend no longer to be surrounded by lacunæ, and their cytoplasm is found multipolar or stellate. Apparently an early stage of this regressive process is represented by unmasking of the collagen fibers and an acidophilic staining tendency of the ground substance.

In sections stained with hematoxylin, such ground substance as is undergoing calcification will at least look dusty, in consequence of the presence of calcareous granules in it. When the calcification is more pronounced, the granules may be particularly conspicuous around lacunæ, and also at the periphery of the cartilage lobules, especially where the latter border upon interlobular vascular spaces. Where the calcareous status is quite pronounced, the cartilage cells may be found to have undergone necrobiosis or even to have disappeared completely. Heavily calcified areas, especially where they border upon the vascular spaces, may even undergo ossification by process of metaplasia. (See Fig. 53.)

In attempting to evaluate the benignity of a cartilage tumor, one should concentrate on the cellular elements and specifically on those in the viable and not too heavily calcified areas. Also, one should avoid tissue from the immediate sites of fractures. In representative areas of a clearly benign enchondroma the cartilage cells will be found consistently small. Their cytoplasm is pale and often more or less vacuolated, and its outlines are frequently indistinct. Their nuclei, too, are consistently small and are roundish and dark-staining. Indeed, practically all of the cartilage cells of a benign enchondroma present essentially this appearance, whether or not they lie in lacunæ and irrespective of the size of the latter if they do. Scanning many preserved fields from as many parts of the lesion as possible, one may find cartilage cells which, though small, contain 2 nuclei. However, some lesions show practically no cells of this kind, while in others most of the fields will show none, but an occasional field will show one or two or even several. Such binuclear cartilage cells are cells in process of amitotic division, and indeed a clearly benign enchondroma does not show cartilage cells in mitosis. What stamps the

***Figure 53***

*A*, Photomicrograph (× 80) showing the histologic architecture of the lobules of cartilage in an enchondroma. Note that, in this lesion, the cartilage is undergoing calcification and ossification, especially about the periphery of the lobules. The tissue represented in this illustration comes from the spottily calcified femoral lesion shown in Figure 51-*G*.

*B*, Photomicrograph (× 250) showing the histologic pattern usually presented by the cartilage in a solitary enchondroma, especially of a short tubular bone. The cartilage is not highly cellular, and the intercellular material is somewhat edematous. Many of the cells have retracted in their lacunæ, and in many, both the nucleus and the cytoplasm appear drawn out. In the field shown, there are clearly no cells with double nuclei.

*C*, Photomicrograph (× 250) showing the histologic pattern of a phalangeal enchondroma in which there is heavy calcareous dusting of the intercellular material of the lesional cartilage. Again, the tissue is not highly cellular, and the cells are almost entirely uninuclear.

*D*, Photomicrograph (× 250) showing the histologic pattern usually presented by a solitary enchondroma which is very heavily calcified. Note that, despite the heavy calcification, cartilage cells are still apparent in the tissue field.

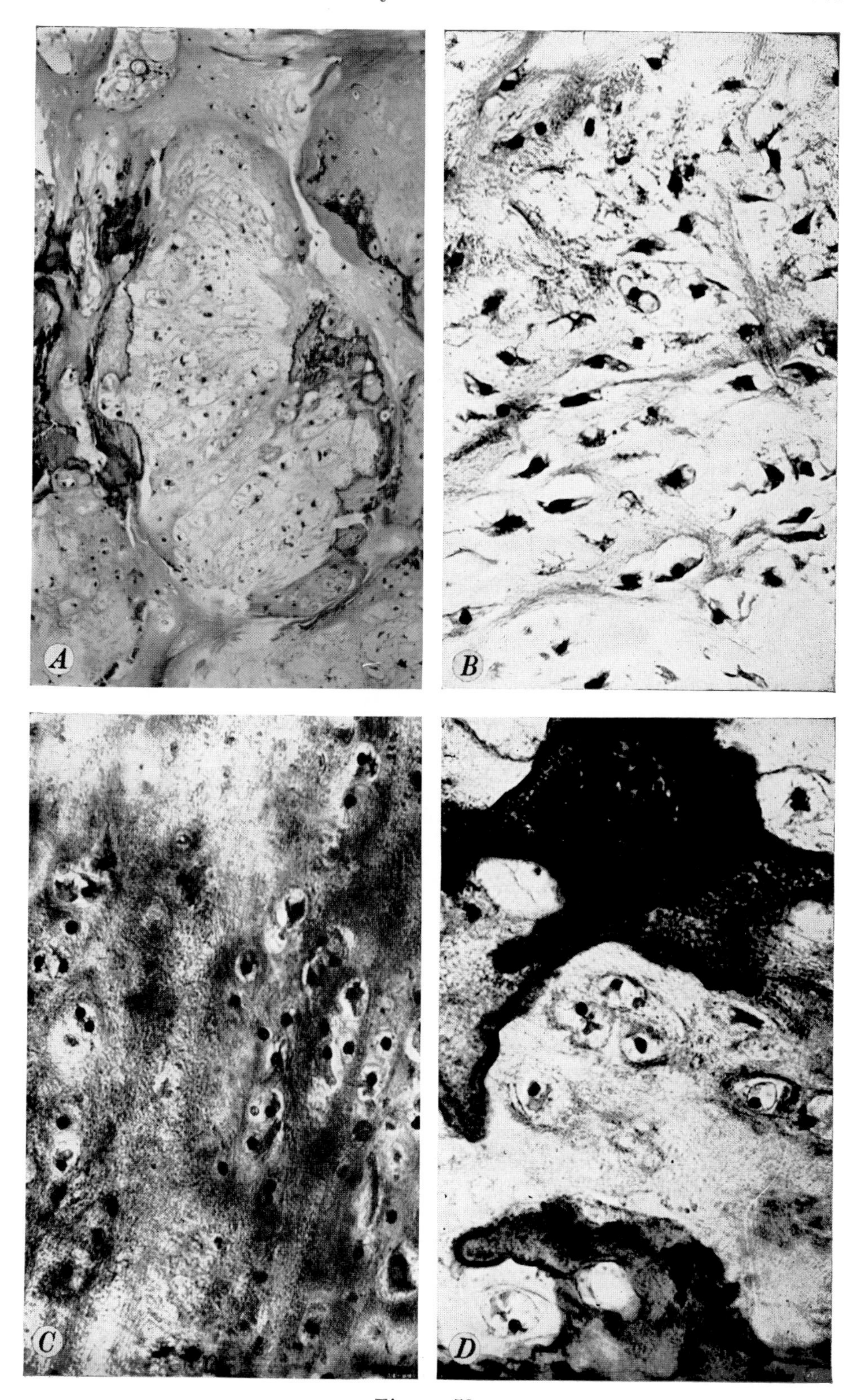


*Figure 53*

lesion as benign cytologically is the fact that the viable cartilage cells are uniformly rather small and very preponderantly uninuclear.

## MALIGNANT TRANSFORMATION OF AN ENCHONDROMA

As already noted, a solitary enchondroma sometimes undergoes malignant transformation. This rarely happens in cases in which the enchondroma is in a phalanx, metacarpal, or metatarsal bone. It is most likely to happen in cases in which the enchondroma is in a long tubular bone. However, currently, there seems to be a trend to exaggerate the tendency of benign enchondroma of long bones toward malignant transformation.

As a benign growth, the lesion may have been present for many years and may even have been entirely symptomless until there was a change in its nature. Prior to its reviviscence and malignant transformation, the enchondroma may even have become extensively calcified and ossified. The evolution of a chondrosarcoma out of a benign enchondroma, though sometimes rapid, is usually a very slow process. Early in this evolution, cytologic evidence of change in the direction of malignity is already present. However, at this stage, the significant cytologic aberrations are often by no means obvious, and furthermore are usually present only in scattered fields. To recognize them, one has to take due cognizance of the characteristic cytologic pattern of the benign lesion as described above and watch for such deviations from the pattern as increased cellularity, the presence of more than an occasional binuclear cell, and a general plumping up of the nuclei. If one finds, even if only in scattered areas, many microscopic fields showing several or more binuclear cartilage cells and especially any giant cartilage cells containing large nuclei, several nuclei or a number of chromatin clumps, the growth is no longer a clearly benign enchondroma. It may not be until much later, however, that the histologic picture of the lesion is that of a crudely obvious chondrosarcoma (see Fig. 54). For further

### *Figure 54*

*A*, Photograph showing the sagittally cut surface of the upper end of a humerus presenting a chondrosarcoma early in the course of its evolution from a calcified and ossified enchondroma. It can be seen that the surgical and anatomic neck of the bone is somewhat expanded, and there are also indications that the articular surface is finely ridged and knobbed. Small foci of cartilage can be seen in the central part of the affected area, although, on the whole, this part of the lesion is highly calcified and ossified. Peripherally, a cuff of hyaline cartilage, of irregular thickness, can be noted, and it was certain areas of this cuff that revealed clearly the sarcomatous histologic character of the lesion (see *D*).

*B*, Roentgenograph of the affected portion of the humerus shown in *A*. The relative radiolucency at the periphery represents the peripheral cuff of hyaline cartilage. The relative radiopacity of the central part of the lesion reflects calcification and ossification apparently dating back to the benign enchondromatous stage of the lesion.

*C*, Photomicrograph (× 250) showing the histologic pattern of a typical field from the biopsy specimen obtained 10 months before the tumor illustrated in *A* and *B* had been resected. Note that at that time the cartilage cells were still relatively few and the nuclei relatively small. Several of the cartilage cells have double nuclei. Originally, the lesion was regarded as a benign enchondroma, but the presence, as in this case, of more than an occasional cell with a double nucleus, in all tissue fields from the lesion, even under high power, should make one suspect that the lesion may be in course of transition to malignancy (see *D*).

*D*, Photomicrograph (× 200) showing the histologic pattern, in scattered fields, of the cartilage at the periphery of the specimen illustrated in *A*. Now, 10 months after the original biopsy (compare with *C*), the lesional tissue is relatively more cellular, the nuclei are generally plumper, and many more cells show multiple nuclei. On the basis of even scattered fields like this in a cartilage tumor thought to be benign, the lesion can be regarded as having already made the transition into a chondrosarcoma.

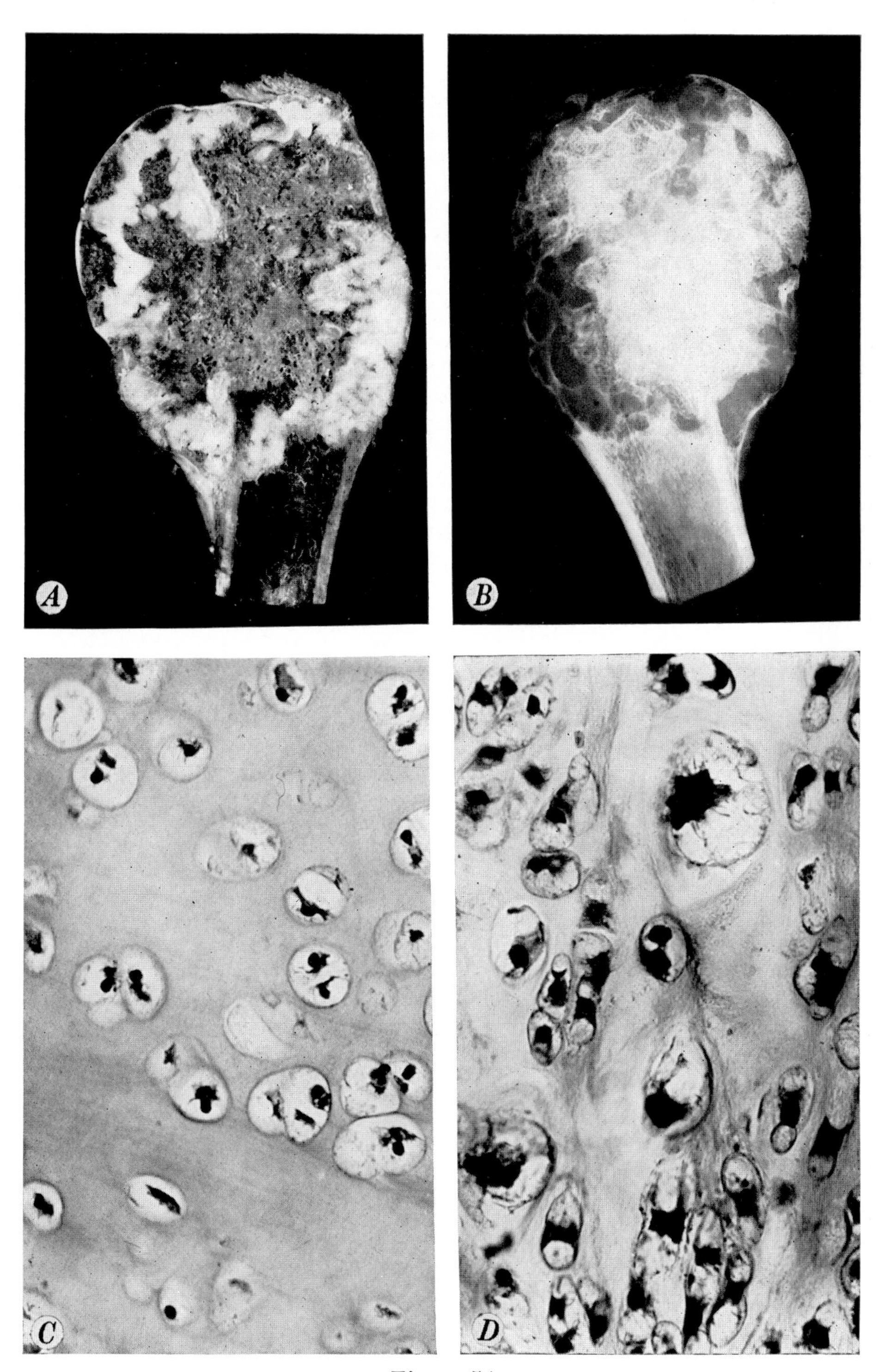


*Figure 54*

details on the transition of an enchondroma into a chondrosarcoma, see the chapter on Chondrosarcoma, page 326.

## DIFFERENTIAL DIAGNOSIS

Questions relating to differential diagnosis, insofar as they apply to a solitary enchondroma in a phalanx or in a metacarpal or metatarsal bone, have already been discussed in connection with the roentgenographic findings (p. 172). A solitary enchondroma of a long bone which extends into the epiphysial end of the bone and in which the lesional cartilage is neither calcified nor ossified might be mistaken for a giant-cell tumor or possibly a benign chondroblastoma on the basis of the clinical roentgenograph (see Figs. 52-*B* and *E*). An enchondroma which is restricted to the shaft of a long bone and in which the lesional tissue is likewise not calcified or ossified may again raise problems of clinical differential diagnosis. On the basis of the roentgenographic appearances, one might think that the lesion in question was a focus of fibrous dysplasia or even a solitary bone cyst. Thus, in such a case, too, the definitive diagnosis may have to await tissue examination (see Figs. 51-*F* and *H*).

**Bone Infarct.**—Whether asymptomatic or not, a relatively large and heavily calcified enchondroma or cartilage rest may have to be differentiated from a bone infarct. Anatomically, the differentiation is not difficult, since, no matter how heavily calcified the cartilage lesion may be, it still shows the presence of cartilage cells histologically. A bone infarct does not show them, the radiopacity it produces being due to calcification of the necrotic marrow and of the disintegrating necrotic osseous tissue. However, the differentiation is usually not difficult even on a roentgenographic basis. Specifically, in a heavily calcified cartilage growth, the radiopacities are, on the whole, small, rounded, and more or less agglomerated into a rather circumscribed, spottily radiopaque area. In a case of bone infarction, on the other hand, the radiopacity is not likely to be well circumscribed, and there are often curlicue radiopaque streaks extending away from the main area of radiopacity (see Fig. 55).

## PROGNOSIS AND TREATMENT

In general, the treatment of choice for solitary benign enchondroma of bone is surgical. Probably only those lesions need to be treated which are causing clinical complaints or whose removal may appear desirable for cosmetic or practical reasons (notably in connection with lesions in carpal phalanges). In principle, the surgical treatment consists of curettement (perhaps followed by chemical cauterization) and, in addition, under appropriate circumstances, collapse of the distended part

### *Figure 55*

*A*, Roentgenograph showing a large area of bone infarction in the upper end of a tibia of a woman 64 years of age. The lesion was asymptomatic. The tibia was the only bone affected, and the cause of the bone infarction was never ascertained. Note the rather uniform and dense radiopacity of the affected area, and the curlicue radiopacity extending down the shaft.

*B*, Photomicrograph (× 65) showing intense calcification (calcareous detritus) of the intertrabecular marrow. Note also that the osseous tissue is not viable, lacking bone cells in the lacunæ, and that it is undergoing disintegration.

*C*, Roentgenograph of a highly calcified enchondroma in the upper end of a tibia of a man 40 years of age. Note that the lesional area shows numerous small, more or less agglomerated radiopacities, in contrast to what is seen in the bone infarct shown in *A*.

*D*, Photomicrograph (× 65) showing the histologic pattern of the tissue curetted from *C*. Note that the basic character of the lesional tissue as cartilage is still clearly apparent.

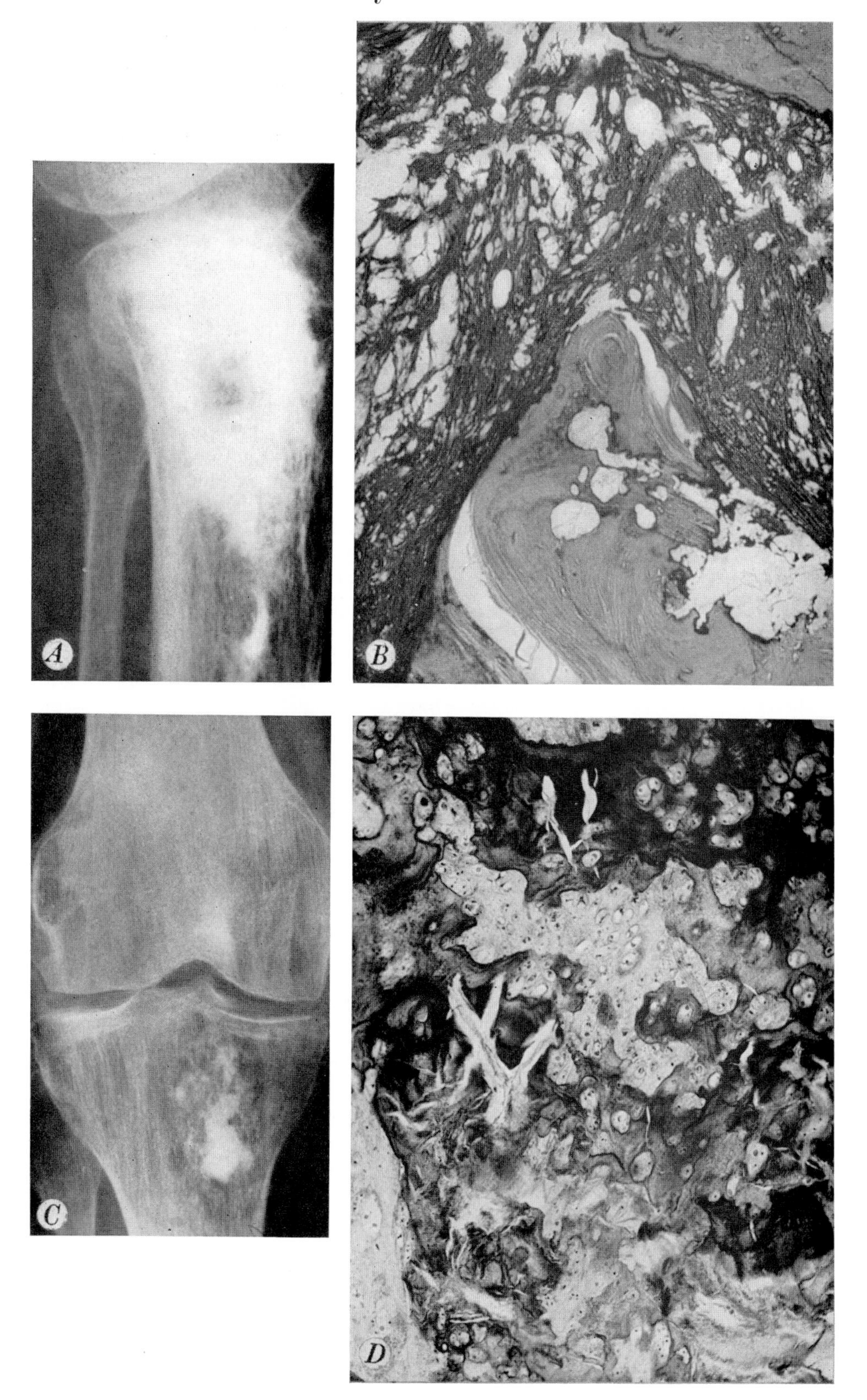


*Figure 55*

of the cortical wall, the introduction of bone chips, or the insertion of bone grafts. A surgeon confronted with a clinically troublesome enchondroma in a long tubular bone must, as indicated, be particularly aware of the possibility of sarcomatous degeneration. Nevertheless, for most enchondromas in such a location, curettage and the use of bone chips or a bone graft will prove adequate. A recurrence, with or without clear-cut evidence of malignant transformation, is an indication for considering more drastic surgery. What this should consist of will depend, of course, upon the case as a whole and upon the precise location of the lesion. Certainly, in some of these cases, at least segmental resection of the affected portion of the bone and its replacement by a massive bone graft or a metallic prosthesis is indicated.

## MULTIPLE ENCHONDROMATOSIS

Multiple enchondromatosis is characterized by the presence of circumscribed foci and/or large masses of cartilage in the interior of at least several and sometimes many bones of the affected person. Even if numerous bones are affected, the involvement tends to be heavier on one side of the body than on the other. The disorder is of rather infrequent occurrence, and apparently not hereditary. In contrast to solitary enchondroma, multiple enchondromatosis apparently represents a deep-rooted anomaly of skeletal development, and specifically a cartilage dysplasia of the bones. Also, lesional cartilage from a case of multiple enchondromatosis tends to be much more cellular than lesional cartilage from a solitary enchondroma. Indeed, in this connection, it is often possible to decide histologically, even on the basis of a single tissue section, whether the tissue came from a solitary enchondroma or from one of the lesions in a case of multiple enchondromatosis.

In some cases, the skeletal involvement becomes more or less stabilized after puberty. In others, the involvement is progressive, and, by the time early adulthood is reached, monstrous deformities may have developed, particularly in relation to the bones of the hands and feet. Not infrequently, also, the cartilage within one or another affected bone undergoes chondrosarcomatous transformation. This complication is by no means confined to the cases in which the skeletal involvement is widespread and pronounced. Furthermore, it is not unusual for a patient affected with enchondromatosis to present multiple hemangiomata, along with phlebectasia, in various soft parts.

**Nomenclature.**—The name "dyschondroplasia" is frequently used for the disorder. It was introduced by Ollier, and, on account of his contribution to the understanding of the condition, the latter is also often denoted as "Ollier's disease." However, the term "Ollier's disease" is often restricted to cases showing heavy involvement of limb bones on one side of the body, in accordance with the findings in the cases described by Ollier himself. The term "dyschondroplasia" is a good name, in a way, since it suggests correctly that one is dealing with a developmental defect relating to cartilage. However, the name can be a source of confusion because the term "hereditary deforming chondrodysplasia" has been used, and is still often used, for cases of hereditary multiple exostosis (p. 150), which is a disorder entirely unrelated to the condition in question here. The writer favors the name "multiple enchondromatosis" in spite of his recognition of one objection to it—an objection bearing on the question of pathogenesis. Specifically, the name fails to allow for the fact that, while much of the proliferating cartilage develops from within the bone, as the name implies, some of it develops beneath the periosteum and penetrates into the bone. The name does have the advantage of covering all cases of the disorder, irrespective of the extent or precise distribution of the involvement, and of contrasting the disorder with multiple exostosis. The term

"Maffucci's syndrome" has been applied to cases of multiple enchondromatosis (or "dyschondroplasia") associated with hemangiomata.

## CLINICAL CONSIDERATIONS

As noted, skeletal enchondromatosis is of rather infrequent occurrence. It is generally stated that it predilects males. In the writer's own experience, covering about 15 cases, there was no significant sex difference in incidence. It is usually during childhood that the condition first gives rise to clinical manifestations. The cases in which the skeletal involvement is widespread come to notice particularly early—generally when the affected child is about 2 years old.

**Skeletal Distribution.**—Like solitary enchondroma, the condition of skeletal enchondromatosis affects only bones preformed in cartilage. On this basis, certain parts of the skull (parts of the base and some bones of the face) ought to be vulnerable. However, their involvement is apparently rare and certainly not part of the characteristic clinical picture of the condition.

It is clearly recognized that the extent of implication of the skeleton may vary widely from case to case. At one end of the scale are the cases in which the disorder is limited to some bones of one upper or lower limb or even to a few short tubular bones of the hand or foot of the limb in question (see Fig. 56). Then there are the cases of more extensive but still solely (or at least predominantly) unilateral involvement. In these, the disorder has affected the bones of a limb and the adjacent part of the trunk, or of both limbs on the same side, and perhaps also a few bones (particularly hand or foot bones) on the other side. At the other end of the scale are the cases in which there is heavy implication of the limb bones, often along with trunk bones, on both sides. However, even in these cases, as already stated, the disorder is likely to be somewhat more severe on one side of the body than on the other.

**Clinical Emergence and Course of the Disorder.**—The complaints which lead to discovery of the disorder vary with the distribution of the lesions and the extent to which they have weakened or deformed the affected bones in the particular case. Pathologic fracture of an affected bone may be a presenting feature, but is not a common one. Also, the patients rarely complain of pain in connection with the disorder.

When an upper limb is involved, the most common complaint is of slowly increasing swelling of some fingers, due to bulging out of the phalanges by the enchondromata. Sometimes, with involvement of an upper limb, the presenting feature may not be the swelling of the fingers so much as deformity of the forearm. This is usually a bowing deformity associated with ulnar deviation of the hand and/or restriction of rotary motion of the forearm. The forearm deformity is usually the result of discrepancy in growth between the radius and ulna at their lower ends, the ulna being shorter than the radius, so that the latter becomes bowed and its head may even protrude abnormally at the elbow. This deformity is reminiscent of that seen in the forearm in many cases of multiple exostosis (p. 154). When a lower limb is involved, while swelling of the pedal phalanges may be the presenting complaint, the latter is more often that of knock-knee. This is due to deformity and retarded growth of the femur and tibia, from the presence of enchondromata in them. Of course, in the severe cases, showing involvement of both limbs on one side or all four limbs, the presenting complaints will vary correspondingly.

The retarded growth of affected limbs stands out particularly clearly in relation to the lower extremities. It is most striking in those cases in which one lower limb is heavily affected, while the opposite one is involved only slightly if at all. In these cases, of course, the patient limps. At the age of 2 or 3 years, the discrepancy in length between the two lower extremities may already amount to as much as 2 to 4 cm. In adolescents or young adults, discrepancies as large as 10 to 25 cm. have sometimes been noted. Pronounced discrepancy in length between the two lower limbs is often associated with a compensatory scoliosis and sharp tilt of the pelvis. Even in the cases in which the lesions are more nearly symmetrically distributed over the two sides of the body, the limb bones may be more extremely shortened on one side, in consequence of their severer involvement on that side. Cases of widespread enchondromatosis surviving into adult life may come to show, as already noted, monstrous deformities of the hands and feet (especially the former).

**Nonskeletal Manifestations.**—As indicated, multiple hemangiomata are observed in some cases of skeletal enchondromatosis, and such cases are sometimes denoted as instances of the *Maffucci syndrome.* Indeed, hemangiomata represent the most common extraskeletal aberration associated with skeletal enchondromatosis. They were present in 3 of the cases studied by the writer, and the literature contains reports on about 25 cases in which hemangiomata were found in association with skeletal enchondromatosis. The paper by Carleton and associates is particularly illuminating in this connection. In any particular case, many of the hemangiomata may measure 5 cm. or even more in diameter. They usually appear as soft, lobulated or nodular tumors in the deeper layers of the skin or in the subcutaneous tissues, but sometimes extend even deeply into the muscles. The more superficially located ones may impart a bluish discoloration to the skin.

The hemangiomata are ordinarily painless and do not give rise to capillary pulsation or murmurs. Their presence is sometimes associated with superficial phlebectasia. The hemangiomata may occur in the soft tissues overlying affected bones or in the soft tissues overlying unaffected bony parts. Furthermore, they may be found in the abdominal wall or in the intercostal spaces, and, at autopsy, have even been noted in internal organs. Many of the vascular tumors may eventually contain phleboliths and hence come to stand out roentgenographically through the presence of small, roundish radiopacities within them. The hemangiomata apparently represent a vascular anomaly associated with, but independent of, the skeletal aberration. In this respect, they correspond, for instance, to the abnormal skin pigmentation observed in many cases of fibrous dysplasia of bone.

***Figure 56***

*A*, Roentgenograph of a hand of a man 20 years of age affected with multiple enchondromatosis limited to the phalanges of the fifth finger of that hand. He had been aware since he was 11 years old of a slowly progressive but painless enlargement of that finger. The absence of involvement of other skeletal parts was confirmed by roentgenographic examination.

*B*, Roentgenograph of a hand of a boy 13 years of age affected with multiple enchondromatosis of somewhat greater extent. The bones involved were a number of phalanges of the third, fourth, and fifth fingers, corresponding metacarpal bones of that hand, and the lower end of the ulna. From the time when the boy was 6 years old, it had been noted that there were painless swellings on the fourth finger, and that the lower end of the forearm was undergoing enlargement, associated with limitation of supination and pronation.

*C*, Roentgenograph of a hand of a boy 13 years of age affected with multiple enchondromatosis of still greater extent but still limited to the bones of that upper limb. From the time when the boy was 4 years old, painless, slowly progressing swellings were evident on the fingers. A skeletal survey in this case also showed the presence of lesions in the radius and ulna of the limb in question.

*D*, Photograph of the hand illustrated in Figure *C*.

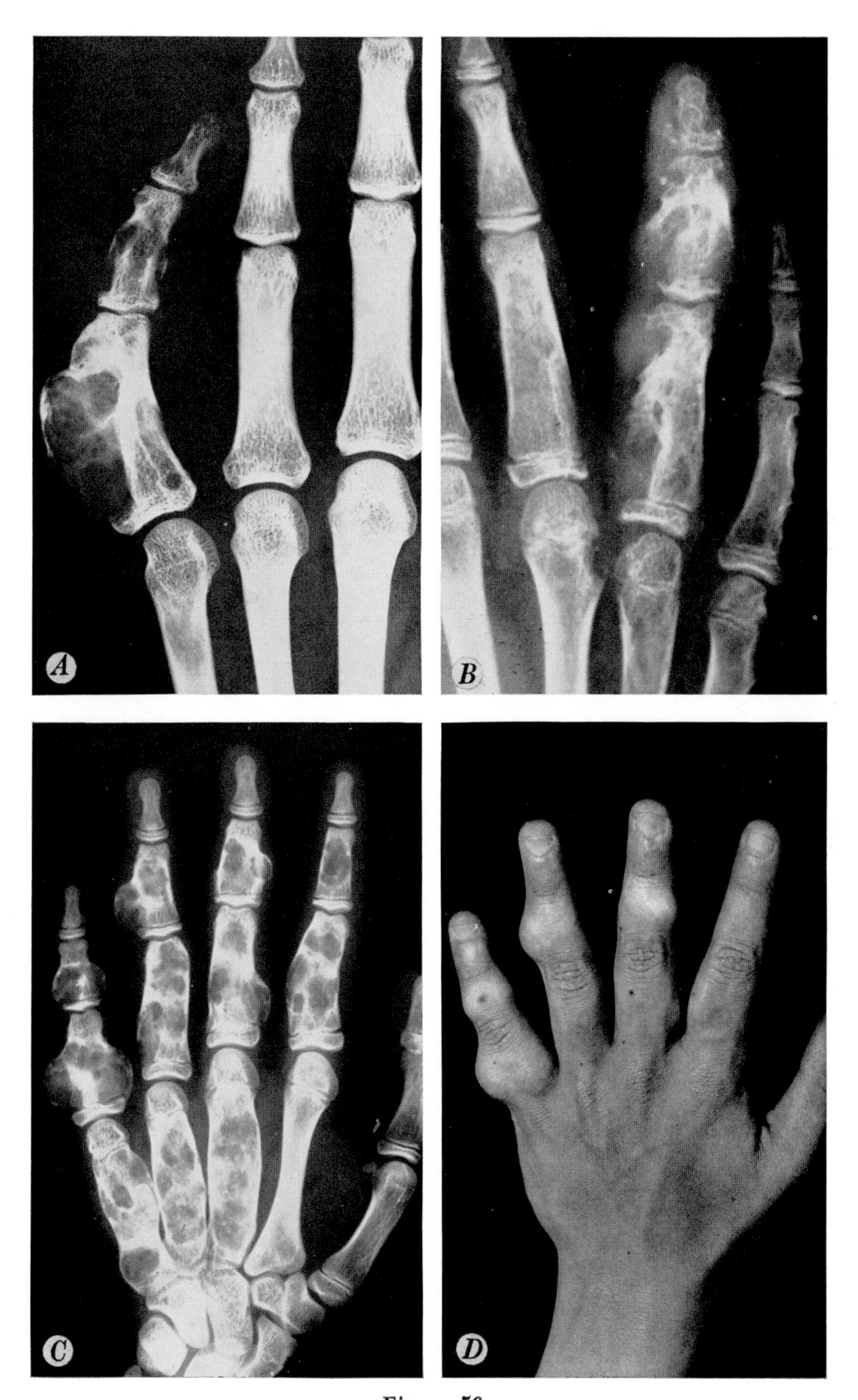


*Figure 56*

In cases showing heavy involvement of one side of the body, a slight amount of flattening of the face on that side has sometimes been observed. Other abnormalities also occasionally mentioned include vitiligo and multiple pigmented nevi. In one reported case of skeletal enchondromatosis, a severe anemia supervened, presumably due to crowding out of the bone marrow by the cartilage, and this was held to have contributed to the fatal outcome.

## ROENTGENOGRAPHIC FINDINGS

First, it can be stated that, in any particular case, many more bones are usually found affected roentgenographically than appear to be involved on physical examination. Also, on the whole, skeletal enchondromatosis is not particularly difficult to diagnose on a roentgenographic basis. It will be observed that, in young subjects, affected long bones, when not too severely involved, may retain their normal contour. On the other hand, they may show some bulging of the contour (especially on one side), particularly in one or both metaphysial regions. Especially in these regions, the bulged long bones are likely to present more or less radiolucent areas interspersed by one or several septa running approximately in the long axis of the bone. As the subjects become older, such striped radiolucent areas occasionally come to involve the epiphysial regions also. Furthermore, in one or both iliac bones the roentgenographs may show rarefied areas traversed by septa which, in these bones, may be arranged in somewhat fan-like striations. From the point of view of pathology, the more light-permeable regions between the septa are to be interpreted as containing cartilage, and the septa themselves as densified osseous trabeculæ (see Fig. 57).

In the phalanges and the metacarpal and metatarsal bones, the enchondrotic involvement is usually manifest in oval or roundish areas of rarefaction, without striping, but sometimes delimited in part by a marginal zone of radiopacity. As noted, the enchondromata commonly thin and bulge out the cortex, or even destroy the latter. Finally, it may be pointed out that within large areas of enchondromatous rarefaction there may be some radiopaque spots indicating sites at which the cartilage has undergone calcification.

## PATHOLOGIC FINDINGS AND PATHOGENESIS

**Gross Pathology.**—A moderately affected long bone (for instance, a femur) of an adult patient is usually found somewhat shortened and bowed. It is usually also found somewhat broadened in the metaphysial regions. In longitudinal section, these regions will be found occupied by numerous pea-sized to bean-sized

*Figure 57*

*A*, Roentgenograph showing involvement of the upper parts of the femora of a girl 7 years of age affected with multiple enchondromatosis widely distributed over the skeleton. The child was slow in learning to walk, and the observation that she was knock-kneed led to discovery of the enchondromatosis. Note that the extent of the involvement is greater on the left side than on the right. Note also the presence of radiolucent areas interspersed by septa —a finding rather characteristic of the *x*-ray picture of affected long bones. Lesions are also present in the innominate bones, but the latter are not so strikingly involved as the femora.

*B*, Roentgenograph showing the appearance of the lower ends of the femora and upper ends of the tibiæ and fibulæ from the case illustrated in *A*. Again, the involvement is more severe on the left side than on the right. In this case, the lesions in the other affected long and short tubular bones were likewise more striking on the left than on the right.

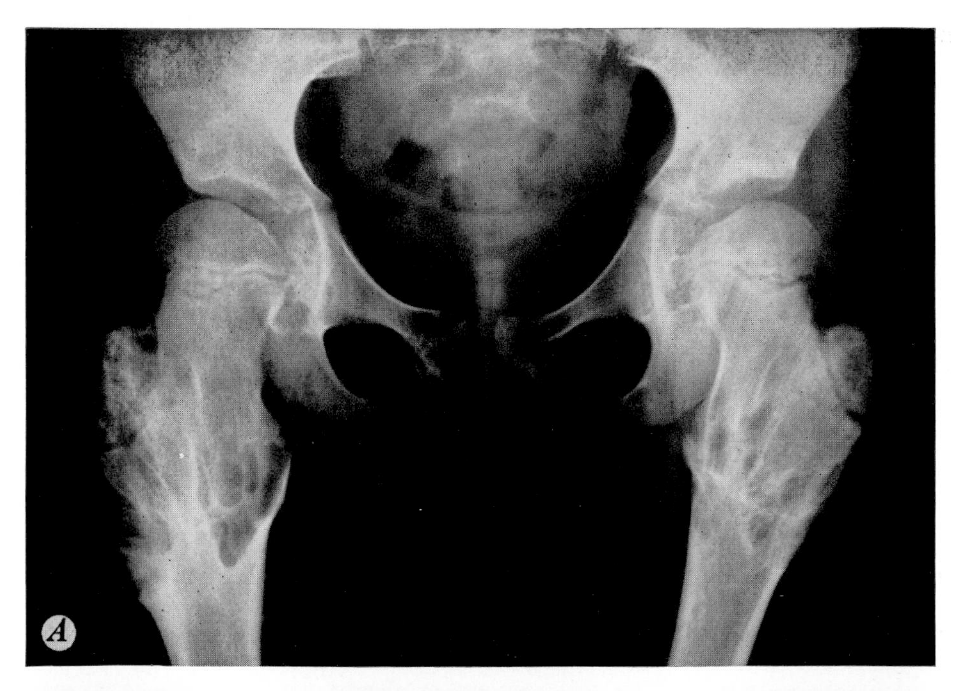


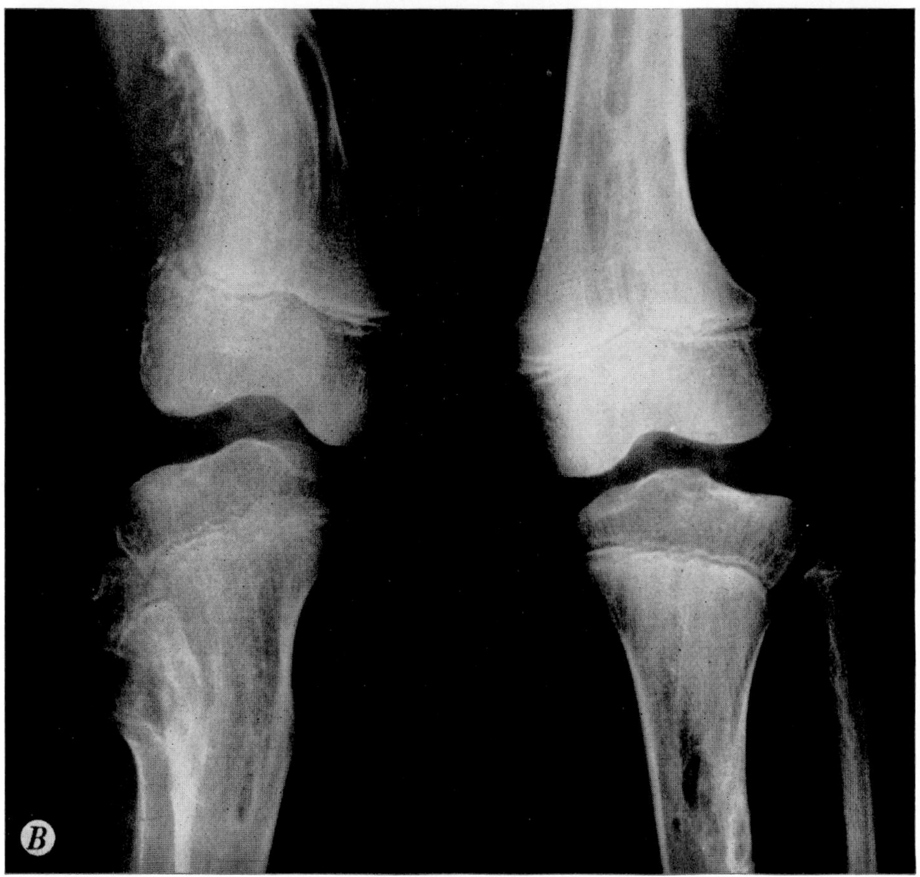


*Figure 57*

glassy, gray-white, discrete or confluent cartilage masses separated by bony septa. One may also encounter cartilage masses several centimeters in diameter, and the cartilage tissue may even appear as a solid rod down the middle of the shaft. In the broadened metaphysial regions in such a case, the cortex is not necessarily bumpy. However, cartilage will be found abutting upon the inner surface of the cortex in many places. In the ends of the bone, cartilaginous foci may be absent. If present, they are ordinarily neither large nor numerous. It will also be noted that nothing remains of the former epiphysial cartilage plates in the adult, for the epiphyses of the affected bone fuse normally with the shaft.

In a more severely affected femur, the extent of the cartilaginous invasion of the interior is much greater, and the cartilage may even substantially fill one or both epiphysial ends of the bone. Furthermore, the contour of the bone is likely to be found distorted over a large extent, and to present many distinct bumps. Also, the articular cartilages themselves may show evidences of cartilage proliferation, their surfaces presenting a warty, nodular appearance. In any case, it is interesting to note that no matter how severely the ends of a bone are affected, the synovium of the articular capsules shows no evidence of cartilage metaplasia.

The findings in affected phalanges are well exemplified in a finger studied by the writer. It had been amputated because it had become unwieldy and inconvenient, though it was by no means as severely affected by the disorder as fingers can be. This finger presented 3 main bulges, of which the distal one was the smallest and the proximal one the largest. When it was cut longitudinally, the bulged, expanded phalanges presented an almost solidly cartilaginous composition. The cartilage was composed of closely set lobules or facets of hyaline cartilage tissue, but showed, here and there, some small areas of ossification. In some of the distended areas, there was no delimiting bone beneath the periosteum, while in others there was merely a paper-thin cortical shell. Also striking was the fact that when the articular surfaces of the phalanges were inspected they were found to be bumpy and warty instead of smooth, suggesting that the articular cartilages, too, had been proliferating (see Figs. 58-*A* and *B*).

In an affected lower limb, for instance, in which both the femur and the tibia are heavily involved, the fibula may not appear involved from the outside. However, when split open, it will usually show at least some scattered cartilage foci in the metaphysial regions. In a case in which the disease has heavily affected the upper and lower limb on one side of the body, or even all four limbs, trunk bones, too, are found involved. Thus the ribs not infrequently show cartilage foci at some distance from the costochondral junction. The sternum, too, usually shows en-

***Figure 58***

*A*, Photograph of a longitudinally sectioned finger from a case of skeletal enchondromatosis. The finger was removed because of functional inconvenience. Note the cartilage occupying the interior of the expanded phalangeal bones, and note also the bumpiness of the articular surfaces of these bones.

*B*, Photograph of a tibia removed at autopsy in a case of skeletal enchondromatosis. Note the broadening of the upper and lower portions of the shaft. The sectioned bone (right) shows a considerable amount of cartilage in the interior. These accumulations of cartilage are present even in the midportion of the shaft. (Reproduced from article by Carleton *et al.*, Quart. J. Med., *11*, 203, 1942.)

*C*, Photomicrograph (× 25) showing the histologic pattern of the cartilage occupying the interior of the phalanges illustrated in *A*. Note that the cartilage is more cellular than the cartilage ordinarily is in cases of solitary enchondroma.

*D*, Photomicrograph (× 75) showing in greater detail the cartilage topography illustrated in *C*.

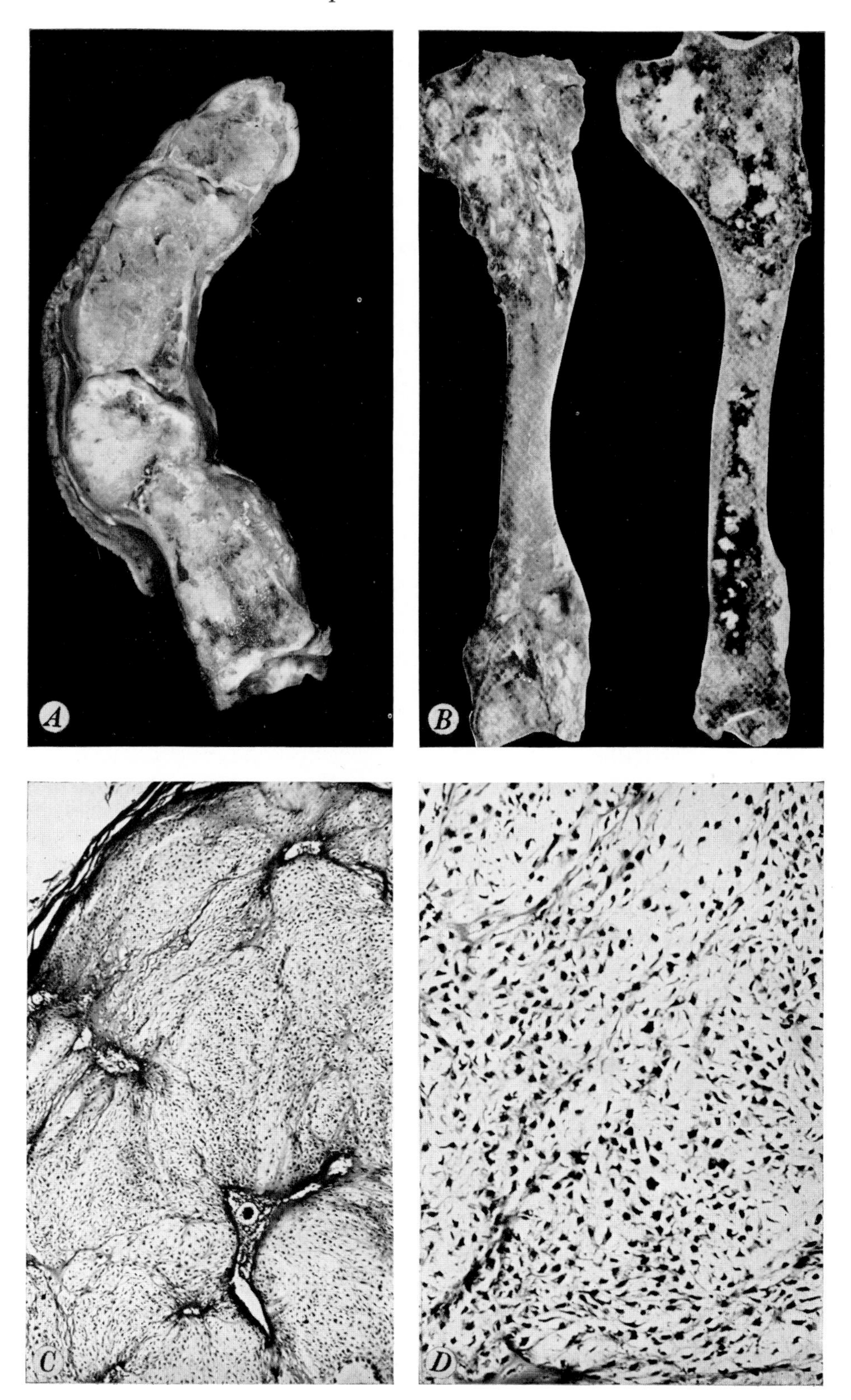


*Figure 58*

chondromata. Small enchondromata may likewise be noted in vertebral bodies, sometimes in connection with, and sometimes remote from, the intervertebral disks. The pelvic bones are not infrequently rather heavily affected, showing cartilage masses in the marrow spaces between the cortical tables, which are expanded in places.

**Pathogenesis.**—The question of the source of the cartilage in the interior of the bones in skeletal enchondromatosis is discussed by Speiser on the basis of the autopsy findings in the case of a boy $4\frac{1}{2}$ years old. He states that it is the periosteum, the epiphysial cartilage plates (or their cartilaginous analogues at synchondroses) or, in appropriate bones, both together, that give rise to the cartilage formations of enchondromatosis. He says, furthermore, that the cartilage nests originating from the periosteum grow from the cambium layer. In his case, the cambium-cartilage nests were widely distributed over the bones, were relatively small, and tended to grow inward, invading the marrow cavity. As to the participation of the epiphysial cartilage plates in the formation of the enchondromata, Speiser found that some of those originating from the plates could still be traced to the latter by stalks, although these stalks might be very thin. The enchondromata regarded as issuing from the plates were much larger but less numerous than those of periosteal origin.

In supporting the idea that epiphysial cartilage plates are a source of the enchondromata, Speiser's study brings partial confirmation to the conception of the pathogenesis of enchondromata developed by Virchow and espoused by many followers. Obviously, however, he does not hold, as Virchow did, that epiphysial cartilage plates are the sole source of the enchondromata. In maintaining that the periosteum is another source of the enchondromata, Speiser raises some interesting questions in regard to the possible relations between multiple enchondromatosis and multiple exostosis. However, as is brought out elsewhere (p. 166), these two conditions are to be regarded as quite independent disease entities.

**Microscopic Pathology.**—Much of what has been said about the histology of the cartilage tissue in solitary enchondroma of bone is applicable in a general way to the histology of this tissue in cases of multiple enchondromatosis. However, there is likely to be less calcium impregnation of the matrix of the cartilage of the lesional tissue from a case of multiple enchondromatosis than in the lesional tissue of a solitary enchondroma. A much more important difference, as already noted, is that the cartilage of the lesional tissue is much more cellular in cases of enchondromatosis. Furthermore, the cartilage cell nuclei tend to be slightly larger than they are in lesional tissue from a solitary enchondroma. Also, more than an occasional cell will show double nuclei. Indeed, on the basis of these differences in the histologic picture, it is possible for a pathologist to state with some confidence whether a cartilage lesion under inspection comes from a case of solitary enchondroma or from one of multiple enchondromatosis. These findings in enchondromatosis are in line with the rather persistent cartilage proliferation occurring in the disorder. Altogether, in fact, one may regard the lesional tissue in cases of skeletal enchondromatosis as being in a precancerous state (see Figs. 58-*C* and *D*).

***Figure 59***

*A*, Photomicrograph (× 6) showing the topography of a focus of cartilage in a femur from a case of enchondromatosis. Note the lobular arrangement of the cartilage. Note also that, about the periphery of the darker-staining lobules of cartilage, there are lobules which have stained more lightly. In these lighter areas, the lesional cartilage is undergoing chondrosarcomatous transformation (see *B*).

*B*, Photomicrograph (× 65) showing, in greater detail, the histologic pattern of the evolving chondrosarcoma illustrated in *A*. Note at the left and at the upper right that the cartilage matrix is loosened up and that many of the cartilage cells have abnormally large and bizarre nuclei.

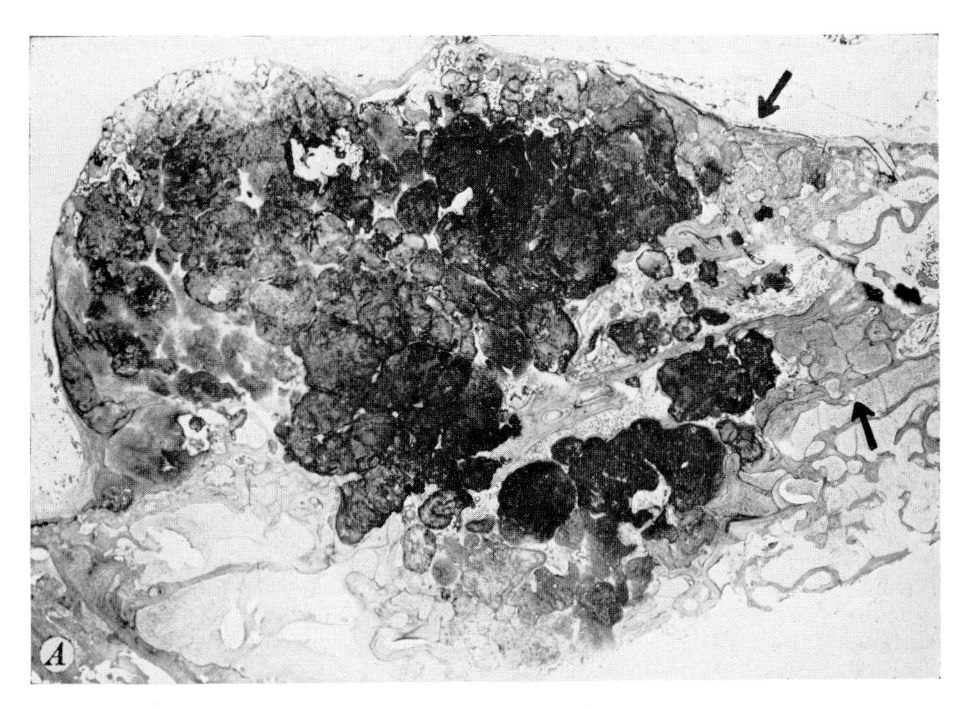


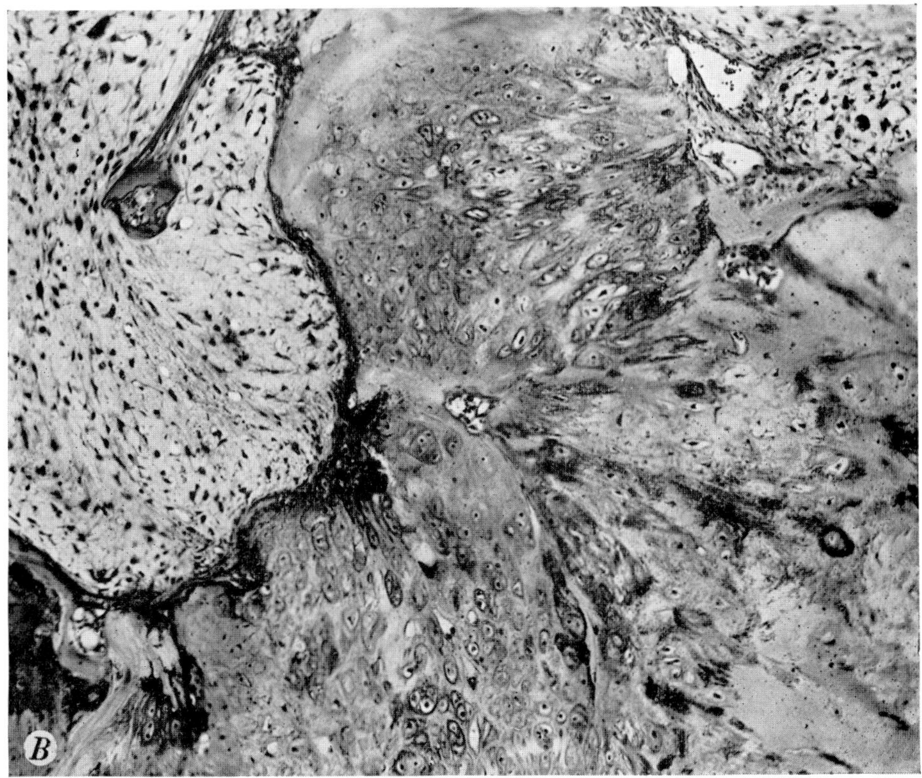


***Figure 59***

## CHONDROSARCOMA AS A COMPLICATION

A chondrosarcoma appearing in one or more of the affected bones is a rather common complication in cases of multiple enchondromatosis. This complication rarely occurs before adulthood, however, and most often appears during middle life. It is difficult to estimate its true incidence, but this is probably somewhere around 50 per cent, at least, in any group of cases representing all ages and all stages of the disorder. At any rate, this was the incidence in our group of cases as a whole. However, the majority of the patients in this group were still young. Therefore, it is likely that some of them will develop chondrosarcomas by the time they reach middle life. Thus the true incidence of chondrosarcoma in this group will probably be higher when all the returns are in.

It should be noted that the development of chondrosarcoma is by no means confined to the pronounced cases. Thus, the writer has seen it develop in a first metatarsal bone of a young woman in whom the enchondromatosis involved only this bone, the phalanges of the corresponding big toe, and, to a slight degree, the homolateral tibia. Also, he has seen it develop in an ulna of a youth in whom the enchondromatosis was present in addition only in some of the homolateral phalanges and metacarpal bones. On the other hand, he has studied the case of an elderly woman in whom the enchondromatosis was widespread in the skeleton and in whom a chondrosarcoma developed in a severely affected femur. When it does develop, the chondrosarcoma breaks out of the bone and invades the neighboring soft parts. Cytologically, its character is the same as that of a chondrosarcoma appearing under any other conditions (see p. 320). As the chondrosarcoma becomes more obviously malignant, its cells show progressive atypism. They then stand out in bold relief from the cells of such cartilage tissue within the affected bone as has not yet undergone sarcomatous transformation (see Fig. 59).

## TREATMENT

No form of medical treatment is known for enchondromatosis. It is doubtful whether radiation therapy is of any value, either. Certain surgical procedures have been useful in some cases, in accordance with various indications. For instance, for knock-knee deformity, osteotomy of the femur, and sometimes also of the tibia, has been practiced, even in young children. In late childhood and adolescence, important discrepancies in length between the lower limbs are an indication for surgical arrestment of epiphysial growth on the less affected or normal side. Fortunately, in some cases, the disorder ceases to progress after general body growth comes to an end. In others, however, it does not cease, and many of the bones, particularly of the hands and feet, may become monstrously deformed. If one or more affected fingers, for instance, become very large and unwieldy, it may be best to ablate them. The emergence of a chondrosarcoma of course requires treatment in harmony with the gravity of this complication.

### REFERENCES

Burack, P. I.: Ossifying Enchondroma of the Head of the Humerus, Bull. Hosp. Joint Dis., *1*, 3, 1940.

Buschbeck, H.: Beitrag zur Kenntnis röntgenologisch sichtbarer (bisher als Enostosen beschriebener) Gebilde in der Femurspongiosa, Fortschr. a. d. Geb. d. Röntgenstrahlen, *46*, 53, 1932.

Carleton, A., Elkington, J. St. C., Greenfield, J. G., and Robb-Smith, A. H. T.: Maffucci's Syndrome (Dyschondroplasia with Haemangeiomata), Quart. J. Med., *11*, 203, 1942.

Dahle, M.: Chondrodysplasia (Ollier's Disease)—Multiple Enchondromatosis? Acta chir. scandinav., *83*, 329, 1940.
Exner, G.: Chondromatose—Dyschondroplasie—Ollier'sche Wachstumsstörung, Fortschr. a. d. Geb. d. Röntgenstrahlen, *73*, 454, 1950.
Fairbank, H. A. T.: Dyschondroplasia, J. Bone & Joint Surg., *30-B*, 689, 1948.
Ferguson, A. B., Jr.: Calcified Medullary Defects in Bone, J. Bone & Joint Surg., *29*, 598, 1947.
Fevre, M., and Alptekin: Maladie d'Ollier. Syndrome de Kast, Rev. chir. orthop., *40*, 15, 1954.
Hunter, D., and Wiles, P.: Dyschondroplasia (Ollier's Disease), Brit. J. Surg., *22*, 507, 1935.
Jaffe, H. L., and Lichtenstein, L.: Solitary Benign Enchondroma of Bone, Arch. Surg., *46*, 480, 1943.
Kast, and Recklinghausen: Ein Fall von Enchondrom mit ungewöhnlicher Multiplication, Virchows Arch. f. path. Anat., *118*, 1, 1889.
Laurence, W., and Franklin, E. L.: Calcifying Enchondroma of Long Bones, J. Bone & Joint Surg., *35-B*, 224, 1953.
Mason, M. L.: Tumors of the Hand, Surg., Gynec. & Obst., *64*, 129, 1937.
Menne, F. R., and Frank, W. W.: So-called Primary Chondroma of the Ethmoid, Arch. Otolaryng., *26*, 170, 1937.
Ollier, L.: De la Dyschondroplasie, Bull. Soc. de chir. de Lyon, *3*, 22, 1900.
Scherer, E.: Exostosen, Enchondrome und ihre Beziehung zum Periost, Frankfurt. Ztschr. f. Path., *36*, 587, 1928.
Speiser, F.: Ein Fall von systematisierter Enchondromatose des Skeletts, Virchows Arch. f. path. Anat., *258*, 126, 1925.
Strang, C., and Rannie, I.: Dyschondroplasia with Haemangiomata (Maffucci's Syndrome). Report of a Case Complicated by Intracranial Chondrosarcoma, J. Bone & Joint Surg., *32-B*, 376, 1950.
Umansky, A. L.: Dyschondroplasia with Hemangiomata (Maffucci's Syndrome). Bull. Hosp. Joint Dis., *7*, 59, 1946.
Virchow, R.: Ueber die Entstehung des Enchondroms und seine Beziehungen zur Enchondrosis und Exostosis cartilaginea. Monatsberichte d. kgl. preuss. Akad. d. Wissenschaften for 1875, p. 760.

Chapter

# 12

# Juxtacortical Chondroma

THE name *juxtacortical chondroma* refers to a benign cartilage growth which develops in relation to the periosteum and/or immediate parosteal connective tissue of a bone, tends to invade the underlying bone cortex, but usually does not break through the cortex into the medullary cavity of the bone. Other names by which the lesion has been denoted are: "eccentric chondroma" (see Roberts) and "periosteal chondroma" (see Mason, and Lichtenstein and Hall). The term "juxtacortical chondroma" seems preferable because it is not only flexible in respect to the site of origin of the lesional cartilage, but also emphasizes the orientation of the lesional tissue to the neighboring bone cortex.

The juxtacortical chondroma is encountered only occasionally. It usually appears as a solitary lesion, but sometimes more than a single lesion is present in a given subject. Particularly if the lesional cartilage is not calcified, the *x*-ray picture of a juxtacortical chondroma may raise problems of differential diagnosis. Cartilaginous growths oriented primarily to the capsules of joints are also occasionally encountered. These para-articular chondromas will be found discussed in connection with tumorous lesions appearing in and around joints (see p. 567).

## CLINICAL CONSIDERATIONS

**Incidence.**—As indicated, the juxtacortical chondroma is not at all a common lesion. The writer's experience with the lesion covers only 9 cases. There appears to be no sex difference in its incidence. As to age incidence, the subject is more likely to be a young or middle-aged adult than a child.

**Localization.**—A juxtacortical chondroma does not tend to exceed 3 or 4 cm., and is often only 1 or 2 cm. in its greatest dimension. In 7 of the 9 cases studied by the writer, the lesion was solitary, while in the other 2 there were multiple lesions. In one of the latter cases, a chondroma was oriented to the lower part of the shaft cortex of the right fibula, and this was the presenting lesion. However, another focus of juxtacortical chondroma was found abutting upon the shaft cortex of the right radius, but this lesion was asymptomatic. In the second of the 2 cases presenting multiple lesions, the symptomatic lesion (among the largest seen) was oriented to the proximal phalanx of the third left finger. In addition, several other phalanges of the same hand showed declivities produced in the cortex by pressure from small foci of abutting cartilage. In the cases presenting the condition in solitary form, the lesion was again oriented to the shaft cortex of either a short or a long tubular bone.

**Clinical Complaints and Findings.**—On the whole, these are not striking. As a rule, the presence of a small, slowly enlarging, and sometimes entirely painless local swelling or mass has been noted for months or even years. When some pain is present, it is usually of a dull, aching character. The mass, which is usually firm and nonmovable, is sometimes not even tender to pressure. In an occasional instance, it remains small for many years and then begins to undergo perceptible enlargement. Thus, in one case, in which the lesion was oriented to a phalanx, the patient had been aware for 15 years of a small, painless local swelling which then grew considerably in the ensuing 7 years. It finally reached the size of a small hen's egg but nevertheless remained painless.

## ROENTGENOGRAPHIC FINDINGS

In a case in which the roentgenographic changes are not very striking, the *x*-ray picture may reveal the juxtacortical cartilage mass only as a very faint soft-tissue shadow, 1 or 2 cm. in length. This mass will be found overlying a shallow cortical indentation with a somewhat sclerotic base. In one or another case in which the *x*-ray changes are more pronounced, the defect in the cortex may be quite deep though still closed off from the medullary cavity by a border of sclerotic bone. A ledge or buttress of periosteal new bone may also be visible, especially at the proximal end of the defect. In such cases, the cartilaginous soft-tissue mass, which may or may not extend much beyond the limits of the cortical defect, may show foci of radiopacity. These foci represent areas in which the lesional cartilage is undergoing calcification and/or ossification. If present, these constitute an important guide to the roentgenographic diagnosis of the lesion. In an occasional case, too, the juxtacortical cartilage mass, especially if it is of large size, is outlined, in part or throughout, by a thin shell of radiopacity. This represents an osseous capsule which has developed about the periphery of the cartilage mass through a process of metaplasia (see Fig. 60).

Altogether, then, the roentgenographically visible changes produced by a juxtacortical chondroma fall into three groups: those representing the cartilaginous soft-tissue mass; those representing secondary changes going on within this mass; and those reflecting the erosion of the adjacent underlying cortex by pressure from the growing cartilage mass, along with any local reactive changes which may have been incited in the cartilage. In considering the *x*-ray diagnosis of juxtacortical chondroma, one sometimes has to distinguish the lesion from such other conditions as the fibrous cortical defect, or a pigmented villonodular tenosynovitis (giant-cell tumor of a tendon sheath) which has invaded the underlying bone cortex. The questions of differential diagnosis pertaining to these lesions and a number of others are discussed below (p. 200).

## PATHOLOGIC FINDINGS

**Gross.**—When approached surgically, the lesional cartilage is found to have an outer covering of fibrous tissue of variable thickness. On excision, the cartilage is seen to be hyaline, blue-white or dull white, and, as a rule, subdivided into small lobules. If calcific foci are present in it, these appear yellowish white and feel gritty. After removal of the lesional tissue, the underlying cortex is found to be sclerotic, as probably already suggested by the *x*-ray picture. In several specimens studied, the site of the lesion was the site of insertion of ligamentous or tendinous tissue into the bone. In these cases, the lesional cartilage undoubtedly developed by metaplasia in the ligamentous or tendinous connective tissue at the site of its insertion into the bone. Since these sites are not actually covered by periosteum, it is obvious that one cannot always speak of the lesional cartilage as developing beneath the periosteum.

**Microscopic.**—Sections of the lesional tissue reveal clearly the division of the cartilage into small lobules. The cartilage cells tend to lie in rather large lacunæ. Many of the cartilage cells are likely to be nonviable, and those cells which are viable are, on the whole, uninuclear. The nuclei are not particularly large and show no atypism. This is true even in regard to those occasional cartilage cells which are binuclear. In one lesion or another, the cartilage matrix may be more or less edematous or collagenized in places, may show spotty calcification, or may even be found ossified here and there (see Fig. 61).

On the whole, the cartilage of a juxtacortical chondroma is more cellular than cartilage from a solitary enchondroma of a phalanx, metacarpal, or metatarsal bone. On the other hand, it is usually not more cellular than cartilage coming from a solitary enchondroma of a long bone. In any event, experience has shown that, in evaluating histologically a cartilage lesion not contained *within* a bone, even fairly high cellularity does not in itself necessarily indicate that the lesion is no longer benign. This is an empirical observation which the writer has found useful in avoiding the "overdiagnosis" not only of a juxtacortical chondroma, but also of other extra-osseous cartilage growths such as a para-articular chondroma (p. 567) or of actively proliferating cartilage foci in a case of synovial chondromatosis (p. 564). Evaluation of an extra-osseous cartilage lesion in respect to malignancy must include appreciation of the size of the cartilage growth, in addition to the histologic appearance of the tissue. Large size of the lesion is just as ominous as high cellularity of the constituent tissue. An impression of malignancy in connection with large extra-osseous cartilage lesions is reinforced by such histologic

***Figure 60***

*A*, Roentgenograph showing a small defect produced in the cortex of the upper part of a humeral shaft by a juxtacortical chondroma. The patient was a woman 49 years of age who had complained of mild local pain of 6 months' standing. Note that the lesional area is outlined by a narrow margin of radiopacity. At the surgical intervention, after the lesional cartilage was removed, the underlying cortex, though thinned and eroded, was found still sealed off from the marrow cavity.

*B*, Roentgenograph showing the alterations produced by a juxtacortical chondroma which abuts on, and has eroded the shaft cortex at the lower end of a femur. The patient was a woman 55 years of age who had complained of a constant dull, aching local pain, of 4 months' standing. Note the irregularity of the cortex in the lesional area and the barely visible soft-tissue mass. At the surgical intervention, a cartilage mass measuring 3 cm. in length and about $1\frac{1}{2}$ cm. in thickness was found beneath the periosteum.

*C*, Roentgenograph showing a large cortical defect produced in a fibula by a juxtacortical chondroma. The patient was a girl 4 years of age in whom a small, hard, nonmovable painless mass was palpated in the fibular area in question. Note the buttress-like ledge resulting from the deposition of periosteal new bone at the upper margin of the cortical defect. Note also the sclerosis of the eroded fibular cortex, and the faint radiopacities in the hollow of the defect, which are due to calcification going on within the lesional cartilage.

*D*, Roentgenograph showing the alterations produced by a juxtacortical chondroma oriented to the cortex of the lower end of the homolateral radius in the patient presenting the fibular lesion illustrated in *C*. This juxtacortical chondroma was entirely asymptomatic, the lesion having been discovered in the course of a roentgenographic survey of the skeleton.

*E*, Roentgenograph showing a large juxtacortical chondroma which is eroding the cortex of the proximal phalanx of the third finger of a hand. The patient was a man 50 years of age who had been aware for the past 22 years of a hard, painless mass in the region in question. It was only during the 7 years just preceding admission for removal of the cartilage growth that he noted any considerable increase in size of the lesion. Note that the cortex of the middle phalanx of the fourth finger is likewise altered. However, there were no complaints relating to the juxtacortical chondroma in that area.

*F*, Roentgenograph of a large juxtacortical chondroma abutting upon the cortex of a fifth metatarsal bone. The patient was a man 37 years of age who gave no complaints except of a local swelling, of 6 months' standing, in the area in question. Note the radiopacities produced by calcification and ossification going on in the lesional cartilage.

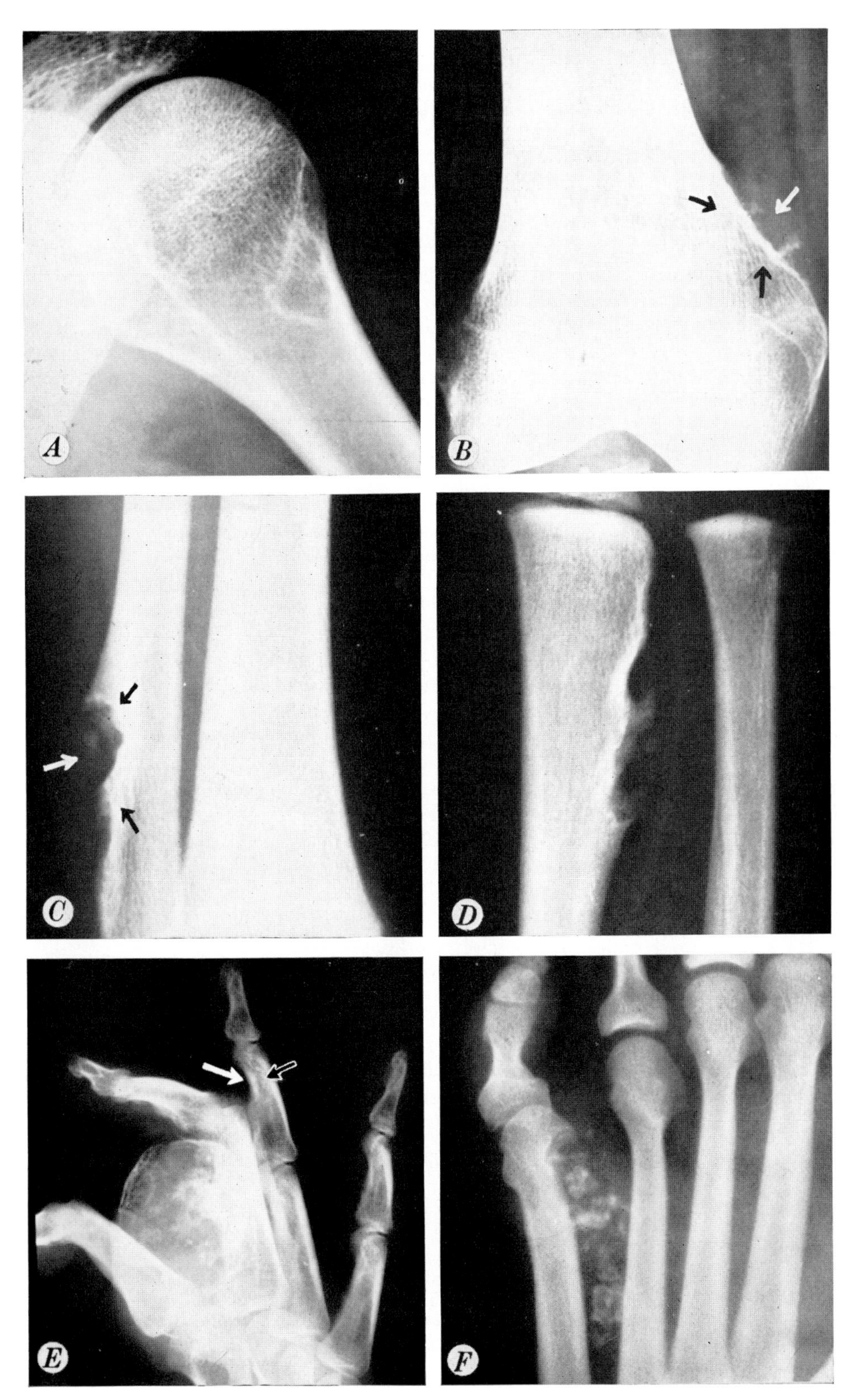


*Figure 60*

findings as general plumpness of the cell nuclei, and the presence of many cells with double nuclei and some with large, bizarre nuclei. However, in relation to an extra-osseous cartilage growth, even these traits often do not have the same serious prognostic significance that they do in relation to a cartilage lesion appearing within a bone.

## DIFFERENTIAL DIAGNOSIS

**Fibrous Cortical Defect.**—The fibrous cortical defect (p. 76) is a very common lesion. It is usually located in the cortex of the metaphysial region of a long bone—most often the distal metaphysis of a femur—and the lesional tissue erodes the cortex at its site. In the *x*-ray picture, the eroded cortex at the lesional site usually shows a smooth or scalloped sclerotic border (see Figs. 19-*A* and *B*, p. 77). It is such an *x*-ray picture that creates what possibility there is of misinterpreting a fibrous cortical defect as a juxtacortical chondroma or vice versa. In a long bone of an otherwise normal young child, a small metaphysial area of cortical erosion, with or without a visible overlying soft-tissue shadow, is overwhelmingly more likely to be ascribable to a fibrous cortical defect than to a juxtacortical chondroma. In an adult, on the other hand, such an area of cortical erosion might well represent a juxtacortical chondroma. This is so because the fibrous cortical defect is an ephemeral lesion which has usually disappeared spontaneously by the time the subject is 8 or 10 years of age. Histologically, there is no likelihood of confusion between the two conditions. The lesional tissue of a fibrous cortical defect consists not of cartilage, but of whorled bundles of fibrous connective tissue often containing some multinuclear giant cells. (See Fig. 20-*A*, p. 79.)

**Pigmented Villonodular Tenosynovitis.**—Once in a while, a pigmented villonodular tenosynovial lesion, the so-called giant-cell tumor of tendon sheaths (p. 545), produces pressure erosion of the cortex of a bone neighboring upon it. This is especially likely to occur in connection with large villonodular tenosynovial lesions of fingers or toes—particularly the latter. In the *x*-ray picture, the soft-tissue mass representing a pigmented villonodular lesion of the tendon sheath is likely to appear lobulated. It never contains any foci of radiopacity such as might be produced by a juxtacortical chondroma which has undergone focal calcification or ossification.

In a case in which a pigmented villonodular tenosynovial lesion is eroding the cortex of a phalanx, for instance (see Fig. 173, p. 551), the patient is usually a middle-aged adult, and the history generally records a swelling of at least several years' standing. Though there might be some problem in trying to distinguish on clinical and roentgenographic grounds between such a case of pigmented villonodular tenosynovitis and an instance of juxtacortical chondroma, there is none on pathologic grounds. A villonodular lesion consists of a lobulated mass of tissue which may range in color from whitish grey through yellowish to reddish brown. In a particular specimen, the coloring is usually mottled, rather than uniform throughout. Histologically, these lesions show a substratum of collagenizing spindle

### *Figure 61*

*A*, Photomicrograph (× 35) showing the topography of a juxtacortical chondroma which has developed beneath the periosteum and is eroding the cortex. Note the periosteum at the top of the picture, the cortex to the right, and the cartilage mass occupying most of the center and left of the picture.

*B*, Photomicrograph (× 35) showing the topography of a juxtacortical chondroma which has developed at the site of insertion of a ligament into the cortex. Note the cartilage at the top and right of the picture, the ligamentous fibers at the left, and the cortical bone in the lower part of the picture.

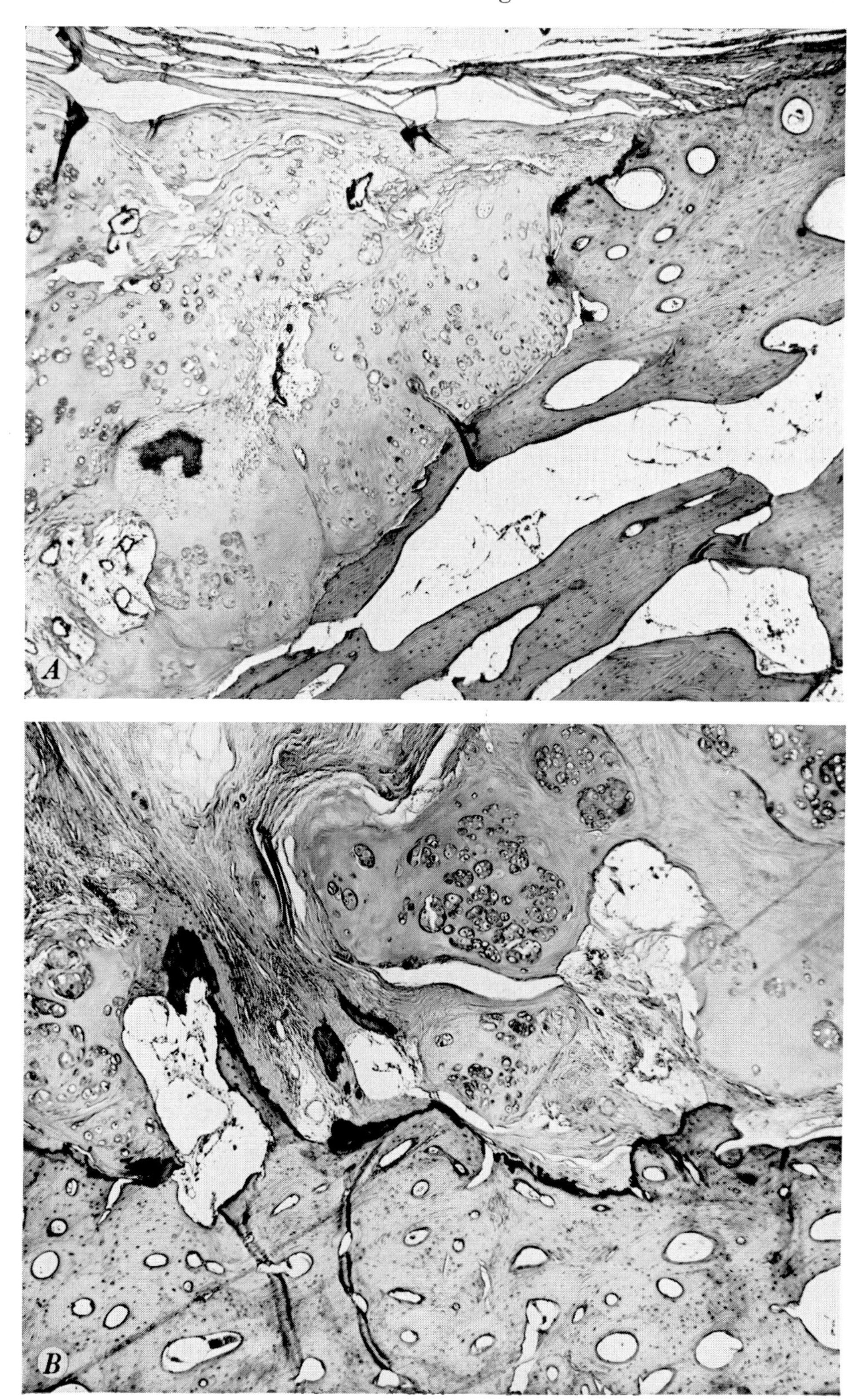

***Figure 61***

cell connective tissue with various amounts of multinuclear giant cells containing cholesterol or hemosiderin pigment.

**Other Differential Diagnostic Considerations.**—Occasionally, a small area of cortical erosion is produced by pressure from still another type of lesion. The writer has seen several cases in which erosion of the cortex of the lower end of a tibia has been produced by a nonspecific tenosynovitis in the region of the ankle. In a case described by Fisk, a ganglion had produced, in the cortex of the lower end of a tibia, a large defect simulating roentgenographically one which might have been produced by a juxtacortical chondroma.

In cases of neurofibromatosis, it is not unusual for a neurofibroma developing in the periosteum or in the juxtacortical connective tissue to produce erosion of the adjacent bone cortex (see Fig. 74, p. 245). In these cases, however, the patient usually presents clear-cut stigmata of neurofibromatosis such as smaller or larger brownish patches of skin pigmentation, numerous neurofibromata of the skin, palpable thickening of the larger peripheral nerves, and, not infrequently, even scoliosis. In the presence of such generalized evidence of neurofibromatosis, a cortical bone defect would have to be regarded as a manifestation of that disease, rather than of a juxtacortical chondroma.

## TREATMENT

In principle, the treatment appropriate for juxtacortical chondroma is surgical extirpation of the cartilaginous soft-tissue mass, together with the overlying fibrous covering, and curettage of the bone cortex where the cartilage mass has eroded it. If the lesion is oriented to the cortex of a long bone, a block resection of the cartilaginous tumor, together with the underlying cortex, may be done instead, unless this procedure would create the danger of a fracture. The possibility of recurrence under these circumstances is negligible. There were no recurrences in the cases studied by the writer.

### REFERENCES

Fisk, G. R.: Bone Concavity Caused by a Ganglion, J. Bone & Joint Surg., *31-B*, 220, 1949.

Jaffe, H. L.: Juxtacortical Chondroma, Bull. Hosp. Joint Dis., *17*, 20, 1956.

Lichtenstein, L., and Hall, J. E.: Periosteal Chondroma: A Distinctive Benign Cartilage Tumor, J. Bone & Joint Surg., *34-A*, 691, 1952.

Mason, M. L.: Tumors of the Hand, Surg., Gynec. & Obst., *64*, 129, 1937.

Roberts, R. E.: Some Observations on Osteochondromata, Chondromata and Cystic Diseases of Bone, Brit. J. Radiol., *10*, 196, 1937.

Chapter

# 13

# Chondromyxoid Fibroma

THE *chondromyxoid fibroma* is a rather uncommon benign tumor of bone. It is observed mainly in older children and young adults, and one of its most frequent sites is the tibia. Histologically, it is a lesion which is likely to cause diagnostic difficulties and, in particular, to create the false impression of being a malignant tumor rather than a benign one. Indeed, there is an almost paradoxical incongruity between its ominous cytologic appearance (more striking in some lesions than in others) and its generally benign clinical course. This ominous appearance is created especially by the fact that, in the course of cytologic evolution of the tumor tissue, considerable intercellular mucin-like material (myxoid) develops between the small, roundish basic tumor cells, and that many of the latter come to show large and even bizarre nuclei. In a given lesion also, in part or throughout, the myxoid intercellular material may become collagenized, and such tumor tissue takes on the cytologic aura of cartilage. In such chondroid areas, the tumor cells may even come to lie in lacunæ.

The lesion is basically a connective-tissue growth. In formulating the name "chondromyxoid fibroma" for it, we were seeking a term which would best express its histologic characteristics and signalize its distinctiveness. However, one can understand how a chondromyxoid fibroma presenting chondroid and, in particular, showing myxoid fields containing cells with giant and/or bizarre nuclei can be misinterpreted histologically as a chondrosarcoma or a chondromyxosarcoma of bone. Clinically, in any case, the mildness of the complaints, the slowness of the lesion's evolution, the absence, as a rule, of alarming roentgenographic features, and the rarity of recurrence after mere curettement of the lesion all refute any impression of malignity that may be created by the histologic picture. Indeed, the chondromyxoid fibroma represents the type of bone lesion in regard to which it is particularly important not to lose sight of the roentgenographic appearance and clinical behavior in evaluating the histologic findings.

## CLINICAL CONSIDERATIONS

**Incidence.**—The writer's experience with the chondromyxoid fibroma covers about 25 cases. As to sex incidence, the cases were about equally distributed between males and females. As to age incidence, about a third of the patients were in the second decade and about a third in the third decade of life. Thus, adolescents and young adults appear to be predilected. Furthermore, none of the patients in our series were very young children or old adults.

**Localization.**—Preponderantly, the lesion involves some bone of a lower limb. Among these bones, we found the tibia to be strongly predilected, this being the bone affected in about half of the cases in which a bone of a lower limb was involved. In the other half, the lesion was in a femur, fibula, metatarsal bone, or calcaneus. Sporadically, the writer has also observed the lesion in a humerus, rib, ilium, and mastoid. Its occasional occurrence in still other bones cannot be excluded. When a long tubular bone is affected, as is most commonly the case, the lesion is usually located at one end of the shaft, ordinarily does not involve the actual epiphysial end of the bone, and generally does not extend across the full width of the shaft.

**Clinical Complaints.**—The complaints are usually mild, and ordinarily of at least some months' standing before the patient seeks treatment. Occasionally, also, one encounters an instance in which there have been no complaints prior to discovery of the lesion. Thus, the lesion sometimes comes to light only because a bone or joint part was examined roentgenographically after a local trauma. In 2 cases studied by the writer in which the lesion was in a rib, it was discovered in the course of a routine *x*-ray examination of the chest. When there are complaints, the most common one is local pain, which is intermittent and not very distressing. In addition, when first seen, many patients state that they have already been aware for some time of a palpable mass at the affected bone site. Such a mass may even

## *Figure 62*

*A*, Roentgenograph showing a roundish, somewhat trabeculated, and slightly marginated, relatively radiolucent defect produced by a chondromyxoid fibroma in the lower part of a femoral metaphysis. The patient was a boy 18 years of age. The clinical complaint was mainly local swelling, which resulted from slight bulging of the contour of the bone in the area in question. A follow-up examination 7 years after local curettement showed the lesional area to be completely filled in.

*B*, Roentgenograph showing a chondromyxoid fibroma in the upper metaphysis of a tibia—a common site for the lesion. The patient was a boy 12 years of age. The presenting feature was the discovery, by the patient's mother, of a local swelling on the bone. Note that the lesion is eccentrically located, that its inner border is outlined by a margin of sclerotic bone, and that the cortex is thinned and, in part, completely lacking. The *x*-ray picture in this case represents a classic example of the lesion in the site in question, and almost justifies by itself the diagnosis of chondromyxoid fibroma.

*C*, Roentgenograph showing a chondromyxoid fibroma in the lower metaphysis of a fibula. The patient was a girl 11 years of age who had suffered a sprain in the region of the ankle 6 months before this *x*-ray picture was taken. At the time of the injury, the ankle was not studied roentgenographically, but the great likelihood is that the lesion was already present then. Note that in this narrow tubular bone the lesion extends almost across the entire width of the bone. Note also that the lesional area is radiolucent and slightly marginated, and that the cortex of the bone, proximal to the lesion, is thickened in consequence of periosteal new bone deposition.

*D*, Roentgenograph showing a chondromyxoid fibroma in a calcaneus. The patient was a girl 13 years of age who, for some months, had complained of pain on walking, and then noticed a local swelling. In this case, there was a recurrence ascribable to incomplete curettement at the original surgical intervention. The second curettement, 9 months later, led to prompt filling in of the lesional area, and cure.

*E*, Roentgenograph showing a large chondromyxoid fibroma in a first metatarsal bone. The patient was a woman 42 years of age who was aware of local swelling of the bone for 20 years. The affected bone was not tender, but there was some pain on walking. The lesional area was solidly filled with a whitish cartilage-like tissue which presented the characteristic cytologic pattern of a chondromyxoid fibroma. The presence of the lesion in the bone for so long a time undoubtedly accounts for the intense reactive sclerosis about it, the extension into the actual epiphysis of the bone, and the trabeculated appearance presented by the lesional area.

*F*, Roentgenograph showing an intracortical chondromyxoid fibroma in a humerus. The patient was a young woman who had noticed merely a local swelling of the bone. Note that the cortex in the vicinity of the lesion is quite thick, and that the lesion has not penetrated the medullary canal. Because of the unusual location of the lesion, the possibility of chondromyxoid fibroma was not even considered on the basis of this *x*-ray picture, and the definitive diagnosis had to await tissue examination.

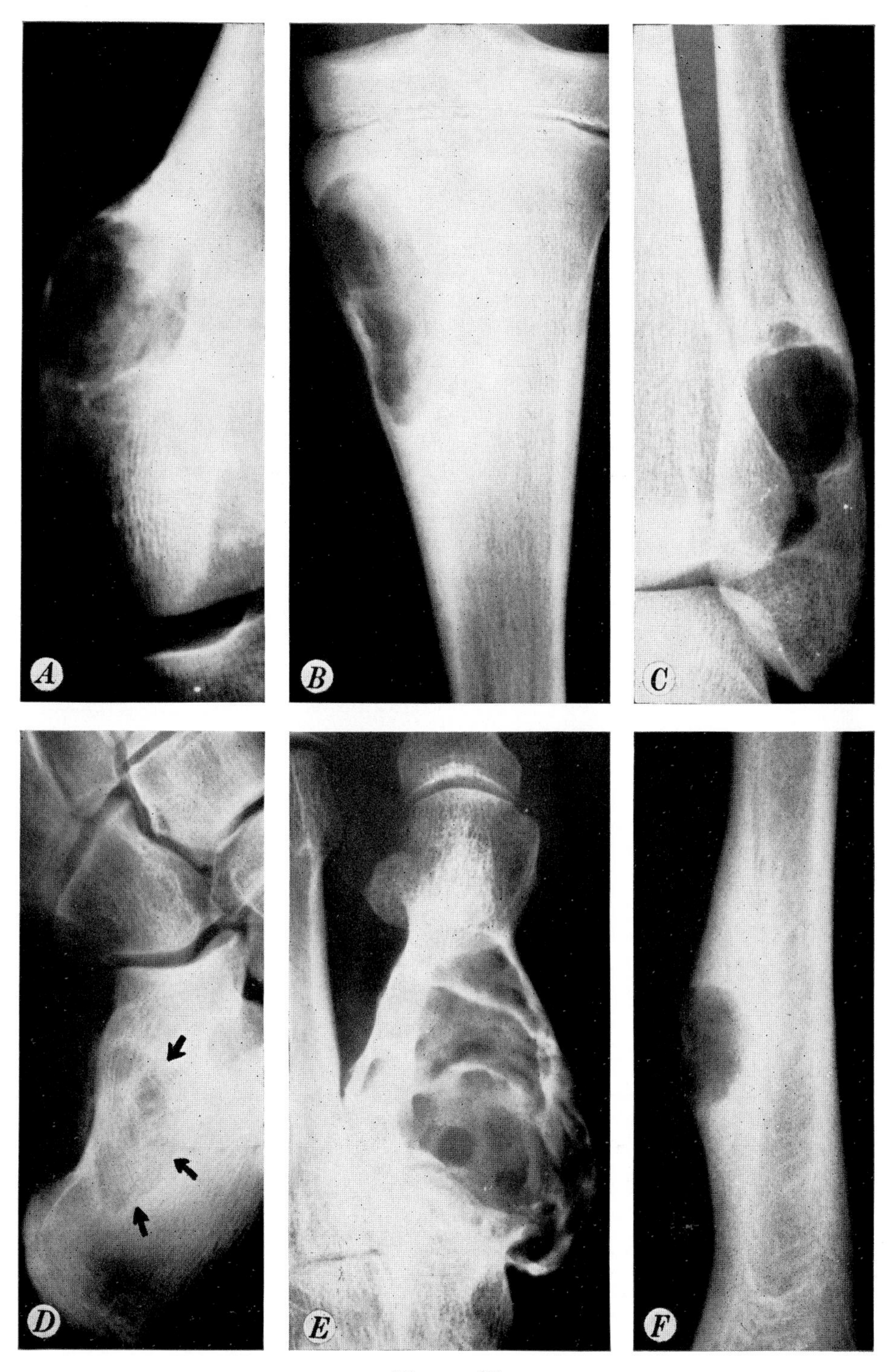


*Figure 62*

have been the presenting complaint, but in any case the mass is not likely to be very tender to palpation. As with bone tumors in general, some patients give a history of previous injury, but in no case seen by the writer could any causal connection between this injury and the onset of the lesion be proved.

## ROENTGENOGRAPHIC FINDINGS

In an affected tibia or femur, for instance, a chondromyxoid fibroma is usually found at one end of the shaft, not extending across the full width of the shaft, and only rarely encroaching upon the actual epiphysial end of the bone. In a narrow long bone (a fibula, for example), the lesion is likely to extend across the full width of the affected part of the shaft. Exceptionally, too, in a tubular bone, the lesion may extend into the actual epiphysial end of the bone, but it was not found to have done so in any case in which the cartilage plate still existed and the epiphysis had not yet fused with the shaft. There can be little doubt that a chondromyxoid fibroma nearly always begins in the interior of a bone, though it may be eccentrically located. However, in 2 cases studied by the writer in which the lesion was in a long bone, the lesion seemed to have originated within the cortex or in relation to it, and had not entered the medullary cavity of the bone at the time when the lesion was studied (see Fig. 62).

Whether the lesion is located in a tubular bone or in some other bone, the disease focus usually appears oval but is sometimes roundish. In one or another instance, it may measure as much as 7 or 8 cm. in its longest dimension, and 4 or 5 cm. across. The area of the lesion appears relatively radiolucent, on the whole. The contour of the bone in the affected area is often bulged. The bulging is usually associated with thinning, at least, of the overlying cortex. Indeed, in one case or another, much of the regional cortex may be found to have disappeared altogether. However, even when this is the case roentgenographically, the surgeon finds that the lesion has not broken through the bulged periosteum, but is contained by the latter. On the other hand, in some cases, the expanded area may be demarcated externally by a thin or even thick shell of periosteal new bone. On the medullary side, at least, the lesional area is likely to be found bordered by a margin of sclerosed bone. This margin may be distinctly grooved, and the lesional area occasionally presents coarse trabeculation, roentgenographically, especially if it is also delimited externally by a shell of periosteal new bone. In addition, the otherwise uninvolved part of the bone may show some thickening of the cortex for a short distance beyond the lesion, further along the shaft.

### *Figure 63*

*A*, Photomicrograph (× 30) showing the topography of a chondromyxoid fibroma in a tissue area in which there is considerable intercellular myxoid material. Note the vague lobulated pattern of the tissue, the numerous vessel spaces between the lobules, and the greater cellularity of the tissue at the periphery of the lobules. (For further detail, see *B* and *C*.)

*B*, Photomicrograph (× 225) showing, under higher magnification, the appearance of the tissue in the central part of a lobule of *A*. The tumor cells have indistinct cytoplasmic borders, and many of the cells show cytoplasmic processes. The intercellular matrix is vacuolated.

*C*, Photomicrograph (× 150) showing cytologic features frequently encountered in the more cellular areas at the periphery of the lobules. Note that many of the cells have prominent hyperchromatic nuclei, and that, in the upper part of the picture, there is a very large cell showing multiple nuclei. It is particularly tissue fields like this that contribute to the impression of ominousness given by the histologic picture.

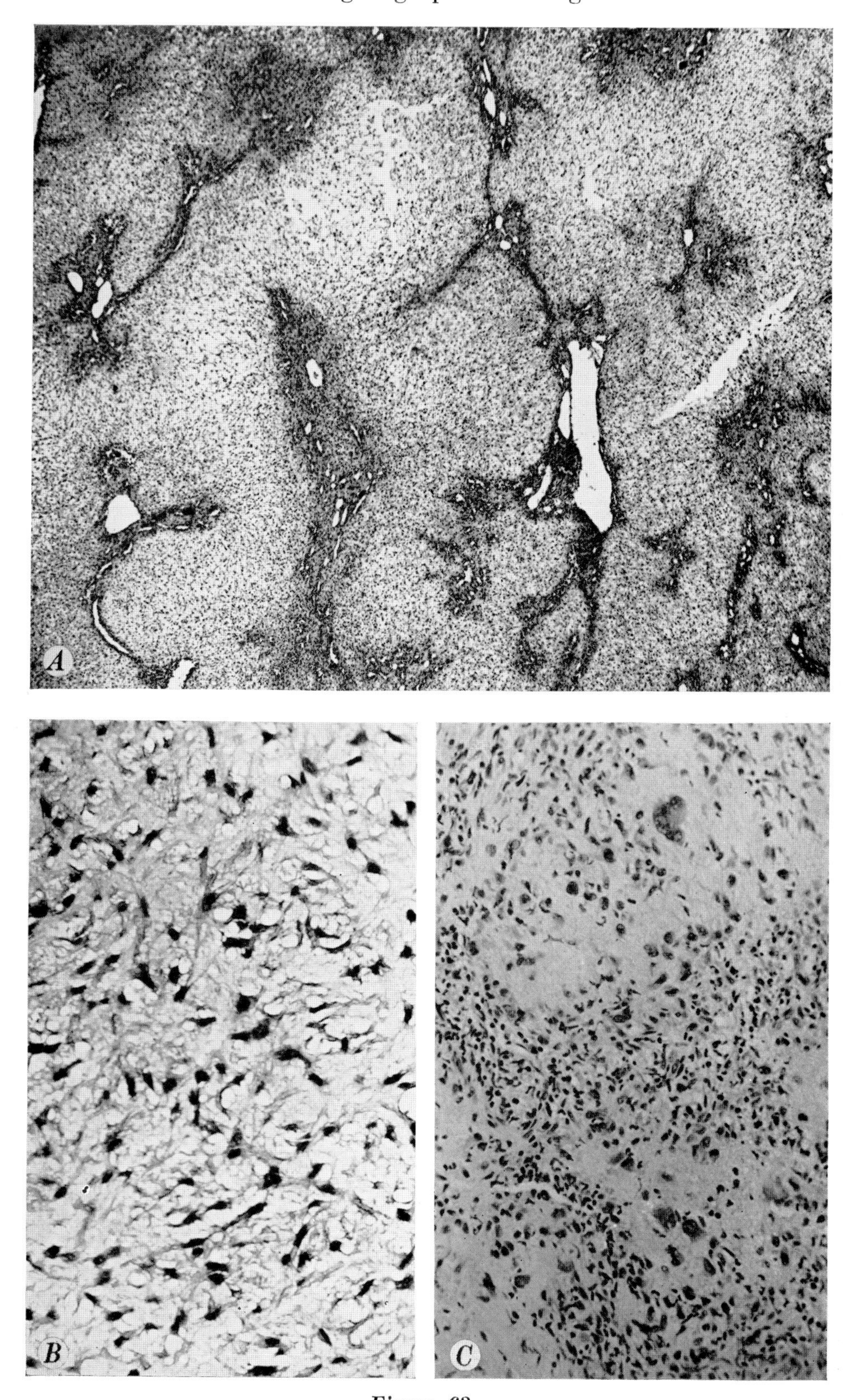


*Figure 63*

This general description of the roentgenographic picture in cases of chondromyxoid fibroma as it appears in a long bone also applies, more or less closely, to localizations in other bones. That is, in these bones, too: The lesion has usually expanded the local contour of the bone; the lesional area is relatively radiolucent; it is likely to be marginated; and it is sometimes trabeculated.

## PATHOLOGIC FINDINGS

**Gross.**—Even when, in one place or another in a given lesion, the roentgenograph has shown the absence of a demarcating cortical shell, the surgeon, when entering the lesion, will find, as already noted, that the tumor is still contained by the periosteum and the overlying parosteal connective tissue. Insofar as it is chondroid, the lesional tissue is found to be whitish, rather glistening, and firm but compressible. In essentially myxoid areas, on the other hand, the tissue is rather grayish white in color and distinctly not glistening. In any case, however, the tissue of a chondromyxoid fibroma lacks the blue-white luster and the faceted pattern of clear-cut cartilage. Also, the tissue does not appear slimy, even though a considerable amount of intercellular myxoid matrix may be apparent microscopically.

**Microscopic.**—Such variations as one may find in the histologic pattern of a chondromyxoid fibroma, from lesion to lesion or from area to area in a given lesion, are largely governed by the extent to which the lesional tissue is myxoid or chondroid. In myxoid fields, examination of the tissue under very low magnification will show that it has a vaguely lobular general pattern. In the more central parts of the lobules, the cells are likely to be widely separated by an intercellular mucin-like substance. At the periphery of the lobules, the cells are less widely separated, and between the lobules themselves there are usually numerous blood channels (see Fig. 63).

On examination under higher power, myxoid fields will show that, on the whole, the tumor cells have only indistinct cytoplasmic borders, though some of the cells will show branching fibrillar cytoplasmic processes. The cell nuclei are mainly ovoid and of moderate size, though some cells may have rather large single nuclei and some even multiple nuclei. The intercellular material is likely to be quite vacuolated. When sections are stained for the demonstration of mucin, the intercellular material does not give the mucin response. Indeed, it seems that the myxoid character of the intercellular material is attributable rather to its aqueous content than to mucin. Furthermore, when stained for fat, the myxoid tumor fields fail to give evidence of lipid.

### *Figure 64*

*A*, Photomicrograph (× 90) showing a stage in the transformation of a myxoid into a chondroid tissue area. Note that, in the upper part of the picture, the tissue is still myxoid but collagen fibers are appearing in the intercellular material. Below this myxoid area, the tissue has advanced further in the direction of chondroid transformation.

*B*, Photomicrograph (× 90) showing two adjacent lobules of tissue in which the chondroid appearance is still more distinct.

*C*, Photomicrograph (× 225) showing the histologic details in a chondroid area. Many of the tumor cells lie in lacunae.

*D*, Photomicrograph (× 125) showing a field in a chondromyxoid fibroma in which there is a group of polyhedral cells (left middle) resembling the cells of a benign chondroblastoma. Note, however, that, between these basic cells of the chondromyxoid fibroma, vacuolated intercellular material has appeared in many places. In a clear-cut benign chondroblastoma, myxoid transformation of the intercellular material does not occur.

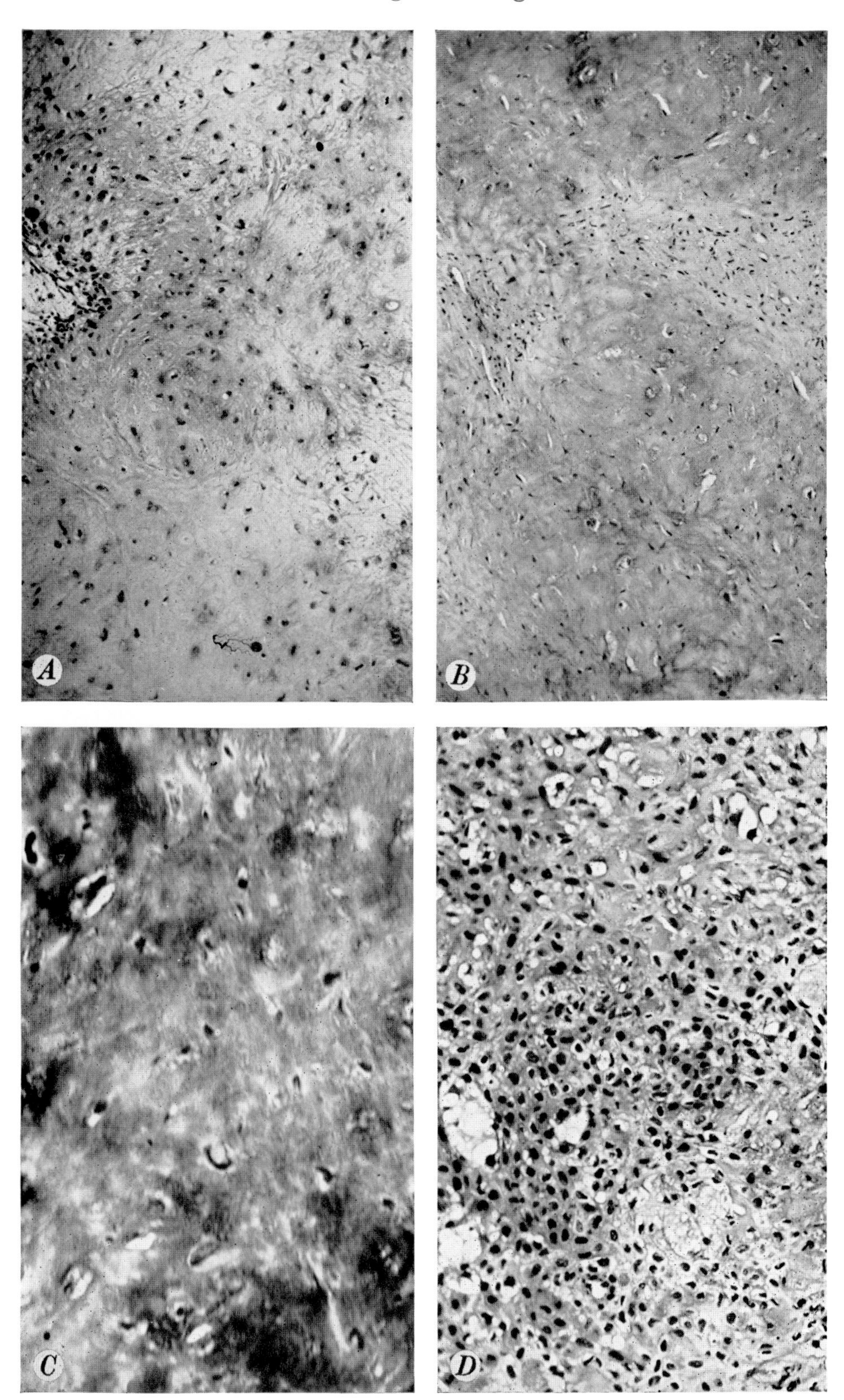


*Figure 64*

At the periphery of the myxoid lobules, where the tumor cells are more closely compacted, one is likely to see some cells with particularly prominent nuclei. Such cells may present large, plump nuclei, strikingly hyperchromatic nuclei, and even large double or multiple nuclei. Also, about the vessels at the periphery of the lobules, one may observe evidence of blood extravasation and sometimes even some multinuclear giant cells, some hemosiderin-laden macrophages, a sprinkling of small mononuclear cells, and an occasional polymorphonuclear leukocyte.

Sooner or later, in a chondromyxoid fibroma, the myxoid tissue areas apparently undergo more or less collagenization of their intercellular material. In the course of this, the originally myxoid intercellular substance loses its loose, vacuolated structure and gradually comes to appear more homogeneous. Indeed, the intercellular material now takes on an appearance suggestive of the intercellular substance of cartilage; that is, it takes on a chondroid aura. The tumor cells may even come to lie in lacunæ, and this appearance, too, may create the impression that such areas represent cartilage. Furthermore, in the chondroid tissue areas, one no longer sees the rather lobulated pattern presented microscopically by the tumor tissue in the myxoid areas. In one or another chondromyxoid fibroma, the chondroid tissue areas may even predominate. However, in other cases, such chondroid areas are hardly seen at all, while in still others one finds areas demonstrating transition stages from previously myxoid tissue (see Fig. 64).

Finally, it should be pointed out in relation to the histopathology of chondromyxoid fibroma that one may encounter, in some of the lesions, sporadic microscopic fields in which smaller or larger groups of cells resemble those characteristic of benign chondroblastoma. The tumor cells in these fields are roundish or polyhedral, but such fields merge smoothly into myxoid areas characterized by drawn-out cells interspersed with considerable loose intercellular material (Fig. 64-*D*). Against the interpretation of such roundish or polyhedral cells as being identical with the basic cell of the benign chondroblastoma is the fact that one does not see, within these tissue fields, evidence of spotty calcification such as is characteristic of benign chondroblastoma (see also Fig. 10). In a benign chondroblastoma, on the other hand, calcified areas which have become necrotic may undergo organization in the direction of chondroid tissue, but that fact, too, should not be taken as representing a morphologic interrelationship between the two lesions.

**Recurrence and Malignant Transformation.**—That a chondromyxoid fibroma often presents an ominous cytologic appearance, which one must learn to discount because of the established generally benign clinical behavior, has been sufficiently stressed. However, the writer has now seen one example of a recurrence of a chondromyxoid fibroma, apparently after inadequate removal of the lesion. In this case, the lesion appeared in a calcaneus of a boy 13 years of age. About 9 months after the original curettement, the lesion recurred. Recurettement of the lesion was not followed by a new recurrence.

On the other hand, in a case in which the lesion was in the upper end of a fibula of a boy 17 years of age, removal of the lesion was followed shortly by a recurrence. A second recurrence (about one and a half years after the original intervention) showed that the character of the lesion had changed and that one was now dealing with an indubitable chondrosarcoma. Such behavior by a chondromyxoid fibroma is certainly rare and does not invalidate the general finding that the lesion nearly always runs a benign clinical course.

## DIFFERENTIAL DIAGNOSIS

The problems of differential diagnosis relating to chondromyxoid fibroma fall into two categories. On the one hand, there are the problems of clinical (and particularly roentgenographic) differential diagnosis and, on the other, the problems of anatomic differential diagnosis.

On the whole, the roentgenographic picture of a chondromyxoid fibroma has a certain distinctiveness, at least when the lesion is restricted to the metaphysial region of a long bone shaft and has attained a considerable size. Under these circumstances, which are the ordinary ones, one can usually exclude rather easily, on the basis of the *x*-ray picture, the diagnostic possibility of a solitary bone cyst. The possibility of a benign chondroblastoma can almost always likewise be excluded on a roentgenographic basis, if the lesion does not involve the epiphysis along with the metaphysis. Sometimes, however, even when the lesion is in a long bone, and certainly when it is in other sites, its clinical recognition on the basis of the roentgenographic appearance may be difficult. Thus, in the case of a lesion confined to the cortex of a long bone, one might even reject the possibility of a chondromyxoid fibroma in attempting to make a differential diagnosis.

In regard to anatomic considerations, there can be no doubt that cases reported in the literature under the heading of "myxoma" or "central myxoma" but involving bones other than jawbones are mainly misinterpreted instances of chondromyxoid fibroma. Certainly, as already noted, the tissue of chondromyxoid fibroma is not at all mucoid or gelatinous in its gross appearance, as a myxoma is, and does not give the mucin reaction which one also expects of myxomatous tissue. Furthermore, such experience as the writer has had with the lesion called "myxoma of the jawbone" shows that, whatever the latter lesion may actually represent, its cytologic picture likewise does not correspond to that of the lesion we call chondromyxoid fibroma of bone. Indeed, the pseudolobulation of the tissue and the presence of chondroid areas serve to differentiate the latter from the so-called "myxoma of jawbones" (see p. 435).

That a chondromyxoid fibroma is likely to be misdiagnosed as a chondrosarcoma or at least as an enchondroma of an aggressive type has already been indicated. This confusion stems in part from the suggestive cartilaginous character of the tumor tissue in the gross. It is furthered by the cytologic appearance of the chondroid intercellular matrix, but more specifically by the presence in the tumor of smaller or larger numbers of cells with large nuclei, double nuclei or even bizarre nuclei. By the same token, when the intercellular matrix is less obviously chondroid and is predominantly myxoid, one can readily understand also why a diagnosis of myxosarcoma or myxochondrosarcoma may sometimes be entertained. However, experience with the chondromyxoid fibroma will lead one to recognize that its tissue pattern as a whole permits one to state that the lesion is benign, even though it presents disturbing cytologic details. Altogether, the chondromyxoid fibroma is the kind of lesion for whose proper identification one has to call upon a sort of sixth sense to amalgamate a number of minute, evanescent impressions into a distinctive whole.

## TREATMENT

Thorough curettage, including, when practical, even removal of the neighboring condensed bone, is the treatment of choice. If the lesion was large and the resultant defect is considerable, the latter may be filled with bone chips or a bone graft.

## REFERENCES

Copello, O.: Mixoma del metatarsiano, Bol. y trab. de la Soc. de cir. de Buenos Aires, *19*, 1151 1935.

Dahlin, D. C.: Chondromyxoid Fibroma of Bone, with Emphasis on its Morphological Relationship to Benign Chondroblastoma, Cancer, *9*, 195, 1956.

Dahlin, D. C., Wells, A. H., and Henderson, E. D.: Chondromyxoid Fibroma of Bone, J. Bone & Joint Surg., *35-A*, 831, 1953.

Freund, E.: Unusual Cartilaginous Tumor Formation of the Skeleton, Arch. Surg., *33*, 1054, 1936.

Goorwitch, J.: Chondromyxoid Fibroma of Rib: Report of an Unusual Benign Primary Tumor, Dis. of Chest, *20*, 186, 1951.

Herfarth, H.: Ein zentrales Myxom der Tibia, Arch. f. klin. Chir., *170*, 283, 1932.

Jaffe, H. L., and Lichtenstein, L.: Chondromyxoid Fibroma of Bone: A Distinctive Benign Tumor Likely to be Mistaken Especially for Chondrosarcoma, Arch. Path., *45*, 541, 1948.

Lichtenstein, L., and Kaplan, L.: Benign Chondroblastoma of Bone: Unusual Localization in Femoral Capital Epiphysis, Cancer, *2*, 793, 1949.

Wrenn, R. N., and Smith, A. G.: Chondromyxoid Fibroma, South. M. J., *47*, 848, 1954.

Chapter

# 14

# Adamantinoma of Limb Bones

THE so-called *adamantinoma of limb bones* is a peculiar tumor of rare occurrence found almost exclusively in relation to the tibia. It derived its name from the fact that its cytologic pattern mimics that of the familiar adamantinoma (or better, ameloblastoma) of jawbones. Of the cases (approximately 30) which have been reported since Fischer originally described the lesion in 1913, there seem to be only 3 in which the bone affected was not a tibia. The writer's personal experience with the lesion covers 8 cases, 2 of which were reported by Wolfort and Sloane. In 7 of these cases, the lesion was in a tibia, and in 1 it was in a radius. The total experience with so-called adamantinoma of limb bones indicates that, because of local invasiveness and tendency to recurrence, the affected limb nearly always has to be amputated eventually. Furthermore, in one of the cases studied by the writer, pulmonary metastases eventually appeared, leading to death of the patient. The literature (see Baker, Dockerty, and Coventry) contains at least 8 other instances of metastasis and fatal termination in cases of the kind in question. (For discussion of adamantinoma or ameloblastoma of jawbones, see p. 442.)

Until recently there was general agreement that the so-called adamantinoma of limb bones was an epithelial tumor primary at the site of its development. In conformity with this idea, it was held that the tumor developed out of misplaced epithelium, though there were differences of opinion as to how and when the misplacement of the epithelium occurred. Recently, however, the basic epithelial nature of the lesion has itself been questioned. In fact, some workers (see Hicks, and Lederer and Sinclair) now hold that it represents a connective-tissue growth, and specifically a specialized mesodermal tumor akin to the synovioma (synovial sarcoma). Changus *et al.*, in turn, have suggested that the lesion actually represents a malignant vascular tumor (malignant angioblastoma) rather than an epithelial tumor. These questions are considered further in relation to the nature and genesis of the lesion (p. 220).

## CLINICAL CONSIDERATIONS

**Incidence.**—As to age, small as their number is, the cases present a wide range. However, about half of the patients were adolescents or young adults at the time when they first came for treatment. So far, no cases have been reported in very young children. In the writer's series, the youngest patient was 8 and the oldest 57 years of age.

**Localization.**—The strongly predilective involvement of the tibia has already been noted. In that bone, and in the few other long bones found affected, the lesion was nearly always in the shaft. More precisely, within a long bone shaft the lesion is frequently located in the midportion but may lie more toward one or the other end of the shaft. It may even finally extend into the epiphysial end of the bone, but a purely epiphysial location is certainly rare, to say the least.

**Clinical Complaints.**—It is interesting that although the lesion is often already of considerable size when the patient first seeks treatment for it, the antecedent complaints are usually rather mild. Often they consist of local, intermittent, dull, aching pain, which may be of long standing. Along with this, a local swelling is usually complained of, or has at least been noticed. Not infrequently, despite mild antecedent complaints, it is a pathologic fracture that first leads to the patient's hospitalization.

**Role of Trauma.**—In view of the lesion's usual location in a tibial shaft, it is not surprising that local trauma is frequently mentioned in the histories and associated with the onset of the complaints. The cited latent period between the inculpated trauma and the appearance of complaints has been merely weeks in some cases and years in others. However, the case histories fail to furnish details (and especially roentgenographic evidence) indicating that the lesion appeared and developed after the trauma in a previously intact bone. Indeed, the adamantinoma was probably already present at the time of the trauma. Furthermore, the provocative rôle of trauma is challenged by the fact that in some cases the patients give no history of local trauma at all. Also, doubt is cast on it by the rarity of adamantinoma of the tibia in comparison with the great frequency of trauma to the leg. Finally, the writer does not know of a single case in which it can be unequivocally established that an adamantinoma developed at the site of a tibial trauma even so severe as to cause a fracture (simple or compound) in a previously normal bone.

## ROENTGENOGRAPHIC FINDINGS

In some cases of adamantinoma of the tibia, the roentgenograph might suggest the diagnosis. The *x*-ray picture seen in these cases is familiar because it corresponds to the one sometimes used in articles to illustrate the lesion. The picture

***Figure 65***

*A*, Roentgenograph showing an adamantinoma of a tibia, confined essentially to the cortex of the bone. The patient was a boy 16 years of age whose difficulty was local swelling and some pain of several months' standing. No history of antecedent trauma was given. Note that the lesion shows up as a well-marginated multilocular rarefaction shadow in the cortex. This *x*-ray picture represents what is often thought to be the classic example of the lesion in its usual tibial location, and this appearance justifies serious consideration of the possibility of adamantinoma. A shadow simulating this appearance might also be produced by a non-ossifying fibroma, for instance. In such a case, however, the patient would be likely to be somewhat younger, and the lesion farther toward one end of the shaft.

*B*, Roentgenograph showing a large adamantinoma of a tibia, with a pathologic fracture through the lesional area. The patient was a girl 17 years of age. She had been complaining of mild pain in the leg for 4 months, but the lesion was not discovered until she sustained a pathologic fracture from a fall while skating. The appearance in the upper half of the picture is not inconsistent with the idea that the lesion is burrowing into the tibia from the outside. However, there is certainly nothing obviously suggestive of adamantinoma about the picture as a whole.

*C*, Roentgenograph showing an adamantinoma in the lower part of a tibial shaft. The patient was a man 48 years of age whose complaints were of 5 months' standing when this picture was taken. The initial complaint was of a local swelling. Subsequently, there was some pain, but only on weight bearing. There was no history of antecedent trauma. In the view shown, the lesion presents as an essentially intramedullary growth. However, from the lateral *x*-ray view in this case, one might gain the impression that the lesion may have extended into the tibia through the posterior surface of the cortex. The photograph of the gross specimen from this case is shown in *D*.

*D*, Photograph showing the gross appearance of the adamantinoma of the tibia illustrated in *C*. The tumor mass is well circumscribed and clearly delineated from the neighboring bone. The tissue of the tumor mass appears white and somewhat nodular. Above the center, a small area of cystic softening can be noted.

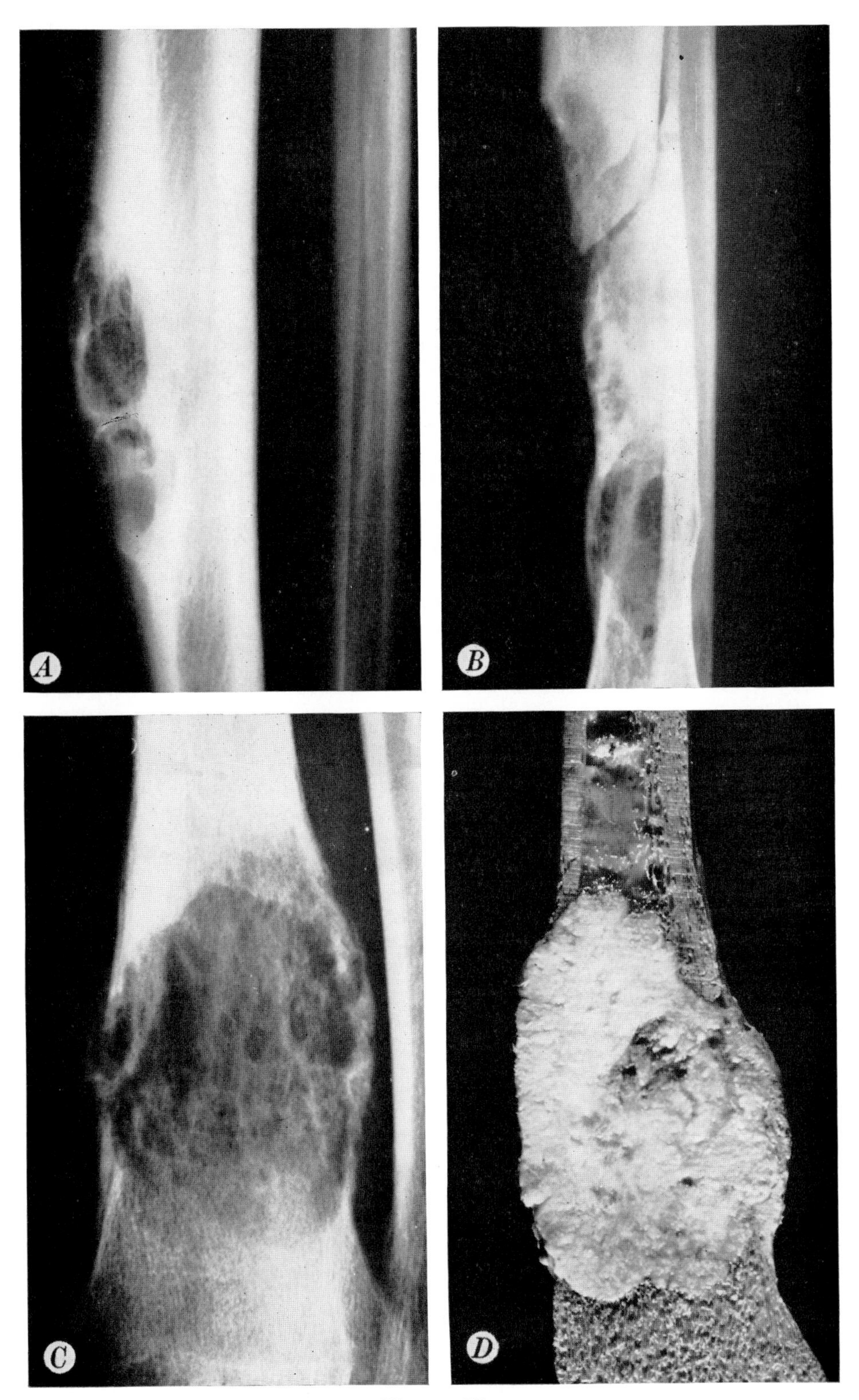


*Figure 65*

is characterized by a relatively large, rather radiolucent, and somewhat "bubbly" or trabeculated area of abnormality involving part of the shaft cortex. Furthermore, in these cases the lesion seems not to involve the medullary cavity of the bone in the affected area. Externally, the contour of the bone is somewhat bulged and the local cortex below and above the lesional area is likely to be thickened. Indeed, it is from pictures like these that the writer is inclined to infer that the adamantinoma starts its development in relation to the external surface of the cortex and erodes and burrows into the latter before reaching the medullary cavity.

In other cases, though the lesion already involves the medullary cavity in some places, it can still be seen that, at least in some parts of the affected bone, the tumor is still burrowing into the cortex from the outside. Such cases, too, support the idea that the tumor tissue enters the medullary cavity from the outside—that is, that the adamantinoma of limb bones is not primarily a central lesion. In still other cases, it will not be possible to demonstrate that the tumor reached the interior of the bone from the surface, since it presents as an essentially intramedullary growth at the time when it is first seen. Specifically, in such cases the lesional area shows up as a variably radiolucent and vaguely trabeculated central focus of rarefaction which has caused local bulging of the bone contour. (See Fig. 65.)

## PATHOLOGIC FINDINGS AND PATHOGENESIS

**Gross Pathology.**—When first seen, an adamantinoma of a limb bone is usually a fairly large lesion. Its longitudinal extent is often as much as 7 or 8 cm. and sometimes more. When not modified by secondary change, the lesional tissue is rather tough, firm, and gray white or even glistening white. Also, the tumor tissue is likely to appear vaguely lobular and nodular in the gross. In one or another case, the tumor tissue may present areas of cystic and/or hemorrhagic softening. (See Fig. 65-*D*.)

**Microscopic Pathology.**—In comparing different cases of so-called adamantinoma of limb bones, one may find a good deal of variety in the details of the histologic pattern. On the one hand, there is the pattern in which the tumor cells of the lesional tissue tend rather strongly to show an alveolar or tubular arrangement. In the cases in which this is particularly conspicuous, the histologic resemblance of the limb bone lesion to the adamantinoma of jawbones is striking. In other lesions, however, a good deal of collagenizing connective tissue appears between the tumor cells. Under such circumstances, these cells tend to spindle out and, at least in many areas, the alveolar and tubular arrangement of the tumor cells may be absent or very inconspicuous. It is understandable that a lesion presenting such a pattern, with its sarcomatoid aura, might indeed be interpreted as a sarcoma, and specifically as a synovial sarcoma. Another variation in the pattern is that in which sparse but well-formed alveoli are interspersed with large tracts of spindle-

***Figure 66***

*A*, Photomicrograph (× 65) showing the topography of a tibial adamantinoma which simulates appearances encountered in some adamantinomas of jawbones. In the upper left-hand part of the picture, alveolar and tubular structures can be observed. In the lower central part, large sheets of cells in syncytial arrangement are prominent. In the lower right-hand part of the picture, the tumor cells are found in more or less solid cords.

*B*, Photomicrograph (× 125) from an area in *A* showing nests of somewhat drawn out or stellate cells. At the periphery of these nests, the cells show palisading, as stands out well in the lower right part of the picture.

*C*, Photomicrograph (× 125) from an area in *A* presenting alveolar and tubular structures. Note that the tumor cells are cuboidal or columnar in shape.

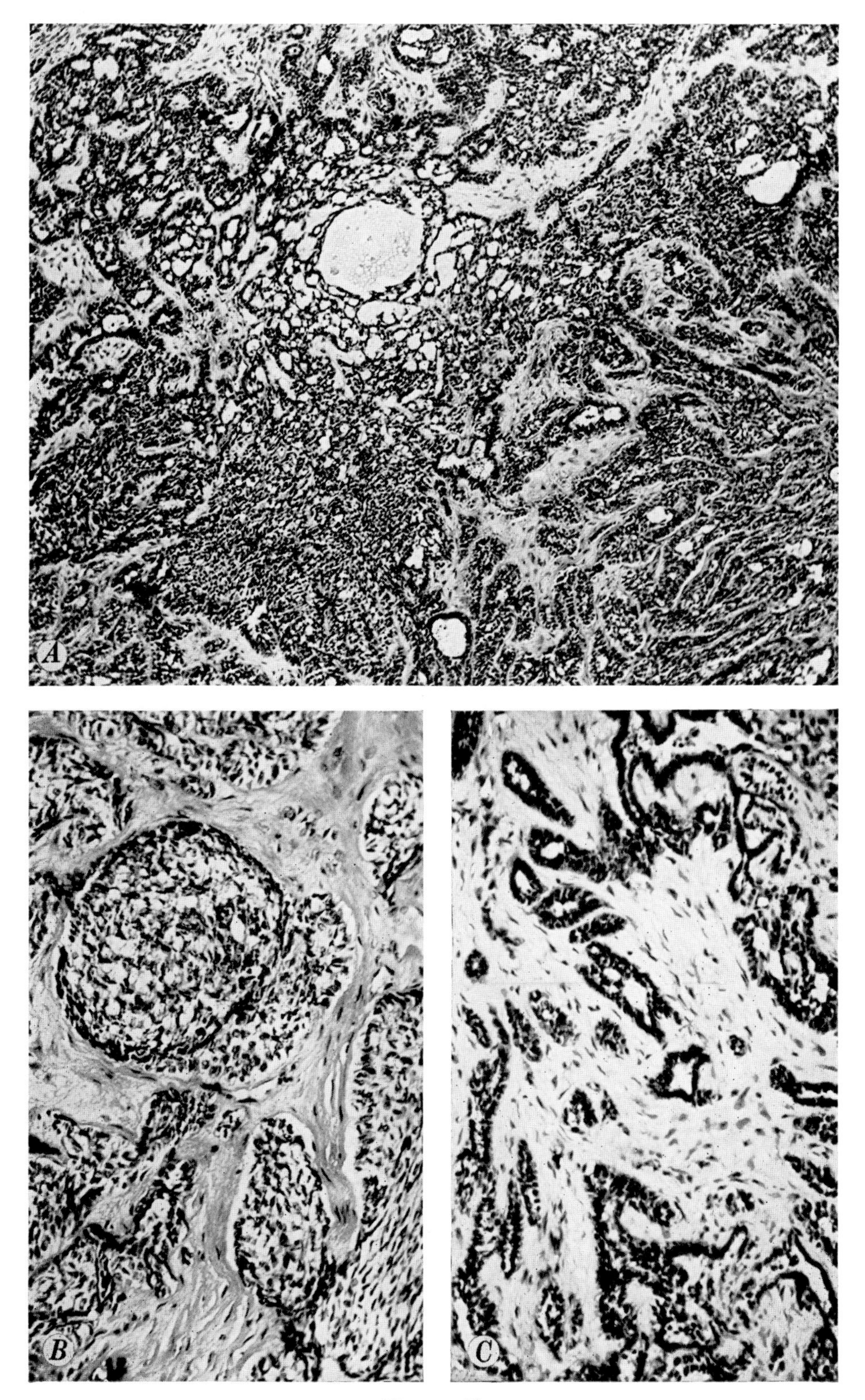


***Figure 66***

shaped cells. Still another variation is introduced by squamous transformation of the tumor cells, even to the extent of forming epithelial pearls in many places. Some degree of squamous transformation of the tumor cells may be found even in an adamantinoma which has a predominantly sarcomatoid histologic pattern. Again, in an occasional lesion, squamous transformation is so prominent as to give the lesion the cast of a squamous cell carcinoma.

In a lesion whose tissue pattern resembles the one frequently seen in cases of adamantinoma of jawbones, one notes that, in addition to alveolar and tubular structures, many places show tumor cells closely compacted into sheets or cords. The cells in these sheets and cords are darkly staining polygonal or spindle-shaped cells which often become syncytial or stellate toward the center and usually show palisading at the periphery of the sheet or cord. In the areas presenting the alveolar and tubular structures, the tumor cells are found arranged around spaces which may be small and rounded, large and branching, or even quite drawn out and tubular. The cells lining the spaces are cuboidal or columnar in shape, and the lining layer is frequently more than one cell thick. The appearance of these spaces with their tumor cell linings suggests that of glandular structures lined by epithelial cells. Nevertheless, if one examines the tissue fields in which the tumor cells are still present in syncytial sheets or cords, one gains the impression that the alveoli and tubules evolve out of local degenerative changes. Specifically, one can defend the idea that they come into being through liquefaction of the more centrally placed cells in the sheets or cords. (See Fig. 66.)

In other limb bone adamantinomas, as already noted, the development of considerable amounts of collagen between the tumor cells may result in spindling of these cells over large areas of the lesional tissue. Elsewhere in this tissue, however, the tumor cells are likely still to be present in compact cords and, here and there, lumina appear in the cords so that the impression of alveoli is again created. In a case in point studied by the writer, what was even more striking than the formation of spaces was the squamous transformation of small nests of cells in the center of the cords of tumor cells. In connection with many of these cell nests, one could even note the presence of intercellular bridges. However, it is only in an occasional case that one observes squamous metaplasia of such a high degree that numerous large epithelial pearls are seen in many areas of a tissue field. (See Fig. 67.)

As noted, one may also encounter a limb bone adamantinoma in which the histologic pattern shows numerous alveoli set between large tracts of drawn out spindle cells. The alveoli are usually lined by tall cuboidal or columnar cells. Such pictures give the impression that one is dealing with glandular alveoli lined by epithelial cells. It would not be plausible to contend that the alveolar spaces in such a lesion came into being through the development of clefts or spaces in the spindle cell

***Figure 67***

*A*, Photomicrograph (× 125) showing the histologic appearance of a tibial adamantinoma in which the tumor cells are compressed and tend to be strung out. Spindling of the tumor cells is conspicuous on the right-hand side of the picture. On the left-hand side, the cells, though strung out for the most part, still create the impression of tubules and even solid nests. The section was prepared from tissue removed in the case illustrated in 65-*B*.

*B*, Photomicrograph (× 125) showing the histologic appearance of the tissue in another field than that shown in *A*. In this field, solid nests of cells predominated and, in the center of many of the nests, the cells show the beginning of squamous transformation.

*C*, Photomicrograph (× 125) showing striking squamous transformation of the tumor cells from another adamantinoma of a tibia. The patient in this case was a man 43 years of age who had complained of a tender and painful swelling over the midportion of the right tibia for 1 year.

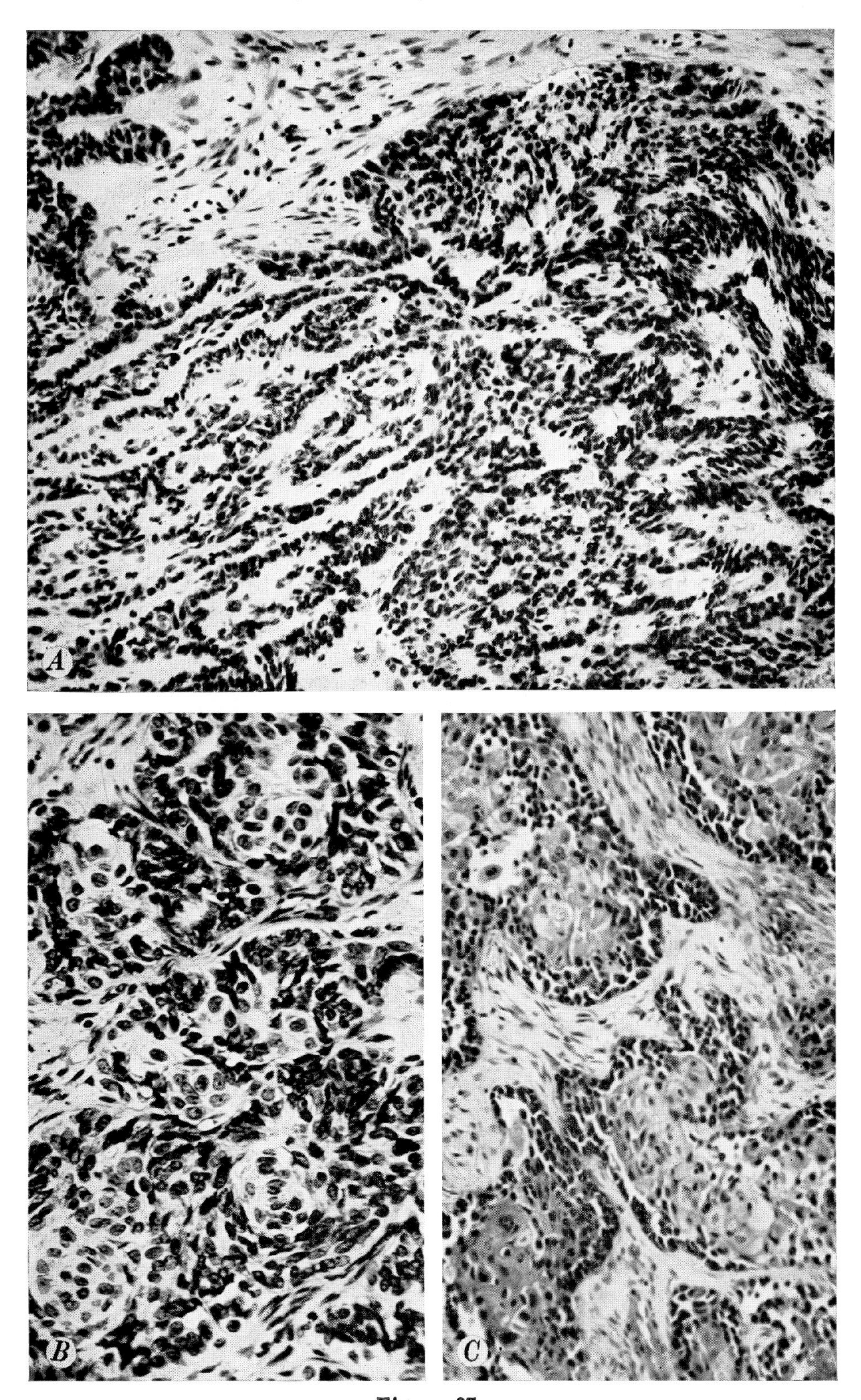


***Figure 67***

stroma, and that the spindle cells lining the clefts became differentiated in the direction of cuboidal cells, and/or columnar cells as, for instance, in a synovioma.

**Metastasis.**—As cases of adamantinoma of limb bones accumulated in the literature, it became clear that the lesion not only tended to recur if an amputation was not performed, but sometimes even metastasized. Furthermore, if the amputation was delayed, metastases sometimes showed up later in spite of it. It should not be inferred, however, that metastasis will necessarily take place even if the amputation is delayed for years. In a pertinent case studied by the writer, an adamantinoma of a tibia had been present for 19 years without having metastasized. It is known that the patient had 2 courses of *x*-radiation for the lesion, but information about the exact dosage is lacking. Though the radiation may have held the lesion in check, it certainly did not destroy it. Indeed, after remaining dormant for 19 years, the adamantinoma began to grow rapidly, and the limb was finally ablated. Anatomic examination of the tibia showed the presence of viable tumor tissue whose cells were disposed in nests, cords and alveoli and presented squamous differentiation in some places. A follow-up about 1½ years after the amputation revealed that the patient was well and still showed no evidences of metastasis.

In another case studied by the writer, pulmonary metastases appeared and the patient died 6 years after amputation of the affected limb. The amputation was done 2 years after the diagnosis of adamantinoma of the tibia had been established through study of tissue obtained by curettage of the lesion. In the interim between the initial curettage and the amputation, the lesion had been irradiated and also curetted again because of recurrence. About a year after the amputation, the patient already began to have pulmonary difficulties—spontaneous pneumothorax and hemoptysis—and she died 5 years later. That is, death occurred 8 years after the diagnosis had been established through study of the tissue originally curetted from the lesion. At autopsy, the right lung was found to be the site of a huge tumor. There was also tumor tissue in the intercostal spaces which was compressing and destroying many adjacent ribs on the right side, and tumor tissue also extended into the diaphragm.

As to the cases reported in the literature, about 25 per cent ultimately showed metastases. In these cases the interval between diagnosis of the lesion as an adamantinoma and the appearance of metastases ranged from 1 to 8 years. In addition to pulmonary metastases, some of these cases showed metastases to the regional inguinal lymph nodes, sometimes before the lungs were found to be involved.

**Nature and Genesis.**—The nature and genesis of the so-called adamantinoma of limb bones present intriguing and as yet unsettled problems. Among these is the question of whether the lesion starts its development outside of the bone (nearly always the tibia) and then comes to erode into the bone, or starts centrally—that is, within the interior of the affected bone. Another question is whether the lesion is an epithelial growth and, if so, whether it is related to the adamantinoma of jawbones or represents a basal cell carcinoma. Still another question is whether the lesion is a mesodermal rather than an epithelial growth, and specifically whether it is a synovial sarcoma (malignant synovioma), or a malignant vascular tumor (malignant angioblastoma).

In regard to site of origin, the writer believes that the lesion starts its development in relation to the outer surface of the cortex and not in the medullary cavity of the bone, though it usually comes to penetrate into the interior of the bone. This idea is definitely supported by the fact that, in some cases, the *x*-ray picture shows the lesion still confined to the cortex and sparing the medullary cavity. Furthermore, on the assumption that the lesion is a primary epithelial growth, its point of departure would naturally be outside of the bone. Under these circumstances, if the lesion involves the medullary cavity, the tumor tissue must have reached it by eroding through the cortex.

We come now to the direct question of whether the lesion is of epithelial nature. The original conception in this connection (see Fischer) was that the tumor arose from local dermal epithelium misplaced by bud-like ingrowth toward the tibia during embryonal development. The misplacement was held to occur at such an early stage of embryonal development that the epithelium was still multipotential and could differentiate along the lines of dental epithelium. Indeed, this hypothesis served to explain why, in some of the cases of so-called adamantinoma of limb bones, the histologic pattern strongly mimics that of adamantinoma of jawbones. Acceptance of this interpretation also implies acceptance of the idea that the misplaced epithelium retains its capacity for specialized differentiation even over a period of 10, 20, or 30 years or more before it becomes activated to undergo tumorous proliferation. These various corollaries make it difficult to accept the idea that the lesion evolves out of epithelium misplaced early in embryonal life.

On the other hand, there are those (see Ryrie) who, though agreeing that the lesion arises from misplaced epithelium, maintain that the displacement occurs during postnatal life. The displacement is held to have a traumatic basis. Specifically, shearing injury is thought to displace epithelium from the skin or its appendages into the periosteum. However, something more than traumatic displacement of mature epithelium is needed to produce a lesion presenting the histologic pattern of an adamantinoma of a limb bone. This is shown by the fact that an adamantinoma is not the lesion which develops when mature epithelium is known to have been displaced under conditions of trauma. For instance, when, as happens occasionally, epithelium comes to be traumatically displaced into a phalanx or a calvarium, the lesion which evolves is an epithelial-lined inclusion cyst and not an adamantinoma.

To explain this discrepancy, it has been maintained (see Willis) that an adamantinoma of a tibia actually represents a basal cell carcinoma which has arisen from traumatically displaced hair follicles and which is invading the bone. The fact is that a particular limb bone adamantinoma, while mimicking the histologic architecture of a jawbone adamantinoma, may, at the same time, mimic that of a basal cell carcinoma. In other cases, however, the limb bone adamantinoma bears little if any resemblance to a basal cell carcinoma. Furthermore, the high incidence of metastasis in cases of adamantinoma of limb bones seems to constitute a strong argument against interpreting the lesion as a mere bone-invading basal cell carcinoma.

We now come to the idea held by some (see Hicks and also Lederer and Sinclair) that the so-called adamantinoma of limb bones should be regarded as a connective-tissue growth exhibiting complex synovial differentiation, rather than as an epithelial growth. On the basis of this conception, the lesion represents a synovial sarcoma (synovioma) which may either have invaded the bone from the outside or started its development in the medullary cavity of the bone. There can be no doubt that on casual histologic examination a synovioma showing clefts and spaces lined by cuboidal cells may suggest an adamantinoma. However, most synoviomas show relatively few such spaces, and most of the tumor tissue of a synovioma appears like that of a frank fibrosarcoma (see p. 576). In fact, it is usually difficult to distinguish a synovial sarcoma from an ordinary fibrosarcoma histologically unless one encounters the spaces lined by cuboidal cells.

The hypothesis identifying the adamantinoma of limb bones with the synovial sarcoma is intriguing because it does away with the apparent paradox of an epithelial tumor developing in relation to bone. Nevertheless, on the positive side, this hypothesis is undermined by the much greater clinical gravity of the synovial sarcoma and by the tendency of the resemblance to become less striking as one compares many different sections from a number of cases of each of these lesions. Thus, an adamantinoma of the tibia often shows rather well developed squamous differentiation here and there in its lesional tissue, which is not in accord with what one sees in synovial sarcoma.

Finally, we come to the idea, recently suggested by Changus *et al.*, that the so-called adamantinoma of limb bones is actually a tumor derived from angioblasts—that is, from primitive vascular mesenchymal cells. They believe that the so-called adamantinomas of limb bones reveal histologic tissue patterns analogous to those to be observed in the primitive mesoderm during the course of evolution of the blood vessels. In accordance with this conception, they think that the term "adamantinoma of limb bones" should be dropped and the lesion in question denoted as the "malignant angioblastoma of bone." Acceptance of this idea already seems to meet a serious obstacle in the fact that adamantinomas of limb bones occur almost solely in the tibia. On the histologic side, the frequent finding of some degree of squamous differentiation of the tumor cells of the lesion is not compatible with the "angioblastic" theory.

These doubts about the idea that the adamantinoma of limb bones is a mesodermal tumor (synovial sarcoma or malignant angioblastoma) throw one back upon the conception of it as an epithelial tumor. It must be admitted that this conception, too, leaves a number of unanswered questions. Nevertheless, one cannot ignore the suggestive epithelial nature of the lesional tissue as manifested on histologic examination of adequate material from a number of lesions.

## DIFFERENTIAL DIAGNOSIS

Some of the problems relating to the histologic differential diagnosis of the adamantinoma of limb bones were already touched upon in the discussion of the nature and genesis of the lesion. In any event, the histologic diagnosis of a lesion in a limb bone as an adamantinoma should be made only after careful exclusion of alternative possibilities. Although, in a given tumor, many different arrangements of the tumor cells are usually represented, there is often a predominant one. If the areas examined show a striking alveolar arrangement of the tumor cells, the lesion might be misinterpreted as a metastatic adenocarcinoma. However, one should be particularly wary about such a diagnosis, especially if the patient is an adolescent or a young adult and if the lesion is oriented toward the middle of the tibial shaft. If the sections show the tumor cells mainly in plexiform arrangement, the lesion may be misdiagnosed as a sarcoma or possibly as an "endothelioma." On the other hand, a lesion in which the epithelial cells show considerable squamous-cell differentiation may be mistaken for an epidermoid carcinoma.

From the clinicoroentgenographic point of view, it is only when the adamantinoma is intracortical and presents as a sort of multiloculated rarefaction shadow that one might suspect the correct diagnosis before tissue examination. However, in a young subject, a rather similar *x*-ray shadow may be produced by a non-ossifying fibroma (see Fig. 22-*B*). While the non-ossifying fibroma usually occurs in youthful subjects, it is more likely to be located in the metaphysial part of the shaft than in a midshaft area. Occasionally, too, a chondromyxoid fibroma (p. 205) may be restricted to the bone cortex and, if located in a tibia, present problems of differential diagnosis from limb bone adamantinoma.

## TREATMENT

If surgically feasible, the appropriate treatment at the initial intervention might well be wide block resection of the affected bone part and its periosteal cover.

However, even in cases in which this would be practical, the surgeon is not likely to know, at the initial intervention, that he is dealing with an adamantinoma. This is so because the lesion is ordinarily diagnosed only after histologic study of tissue from it. Thus, in most cases, the initial procedure has been curettage. Curettage is rarely an adequate procedure in these cases, being almost invariably followed by a recurrence. Indeed, in most cases, the limb affected eventually has to be amputated. Irradiation therapy is ineffective against the tumor.

Sufficient cases have been followed long enough to show that if amputation is carried out rather promptly, the patient is likely to remain well, and specifically will not develop metastases. The incidence of metastasis is, as already noted, about 25 per cent. This high rate is due, at least in part, to delay in amputation.

## REFERENCES


Anderson, C. E., and Saunders, J. B. de C. M.: Primary Adamantinoma of the Ulna, Surg., Gynec. & Obst., *75*, 351, 1942.

Baker, P. L., Dockerty, M. B., and Coventry, M. B.: Adamantinoma (So-called) of the Long Bones, J. Bone & Joint Surg., *36-A*, 704, 1954.

Changus, G. W., Speed, J. S., and Stewart, F. W.: Malignant Angioblastoma of Bone. A Reappraisal of Adamantinoma of Long Bone, Cancer, *10*, 540, 1957.

Fischer, B.: Über ein primäres Adamantinom der Tibia, Frankfurt. Ztschr. f. Path., *12*, 422, 1913.

Halpert, B., and Dohn, H. P.: Adamantinoma in the Tibia, Arch. Path., *43*, 313, 1947.

Hebbel, R.: Adamantinoma of the Tibia, Surgery, *7*, 860, 1940.

Hicks, J. D.: Synovial Sarcoma of the Tibia, J. Path. & Bact., *67*, 151, 1954.

Lederer, H., and Sinclair, A. J.: Malignant Synovioma Simulating "Adamantinoma of the Tibia," J. Path. & Bact., *67*, 163, 1954.

Mangalik, V. S., and Mehrotra, R. M. L.: Adamantinoma of the Tibia, Brit. J. Surg., *39*, 429, 1952.

Marzet, A.: Un cas d'adamantinome du tibia, Mém. Acad. de chir., *80*, 190, 1954.

Morgan, A. D., and Mackenzie, D. H.: A Metastasising Adamantinoma of the Tibia, J. Bone & Joint Surg., *38-B*, 892, 1956.

Ryrie, B. J. :Adamantinoma of the Tibia: Aetiology and Pathogenesis, Brit. M. J., *2*, 1000, 1932.

Willis, R. A.: *Pathology of Tumours*, London, Butterworth & Co., Ltd., p. 280, 1948.

Wolfort, B., and Sloane, D.: Adamantinoma of the Tibia, J. Bone & Joint Surg., *20*, 1011, 1938.

Chapter

# 15

# Benign Vascular Tumors

THE *benign vascular tumors* of bone are almost always hemangiovascular rather than lymphangiovascular lesions. Indeed, *lymphangioma* of bone (whether appearing in a single bone site or in numerous bone sites) is so rarely encountered that the pertinent literature is limited to a few reported cases. By comparison, *hemangioma* of bone is not at all unusual. However, one's evaluation of the actual incidence of hemangioma of bone will depend on one's interpretation of the so-called hemangiomas of vertebræ. Specifically, it will depend on one's conception of the very common, usually small, often multiple, and nearly always asymptomatic vertebral vascular lesions generally classed with the hemangiomas. The writer feels that these asymptomatic vertebral vascular lesions probably represent for the most part mere focal varicosities rather than true hemangiomas. If they are excluded from the category of hemangiomas, then hemangioma of bone in general would have to be regarded as a rather uncommon condition. However, in accordance with custom, these asymptomatic vertebral vascular lesions will be discussed in this chapter as hemangiomas.

As to hemangiomas in other bone sites, it is probably hemangioma of the calvarium that is most common and has attracted most attention. Only occasionally does one encounter a solitary hemangioma in still another skeletal part. Even more rare are the cases of hemangioma of bone in multiple sites. Still more unusual are those cases in which multiple vascular bone lesions are found associated with hemangiomas of overlying soft parts and even of internal organs.

## VERTEBRAL HEMANGIOMA

In the field of vertebral hemangioma, we have to consider, as already indicated, the asymptomatic vertebral vascular lesions which are commonly encountered as incidental findings at autopsy, and, on the other hand, those vertebral vascular lesions which give rise to clinical complaints. The former lesions are represented by small, dark red foci of vascularity in one or a number of vertebral bodies of a vertebral column removed at autopsy. They are encountered most commonly in the lower thoracic or upper lumbar part of the column. Their nature as actual hemangiomas may be questioned, as noted above. Indeed, such lesions may well represent merely focal areas of capillary angiectasis following in the wake of focal bone marrow atrophy. In contrast, those vertebral vascular lesions which give rise to clinical complaints are relatively large lesions. Usually, furthermore, it is only one vertebra that is involved in a given patient. One could defend the idea that it is only these large and relatively uncommon vertebral vascular lesions that actually represent vertebral hemangiomas.

### CLINICAL CONSIDERATIONS

**Incidence.**—As has already been implied, there is a wide disparity between the *anatomic* and the *clinical* incidence of vertebral hemangioma. Its remarkably high anatomic incidence was clearly demonstrated by Schmorl. His findings in this connection are also summarized in the articles by his co-workers, Junghanns and Töpfer. These anatomic investigations have shown that one or more vertebral hemangiomas which had been clinically silent were present in 409 (10.7 per cent) of 3,829 vertebral columns routinely removed at autopsy and split longitudinally for gross inspection. The writer, too, has encountered the lesion rather often in autopsy material. He estimates that he observed it in 1 of every 10 to 15 autopsies in which the dorsolumbar part of the vertebral column had been removed and cut into serial segments on the band saw. In contrast, the cases of vertebral hemangioma associated with clinical complaints are so infrequent that the personal experience of an author discussing the subject rarely covers more than a few instances.

As to sex incidence, vertebral hemangioma, whether producing clinical complaints or noted only as an incidental finding at autopsy, apparently predilects females. As to age incidence, one can say that in general the condition is observed most often in persons beyond middle age. However, if only those cases are considered in which the condition led to clinical difficulties, it will be found that, in this group, younger adults predominate.

**Clinical Complaints.**—When a vertebral hemangioma produces clinical complaints, these usually consist at first of local pain, associated with muscle spasm and rigidity of part of the column. Sensory changes may be present, there may be radicular pain, and eventually signs of partial paraplegia may appear. These severer complaints result from the fact that the posterior cortex of the affected vertebral body has bulged and has narrowed the canal. Furthermore, hemangiomatous tumor tissue may have broken through the cortex and extended between the bone and the dura, producing pressure in this way also upon the spinal cord and nerve roots.

These various clinical complaints are such as might likewise be encountered in connection with some other bone tumor primary in the vertebral column or metastatic to it, or a tumor within the spinal cord. However, the roentgenographic findings at this stage are helpful in the differentiation and are likely to suggest a clinical diagnosis of vertebral hemangioma if that is the lesion which is present. Should the hemangiomatously affected vertebra have collapsed by the time the case is studied, complete paralysis of the extremities below the level of the lesion is likely to supervene. After the collapse, the roentgenographic findings may no longer be helpful in establishing the clinical diagnosis.

## ROENTGENOGRAPHIC AND PATHOLOGIC FINDINGS

**Roentgenographic Findings.**—Asymptomatic vertebral hemangiomas of the conventional small size rarely show up at all in clinical roentgenographs. Indeed, the writer has noted that even when a vertebral column removed at autopsy was halved in the sagittal plane and found to show one or more small hemangiomas, roentgenographs of the hemisected column often still failed to reveal them. Of course, when a body containing a hemangioma is sliced in slabs only a few millimeters thick, and these are then roentgenographed, the lesion does show up—often quite strikingly.

On the other hand, relatively large vertebral hemangiomas are likely to show up in the clinical roentgenographs. Under favorable technical conditions, a large hemangioma appears as a focus of coarse, porous rarefaction traversed by sparse but thick trabeculæ which run mainly in the longitudinal axis of the affected body. Along with these findings, there may be evidence of some bulging of the cortex of the body and modification of the adjacent intervertebral disk spaces. However it must be realized that such a picture may also be produced by some other type of lesion in a vertebral body. Thus a myeloma or lymphoma in a vertebral body may present much the same roentgenographic appearance if the lesion is in an early stage of its evolution and has not yet produced a large area of osteolysis. At any rate, in arriving at a roentgenographic diagnosis of vertebral hemangioma, it is necessary to rule out carefully various other possibilities. (See Fig. 68.)

**Gross Pathology.**—Grossly, a vertebral hemangioma stands out from the surrounding tissue as a brownish red or dark red or even purple stippled area. Palpation reveals that the area in question is not so rich in osseous trabeculæ as it would normally be. If the lesion abuts upon the cortex, the latter too may be thinned. As pathologico-anatomic studies have also shown (see Makrycostas), it is mainly in the lower thoracic and upper lumbar part of the column that vertebral hemangiomas are encountered. The cervical part and the sacral part of the column are only occasional sites of the lesion. As already noted, asymptomatic vertebral hemangiomas are much more likely to be multiple than single. Indeed if, when bisected longitudinally, a vertebral column reveals a hemangioma in one body, sectioning of the halves of the column at different levels is likely to reveal one or a few additional hemangiomas in other bodies.

The hemangioma almost always arises in, and is almost always restricted to, the body of the vertebra. Occasionally it may be found involving also the adjacent part of the arch and/or transverse process. In a rare instance it may even be limited to one of these areas. As to the precise location of the hemangioma within the affected body, there is no particular uniformity. It may lie centrally; it may abut upon the anterior cortex; it may be oriented toward the upper or lower disk; or it may lie against the posterior cortex, though it does not often do this.

The great majority of the asymptomatic hemangiomas are not more than 1 cm. or $1\frac{1}{2}$ cm. in their greatest dimension. Small ones measuring 3 to 4 mm. in greatest

***Figure 68***

*A*, Photograph showing the gross appearance of an asymptomatic vertebral hemangioma encountered as an incidental finding at autopsy. The subject was a woman 49 years of age. The focus of vascularity is located in one of the lower thoracic vertebral bodies. A photomicrograph of this lesion is shown in Fig. 69-*A*.

*B*, Roentgenograph of the segment of sagittally sectioned vertebral column shown in *A*. Note that the vertebral body corresponding to the one presenting the gross focus of vascularity fails to reveal that focus in the *x*-ray picture.

*C*, Roentgenograph of a hemisected vertebral body showing faintly a roundish and somewhat radiolucent area through which some thick, pillar-like trabeculæ run in the longitudinal axis. A roentgenograph of this vertebral body before it was sectioned did not suggest the presence of the hemangioma at all.

*D*, Roentgenograph of a thin slice cut from the hemisected body illustrated in *C*. The hemangiomatous area now shows up strikingly.

*E*, Roentgenograph showing a symptomatic hemangioma in the 11th thoracic vertebra. The patient was a woman 22 years of age. For several months prior to the time when this *x*-ray picture was taken, she complained of some mild pain referred to the back. An episode of severe pain in the back, associated with sudden weakness in the legs and other signs of mild paraplegia, led to the discovery of the hemangioma. Note that the contour of the affected vertebral body is somewhat bulged. Note also its altered internal architecture, which presents a finely porous, honeycomb-like pattern. Tissue removed from the lesional area is illustrated in Fig. 69-*C*.

*F*, Roentgenograph showing a hemangioma in the 3rd lumbar vertebra of a woman 40 years of age. The clinical complaint was of pain referred to the back. The affected vertebral body has retained its normal contour, but the coarse, porous, honeycomb rarefaction rather characteristic of vertebral hemangioma is clearly apparent.

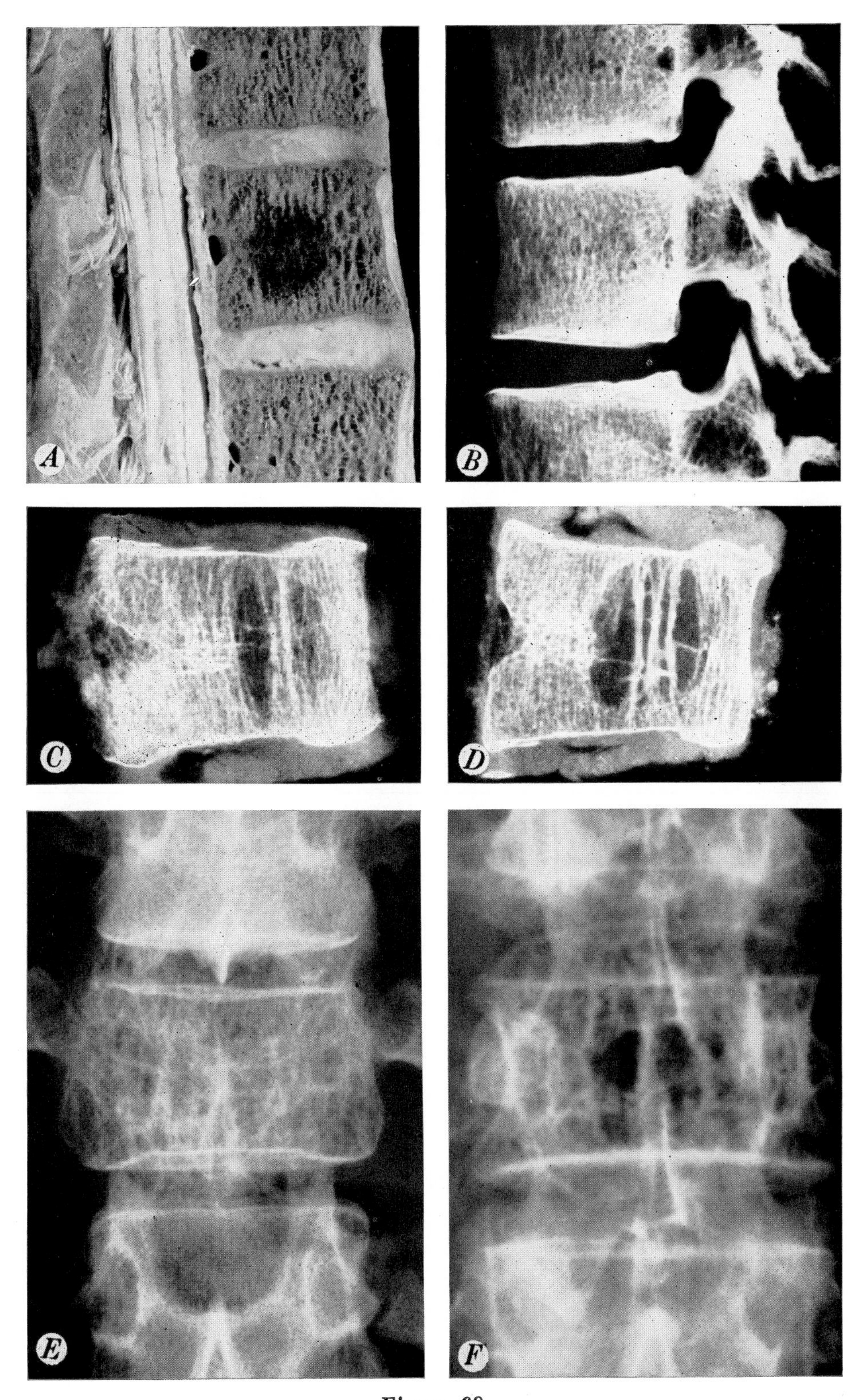


*Figure 68*

diameter are also fairly frequently encountered. A very large hemangioma giving rise to clinical manifestations may fill out almost the entire vertebral body and expand the cortex over at least part of its extent. Even if the bulging is not pronounced, the cord may be found compressed if the lesional tissue traverses the attenuated cortex and extends to the dura.

**Microscopic Pathology.**—Histologic examination shows that the blood channels composing the hemangioma vary in size, some being quite large and considerably dilated. Their walls are always thin. The vascular channels are found set in a substratum of fatty marrow which is usually somewhat edematous or gelatinous. Microscopic study also shows that much of the original osseous tissue at the site of the lesion has been resorbed. However, some of the osseous trabeculæ still present are likely to be of abnormal thickness. These thick trabeculæ run mainly in the longitudinal direction, and their thickness apparently compensates, at least in part, for the static insufficiency of the area.

The vessels in the lesional area are lined only by a single layer of endothelial cells. These vessels tend to be engorged. They may even contain thrombi, either fresh or in some stage of organization. In consequence of the thrombosis, one notes evidences of hemorrhage in the fatty supporting marrow, and this may explain why the latter is also somewhat edematous or gelatinous. It is interesting that phleboliths (calcified thrombi) such as are often seen in soft-tissue hemangiomas are not to be observed. Nor does one see evidence, such as is found in muscle hemangiomas, for instance, of proliferative activity associated with the actual formation of new vessel channels. Peripherally, the vertebral angiomatous area is not delimited by a connective-tissue capsule. Indeed, the fatty marrow substratum of the lesion either abuts abruptly upon, or merges gradually into, the cellular marrow of the neighboring spongy marrow spaces. (See Fig. 69.)

The fact that the vertebral hemangioma presents a substratum of fatty marrow raises the question of the possible relation of that lesion to the so-called "lipoma of vertebral bodies." The latter lesion has been noted as an incidental autopsy finding in the lumbar or sacral part of the column in elderly persons. In any particular case, a single vertebral body or several bodies may show the lesion. It stands out from the surrounding marrow by its yellow color, is usually irregular in shape, and may be as much as 1 to 1½ cm. in its greatest diameter. The lesion is apparently more likely to be in the central than in the marginal part of the affected body and does not tend to bulge the contour of the bone.

Histologically, the lesion in question is composed essentially of compacted fat cells, but since there is no delimiting capsule, the fat cells at the periphery merge smoothly with the surrounding cellular marrow. Sparse bony trabeculæ may traverse the lesional fatty tissue. These are not necessarily thinned, but are certainly never thickened. Since some of these so-called vertebral lipomas are rather vascular, and since they are also observed in association with so-called vertebral angiomas, Makrycostas thought that the vertebral "lipoma" may possibly represent

***Figure 69***

*A*, Photomicrograph (× 3) showing the histologic pattern of the hemangiomatous focus illustrated in Fig. 68-*A*. The scattered small, dark dots in the lesional area represent engorged capillaries.

*B*, Photomicrograph (× 3) of a hemangiomatous focus occupying the anterior half of a lumbar vertebra. The engorged capillaries are set in a substratum of fatty marrow.

*C*, Photomicrograph (× 65) showing the histologic pattern of the hemangiomatous tissue removed at surgical intervention in the case of the symptomatic hemangioma in the 11th thoracic vertebra illustrated in Fig. 68-*E*.

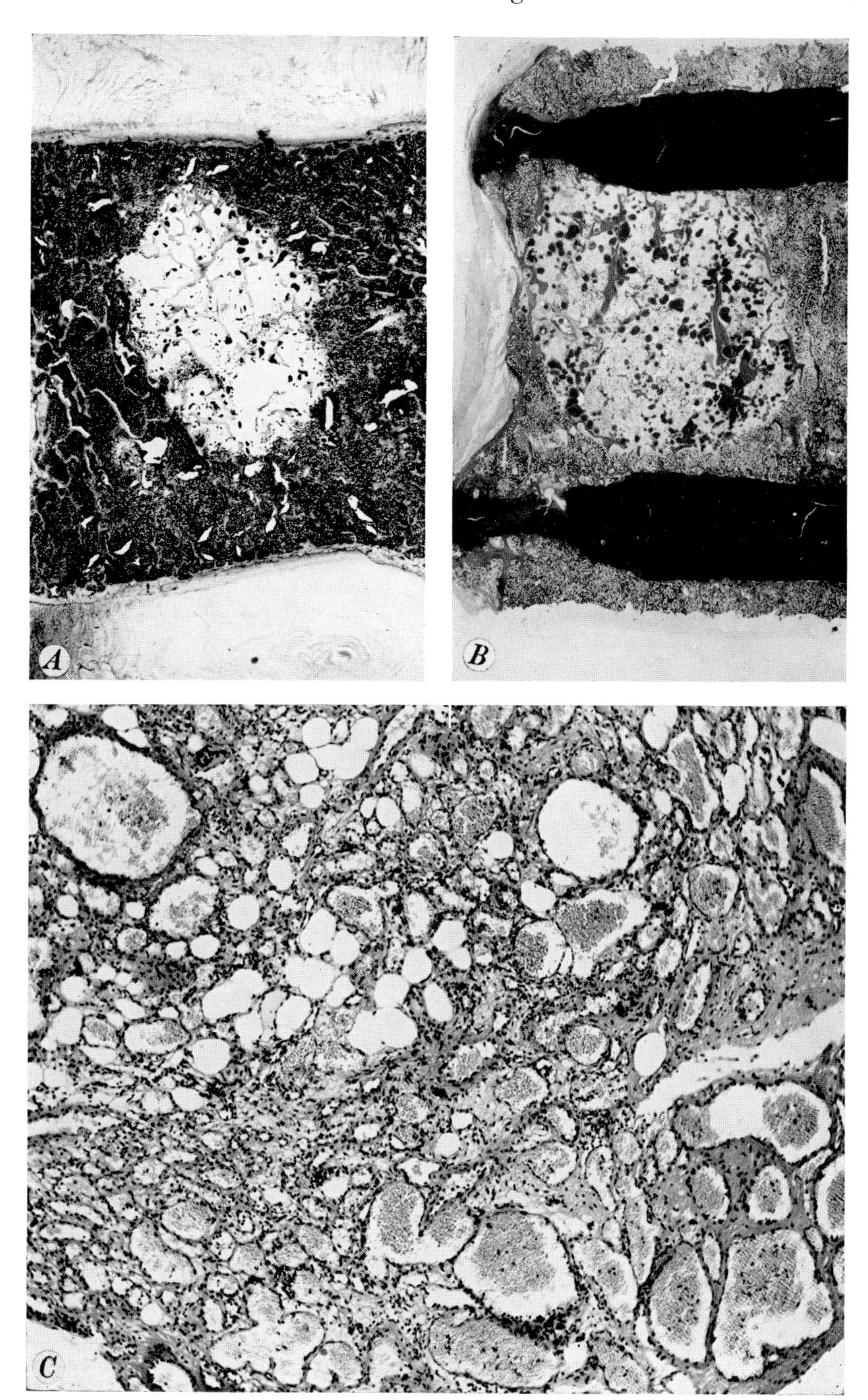


*Figure 69*

an end stage in the devolution of a vertebral "angioma." At any rate, whether this is their mode of genesis, or whether they represent merely focal areas of pronounced fatty atrophy of the marrow at the site of their development, these lesions ought not to be regarded as lipomas—that is, fat-tissue tumors in the true sense.

Indeed, the literature yields no convincing reports of a true lipoma (that is, a circumscribed and encapsulated tumor composed of fat tissue) in the interior of a bone, whether a vertebral body or some other bone. It is true that occasional references to lipoma of bone in other sites than the vertebral column are encountered in the literature. However, with few exceptions, these reported instances relate to lipomas involving only the periosteum of the bone, and not necessarily even arising from the periosteum.

On the basis of histologic appearances, there is little likelihood of misinterpreting tissue from a vertebral hemangioma as representing any other kind of lesion. Tissue removed from an aneurysmal bone cyst presents a histologic pattern quite different from that of a hemangioma. (See Fig. 14.) Clinically, however, and particularly on the basis of the $x$-ray picture, an aneurysmal bone cyst involving part of the vertebral column is not infrequently misinterpreted as an expansile hemangioma.

### TREATMENT

The question of treatment for vertebral hemangioma arises only in those cases in which a large and usually solitary lesion is producing clinical difficulties. When it is suspected that a noted collapse of a vertebral body has been due to a hemangioma, prompt laminectomy is indicated if a compression myelopathy is present. Laminectomy should be followed by radiation therapy to the affected part of the column. On the other hand, if the affected vertebral body has not collapsed, and signs of pressure on the nerve roots and/or cord are still mild, $x$-ray therapy is the treatment of choice. Doses of about 3,000 r into the center of the lesion are usually given. Some hold, however, that the myelopathy may advance to an irreversible stage before the effects of radiation therapy can make themselves adequately felt, and advocate laminectomy initially for these cases also.

## CALVARIAL HEMANGIOMA

The calvarial hemangioma is another distinctive vascular lesion encountered in relation to the skeleton. It may appear in any bone of the calvarium and nearly

***Figure 70***

*A*, Roentgenograph showing, in flat projection, a calvarial hemangioma in a frontal bone. The patient was a woman 29 years of age who had been aware since childhood that she had a swelling in that area. Note that the characteristic "sunburst" appearance (see *B*) is at least suggested in this clinical roentgenograph.

*B*, Roentgenograph of the surgical specimen removed from the calvarium in the case illustrated in *A*. The picture shows the specimen in flat projection and slightly magnified. In this picture there is a striking "sunburst" effect, produced by the osseous spicules radiating outward from the lesional area.

*C*, Clinical roentgenograph showing, in lateral projection, the hemangioma in the case in question. Note the radiopaque spicules running at right angles to the surface of the calvarium in a "sunray" pattern.

*D*, Roentgenograph of the extirpated specimen, taken with the specimen on end, so as to accentuate the "sunray" effect. (Compare with *B*.)

*E*, Roentgenograph (almost 3 times natural size) of a thin slice of the hemangioma specimen in this case. Note the details of the "sunburst" effect produced by the spicules of osseous tissue radiating at right angles to the surface of the involved area of the calvarium. Note also the presence of small osseous projections from the inner table.

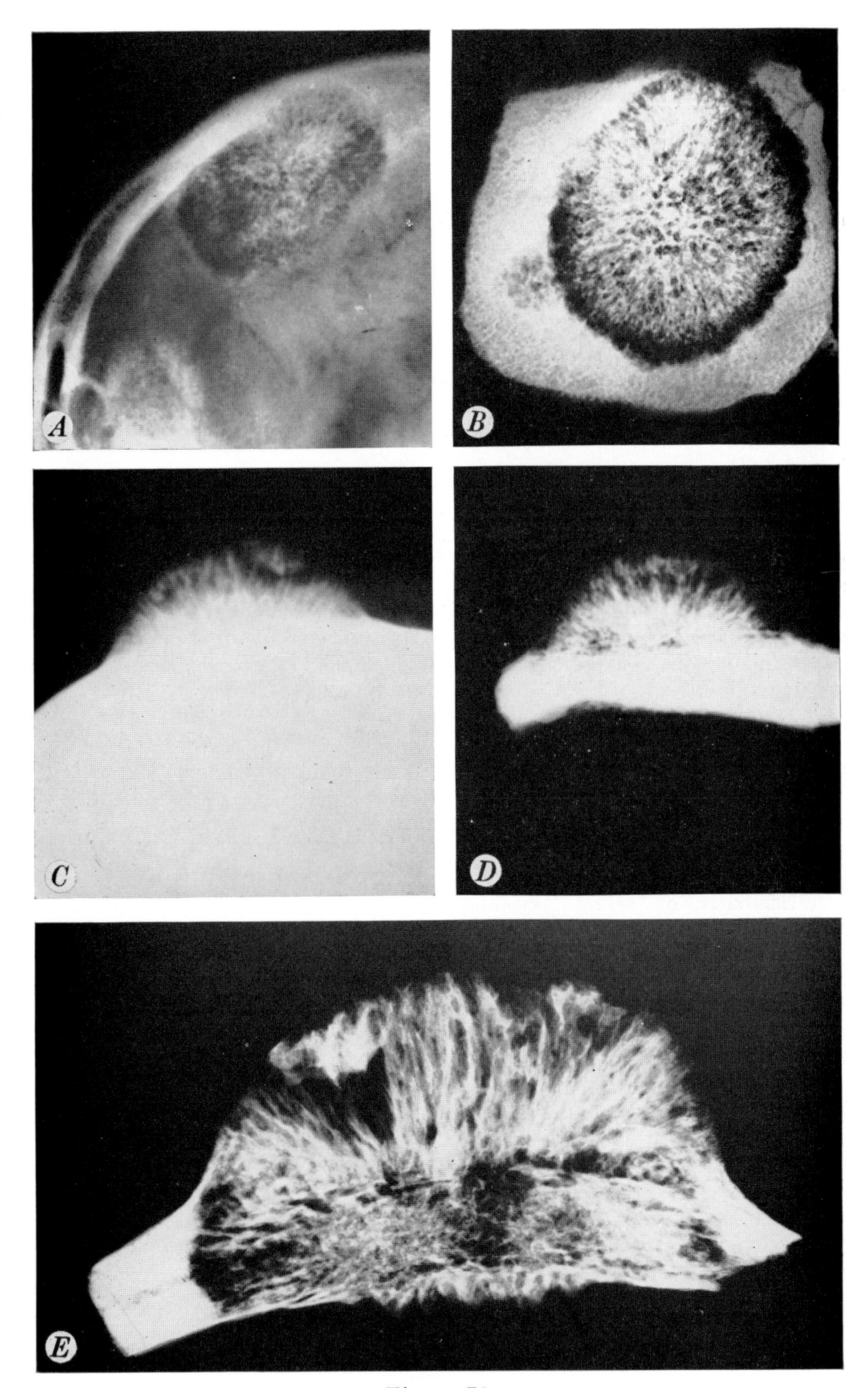


*Figure 70*

always presents as a solitary growth involving only a part of the bone affected. However, it has been known to appear in multiple form. Specifically, Erös reported an instance in which, in addition to the main lesion, which was in the right half of the frontal bone, there were a number of very small ones elsewhere in the calvarium. Although the definitive diagnosis usually rests upon tissue examination, the roentgenographic appearance is often strongly suggestive of the condition. What makes the picture striking is the so-called "sunburst" or "sunray" effect presented by the *x*-ray picture of the lesional area.

## CLINICAL CONSIDERATIONS

The calvarial hemangioma is of infrequent occurrence. The patient may be a child, but is more often a mature or even elderly adult. The usual history is that a slowly enlarging bump or protuberance has been noticed for at least some years. In one case from which material was studied by the writer, the patient was a man 47 years of age who had been aware of a small bony bump over the left orbital ridge for 12 years. During most of this time, the swelling had been enlarging very slowly, but for the last 1½ years its growth had been somewhat more rapid. In another case, the patient was a woman 29 years of age who had been aware since childhood of a small bump in the left frontal area. In this case, too, the lesion grew very slowly for many years, but for the past 7 years it had been growing somewhat more rapidly.

In general, the protuberance does not tend to exceed several centimeters in its greatest dimension at the time when the patient seeks definitive treatment. The protruding mass is bony hard and usually not tender. As a rule, the skin over it is freely movable and not grossly discolored. In an occasional case there may also be a complaint of local fullness or a sense of pressure. In addition, the patient may give a history of periodic vomiting. However, the general physical and neurological examinations are likely to yield essentially negative findings.

## ROENTGENOGRAPHIC AND PATHOLOGIC FINDINGS

**Roentgenographic Findings.**—As to the roentgenographic picture, the characteristic "sunburst" or "sunray" appearance presented in most cases of calvarial hemangioma has already been noted. In a flat projection of the lesion, the picture is that of osseous spicules tending to radiate from the center of the lesional area toward the periphery, so as to produce the "sunburst" effect. In a lateral projection showing the protuberance clearly, one sees numerous radiopaque spicules running at right angles to the surface of the calvarium, in a "sunray" pattern. (See Fig. 70.)

As to roentgenographic differential diagnosis, it is to be noted that the "sunburst" effect may simulate the picture of a sclerosing osteogenic sarcoma in partic-

### *Figure 71*

*A*, Photograph (almost 3 times natural size) of the hemisected specimen from the case also illustrated in Fig. 70. The highly vascular character of the lesional area is clearly apparent.

*B*, Photograph of the specimen shown in *A*, after all the soft tissue had been macerated away to bring out the details of the osseous architecture in the lesional area. (Compare with Fig. 70-*E*.)

*C*, Photomicrograph (× 15) of part of an area from a calvarial hemangioma. Note the numerous thin-walled, engorged blood channels between the trabeculæ of osseous tissue.

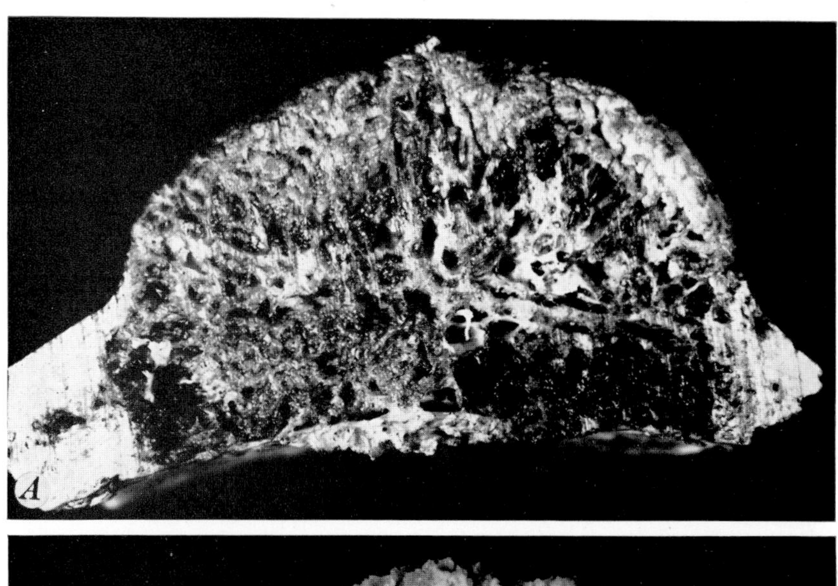


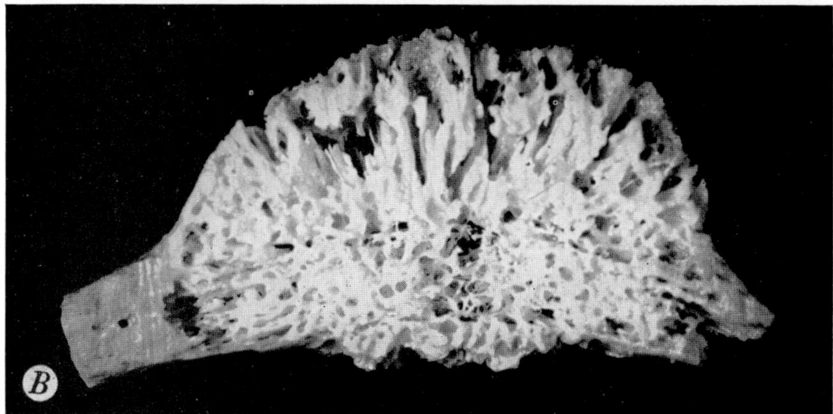


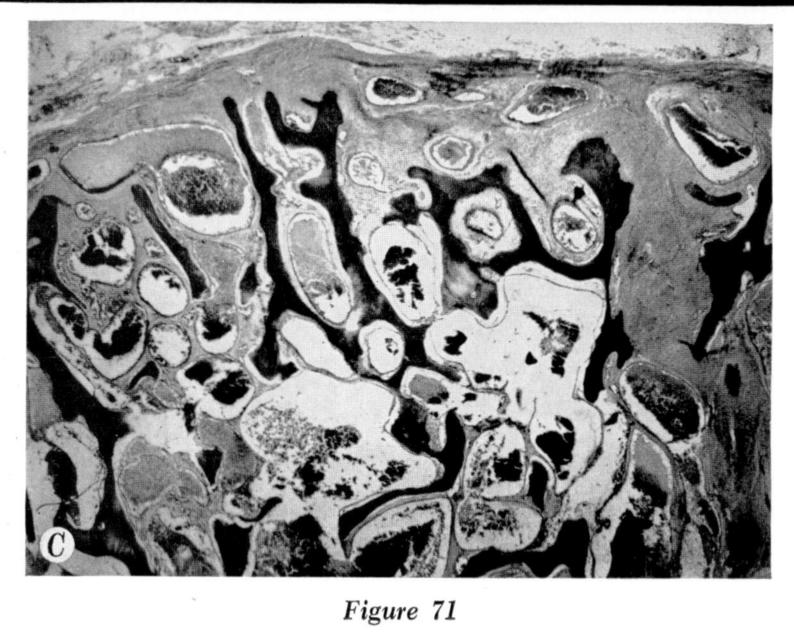


*Figure 71*

ular. Practically, however, the long history and slow growth of the calvarial hemangioma should weigh heavily against possible interpretation of the lesion as an osteogenic sarcoma. Confusion with the hyperostosis and spicule formation that sometimes develops in a calvarial area in association with a meningioma is much less likely (see Sosman and Putnam).

**Pathologic Findings.**—It seems clear that the hemangioma starts its development in the diploic spaces of the affected part of the calvarium. As it grows, it gradually induces local alterations in the architecture of the diploic osseous tissue and erosion of the inner and outer compact tables. Expansion of the affected area from pressure against the yielding tables is ordinarily more pronounced toward the outer than toward the inner surface. It is this external expansion, of course, that accounts for the bulge palpable clinically in the affected area.

Very few calvarial hemangiomas have been described in anatomic detail. As to variations in size, the lesion reported by Pich measured 1.5 cm. in thickness and 2.5 cm. across; the one described by Sommer measured 7 cm. in thickness and even more than this across; and the one described by Bucy and Capp was intermediate in size between these two. A lesion which had been removed intact in its setting and which was studied in detail by the present writer measured 2.5 cm. in thickness and 3.5 cm. across in its widest area.

On gross inspection, a calvarial hemangioma also stands out from the surrounding unmodified part of the calvarium by its gray red or even livid dark red color. Even if the lesional area is much bulged, it will usually be found that the pericranium has not been transgressed and that it can be stripped from the bone. Ordinarily the dura, too, is not invaded and can likewise be stripped away. However, the writer has studied a specimen in which, over a small area, the dura had been penetrated and had become intimately adherent to the lesional area.

When a hemangioma specimen is hemisected, its cut surface presents smaller or larger dark red engorged vascular spaces supported in a meshwork of osseous trabeculæ. Especially toward the outer surface, the trabecular structure is likely to be coarse, and the individual trabeculæ tend to be thick and to run more or less at right angles to the surface. Deeper in the lesion, the trabecular structure tends to appear more uniformly honeycombed. The details of the osseous architecture in the lesional area stand out particularly well in a roentgenograph of the cut specimen, or in the actual cut specimen if all the soft tissue has been macerated away.

It is the intermingling of thin-walled, engorged small or large blood spaces with a supporting osseous trabecular structure that distinguishes most calvarial hemangiomas anatomically from vertebral hemangiomas. Indeed, in vertebral hemangiomas, as already noted, osseous tissue is ordinarily very sparse in the lesional area,

***Figure 72***

*A*, Photograph (somewhat enlarged) of a primary hemangioma involving a clavicle. The contour of the affected part of the bone is very much expanded. The vascular character of the lesional tissue is apparent even to the naked eye. (This photograph was kindly supplied by Dr. C. Howard Hatcher of the Department of Orthopedics of the University of Chicago.)

*B*, Roentgenograph showing a large hemangioma in the soft tissues of the calf of a leg. The patient was a man 36 years of age. The hemangiomatous character of the lesion is betrayed by the numerous roundish radiopacities (representing calcified phleboliths) in the soft tissue mass. Note that the fibula is being invaded by the lesional tissue. This involvement of the bone is apparently secondary, however, to hemangiomatous involvement of the local ligamentous tissue and/or periosteum.

*C*, Roentgenograph showing a large hemangioma, again located in the soft tissues of the calf of a leg. The patient was a girl 17 years of age. In this case the local bones are not modified, apparently because the local ligamentous tissue and periosteum were not affected

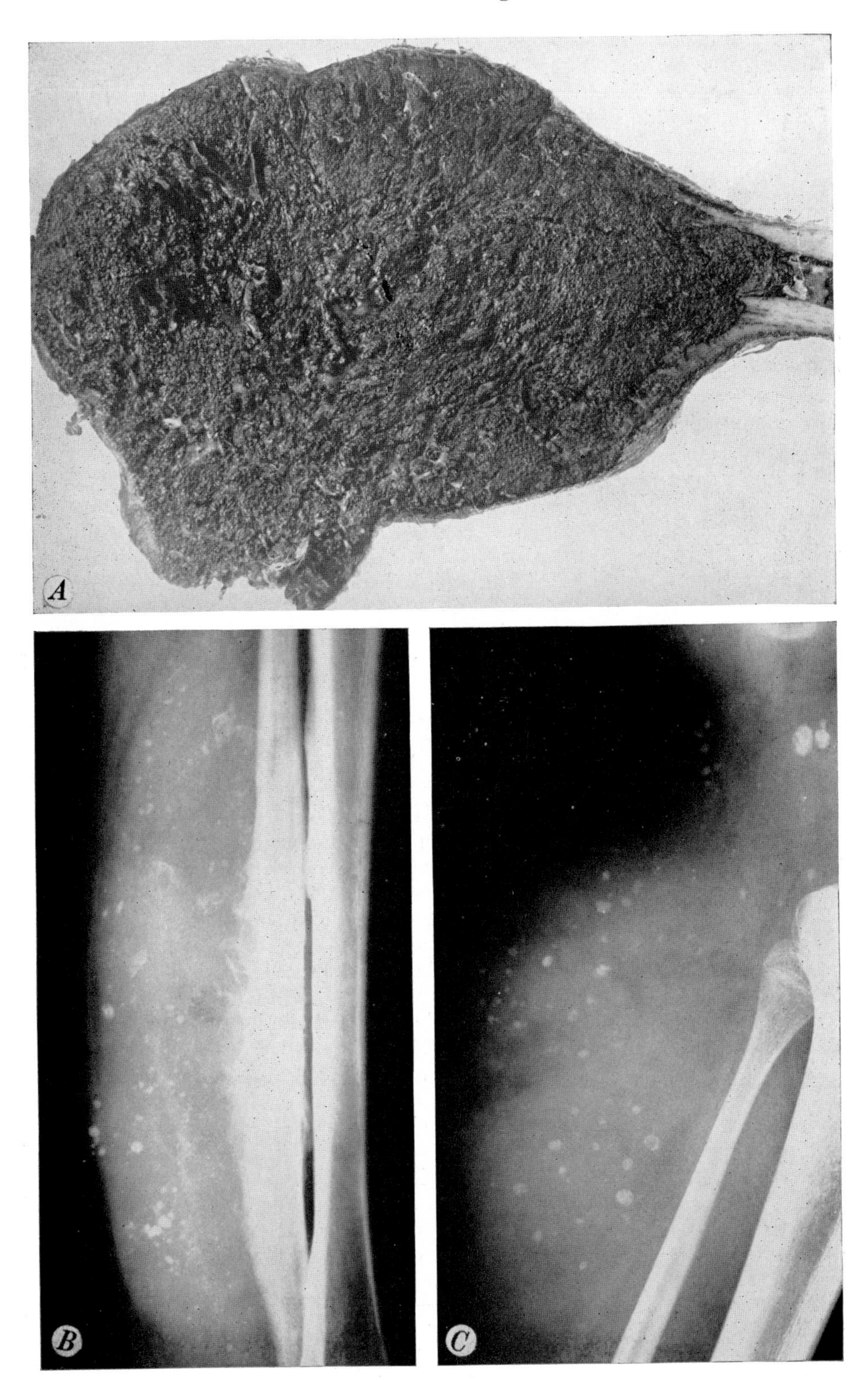


*Figure 72*

though the few trabeculæ present are usually thick. Why there should be this difference is not clear. There can be no doubt, however, that, in the calvarial lesions, the osseous trabeculæ present between individual blood channels or groups of them represent a secondary deposit in the supporting stroma of the lesion. That is, the osseous framework between the vessels represents newly formed osseous tissue. In some areas, engorged vessels lined merely by endothelium abut on the osseous trabeculæ, while in other areas they are separated from them by a connective-tissue stroma. (See Fig. 71.)

### TREATMENT

The treatment of choice for calvarial hemangioma seems to be *x*-ray therapy. This can be expected to check the course of growth of the lesion, but the osseous deformity present will, of course, remain. On this account (and possibly also to avoid radiation damage to local soft parts), excision of the lesion with some of the surrounding calvarium has been carried out in some cases.

## HEMANGIOMA IN OTHER SKELETAL SITES

It is only rarely that one encounters a hemangioma which has originated within a bone other than a vertebra or a calvarial bone. The rarity of hemangioma *primary* in bone sites other than the vertebral column or the cranium is illustrated by the fact that Bucy and Capp were able to find only 15 such cases in a survey of the literature to 1930. To these they added 4 from various personal sources. The more recent literature, too, contains but very few reports of additional cases of this kind.

In the cases in question, the lesion shows no tendency toward predilection of any particular bone or type of bone. Indeed, in one case or another, a primary hemangioma has been observed in a long bone, clavicle, scapula, ilium, or some hand or foot bone. One does not find the lesion predilecting any particular age group, either. The case history and the objective clinical findings are such as may be noted in connection with other benign tumors also. Even the *x*-ray picture may fail to be helpful, though sometimes it does give a clue to the character of the lesion.

In a long bone the lesion is likely to be located toward one end of the shaft. Characteristically, in the *x*-ray picture the contour of the bone in the affected area is found bulged out but not interrupted anywhere. The area may present a "loculated" appearance, the loculæ tending to be small and their partitions delicate. In the presence of persisting cortical bone, the loculation will not be uniform. If none of the original osseous tissue persists in the area and the loculæ are very delicate, the area may present, roentgenographically, the appearance of a fine honeycomb. This results from the formation of numerous thin trabeculæ of new bone between the blood sinuses. Furthermore, should these trabeculæ have coarsened in the peripheral part of the growth and come to be arranged more or less at right angles to the surface, a hemangioma in a tubular bone may even present the "sunburst" appearance already noted in connection with the calvarial lesion.

On the other hand, in a flat bone such as a scapula or an ilium, a "sunburst" *x*-ray picture may be presented almost from the start. Even in such a bone, however, in the early phases of the evolution of the lesion, the *x*-ray picture may not suggest the diagnosis. Specifically, the lesion may show up only as a more or less uniform rarefaction shadow, or as a coarsely trabeculated one. Altogether, then, while there are certain roentgenographic features suggesting the diagnosis in these cases of hemangioma, it is probable that the diagnosis will actually be made only on the basis of examination of tissue from the lesion.

When the diagnosis has been established, the treatment of choice in these cases is *x*-ray therapy. After *x*-ray treatment of the hemangioma, one can usually note a marked increase in the density of the lesional area. Occasionally, however, even without *x*-ray therapy, a hemangioma in an extracranial or extravertebral site may become static and undergo a certain degree of spontaneous sclerotization.

More often than not, when a bone of an extremity is the site of a vascular growth, the latter represents a *secondary* involvement in the sense that it has reached the bone by extension from the overlying soft parts. It is true that one frequently observes extensive hemangiomatous involvement of the musculature of part of a limb without any evidence of invasion of the regional bone or bones. Often the vascular growth in the overlying soft tissue does not even deform the contour of the neighboring bone or bones through pressure. Occasionally, however, even if the soft-part hemangioma is small, it may produce a local pressure deformity in the contour of the bone if the lesion is growing in a confined space. In a bone area showing such a local pressure deformity, the outline of the bone remains smooth, indicating that the bone has merely been molded, and not actually invaded, by the hemangioma.

On the other hand, when the presence of a hemangioma of muscle is associated with hemangiomatous involvement of the local ligamentous tissue and/or periosteum, one does find evidence of invasion of neighboring bone. This may take the form of extensive erosion of the bone cortex, and even actual penetration of the hemangiomatous tissue into the interior of the affected bone part or parts may be demonstrable in one case or another. In any event, in such cases, the fact that one is dealing essentially with a hemangioma of the soft parts is usually made evident by the presence of small, roundish opacities, representing calcified thrombi (phleboliths) in the *x*-ray picture of the involved area. (See Fig. 72.)

## HEMANGIOMATOSIS

Occasionally one encounters a case in which extensive hemangiomatosis of the soft parts of one or another limb is associated with the presence of vascular tumors in one or a number of bones of that extremity, and, in a limb so affected, local skeletal overgrowth is not uncommon. In one such case observed by the writer, the patient, a woman 58 years of age, presented extensive hemangiomatosis of the soft parts of the left upper and lower limbs, the involvement being most striking in the upper extremity and shoulder region. The condition had been present since birth and was progressive. *X*-ray examination showed that not only the soft parts, but also most of the bones of the upper limb were involved.

In another pertinent case, in which the patient was a man 32 years of age, the subcutaneous tissues and muscles overlying the left innominate bone and the left femur had been the site of a pronounced hemangiomatosis, again since childhood, and the femur itself was also involved. In the case of a girl 17 years of age who presented numerous small nodular hemangiomatous tumors in the soft tissues of the lower back, right thigh, and left thigh and leg, there was also overgrowth of the bones of the left lower extremity to the extent of 9 cm. In addition, this patient presented roentgenographic evidence of hemangiomatosis of the spleen.

Finally, there are rare instances of what may be denoted as skeletal hemangiomatosis, sometimes associated with hemangiomatosis of overlying soft parts and even of various internal organs. In such a case, the vascular bone tumors constitute merely the skeletal aspect of a systematized neoplastic disease of the vasoformative tissues. However, this is not the only interpretation that has been offered for such cases. Specifically, some do not accept the various lesions in these cases as multiple independent vascular tumors, holding instead that there is only one primary lesion, and that the other foci represent metastases. This conception is maintained by some even in cases in which the histologic pattern of the lesion in the various sites has proved to be that of a "benign" rather than a "malignant" vascular tumor. It is to such cases that the self-contradictory designation of "benign metastasizing hemangioma" is sometimes applied.

In this connection, Köhlmeier reports a case in which, along with numerous hemangiomas in the spleen and a hemangiomatous soft tissue tumor about the left ilium, there were numerous hemangiomatous sclerotized foci in the calvarium and vertebral column, and the sternum and left femur were also involved. Ritchie and Zeier report a case of widespread hemangiomatosis of the skeleton, associated with cystic hemangiomatosis of the spleen. Roentgenographically, the skeletal lesions in this case took the form of multiple irregular multilocular and monolocular "cystic" rarefaction shadows of fairly large size. These were found distributed through the shafts of various tubular bones, and were present also in the calvarium, the ribs, and the innominate bones.

## LYMPHANGIOMA

Lesions which might be held to represent lymphangioma of bone are very rare indeed. The writer himself has not yet encountered a case which he felt should be interpreted in this way. However, the case reported by Bickel and Broders might well be an instance in point. In this case of relatively localized lymphangioma apparently beginning within the affected bone, the lesion involved mainly the left innominate bone. The patient, a girl, was 5 years old at the time when the condition began to cause clinical difficulty. At that time roentgenographic examination showed that a substantial part of the ilium was the site of an osteolytic process. Within a period of some months, progressive destruction of the affected bone area occurred. The diagnosis of lymphangioma was made on the basis of histologic study of tissue obtained by biopsy. Osseous tissue and overlying soft tissue removed from the lesional area were found to show numerous lymphatic channels and sinuses set in a substratum of fat, connective tissue, and muscle. The lesion was treated by *x*-ray therapy, but the process was not contained. Indeed, it came to extend into other portions of the innominate bone and eventually appeared to be involving the sacrum and contiguous lumbar vertebræ.

Instances of widespread involvement of the skeleton by lymphangiomas and/or lymphangiectases have been reported by Harris and Prandoni and by Cohen and Craig. The case reported by the latter authors is particularly illuminating because it included gross and microscopic anatomic findings relating to many of the bones. Roentgenographically, some of the affected bones presented expansion of their contours and considerable rarefaction, in association with a finely multilocular "soap bubble" appearance. Histologic examination of the porotified bones indicated that the destruction of their osseous tissue was the result of pressure from enlarging lymph vessels. It was also evident that the intra-osseous lymph channels were communicating with lymph channels in neighboring soft tissues beyond the affected bones.

### REFERENCES

Ackermann, A. J., and Hart, M. S.: Multiple Primary Hemangioma of the Bones of the Extremity, Am. J. Roentgenol., *48*, 47, 1942.

Anspach, W. E.: Sunray Hemangioma of Bone: With Special Reference to Roentgen Signs, J.A.M.A., *108*, 617, 1937.

Baldini, G., and Ferri, L.: Sui tumori angioblastici dell'osso; considerazioni anatomo-radiologiche sull'emangioma osseo primitivo del cranio, Radiol. med., *42*, 561, 1956.

Bickel, W. H., and Broders, A. C.: Primary Lymphangioma of the Ilium, J. Bone & Joint Surg. *29*, 517, 1947.
Bucy, P. C., and Capp, C. S.: Primary Hemangioma of Bone: With Special Reference to Roentgenologic Diagnosis, Am. J. Roentgenol., *23*, 1, 1930.
Cohen, J., and Craig, J. M.: Multiple Lymphangiectases of Bone, J. Bone & Joint Surg., *37-A*, 585, 1955.
Cushing, H.: Surgical End-results in General, with a Case of Cavernous Hemangioma of the Skull in Particular, Surg., Gynec. & Obst., *36*, 303, 1923.
Erös, G.: Multiples Hämangiom der Schädelknochen, Zentralbl. f. allg. Path. u. path. Anat., *43*, 532, 1928.
Ferber, L., and Lampe, I.: Hemangioma of Vertebra Associated with Compression of the Cord, Arch. Neurol. & Psychiat., *47*, 19, 1942.
Foster, D. B., and Heublein, G. W.: Hemangioma of Vertebra Associated with Spinal Cord Compression, Am. J. Roentgenol., *57*, 556, 1947.
Geschickter, C. F., and Maseritz, I. H.: Primary Hemangioma Involving Bones of the Extremities, J. Bone & Joint Surg., *20*, 888, 1938.
Ghormley, R. K., and Adson, A. W.: Hemangioma of Vertebræ, J. Bone & Joint Surg., *23*, 887, 1941.
Goidanich, I. F., and Venturi, R.: Emangioma cavernoso della tibia, Chir. d. org. di movimento, *43*, 295, 1956.
Harris, R., and Prandoni, A. G.: Generalized Primary Lymphangiomas of Bone, Ann. Int. Med., *33*, 1302, 1950.
Hitzrot, J. M.: Haemangioma Cavernosum of Bone, Ann. Surg., *65*, 476, 1917.
Junghanns, H.: Über die Häufigkeit gutartiger Geschwülste in den Wirbelkörpern (Angiome, Lipome, Osteome), Arch. f. klin. Chir., *169*, 204, 1932.
Karshner, R. G., Rand, C. W., and Reeves, D. L.: Epidural Hemangioma Associated with Hemangioma of the Vertebræ, Arch. Surg., *39*, 942, 1939.
Kleinberg, S.: Angioma of the Foot, J. Bone & Joint Surg., *24*, 367, 1942.
Köhlmeier, W.: Zur Kenntnis der Angiome des Knochens, Wien. klin. Wchnschr., *50*, 274, 1937.
Lindqvist, I.: Vertebral Hemangioma with Compression of the Spinal Cord, Acta radiol., *35*, 400, 1951.
Makrycostas, K.: Über das Wirbelangiom, -lipom und -osteom, Virchows Arch. f. path. Anat., *265*, 259, 1927.
Perman, E.: On Haemangiomata in the Spinal Column, Acta chir. scandinav., *61*, 91, 1926.
Pich, G.: Über das Osteoangiom des Schädeldaches, Beitr. z. path. Anat. u. z. allg. Path., *101*, 181, 1938.
Ritchie, G., and Zeier, F. G.: Hemangiomatosis of the Skeleton and the Spleen, J. Bone & Joint Surg., *38-A*, 115, 1956.
Schmorl, G.: Die pathologische Anatomie der Wirbelsäule, Verhandl. d. deutsch. orthop. Gesellsch., Kong. 21, p. 3, 1927.
Sherman, M. S.: Capillary Hemangioma of Bone, Arch. Path., *38*, 158, 1944.
Sommer, G.: Über das primäre kavernöse Hämangiom der Schädelknochen, Beitr. z. klin. Chir., *168*, 101, 1938.
Sosman, M. C., and Putnam, T. J.: Roentgenological Aspects of Brain Tumors—Meningiomas, Am. J. Roentgenol., *13*, 1, 1925.
Thomas, A.: Vascular Tumors of Bone, Surg., Gynec. & Obst., *74*, 777, 1942.
Töpfer, D.: Über ein infiltrierend wachsendes Hämangiom der Haut und multiple Kapillarektasien der Haut und inneren Organe: Zur Kenntnis der Wirbelangiome, Frankfurt. Ztschr f. Path., *36*, 337, 1928.

Chapter

# 16

# Bone Lesions Associated with Neural Tumors

OCCASIONALLY a bone lesion develops on the basis of a solitary neural tumor. The neural tumor may have started its development in the medullary cavity of the affected bone part or in the periosteum and/or adjacent soft tissues. Thus, a few clear-cut instances of a *neurilemmoma* producing a tumorous bone lesion have been recorded. Even rarer must be the cases in which a bone lesion has been produced by a *solitary neurofibroma.*

On the other hand, the so-called *neurofibromatosis of Recklinghausen* is quite likely to be associated with skeletal aberrations of various kinds. Those which concern us in particular in connection with neurofibromatosis are: (1) the cortical defects due to pressure erosion from proliferating neurofibromatous tissue in the periosteum and/or overlying soft parts, and (2) central lesions resulting from expansive growth of neurofibromatous tissue in the medullary cavity of an affected bone part. However, the skeletal manifestations of neurofibromatosis are so protean that it seems worth while to give some consideration also to certain of the other skeletal aberrations encountered in connection with this disorder.

The finding of a bone lesion conditioned by a *glomus tumor* is very rare indeed. Actually, a glomus tumor is preponderantly a vascular rather than a neural lesion. However, the arteriovenous anastomotic complex constituting the normal glomus does have a wrapping of unmyelinated neural filaments. Therefore, it may not be too inappropriate to include in this chapter the occasional finding of a bone lesion conditioned by a glomus tumor.

A unique case of *ganglioneuroma* occurring in multiple bone sites has been reported by Wilber and Woodcock. Even if it should turn out that the intra-osseous ganglioneuromas in this case are not primary lesions but represent metastases from an occult ganglioneuroma of the sympathetic nervous system, the case is still unusual.

## NEURILEMMOMA OF BONE

A neurilemmoma is a rather specific benign tumor arising from the sheath of a nerve, and most probably from the Schwann cells of the sheath. Though the neurilemmoma in general is not an uncommon tumor, it is one which, as already indicated, only rarely develops in relation to a bone. As to localization, so few cases of neurilemmoma involving bone have been encountered that it is not possible to make any generalizations on this point. Peers has described a case in which the lesion had arisen in the medullary cavity of the shaft of an ulna. Gross, Bailey, and Jacox discuss one in which it developed in the medullary cavity of the shaft of a humerus. DeSanto and Burgess have reported 2 instances of neurilemmoma of bone. In one case, they thought it arose within the cortex of the midshaft of an ulna. In the other case, the tumor involved part of the sacrum but clearly had started not within the bone, but in the dorsal root of the 5th right lumbar nerve, from which it invaded the right sacral wing. Schroff has described a neurilemmoma which originated in a ramus of a mandible. The writer's personal experience with neurilemmoma involving bone relates to 2 cases. In one of them, the lesion was in the interior of a patella and was about 1 cm. in diameter. In the other, the lesion was in the sacrum, and a considerable part of this bone was found expanded and cystified.

Most of the patients have been mature adults, and the majority have been females. The complaints are ordinarily neither severe nor specific. They tend to be of rather long standing, since the lesion ordinarily grows rather slowly. Thus it is not unusual for the patient to give a history of local complaints dating back one year or even several years. Indeed, in the case seen by the writer in which the sacrum was involved, the complaints dated back 20 years. The complaints vary, of course, with the particular skeletal area implicated. A neurilemmoma in the shaft of a long bone, for instance, usually produces some local bone swelling and aching, and may even be the cause of repeated pathologic fractures. A neurilemmoma involving the sacrum is likely to produce low back pain and to be associated with neurological aberrations suggesting a sciatic syndrome.

Like the clinical complaints, the *roentgenographic findings* are nondescript. Most often, the lesion does not attain a size of more than a few centimeters in its largest dimension. An intramedullary neurilemmoma may present as a clear-cut rarefaction shadow often bordered by a thin zone of sclerosis, and may be mistaken for a bone cyst. Sometimes a central lesion is larger and appears as a multiloculated rarefaction shadow expanding and even perforating the cortex in some area. A neurilemmoma taking its departure from the periosteum shows a picture representing erosion or even penetration of the bone from the outside by the lesion. At any rate, on the basis of the *x*-ray findings, one rarely thinks of a bone lesion as possibly being a neurilemmoma, so that the diagnosis usually has to wait upon tissue examination. (See Fig. 73.)

On *gross examination*, an osseous neurilemmoma which has been exposed surgically rarely permits one to establish the relation of the tumor to the nerve of origin. This is so because, when the nerve of origin is small, it is difficult to identify it. Indeed, the nerves of the periosteum, though numerous, are delicate, as are also those which may be found in the nutrient canals and even in the marrow spaces in association with blood vessels. Thus the nerve from which a neurilemmoma develops in relation to a bone is likely to be a small one. It is true that within the neural canal of the sacrum it might arise from a fairly large nerve. However, in regard to such a location, the identification of the nerve would be difficult for practical surgical reasons.

Be that as it may, the tumor tissue proper is ordinarily soft, friable, myxomatous, and of a mixed pinkish gray and yellowish color. A very large neurilemmoma is likely to undergo extensive degeneration and cystification. This was so in the case, seen by the writer, in which the neurilemmoma involved much of the sacrum. The posterior wall of the sacrum was bulged and a large cavity was present within the body of the sacrum. From the wall of this cavity, a considerable amount of yellowish brown tissue was curetted which presented the histologic pattern characteristic for neurilemmoma.

On *microscopic examination*, the lesional tissue of a neurilemmoma is found to be composed, in varying proportions, of spindle-cellular areas (the type A or fibrillar tissue of Antoni) and loose-meshed edematous areas (the type B or reticulated tissue of Antoni). The tissue of type A is composed of cells having elongated nuclei and elongated cell bodies. Between the cells there is an abundance of long, slender, straight or serpentine reticulum fibers. A characteristic feature of the type A tissue nearly always observable is the so-called "palisading" of nuclei. This "palisading" effect is due to the alignment of nuclei in a sort of border around areas in which masses of reticulum fibers are banded together in parallel array. In some places,

16

the type A tissue may present a whorled nodular pattern producing the organoid appearance of so-called Verocay bodies. Intermingled with the tissue of type A is that of type B, which probably results from degeneration of the former. The tissue of type B is loose-meshed, and its fibers and cells run every which way, at random. Within the irregular network of cells and fibers there is intercellular fluid, and in places this fluid may have collected to form microcystic spaces. Because of the extensive degeneration which a neurilemmoma in a bone is likely to undergo, tissue of type B usually predominates in it. Such nonspecific features as the presence of dense collagen sheaths about the numerous capillary vessels, evidence of old hemorrhage, and the finding of foam cells need only be mentioned.

The *treatment* of neurilemmoma of bone can be guided by the fact that this tumor is essentially a benign one. Furthermore, it rarely recurs after thorough removal. Whether it ever undergoes malignant degeneration is still a moot question. The neurilemmoma of the ulna described by Peers seems to show some evidence of sarcomatous transformation. However, it is safe to say that if, in a case of neurilemmoma of bone, the tumor tissue has been thoroughly curetted out, or if the affected area is removed by block resection, even recurrence is unlikely.

## NEUROFIBROMATOSIS

The so-called neurofibromatosis of Recklinghausen is a hereditary and familial disorder in which the basic aberration is a maldevelopment of neural tissue, affecting particularly the peripheral nerves. However, neurofibromatosis so often implicates other tissues (notably the skin, subcutis, and skeleton) that a patient presenting the disorder in its most florid form may be a veritable museum of abnormalities.

The alterations in the nerves are based upon diffuse and haphazard proliferation of the Schwann sheath cells and also of the nerve fibers themselves. In consequence of the proliferative changes, nerve trunks become thickened and nodulated, and nerve terminations become the site of localized or diffuse proliferative overgrowth.

The typical clinical stigmata of the disorder are: patchy, brownish pigmentation of the skin; encapsulated or plexiform neurofibromata palpable as swellings along the course of the peripheral nerve trunks, especially of the extremities; and discrete neurofibromatous nodules in the skin (or patches of diffuse neurofibromatous thickening of the skin) resulting from involvement of the peripheral terminations of nerves.

The disorder usually begins to be manifest early in childhood. In certain cases, however, no neurofibromata may be palpable, at least for some years after birth,

***Figure 73***

*A*, Roentgenograph showing alterations produced in a sacrum by a neurilemmoma. The affected part of the bone casts a multiloculated shadow. The patient was a man 58 years of age. There had been complaints of intermittent attacks of pain in the back for over 20 years, but more recently the pain had become persistent and was radiating. At the surgical intervention, the contour of the posterior aspect of the sacrum was found expanded, and when the lesional area was entered, a large cavity was found within the body of the bone. This cavity was lined by a thick, irregular layer of soft, lobulated, yellowish brown tissue. In many places, this tissue presented the histologic pattern (see *B*) characteristic for neurilemmoma.

*B*, Photomicrograph (× 125) showing the histologic pattern found in the better preserved areas of tissue curetted from the wall of the cystified sacrum illustrated in *A*. The pattern in this field is that of the so-called type A or fibrillar tissue of Antoni. Note the "palisading" of the nuclei in various parts of the field.

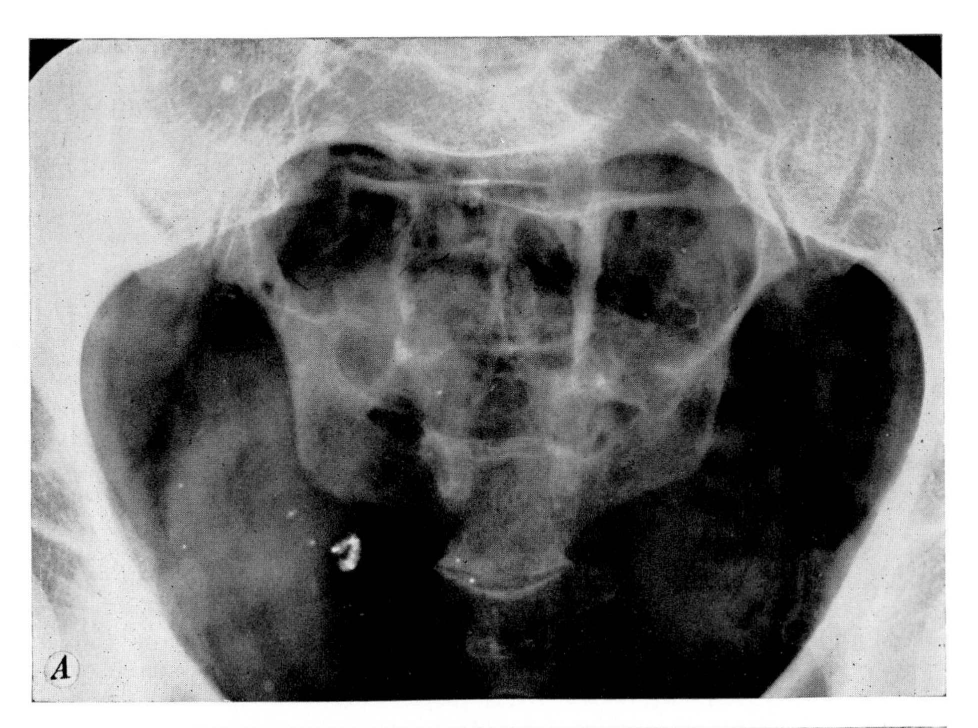


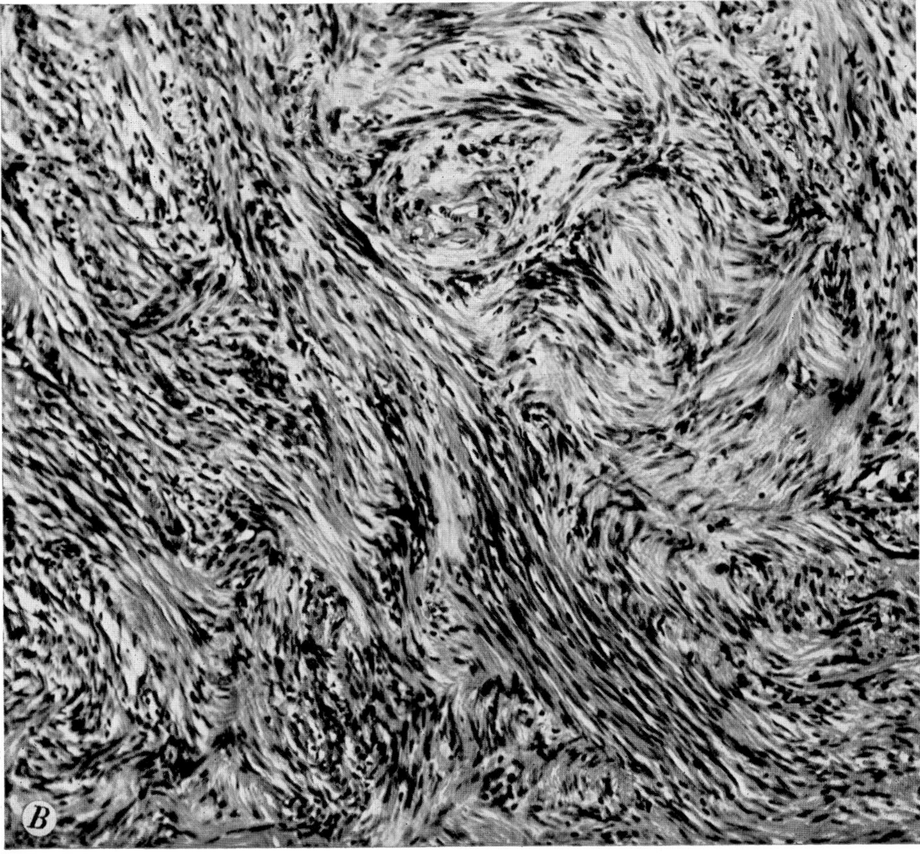


*Figure 73*

and the cutaneous manifestations may be limited to the presence of areas of pigmentation. Both in the cases presenting the typical stigmata and in those showing merely cutaneous pigmentation, various skeletal abnormalities (see below) are often encountered. Indeed, Grenet and associates have even described, as representing an abortive form ("forme fruste") of Recklinghausen's neurofibromatosis, cases in which the manifestations seemed to be limited to cutaneous pigmentation and skeletal involvement, and in which the latter occupied the foreground of the clinical picture. In their opinion, the idea that this cutaneo-osseous syndrome belongs within the category of Recklinghausen's disease is supported by the fact that among the antecedents of these subjects one can usually find complete and typical cases of the disorder.

## SKELETAL ALTERATIONS

As already stated, skeletal aberrations of various kinds are encountered rather frequently in connection with neurofibromatosis. In 1901, Adrian had already devoted considerable attention to them and gave numerous references to the earlier literature. More recently, they have been summarized and discussed by Brooks and Lehman, Friedman, Holt and Wright, McCarroll, and the present writer, among others. It should be borne in mind, however, that the skeleton is not involved in all cases of neurofibromatosis. The actual proportion of cases in which at least some changes in the bones are present is by no means clear, since roentgenographic surveys of the skeleton are not likely to be undertaken in all cases of the disease. In the cases in which bone changes are found, these are by no means uniform, and even in a case in which the skeletal involvement is pronounced, not all the possible abnormalities are likely to be represented.

Some of the skeletal abnormalities observed represent the direct destructive effect of neurofibromatous tissue proliferation acting upon one or another bone part. Others apparently represent aberrations of skeletal development and growth, either localized or systemic, and reflect the fact that neurofibromatosis is a disorder

***Figure 74***

*A*, Roentgenograph showing a long, furrow-like erosive defect in the cortex of a tibia in a case of neurofibromatosis. The patient was a boy 10 years of age who presented numerous patches of *café au lait* skin pigmentation and also numerous neurofibromata palpable in the skin. Furrow-like cortical erosive defects were also observed in various other long bones.

*B*, Roentgenograph showing a deep concavity in the cortex of the upper metaphysis of a tibia in the case of a child 1 year of age affected with neurofibromatosis. The infant presented diffuse soft-tissue hypertrophy of the corresponding foot and lower part of the leg, and several patches of skin pigmentation. The erosion of the cortex of the tibia was discovered in the course of a general skeletal survey.

*C*, Roentgenograph showing the lower end of a femur of a girl 18 years of age who had numerous stigmata of neurofibromatosis. Note the oblique band of relative radiopacity, along each side of which the bone appears relatively radiolucent. The radiolucencies reflect erosion of the bone cortex (see *D*). In this case, many other bones too showed roentgenographic aberrations from the normal.

*D*, Photograph of the sagittally sectioned lower end of the femur and adjacent part of the tibia from the case illustrated in *C*. The lower extremity in question was amputated on account of the development of a sarcoma (malignant schwannoma) in the neurofibromatously altered common peroneal nerve. Note that the thick mass of tissue present posteriorly has eroded so deeply into the local cortex that the latter has been practically destroyed. The lesional tissue producing the defect in the cortex was tough collagenous fibrous tissue in which many nerves showing haphazard schwannian overgrowths were emneshed.

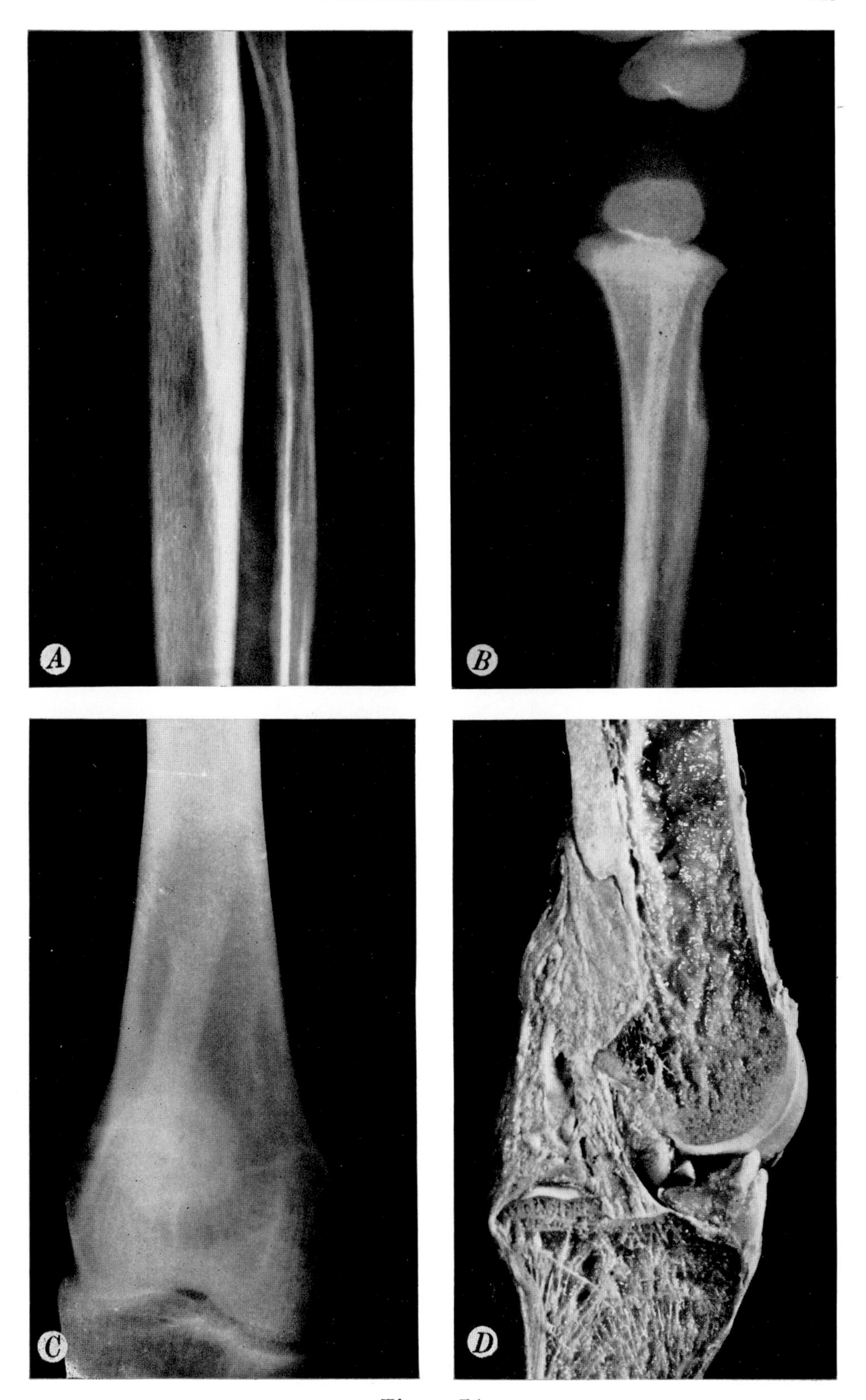


*Figure 74*

deeply rooted in the germ plasm. In respect to still other skeletal abnormalities observed, the relation to the disorder is not understood, and we know only that they are often found together with neurofibromatosis.

At any rate, the skeletal aberrations found in one case or another include: (1) cortical bone defects due to pressure erosion from proliferating neurofibromatous tissue in the periosteum and overlying soft parts; (2) central "cystic" lesions of bone, resulting from expansive growth of neurofibromatous tissue in the medullary cavity of an affected bone part; (3) scoliotic distortions of the thoracic cage; (4) striking bowing deformity (especially of the tibia and/or fibula) associated with pseudarthrosis; (5) abnormal length or abnormal shortness of bones (especially long bones); (6) localized abnormality of the gross internal architecture of a bone or bone part; (7) general gracility of the skeleton or of individual bones; (8) absence (complete or partial) of limb bones; and (9) spina bifida, luxation of the hip, club foot, and other local anomalies.

In *tuberous sclerosis*—a disorder based on the development of numerous sclerotic areas in various parts of the cerebrum—the occasional occurrence of bone lesions has also been noted. Thus Ackermann describes a case in which numerous rather large, multiloculated, cyst-like skeletal lesions were observed roentgenographically, particularly in the innominate bones and the upper ends of the femora. In the 2 cases reported by Hall, the bone lesions seen roentgenographically were less dramatic. Some writers have related the bone lesions of tuberous sclerosis to those of neurofibromatosis. However, so little information is available about the actual pathology of the bone lesions in tuberous sclerosis that a decision about their nature must be held in abeyance.

As to the bone lesions appearing in connection with neurofibromatosis, those which seem to be the most strictly pertinent to the present chapter are the erosive cortical defects and the central "cystic" bone lesions. However, among the almost bewilderingly numerous other associated skeletal abnormalities, scoliotic deformity of the thorax and pseudarthrosis of the tibia and/or fibula are sufficiently common to deserve some consideration also.

**Erosive Lesions of the Cortex.**—Proliferating neurofibromatous tissue in the periosteum and/or adjacent soft tissues not infrequently causes the development of smaller or larger defects in the underlying bone cortex. In any particular case, one or a number of bones may show such defects. Roentgenographically, the defects may appear as small, superficial, pit-like indentations of the cortical surface, as narrow furrow-like excavations, or as deep concavities in the cortex, sometimes even penetrating the latter completely. These pits, furrows, and concavities usually

***Figure 75***

*A*, Photomicrograph (× 65) showing the histologic pattern of tissue removed from an erosive cortical defect in a case of neurofibromatosis. Note the hypertrophied nerve filaments imbedded in a fatty fibrous connective-tissue substratum.

*B*, Roentgenograph showing a sacrum presenting multilocular cyst-like changes in a case of neurofibromatosis. The patient was a boy 9 years of age who showed abnormal skin pigmentation and numerous intracutaneous and subcutaneous neurofibromata proved by biopsy. He had complained of severe sciatic pain, and presented a soft, tender tumor mass, about 7.5 cm. in diameter, over the left sacro-iliac region. This soft-tissue mass extended out of the sacrum. Three years previously, a roentgenograph of that bone had revealed essentially the same loculated appearance as the one illustrated, and tissue removed from the sacral lesion at that time was clearly neurofibromatous. At the time of the current admission, it was thought that the neurofibromatous tissue which had produced the *x*-ray changes shown had undergone sarcomatous transformation. However, since the lesion was not re-biopsied, this point was not established unequivocally.

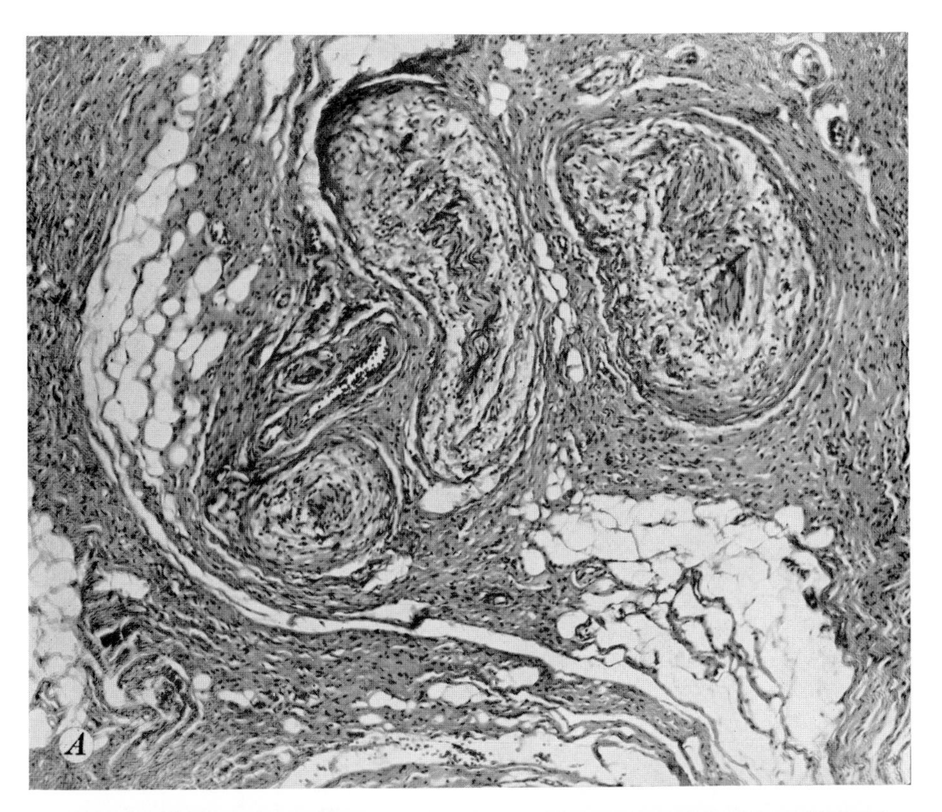


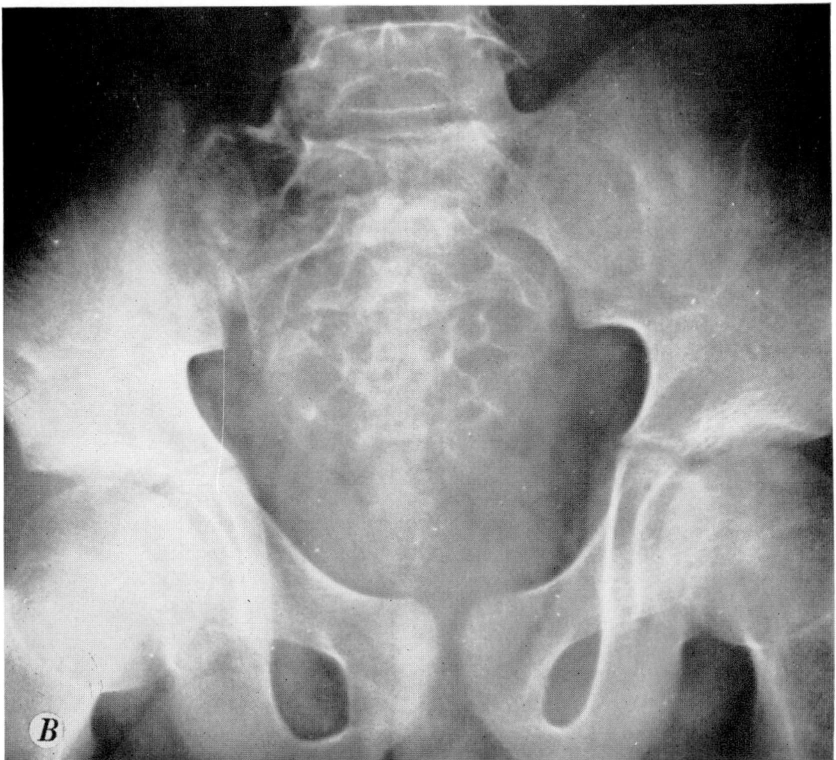


*Figure 75*

show sclerotic borders. Furthermore, if a number of smaller or larger defects are scattered around the circumference of a given cortical area, the affected bone part may even present a multiloculated appearance roentgenographically.

The writer was able to study the anatomic correlates of such roentgenographic cortical changes in the bones of a lower limb amputated because one of the neurofibromatously affected main nerves had become the site of a sarcoma. In this case, the *x*-ray picture of the lower end of the femur presented an oblique band of relative radiopacity, along each side of which the bone appeared relatively radiolucent. Dissection showed that these roentgenographic abnormalities were to be related to a neurofibromatous tumor mass involving the periosteum and also the overlying fatty connective tissue on the posterior surface of the femur. Apparently through pressure erosion, the neurofibromatous tumor mass had gouged out the regional cortex of the femur. The oblique radiopaque ridge represented a strip of cortex which had not yet been eroded. The tissue composing the neurofibromatous tumor mass was of whitish color and tough and firm, and measured 2.5 cm. across at its widest point. Nowhere did it actually penetrate through the cortex into the spongiosa of the femur. (See Fig. 74 and Fig. 75-*A*.)

Toward the upper end of the tibia in this case, the cortex showed a long furrow-like defect roentgenographically. Anatomically, this defect, too, could be correlated with neurofibromatous thickening of the periosteum and neighboring fat along an area which, in the region of the furrow, was about 0.5 cm. in thickness. In many places, the fibula, also, was surrounded by thickened tissue representing neurofibromatously altered periosteum and surrounding fat. The surface of the fibula, too, appeared pitted and ridged in some places, and again it was clear that the irregularity of its surface was the result of pressure erosion from the outside. Like the femur, both the tibia and the fibula were sectioned longitudinally, and they, too, failed to reveal any neurofibromatous tissue in their medullary cavities.

As to *differential diagnosis*, it is clear that in the presence of various stigmata of neurofibromatosis (areas of skin pigmentation, nodules in the skin and along the peripheral nerves, etc.) the presence of cortical erosions is to be related to that disorder. However, cortical erosions sometimes resembling roentgenographically those seen with neurofibromatosis are seen much more often in other connections.

The most common form in which they are encountered is that which has been discussed in the chapter dealing with the so-called *fibrous cortical defect* and the *non-ossifying fibroma* (p. 76). These erosive cortical lesions are often completely asymptomatic and are encountered mainly in children. The subjects are usually otherwise well, and the cortical erosions often disappear spontaneously in the course of a few years. The tissue whose proliferation produces the cortical defects and erosions in these cases is basically connective tissue which has invaded the bone from the periosteum. It often presents a sprinkling of multinuclear giant cells among the spindle connective-tissue cells, sometimes along with cholesterol-bearing foam cells and/or cells containing hemosiderin pigment. Thus the lesional tissue of the fibrous cortical defect or the non-ossifying fibroma bears no histologic resemblance to the tissue producing the cortical erosions in cases of neurofibromatosis.

Once in a while, too, a *juxtacortical chondroma*, particularly if the lesional cartilage is not calcified, produces an *x*-ray picture (see Fig. 60) which might suggest a cortical erosion appearing in connection with neurofibromatosis. The lesional tissue is, of course, cartilage, and in these cases, too, the patients are without any cutaneous and neural stigmata of neurofibromatosis.

**Intramedullary Lesions.**—Central or intramedullary cyst-like rarefactions of bone are also occasionally observed roentgenographically in connection with neurofibromatosis. The principal question raised by these *x*-ray findings centers around the problem of whether they necessarily represent local lytic destruction of osseous tissue by neurofibromatous tissue proliferation within the marrow cavity of the affected bone part. In the cases reported by Friedman and by Uhlmann and Grossman, the abnormal *x*-ray shadow was related, on the basis of tissue examination, to the presence of proliferating neurofibromatous tissue at the affected bone site. In any event, it is clear that central bone lesions produced by the growth of neurofibromatous tissue in the marrow cavity of an affected bone part are rare. (See Fig. 75-*B*.)

Finally, a few cases interpreted as representing neurofibromatosis have been reported in which many bones presented large multiloculated rarefaction shadows roentgenographically. Actually, it has not been established histologically that the bone lesions in these cases were the result of local overgrowth of neurofibromatous tissue at the site of the bone rarefactions. Two cases described by Holt and Wright are of great interest in this connection. In one case, the patient was an infant 4 months of age who, already at that time, was held to be affected with neurofibromatosis. A skeletal survey showed numerous cystic lesions in the metaphyses of many of the long bones. About a year later, another roentgenographic survey revealed that the skeletal abnormalities previously observed had apparently undergone spontaneous regression. In the other case, the patient, again an infant, was stated to have shown stigmata of neurofibromatosis from birth. A skeletal survey made when the infant was 6 weeks of age revealed radiolucent lesions widely distributed over the bones. Three of the bone lesions were subjected to biopsy, but none of the tissue removed showed evidence of neurofibromatosis. When the infant was 8 months of age, a new skeletal survey revealed that in this case, too, the osseous defects had already undergone remarkable spontaneous regression. Certainly the spontaneously disappearing multilocular cyst-like lesions in these infants did not have their basis in the proliferation of actual neurofibromatous tissue within the affected bones.

The writer has had the opportunity of studying 3 pertinent cases in which similar multiloculated rarefactions were observed in the skeletons of infants not affected with neurofibromatosis and in which, again, these lesions either disappeared spontaneously or substantially regressed in the course of a year or so. In all 3 cases, the writer studied biopsy material removed from one or more bone lesions. In all instances, the lesional tissue was spindle cell connective tissue which failed to present the histologic pattern characteristic of proliferating neurofibromatous tissue. The basic nature of the condition in these cases is still unknown. Details concerning 1 of these 3 cases are given in the article by Zeisel and Helbig.

In older children, too, one occasionally encounters a case in which many bones, especially long bones, show multiloculated rarefaction shadows roentgenographically in their metaphysial regions. When such lesions are biopsied, they present the histologic pattern of whorled bundles of spindle-shaped cells interspersed with some small multinuclear giant cells, and some of the tissue areas may also contain foam cells. Such cases (see Figs. 22-*C* and *D*) apparently represent instances of disseminated non-ossifying fibroma—a condition which likewise still requires a good deal of clarification. The bone lesions in these cases, too, may undergo spontaneous resolution.

Should a patient presenting disseminated non-ossifying fibroma lesions show, in addition, patches of brownish skin pigmentation but no neurofibromata, it is possible that the case in question might nevertheless be interpreted clinically as an instance of neurofibromatosis dominated by bone lesions—that is, as an abortive form ("forme fruste") of neurofibromatosis. Furthermore, such a case may even be misinterpreted as an instance of fibrous dysplasia of bone. The histologic tissue pattern is, of course, inconsistent with that diagnosis, too. Actually, much of the confusion that exists in the literature about the possible interrelation between neurofibromatosis and fibrous dysplasia stems from the erroneous interpretation of cases of disseminated non-ossifying fibroma as instances of either neurofibromatosis or fibrous dysplasia. (See articles by Thannhauser, Jaffe, and Albright.)

**Scoliosis.**—Discrepancy in the length of the lower limbs in a case of neurofibromatosis may in itself be the cause of scoliosis. However, even without this agency, severe distortion of the thoracic cage, centering principally around curvature of the column, is not infrequently seen in this disorder. This curvature usually involves rotational torsion of part of the column (most often the thoracic part) and is associated with sharp angulation. The *x*-ray picture in such cases of pronounced kyphoscoliosis usually reveals wedging of several adjacent vertebral bodies in the angulated area. However, on account of the distortion and the resultant overlapping of shadows, it is likely to be difficult to obtain a clear, detailed picture of the osseous alterations.

Gould ascribed the kyphoscoliotic deformity to osteomalacic softening, and the conclusions which he drew from his case were often invoked to explain the deformity of the column. However, this is certainly not an acceptable explanation. A deformed column examined anatomically by Inglis showed striking compression of the anterior portions of the 10th and 11th thoracic vertebræ, and fusion of these vertebræ. There was also considerable degeneration of the intervertebral disks between the 10th and 11th and the 11th and 12th bodies. Histologically, he found no evidence of osteomalacia and no recognizable neurofibromatous tissue within the altered vertebral bodies. The writer, too, has dissected a severely deformed vertebral column which he removed at autopsy in a case of neurofibromatosis and likewise failed to find any tangible explanation for the deformity.

Kessel, however, points out that in most of the reported instances of deformity of the vertebral column appearing in association with intrathoracic meningocele, the patients were also affected with neurofibromatosis. In such cases, the distended sacculated dura tends to bulge through the large intervertebral foramina and to deform and hollow out the regional vertebral bodies. However, the aneurysmal action of an undisclosed meningocele is probably only an occasional cause of the deformity of the column in cases of neurofibromatosis. Altogether, it is clear that there is need for further study directed toward finding the basis for the deformation of the vertebral column that one encounters so often in cases of neurofibromatosis.

**Pseudarthrosis.**—Not infrequently a child is born with a bowing deformity of the lower part of the leg, due to curvature of the tibia and often also of the fibula. The affected infant may also show large patches of brown pigmentation of the skin,

***Figure 76***

*A*, Roentgenograph showing bowing of the tibia and fibula and cystlike rarefactions in the shaft of the tibia in a child who subsequently developed a fracture and pseudarthrosis (see *B*). At the time when this picture was taken, the boy was 8 months of age. A bowing deformity of the leg had already been noticed when he was 1 month old. The skin showed several areas of *café au lait* pigmentation over the right side of the chest posteriorly and over the left buttock. There were no palpable nodules in the skin or along the course of the nerves. Also, the parents showed no stigmata of neurofibromatosis.

*B*, Roentgenograph showing a fracture of the tibia and fibula which developed one and a half years after the picture shown in *A* was taken. The fractured limb was immobilized, but the fracture ends did not unite. An open reduction was then carried out and a bone graft was inserted, but nonunion persisted. Tissue removed at that intervention was examined histologically (see *C*).

*C*, Photomicrograph (× 125) showing neurofibromatous tissue removed from the interior of the cystically rarefied and pseudarthrotic tibia illustrated in *B*. Note the irregular bundles of spindle cells representing proliferating schwannian cells.

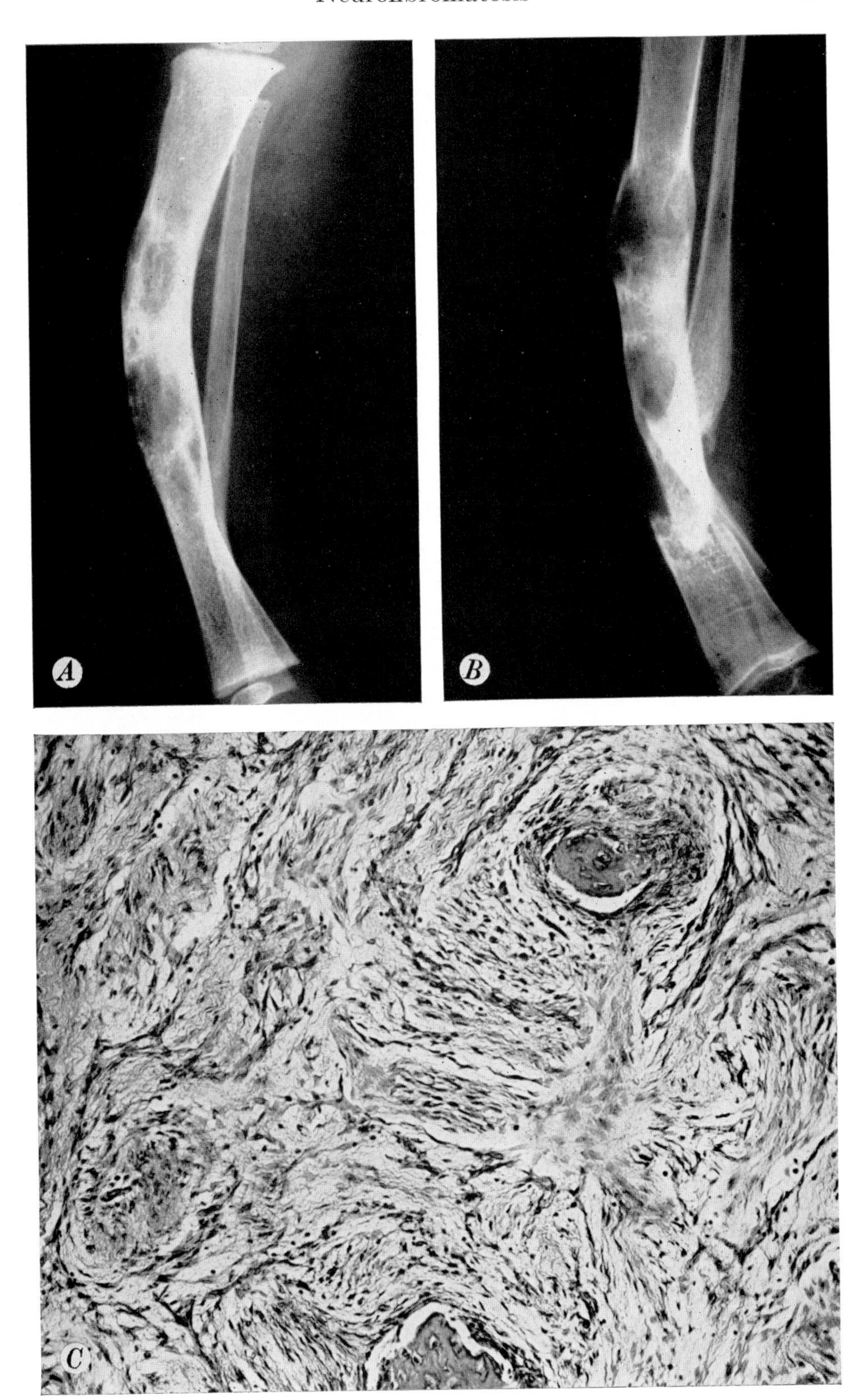


*Figure 76*

and this pigmentation may be the only stigma of neurofibromatosis present as yet. The congenitally bowed tibia may show one or more radiolucent shadows in the shaft, particularly in the convexity of the curvature. A fracture may develop somewhere in the region of the curvature of the tibia and/or fibula, but healing is unlikely to take place and a pseudarthrosis ensues. If, in such a case, a surgical intervention is undertaken to correct the deformation of the leg bones before a fracture has occurred, a pseudarthrosis also usually ensues. Furthermore, in these cases it is almost impossible to abolish the pseudarthrosis once it has developed. Indeed, repeated operative intervention using bone grafts for this purpose is nearly always followed by their resorption, and the gap between the bone ends seems even to enlarge. Occasionally the shortened affected limb comes to be such an impediment that amputation becomes advisable. On the other hand, if the patient can be tided over childhood, the chances of bridging the pseudarthrotic gap or gaps with bone grafts seem to improve. (See Fig. 76.)

The pathogenetic mechanism underlying the bowing and pseudarthrosis is by no means established. In an occasional case (see Green and Rudo), intra-osseous neurofibromatous tissue was reported as being present at the site of the bone deformity, and its proliferative growth has been held responsible for the nonunion and pseudarthrosis following upon fracture. In the case reported by Jacobs, Kimmelstiel, and Thompson, the tissue removed from between the fracture ends was likewise interpreted histologically as being of neurofibromatous nature. Still, it is often difficult to be certain that the tissue removed from the site of the pseudoarthrosis actually is neurofibromatous. In fact, much more often than not, the writer has been unable to identify the tissue removed from the site of a pseudarthrosis in any more specific way than as connective tissue. Furthermore, like Holt and Wright, the writer also studied an amputation specimen from a severely deformed pseudarthrotic leg in a case of neurofibromatosis and, like them, he was unable to identify neurofibromatous tissue in or near the site of the pseudarthrosis. Thus, while neurofibromatous tissue can be identified in the deformed bone or in the vicinity of the pseudarthrosis in some cases, it is not clearly established that its presence is directly responsible for the bone deformity, fracture, and nonunion. It is much more likely that this skeletal complex represents one expression of the mesodermal defect associated with the deep-rooted neuro-ectodermal defect underlying the disorder of neurofibromatosis as a whole.

***Figure 77***

*A*, Roentgenograph showing a multiloculated appearance of the distal half of the terminal phalanx of a finger, produced by a glomus tumor which developed in the interior of the affected bone. The patient was a woman 28 years of age who had been suffering for 4 years from attacks of sharp, stabbing pain in that finger, associated with vesiculation of the local skin. (Reproduced from the article by Lattes and Bull.)

*B*, Roentgenograph showing a small, roundish area of radiolucency in the terminal phalanx of a finger, produced by a subungual glomus tumor which had hollowed out the bone area in question. The patient was a woman 36 years of age who suffered from stabbing pain in the finger, initiated by changes in weather, temperature, or local pressure. (Reproduced from the article by Lehman and Kraissl.)

*C*, Photomicrograph (× 65) showing the histologic tissue pattern of the glomus tumor abutting upon attenuated cortical bone in the case illustrated in *A*.

*D*, Photomicrograph (× 125) showing in greater detail the histologic pattern of the glomus tumor which had eroded into the terminal phalanx of a thumb in the case observed by the writer. The lesional tissue in this case showed mainly overgrowth of the polyhedral pericyte-like muscle cells.

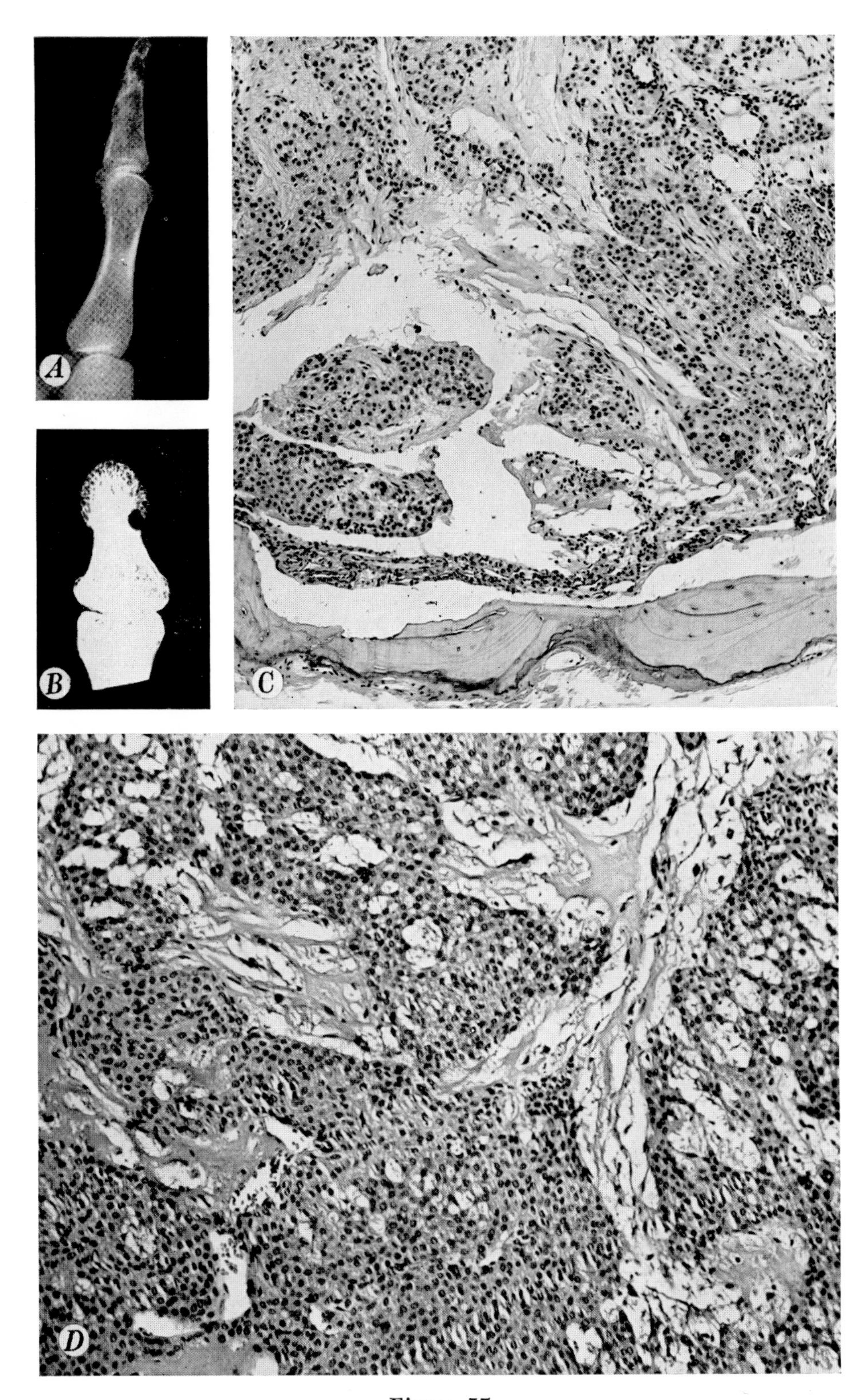


*Figure 77*

## GLOMUS TUMOR OF BONE

A normal glomus is a minute globoid organelle representing an arteriovenous anastomotic complex wrapped in unmyelinated neural filaments. The walls of the arterioles in the glomus contain variable numbers of polyhedral (epithelioid) cells which have been interpreted as being modified smooth-muscle cells and akin to the so-called "pericytes" of Zimmermann. Hence the name "neuromyo-arterial glomus" for these ball-shaped organoid structures, whose function seems to be related to the local control of blood flow.

The tumors which apparently occasionally develop out of the normal glomus bodies present the constituent elements of the normal glomus in varying amounts and arrangements. Some may have a preponderance of vessels, many quite thick-walled, and show a minimum of the polyhedral epithelioid cells and hence are sometimes referred to as glomangiomas. Others show mainly overgrowth of the polyhedral pericyte-like muscle cells about the vessels, many of which may be thin-walled, and the lesion may then come to resemble cytologically the so-called hemangiopericytoma. Between these two extremes there are glomus tumors presenting the more conventional pattern.

The appearance of *osseous lesions* in connection with glomus tumor is rare. Nevertheless, several instances of intra-osseous glomus tumor have been reported. In these cases, the tumor was situated in the terminal phalanx of a finger, and more particularly in the terminal half of the phalanx. Roentgenographically, the affected bone area showed a rarefaction shadow which (if considered independently of the clinical findings) could have suggested an enchondroma or possibly an epithelial inclusion cyst in the phalanx. Clinically, in these cases, the affected finger had been painful for several years. In the case described by Iglesias de la Torre and associates, the affected index finger did not show anything remarkable on inspection. In the case described by Lattes and Bull, the end of the affected thumb was slightly enlarged, the skin was thickened and discolored, and the nail was also enlarged. (See Fig. 77.)

In the cases in question, the glomus tumor probably arose out of an originally normal glomus organelle in the interior of the affected bone. That glomera are normally present in large numbers on the ventral surfaces of the hands and feet and particularly in the nail bed is well known. However, if one studies histologically the terminal ends of fingers or toes, one occasionally also finds normal glomera in the medullary cavity of the terminal phalanx. This fact lends support to the idea that the glomus tumor present in the terminal phalanx in the cases cited developed out of an intramedullary glomus organelle.

Occasionally, also, a subungual glomus tumor can come to hollow out a terminal phalanx by pressure erosion. Lehman and Kraissl have reported 2 cases in point. In a case studied by the writer, the distal phalanx of a thumb showed roentgenographically, near its tip, a defect about 0.5 cm. in diameter. This hollow formed the bed of a glomus tumor which, developing under the nail, had caused pressure erosion of the underlying bone and given rise to the pain complex characteristic of the glomus tumor in almost any site.

Glomus tumors developing in relation to bones, like glomus tumors elsewhere, are benign lesions, and no recurrence is to be expected if the lesional area is resected or thoroughly curetted.

### REFERENCES

Ackermann, A. J.: Pulmonary and Osseous Manifestations of Tuberous Sclerosis, with some Remarks on their Pathogenesis, Am. J. Roentgenol., *51*, 315, 1944.

Adrian, C.: Ueber Neurofibromatose und ihre Komplikationen, Beitr. z. klin. Chir., *31*, 1, 1901.

ALBRIGHT, F.: Polyostotic Fibrous Dysplasia: A Defense of the Entity, J. Clin. Endocrinol., *7*, 307, 1947.
BROOKS, B., and LEHMAN, E. P.: The Bone Changes in Recklinghausen's Neurofibromatosis, Surg., Gynec. & Obst., *38*, 587, 1924.
DESANTO, D. A., and BURGESS, E.: Primary and Secondary Neurilemmoma of Bone, Surg., Gynec. & Obst., *71*, 454, 1940.
FRIEDMAN, M. M.: Neurofibromatosis of Bone, Am. J. Roentgenol., *51*, 623, 1944.
GOULD, E. P.: The Bone Changes Occurring in von Recklinghausen's Disease, Quart. J. Med., *11*, 221, 1918.
GREEN, W. T., and RUDO, N.: Pseudarthrosis and Neurofibromatosis, Arch. Surg., *46*, 639, 1943.
GRENET, H., DUCROQUET, R., ISAAC-GEORGES, P., and MACÉ, M.: Forme fruste pigmentaire et osseuse de la neurofibromatose, Presse méd., *42*, 2060, 1934.
GROSS, P., BAILEY, F. R., and JACOX, H. W.: Primary Intramedullary Neurofibroma of the Humerus, Arch. Path., *28*, 716, 1939.
HALL, G. S.: Tuberose Sclerosis, Rheostosis, and Neurofibromatosis, Quart. J. Med., *9*, 1, 1940.
HOLT, J. F., and WRIGHT, E. M.: The Radiologic Features of Neurofibromatosis, Radiology, *51*, 647, 1948.
IGLESIAS DE LA TORRE, L., GOMEZ CAMAJO, M., and PALACIOS, G.: Consideraciones clínicas, anatómicas, radiológicas y quirúrgicas del Glomus Tumoral de Masson, Cir. ortop. y traumatol., Habana, *7*, 11, 1939.
INGLIS, K.: The Nature of Neurofibromatosis and Related Lesions, with Special Reference to Certain Lesions of Bones, J. Path. & Bact., *62*, 519, 1950.
JACOBS, J. E., KIMMELSTIEL, P., and THOMPSON, K. R., JR.: Neurofibromatosis and Pseudarthrosis, Arch. Surg., *59*, 232, 1949.
JAFFE, H. L.: Fibrous Dysplasia of Bone: A Disease Entity and Specifically not an Expression of Neurofibromatosis, J. Mt. Sinai Hosp., *12*, 364, 1945.
KESSEL, A. W. L.: Intrathoracic Meningocele, Spinal Deformity, and Multiple Neurofibromatosis, J. Bone & Joint Surg., *33-B*, 87, 1951.
LATTES, R., and BULL, D. C.: A Case of Glomus Tumor with Primary Involvement of Bone, Ann. Surg., *127*, 187, 1948.
LEHMAN, W., and KRAISSL, C.: Glomus Tumor within Bone, Surgery, *25*, 118, 1949.
MCCARROLL, H. R.: Clinical Manifestations of Congenital Neurofibromatosis, J. Bone & Joint, Surg., *32-A*, 601, 1950.
MURRAY, M. R., and STOUT, A. P.: Schwann Cell versus Fibroblast as the Origin of the Specific Nerve Sheath Tumor, Am. J. Path., *16*, 41, 1940.
PEERS, J. H.: Primary Intramedullary Neurogenic Sarcoma of the Ulna, Am. J. Path., *10*, 811, 1934.
SCHROFF, J.: Solitary Neurofibroma of the Oral Cavity (Neurilemmoma; Neurinoma), J. Am. Dent. A., *32*, 199, 1945.
STALMANN, A.: Nerven-, Haut- und Knochenveränderungen bei der Neurofibromatosis Recklinghausen und ihre entstehungsgeschichtlichen Zusammenhänge, Virchows Arch. f. path. Anat., *289*, 96, 1933.
THANNHAUSER, S. J.: Neurofibromatosis (von Recklinghausen) and Osteitis Fibrosa Cystica Localisata et Disseminata (von Recklinghausen): A Study of a Common Pathogenesis of Both Diseases, Medicine, *23*, 105, 1944.
UHLMANN, E., and GROSSMAN, A.: Von Recklinghausen's Neurofibromatosis with Bone Manifestations, Ann. Int. Med., *14*, 225, 1940.
WEBER, F. P.: Cutaneous Pigmentation as an Incomplete Form of Recklinghausen's Disease, with Remarks on the Classification of Incomplete and Anomalous Forms of Recklinghausen's Disease, Brit. J. Dermat., *21*, 49, 1909.
WILBER, M. C., and WOODCOCK, J. A.: Ganglioneuromata in Bone, J. Bone & Joint Surg., *39-A*, 1385, 1957.
ZEISEL, H., and HELBIG, G.: Polyostische, polytope, fast systematisierte Skeletaffektion mit parossalen Herden beim Säugling, Ztschr. f. Kinderh., *76*, 379, 1955.

Chapter

# 17

# Osteogenic Sarcoma

In general, an *osteogenic sarcoma* may be defined as a specialized connective-tissue sarcoma which forms neoplastic osteoid and osseous tissue in the course of its evolution. In the main, the osteoid and osseous tissue arises from the sarcomatous connective tissue directly, but in rapidly growing tumor areas it may also be formed by way of a chondroid or cartilaginous intermediary stage. There is considerable variation among the osteogenic sarcomas in respect to ossification, some of them showing relatively little osteogenesis and others a good deal of it.

An osteogenic sarcoma of bone may start its development: (1) in the interior of the affected bone or (2) on the bone surface in relation to the periosteum and/or immediate parosteal connective tissue. However, when one speaks of osteogenic sarcoma of bone, it is usually the central lesion that one has in mind, and it is this *common* form of osteogenic sarcoma (also denoted as "osteosarcoma") that constitutes the subject of the present chapter. The osteogenic sarcoma which starts its development in relation to the surface of the bone is designated by the writer as the *juxtacortical osteogenic sarcoma* (p. 279). This form of osteogenic sarcoma is relatively uncommon, has a much better prognosis than the central osteogenic sarcoma, and is sufficiently distinctive in other ways also to warrant discussion as a separate clinicopathologic entity.

Furthermore, in the delimitation of osteogenic sarcoma of bone, it should be noted that a malignant connective-tissue sarcoma occurring in a bone and not giving evidence of osteogenesis (either at its original site or in any metastases) is to be interpreted as a *fibrosarcoma of bone* (p. 304) rather than as an osteogenic sarcoma. Osteogenic sarcoma of bone is also to be distinguished from *chondrosarcoma of bone* (p. 314), since a chondrosarcoma develops out of cartilage directly and remains essentially a malignant tumor of cartilage. That is, no matter how much cartilage a given sarcoma may show, if the cartilage is being formed by way of sarcomatous connective tissue, the lesion represents an osteogenic sarcoma and not a chondrosarcoma. Indeed, even if it has considerable cartilage, such a lesion will also show, in various areas, neoplastic osteoid and osseous tissue being formed out of the sarcomatous stroma.

From the historical point of view, it is of interest that the Registry of Bone Sarcoma defined osteogenic sarcoma as a sarcoma derived from tissue presumably intended to form bone, irrespective of whether it eventually does so. (See Codman and also Ewing.) On the basis of this definition, one can understand why, in its original classification of the bone sarcomas, the Registry gave no special recognition to chondrosarcoma and fibrosarcoma of bone. However, while retaining its original definition of osteogenic sarcoma, the Registry, in its revised (1939) classification, did give recognition to chondrosarcoma as a tumor entity distinct from osteogenic sarcoma. Nevertheless, it still included under osteogenic sarcoma the lesion which the writer and others prefer to call fibrosarcoma of bone—a connective-tissue sarcoma which, as noted, fails to express any bone-forming capacity. However, if such a sarcoma does not form bone at any time in the course of its evolution, what evidence is there that it has arisen from "osteogenic" and not from neutral or supporting connective tissue?

## CLINICAL CONSIDERATIONS

**Incidence.**—Osteogenic sarcoma is the most common of the primary malignant tumors of bone. As to sex of the patients, males seem to be predilected over females, approximately in the proportion of 2 to 1. As to age distribution of the cases, about three-fourths of the patients in any representative series are between 10 and 25 years, some below 10 though few below 5, and most of the rest between 26 and 40 years of age. Occasionally, a patient with an osteogenic sarcoma is in his fifties. However, before an osteogenic sarcoma in a person who is no longer young is accepted as having developed *de novo*, one should carefully exclude the possibilities of its having evolved at a site of pre-existing bone disease (Paget's disease in particular) or at a site of bone damage from a noxious agent (for instance, a radioactive substance ingested years before). A very rare finding of some clinical interest is the occurrence of osteogenic sarcoma in 2 or more offspring of the same parents.

**Localization.**—It is the long bones of the limbs that are the most common sites of osteogenic sarcoma, the lesion being in a femur in more than half of all cases, and in a tibia or a humerus in many of the others. All other localizations taken together account for only a small minority of the cases in any large series. In a long bone, the tumor is usually found to involve one end of the shaft and often at least part of the adjacent epiphysial area in addition. When a femur is involved, the lesion is more likely to be in the lower part of the bone, and, when a tibia or a humerus is involved, in the upper part of the bone. On the other hand, an osteogenic sarcoma of a long bone is occasionally situated well along toward the middle of the shaft.

**Clinical Complaints and Findings.**—The cardinal, and nearly always the initial, complaint in cases of osteogenic sarcoma is local pain. When the tumor is in a long bone of a limb, the patient generally reports that the relevant pain was at first slight and intermittent, though aggravated by use of the part. Within a matter of weeks, the pain definitely becomes more severe and persistent, and is usually already associated with the presence of a local swelling. If the tumor has extended to the articular capsule, it is likely that there will be some limitation of motion of the joint, and some accumulation of fluid in it. In the cases in which the tumor is in a bone of a lower limb, there is also often a complaint of lameness. Aside from the pain and local swelling, tumors in other locations than long bones give rise to complaints referable to their special sites—sciatic pain, for instance, if the tumor involves an ilium.

In the cases admitted to our hospital, these various complaints were usually of only a few months' standing. Occasionally, however, they had been present for as little as 1 month or as long as 8 months or so. The local visible and palpable tumor mass, in the usual case as seen now, is not very large. Its firmness varies in accordance with the intensity of ossification of the lesion. In any case, the tumorous area is found rather sensitive to pressure. The overlying skin sometimes feels abnormally warm, especially when the local tumor mass is rather large and relatively soft. Occasionally, also, in these cases the superficial veins of the area are found prominent. Not often has a patient with an osteogenic sarcoma already shown a pathologic fracture at the time of admission to our hospital. When such a fracture does occur, it is usually in the case of a rapidly growing tumor showing relatively little ossification.

The general health of the patient is usually still good at the time of admission for treatment. Occasionally, a patient does report a considerable loss of weight at that time, and in such cases pulmonary metastases are sometimes already demonstrable, and the subsequent duration of life is usually only a matter of months.

**Serum Alkaline Phosphatase.**—An increase in the alkaline phosphatase value is the only abnormal blood chemistry finding pertinent to osteogenic sarcoma. Such an increase may or may not be present at the time when the patient is first admitted to the hospital for treatment. Usually, even when increased values are found, they are not strikingly high—ordinarily not more than about twice the normal. Especially in the cases in which the initial serum phosphatase values are significantly high, these drop sharply after amputation, though not always to the level normal for the age of the subject. Radiation therapy against the local lesion, when given in adequate dosage, likewise results in reduction of the phosphatase value. However, as metastases appear, the value tends to rise again, at least to levels above those found on admission. Finally, in the cases in which the phosphatase value is already strikingly high on admission, the clinical course tends to be particularly rapidly fatal. (See the articles by Woodard and Higinbotham, and Jaffe and Bodansky.)

**The Question of Antecedent Trauma.**—There has been much discussion of the possible role of trauma in the instigation of osteogenic sarcoma. In fully 70 per cent of our cases, there was no history of trauma relating to the onset of the local complaints. In the remaining cases, some kind of trauma, supposedly relevant, was mentioned. It was rarely a severe trauma leading to serious bruising of the local soft parts. Usually, the supposedly relevant trauma in these cases was merely deduced from the fact that pain at the site where the tumor developed was felt for the first time during the activity of work or sport. Thus, some patients first noted the pain while lifting a weight, or bumping the part while at work. Others noted it while playing basketball or football, skating, or riding a bicycle, or in the course of a fall connected with such an activity.

However, to prove the relevance of trauma in this minority group of cases, one would have to have a roentgenograph of the affected part showing that no tumor was present in it at the time. In the ordinary course of events, this is an almost impossible requirement to fulfill. Indeed, it is often only weeks or months after the trauma that the painful part is first roentgenographed. In several of our cases, roentgenographs were taken a week or two after the inculpated trauma, and then already showed an unequivocal and well developed tumor. Furthermore, the writer has

***Figure 78***

*A*, Roentgenograph showing a sclerosing osteogenic sarcoma in the upper part of the shaft of a tibia. As anatomic examination also revealed, the tumor is essentially confined to the interior of the bone and, though it is disrupting the cortex on the medial side, it has not extended through the cartilage plate into the epiphysis. The patient was a boy 10 years of age whose complaints consisted of some local pain and a limp, of about 6 weeks' standing.

*B*, Roentgenograph of a sclerosing osteogenic sarcoma involving the lower part of a femur and extending widely beyond the limits of the bone. The sectioned amputation specimen brought out even more clearly that the tumor was also invading the condyles of the bone and had even reached to the articular cartilage in some places (see also Fig. 82-*B*). The patient was a man 21 years of age who had had pain referable to the affected femur for 3 months, and also noted a swelling of the lower part of the thigh.

*C*, Roentgenograph showing a large, bulky, but only moderately ossified osteogenic sarcoma in the lower end of a femur. The sectioned amputation specimen revealed that the tumor tissue in the relatively radiolucent area, in particular, was only meagerly ossified and extensively telangiectatic. The patient was a girl 15 years of age whose difficulties were of only 2 months' standing. Her principal complaint was of sharp and almost constant pain in the knee area, and she had noted a rapidly increasing swelling in the lower end of the thigh.

*D*, Roentgenograph showing an essentially osteolytic osteogenic sarcoma in the upper part of the shaft of a femur. Note the lack of significant radiopacity in the lesional area. The patient was a girl 16 years of age who complained of pain in the hip region of about 1 month's standing.

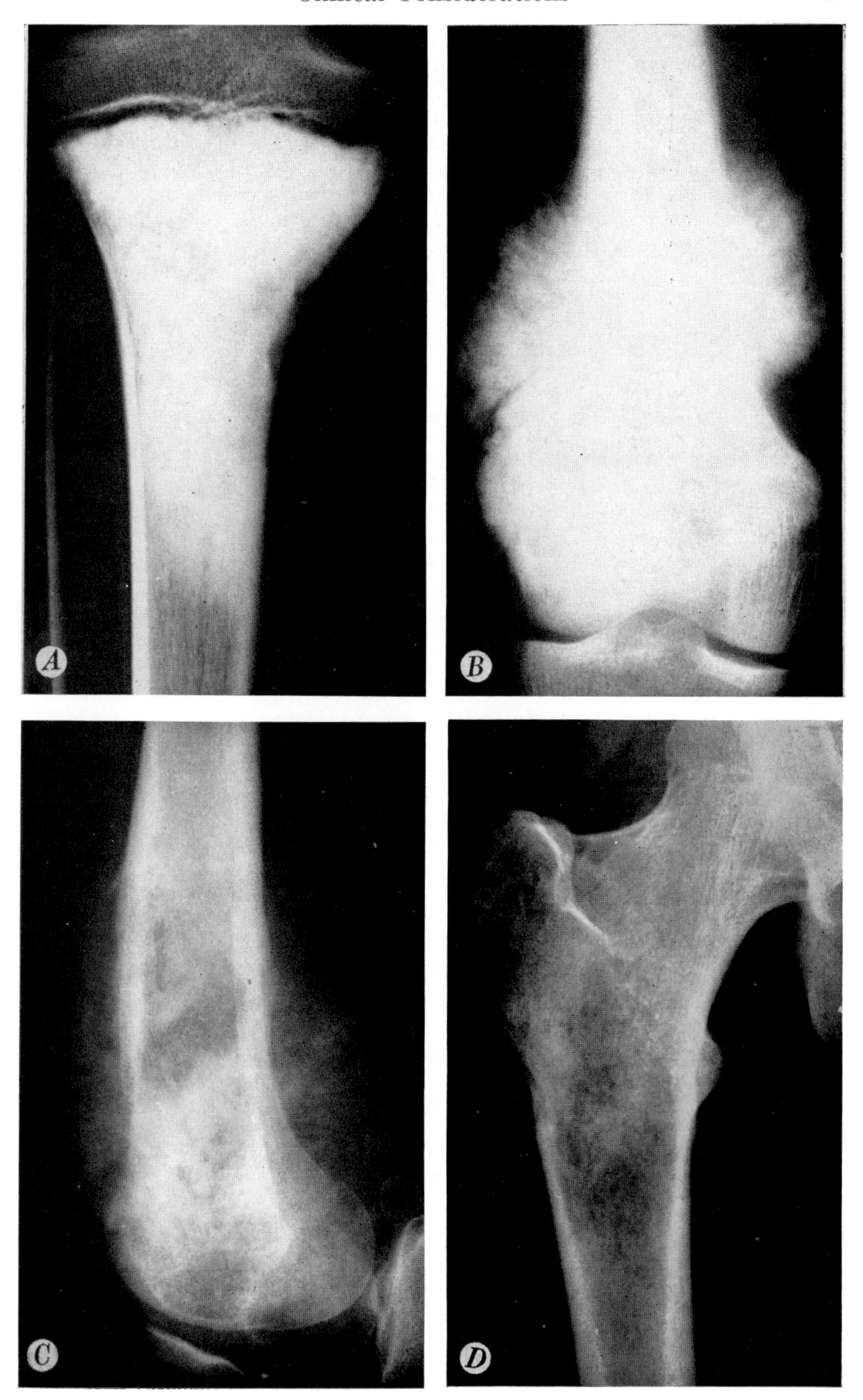


*Figure 78*

seen the case of a young girl who injured a knee area and in whom a roentgenograph taken only a few hours later revealed an osteogenic sarcoma at the lower end of a femur. It is hardly to be doubted that in these latter cases the tumor was already present when the trauma occurred, and that the trauma merely called attention to it. In summary, then, there was not one among our cases of primary osteogenic sarcoma of bone in which a definite causal relation between trauma (without fracture) and the appearance of the sarcoma could actually be established.

Furthermore, it seems obvious that if trauma were an important factor in the causation of osteogenic sarcoma, it ought to be of common occurrence in the wake of fractures. Though there is an occasional report of such an occurrence, these reports do not seem to stand up under critical analysis. The writer himself has never seen an unequivocal case in which an osteogenic sarcoma developed at the site of a fracture in an otherwise normal bone.

## GROSS PATHOLOGY

**Terminology in Relation to General Pathologic Features.**—As already indicated the osteogenic sarcoma lesion discussed in this chapter is the one which starts its development in the interior of the affected bone. However, when first seen, the lesion has usually penetrated the cortex somewhere, to lie beneath the periosteum, or has even perforated the latter in some places and gone on growing beyond it. Furthermore, such an osteogenic sarcoma may show relatively little, moderate, or very considerable ossification. In our series of cases, about one-quarter of the lesions were slightly ossified, about one-quarter were moderately ossified, and about one-half were heavily ossified and often even considerably eburnated. In reference to the intensity of ossification shown by the tumor, certain qualifying terms have come into use. Specifically, the highly ossified ones are commonly described as "sclerosing osteogenic sarcomas." Those showing relatively little ossification are commonly termed "osteolytic osteogenic sarcomas." (See Figs. 78 and 79.)

The degree of ossification seems to have little to do with the size or stage of development of the lesion. That is, a tumor which is still small and mainly confined within the limits of the bone may be slightly or highly ossified, and a tumor which is large and has erupted widely beyond the bone limits may likewise be so. On the whole, the less ossified the tumor, the more likely it is to show necrosis, cystification, and telangiectasis as secondary features of its pathologic anatomy. However, even highly ossified tumors occasionally show considerable telangiectasis, particularly in their more peripheral portions. In the older literature on osteogenic sarcoma, the term "malignant bone aneurysm" is sometimes encountered. This term was usually employed to specify the bulky and extensively hemorrhagic and telangiectatic tumors showing very little ossification. Such bulky, degenerated osteogenic sarcomas are rarely encountered today, since the patient now usually comes under definitive medical care before the lesion reaches such a stage.

***Figure 79***

Photograph of an osteogenic sarcoma in a femur illustrating many characteristic features of the tumor. The patient was a boy 17 years of age who began to complain of pain in the thigh 2 months before the amputation was done. On the left, one can note that the periosteum has been elevated by tumor tissue which, as yet, is relatively uncalcified. To the right, one observes a bulky tumor mass overlying an area in which part of the cortex has been destroyed. Except at the periphery, much of this extra-osseous tumor mass is ossifying and hence appears whitish. The tumor tissue in the interior of the bone is in part (lower half) highly ossified, and in part (upper half) permeated by large vascular channels.

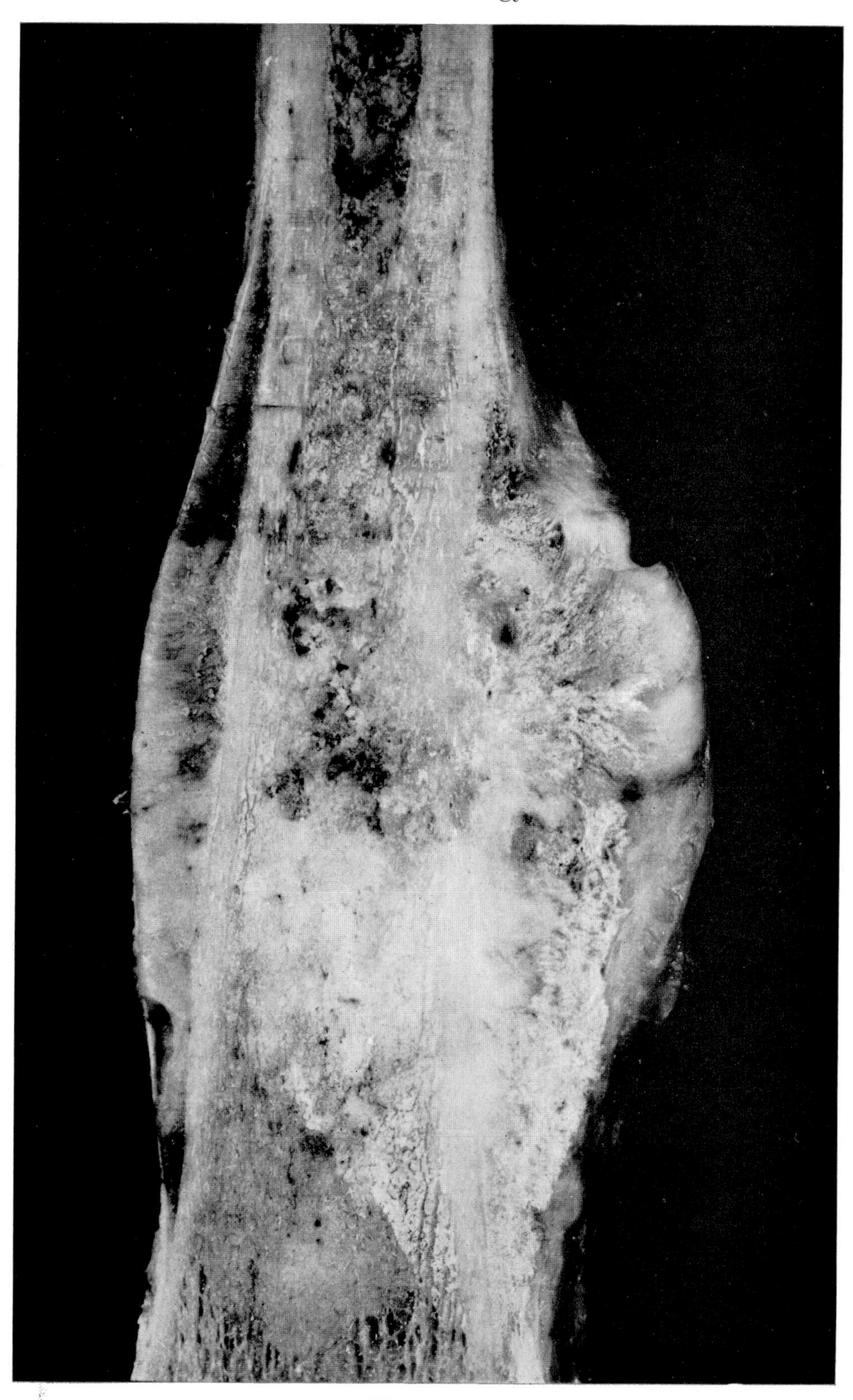

*Figure 79*

Against the background of these general orienting remarks, one can see certain objections to subdividing osteogenic sarcoma (as some still do) into the categories of: (1) medullary and subperiosteal, (2) telangiectatic, (3) sclerosing, and (4) periosteal. In the first place, as noted, those osteogenic sarcomas (relatively few) which originate in the periosteum, or at any rate in the immediate parosteal connective tissue, represent a special kind of osteogenic sarcoma (the *juxtacortical osteogenic sarcoma*, p. 279), and not a mere variant of the conventional, central osteogenic sarcoma. As to a "sclerosing" type, it is true, as also pointed out, that at least half of the osteogenic sarcomas in any large collection will be found heavily ossified. However, ossification is merely a trait of which a given osteogenic sarcoma may show more or less. As likewise indicated, the same statement applies to the so-called "telangiectatic" type of osteogenic sarcoma. Indeed, telangiectasis represents merely a secondary degenerative change which may be observed in both poorly ossified and highly ossified osteogenic sarcomas, and bulky telangiectatic lesions are now rarely seen. As to the "medullary and subperiosteal" type, we have already pointed out that, in our opinion, all osteogenic sarcomas of bone, except the distinctive juxtacortical lesion, start in the medullary cavity, although, when examined anatomically, they have usually already extended at least somewhat beyond the cortex of the affected area.

**Gross Pathologic Findings.**—The gross appearance of a central osteogenic sarcoma is best described as presented in a long bone of a limb. As noted, the tumor usually is found involving one end of the shaft and at least part of the adjacent epiphysial area, though sometimes it is situated well along toward the middle of the shaft. The tumor is likely to measure between 10 and 20 cm. in longitudinal extent. At the end directed toward the middle of the shaft, it generally terminates in a more or less dome-shaped plug in the medullary cavity. This plug ordinarily represents the limit of longitudinal advance of the tumor, both inside and around the bone. At the opposite end—that is, in the direction of the joint—the delimitation of the tumor is far less precise. If, in one longitudinal slice, it is not found extending into the epiphysial area (and through the plate if the latter is still present), a parallel slice through another plane may show it extending into the end of the bone, and in fact somewhere even reaching to the articular cartilage. Furthermore, a tumor extending into the end of the bone may, at one point or another, especially along the line of attachment of the joint capsule, penetrate the latter and invade the synovium or even the articular space to some degree.

***Figure 80***

*A*, Photograph showing a substantially ossified osteogenic sarcoma in the lower part of the shaft of a femur. Note that the tumor has not advanced into the epiphysis, though it extends to the epiphysial cartilage plate. Posteriorly, however, the tumor has penetrated the cortex and bulged the periosteum somewhat. The tumor tissue in the marrow cavity is hard and eburnated and ends proximally in a dome-shaped plug.

*B*, Roentgenograph of a slice of the tumor shown in *A*. Note that, in accordance with its heavy ossification, much of the tumor tissue in the interior of the bone shaft is radiopaque. Note also that the cortex has been penetrated on the right. The area in question corresponds to what is seen on the left in *A*.

*C*, Photograph showing a rather meagerly ossified osteogenic sarcoma in the lower part of a femur. The patient was a boy 16 years of age who had had pain in the knee area for 4 months prior to the amputation. The tumor tissue felt soft and fleshy, but was streaked with white where calcification and ossification had been going on in it.

*D*, Roentgenograph of a slice of the tumor shown in *C*. In accordance with the meagerness of its ossification, much of the tumor tissue in the interior of the bone is not radiopaque.

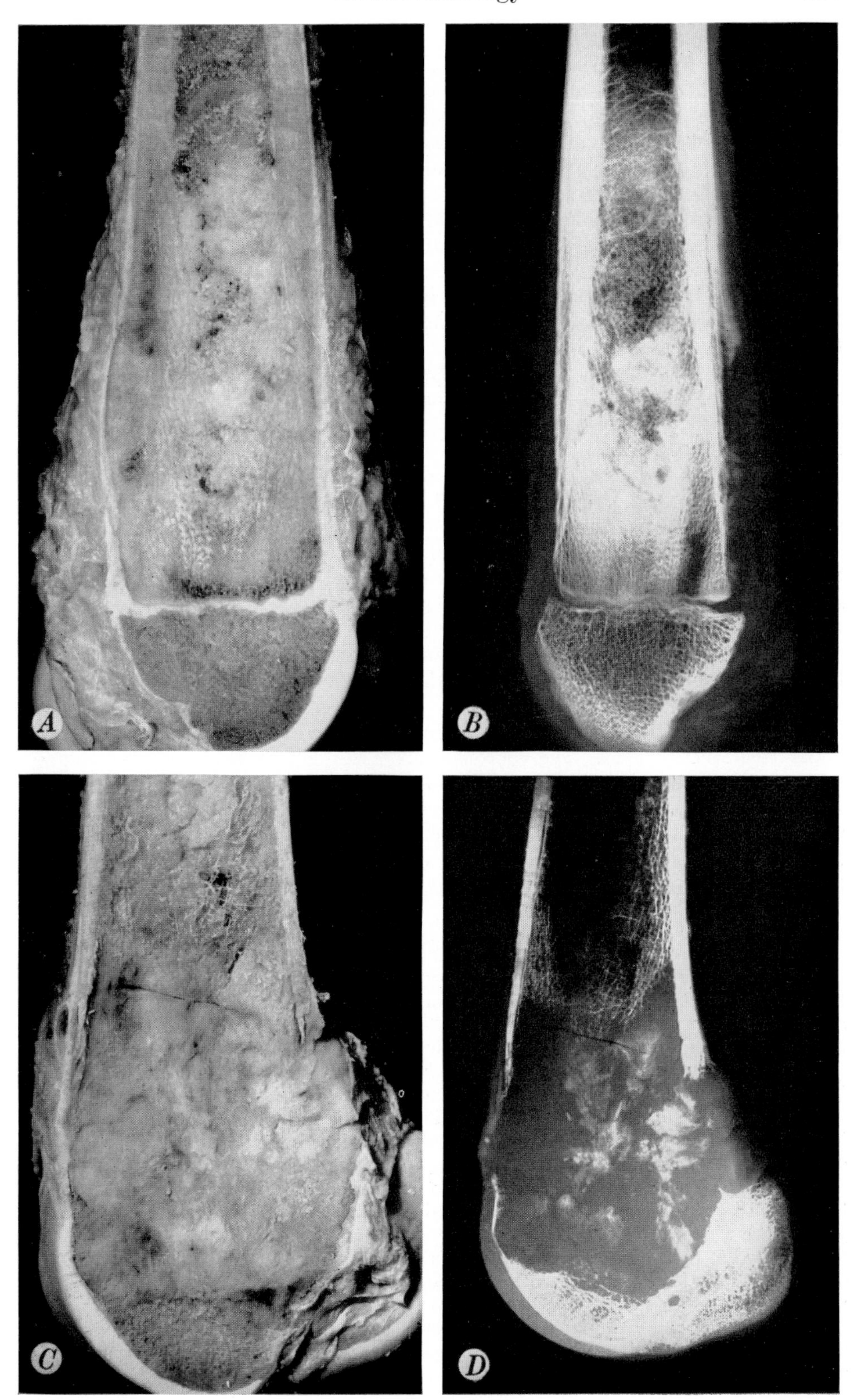


*Figure 80*

If the tumor tissue has penetrated the cortex in only a limited area and is still confined there by the periosteum, the contour of the affected area will, of course, show only slight modification. If there has been extensive penetration of the cortex and also of the periosteum, so that the bone in the affected area is widely encuffed by tumor tissue, aside from containing it, the circumference of the entire affected area is naturally much enlarged, either uniformly or in coarse bulges. However, as already indicated, the extent to which an osteogenic sarcoma, when seen, is confined within the limits of the bone or lies outside of the cortex and periosteum is not related to the degree of ossification shown by the individual tumor.

In an osteogenic sarcoma which is small and still mainly confined within the medullary cavity of the bone, and which shows relatively little ossification, the tumor tissue tends to be rather firm and elastic and whitish on the whole, but also to show gritty yellowish dots and streaks where it is undergoing ossification. On the other hand, in a large, meagerly ossified lesion which has erupted extensively out of the bone, the tumor tissue will probably be found more or less necrotic, cystified, and telangiectatic. Furthermore, one finds that, in these latter lesions, the cortex has undergone extensive destructive resorption and perhaps been so weakened that a pathologic fracture has resulted.

In a small, confined, and highly ossified lesion, the tumor area is dense, compact, and eburnated practically throughout. In a large and highly ossified lesion, on the other hand, the most densely ossified portion of the tumor will be found in the interior of the affected bone area, while the tissue overlying the cortex, though quite sclerotic on the whole, will show at least some parts, especially near the periphery, which, as yet, are ossified only slightly if at all. In such a lesion, the highly ossified areas tend to have a yellow-white color and to be so eburnated as almost to have the hardness of cortical bone; the less ossified areas tend to be less yellow and more white and to have a rather gritty-rubbery consistency; and the least ossified areas tend to be white and of a chondroid or fleshy consistency. As histologic examination makes clear, highly ossified and eburnated areas in the interior of the affected bone part are the result of the superposition of ossified tumor tissue upon pre-existing spongy trabeculæ, with consequent obliteration of the spongy marrow spaces. The presence of densely ossified areas of tumor tissue outside of the cortex can be shown to be due to the intermingling of actively ossifying tumor tissue with reactive nontumorous new bone of periosteal origin.

***Figure 81***

*A*, Photograph showing an osteogenic sarcoma which had started in the upper end of a tibia. After breaking out of the bone, the tumor grew in the interosseous space and also around the upper end of the fibula. The patient was a boy 15 years of age who gave a history of pain and swelling around the knee for a period of about 6 months.

*B*, Roentgenograph of a sagittally cut slice from the specimen shown in *A*. Note that in the epiphysial end of the bone much of the tumor area casts a relatively radiolucent shadow. In this area the tumor tissue was soft and mainly necrotic and telangiectatic. The remaining part of the tumor tissue in the tibia is heavily ossified, as is the tumor tissue in the interosseous space and around the fibula.

*C*, Photograph of an osteogenic sarcoma in the lower end of a femur. Part of the tumor tissue is well ossified and part of it is soft and telangiectatic. The patient was a man 53 years of age whose difficulties relating to the lesion were of 9 months' standing. A skeletal survey failed to reveal the presence of Paget's disease, and the case had to be accepted as one of the unusual instances in which an osteogenic sarcoma starts *de novo* in a person of middle age.

*D*, Roentgenograph of a slice from the tumor shown in *C*. Note that in the upper part of the lesional area the tumor tissue is radiopaque, and that in the telangiectatic area it is relatively radiolucent.

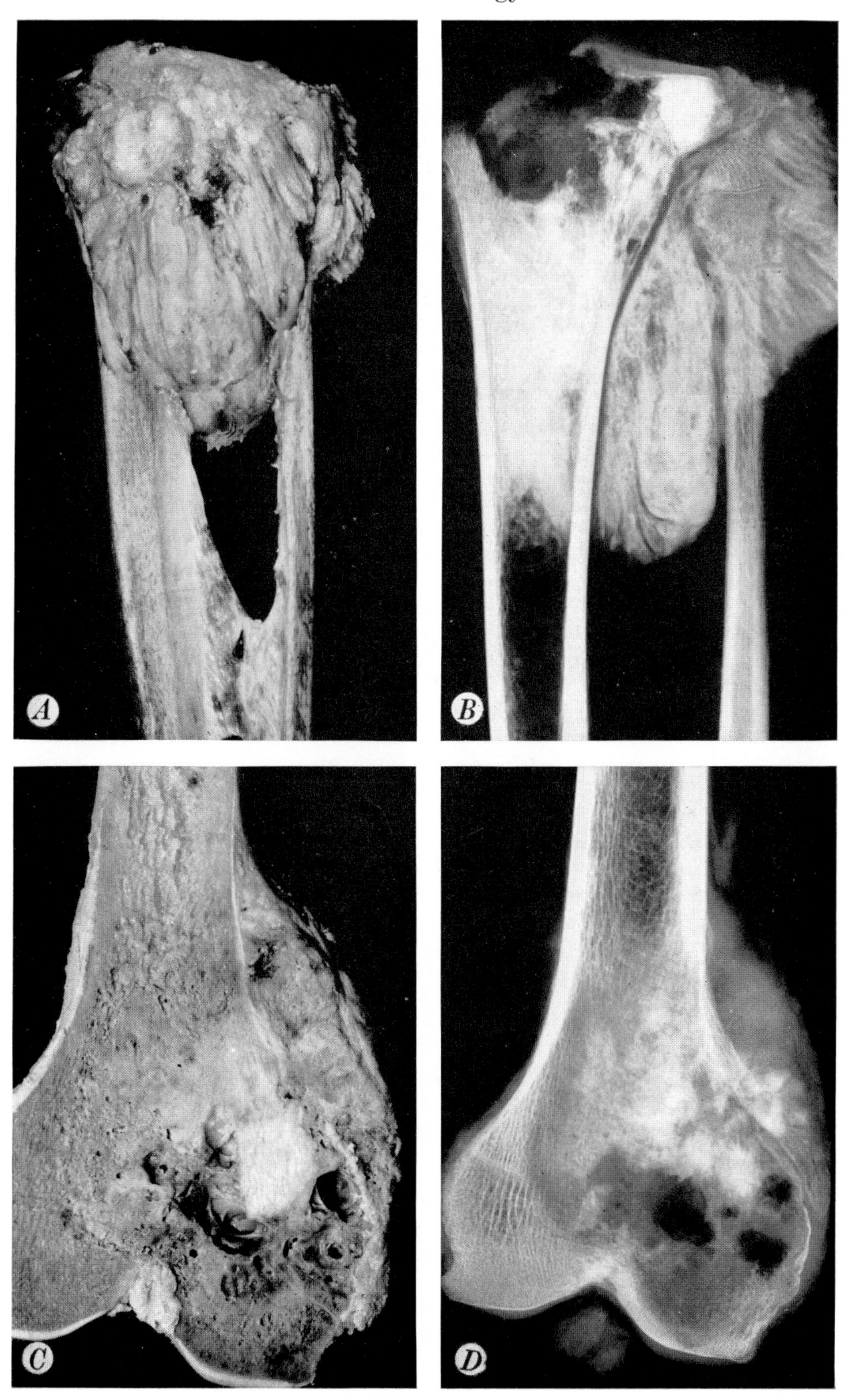


*Figure 81*

It should also be noted, however, that between the relatively slightly and the relatively heavily ossified lesions, as delimited above, there are those which are intermediate in respect to ossification. Thus, one may encounter small lesions in which the tumor mass is more or less evenly divided off into a highly sclerotic and ossified section and a soft, cellular, non-ossified and telangiectatic section. One also encounters tumors in which, though they have attained large size through growth both in the interior of the bone and around it, the tumor tissue is still rather firm and gritty cellular tissue everywhere, though showing no densely ossified and sclerotic areas. Such tumors, too, may present larger or smaller areas of telangiectasis and hemorrhage. (See Figs. 80 and 81.)

**Metastasis.**—Spread of the sarcoma from the original bone site to the regional lymph nodes seems to be of rare occurrence, but has been reported. In those of our cases in which the affected limb was removed by amputation or disarticulation, we have regularly examined such nodes without finding evidence that they were involved.

Distant metastasis seems to occur mainly, if not exclusively, by the hematogenous route. Metastases to the lungs are consistently found in cases which have terminated fatally. At autopsy, these metastases usually present themselves in the form of numerous smaller and larger discrete soft or gritty gray or yellowish nodules scattered throughout both lungs. Occasionally, however, the metastases may be practically limited to one lung, the thoracic cavity on that side being massively filled by tumor tissue. Pulmonary metastases are often the only metastatic finding. However, occasionally, one or more skeletal metastases are observed along with them (and perhaps with other visceral metastases). If foci of skeletal metastasis do appear, they are most likely to be found in the vertebral column, the skull, and/or the pelvic bones.

**Primary Multicentric Osteogenic Sarcoma.**—The cases which fall into this category are those in which foci of osteogenic sarcoma develop in multiple and even numerous skeletal sites more or less simultaneously and apparently *de novo*. Thus, cases in which multicentric foci of osteogenic sarcoma have become engrafted upon bones affected with Paget's disease (a not unusual circumstance) do not belong among the instances of primary multicentric osteogenic sarcoma. Naturally, one also excludes from this category the cases in which multiple skeletal foci of osteogenic sarcoma represent metastatic spread from one of the individual tumors.

Several remarkable instances of primary multicentric osteogenic sarcoma occurring in young children have been described (see Halpert *et al.*, Busso and Schajowicz, and Moseley and Bass). The distribution of the skeletal involvement as observed roentgenographically was essentially the same in these various cases. In particular, the skeletal surveys revealed multiple areas of intense radiopacity, widely distributed over the skeleton and present more or less bilaterally and symmetrically. In the long and short tubular bones, the radiopaque areas of osteogenic sarcoma formation were especially prominent in the metaphyses of the affected bones, though some of the epiphysial areas were also found involved. In one case or another, radiopaque tumor foci were present also in ribs, the clavicles, innominate bones, vertebræ, skull, and even some of the round bones of the carpus and tarsus. In some of the affected skeletal sites, the tumor tissue had remained confined within the limits of the bone. In others, however, it had broken out and extended into the adjacent soft tissues. In the case reported by Moseley and Bass, there was no roentgenographic evidence of pulmonary metastasis, despite the extensiveness of the skeletal involvement. The clinical course pursued in these various cases was consistently a rapid one with fatal termination.

A case of primary multicentric osteogenic sarcoma in an adult not affected with Paget's disease was described by Price and Truscott. A roentgenographic survey revealed densely radiopaque foci of tumor formation widely distributed over the skeleton. In most places the tumor bone was so highly ossified and so poor in cells that it was difficult to be certain that the lesional tissue actually represented osteogenic sarcoma. Also of interest in connection with this case is the fact that, at autopsy, the lungs were found free of metastases.

## ROENTGENOGRAPHIC FINDINGS

Often (perhaps in half of the cases of any series) the roentgenographic findings at the site of the lesion permit one to make an almost unequivocal preoperative diagnosis of osteogenic sarcoma. These are the cases in which particularly pronounced and extensive calcification and ossification have occurred in the tumor tissue. In these instances, the shadow cast by the affected bone area and by any tumor tissue beyond the limits of the bone proper is densely radiopaque, at least to a very large extent. Even by the relatively inexperienced observer, such lesions are identified readily from their roentgenographs as classic examples of the so-called sclerosing osteogenic sarcoma of bone. (See Fig. 78-*A* and *B*.)

Occasionally, in a case of this type, the area of radiopacity does not even clearly transgress the cortex, though the shadow of the cortex may merge in some places with the radiopaque shadow of the tumor in the interior of the bone. More often, however, the *x*-ray picture shows that the cortex has plainly been transgressed, at least over a limited extent. In the region of penetration the shadow of the cortex is then fuzzy, though its original outline can usually still be traced. Overlying it is the shadow cast by the calcifying and ossifying tumor tissue which has extended under and even through the periosteum and by any new (nontumor) bone which the irritated periosteum has managed to deposit. Among the cases of this type, the shadow beyond the limits of the cortex in the affected bone area varies rather widely in respect to size, extensiveness, and density. In general, the greater the tumor area within the bone, and the more widespread the cortical transgression, the more conspicuous is the extracortical shadow.

This shadow, in an occasional case, may show transverse or radiating ("sunburst") striations. As histologic examination reveals, such striations represent osseous trabeculæ coursing transversely through less heavily calcified and ossified extracortical tumor tissue. Furthermore, in regard to periosteal activity, one can often note some new bone apposition somewhere on the cortex immediately above (and less often, also below) the roentgenographic limits of the main tumor mass. Here the bone deposit takes the form of a thin shell or even striæ, following the long axis of the bone, and histologic examination may reveal little or no tumor tissue between the delineated striæ of periosteal new bone. (See Fig. 82.)

We come now to the other cases—those in which the *x*-ray picture falls short, to a lesser or greater degree, of that described above as typical for so-called sclerosing osteogenic sarcoma. In regard to those in which moderate ossification is present (about a quarter of all cases), a diagnosis of osteogenic sarcoma can still be made with reasonable confidence on the basis of the roentgenographic findings. In these cases, a good deal of radiopacity reflecting calcification and ossification within the lesional area is to be seen, though this does not dominate or monopolize the lesional shadow as a whole. (See Fig. 78-*C*.)

There remain to be considered those cases (again representing about a quarter of any series) in which the *x*-ray picture of the lesion tends to be ambiguous, so that the decision that the lesion really is an osteogenic sarcoma usually has to await anatomic study. (See Fig. 78-*D*.) In such cases (as others have also stressed), it is not necessarily the size of the lesion, its position in relation to the bone, nor the matter of radiopacity that by itself creates diagnostic difficulty, but rather the sum total of deviation from the $x$-ray picture typical of sclerosing osteogenic sarcoma. (See articles by Luck, by MacDonald and Budd, and Pendergrass, Lafferty, and Horn.)

In summary, osteogenic sarcoma, in most cases, is relatively easy to diagnose on the basis of the $x$-ray picture. Difficulties are created largely by those cases in which ossification is slight and the $x$-ray picture therefore ambiguous. On the other hand, when radiopacity is moderate (that is, fairly well developed, though not dominating the lesional shadow as a whole), a diagnosis of osteogenic sarcoma can already be made with reasonable confidence from the $x$-ray picture. In regard to the highly ossified and eburnated tumors (that is, frankly sclerosing osteogenic sarcomas), the preoperative diagnosis on the basis of the $x$-ray picture becomes even more certain. However, in studying and evaluating the roentgenographic picture in any particular case, even if the lesion shows moderate or intense radiopacity, one must, of course, consider this picture within the framework of the case as a whole. Thus, if the patient is a child or at most a young adult, if the lesion is a solitary one lying toward one end of a long bone, and if the shadow it casts is strikingly radiopaque, anatomic examination will almost always establish the tumor as an osteogenic sarcoma. On the other hand, if the patient is a mature or older adult, the possibility that one may be dealing with some other tumor (for instance, an osteoplastic carcinoma metastasis) has to be explored, even if the lesion is oriented toward the end of a long bone and casts a strikingly radiopaque shadow.

## MICROSCOPIC PATHOLOGY

The histologic pattern presented by an osteogenic sarcoma may vary considerably in detail from lesion to lesion and from area to area within the same lesion. The differences are in accord with the fact that some osteogenic sarcomas show relatively little and others considerable osteogenesis, and that even a lesion of the latter type may contain large areas which are poorly ossified. The full gamut of the histologic patterns presented by the sarcomatous connective-tissue stroma can be followed best in the "osteolytic" tumors or in meagerly ossified parts of the so-called "sclerosing" ones. For observing to the fullest extent the histologic changes in the course of which the sarcomatous stromal tissue becomes converted into tumor osteoid and bone, one turns to the essentially sclerosing tumors. (See Figs. 83 and 84.)

Within an unossified tumor area the cells of the stroma may be predominantly spindle-shaped, or may present a highly variegated anaplastic morphology, and/or may be roundish and lie in lacunæ so that they suggest cartilage cells. In the anaplastic areas, most of the cells contain 2 or more large and sometimes bizarre hyperchromatic nuclei, and the large cells particularly may even be crowded with such

***Figure 82***

*A*, Roentgenograph of a slice from a femur which is the site of a sclerosing osteogenic sarcoma. Note the transverse "sunray" streamers of radiopacity on the left, representing ossification which has taken place in the extra-osseous tumor tissue (see *C*).

*B*, Roentgenograph of a slice from another femur which is the site of a sclerosing osteogenic sarcoma. Note the "sunburst" effect produced by the streamers of ossification in the extra-osseous tissue.

*C*, Photomicrograph (× 35) showing the histologic pattern to which the "sunray" effect in *A* corresponds. Note the bone cortex on the left, beyond which there is rather highly vascular and cellular tumor tissue permeated by osseous trabeculæ running more or less at right angles to the cortex.

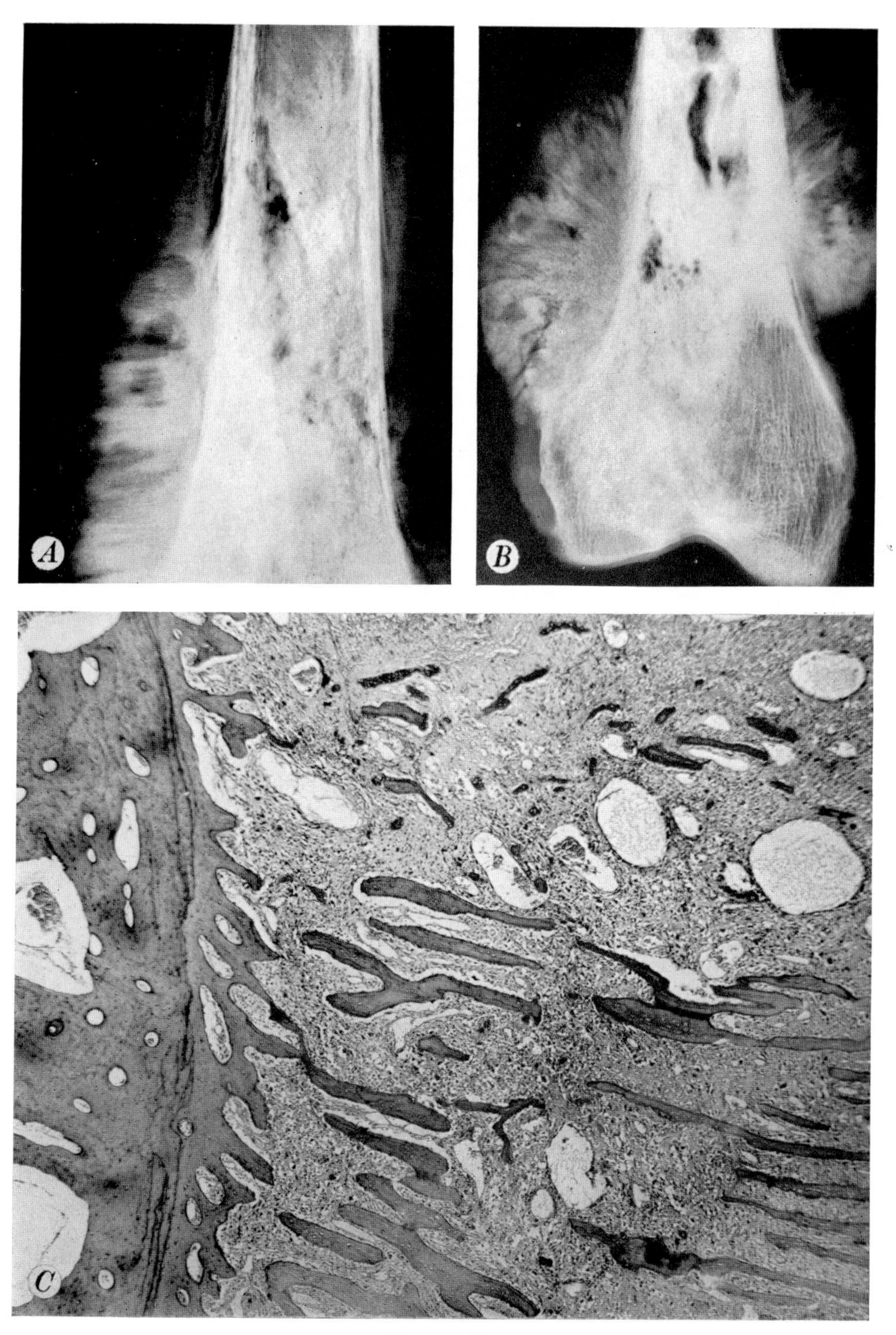


*Figure 82*

nuclei, appearing as veritable sarcoma giant cells. In the chondroid areas, one can note transition forms which indicate that the tumor cartilage has been created directly through differentiation of the sarcomatous spindle cells.

Where the sarcomatous stromal tissue is beginning to undergo ossification, one notes the appearance of intercellular fibrillar collagenous material, at first mainly between small groups of the stromal cells. Where there has been further advance toward ossification, one notes increase of the intercellular substance in the form of streamers which tend to break up the cell clusters so that individual cells become more widely separated. Many of the sarcomatous stromal cells become enmeshed in the ground substance, and one then sees sheets and trabeculæ of tumor osteoid. Further along the line of evolution, the osteoid trabeculæ and the sheets of osteoid show deposits of calcium in the intercellular matrix, inaugurating the appearance of actual tumor bone. It is of interest to note that, after becoming incarcerated in the trabeculæ of tumor osteoid and tumor bone, the originally plump sarcomatous stromal cells tend to become smaller. Indeed, as Phemister already pointed out, the more ossified the tumor bone trabeculæ become, the smaller and more sparse, on the whole, are the tumor cells contained within them, and the more closely do these cells approach in appearance the osteocytes of nontumor bone. That is, this process of incarceration tends to have a "normalizing" influence, as it were, upon the appearance of the tumor cells which have become the osteocytes of the tumor bone.

If the lesion is one whose sarcomatous stroma does not lay down much tumor osteoid and bone, the original osseous tissue at the site of its growth is subjected from the beginning mainly to resorption and dissolution. Specifically, as the tumor tissue fills the marrow spaces and surrounds the original spongy trabeculæ, these tend to be irregularly gnawed out and broken up, and many are resorbed altogether, while at the same time the cortex, too, is substantially resorbed and destroyed. On the other hand, if the lesion is one in which the deposition of neoplastic osseous tissue is considerable, the intertrabecular marrow spaces come to contain much tumor bone and the original spongy trabeculæ become encased by it, yielding slowly to it by a process of gradual substitution. In such a case the process of erosion and destruction of the original cortex, too, is slower than in a case in which the osteogenic potentiality of the sarcoma is relatively slight.

In an individual case, before the tumor tissue has yet extended through the cortex, the lesional area may already show some new bone laid down under the periosteum. Such a deposit, which represents merely a reaction to periosteal irritation, varies in thickness. It consists of loosely woven radiating bone trabeculæ interspersed with moderately vascular loose-meshed connective tissue apparently quite free of tumor cells. After the sarcomatous stromal tissue has spread beyond the

***Figure 83***

*A*, Photomicrograph (× 100) showing the tissue pattern to be found in an area of an osteogenic sarcoma where the sarcomatous stroma is highly anaplastic and as yet uncalcified. Note the numerous sarcoma giant cells.

*B*, Photomicrograph (× 100) showing the tissue pattern to be found in an area where the sarcomatous stromal cells are differentiating in the direction of cartilage cells.

*C*, Photomicrograph (× 125) showing streamers of intercellular material which have developed between the stromal cells and which are entrapping some of these cells. As the intercellular material increases in amount, it becomes calcified and thus inaugurates the formation of tumor bone.

*D*, Photomicrograph (× 75) showing the emergence of tumor bone in the sarcomatous stroma. Note that sarcomatous stromal cells are being enmeshed in the intercellular material. Note also that, where tumor bone has appeared, the enmeshed cells are small and have become the osteocytes of the tumor bone.

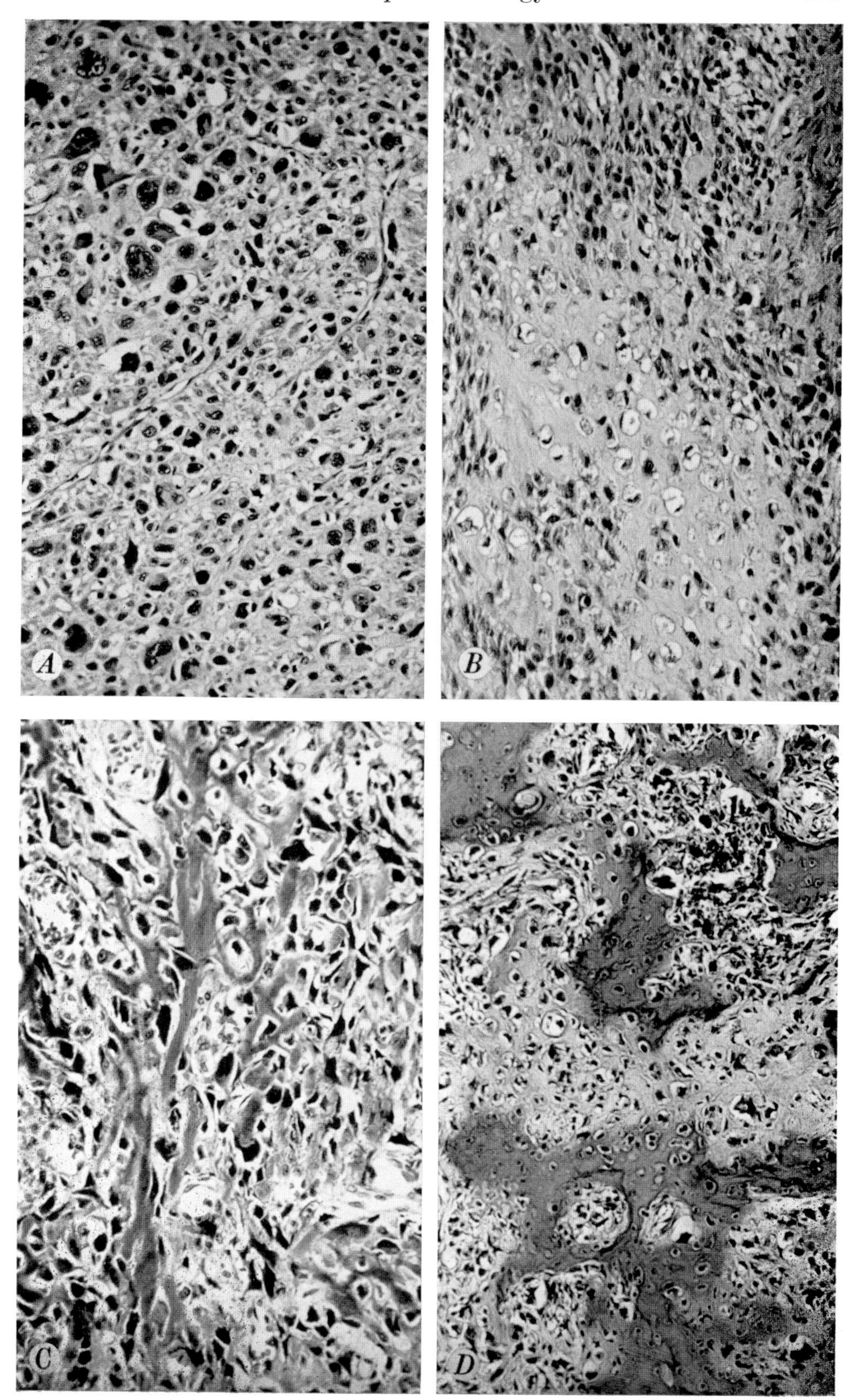


*Figure* 83

limits of the cortex, the bone found under the periosteum represents mainly tumor bone. In an individual case, one may even find a considerable amount of tumor bone under the periosteum, distending it, sometimes tremendously, and even penetrating it, perhaps in many places. It is when the trabeculæ in this subperiosteal tumor tissue run at right angles to the longitudinal axis of the bone that the *x*-ray picture presents the "sunburst" pattern already mentioned.

Finally, it should be noted that most osteogenic sarcomas are rather vascular. They are more so in some portions than in others, the still cellular stromal tissue being interspersed with smaller or larger sinuous thin-walled blood channels bordered by tumor cells. In some parts in particular, one may note engorged vascular channels lying close together. Viable tumor cells usually border them, and some tumor cells may also be found admixed with the blood in the spaces. Such telangiectatic areas may be near, or independent of, areas in which the tumor tissue is undergoing anemic or even hemorrhagic necrosis.

**Phosphatase Activity in the Tumor Tissue.**—The tissue from an osteogenic sarcoma regularly shows high concentrations of *alkaline* phosphatase on histochemical analysis. The phosphatase activity is greatest in the peripheral, that is, the most rapidly growing, portions of the tumor. It is most concentrated about the blood vessels. In the more static areas, represented by highly sclerotized or necrotic portions of the tumor, the alkaline phosphatase activity, though still considerable, is much less pronounced. The entrance of phosphatase from the tumor tissue into the blood stream is reflected in the elevation of the serum alkaline phosphatase value. As to *acid* phosphatase activity, it has been found that osteogenic sarcoma tissue does not show this. In contrast, it is worth noting that giant-cell tumors, and specifically the actual giant cells, do show it to a considerable degree.

## DIFFERENTIAL DIAGNOSIS

As already implied, the diagnosis of osteogenic sarcoma is often not difficult. Specifically, one is almost certainly dealing with an osteogenic sarcoma if the lesion is a substantially radiopaque tumor which has broken out, or is breaking out, from the interior of the shaft end of a long limb bone and the patient is between 10 and 25 years of age. If the age of the patient is within these limits, and if the stated conditions relating to location and manner of advance of the lesion are also fulfilled, the tumor is still likely to be an osteogenic sarcoma, even if the lesional area is only spottily radiopaque.

The problems of differential diagnosis are mainly the problems of distinguishing between: (1) conventional (central) osteogenic sarcoma and *juxtacortical osteogenic sarcoma;* (2) "osteolytic" osteogenic sarcoma (*i.e.*, an osteogenic sarcoma forming

### *Figure 84*

*A*, Photomicrograph (× 35) showing the histologic pattern often presented by the spongiosa of a bone affected with sclerosing osteogenic sarcoma. Note that there is a considerable amount of tumor bone in the intertrabecular spaces, but that the original trabeculæ of spongy bone largely remain.

*B*, Photomicrograph (× 125) showing in greater detail an original spongy trabecula with tumor tissue above and below it. Note that the tumor bone being formed in the sarcomatous stroma becomes attached to the nontumor bone.

*C*, Photomicrograph (× 75) showing the histologic appearance presented by a spongy bone area in which the growth of the sarcomatous tissue has largely destroyed the original spongy bone. Note, somewhat below the middle of the picture, 2 fragments of original spongy bone which are still persisting in the ossifying tumor tissue.

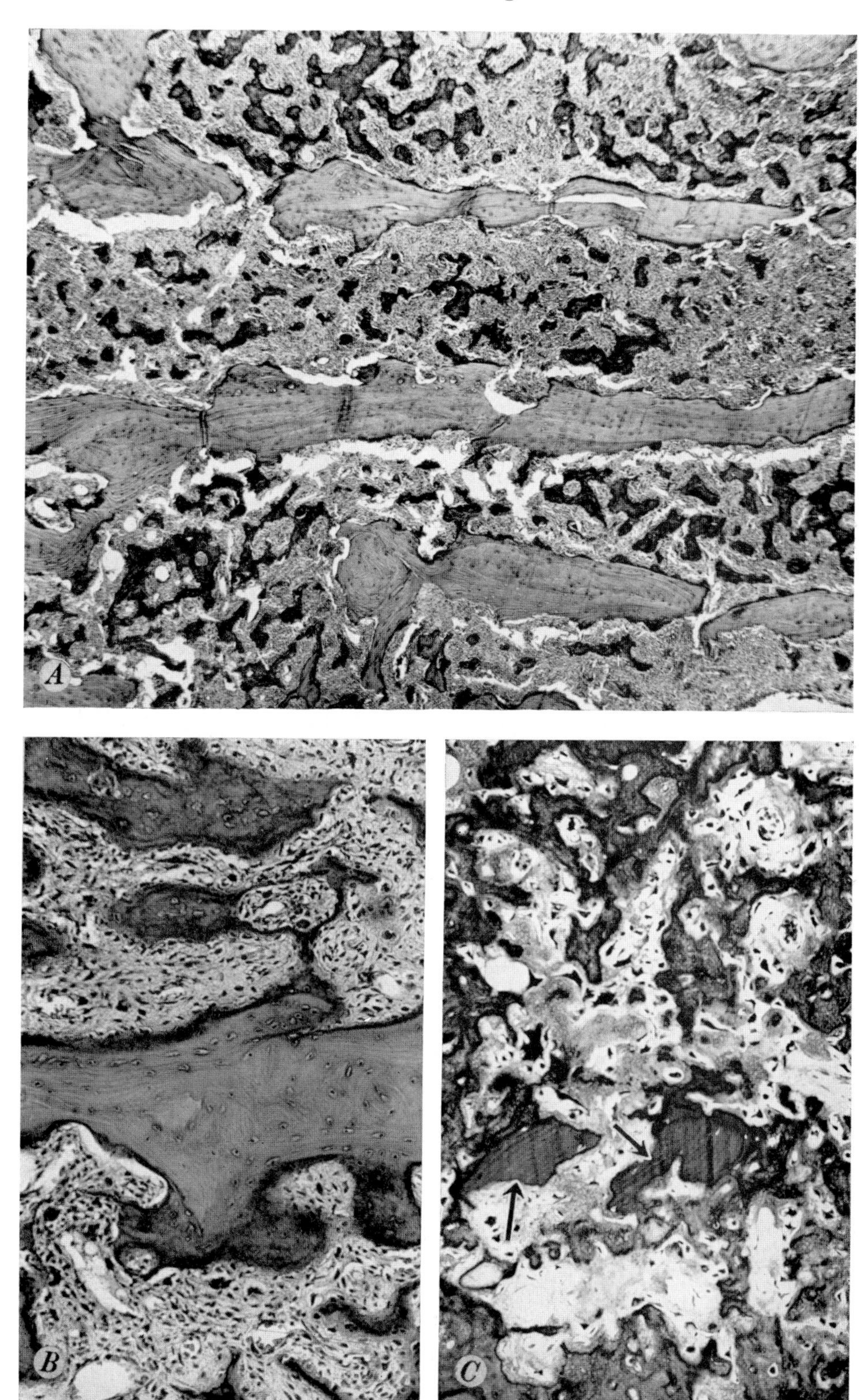


*Figure 84*

relatively little tumor osteoid and bone) and *fibrosarcoma of bone* (*i.e.*, an essentially non-bone-forming connective-tissue sarcoma); (3) osteogenic sarcoma and *chondrosarcoma;* and (4) osteogenic sarcoma and a *highly ossified focus of fibrous dysplasia* or some other benign lesion which may show heavy radiopacity of the lesional tissue.

**Juxtacortical Osteogenic Sarcoma.**—This tumor entity is discussed in the following chapter (p. 279). In respect to differentiation between it and the conventional osteogenic sarcoma, the following points are relevant: As already indicated, the juxtacortical osteogenic sarcoma develops in relation to the periosteum and/or immediate parosteal connective tissues, instead of originating within the affected bone, as the conventional osteogenic sarcoma does. From the clinical point of view, these two bone-forming sarcomas differ in that the juxtacortical osteogenic sarcoma has a much better prognosis.

The earlier stages of the juxtacortical osteogenic sarcoma lesion are represented roentgenographically by the presence of a more or less radiopaque shadow in the soft tissues overlying the cortex of the neighboring bone. The parosteal mass varies in size and shape from case to case, and, in respect to opacity, it may be uniform or streaky. In the course of time, growth of the lesion (without intervention) or regrowth after attempts at removal is reflected roentgenographically in a large irregular tumor mass which finally may encircle, more or less, the bone in its vicinity. This tumor mass may be heavily radiopaque. Furthermore, at this later stage there may be evidence of erosive destruction of the local cortex in some areas, or even of invasion of the marrow cavity by the tumor tissue. Of course, if the lesion is already at this end stage when one sees it for the first time, it is sometimes not possible to say with certainty that the lesion started as a juxtacortical growth which had come to invade the bone secondarily.

**Fibrosarcoma of Bone.**—Frankly malignant fibrosarcoma of bone (p. 304) and "osteolytic" osteogenic sarcoma are occasionally confused. Since they are both basically connective-tissue sarcomas, the distinction between them resides in the fact that, in the osteogenic sarcoma the sarcomatous stroma forms tumor osteoid and osseous tissue, while in the fibrosarcoma it does not.

Microscopic examination of tissue sections from a frankly malignant fibrosarcoma will reveal a connective-tissue growth whose stromal cells, though they may be spindle-shaped in some areas, are on the whole polymorphous. Many of these cells will show giant nuclei or multiple nuclei, and many cells in process of mitotic division also will be observed. Furthermore, search of the tissue will fail to reveal any evidence of osteoid or bone formation in the tumoral stroma. However, ample sampling of the specimen may be necessary to establish the fact that neoplastic osteoid or osseous tissue is not being laid down somewhere in the lesion, and thus eliminate the possibility that one is dealing with an osteogenic sarcoma which is merely failing to lay down much tumor bone. On the other hand, it must be recognized that a biopsy specimen representing a random sampling of an individual osteogenic sarcoma may fail to show the presence of tumor osteoid and osseous tissue. This may lead to misinterpretation of the lesion as a fibrosarcoma of bone, the examiner not appreciating that he was dealing merely with a still unossified area of an osteogenic sarcoma.

**Chondrosarcoma.**—As already indicated, a chondrosarcoma of bone is a malignant cartilage tumor which is characterized not only by its direct derivation from cartilage cells, but also by its tendency to maintain its essentially cartilaginous nature throughout its evolution. By this definition, chondrosarcoma (p. 314) is set apart from osteogenic sarcoma, since any cartilage present in the latter tumor has been formed from the basic sarcomatous connective tissue. There can be little doubt that when the term "osteochondrosarcoma" or "chondro-osteosarcoma" is applied to a lesion, the latter is usually an osteogenic sarcoma containing considerable amounts of cartilage rather than actually a chondrosarcoma.

Any confusion that may arise between chondrosarcoma and osteogenic sarcoma relates only to so-called "central chondrosarcoma"—that is, to a chondrosarcoma which begins its development in the interior of a bone. However, in anatomic detail, as well as clinically and roentgenographically, a "central chondrosarcoma" usually presents definite differences from osteogenic sarcoma. The age of a patient affected with chondrosarcoma is usually between 25 and 50. Roentgenographically, a central chondrosarcoma of a long bone which has evolved from a pre-existing solitary enchondroma frequently shows up as an area of irregular, mottled radiopacity in the interior of the bone, associated with some local bulging of the bone contour and with thickening and perhaps fuzziness and/or perforation of the cortex. On the other hand, a central chondrosarcoma which has arisen *de novo* may fail to show such mottled radiopacity, though there will be some local distention of the bone contour, and the regional cortex may be found thinned in some places and perhaps thickened in others.

In any event, whether the central chondrosarcoma has developed *de novo* or from a pre-existing cartilage growth, the tumor, if left to run its natural course, will ultimately break out of the confines of the cortex, and a definite mass will be visible roentgenographically beyond the limits of the altered cortex. If the affected bone is sectioned in its long axis, it will be found, whether the tumor is bulky or not, that the pathologic tissue in the interior of the bone, and any which is outside of the limits of the cortex, is composed of smaller or larger faceted islands of cartilage. If radiopacities are visible roentgenographically in the lesional area, these will turn out to have represented areas in which the tumor cartilage is heavily calcified or even ossified.

**Fibrous Dysplasia.**—It is only in relation to an occasional solitary focus of fibrous dysplasia that any danger of confusion with osteogenic sarcoma arises. It is more likely to arise in regard to those solitary fibrodysplastic lesions in which the replacement tissue in the lesional area is rather on the osseous side of the fibro-osseous complex (Fig. 40-*D*) than on the fibrous side. Whether the replacement tissue tends toward the osseous or toward the fibrous side, lesions of fibrous dysplasia do not tend to perforate the cortex, though they often thin the cortex and expand the contour of the affected bone part. Furthermore, the fibrous stroma shows no evidences of atypism or remarkable plumpness of the cells such as would indicate that the stroma is sarcomatous. Nevertheless, there can be no doubt that, in an occasional instance, a solitary focus of fibrous dyplasia is still misinterpreted as an osteogenic sarcoma, though not so often as it used to be.

**Other Lesions Raising Diagnostic Problems.**—A *primary reticulum cell sarcoma of bone* (p. 416) occasionally presents an *x*-ray picture suggestive of osteogenic sarcoma. This is most likely to happen if the tumor is located toward the end of a long bone and has provoked a good deal of reactive osteosis, so that patchy radiopacity is conspicuous in the lesional area. If the subject is still relatively young, that fact may seem to support this erroneous impression, but this is corrected by study of a biopsy specimen. Occasionally, also, a focus of *osteoplastic carcinoma metastasis* creates an *x*-ray picture which might be held to represent an osteogenic sarcoma. Indeed, the writer has seen a number of instances in point in which a clinically silent prostatic or bronchogenic cancer had metastasized to a long bone and the bone lesion was believed to be an osteogenic sarcoma until examination of a biopsy specimen revealed its true nature (see Fig. 187). Once in a while, too, in one of the rare cases in which an *acute osteomyelitis* has developed in the shaft of a long bone *of an adult*, the *x*-ray picture may suggest that of an osteolytic osteogenic sarcoma. Finally, it may be worth noting that, before the concept of *osteoid-*

*osteoma* was delimited, an occasional instance of this condition, too, was misinterpreted as osteogenic sarcoma. These were cases in which the lesion was oriented to the bone cortex and provoked massive thickening of the latter which looked ominous in the *x*-ray picture and led to amputation of the affected extremity.

## PROGNOSIS AND TREATMENT

Surgery is currently the generally accepted therapeutic procedure against an osteogenic sarcoma in an accessible site. It is generally held that the amputation should be done as soon as the diagnosis has been established through histologic examination of tissue obtained by needle punch or incision. As to the proper level for the amputation, one can usually clear the tumor if this is done 4 or 5 inches above the roentgenographically established upper limit of the lesion. However, one is on much safer ground if one carries out the amputation even higher up. For example, the writer has seen several instances of osteogenic sarcoma of the lower end of the femur in which, had not a disarticulation at the hip been done, there would certainly have been a local recurrence in the stump. This was shown by the fact that examination of the ablated limb revealed a focus of tumor tissue in the upper end of the disarticulated femur, separated from the tumor tissue in the lower end by a large area of apparently uninvolved femoral shaft. For an osteogenic sarcoma in the upper end of a femur, the procedure practiced is often more radical than a disarticulation at the hip joint, a hemipelvectomy being done. For an osteogenic sarcoma at the upper end of a humerus, an interscapulothoracic amputation is commonly practiced. When the primary lesion is in a site which does not permit amputation, palliative radiation therapy becomes the only possibility.

However, osteogenic sarcoma is a tumor having an extremely high mortality rate, no matter how soon after the establishment of the diagnosis the surgeon ablates the affected part. Indeed, in the writer's experience, the 5-year survival rate is not much above 5 per cent, at best, in cases treated primarily by surgery. The writer is aware that the literature contains many reports that at least 20 per cent of the patients survive for the crucial 5-year period after amputation or disarticulation, and that some reports even give the survival rate for this period as 30 per cent. It is to be suspected that when survival rates of 20 and 30 per cent or more have been reported, the material has included lesions other than conventional (central) osteogenic sarcoma. In particular, such reports undoubtedly include some cases of: juxtacortical osteogenic sarcoma, chondrosarcoma, low grade fibrosarcoma of bone (p. 310), and even instances of monostotic fibrous dysplasia.

Prognostic significance has sometimes been attached to the intensity of ossification shown by the osteogenic sarcoma, but the fact is that, as a rule, the disease reaches its fatal termination after amputation or disarticulation about as quickly when this tumor is a highly ossified one as when it is not. A large proportion of the patients are already dead within a year from the onset of their first clinical complaints, and most of the rest shortly after 2 years. Only an occasional patient survives into the fourth or even fifth year from the onset of the complaints before succumbing. Indeed, it is to be deduced from the rapidity with which the course is ordinarily run that a large proportion of patients with osteogenic sarcoma already have pulmonary metastases, though not yet roentgenographically visualizable ones, by the time the diagnosis is made and amputation done. In contrast to ossification, location has some importance in the prognosis. In particular, so far as location in limb bones is concerned, the prognosis is somewhat less grave when the lesion is distal than when it is close to the trunk of the body. Indeed, an osteogenic sarcoma appearing *de novo* in the upper end of a femur or humerus is almost inevitably fatal. In the case of an osteogenic sarcoma in a foot bone or in the lower end of a tibia, the prognosis is not so baleful.

The doleful prognosis in cases of osteogenic sarcoma promptly treated by amputation or disarticulation justifies careful consideration of other methods of treatment. Ferguson and also Cade have advocated deferment of amputation or disarticulation for the lesion until some time after it has been treated by heavy irradiation. These workers maintain that this form of therapy will raise the survival rate very appreciably above the 5 or at most 10 per cent to be expected under purely surgical therapy.

Cade advocates first treating the lesion by means of a supervoltage $x$-ray machine and delivering about 8,500 r over a period of about 8 to 10 weeks. If pulmonary metastases do not show up within a period of 6 months or so after the course of $x$-ray treatment is completed, the affected limb, sooner or later, is amputated or disarticulated in accordance with the site of the tumor. If additional experience with this therapeutic routine should confirm the indications that it does sharply raise the survival rate, it would represent the best available procedure known as yet for the treatment of osteogenic sarcoma.

As indicated in connection with metastasis of osteogenic sarcoma (p. 266), pulmonary metastases are often the only ones found at autopsy. Furthermore, in some cases the pulmonary metastases are found limited to one lung. These facts have encouraged thoracic surgeons to undertake pulmonary surgery in suitable cases with some hope of occasionally saving a patient. Experience is accumulating in regard to cases in which a limb was ablated because of an osteogenic sarcoma, and in which a solitary focus of pulmonary metastasis (or a solitary focus and some neighboring daughter foci) subsequently appeared and was removed. In some of these cases, wedge resection or radical lobectomy was followed by a survival period of 5 years or more (see Goldenberg and also Cahan). The reasonable explanation for the apparent cure in such cases is that the focus of pulmonary metastasis removed had been the only one present, and that it was removed before further pulmonary seeding from it could take place.

## REFERENCES


Busso, M. G., and Schajowicz, F.: Sarcoma osteogénico a localización múltiple, Rev. ortop. y traumatol., *15*, 85, 1945.

Cade, S.: Osteogenic Sarcoma, J. Roy. Coll. Surgeons, Edinburgh, *1*, 79, 1955.

Cahan, W. G.: Personal Communication.

Carroll, R. E.: Osteogenic Sarcoma in the Hand, J. Bone & Joint Surg., *39-A*, 325, 1957.

Case Records of the Massachusetts General Hospital (Osteogenic Sarcoma of Humerus, with Ossifying Metastases in the Regional Nodes), New England J. Med., *225*, 953, 1941.

Codman, E. A.: *Bone Sarcoma:* An Interpretation of the Nomenclature Used by the Committee on the Registry of Bone Sarcoma of the American College of Surgeons, New York, Paul B. Hoeber, Inc., 1925. (See p. 23.)

Coventry, M. B., and Dahlin, D. C.: Osteogenic Sarcoma, J. Bone & Joint Surg., *39-A*, 741, 1957.

Engfeldt, B.: Biophysical Studies on Bone Tissue. VI. Biophysical Studies on Bone Tissue from Osteogenic Sarcoma, Cancer, *7*, 815, 1954.

Ewing, J.: A Review of the Classification of Bone Tumors, Surg., Gynec. & Obst., *68*, 971, 1939.

Ferguson, A. B.: Treatment of Osteogenic Sarcoma, J. Bone & Joint Surg., *22*, 92 and 916, 1940.

Finlayson, R.: Osteogenic Sarcoma with Multiple Skeletal Tumours, J. Path. & Bact., *66*, 223, 1953.

Goldenberg, R. R.: Osteogenic Sarcoma of the Tibia with Pulmonary Metastasis. Report of a Case with Ten-Year Survival, J. Bone & Joint Surg., *39-A*, 1191, 1957.

Halpert, B., Russo, P. E., and Hackney, V. C.: Osteogenic Sarcoma with Multiple Skeletal and Visceral Involvement, Cancer, *2*, 789, 1949.

Higinbotham, N. L., and Coley, B. L.: The Methods and Effects of Preoperative Irradiation in the Treatment of Osteogenic Sarcoma, Am. J. Roentgenol., *47*, 902, 1942.

Hodges, P. C., Phemister, D. B., and Brunschwig, A.: *The Roentgen-Ray Diagnosis of Diseases of the Bones and Joints*, New York, Thomas Nelson & Sons, 1938. (See p. 181.)

JAFFE, H. L.: Osteogenic Sarcoma of Bone, Clinical Orthopaedics, *7*, 27, 1956.
——————: Tumors of the Skeletal System. Pathological Aspects, Bull. New York Acad. Med., *23*, 497, 1947.
JAFFE, H. L., and BODANSKY, A.: Diagnostic Significance of Serum Alkaline and Acid Phosphatase Values in Relation to Bone Disease, Bull. New York Acad. Med., *19*, 831, 1943.
JAFFE, H. L., and SELIN, G.: Tumors of Bones and Joints, Bull. New York Acad. Med., *27*, 165, 1951.
LUCK, J. V.: A Correlation of Roentgenogram and Pathological Changes in Ossifying and Chondrifying Primary Osteogenic Neoplasms, Radiology, *40*, 253, 1943.
MACDONALD, I., and BUDD, J. W.: Osteogenic Sarcoma: II. Roentgenographic Interpretation of Growth Patterns in Bone Sarcoma, Surg., Gynec. & Obst., *82*, 81, 1946.
MOSELEY, J. E., and BASS, M. H.: Sclerosing Osteogenic Sarcomatosis, Radiology, *66*, 41, 1956.
PENDERGRASS, E. P., LAFFERTY, J. O., and HORN, R. C.: Osteogenic Sarcoma and Chondrosarcoma: With Special Reference to the Roentgen Diagnosis, Am. J. Roentgenol., *54*, 234, 1945.
PHEMISTER, D. B.: A Study of the Ossification in Bone Sarcoma, Radiology, *7*, 17, 1926.
POPPE, E.: Osteogenic Sarcoma—Along What Lines should it be Treated?, Acta radiol., *31*, 335, 1949.
PRICE, C. H. G.: The Grading of Osteogenic Sarcoma, Brit. J. Cancer, *6*, 46, 1952.
PRICE, C. H. G., and TRUSCOTT, D. E.: Multifocal Osteogenic Sarcoma, J. Bone & Joint Surg., *39-B*, 524, 1957.
ROBERTS, C. W., and ROBERTS, C. P.: Concurrent Osteogenic Sarcoma in Brother and Sisters, J.A.M.A., *105*, 181, 1935.
SCOTT, R. K.: Pre-operative Radiotherapy in the Treatment of Osteogenic Sarcoma: A Preliminary Communication, M. J. Australia, *36(2)*, 304, 1949.
WOODARD, H. Q., and HIGINBOTHAM, N. L.: The Correlation between Serum Phosphatase and Roentgenographic Type in Bone Disease, Am. J. Cancer, *31*, 221, 1937.

Chapter

# 18

# Juxtacortical Osteogenic Sarcoma

THE *juxtacortical osteogenic sarcoma* is a distinctive bone-forming connective-tissue tumor which develops in relation to the surface of a bone and specifically in relation to the periosteum and/or the immediate parosteal connective tissue. As the term "juxtacortical" implies, it is a tumor which, at least at first, is merely oriented and attached to the regional bone cortex. In this respect the lesion is to be distinguished from the *conventional* osteogenic sarcoma of bone, which originates centrally—that is, within the affected bone. From the clinical point of view, also, it is worth while to distinguish between these two types of osteogenic sarcoma because of the much better over-all prognosis of the juxtacortical type.

It is true that some juxtacortical osteogenic sarcomas are aggressively malignant from the start, present a histologic pattern in accord with this fact, and readily break into the regional bone and metastasize. However, most of the juxtacortical osteogenic sarcomas are of rather low grade malignancy, tending not to metastasize for many years though they recur again and again after attempts at local excision. In these latter cases, the tissue removed from the lesion at the original intervention or even in connection with one or more recurrences is likely to be underrated in respect to its malignant potentialities because of a deceptively "benign" histologic appearance. Indeed, the lesion is likely to be regarded, at least for some while, as a peculiar or atypical osteochondroma or as a relatively innocuous focus of metaplastic parosteal ossification somewhat akin to a focus of myositis ossificans. However, if one pays adequate attention to the cytologic details of the spindle cell stroma between the osseous elements of the lesional tissue, one cannot fail to be impressed by the sarcomatous aura it presents, at least in many areas. In any event, repeated recurrences tend to be associated with accelerated growth of the lesion and with the emergence of a histologic tissue pattern pointing more clearly in the direction of a sarcoma. Ultimately a juxtacortical osteogenic sarcoma of this type, too, may come to erode the cortex of the regional bone and even invade the marrow cavity. However, even in cases in which an amputation has been done after this has already happened, the prognosis is still not completely unfavorable.

**Nomenclature.**—The Bone Sarcoma Registry classification of 1939 (see Ewing) included under the general heading of osteogenic sarcoma the category of "parosteal (or capsular) osteogenic sarcoma." There can be no doubt that this subcategory of osteogenic sarcoma was meant to include cases such as are being discussed in the present chapter. Hatcher, in a presentation before the American Orthopaedic Association in 1947, stressed the need for a clearer delimitation of these lesions, which he grouped together under the tentative heading of "Extra-Skeletal Ossification Simulating Sarcoma." It was with this need in mind that we subsequently evaluated the pertinent cases in our files and denoted the lesion as the "juxtacortical osteogenic sarcoma" (see Jaffe and Selin). The term "parosteal osteoma" has also been used for the lesion in question, but seems undesirable because it suggests benignity even though the proposers of this term (see Geschickter and Copeland) did realize the malignant potentialities of the lesion. As a distinctive entity, the lesion has also been denoted by the name of "parosteal osteogenic sarcoma" (see Dwinnell, Dahlin, and Ghormley).

## CLINICAL CONSIDERATIONS

**Incidence.**—The juxtacortical osteogenic sarcoma is a relatively uncommon lesion. Neither sex seems to be strikingly predilected. The age range of the patients is fairly wide. In our collected series of 18 cases, the age distribution was spread rather evenly between 15 and 55 years, and half of the patients were over 30 years of age. In this respect there is something of a contrast to what one finds in connection with the conventional (central) osteogenic sarcoma, whose victims are mainly under 25 years of age.

**Location.**—By far the most common site of origin of the lesion is the peri- and/or parosteal connective tissue adjacent to the cortex of the lower part of the femoral shaft. Indeed, in at least half of the cases the lesion is in this location. In the other cases the lesion is usually oriented to the cortex of some other long tubular bone (most often the tibia or the humerus) and generally likewise toward the end rather than the midshaft area. Occasionally also the lesion develops about some other bone than a long tubular bone. For instance, in one case seen by the writer, the site was the coracoid process of the scapula. (See Fig. 85.)

**Clinical Complaints and Findings.**—In the cases of juxtacortical osteogenic sarcoma which are slow in revealing their malignant potentialities, the clinical complaints are relatively mild and have been present for a long time before the patient first seeks treatment. This is especially likely to be true when the lesion is located in relation to the cortex of the lower end of the femur. In these cases the patients often indicate that for several years they have noted some limitation of flexion of the knee, associated with slight discomfort. These complaints may even only be noted in connection with activities making somewhat excessive demands upon the joint in question, such as professional dancing, exhibition skating, or exceptionally frequent stair climbing.

If, in these cases, the lesion is oriented to the posterior surface of the femoral cortex, the patient is sometimes not even aware of the presence of a local tumor

### *Figure 85*

*A*, Roentgenograph showing a juxtacortical osteogenic sarcoma oriented to the lower end of a femur. The lesion appears as a somewhat lobulated and densely radiopaque shadow adherent to the cortex posteriorly and also straddling the bone. The cortex itself is intact. The patient was a girl 19 years of age whose principal complaint was that for several years she had been having difficulty in flexing the knee. A hard, nonmovable, nontender tumor mass was palpable in the lesional area. Tissue examination (see Fig. 89) showed the lesion in this case to be of low malignancy, as were the other lesions also illustrated in this plate.

*B*, Roentgenograph showing a juxtacortical osteogenic sarcoma oriented to the cortex of the upper end of a humerus. Note again the lobulated, radiopaque tumor shadow abutting on the cortex of the bone. The patient was a woman 26 years of age who had become aware of a local swelling. This had been present for 3 years before it became somewhat painful and made her seek medical care.

*C*, Roentgenograph showing a juxtacortical osteogenic sarcoma oriented to the upper end of a tibia. The patient was a man 49 years of age.

*D*, Roentgenograph of a juxtacortical osteogenic sarcoma abutting on the medial aspect of the lower end of a tibia and encircling the regional part of the fibula. The patient was a man 40 years of age who had become aware of a progressive swelling in the ankle region which was neither painful nor tender. He stated that he had begun to notice the swelling after sustaining a trivial local injury about 6 months before this *x*-ray picture was taken.

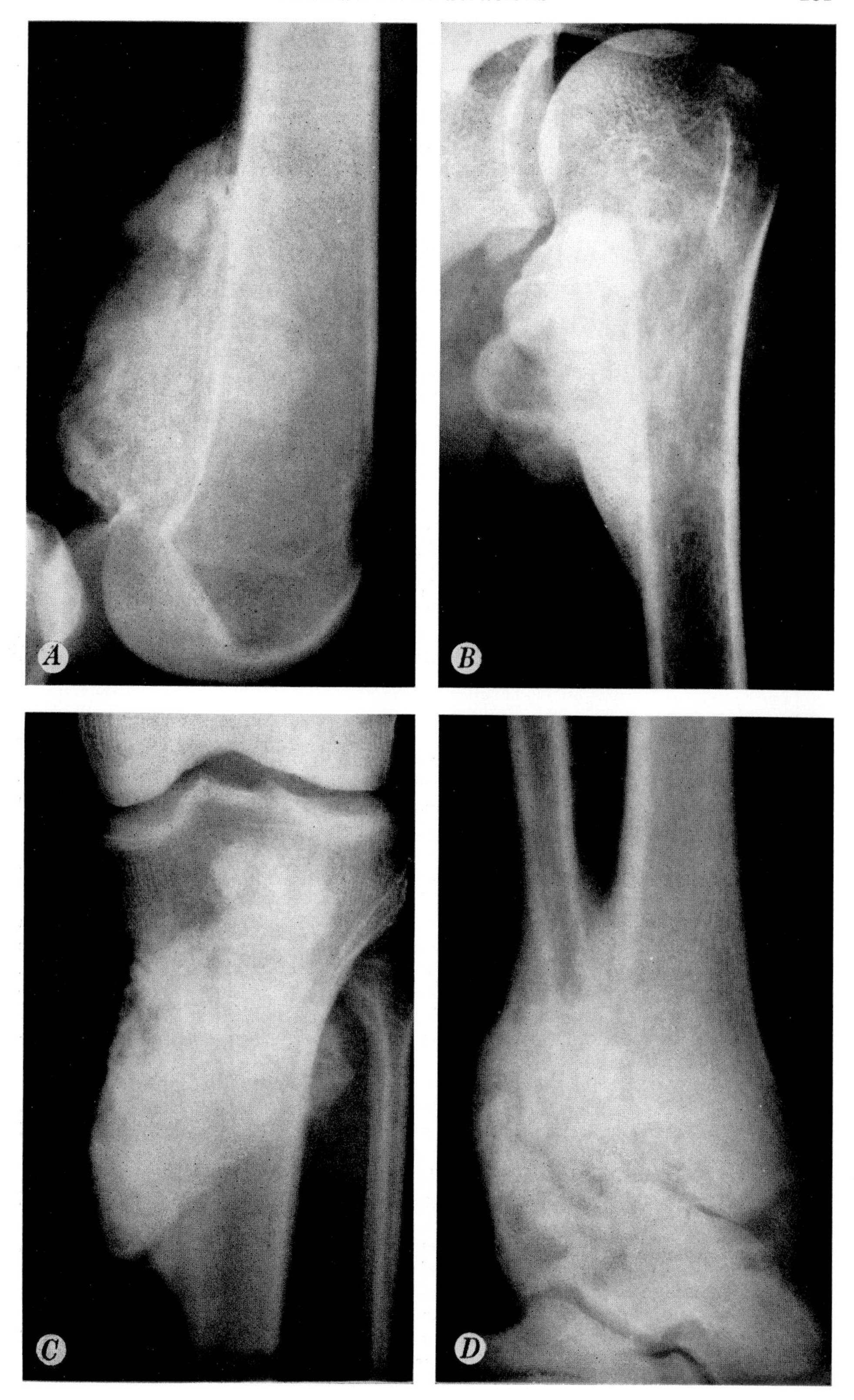


*Figure* 85

mass. On the other hand, if the lesion is oriented to either side or to the anterior aspect of the femoral cortex, the presence of a local mass may constitute the presenting complaint. When the lesion is oriented toward such a superficial site as the upper or lower end of a tibia or the upper end of a humerus, the presence of a tumor mass is quite likely to be the initial complaint. Palpation of the mass reveals that it is bony hard, perhaps lobulated, and usually nontender. It is firmly fixed to the cortex of the adjacent bone, but the overlying skin is freely movable.

If left to itself, the tumor mass in such cases continues to grow, but usually only very slowly. An attempt at local excision is usually followed by a recurrence. In such cases the patient may report that the original surgical intervention was followed by one or more subsequent interventions at intervals of 6 months to a year or so, necessitated by recurrences. Indeed, recurrence in more exuberant form after each attempt at excision seems to be quite usual. In this connection, in one of the cases studied by the writer, in which the lesion was oriented to the lower part of a femur, there were 4 attempts at excision of the lesion, necessitated by recurrences, in the course of 4 years. In another case in which the lesion had a similar location, there were 3 recurrences and new interventions in the course of 6 years after the original attempt at local excision. In both of these cases, amputation was finally undertaken, and in both instances the patients have remained free of complaints referable to the condition.

While in most cases of juxtacortical osteogenic sarcoma (about 75 per cent) the clinical course is protracted and metastases appear late if at all, there are some cases which tend to run a rapid and baleful course. These cases belong to the smaller

***Figure 86***

*A*, Roentgenograph of a juxtacortical osteogenic sarcoma located in relation to the posterior cortex of the lower end of a femur. The tumor area is heavily radiopaque, and the tissue removed when the lesion was originally excised presented indubitable histologic evidence of malignancy, although it was underrated at the time by the writer as representing a focus of myositis ossificans. The patient was a woman 52 years of age. Within 4 months after the attempted local excision, there was a recurrence and another attempt at local excision was made. Three months after this there was another recurrence, and after that the limb was ablated. In the amputation specimen it could be seen that the tumor had invaded the interior of the femur. Histologically, much of the tumor tissue now appeared highly anaplastic. Death ensued from metastases.

*B*, Roentgenograph of a juxtacortical osteogenic sarcoma abutting on the cortex of a tibia. The lesional area is not heavily radiopaque, and the tissue removed when the lesion was originally excised was underrated in this case too in respect to its malignant potentialities. There was a rapid recurrence, the lesion was again excised, and it now showed indubitable evidence of malignancy (see Fig. 90). Another recurrence took place in the course of a few weeks. An amputation was now done, but the patient, a man 22 years of age, died of metastases about 6 months later.

*C*, Roentgenograph showing the appearance of a juxtacortical osteogenic sarcoma in a case in which, in the course of 6 years, 3 attempts at local excision of the tumor had been made. A midthigh amputation was then done, and the tumor was found to have invaded the femur. The patient, a woman 33 years of age at that time, has now been free of any further local difficulties and in good general health for 2 years.

*D*, Roentgenograph of a juxtacortical osteogenic sarcoma of a femur in the case of a girl 20 years of age. The picture shows the appearance of the lesional area after 4 attempts at excision of the lesion, necessitated by recurrences in the course of 4 years. An amputation through the thigh was then carried out, and the most recent follow-up showed that the patient had remained well and free of metastases for 4 years. This is particularly interesting in view of the fact that, at the time of the amputation, the tumor had been found to have invaded the femur and that the tumor tissue removed at the successive interventions showed increasing amounts of fibrosarcomatous stroma.

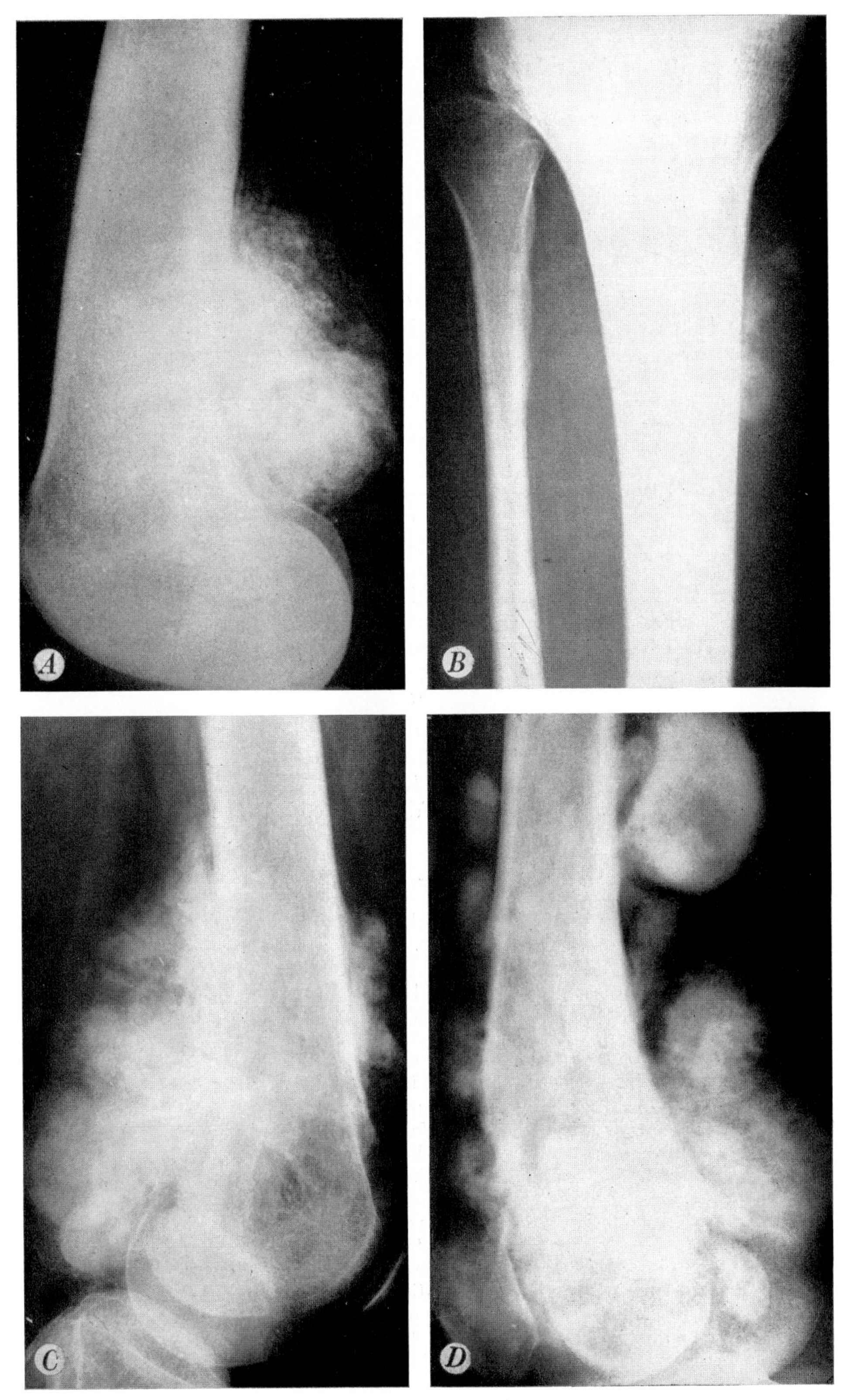


***Figure 86***

group in which the tissue removed in the first attempt at local excision of the lesion already presents an obviously sarcomatous histologic pattern. After excision of the lesion there is usually a prompt recurrence, and the histologic pattern of the tissue of the recurrence is even more frankly sarcomatous. The lesion tends to invade the regional bone rather promptly, and, even if an amputation is carried out after the first or second recurrence, death from pulmonary metastases usually ensues within a year or so after the condition first comes under clinical observation. The clinical course and histologic tissue findings in these cases correspond more or less closely to what is observed in connection with the fully malignant bone-forming connective-tissue sarcomas (osteogenic sarcomas) which develop in the soft parts of a limb and are not oriented to a bone at all (see Fine and Stout).

In one of the cases studied in which the juxtacortical osteogenic sarcoma was aggressively malignant from the start, the lesion was oriented to the lower end of a femur and the patient was a woman 55 years of age whose only complaint was of a local tumor mass of about 6 months' standing. An attempt at local excision was followed within 3 months by a massive recurrence and invasion of the local bone. The affected limb was then amputated, but death from widespread metastases occurred 18 months after the amputation. In another case in which the lesion was oriented to the lower end of a femur, the patient was a woman 52 years of age whose chief complaint was of vague local pain of rather short duration. An attempt at local excision of the lesion was followed by recurrence in 4 months, after which another attempt at local excision was made. This was followed by another recurrence in 3 months. The limb was then amputated, the tumor having invaded the femur, but the patient died from metastases 16 months after the operation. In this case, too, tissue removed at the original intervention already had the aura of an osteogenic sarcoma (though the diagnoses made at the time included "a peculiar exostosis" and "myositis ossificans"). Lesional tissue removed at the successive interventions showed more and more clearly the pattern of a full-blown bone-forming connective-tissue sarcoma, which in this case had taken its departure from the soft tissues abutting on the cortex of the lower end of the femur.

***Figure 87***

*A*, Roentgenograph showing a juxtacortical osteogenic sarcoma of low malignancy attached to the cortex of the lower end of a femur. The patient was a man 20 years of age who, for 2 years, had experienced some difficulty in flexing the knee. A biopsy of the lesion was done, and an amputation was carried out about a week later, since the location of the lesion was such that a complete excision was impossible and experience had taught that recurrence was hence inevitable.

*B*, Photograph of the femur and the adherent juxtacortical osteogenic sarcoma after removal of the overlying soft parts. Note the lobulated appearance of the tumor mass and how this matches up with the *x*-ray picture shown in *A*.

*C*, Photograph of a sagittal section of the femur and adherent tumor mass in this case. The tumor mass blends with the cortex, which has become thickened, but the marrow cavity has not been invaded. The whitish tissue at the lower end of the tumor mass represents an area of cartilage.

*D*, Photograph showing, in cross section, the orientation of the tumor to the cortex at one level. Note that the cortex has not been penetrated by the tumor.

*E*, Photograph showing, in cross section, the orientation of the tumor to the cortex at a level below that shown in *D*, and again indicating that the cortex has not been penetrated. On the right, adjacent to the tumor mass, the periosteum has laid down some new bone on the cortex, presumably in consequence of irritation by traction.

*F*, Roentgenograph of the specimen shown in *E*.

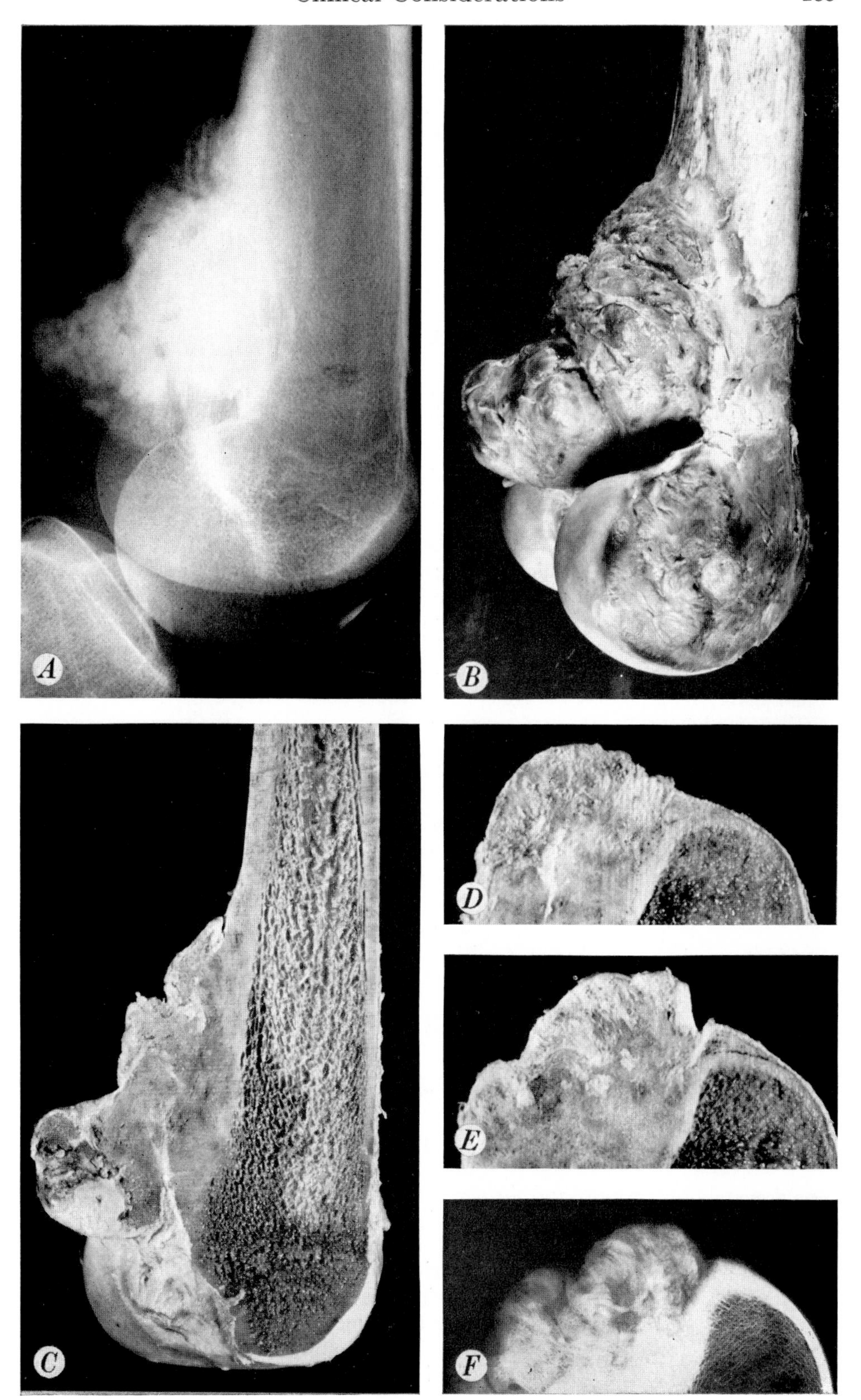


*Figure 87*

## ROENTGENOGRAPHIC FINDINGS

Roentgenographically, a juxtacortical osteogenic sarcoma is likely to present as a rather large, irregular, and densely radiopaque tumor mass adherent to and blending with the regional bone cortex. In some cases, however, the shadow cast by the tumor mass shows only blotchy and streaky radiopacity. In connection with radiopacity, it may be stated in general that if the juxtacortical tumor mass is densely and more or less uniformly radiopaque, the condition is less likely to run a fulminating course than if it is not. However, the writer has also seen a few cases presenting a densely radiopaque tumor mass but nevertheless having a rather rapidly fatal outcome. (See Figs. 85 and 86.)

In any event, if one is not familiar with the juxtacortical osteogenic sarcoma, one might interpret the *x*-ray picture of the still untreated lesion as representing a large and otherwise atypical osteoma or osteochondroma. If the patient has given a history of an antecedent trauma (though such a history is not commonly given or really relevant), the lesion might be interpreted roentgenographically as an ossifying tissue mass appearing in the wake of trauma and hemorrhage involving the soft tissues neighboring on the bone and/or affecting the periosteum. That is, the lesion might be interpreted as something on the order of a post-traumatic myositis ossificans or as what one might call a "post-traumatic periosteoma." On the other hand, instead of being designated as a peculiar osteochondroma or as an unusual focus of post-traumatic ossification, the lesion might possibly be misinterpreted roentgenographically as an osteogenic sarcoma of predominantly periosteal location.

In the course of time, growth of the lesion without surgical intervention, or regrowth after attempts at removal, is represented roentgenographically by a large tumor mass which may more or less encircle the bone in its vicinity. The ossified portions of the tumor mass may appear as large, roundish, discrete or confluent areas of dense radiopacity. At this stage, furthermore, there may be evidence of erosive destruction of the local cortex in some areas, or even of invasion of the marrow cavity of the bone by the tumor tissue. Of course, if the lesion already presents this picture when one sees it for the first time, it may not be possible, on the basis of that picture alone, to say with certainty that the lesion started as a parosteal growth and had come to invade the bone secondarily. In this connection a history of protracted morbidity with recurrences after attempts at local excision becomes very helpful in pointing up the correct diagnosis. If the patient is well over 25 years of age, one has an additional cue along this line.

## PATHOLOGIC FINDINGS

**Gross Pathology.**—Only rarely does one have the opportunity of studying the gross appearance of a juxtacortical osteogenic sarcoma intact in its setting from a case in which the affected limb has been ablated before any attempts at surgical excision of the lesion have been made. In a case in point, the lesion was oriented to the cortex of the lower end of a femur. Roentgenographically, the lesion appeared heavily radiopaque, and the associated clinical disability had been mild and of 2 years' standing. Altogether, the lesion in this case appeared to belong to the group characterized by low malignity.

For the purposes of the examination, the affected area of the femur was shelled out from the overlying soft parts. During this procedure it was found that the course of the popliteal artery was deflected somewhat medially by the growing tumor mass. However, that artery and the companion nerve and veins were not adherent to it. On the other hand, the lower end of the tumor was adherent to, and invading, the knee joint capsule, particularly posteriorly. More proximally, the fascia and fatty tissues were adherent to the tumor mass but could still be stripped from it fairly easily. At the upper end of the tumor, the periosteum of the uninvolved part of the femur merged with the tumor mass.

When the affected femoral area was completely freed from the overlying soft parts, the tumor stood out as a rather lobulated, bony hard mass which was intimately adherent to the cortex posteriorly and also laterally and medially. The mass extended from the intercondylar notch upward for a distance of 8 cm. in its longitudinal dimension. At its widest, just above the condylar area of the femur, the tumor mass measured 7 cm. across. When the specimen was sectioned in the sagittal plane, the cut surfaces showed that the tumor mass was continuous with the posterior cortex of the femur. It was also evident that there was no extension of the tumor tissue into the interior of the bone. In harmony with the surface of the lesion, the interior of the sectioned tumor mass was found bony hard and clearly osseous practically throughout. It is true that at the lower end of the tumor there was an area about 2 × 1 cm. where the tumor tissue was cartilaginous. However, this cartilaginous area was continuous with the tumor tissue which was highly osseous, and certainly the lesion did not present a peripheral cartilaginous cap. The longitudinal cut surface of the tumor also showed some streaks of whitish fibrous tissue. On the basis of gross inspection it was difficult to decide to what extent these represented trapped fascial tissue and to what extent they represented tracts of cellular tumor tissue, which microscopic examination indeed showed them mainly to be. (See Fig. 87.)

As already noted, even in cases characterized by low malignity, if excision has been attempted and the lesion has recurred once or more often, the eventually amputated limb will usually show evidence of invasion of the interior of the regional bone. In a case in point, the patient had become aware of the presence of a mass in the lower part of the thigh 8 years before the amputation was done. An attempt at local excision of the lesion was carried out 4 years before the amputation. The lesion not only recurred, but became much larger, grew painful, and was now associated with flexion deformity and limitation of motion at the knee.

The amputation specimen showed that the lower two-thirds of the thigh was much enlarged, and one could feel a bony hard mass encuffing the lower end of the femur. When the femur and the surrounding bony mass were cut in the sagittal plane, it was noted that, although the posterior cortex of the bone was still clearly defined, a large, hard, bony mass, cystic in some places, had fused with it. The sciatic nerve was caught in this mass. Anteriorly, the cortex of the femur was defective, and the ossified tumor tissue overlying this portion of the femur was continuous with tumor tissue present in the interior of the bone. The latter tissue was ossified on the whole, though it also had softer, fibrous areas and some cystified areas.

A juxtacortical osteogenic sarcoma already presenting indications of full malignancy from the start is likely to be less highly osseous, especially peripherally, than one of low malignancy. That is, in the gross, a good part of the tumor tissue mass may be rather cellular and chondroid. Indeed, especially at or near the periphery of the tumor mass, the tumor tissue may be grayish or whitish in color and relatively slightly ossified. In fact, parts of it there may have the texture of purely fibrous tissue. Other peripheral parts may be of fibrous gritty consistency. Still other more or less peripheral parts may be essentially cartilaginous, though perhaps also showing small gritty areas representing foci of calcification. On the other hand, the more deeply placed tumor tissue—that is, the part of the tumor mass near or abutting on the cortex—is likely to be yellowish white and for the most part quite ossified.

**Microscopic Pathology.**—The histologic findings vary from lesion to lesion in accordance with: 1) whether the lesion in question is essentially of low malignancy or of high malignancy; (2) whether one is studying tissue from the original lesion or from a recurrence; and (3) whether the examination is limited to a single tissue area or includes areas from different parts of the lesion.

Indeed, even in connection with a lesion of low malignancy, parts of the lesional tissue may appear histologically much more innocent than others. This was well exemplified by the histologic findings in the case illustrated in Figure 87. Parts of the lesion were composed of highly compacted trabeculæ of moderately vascular lamellar bone which showed relatively little cellular tissue in the intertrabecular spaces. However, in other areas of the lesion one could find large tracts of rather cellular tumor tissue between the osseous trabeculæ. This cellular tissue was composed of long drawn-out spindle cells with plump nuclei and clearly represented sarcomatous connective tissue. One could also see in many places that the osseous tissue was being formed out of this sarcomatous connective tissue. Indeed, study of sections prepared from many tissue blocks from the lesion in question showed that the latter was basically a bone-forming connective-tissue sarcoma (hence an osteogenic sarcoma). However, in some fields, so much osseous tissue had been formed that the sarcomatous stroma had been relegated to the background, and if a biopsy specimen had been taken from such an area, one might have judged the lesion to be quite innocuous. On the other hand, in other tissue areas the sarcomatous stroma occupied the foreground of the histologic picture, and a biopsy specimen from such an area could not be interpreted otherwise than as a sarcoma. (See Fig. 88.)

The problem of evaluating histologically the malignant potentiality of the lesion is indeed a trying one in most of the cases in which the lesion is of low malignancy. Specifically, one is very likely to underrate the lesion unless adequate attention is given to the spindle stroma of the lesional tissue, especially in areas in which no considerable amount of osseous tissue and/or cartilage has yet been laid down. In such tissue fields the stromal cells have the indubitable appearance of sarcomatous connective-tissue cells. On the other hand, if one concentrates on those tissue fields of the lesion which contain considerable osseous tissue and/or cartilage, the sarcomatous aura of the stroma may not be conspicuous. It is for this reason that, on the basis of tissue removed at the original surgical intervention or after one or more recurrences, the lesion is so often interpreted as an osteoma or an atypical osteochondroma. Sooner or later, however, in the course of examination of tissue from recurrences, the sarcomatous character of the stroma comes to dominate the histologic picture in practically all tissue areas. (See Fig. 89.)

In a juxtacortical osteogenic sarcoma which is fully malignant from the start, the histologic findings are usually unequivocal in this respect if enough tissue areas of the lesion are examined. In some lesional areas the sarcomatous connective-tissue stroma is likely to be abundant and there may even be a good deal of cellular

***Figure 88***

*A*, Photomicrograph (× 7) showing the histologic pattern of tissue taken from the periphery of the specimen illustrated in Fig. 87. Note that on the left-hand side of the picture the tissue is highly ossified and that there is relatively little cellular tissue permeating this osseous tissue. However, on the right-hand side, one sees large tracts of cellular tissue (see *B*) between the trabeculæ of osseous tissue.

*B*, Photomicrograph (× 65) showing in some detail the histologic pattern of the tissue on the right-hand side in *A*. Note that the cellular tissue consists of intertwining bundles of proliferating fibrosarcomatous spindle cells.

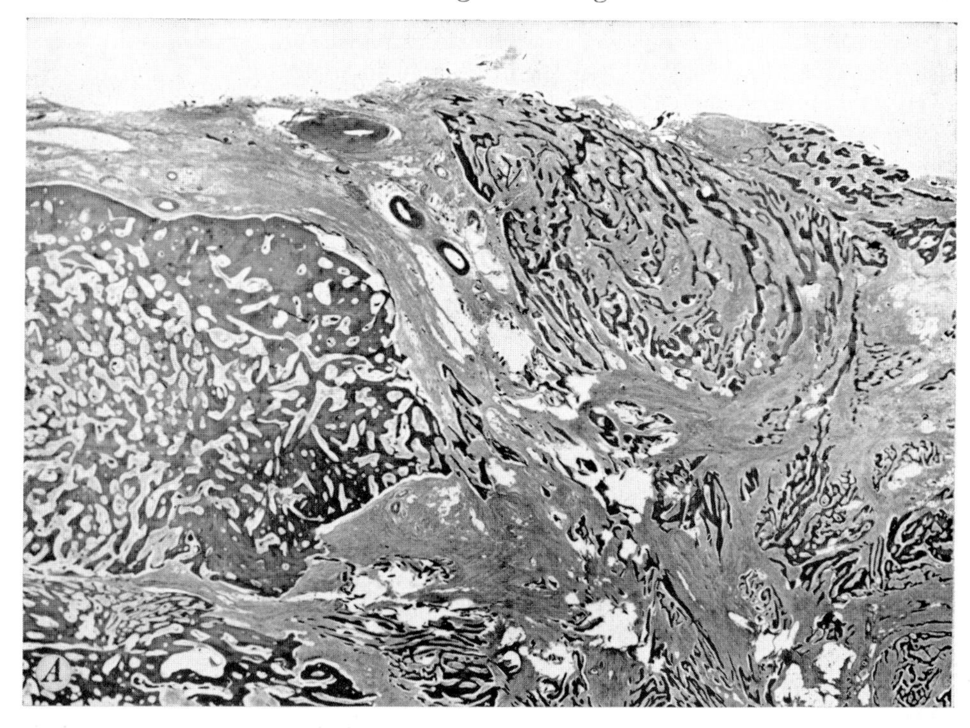


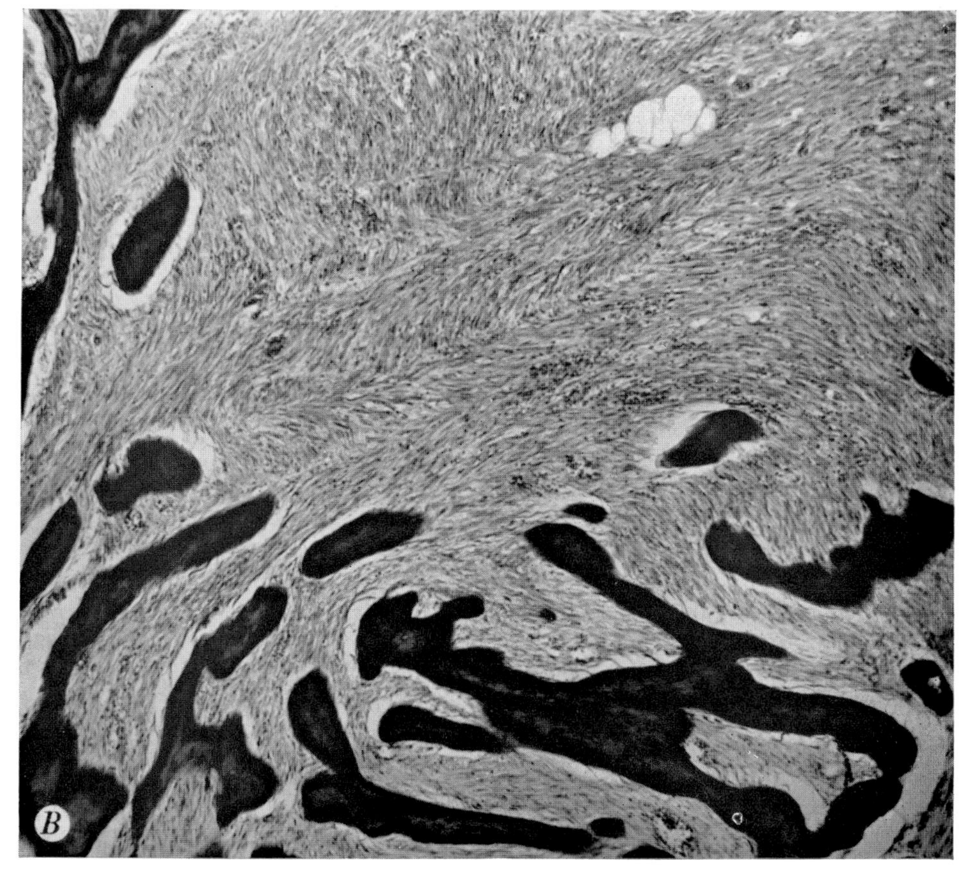


*Figure 88*

pleomorphism. In fact, many of the tumor cells may appear swollen and bizarre, and some may have multiple nuclei, being actual sarcoma giant cells. In such anaplastic fibrosarcomatous areas of the tumor, the inherent osteogenetic capacity of the sarcoma cells is likely not to be expressed. In other tissue areas, however, the sarcomatous stromal cells will be found forming tumor cartilage, osteoid, and bone. The nuclei of the cartilage cells are usually large and plump, and in general the appearance of the cartilage is that characteristic for fully malignant cartilage tissue. Where the sarcomatous stromal cells are producing osteoid and osseous tissue, the latter is laid down in large sheets or in irregular trabeculæ, just as it is in a highly ossified osteogenic sarcoma which has started in the interior of a bone. Furthermore, an occasional lesion may show, in one area or another, fields crowded with multinuclear giant cells. These giant cells are likewise set in a fibrosarcomatous stroma, and the histopathology of such tumor fields, taken by themselves, suggests that of malignant giant-cell tumor. Peripherally, a juxtacortical osteogenic sarcoma of full malignity is usually found to be infiltrating the neighboring soft tissues and muscles. Furthermore, it is usually already found to have broken into the bone. In general, this histologic description applies also to juxtacortical osteogenic sarcomas originally of low malignity which, after repeated recurrences, have finally passed over into full malignity. (See Fig. 90.)

## DIFFERENTIAL DIAGNOSIS

The problems of diagnosis and differential diagnosis relating to juxtacortical osteogenic sarcoma have already been touched upon. The difficulties in this connection arise more from lack of familiarity with the lesion than from actual similarity (roentgenographic and pathologic) between it and other conditions with which it might be confused.

**Myositis Ossificans.**—In the older literature one can find some classic examples of juxtacortical osteogenic sarcoma which have been reported because they were thought to represent peculiar or unusual instances of myositis ossificans. The case reported by Paul and the one reported by Chambers are instances in point. In both these cases the clinical history revealed no direct trauma to the part, the *x*-ray picture showed a large ossifying mass abutting on the regional cortex, and amputation was done because the lesion had recurred in more exuberant form after local excision. Both authors were much puzzled by the clinical course in these cases, but felt that they could resolve their diagnostic dilemma by interpreting them as instances of myositis ossificans exhibiting unusual aggressive qualities.

### *Figure 89*

*A*, Photomicrograph (× 125) showing the histologic pattern presented in one of the tissue areas of the excision specimen removed from the lesion illustrated in Fig. 85-*A*. Note the osseous trabeculæ set in a substratum of loose spindle cells. There is nothing in this pattern to suggest a sarcoma even of low malignancy, and such fields could be duplicated in many areas of the tissue examined. However, other tissue areas in the lesion did show appearances suggestive of a sarcoma (see *C* and *D*).

*B*, Photomicrograph (× 25) of a tissue field showing cartilage formation. The cartilage is developing out of the stroma, which does not present a particularly ominous appearance in this field.

*C*, Photomicrograph (× 125) showing the histologic pattern in an area in which the lesional tissue was essentially fibrous. In such fields the tissue was found to be composed of drawn-out intertwining bundles of spindle cells in the pattern of a well differentiated fibrosarcoma.

*D*, Photomicrograph (× 125) showing the histologic pattern in still another tissue area. Note the evidence of bone formation in the spindle cell fibrosarcomatous stroma.

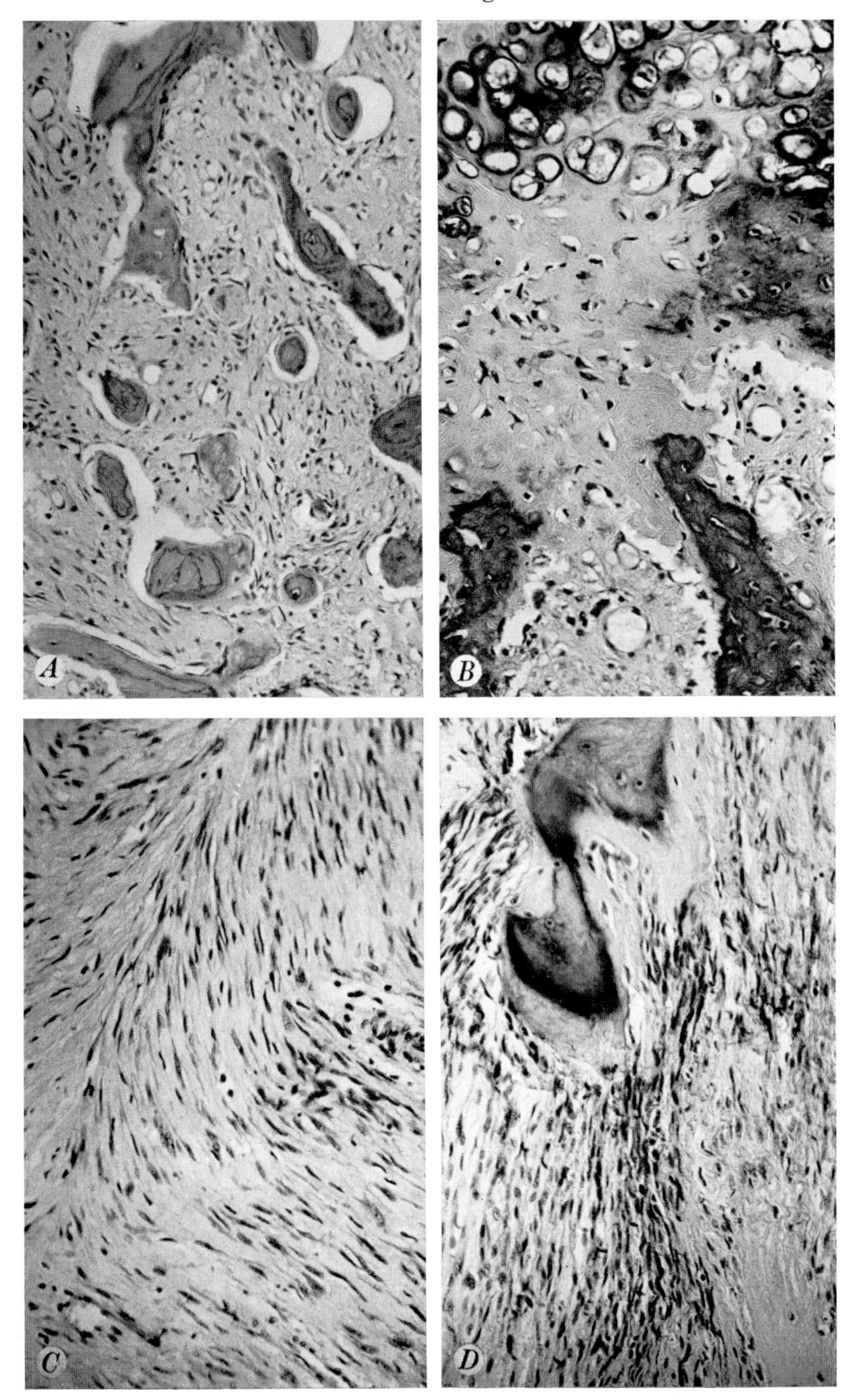


***Figure 89***

Actually, the conventional case of myositis ossificans hardly presents any problem of differential diagnosis from juxtacortical osteogenic sarcoma. Nearly always there is a definite history of a severe local trauma to the part in which the myositis ossificans has appeared. If the part is easily accessible to palpation, a local painful soft-tissue swelling is to be felt soon after the trauma. Furthermore, the skin over the traumatized area usually shows, within a few days, discoloration due to diffusion of blood pigment.

An *x*-ray picture of the part, taken within about a week after the trauma, may not as yet show a radiopaque shadow in the soft parts. However, within another week or so, such a shadow does appear, and in the course of the following weeks it enlarges somewhat and becomes more and more sharply delineated. Indeed, a focus of myositis ossificans usually reaches its maximum size and definitive outline in about 2 months or so from the time of the trauma. The ossified mass in the soft tissues may or may not impinge upon a regional bone part. If it does, its area of attachment is usually not broad unless the periosteum too has been traumatized and there has been hemorrhage into and beneath it. Also, it should be noted that a focus of so-called myositis ossificans is usually not very densely radiopaque and that it is rather clearly set off peripherally from the neighboring soft parts.

Anatomically, too, a focus of myositis ossificans appears well circumscribed peripherally. In fact, the osseous tissue at its periphery is usually the most mature part of the lesion and the part in which its innocent character stands out most plainly. Any muscle about the bony shell of the lesional area is found compressed and otherwise altered, but shows no invasion by tracts of connective-tissue cells extending into it from the ossifying focus. In the interior of the focus one may still see large fields of proliferating spindle cells in which osteoid and even cartilage are being laid down, and one may also note residual degenerating muscle fibers. However, any ominous-looking cytologic fields encountered in the interior of a myositis ossificans focus which might raise the question of malignancy can safely be discounted in view of the fact that the lesion has evolved rapidly and after a trauma, that it is well circumscribed, and that it presents no ominous cytologic features peripherally and is most mature there. (See Fig. 91.)

**Post-traumatic Periostitis.**—Occasionally a person who has incurred an acute and severe trauma to a limb (but no fracture) develops a large, broad-based, ossified mass ("post-traumatic periosteoma") in continuity with the cortex of the regional bone. The condition is probably best interpreted as arising from traumatization of the periosteum and hemorrhage into and beneath it. The writer is familiar with

***Figure 90***

*A*, Roentgenograph of a slice of the resection specimen of the juxtacortical osteogenic sarcoma of high malignancy shown in Fig. 86-*B*. Note that the tumor is invading the cortex and that it is rather heavily ossified, particularly where it abuts on the cortex. Peripherally the tumor tissue is ossified only slightly or not at all.

*B*, Photomicrograph (× 5) showing the tumor and adjacent cortex. Note that at the extreme periphery the tumor tissue shows no evidence of ossification and that signs of the latter increase as one proceeds inward toward the cortex. It is also to be remarked that the vessel canals of the cortex are free of tumor tissue.

*C*, Photomicrograph (× 125) showing the fibrosarcomatous pattern of the unossified tumor tissue at the periphery of the lesion.

*D*, Photomicrograph (× 125) showing the pattern of the tissue just below the unossified peripheral area. Note the streamers of calcific material between the spindle-shaped sarcoma cells. Further inward in the lesional area, the formation of tumor bone is much more clear-cut (see *B*).

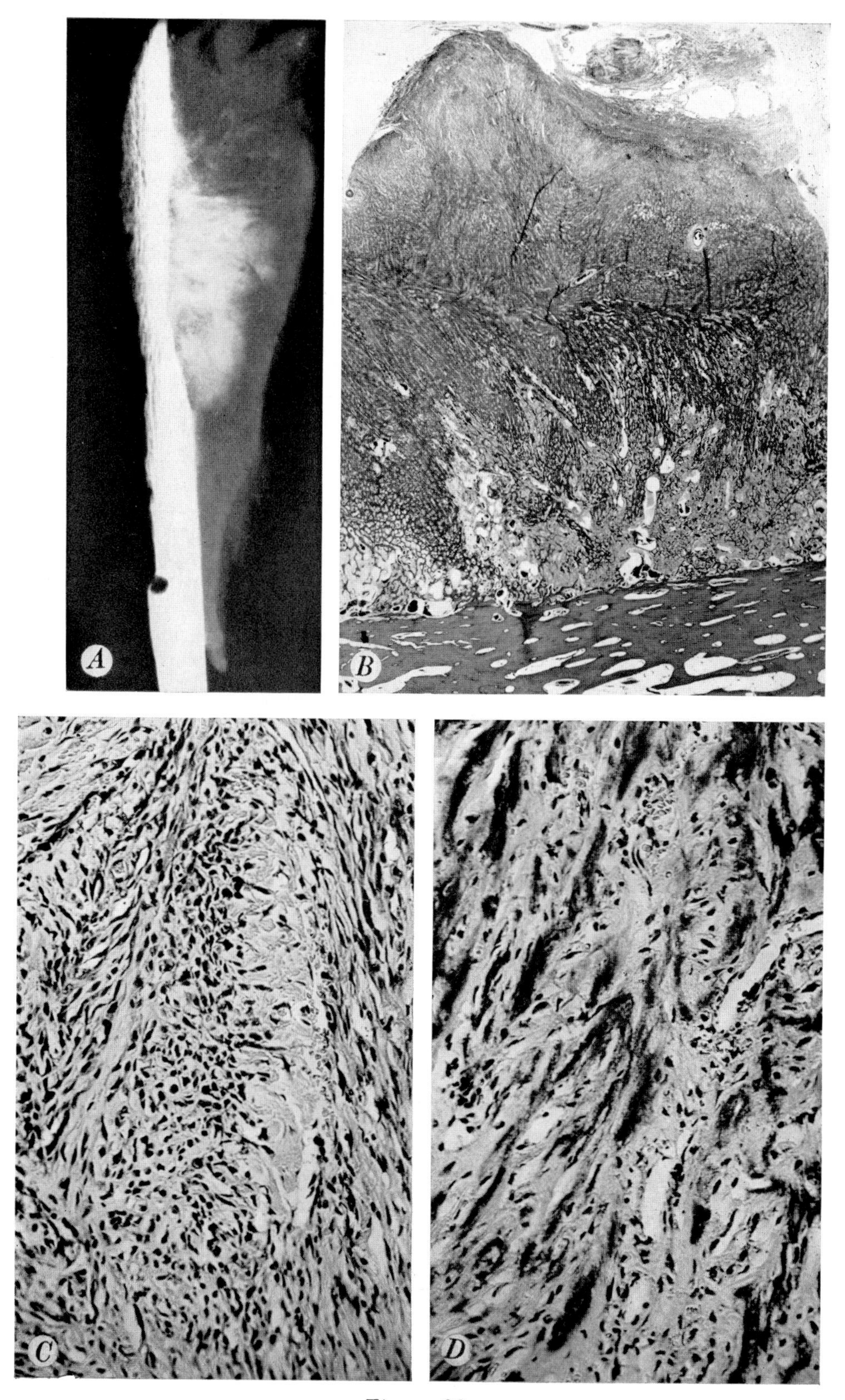


*Figure 90*

several cases in which the condition developed after injury to the thigh in the course of playing football or engaging in some other very strenuous sport activity. Similarly to that of a focus of myositis ossificans starting in the soft parts away from the bone, the $x$-ray shadow of the lesional area 2 or 3 weeks after the trauma is very faint. Subsequently the shadow becomes more and more radiopaque, and it reaches its maximum size within a period of 2 or 3 months. At that stage the radiopaque shadow is likely to have a stratified or lamellated appearance sufficiently peculiar to distinguish it from the picture of a juxtacortical osteogenic sarcoma. Also distinguishing this "post-traumatic periosteoma" from juxtacortical osteogenic sarcoma is the fact that in a matter of a few months more the lesional area gradually decreases in size, becomes more compact, and eventually amalgamates even more completely with the regional cortex. In these cases, too, should tissue be removed from the lesional area within 2 or 3 weeks after the trauma, the histologic tissue pattern might appear ominous, and specifically might make one think that one was dealing with an osteogenic sarcoma. On the other hand, if tissue is removed from the lesion after it has reached its maturity, histologic examination shows that it consists of trabeculæ of new bone well organized peripherally and that it is no longer likely to show much or even any proliferating spindle cell stroma in which osteoid and cartilage are being laid down.

**Osteochondroma.**—There are really very few cases in which there is reason for miscalling a juxtacortical osteogenic sarcoma an osteochondroma, or vice versa. The roentgenographic appearances of both these lesions are nearly always sufficiently distinctive to allow for a differentiation. It is apparently the finding of some cartilage in connection with a juxtacortical osteogenic sarcoma that occasionally leads the pathologist to interpret the lesion as an osteochondroma, albeit a peculiar one. In this connection it should be noted that a juxtacortical osteogenic sarcoma, while it may show some sparse cartilage areas near the periphery, never

***Figure 91***

*A*, Roentgenograph showing the characteristic appearance of a focus of myositis ossificans in the soft tissues of an arm of a boy 12 years of age. About 6 weeks before this picture was taken, he had suffered a severe blow to the arm, which swelled immediately and soon showed local discoloration of the skin. Note the lobulation and clear-cut delineation of the ossified myositic focus.

*B*, Roentgenograph showing part of a femur of a man 26 years of age presenting a post-traumatic periosteoma. The man had suffered an injury to his thigh while playing football about 5 months before this picture was taken. Note the striated and lamellated radiopaque mass adherent to the femur. At the time of the injury there must have been hemorrhage in the vicinity of, and beneath, the periosteum. These post-traumatic periosteomas are characterized by the fact that, after reaching their maximum development in the course of 5 or 6 weeks, they tend to become smaller and more intimately amalgamated with the cortex.

*C*, Roentgenograph of a very large, stalked, densely radiopaque lesion springing from a femur and apparently representing a large osteochondroma containing considerable calcified cartilage. The patient was a boy 19 years of age who had been aware of the presence of a mass in the thigh for about 9 years. The $x$-ray picture might have made one suspect that the lesion was a juxtacortical osteogenic sarcoma. However, on the basis of histologic examination, there could be no confusion with juxtacortical osteogenic sarcoma, since no spindle connective-tissue stroma was present anywhere in the lesional tissue.

*D*, Roentgenograph of a finger of a woman 30 years of age who, for some months, had been aware of some pain and swelling of the area. The tissue removed from the lesional area showed a fully malignant bone-forming connective-tissue sarcoma. The problem of differentiation here is whether the sarcomatous lesion in question is to be interpreted as a juxtacortical osteogenic sarcoma or as a soft-tissue osteogenic sarcoma which has become adherent to the cortex because it was growing in a confined space.

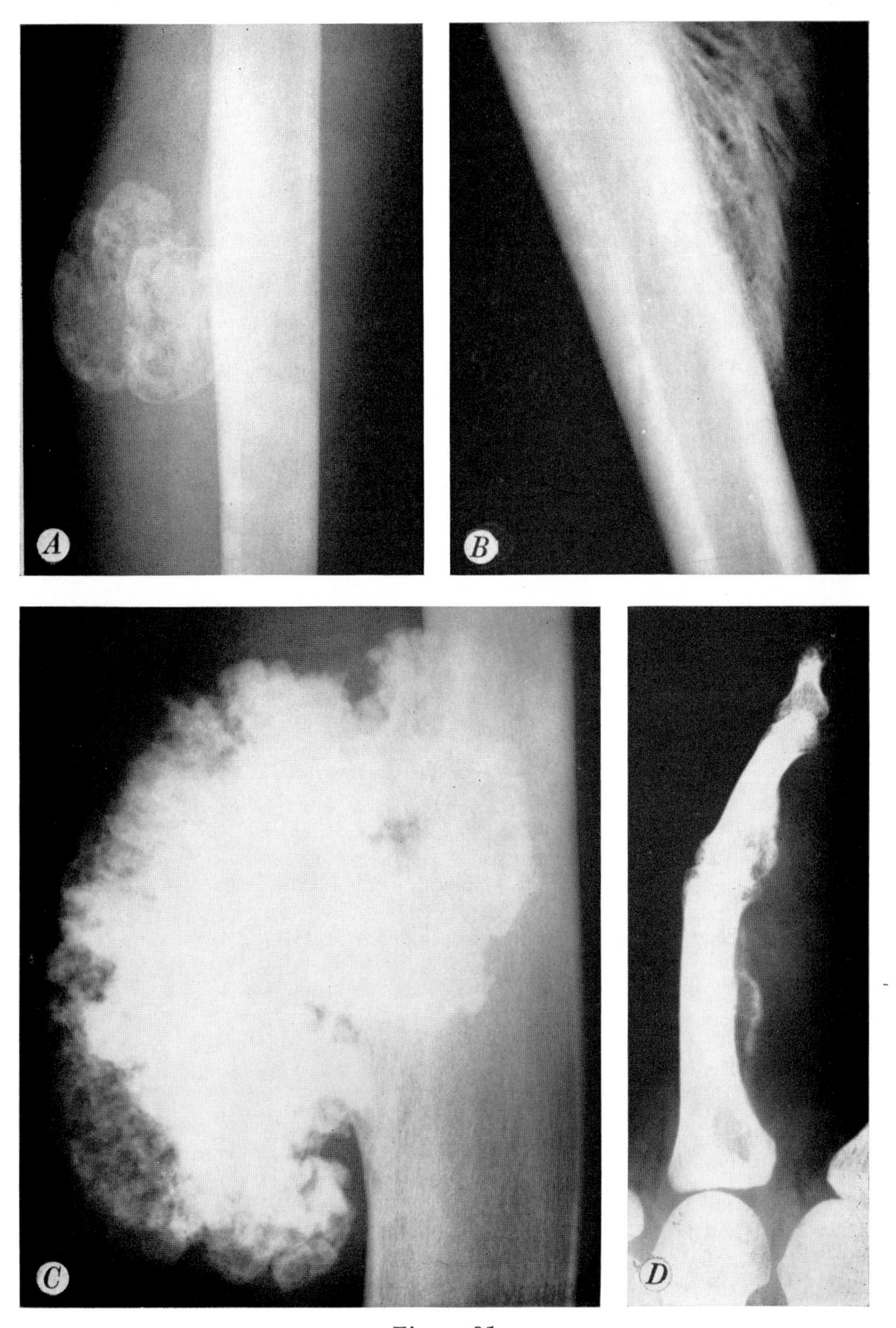


*Figure 91*

presents anything like a clear-cut cartilage cap such as an osteochondroma is likely to show. On the other hand, an osteochondroma (osteocartilaginous exostosis) never presents, anywhere in the lesional tissue, the spindle cell fibrosarcomatous stroma which one can always find in a juxtacortical osteogenic sarcoma even of low malignity. Be that as it may, an osteochondroma which is large and contains considerable amounts of calcified cartilage in its interior might raise the question of differentiation because of the dense radiopaque shadow it casts. However, in such an osteochondroma, too, one fails to find any spindle cell fibrosarcomatous stroma.

**Extraskeletal Osteogenic Sarcoma.**—Fully malignant connective-tissue sarcomas forming cartilage, osteoid, and osseous tissue are sometimes encountered in the soft parts of a limb (see Umiker and Jaffe, and Fine and Stout). In muscular areas these osteogenic sarcomas are not attached to the regional bone and hence offer no possibility of confusion with juxtacortical osteogenic sarcoma. The problem of classification does come up in the occasional instances in which a bone-forming connective-tissue sarcoma is found in the soft parts adjacent to a phalanx, metacarpal, or metatarsal bone—that is, a bone normally having relatively little soft tissue around it. In these cases the sarcoma is growing in a confined space and is usually found adherent to the bone, and it may be impossible to decide either from the *x*-ray picture or from the actual anatomic findings whether the lesion ought to be interpreted as a fully malignant juxtacortical osteogenic sarcoma or a soft-tissue osteogenic sarcoma which has become adherent to the neighboring bone. Fortunately, of course, the distinction here is not of great practical importance.

## TREATMENT

In principle, the treatment for juxtacortical osteogenic sarcoma is amputation of the affected part. The urgency of amputation depends on whether the lesion is initially of high malignancy or of low malignancy. In cases of high malignancy (about 25 per cent), the amputation should be undertaken as soon as possible after the diagnosis has been established. Even if this is done fairly promptly, the ultimate prognosis in these cases is not very good. In the cases of low malignancy, the question of whether the amputation should be done promptly depends upon the practical possibility of carrying out a radical local resection of the lesion. Unfortunately, in regard to the most common location of the lesion—at the lower end of the femur—a complete local excision is seldom feasible and early amputation is indicated.

In any case in which local excision rather than an amputation is attempted, the excision should be made *en bloc*, should include not only the tumor, but also adherent overlying soft parts and the underlying cortex, and should give the lesion itself a wide berth. If, for one reason or another, the excision is incomplete, a recurrence is to be expected within some months and certainly within a year. When there has been a recurrence, there is no longer much chance of eradicating the lesion by local excision. Now amputation is unavoidable, but the prognosis as to survival is still not too bad. In some cases, cures have been obtained by amputation even after 2 or 3 successive attempts at local excision of the tumor had failed to bring this about, though the prognosis worsens with delay.

### REFERENCES

Chambers, T. R.: Myositis Ossificans: Another Unusual Case, Arch. Surg., *16*, 755, 1928.

Dwinnell, L. A., Dahlin, D. C., and Ghormley, R. K.: Parosteal (Juxtacortical) Osteogenic Sarcoma, J. Bone & Joint Surg., *36-A*, 732, 1954.

Ewing, J.: Review of the Classification of Bone Tumors, Surg., Gynec. & Obst., *68*, 971, 1939.
Fine, G., and Stout, A. P.: Osteogenic Sarcoma of the Extraskeletal Soft Tissues, Cancer, *9*, 1027, 1956.
Geschickter, C. F., and Copeland, M. M.: Parosteal Osteoma of Bone, Ann. Surg., *133*, 790, 1951.
Hatcher, C. H.: Extra-Skeletal Ossification Simulating Sarcoma, J. Bone & Joint Surg., *29*, 542, 1947. (Also personal communication.)
Jaffe, H. L., and Selin, G.: Tumors of Bones and Joints, Bull. New York Acad. Med., *27*, 165, 1951. (See p. 169.)
Paul, J. R.: An Unusual Case of Myositis Ossificans, Arch. Surg., *10*, 185, 1925.
Umiker, W., and Jaffe, H. L.: Ossifying Fibrosarcoma (Extraskeletal Osteogenic Sarcoma) of Thigh Muscle, Ann. Surg., *138*, 795, 1953.

Chapter

# 19

# Desmoplastic Fibroma and Fibrosarcoma

THIS chapter is devoted to those central tumors of bone which are composed of fibroblasts or derived from fibroblasts. On the basis of their histologic characteristics, these connective-tissue growths can be separated into two main categories. One category comprises the small group of cases in which the growth is essentially benign. This group is being discussed under the name of *desmoplastic fibroma of bone.* In these cases the fibroblasts of the lesional tissue are almost uniformly small and mononuclear, and the intercellular substance tends to be considerable in amount and highly collagenous in many places. The reasons for calling the lesion in these cases a "desmoplastic fibroma" are given below.

The cases discussed under the heading of *fibrosarcoma of bone* constitute the other category—a much larger one. The cases in this category exhibit a wide range in respect to histologic pattern and aggressiveness. In this connection the fibrosarcomas of bone (like the fibrosarcomas of soft parts) fall roughly into two histologic subdivisions—the *well differentiated* fibrosarcomas and the *poorly differentiated* fibrosarcomas, the latter group including some lesions which are frankly *anaplastic* fibrosarcomas. In a well differentiated fibrosarcoma the tumor cells are still readily identifiable as fibroblasts, but they are much larger than ordinary adult fibroblasts. Though no mitotic figures or relatively few are seen, the microscopic tissue pattern as a whole nevertheless has a sarcomatous aura. In a poorly differentiated fibrosarcoma the lesional tissue shows considerable cellularity, variation in cell size, some nuclear hyperchromatism, and more than an occasional mitotic figure. In the anaplastic examples one is likely to find considerable pleomorphism of the cells (including the presence of sarcoma giant cells) and numerous mitotic figures. Indeed, in such a lesion some tissue areas may appear so anaplastic that they are not easily identifiable as representing a fibrosarcoma at all. In general, also, the clinical behavior of the fibrosarcomas of bone is in harmony with the histologic pattern, the highly anaplastic ones almost invariably metastasizing within a short time.

## DESMOPLASTIC FIBROMA

As already indicated, the term "desmoplastic fibroma of bone" is being used to denote an uncommon benign tumor composed of small fibroblasts in a setting of abundant intercellular material which tends to be rich in collagen fibers. Since the condition seems not to have been discussed as an entity, it is difficult to single out relevant cases in the literature on the bone tumors. In formulating the name "desmoplastic fibroma" for the lesion, the writer wished primarily to indicate the densely fibrous character of the lesional tissue, which makes it resemble the familiar desmoid tumor of the abdominal wall. At the same time it was felt that the qualifying term "desmoplastic" would clearly set the lesion off from "non-ossifying fibroma" of bone (p. 83) and from "chondromyxoid fibroma" of bone (p. 203), whose names likewise include the term "fibroma."

## CLINICAL CONSIDERATIONS

**Incidence and Location.**—In the 5 cases from which the concept of desmoplastic fibroma was evolved, the patients were 9, 10, 19, 21, and 40 years of age, respectively. As to sex, 3 were females and 2 were males. The lesion was in the tibia in 3 cases, the femur in 1, and the scapula in 1. In regard to the cases in which the lesion was in a long bone, it was located at one end of the shaft in 3 and in the mid-shaft area in 1. In none of the cases did the lesion extend into the actual epiphysial end of the bone. In the case in which the lesion was in a scapula, it was located in the vicinity of the glenoid fossa and axillary border of the bone.

**Clinical Complaints.**—The typical history is that there has been slight local functional disability for at least a number of months. This is usually associated with some swelling and mild pain referable to the affected part. Though trauma was mentioned in some of the case histories, there was no case in which it could be established that trauma had a causal relation to the lesion. Indeed, in the cases in which trauma was mentioned, the patients already had local complaints before it occurred

**Roentgenographic Findings.**—In an affected long bone, the lesion is likely to be found at or near the end of the shaft, and within the interior of the bone rather than eccentrically located. In any case, the lesion tends to be already rather large when its presence is discovered. A centrally located lesion in a long bone is likely to present a more or less trabeculated or honeycombed appearance. Also, one can expect to find the contour of the bone in the affected area somewhat expanded and the cortex thinned from the medullary side. If the lesion is located eccentrically in a long bone, the contour of the area likewise tends to be expanded. In harmony with the fact that the fibrous tumor tissue does not undergo osseous metaplasia, the lesional tissue *per se* casts a relatively radiolucent shadow. In some cases, furthermore, the bone about the periphery of the tumor area is thickened so that there is a more or less clearly delimited marginal zone of radiopacity. (See Fig. 92.)

## PATHOLOGIC FINDINGS

**Gross Pathology.**—In connection with desmoplastic fibroma, it is usually only curettements from the lesion that are available for gross examination. The lesional tissue is whitish or grayish white and of a firm and almost rubbery consistency. It is plainly tough, collagenous fibrous tissue which is devoid of grittiness except possibly in some of the tissue fragments coming from the periphery. Furthermore, the lesional tissue may show here and there an occasional tiny fluid-filled locule where it has undergone cystic softening.

On the basis of the gross appearance alone, it might be difficult to distinguish between a desmoplastic fibroma and certain well differentiated fibrosarcomas of low malignancy. In the latter, too, the tissue is likely to appear whitish, tough, and fibrous, and the decision as to whether one is dealing with a desmoplastic fibroma or with such a well differentiated fibrosarcoma has to be made on the basis of the histologic findings. On the other hand, the tissue of a desmoplastic fibroma is usually easy to distinguish grossly from that of a non-ossifying fibroma. The lesional tissue of the latter is brownish or yellowish brown and altogether does not suggest collagenous fibrous tissue. To distinguish grossly between a desmoplastic fibroma and a chondromyxoid fibroma of bone is somewhat more of a problem.

It is true that tissue from the latter lesion likewise tends to be whitish and firm, but even in the gross it has a cartilaginous aura about it rather than the appearance of collagenous fibrous tissue.

**Microscopic Pathology.**—In respect to cellularity, there may be a good deal of variation from lesion to lesion and even within different areas of the same lesion. Whether sparse or fairly numerous in a given tissue field, the fibroblasts tend to be consistently small, their cytoplasm merging with the intercellular collagen fibers. In some tissue sections of the lesion, the cells may appear evenly distributed, while in others they may be compacted here and there and may present a whorled pattern. In any event, the cell nuclei are oval and are not rich in chromatin. The amount and the arrangement of the intercellular collagen may likewise vary considerably in different areas even of the same lesion. In many places the collagen is present in the form of thick, wavy and interlacing bundles. Indeed, here and there the collagen may be so abundant that only sparse fibroblasts are seen and those present are found squeezed between the collagen bundles (see Fig. 93).

The smallness of the fibroblasts and the absence of mitotic division figures attest to the essential benignity of the lesion. It is true that in one case studied by the writer, incomplete removal of the lesional tissue was followed on two occasions by recurrences. However, it is noteworthy that in the recurrences the tissue did not as yet show the more ominous histologic pattern of even a well differentiated fibrosarcoma.

## DIFFERENTIAL DIAGNOSIS

The problems of differential diagnosis relating to desmoplastic fibroma of bone are readily resolved on a histologic basis. A *well differentiated fibrosarcoma* of low malignancy may simulate a desmoplastic fibroma in its *x*-ray picture and even in

***Figure 92***

*A*, Roentgenograph of a lesion in the upper part of a tibial shaft, established by tissue examination as a desmoplastic fibroma. In respect to location and general appearance, this *x*-ray picture might well be interpreted as representing a bone cyst. Actually, however, the lesional area was filled with firm, grayish white collagenous fibrous tissue devoid of any grittiness. (See Fig. 93-*A* for the histologic pattern of the tissue removed from this lesion.) The patient was a girl 9 years of age who was admitted to the hospital because of local pain and a limp of about 3 months' duration.

*B*, Roentgenograph of a lesion in the midshaft area of a tibia, whose nature as a desmoplastic fibroma again could be determined only from tissue examination. The lesional area presents as a rather nondescript focus of patchy radiolucency, such as might be produced by any of several different lesions. The patient was a girl 10 years of age who had been complaining for some months of mild disability referable to the tibia. Curettage of the lesion was followed by a recurrence, and a second curettage by another recurrence, but a third curettage was successful in eradicating the condition. In the course of the recurrences over a period of 6 years, there was no change in the histologic appearance of the lesional tissue.

*C*, Roentgenograph of a rather eccentrically located desmoplastic fibroma involving the lower part of a femoral shaft. The lesional area is radiolucent on the whole, but heavily marginated. The patient was a man 21 years of age in whom the presence of the lesion was discovered incidentally when the leg was *x*-rayed in connection with an accident.

*D*, Roentgenograph of a trabeculated, spottily radiolucent but heavily marginated lesion in a scapula, which represents a desmoplastic fibroma. (When the writer originally studied this lesion, he interpreted it as a well differentiated fibrosarcoma, and the case was reported by Burton under this designation.) Its histologic tissue pattern is shown in Fig. 93-*C*. The patient was a woman 40 years of age whose principal complaint on admission to our hospital was of a slight swelling in the left shoulder region of 1 year's standing.

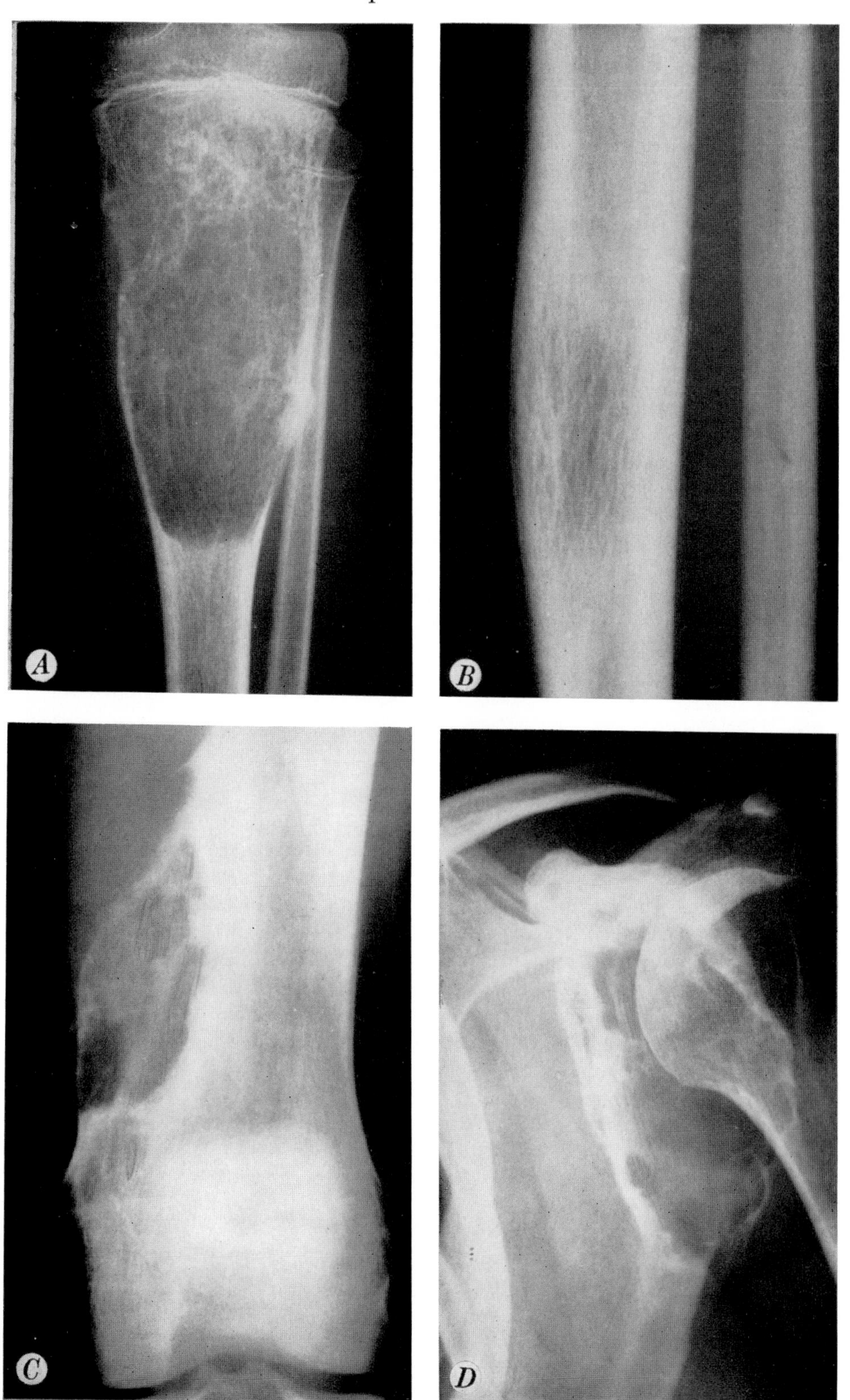


*Figure* 92

the gross appearance of its lesional tissue (Fig. 95-*A*), and the distinction has to be made on the basis of the histologic appearance of the lesional fibroblasts. If their nuclei are relatively large and plump, the lesion is to be designated as a well differentiated fibrosarcoma rather than as a desmoplastic fibroma.

There is little reason for confusing a *non-ossifying fibroma* (p. 83) with a desmoplastic fibroma. The roentgenographic appearance of the two conditions is generally quite different and so, as already indicated, is the gross appearance of the lesional tissue. Histologically, the non-ossifying fibroma presents, in typical and unmodified areas, the pattern of whorled bundles of small spindle-shaped cells, among which are dispersed some small, often elongated, multinuclear giant cells. Also, in some lesions or lesional areas one can observe foam cells containing cholesterol and/or some cells containing hemosiderin pigment. Altogether, the histologic pattern of a non-ossifying fibroma is such that it is more likely to be confused with that of a giant-cell tumor than with that of a desmoplastic fibroma.

In regard to *chondromyxoid fibroma* of bone (p. 203), the *x*-ray picture cannot be depended upon in connection with the differential diagnosis. Grossly, the tissue of a chondromyxoid fibroma does tend to be whitish and firm, though, as already indicated, it does not have the appearance of collagenous fibrous tissue. Microscopically, the characteristic tissue of the chondromyxoid fibroma varies widely, but in none of its forms does it suggest at all the histologic pattern of a desmoplastic fibroma.

Finally, it should be pointed out that even in an occasional lesion representing a solitary focus of *fibrous dysplasia* (p. 126) one may encounter large tissue areas in which the pattern is that of highly collagenous fibrous tissue. However, in other tissue areas from the lesion, the pattern will be that of loose connective-tissue cells in which a good deal of metaplastic ossification is taking place, and this evidence of osteogenesis directs the diagnosis toward fibrous dysplasia.

## TREATMENT

The treatment appropriate for a desmoplastic fibroma is thorough curettage of the lesional area or, even better, segmental resection of the affected bone part if that is feasible. Indeed, in the course of the intervention, the gross character of the lesional tissue is likely to suggest to the surgeon that he is dealing with a benign rather than a malignant lesion. If a segmental resection has been done, a recurrence is not to be expected. If a mere curettage has been carried out, and if this has been incomplete, there is a possibility of recurrence. Even if this does take place, however, an amputation is not indicated if there is no doubt about the correctness of the original histologic diagnosis. Under these circumstances, the second intervention should be merely a segmental resection or a more thorough curettage.

### *Figure 93*

*A*, Photomicrograph (× 125) showing the basic tissue pattern of the desmoplastic fibroma. The tissue represented came from the lesion illustrated in Fig. 92-*A*. Note the small size of the fibroblasts and the thick, wavy bundles of collagen fibers.

*B*, Photomicrograph (× 125) of a more cellular tissue field from the lesion whose basic tissue pattern was shown in *A*. Note again the small size of the fibroblasts.

*C*, Photomicrograph (× 125) illustrating the histologic appearance of a desmoplastic fibroma which was much more heavily collagenous throughout than the one shown in *A*. The tissue illustrated comes from the lesion represented in Fig. 92-*D*.

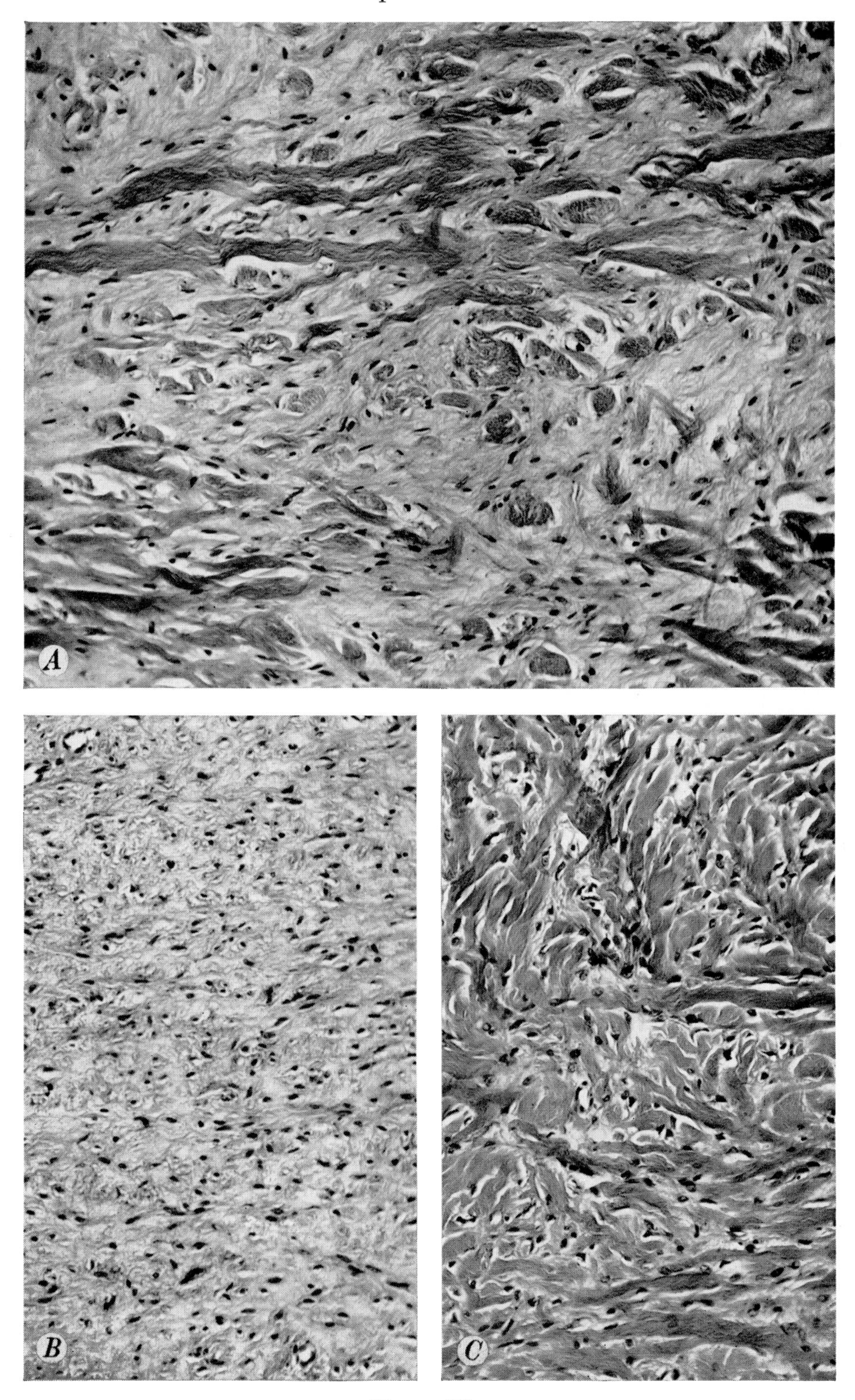


*Figure* 93

## FIBROSARCOMA

A fibrosarcoma of bone may be defined as a fibroblastic connective-tissue sarcoma which starts its development endosteally—that is, in the interior of the affected bone part. As already indicated, there is a certain amount of variety in the histologic pattern of the fibrosarcomas of bone. As also pointed out, however, they can be placed in two general groups—the *well differentiated* and the *poorly differentiated* fibrosarcomas, and among the latter there are some which are so poorly differentiated as to be frankly *anaplastic* fibrosarcomas.

Here we shall deal only with the "primary" fibrosarcomas of bone. That is, we are not concerned here with soft-tissue fibrosarcomas which have broken into the neighboring bone nor with so-called periosteal or parosteal fibrosarcomas which likewise may invade the bone secondarily (p. 503). Also, we shall not consider here the occasional instance of a fibrosarcoma appearing in a bone which is the site of Paget's disease (p. 463) or of fibrous dysplasia (p. 134) or one appearing at a bone site which has been damaged by radiation therapy (p. 479). In passing, it may also be noted that Steiner has reported an instance of fibrosarcoma widely distributed over the skeleton. He conceded that the condition might have been engrafted upon Paget's disease, though he favored the opinion that it represented primary fibrosarcoma appearing simultaneously in many bone sites.

Fibrosarcoma of bone has been slow in gaining recognition as a bone tumor entity. Indeed, until recently it has not been given independent status in classifications of the bone tumors. There can be no doubt that, in the past, lesions actually representing endosteal fibrosarcomas were usually interpreted as osteogenic sarcomas whose inherent capacity to form tumor osteoid and osseous tissue was not being manifested. However, the writer prefers to restrict the term "osteogenic sarcoma" to those malignant connective-tissue sarcomas which actually form neoplastic osteoid and osseous tissue in the course of their evolution. Thus he holds with Hodges, Phemister, and Brunschwig (in contrast to Stout and others) that a fibroblastic connective-tissue sarcoma of bone which evolves *without* laying down neoplastic osteoid or osseous tissue either at the original site of the growth or in its metastases represents a fibrosarcoma rather than an osteogenic sarcoma of bone.

### *Figure 94*

*A*. Roentgenograph showing a well differentiated fibrosarcoma in the lower end of a tibia. The lesion could be thus identified only on the basis of its histologic tissue pattern (see Fig. 96-*A*). The patient was a youth 19 years of age, and the clinical complaints were meager.

*B*, Roentgenograph of a lesion in the upper part of the shaft of a humerus of a boy 9 years of age which turned out to be a poorly differentiated fibrosarcoma (see Fig. 96-*B*). On the basis of the age of the patient, location of the lesion, and general pattern of the *x*-ray picture, one might easily have thought that the lesion was a solitary bone cyst. Actually, the entire lesional area was occupied by tissue which was grayish white in some places or hemorrhagically discolored in others.

*C*, Roentgenograph showing a mottled area of destruction in the upper end of a tibia, produced by a poorly differentiated and rather anaplastic fibrosarcoma. (The photograph of the amputation specimen in this case is shown in Fig 95-*D*, and the histologic pattern of the lesional tissue in Fig. 97-*A*.) The patient was a boy 16 years of age who had noted pain in the leg for about 6 months and local swelling for about 2 months. He died of pulmonary metastases 16 months after the limb was amputated. Histologic examination of numerous metastatic pulmonary foci failed to reveal any evidence of osteogenesis in the tumor tissue.

*D*, Roentgenograph showing striking lytic destruction in the upper end of a femoral shaft, wrought by a rather highly anaplastic fibrosarcoma in a man 53 years of age.

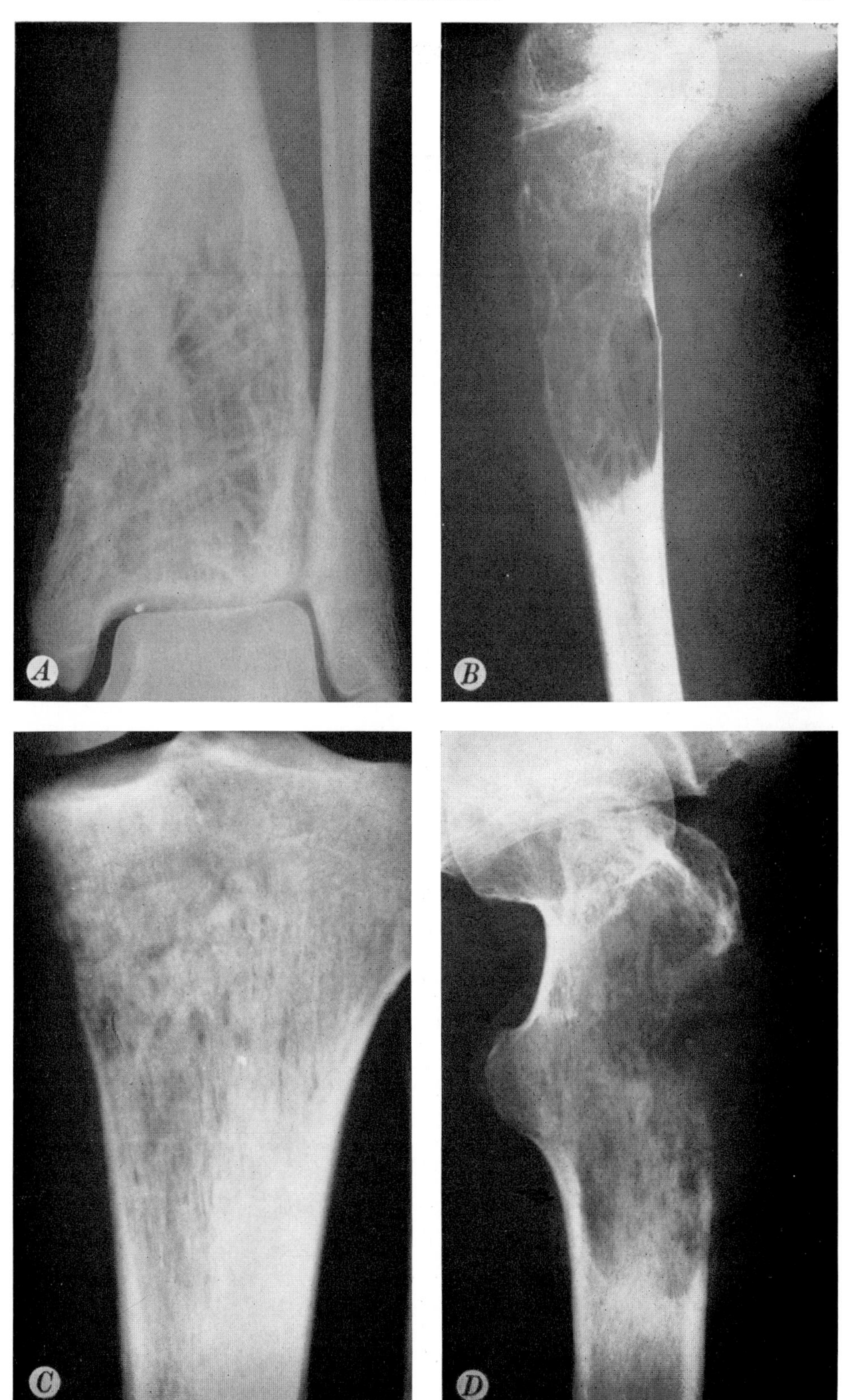


*Figure 94*

Clinically, too, there are differences between these two tumor entities, since, with the exception of the anaplastic fibrosarcomas, the fibrosarcomas of bone run a much more favorable course than the osteogenic sarcomas.

## CLINICAL CONSIDERATIONS

**Incidence and Location.**—The fibrosarcomas of bone in general are not very common. Certainly they are encountered much less frequently than are the osteogenic sarcomas or chondrosarcomas of bone. The age range of the patients is rather wide. However, in most of the cases studied by the writer, the patients were young or middle-aged adults. Among these cases, males predominated over females in the proportion of about 2 to 1, but of course this difference may not be borne out by additional data. It is clear that like most other primary tumors involving bones, the fibrosarcoma strongly predilects the femur and tibia. In the writer's cases, when the lesion did not affect one of these bones, it was more often in some other long bone than in a bone of another kind. When involving a long bone, the tumor was usually oriented toward one end of the shaft and sometimes also extended into the actual end of the bone.

**Clinical Complaints and Course.**—Pain is almost always the presenting and cardinal complaint. Often this is relatively mild at first, but it tends to increase in severity. On the whole, one can say that the pain is likely to have been present for a shorter time and to be more troublesome in the cases in which the fibrosarcoma is of the poorly differentiated or wholly anaplastic type than in the cases in which it is well differentiated. Furthermore, in the former type of case, a definite local swelling is likely to be palpable within a month or two after the pain has first been noticed. Even in the cases in which the fibrosarcoma is well differentiated, a local swelling usually becomes palpable eventually.

Also, it seems worth noting that the patients often relate the onset of their difficulties to a local trauma. It is hard to evaluate the role of the trauma in most of these cases, since months have usually elapsed between the traumatic incident and the time when the affected part is first roentgenographed. It is very likely

### *Figure 95*

*A*, Photograph of the cut surface of an os calcis whose interior is almost completely filled by a tumor which proved to be a well differentiated fibrosarcoma. The tissue is whitish, presents a whorled pattern grossly, and was of a tough, fibrous consistency. The patient was a man 45 years of age who complained of pain in the heel for about 2 years and who also presented a local swelling. The lesion was treated by resection of the entire os calcis, and the patient has remained well and free of local recurrence for 4 years.

*B*, Photograph of a large, recurrent, but well differentiated fibrosarcoma which has broken out of the femur. The patient was a woman 28 years of age who first noted a painless swelling in the thigh about 3 years before the affected limb was amputated. About $1\frac{1}{2}$ years after the onset of her difficulty, the lesion was treated by local excision, but there was a prompt recurrence. The histologic pattern of the tissue from the amputation specimen in this case is illustrated in Fig. 97-*C*.

*C*, Photograph showing a fibrosarcoma which has developed in a metacarpal bone and has broken out of the bone. Histologically, the fibrosarcoma in this case was poorly differentiated and moderately anaplastic, but the patient was cured by the amputation.

*D*, Photograph of the cut surface of a tibia involved by a poorly differentiated and anaplastic fibrosarcoma. Note the tumor tissue in the interior of the bone, and the fact that this tissue has also extended through the cortex. The specimen in question relates to the case whose *x*-ray picture is illustrated in Fig. 94-*C*, and the general histologic pattern of the lesional tissue is shown in Fig. 97-*A*.

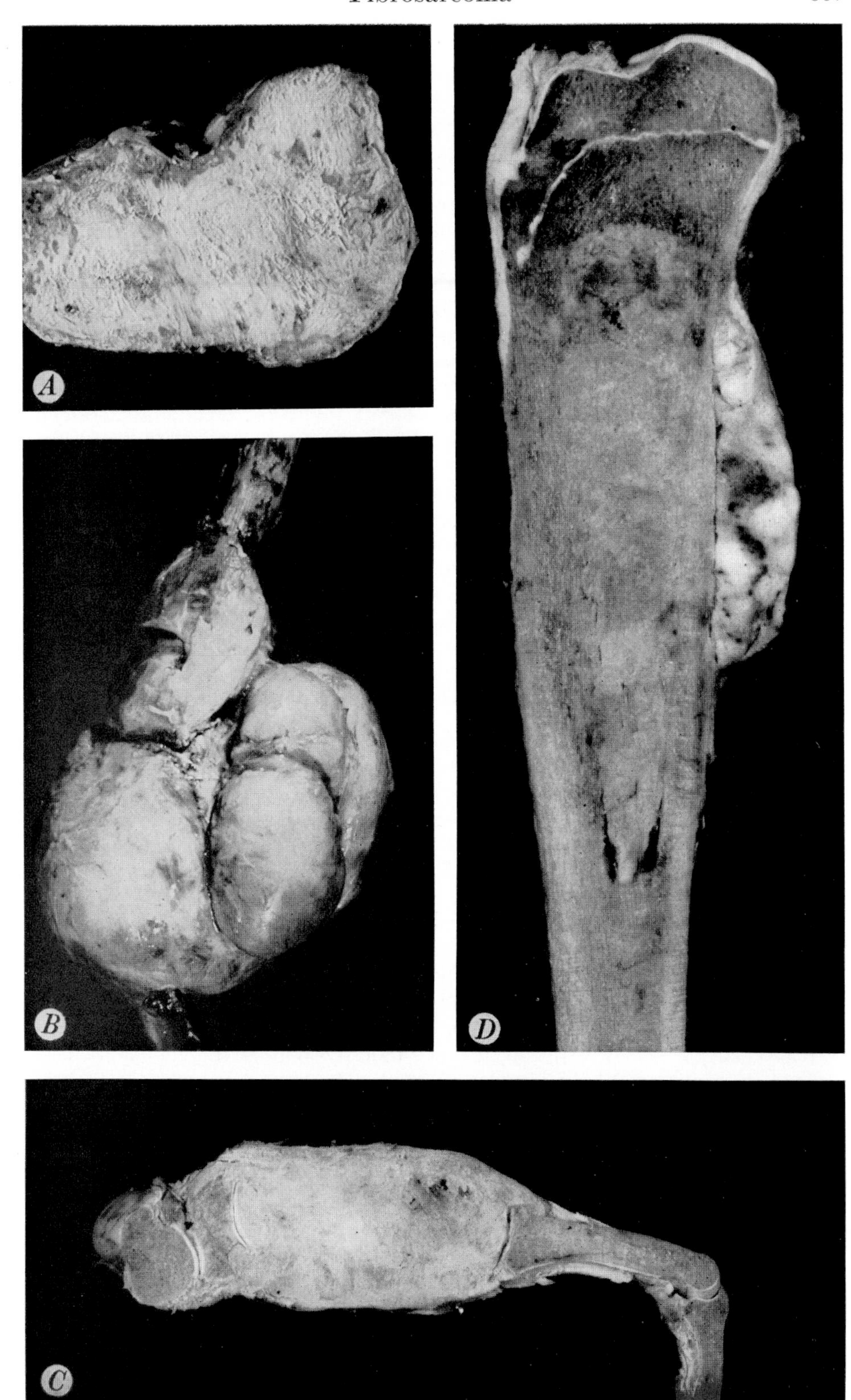


*Figure* **95**

that in most of the cases giving a history of trauma, the presence of the tumor would already have been evident if an *x*-ray picture had been taken promptly. Indeed, in one case studied, the patient had suffered a fracture through the lower end of a tibia, and had the *x*-ray picture which was taken immediately been properly evaluated, it would have led to the conclusion that the fracture was a pathologic fracture occurring through the site of a tumor, and that the trauma had nothing to do with the onset of the tumor.

The clinical course run in cases of fibrosarcoma of bone is quite variable. In some few cases the tumor is of high malignancy, tending to break out of the bone rapidly and to metastasize early. In these cases the clinical course does not differ from the course ordinarily run by an osteogenic sarcoma. Much more often one encounters fibrosarcomas of much lower malignancy, as manifested by slowness in breaking out of the bone and metastasizing. Indeed, some fibrosarcomas of low malignancy fail to metastasize for years even after several attempts at local excision have been followed by recurrences. As already indicated, there is a good deal of correspondence between the clinical course of the condition and the cytology of the tumor tissue. The fibrosarcomas of highest malignancy are usually very poorly differentiated or frankly anaplastic tumors, while those of low malignancy are usually well differentiated tumors. However, in a particular case there is sometimes a certain incongruity between the cytologic appearance and the clinical behavior of the tumor. Notably in a case in which the tumor tissue is poorly differentiated though not frankly anaplastic, the clinical course may be more favorable than one would expect it to be on the basis of the cytologic findings.

## ROENTGENOGRAPHIC FINDINGS

A fibrosarcoma is not infrequently found still contained within the confines of the bone at the time when the lesion is first roentgenographed. This is more likely to be the case when the fibrosarcoma is well differentiated or even poorly differentiated than when it is frankly anaplastic. In any case, while the roentgenographic picture might lead one to consider the diagnostic possibility of fibrosarcoma, this picture is on the whole so equivocal that the definitive diagnosis necessarily rests on tissue examination. (See Fig. 94.)

A fibrosarcoma developing within a bone site destroys the spongy bone in the area and thins the cortex. It also usually bulges the contour of the bone somewhat and not infrequently breaks out of the bone. The motif of the *x*-ray picture is radiolucency. This represents the fact that the lesional tissue of a fibrosarcoma shows no evidence of osteogenesis and is therefore relatively permeable to the *x*-rays. In accordance with the extent of destruction of the spongy bone and

***Figure 96***

*A*, Photomicrograph (× 125) showing the general histologic pattern of a well differentiated fibrosarcoma. The tissue represented came from the lesion illustrated in Fig. 94-*A*. Note the uniform size of the tumor fibroblasts.

*B*, Photomicrograph (× 125) showing the histologic pattern of a poorly differentiated and somewhat anaplastic fibrosarcoma. Note the irregularity in the size of the tumor cells, and the presence of some cells with multiple nuclei. The tissue represented came from the lesion illustrated in Fig. 94-*B*. On the basis of the tissue pattern shown, a disarticulation at the shoulder joint was originally advised as the appropriate treatment in this case, but was refused by the patient's family. In the course of the succeeding 9 years, there were numerous attempts to deal with the lesion by local excision, on account of repeated recurrences, and finally the lesion metastasized.

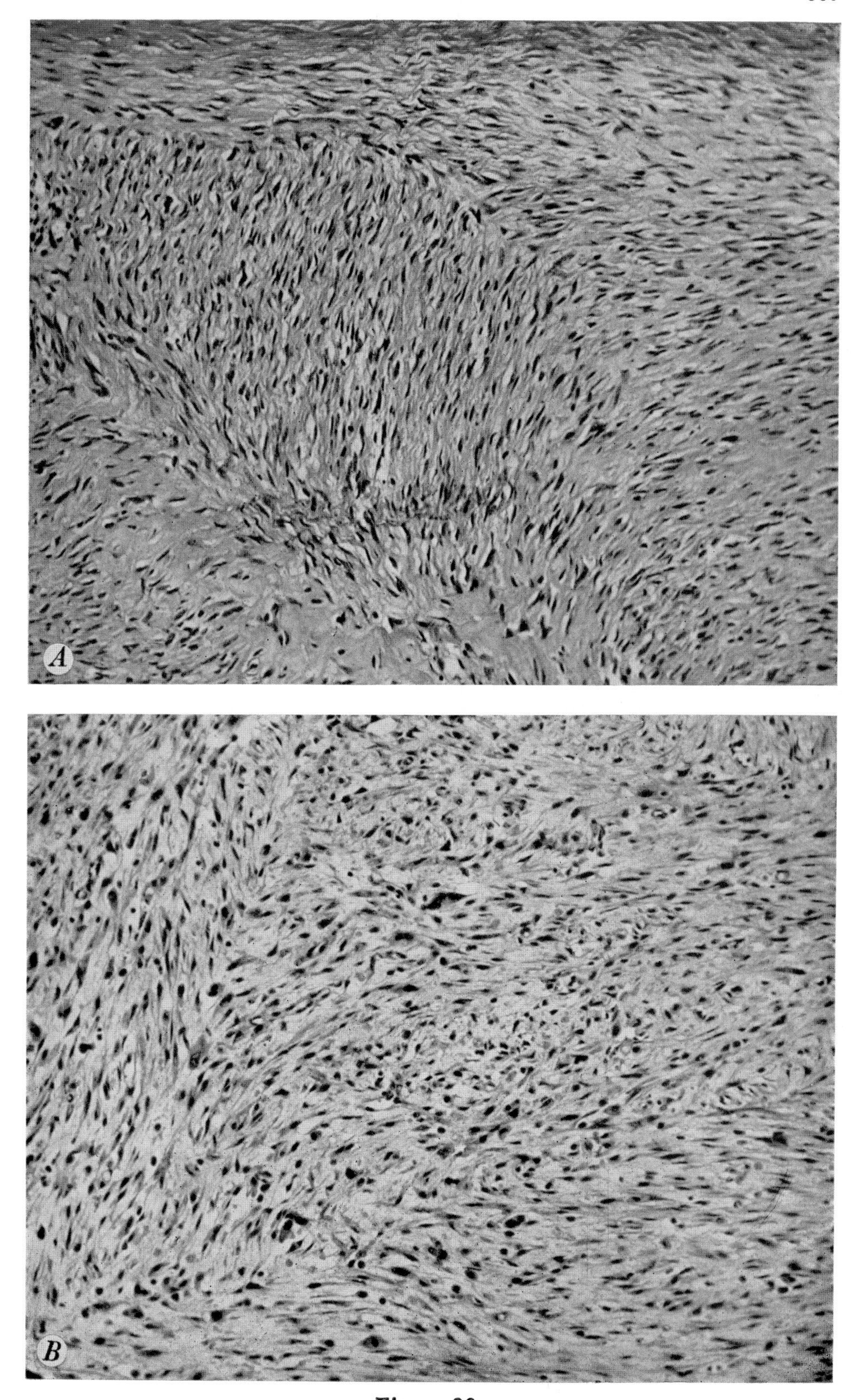


*Figure 96*

thinning and/or destruction of the cortex, the lesional area may show up as: a focus of coarsely mottled radiolucency; a focus of clear-cut multiloculated radiolucency; a smaller or larger area of more or less uniform radiolucency; or a focus of striking radiolucency associated with frank obliteration of part of the cortex. This range of variety in the *x*-ray picture can easily lead to roentgenographic misinterpretation of the lesion in one case or another as: a Ewing sarcoma, an inflammatory bone lesion, a bone cyst, a giant-cell tumor, or (if the picture is one of violent bone destruction) an "osteolytic" osteogenic sarcoma.

## PATHOLOGIC FINDINGS

**Well Differentiated Fibrosarcoma.**—The tumors in this category are lesions of low malignancy. Grossly, the tumor tissue appears grayish white and firm, and in some lesions or lesional areas it may even be rather collagenous. These tumors grow slowly and do not readily break out of the bone. If incompletely excised or merely curetted, they recur, but they tend not to undergo much change in their cytologic character and may not metastasize even after several recurrences. However, occasionally they do change their histologic character. It would seem that in the case described by Hall, Bersack, and Vitolo, the lesion was originally a well differentiated fibrosarcoma (though not a benign fibrous tumor as they thought) and that after some years it became a highly anaplastic fibrosarcoma. (See Fig. 95.)

Microscopically, in a well differentiated fibrosarcoma the fibroblasts are found to be long and spindle shaped, and the nuclei, too, are quite elongated. Some of the nuclei are likely to be rather plump, and altogether they are much larger than those of a desmoplastic fibroma. There may be a considerable amount of collagen fibers between the cells, and the cells and fibers may present the appearance of whorled and interlacing bundles. In any case, what is characteristic of the cytology of the well differentiated fibrosarcoma is a general uniformity of the cells and nuclei and the practically complete absence of mitotic figures.

In regard to microscopic differential diagnosis, a fibrosarcoma should not be considered well differentiated if it shows even moderate anaplasia of the tumor cells (some cells with multiple nuclei), striking hyperchromatism of the nuclei, or more than a rare nucleus in mitotic division. On the other hand, there may be some question, in a given case, as to whether the lesion should be interpreted as a well differentiated fibrosarcoma or as a desmoplastic fibroma. Since a well differentiated fibrosarcoma may be rather collagenous, the decision between the two lesions rests upon the size and appearance of the cells and particularly of their nuclei. On the whole, one can say that the nuclei of the fibroblasts of a well

### *Figure 97*

*A*, Photomicrograph (× 125) showing the general histologic pattern of a frankly anaplastic fibrosarcoma. The tissue represented came from the lesion illustrated in Fig. 94-*C*. Note the great irregularity in the size of the cells, and the presence of numerous tumor giant cells.

*B*, Photomicrograph (× 250) showing the histologic pattern presented by tissue from a focus of pulmonary metastasis in the case illustrated in *A*. There is even greater anaplasia in this tumor tissue than in the tumor tissue of the primary lesion in the tibia.

*C*, Photomicrograph (× 250) showing the pattern of a well differentiated fibrosarcoma, for comparison with *B*. Note the relatively uniform size of the tumor fibroblasts. The tissue represented came from the lesion illustrated in Fig. 95-*B*.

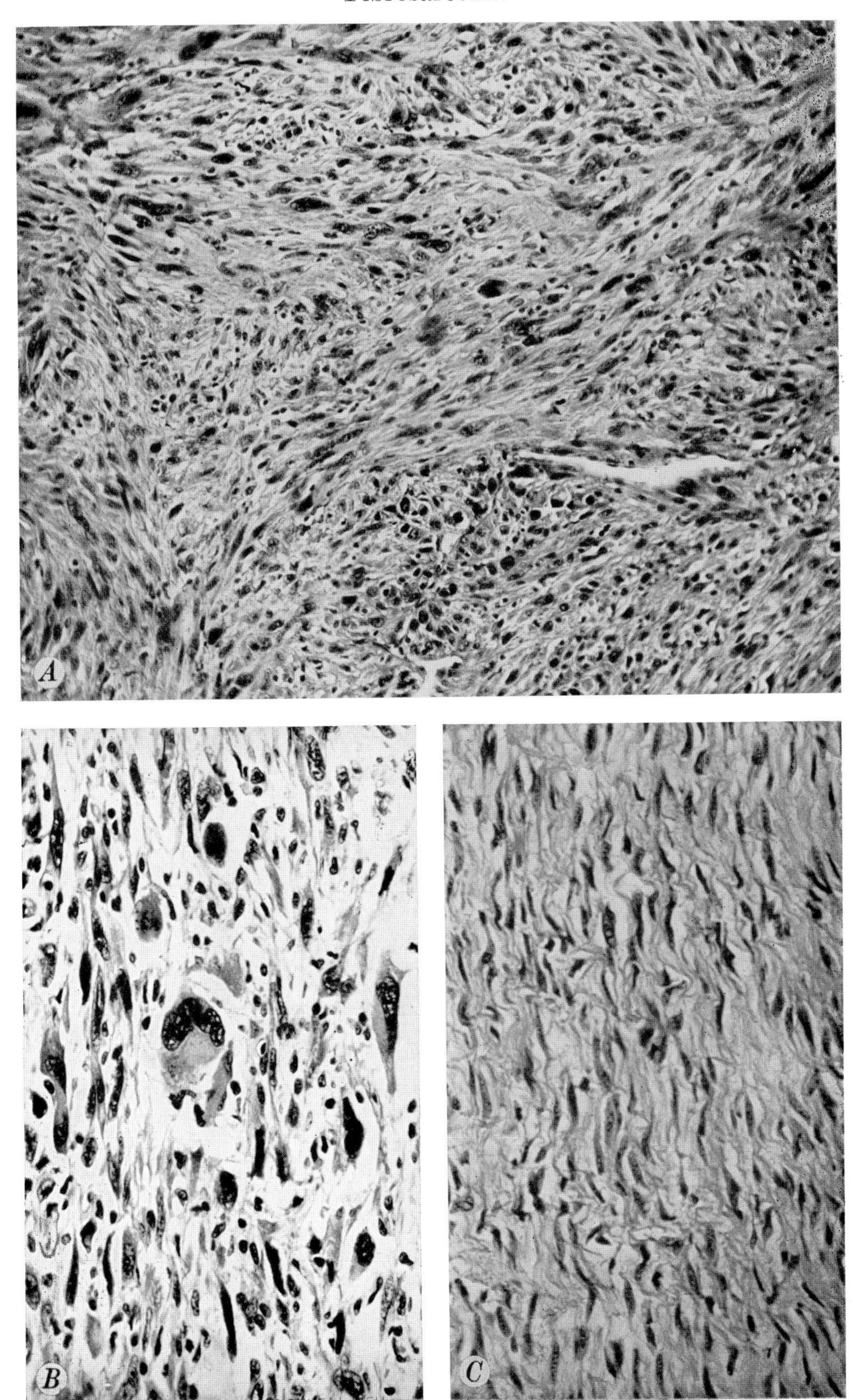


***Figure 97***

differentiated fibrosarcoma are about twice as large as those of a desmoplastic fibroma, though the cells and nuclei of the well differentiated fibrosarcoma still show no evidences of anaplasia. (See Fig. 96.)

**Poorly Differentiated Fibrosarcoma.**—Grossly, though the tumor tissue from a lesion in this category may appear whitish throughout, it usually feels softer and more cellular than the tumor tissue from a well differentiated fibrosarcoma. Also, the poorly differentiated fibrosarcomas tend to break out of the bone and to spread beyond the limits of the cortex, sometimes rather rapidly.

Histologically, these fibrosarcomas of bone are the ones which show at least some cellular atypism in their tissue pattern, and in some of them the atypism is pronounced. In particular, all of them show, to a lesser or greater extent: excessive cellularity of the lesional tissue; lack of uniformity in size of the cells; hyperchromatism of the cell nuclei; and the presence of cells with multiple and/or bizarre nuclei and of cells in mitotic division. Those among them which show considerable atypism and anaplasia along these lines generally prove, in their clinical course, to be of high malignancy, the patient dying of metastases even if an amputation is promptly done. However, a mild or moderate degree of atypism is not necessarily inconsistent with long survival and cure if the lesion is promptly and appropriately treated.

The diagnosis of a fibrosarcoma is generally made on the basis of examination of a biopsy specimen. Particularly in relation to a rather anaplastic lesion, it may be difficult to decide from the biopsy specimen whether one is dealing with a fibrosarcoma or with an extremely "osteolytic" osteogenic sarcoma which happens to show no tumor osteoid or osseous tissue in the area examined. Since in either case the lesion is a fully malignant tumor and amputation is the usual treatment when it appears in a limb bone, a detailed study of the specimen is possible to settle the question. To establish the lesion as a fibrosarcoma, ample sampling of the specimen must show the absence of osteogenesis in all tissue areas studied histologically. Those who deny the existence of fibrosarcoma of bone as a tumor entity claim that occasionally an osteogenic sarcoma fails to show evidence of osteogenesis in its primary site, but will show it in its metastases. To the writer, it seems probable that in such cases the primary lesion would have shown osteogenesis and been recognized as an osteogenic sarcoma had it been adequately sampled. (See Fig. 97.)

## TREATMENT

The appropriate treatment for fibrosarcoma is surgery, but the particular procedure suitable in a given case depends upon the histologic appearance of the lesional tissue as revealed by study of biopsy material. If the fibrosarcoma shows itself to be a poorly differentiated one, the procedure should be amputation or disarticulation in accordance with the specific location of the lesion in the affected limb bone. However, if the lesion is so poorly differentiated as to be frankly anaplastic, the patient is almost sure to succumb to metastases despite such intervention. On the other hand, a lesion which is poorly differentiated but not frankly anaplastic offers a reasonably hopeful prospect for cure by amputation or disarticulation. In regard to a well differentiated fibrosarcoma, segmental resection of the affected bone area not infrequently suffices to bring about a cure. However, in case of a recurrence, amputation should be seriously considered unless favorable local conditions permit a fresh wide excision of the tumor area. In any event, fibrosarcomas are resistant to radiation therapy, and the latter should therefore be used only as a palliative measure against a lesion in a site for which surgery is not practical.

## REFERENCES

BURTON, M. E.: Well-Differentiated Fibrosarcoma of the Scapula, Bull. Hosp. Joint Dis., *15*, 85, 1954.

GILMER, W. S., JR., and MACEWEN, G. D.: Central (Medullary) Fibrosarcoma of Bone, J. Bone & Joint Surg., *40-A*, 121, 1958.

GSCHNITZER, F., and MINERVINI, G. L.: Das zentrale Fibrosarkom des Knochens, Ztschr. f. Orthop., *87*, 76, 1955.

HALL, A., BERSACK, S. R., and VITOLO, R. E.: Fibrosarcoma Arising in an Apparently Benign Fibrous Lesion of Bone, J. Bone & Joint Surg., *37-A*, 1019, 1955.

HODGES, P. C., PHEMISTER, D. B., and BRUNSCHWIG, A.: *The Roentgen-Ray Diagnosis of Diseases of the Bones and Joints*, New York, Thomas Nelson & Sons, 1938. (See p. 181.)

JAFFE, H. L.: Tumors of the Skeletal System: Pathological Aspects, Bull. New York Acad. Med., *23*, 497, 1947.

PACK, G. T., and ARIEL, I. M.: The Desmoplastic Diathesis and its Relationship to Neoplastic Proliferation, Bull. Hosp. Joint Dis., *13*, 1, 1952.

STEINER, P. E.: Multiple Diffuse Fibrosarcoma of Bone, Am. J. Path., *20*, 877, 1944.

STOUT, A. P.: Fibrosarcoma: The Malignant Tumor of Fibroblasts, Cancer, *1*, 30, 1948.

# Chapter 20

# Chondrosarcoma

A *chondrosarcoma* may be defined as a malignant tumor originating from cartilage cells and tending to maintain its essentially cartilaginous nature throughout its evolution. This general definition is pertinent irrespective of the site of the tumor, applying as well to a skeletal as to an extraskeletal chondrosarcoma. In contrast, an osteogenic sarcoma (p. 256) issues from more primitive connective tissue, and any cartilage it may show is formed from the basic sarcomatous spindle cell connective tissue which is also forming neoplastic osteoid and osseous tissue. In addition to this histogenetic and histologic basis for making the distinction between the two lesions, there is the important clinical difference represented by the slower course usually run by chondrosarcoma, and by its generally more favorable prognosis. These various differences between the two lesions were already stressed some time ago by Phemister, and by Lichtenstein and Jaffe. Indeed, currently there seems to be no more doubt that chondrosarcoma of bone should be held apart from osteogenic sarcoma.

A chondrosarcoma which begins its development in the interior of a bone is often denoted as a *central chondrosarcoma,* and one which begins its development in relation to the surface of a bone is frequently designated as a *peripheral chondrosarcoma.* In connection with chondrosarcoma of bone, one also encounters the terms "primary" and "secondary" chondrosarcoma. These terms are intended to distinguish between a chondrosarcoma which has apparently originated *de novo* at a given bone site (*primary chondrosarcoma*) and one which has apparently developed out of a pre-existing benign cartilaginous bone lesion (*secondary chondrosarcoma*).

It is true that there may be difficulty in deciding, especially in respect to central chondrosarcoma, whether a particular lesion represents a primary or a secondary chondrosarcoma. Nevertheless, the secondary development of a central chondrosarcoma through malignant transformation of a solitary enchondroma is not at all unusual when the enchondroma is in a long tubular bone. However, it is quite exceptional when the enchondroma is in a phalanx or a metacarpal or metatarsal bone. In cases of multiple enchondromatosis the eventual appearance of a chondrosarcoma in one or another of the affected bones (including even short tubular bones) is fairly common. Analogously, in cases of hereditary multiple exostosis the emergence of a secondary peripheral chondrosarcoma in relation to one of the affected bones is also a common occurrence. On the other hand, malignant transformation of a solitary osteocartilaginous exostosis is rather rare.

Chondrosarcoma is one of the more common primary malignant tumors of bone, but only about half as common as osteogenic sarcoma. It appears that practically any bone preformed in cartilage may become the site of a chondrosarcoma. However, the long tubular bones (especially the femur) are the most common site for central chondrosarcoma. The peripheral chondrosarcomas tend to be most common in the vicinity of the hip joint (often involving an innominate bone and/or the sacrum) and in the shoulder joint region (often affecting the scapula).

A tumor may still be small and yet present all the histologic earmarks of a fully malignant chondrosarcoma. However, there are few bone tumors whose evaluation can make more exacting demands on experience and judgment than chondrosarcoma sometimes does. One may encounter a very large peripheral chondrosarcoma whose cytologic appearance arouses little if any suspicion of malignancy. The cytologic picture of an evolving central chondrosarcoma may sometimes likewise be underdiagnosed as representing a benign cartilage growth. Indeed, in such cases, only the closest attention to the cytologic details presented by lesional tissue from various areas permits one to decide that the border line from benignity to malignity has been transgressed. Furthermore, the cytologic findings in chondrosarcoma sometimes do not suggest malignancy very strongly even when the idea of malignancy is favored by the fact that the tumor is a recurrent one. In any case, large size or recurrence should be given great weight in connection with the diagnostic interpretation of the histologic picture. Altogether, in evaluating a cartilage tumor which is suspected of being a chondrosarcoma, whichever feature (pathologic or clinical) is the more sinister should be regarded as the more important.

**Nomenclature.**—In addition to what has already been indicated about the nomenclature of chondrosarcoma, there are a few supplementary points to be considered. Some chondrosarcomas (particularly the peripheral lesions) become heavily calcified and may show bone formation through metaplasia of the calcified cartilage or even through endochondral ossification. Such a lesion is sometimes designated as an "osteochondrosarcoma" or as a "chondro-osteosarcoma." These terms introduce confusion because they have also been applied to tumors which are actually osteogenic sarcomas containing considerable amounts of cartilage. The term "myxochondrosarcoma" is sometimes applied to a chondrosarcoma showing a considerable amount of mucoid degeneration of the intercellular matrix. However, in this connection as in the others, it does not seem worth while to load the nomenclature of chondrosarcoma with any qualifying terms expressing merely secondary alterations of the lesional tissue. In regard to the term "myxochondrosarcoma," a word of caution is indicated in addition. When one surveys the literature on lesions so reported, one finds that some of them do not represent chondrosarcoma at all, but rather the relatively innocuous "chondromyxoid fibroma of bone" (p. 203).

## CENTRAL CHONDROSARCOMA

As already indicated, a central chondrosarcoma is one which begins its development in the interior of the affected bone. As also noted, one may or may not be able to deduce, in a particular case, whether the lesion has arisen *de novo* in the bone interior or developed out of a pre-existing cartilage growth. In a case of multiple enchondromatosis, if one or another affected bone area becomes the site of a chondrosarcoma, it is reasonable to conclude that the sarcoma represents a secondary chondrosarcoma. That a solitary enchondroma may have been the precursor lesion for a central chondrosarcoma can also often be reasonably surmised. In this connection, one occasionally encounters in a long bone a well circumscribed and usually highly calcified cartilage lesion revealed originally by biopsy to be benign but ultimately (perhaps years later) found to have become a chondrosarcoma. This evolution is associated with the occurrence of proliferative activity in the lesional area, spotty reduction in radiopacity of the lesional area as a whole, and the appearance of a marginal zone of radiolucency.

However, the writer does not mean to imply that whenever one encounters a central chondrosarcoma showing radiopacity in the *x*-ray picture the lesion was necessarily benign at the start, for a central chondrosarcoma developing *de novo* may likewise show radiopacity due to calcification of the tumor cartilage. On the other hand, one encounters cases of central chondrosarcoma in which the roentgenographic picture gives no evidence of radiopacity and in which one consequently has no basis even for a surmise as to whether or not it evolved from a pre-existing cartilage lesion. Whether all such chondrosarcomas are to be regarded as primary is difficult to say. One must bear in mind that a benign cartilage growth (enchondroma) free of calcification may originally have been present at the site of the chondrosarcoma and been completely replaced by the new growth. Certainly, however, many central chondrosarcomas do evolve *de novo*, and in these cases the lesion is often fully malignant from the start. Some of these, especially when appearing in older children or young adults, may even run a fulminating course.

## CLINICAL CONSIDERATIONS

**Incidence.**—In a representative series of primary bone tumors, the chondrosarcomas are likely to constitute about 10 per cent of the cases. Among the cases studied by the writer, central chondrosarcoma was much more common than peripheral chondrosarcoma. Others, however, have found peripheral chondrosarcoma more common. As to sex of the patients, males and females were about equally represented in our series of 40 cases of central chondrosarcoma, but others have found the incidence higher in males. As to age distribution, the range in this series extended from 11 to 66 years, but the median age was 45. Specifically, only 3 of the patients were below 20 years of age; most of those between 20 and 40 were over 30 years of age, and slightly more than half of all the patients were over 40 years of age.

**Localization.**—In our cases of central chondrosarcoma, about half of the tumors involved a femur. Though in some cases the tumor was in the midshaft area of the femur, it was more often in the upper or lower end of the shaft and not infrequently also extended into the actual end of the bone. The next most common site was the humerus, and in this bone the lesion was nearly always in the proximal part and sometimes even restricted to its epiphysial end. Of the rest of the long bones, it was the tibia that was most commonly affected. Among the bones of the trunk, a rib was occasionally the site of the tumor, as was the ilium, scapula, or sternum.

A short tubular bone is rarely the site of a chondrosarcoma except in a case of multiple enchondromatosis in which the bone in question was one of those affected by the disorder. It seems worth noting also that of 15 cases of enchondromatosis available for study by the writer, 9 showed the development of a chondrosarcoma in one or another affected bone. Not infrequently, indeed, more than one of the affected bones came to show chondrosarcomatous transformation.

**Clinical Complaints and Findings.**—Pain is usually the presenting complaint in cases of central chondrosarcoma. As a rule, the pain is dull and aching, and often it is intermittent, at least at first. While in some cases the patient states that the pain had been present only for some months, it is not unusual to obtain a history of pain of several years' standing. If the lesion is located toward the end of a long bone, the patient may also complain of some restriction of motion or other disability relating to the adjacent joint. A local swelling may be palpable in consequence of some expansion of the contour of the affected bone part or as a result of penetration of the bone cortex by the tumor tissue. The area of swelling is likely to be firm or hard and is usually not very tender, and the overlying skin is rarely reddened or warm.

A short history of pain associated with the presence of a bulky local tumor mass is exceptional. Usually a central chondrosarcoma does not rapidly break out of the bone, but when it does, the lesion is likely to be highly malignant, and the clinical course may be a fulminating one. On the other hand, one occasionally obtains a history in which pain is subordinate to awareness of a tumor mass which has been slowly enlarging for years. This was the clinical picture in several cases of chondrosarcoma of a rib.

As in connection with bone tumors in general, some patients relate their complaints to *trauma* incurred by the affected part. A history of antecedent trauma is much less commonly given in cases of central than of peripheral chondrosarcoma. In the general evaluation of the role of trauma, the fact that many of the patients do not give a history of trauma is more important than the fact that some do. In any event, in cases of central chondrosarcoma, one can hardly ever establish clearly the crucial sequence of: trauma to the part; prompt roentgenographic exclusion of anything suggesting a chondrosarcoma; and the subsequent development of the latter at the site of the trauma. Certainly no causal significance should be attached to a trauma which occurred long (perhaps many years) before the patient sought treatment for the chondrosarcoma.

If one sees a case of central chondrosarcoma which was originally interpreted as a benign cartilage tumor on the basis of its histologic appearance, the history is usually to the effect that recurrence followed within a year after previous curettage of the lesion. If the sarcomatous nature of the lesion was still not recognized at the time of the first recurrence, and a second nonradical intervention was undertaken, the likelihood is that the second recurrence will be evident after an even shorter interval and that the recurrent mass will be larger than it was the first time. Furthermore, tumor tissue from this recurrence will almost certainly show an additional increase in the cytologic manifestations of malignancy if proper weight is given to certain cytologic details (see below) in the evaluation of the lesion.

## ROENTGENOGRAPHIC FINDINGS

Unless a central chondrosarcoma shows at least some spotty or blotchy radiopacity in its *x*-ray picture, one is not likely to suspect that the lesion is a chondrosarcoma or indeed a cartilage tumor at all (see Fig. 98). However, the cases in which it fails to show such radiopacity are definitely in the minority. In such cases the lesion is often represented in the *x*-ray picture by a large area of relative radiolucency. In addition, the area may even appear more or less loculated. The bone contour in the affected region is likely to be somewhat bulged, and the cortex may be thinned and otherwise modified, at least in part.

If the tumor is one which has erupted rapidly from the bone, the latter may not even show clear-cut radiolucency at the site of the lesion. On the other hand, it will show periosteal new bone deposition representing the effects of periosteal irritation resulting from the rapid eruption of the tumor. In addition, one may note an extra-osseous tumor mass, perhaps quite large, which may likewise fail to show any radiopacity such as would represent calcification going on within it.

As implied, a central chondrosarcoma is rather likely to show more or less spotty or blotchy radiopacity. This represents, of course, the fact that in many places the chondrosarcomatous tumor tissue is undergoing calcification of its matrix. Indeed, histologic examination might even reveal some bony metaplasia taking place in the calcified tumor areas. In addition to focal radiopacities, the lesion may show areas of clear-cut radiolucency. Being of slow growth, these calcifying chondrosarcomas do not readily erupt from the bone. At first one may find only some distention of the contour of the affected bone area. In addition, in some places the regional cortex may be found thinned, but in other places it may have become considerably thickened. In a site where the tumor tissue is penetrating and gaining exit through the cortex, the shadow cast by the latter may be fuzzy. If a fracture occurs through such a chondrosarcoma, the tumor gains exit rapidly and the extra-osseous chondrosarcomatous tumor tissue is also likely to show *x*-ray evidence of calcification.

The problem of roentgenographic differential diagnosis in connection with these calcifying chondrosarcomas relates mainly to osteogenic sarcoma and to areas of old bone infarction. If the subject is a mature adult, the factor of age alone should weigh heavily in favor of a diagnosis of chondrosarcoma as against osteogenic sarcoma. A calcified bone infarct in some part of a bone shaft can usually be distinguished from a chondrosarcoma merely through the fact that the regional cortex is neither thinned nor thickened. That is, such an infarct shows no evidence of erosion or penetration of the cortex such as a chondrosarcoma always eventually produces.

Finally, we come to the *x*-ray findings relating to those central chondrosarcomas which have apparently evolved out of pre-existing highly calcified benign enchondromas (see Fig. 99). The shadow cast by the lesion in its benign enchondroma phase tends to be characterized by a more or less well delimited zone of closely compacted and merging foci of radiopacity. A lesion such as this may remain static for years and may never undergo malignant transformation. When it does,

**Figure 98**

*A*, Roentgenograph of a lesion involving the neck and upper part of a femoral shaft and established by tissue examination as a chondrosarcoma. Because of the absence of radiopacity in the lesional area, it is difficult to identify this lesion on a roentgenographic basis. The patient was a woman 33 years of age whose principal complaint was of mild pain, of a few months' standing, referred to the hip area. The lesional area was curetted, and the lesional tissue was underdiagnosed as representing an enchondroma. About one year later there was a recurrence, and the tissue removed from the recurrent lesion was again interpreted as representing an enchondroma. At this point the writer examined the tissue sections from these two interventions and concluded that they showed subtle but clear-cut evidences of chondrosarcoma. A second recurrence took place within a year, and the tissue now presented obvious cytologic evidences of malignancy. A hindquarter ablation was then done, and the patient has remained well and free of recurrence for 6 years.

*B*, Roentgenograph of a large lytic lesion involving the lower end of a femur and again requiring tissue examination for identification as a chondrosarcoma. The lesion had been under clinical observation for almost 9 months, was believed to be a giant-cell tumor, and was treated by irradiation without the guidance of a biopsy examination. Despite this therapy, the lesion increased in size, and the *x*-ray picture illustrated is the preamputation picture. A biopsy was done before the amputation, and the histology of the tissue removed is shown in Fig. 102-*A*. The patient was a man 39 years of age whose disability was of 14 months' standing at the time of the amputation. The amputation level (about the middle of the femur) definitely cleared the tumor so far as the interior of the femur was concerned, but apparently did not clear it in relation to the soft parts and periosteum. Within 6 months after the operation there was a large local recurrence. A disarticulation at the hip joint was then done (a procedure which would have been the more appropriate one at the original intervention), but the patient succumbed to a pulmonary embolism.

*C*, Roentgenograph showing a rather classic picture of a central chondrosarcoma in the neck and upper part of the shaft of a femur. Note the radiopacities in the lesional area and the thickening of the femoral cortex on the medial side. The patient was a woman 50 years of age who was complaining of pain in the hip area in question for about 4 years. For about 6 months before a hemipelvectomy was done in this case, the lesion had been treated by very heavy irradiation, about 10,000 r be ng delivered to the tumor. Despite this treatment, the tumor progressed, and a pathologic fracture occurred. Histologic examination of tissue from the ablation specimen revealed that not only was much of the tumor tissue not necrotic, but active proliferation of the tumor had been going on.

*D*, Roentgenograph showing a highly calcified central chondrosarcoma occupying much of the shaft of a femur. A pathologic fracture was associated with extension of the tumor to the overlying soft parts. The patient was a woman 65 years of age who suffered from pain in the thigh for about 3 years before the femur fractured.

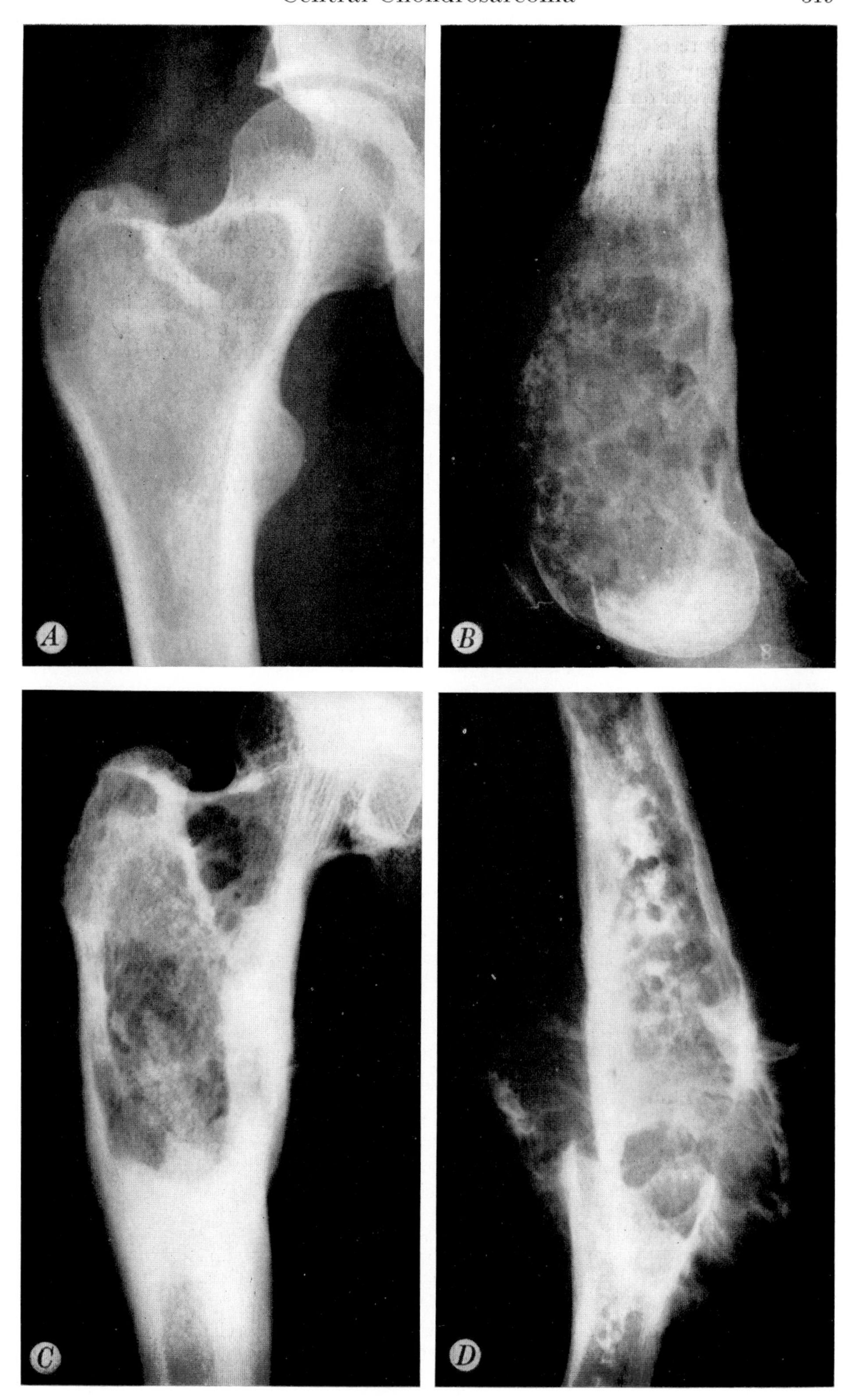


*Figure 98*

its $x$-ray picture comes to show reduction of the radiopacity, or disappearance of much of it, especially around the periphery, and the remaining radiopaque area shows an irregular outline and appears, on the whole, blurred and fuzzy. Also, the sarcoma which has evolved may now be found to have broken out of the bone. In a case in point, in which the lesion was in the upper end of a humerus, 14 months elapsed between the time when the patient was seen because an old calcified focus of cartilage became activated and began to cause him pain and the time when the tumor became fully malignant and broke out of the bone. In the resected portion of the humerus, the tumor tissue in the head of the bone still clearly consisted of cartilage which, in the more central portion, was gritty and calcified. This gritty part of the tumor represented the calcified and ossified portion of the original solitary enchondroma, though cytologic study even of this part of the tumor showed evidence of chondrosarcomatous transformation occurring in previously dormant cartilage tissue.

## PATHOLOGIC FINDINGS

**Gross Pathology.**—Sooner or later, a central chondrosarcoma penetrates the bone cortex and grows beyond the limits of the bone. However, at the time when a particular tumor is examined grossly it may still be largely confined to the bone interior. Even under these circumstances, the contour of the affected bone part is likely to be found slightly distended. Inspection of the outer surface of the cortex will almost certainly reveal that it is thickened, roughened, and pitted. This is the consequence on the one hand of slow infiltrative advance of the tumor tissue along the haversian canals of the cortex and on the other hand of some reactive new bone deposition by the irritated periosteum.

### *Figure 99*

*A*, Roentgenograph of a central chondrosarcoma affecting part of the right 9th rib. Note the radiopacities which help to establish the lesion as a chondrosarcoma. (The photograph of the gross specimen in this case is shown in Fig. 101-*B*.) The patient was a man 53 years of age who had been aware for about 9 years of a painless but slowly enlarging mass in the chest wall. For about 1 year before the tumor was resected, the mass had been growing rather rapidly and was painful. There was no history of antecedent trauma. The presumption in this case is that the lesion was originally an enchondroma and underwent malignant transformation.

*B*, Roentgenograph of a central chondrosarcoma involving the spinous process of the 5th cervical vertebra of a man 56 years of age. Twelve years earlier, an $x$-ray examination made in connection with a local trauma had revealed, in that spinous process, an expanding lesion which, in retrospect, appears to have been an enchondroma. The site of the lesion was not the source of any further difficulty for about 11 years, after which it became painful so that medical advice was sought again and the chondrosarcoma was discovered.

*C*, Roentgenograph of a highly calcified enchondroma in a humerus, which is in the process of transition into a chondrosarcoma. The patient was a man 53 years of age who for years had been known to have a nonsymptomatic focus of radiopacity in the area in question. For 6 months prior to the time when this picture was taken, he complained of some pain in the shoulder. A biopsy was done, but the fact that the lesion was undergoing malignant transformation was indicated by only an occasional microscopic tissue field (see Figs. 103-*A* and *B*).

*D*, Roentgenograph showing the appearance of the humerus illustrated in *C*, 11 months after the biopsy had been taken. Unfortunately, no further surgery had been done in the meantime. Note that the radiopacity has yielded to radiolucency in some areas and that the tumor has violated the cortex and extended out of the bone. The upper end of the humerus was now resected. The photograph of the resection specimen is shown in Fig. 100-*B*. A forequarter ablation would have been preferable to a resection. Indeed, 6 months after the resection there was a recurrence, and one year after that the patient died of metastases.

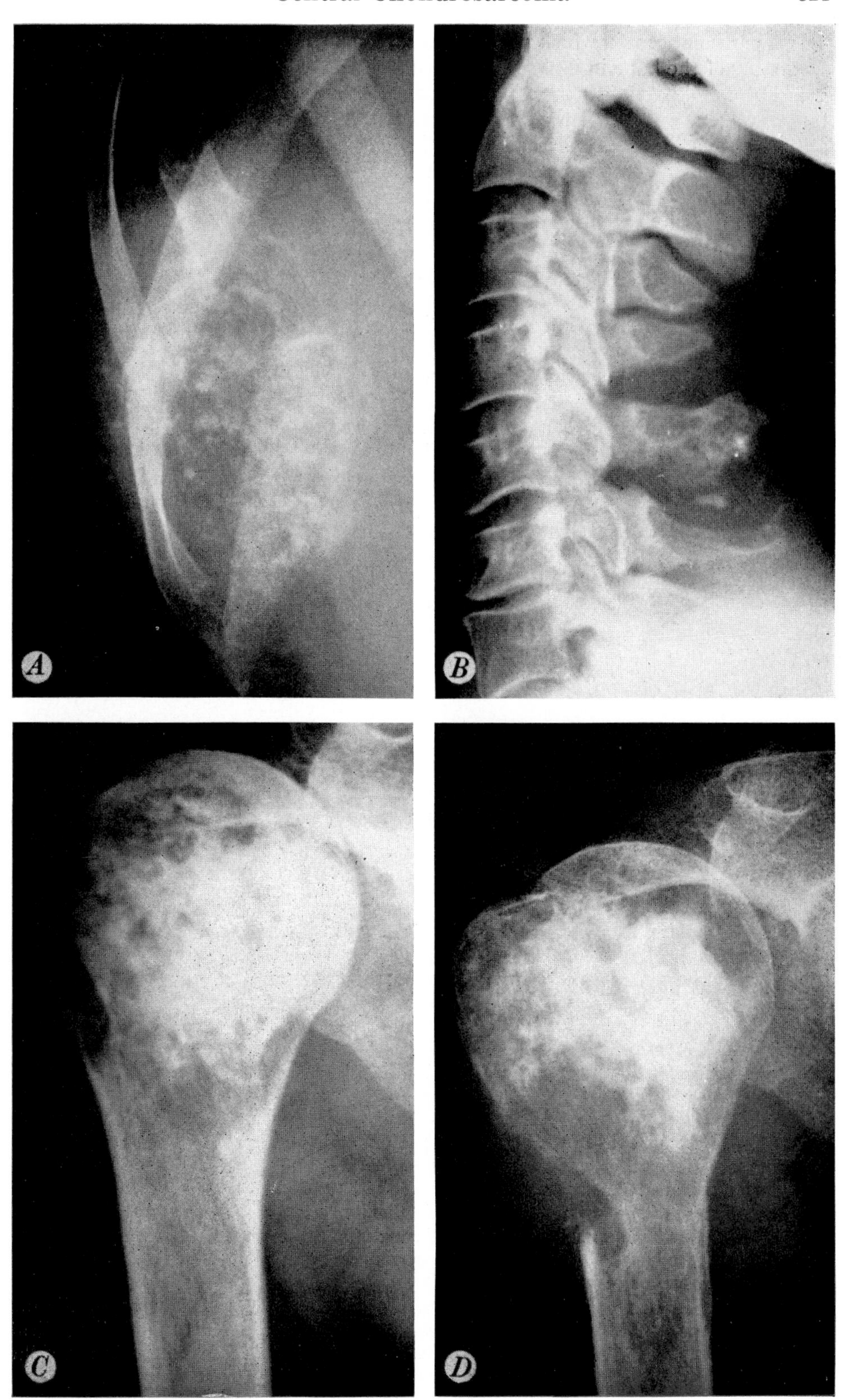


*Figure* 99

In a pertinent case in which the chondrosarcoma was in the upper part of a femur, sectioning of the bone in its long axis revealed that the tumor involved the greater trochanter and part of the neck of the bone, and extended down the shaft for a distance of 17 cm. The tumor was composed of faceted lobules of cartilage mainly grayish to bluish in color. In some areas the tumor cartilage was soft and edematous. In other areas it was speckled with whitish gritty foci representing focal calcification of the tumor tissue. Furthermore, the sectioned specimen showed, even more plainly than mere inspection of the surface of the specimen revealed, that the cortex was being invaded and that in some places it had undergone considerable thickening. This description of the gross appearance of a chondrosarcoma which is still largely confined to the interior of the bone also applies, in a general way, to the various other cases of this kind which were studied by the writer.

On the other hand, a chondrosarcoma may completely destroy a considerable part of the local bone cortex and give rise to a large, protruding tumor mass which is continuous with the tumor tissue in the interior of the bone. There are also cases in which a chondrosarcoma extensively penetrates the local bone cortex, but without completely destroying it, and in which the affected bone area consequently comes to be surrounded by a large, more or less irregularly lobulated tumor mass (see Fig. 100).

In both these types of cases, gross examination of the sectioned specimen shows again that the tumor tissue within and outside of the confines of the bone is composed largely of faceted lobules of grayish white to bluish cartilage tissue. Furthermore, both in the interior of the bone and outside of it, this tumor cartilage may show gritty whitish specks representing focal calcification and/or ossification going on within the tumor cartilage. If the tumor mass outside of the limits of the bone is particularly bulky, larger or smaller areas of tumor tissue may appear as semisoft or gelatinous cartilage or may even have undergone cystic degeneration. Such areas represent merely a nonspecific secondary degenerative change whose incidental character is usually attested by the presence elsewhere of hyaline cartilage.

In a specific case of a bulky, erupted chondrosarcoma, longitudinal sectioning of the specimen demonstrated that the tumor tissue filled the lower end of the femur,

***Figure 100***

*A*, Photograph of the upper end of a longitudinally sectioned femur showing a central chondrosarcoma. Note the faceted appearance of the tumor cartilage, which is somewhat edematous. The medial aspect of the femoral cortex is strikingly thickened. The patient was a man 49 years of age whose complaint was mainly of pain, of 3 months' standing. A disarticulation at the hip joint was done, and the patient has remained well and free of recurrences for 5 years.

*B*, Photograph of the upper end of a longitudinally sectioned humerus showing a central chondrosarcoma which has broken out of the confines of the bone. The sarcoma in this case became engrafted upon an old calcified enchondroma. (See Figs. 99-*C* and *D* for the roentgenographic findings.) Note that much of the tumor in the interior of the bone appears whitish, since it is still calcified. The cytologic features of the lesional tissue in this case are shown in Figure 103.

*C*, Photograph of the lower half of a longitudinally sectioned femur presenting a central chondrosarcoma. The lesion has extended through the cortex without extensively destroying it and has produced a large tumor mass surrounding the bone. The patient was a girl 19 years of age whose history was that for 3 months she had noticed a rapidly increasing tumor mass in the thigh. Note that the extra-osseous tumor mass has undergone cystic and hemorrhagic softening. Although the limb was disarticulated at the hip joint, the patient died 9 months later of pulmonary metastases. The lesion in this case represents one of the occasional examples of a chondrosarcoma running a fulminating course.

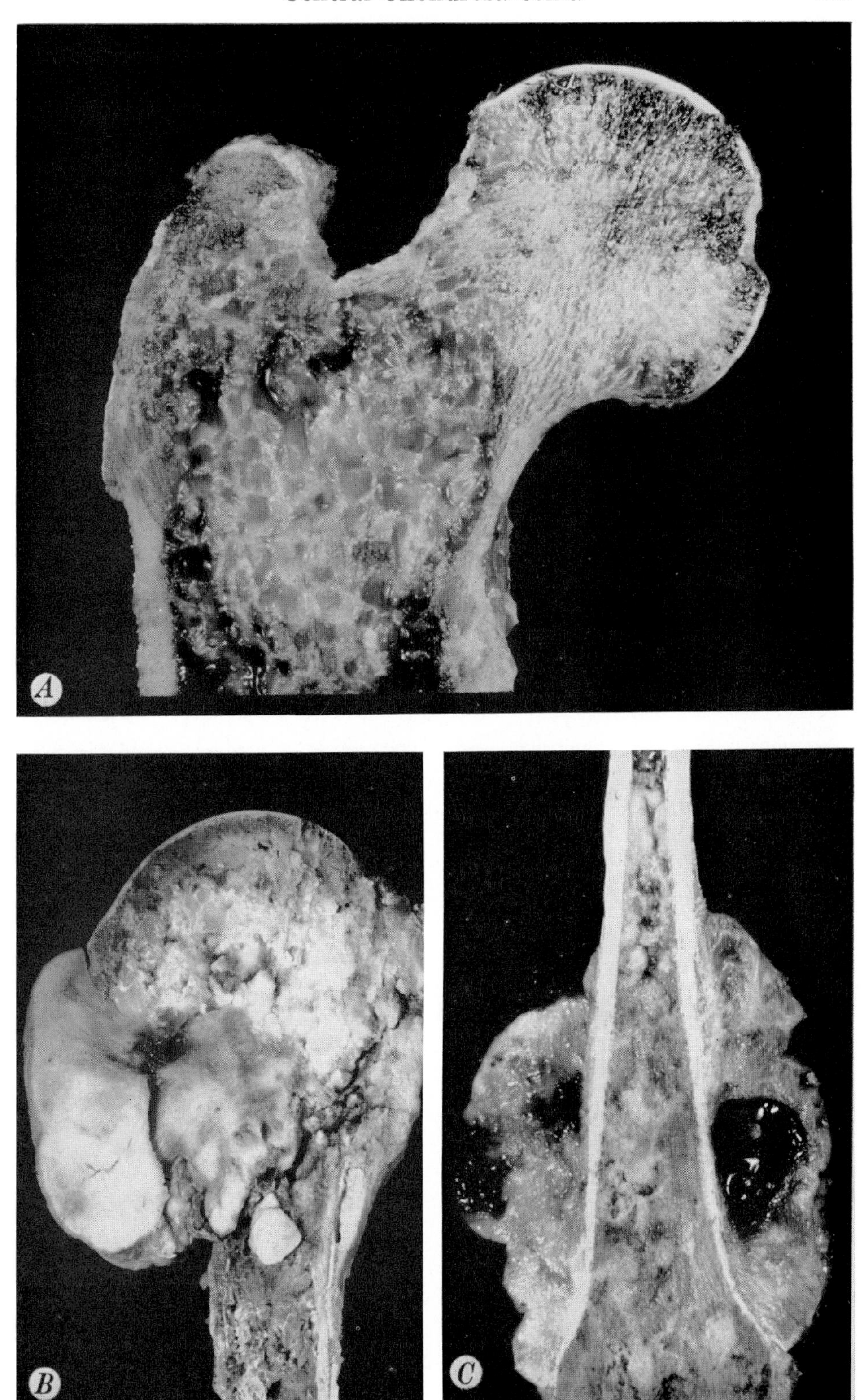


*Figure 100*

surrounded the bone, and extended into the knee joint. Anteriorly, the cortex was found destroyed for some distance beyond the articular cartilage, and in this region somewhat cystified tumor tissue bulged into the anterior compartment of the knee joint. When the patella was retracted and the quadriceps pouch was examined, it was found furthermore that the synovium of the pouch was studded with numerous tiny nodules of whitish tumor tissue. Posteriorly, there was a much larger tumor mass which bulged into the popliteal fossa and forced back the popliteal vessels and sciatic nerve. This posterior tumor mass measured about 10 cm. in its long dimension. For about half this distance, the underlying cortex was substantially destroyed, and in this region the posterior extra-osseous cartilaginous tumor mass merged with the tumor tissue in the interior of the bone. Above this mass the posterior femoral cortex was thickened in consequence of periosteal new bone apposition. At its lower end the mass was continuous with tumor tissue which was projecting from the condylar region of the femur into the posterior compartment of the joint (see Fig. 101).

The findings to be noted when a chondrosarcoma develops in one or another of the affected bones in a case of multiple enchondromatosis were exemplified in an enchondromatous lower limb which had been disarticulated because a sarcoma had developed in the lower end of the femur. The patient was a middle-aged adult and the limb in question had been bumpy, stubby, and shortened from early childhood. When cut open, the bones of the affected limb (especially the femur and tibia) were found almost entirely filled with cartilage plugs and nodules of widely varied size. At the site of the sarcoma the cortex had been perforated and the overlying soft parts showed a large, somewhat gelatinous chondrosarcomatous tumor mass which was continuous with tissue of similar nature in the adjacent bone interior. In contrast, the cartilage filling the upper part of the femur and all of the tibia was free of malignant change both grossly and histologically.

In this case, it had long been clear from the clinical and roentgenographic picture that the patient was suffering from enchondromatosis. Sometimes, however, the fact that a given chondrosarcoma had its foundation in a lesion of enchondromatosis is discovered only fortuitously. Indeed, it is sometimes only because the bones neighboring upon the one bearing the sarcoma are opened in the course of routine dissection of the amputated limb that one discovers that, despite their normal external appearance, they contain cartilage tissue. This finding furnishes the correct orientation as to the anatomic foundation of the chondrosarcoma in the case in question. Furthermore, it seems worth emphasizing that it is not unusual for a chondrosarcoma to develop in one or another of the affected bones in a case of clinically recognized enchondromatosis of very limited extent.

***Figure 101***

*A*, Photograph of a longitudinally sectioned lower half of a femur showing a central chondrosarcoma which has destroyed the cortex in places and extended out of the bone. Note that on the right the tumor has broken into the anterior compartment of the knee joint. Posteriorly the tumor has extended into the popliteal space area and inferiorly it has broken into the posterior compartment of the joint. The tumor tissue appears white and glistening and was composed of smaller or larger facets of cartilage. The patient was a man 29 years of age. He died at another hospital 7 years after amputation, presumably from recurrence and metastases, but no autopsy was secured. The histologic pattern of the lesional tissue in this case is illustrated in Fig. 102-*B*.

*B*, Photograph of a central chondrosarcoma which has developed in the region of the costochondral junction of the 9th right rib. Below, on the left, one can note the presence of tumor tissue in the medullary cavity of the rib. Below, on the right, one notes the chondral cartilage. The pertinent roentgenograph in this case is shown in Fig. 99-*A*, and the legend there gives some clinical facts in the case.

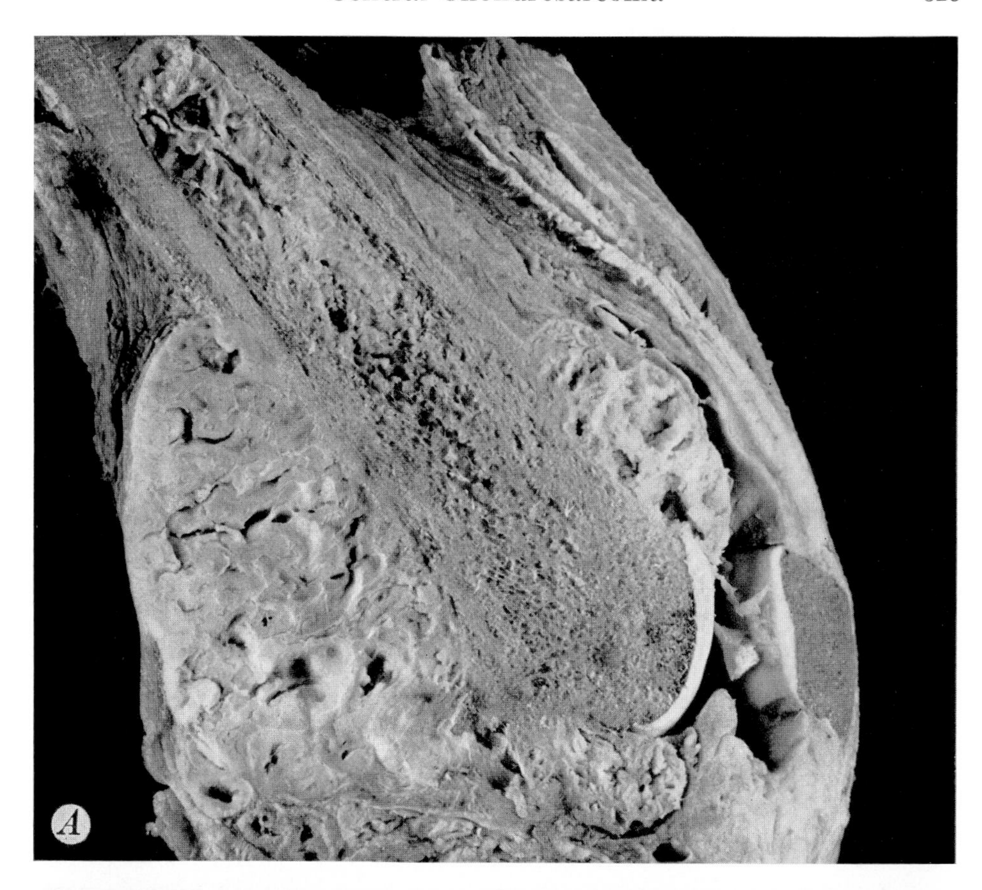


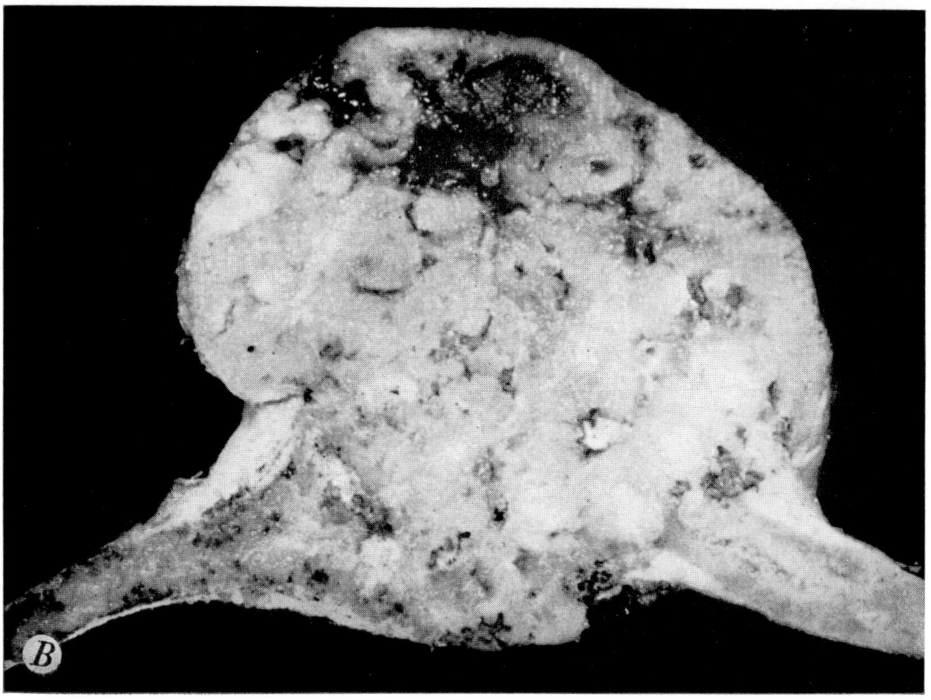


***Figure 101***

**Microscopic Pathology.**—The histologic interpretation of a lesion as a chondrosarcoma gains valuable support from comparison with the histologic findings encountered in relation to the benign cartilage growths. In connection with *solitary enchondroma* (p. 177) it was noted that, while the lesional cartilage may vary from case to case in respect to cellularity, these lesions on the whole are not very cellular. Furthermore, the nuclei of the cartilage cells are consistently small, and few if any of the cells have double nuclei.

In regard to *multiple enchondromatosis* (p. 192) it is well to remember that on the whole the lesional cartilage is much more cellular than in cases of solitary enchondroma. Furthermore, the cartilage cell nuclei tend to be slightly larger than they are in lesional tissue from a solitary enchondroma. Also, in enchondromatosis, more than an occasional cell (and perhaps quite a few cells) will show double nuclei. These findings in enchondromatosis are in harmony with the rather persistent cartilage proliferation occurring in this disorder and bring the histologic pattern of enchondromatosis to the border line of chondrosarcoma.

A *solitary* cartilage growth should be suspect of being a chondrosarcoma if, when viable and not heavily calcified tissue areas are examined, it shows, even in scattered fields: (1) hypercellularity of the tissue; (2) general plumpness of the cell nuclei; and (3) the presence of more than an occasional cell with plump double nuclei. On the other hand, as indicated above, in a lesion from a case of *multiple* enchondromatosis, changes along these lines do not necessarily signify by themselves that the lesion has crossed the border from benignity to malignity.

However, tissue from any type of cartilage lesion should be regarded as chondrosarcomatous if, in addition to the findings listed above, it shows: (1) pronounced irregularity in the size of the cells and their nuclei; (2) the presence of numerous cells with multiple nuclei; (3) pronounced hyperchromatism of the nuclei; or (4) any large or giant cartilage cells with single or multiple nuclei or with clumps of chromatin. Also, some obviously malignant chondrosarcomas show a sprinkling of mitotic division figures, although, in general, cell division in a chondrosarcoma tends to be amitotic. Occasionally a chondrosarcoma even shows areas in which the tumor tissue has undergone dedifferentiation. In such areas this tissue may even have the cytologic appearance of an anaplastic fibrosarcoma. (See Figs. 102 and 103-*D*.)

### *Figure 102*

*A*, Photomicrograph (× 250) showing the histologic pattern of a field typical of the viable tumor tissue of the chondrosarcoma illustrated in Fig. 98-*B*. Note the high cellularity of the tumor cartilage, the general plumpness of the cell nuclei, and the abundance of cells with double nuclei.

*B*, Photomicrograph (× 250) showing the histologic pattern of a field typical of the viable tumor tissue in the amputation specimen of the chondrosarcoma shown in Fig. 101-*A*. Practically all the nuclei are plump, and at least 5 cells with double nuclei can be seen.

*C*, Photomicrograph (× 250) showing the histologic pattern of all viable tumor areas of a recurrence in the amputation stump of a femoral chondrosarcoma. Note the pronounced cellularity of the tumor cartilage and the numerous binuclear cells. The patient was a man 59 years of age who had pain relating to his femur for 5 years before the amputation was done. The amputation level did not clear the tumor in the interior of the femur. The patient subsequently died with complaints suggestive of intravascular propagation of the tumor to the heart and lungs, but no autopsy was done.

*D*, Photomicrograph (× 100) showing the histologic pattern of a metastatic focus of chondrosarcoma in a lung. Even at this relatively low magnification, many binuclear cells can be seen in the upper half of the picture. In the lower half, many giant cells with large nuclei are to be seen. The primary lesion was in the 6th rib. The original surgical intervention was not radical enough, and there were several recurrences during the succeeding 3 years before the lesion metastasized.

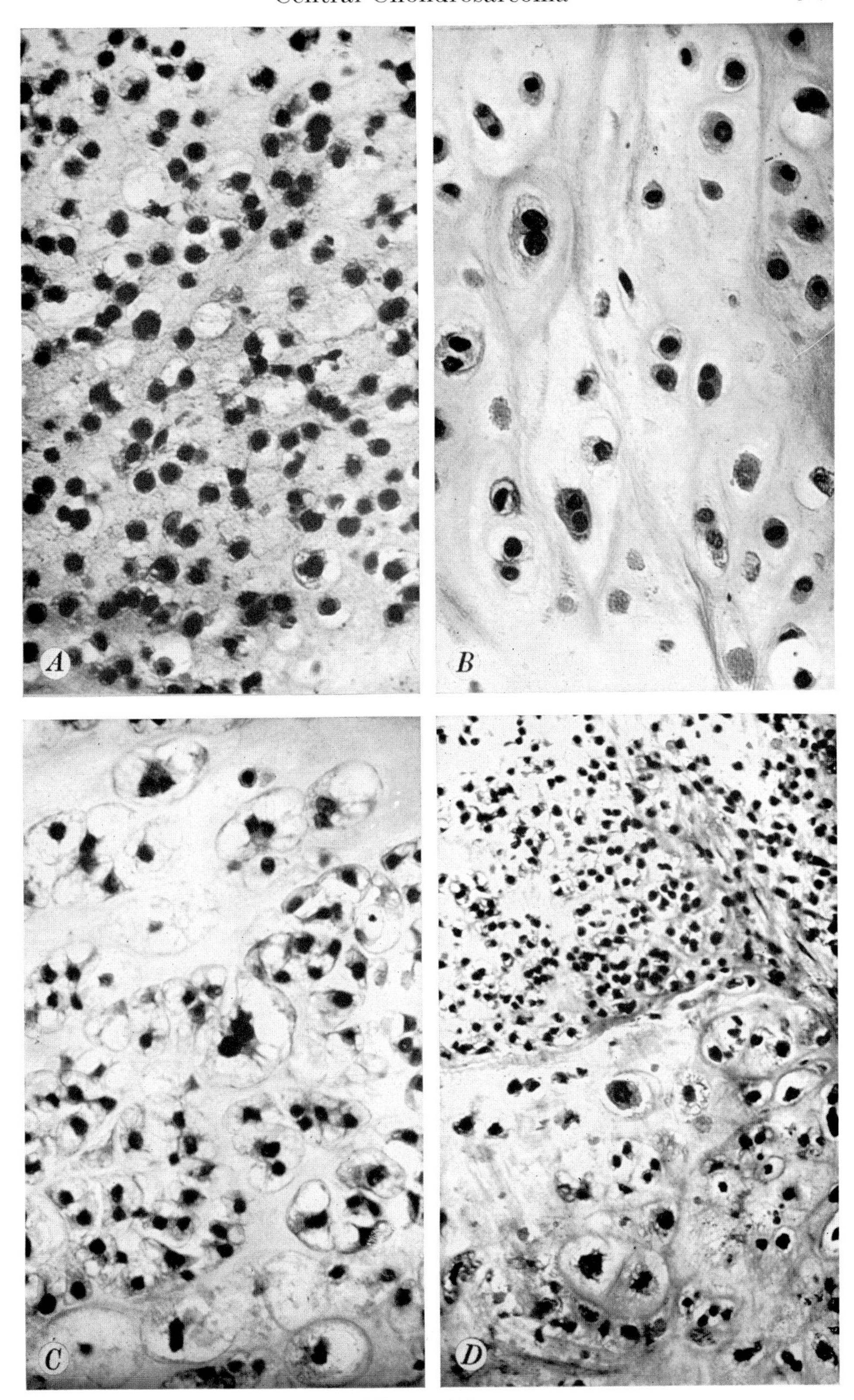


***Figure 102***

The usefulness of the histologic criteria outlined above in making the decision as to whether a particular cartilage growth is benign or malignant has been emphasized by the writer in various published articles on the cartilage tumors. The diagnostic importance of these criteria has recently been emphasized again by others (see O'Neal and Ackerman, and Dahlin and Henderson). The ease with which the histologic diagnosis of chondrosarcoma can be made in a given case depends on the extent to which the various cytologic criteria of malignancy outlined above are represented in the lesional tissue. In some few cases the evidence of malignancy of the tumor is crude and obvious from the start, the tumor tissue showing all the ominous characteristics, including even many mitotic division figures. In a great number of the cases, on the other hand, though various cytologic criteria of malignancy are present, the total picture of malignancy is less striking. For instance, in a particular case the lesional tissue may be found hypercellular and the cell nuclei quite plump and hyperchromatic, but there may be relatively few cells with double nuclei and no cells showing bizarre nuclei or mitotic figures. Again, a chondrosarcoma may reveal itself by its hypercellularity, general plumpness of the nuclei, and the presence in addition of a great number of cells with plump double nuclei. In still another case there may not even be striking hypercellularity, but a considerable number of the cells may nevertheless show plump double nuclei, and an occasional cell may even have a bizarre nucleus.

Finally, it must be emphasized that in some cases the histologic evidence of malignancy is very subtle. This is particularly true for those central chondrosarcomas which are still in the early stages of their evolution out of a highly calcified benign enchondroma. Indeed, the histologic evidence indicating actual transition from benignity to malignity may have to be searched for in the tissue submitted for examination in such a case. This evidence can sometimes easily be overlooked, since it may be present only in a few microscopic tissue fields. Much of the tissue is likely to show merely the pattern of a benign enchondroma. However, detailed examination will reveal here and there some fields in which the cartilage is very cellular and in which the cell nuclei are definitely plump and many of them are even bilobed. If the proper weight is not given to these histologic nuances and the treatment is limited to curettage of the lesion, a recurrence is certainly to be expected. In the recurrence in such a case, the cytologic findings indicating malig-

***Figure 103***

*A*, Photomicrograph (× 250) showing the cytologic pattern present in most of the biopsy specimen removed in the case of the chondrosarcoma (evolving from a calcified enchondroma) illustrated in Fig. 99-*C*. Note that the cartilage is not highly cellular, that the cell nuclei are small, and that no cells with double nuclei are to be seen. From such a cytologic appearance one would conclude that the lesion is benign. However, in a few microscopic fields (see *B*) the cytologic picture deviated from this.

*B*, Photomicrograph (× 250) showing the cytologic pattern in an occasional tissue field from the biopsy specimen also illustrated in *A*. Note that the lesional cartilage is moderately cellular and that practically all the viable nuclei are plump. From such a picture one should suspect that the lesion is a chondrosarcoma.

*C*, Photomicrograph (× 250) showing the cytologic appearance of a tissue field from this case after the lesion had become fully malignant (see also Figs. 99-*D* and 100-*B*). This field comes from the originally highly calcified portion of the chondrosarcoma and shows lysis of the old calcified cartilage and the presence of numerous cartilage cells with plump nuclei.

*D*, Photomicrograph (× 125) showing in this case the histologic appearance of the tumor tissue which had broken out of the humerus. The tumor cartilage has become dedifferentiated, the cells appear drawn out, and the pattern in this area almost suggests an anaplastic fibrosarcoma.

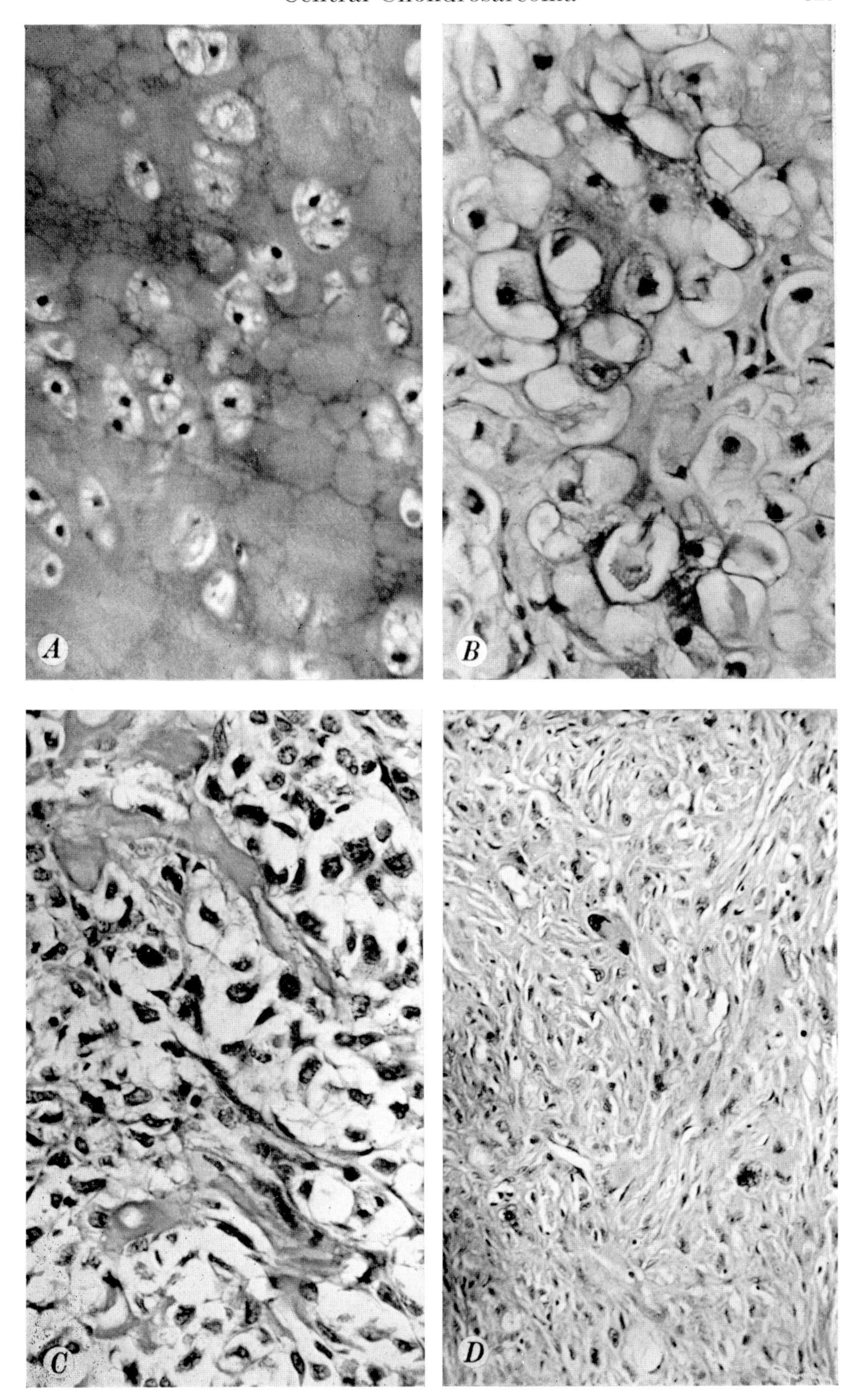


*Figure 103*

nancy will, of course, be more clearly apparent. On the same basis, if a lesion is already a clear-cut chondrosarcoma when first studied, but has been underdiagnosed and treated as a benign lesion, its first recurrence and any subsequent ones will almost certainly present increasingly striking cytologic manifestations of malignancy (see Fig. 103).

**Extension and Metastasis.**—It is only occasionally that one encounters a case of chondrosarcoma which runs a fulminating clinical course. The patients in these cases are usually adolescents or young adults. They usually give a history of a rapidly developing local tumor mass associated with local pain. The interval between the onset of the complaints and the time of admission to the hospital in such cases may be merely 2 or 3 months. Furthermore, under microscopic examination, the lesional tissue will already show full-blown malignity, represented by the presence of numerous cartilage tumor cells with giant and/or bizarre nuclei. Even if a radical surgical intervention is promptly carried out, it is likely that the patient in these cases will be dead of pulmonary metastases within a year or so from the time of discovery of the tumor.

Ordinarily the clinical course is more torpid even if the patient has suffered one or more recurrences because of inadequate surgery. However, a cure may still be effected in some cases after recurrences have taken place, provided that a complete radical intervention ensuring the removal of all tumor tissue is finally done. Nevertheless, in these cases the over-all prognosis is by no means as good as it is in those in which the original intervention was prompt and radical.

If not controlled, a central chondrosarcoma tends to spread by direct extension rather than by hematogenous dissemination of tumor cells. In the course of its spread, the tumor tends to break into the regional venous channels. By intravascular growth and extension, without necessarily adhering very much to the vessel walls, it may reach the heart and lungs. In other cases, while extending into large venous channels, the tumor also gives rise to parenchymal metastases, at least in the lungs. Actually, metastases elsewhere than in the lungs are uncommon in connection with chondrosarcoma. The possibility of lymphatic spread also exists, and the extension of the tumor to lymph nodes, especially regional nodes, has occasionally been reported.

## DIFFERENTIAL DIAGNOSIS

The various questions relating to the differential diagnosis between solitary and multiple enchondroma on the one hand and central chondrosarcoma on the other have been covered in the sections dealing with the roentgenographic and pathologic findings.

In regard to *chondromyxoid fibroma* (p. 208), diagnostic confusion with chondrosarcoma may also arise. This stems in part from the suggestive cartilaginous character of the tumor tissue in the gross. The difficulty is accentuated when, in a particular chondromyxoid fibroma, the lesional tissue reveals on microscopic examination larger or smaller amounts of myxoid intercellular material. Also, where the lesional tissue is undergoing such myxoid degeneration, the suggestion that one is dealing with a malignant tumor of cartilage is reinforced by the finding of some cells with very large hyperchromatic nuclei and cells with 2 or 3 or more nuclei. Experience with the chondromyxoid fibroma will lead one to recognize that its tissue pattern as a whole is that of a benign lesion, even though it presents such disturbing cytologic details. Altogether, however, it must be conceded that, on a purely cytologic basis, there is often good reason for confusion between a chondromyxoid fibroma and a chondrosarcoma. At any rate, in spite of the impression created by such cytologic findings that one may be dealing with a "myxochondrosarcoma," the clinical behavior of a chondromyxoid fibroma is not that of a malignant tumor, and, again unlike the chondrosarcoma, it does not recur even after mere curettement.

Finally, we come to the question, already touched upon, of what distinguishes a chondrosarcoma from an *osteogenic sarcoma*. Ordinarily a chondrosarcoma presents, even grossly, the unmistakable general appearance of a tumor composed of cartilage tissue. This is the fact even though, in one or another chondrosarcoma, much of the basic cartilage tissue may become calcified and ossified. At any rate, cytologically a chondrosarcoma nowhere shows, as do all osteogenic sarcomas properly so called, neoplastic osteoid and osseous tissue evolving directly from a sarcomatous connective-tissue stroma. It is true that, in an individual osteogenic sarcoma, some or even much of the sarcomatous stromal tissue may go through a chondroid or cartilaginous stage before becoming calcified and ossified. However, even under such circumstances, study of the lesion will reveal many places in which the stromal tissue is merging directly into neoplastic osteoid and bone, the tumor thus proving itself to be an osteogenic sarcoma and not a chondrosarcoma.

## TREATMENT

The only form of therapy which offers any prospect of cure in a case of central chondrosarcoma is surgery. Definitive surgery should be preceded by study of a biopsy specimen. In some cases, sufficient diagnostic information can be obtained by a needle biopsy. If it can not, an incisional biopsy should be done. It is safe to delay the definitive surgical procedure until paraffin sections have been prepared, if frozen sections of the biopsy material are not sufficiently clarifying. In planning the definitive surgical procedure, however, it must be borne in mind that the biopsy wound may have been seeded with tumor tissue and that the biopsy area should therefore not be re-entered.

As noted, in the great majority of cases of central chondrosarcoma, the lesion is in a long bone of a limb. In general, the surgical procedure indicated in these cases is amputation, but in an occasional case, segmental resection of the affected part has been found to suffice. In relation to an affected long bone, segmental resection, even if practical, should probably not be attempted unless the lesion is still small and has not extended much if at all beyond the limits of the cortex.

If the tumor has extended into the overlying soft parts, amputation offers the best promise of success. As part of the general principle of giving the lesion a wide margin in any site, the policy of keeping one joint ahead of the growth is a valuable one. Thus, for a tumor in the upper end of a femur which has broken out of the bone, ablation of the limb, together with the hip joint capsule and at least the acetabular area of the innominate bone, would seem better than disarticulation at the hip joint. Correspondingly, for a tumor in the upper end of a humerus which has widely broken out of the bone, a scapulohumeral disarticulation is better than a disarticulation at the shoulder joint alone. On the same basis, if the lesion is in a rib, certainly several inches of the rib on each side beyond the region of apparent involvement, and at least corresponding sections of the rib above and below the affected one, should be sacrificed.

In general, then, the surgical treatment of chondrosarcoma should be definitely on the radical side, and the wider the margin of supposedly normal tissue, the better. As already indicated, a radical procedure offers the best promise of success when it is undertaken at the initial intervention. The hopeful aspect of such surgery (and specifically of the prevention of recurrence by keeping well ahead of the growth) in cases of central chondrosarcoma lies in the fact that, as a rule, the tumor has not yet metastasized at the time of the initial surgical intervention. After an initial surgical intervention, a local recurrence is certainly to be expected if the tumor area has not been well cleared. However, even after one or more local recurrences, radical surgery may still effect a cure, though the hazards of inaccessible local extension and/or metastasis are definitely increased.

Irradiation therapy is hardly of any value, since malignant cartilage tumors are highly resistant to such treatment, tending to continue or resume their growth in spite of it. Irradiation may serve at most as a temporary palliative agent against pain for a chondrosarcoma in a site inaccessible to surgical intervention, and should not be used with any higher expectation.

## PERIPHERAL CHONDROSARCOMA

As already noted, a peripheral chondrosarcoma is one which begins its development in relation to the surface of a bone. More specifically, the writer applies this term to those chondrosarcomas which evolve as a complication in cases of solitary osteocartilaginous exostosis or hereditary multiple exostosis. That is, he excludes from the category of peripheral chondrosarcoma the rare cases of chondrosarcoma developing in the soft parts of patients not suffering from either of these disorders.

The chondrosarcomatous transformation of a solitary osteocartilaginous exostosis is rather unusual, occurring in only about 1 per cent of the cases, at most. On the other hand, the occurrence of a chondrosarcoma in connection with hereditary osteocartilaginous exostosis is fairly common. In a series of 28 cases of that disorder reported by the writer, 3 (nearly 11 per cent) showed this complication. Since the great majority of the patients in this series were still children or adolescents, one must allow for the possibility that, later in life, some of these too will develop this complication. In fact, a complicating chondrosarcoma can probably be expected, sooner or later, in about 25 per cent of cases of multiple exostosis.

In the rare cases in which a chondrosarcoma develops in connection with a solitary exostosis, it can usually be concluded that the sarcoma took its departure from the cartilage cap (or remnants of the cap) of the exostosis. This is likewise the site of origin of the chondrosarcoma in many of the cases of multiple exostosis. However, in some cases of the latter disorder, the sarcoma, while located in the vicinity of an exostotic area, seems not to have developed from the exostosis *per se*. In these cases it may conceivably have evolved out of a cartilage rest lying in the periosteum or between it and the cortex. Finally, it is worth noting that in general, peripheral chondrosarcomas are more torpid growths than central chondrosarcomas, and often come to attain large size.

### CLINICAL CONSIDERATIONS

**Incidence.**—In the writer's experience, cases of peripheral chondrosarcoma were much less common than those of central chondrosarcoma, the ratio being about 1 to 5. The data of Dahlin and Henderson show a similar trend. The experience of others has been different, however. Thus, in the series reported by Coley and Higinbotham there were about the same number of each type, and in the series recorded by O'Neal and Ackerman the peripheral chondrosarcomas predominated.

As to age incidence, while some few patients are adolescents or young adults, most of them are in middle life. However, on the average, the patients showing peripheral chondrosarcomas tend to be somewhat younger than those showing central chondrosarcomas. As to sex of the patients, males seem to be slightly predilected.

**Localization.**—The most common site of peripheral chondrosarcoma is some part of the pelvis and particularly the iliac part of one or the other of the innominate bones. Indeed, probably as much as half of all the peripheral chondrosarcomas involve some part of the pelvic girdle. A large proportion of the other half develop in relation to a scapula or the upper part of a femur or humerus. The few remaining ones are widely scattered in their locations.

**Clinical Complaints and Findings.**—A peripheral chondrosarcoma is often already of large size by the time the patient enters a hospital for treatment. In fact, much more often than not, the patient has been aware for a long time of a slowly enlarging local tumor mass, but paid little attention to it. This might have happened either because the presence of the mass was not associated with appreciable pain or because the patient, being affected with multiple exostosis, thought that the tumor mass was like the protuberances he knew he had on other bones.

Thus, in a case in which a peripheral chondrosarcoma developed from a solitary osteochondroma of a tibia, the patient stated that for 24 years he had been conscious of a tumor mass in the upper part of the leg. Though growing slowly, this mass had attained a huge size by the time the patient was admitted, but even then he was not disabled by the tumor, experiencing at most some local aching and numbness. In regard to a chondrosarcoma which evolved from a solitary costal osteochondroma, the patient stated that for 12 years she had been aware of a painless mass which, though growing slowly, had likewise become quite large.

In a case of multiple exostosis in which a peripheral chondrosarcoma developed in relation to an innominate bone, there was an 8-year history of a slowly progressive tumorous enlargement extending down the thigh and into the pelvis but again not associated with any striking clinical difficulty. In other cases of multiple exostosis, it was again surprising to note the recency and relative mildness of the pain or other complaints in relation to the large size and apparent long duration of the tumor mass. In a case in which the tumor is entirely intrathoracic or intrapelvic, a tumor mass may not even be perceptible to the patient, and the complaints which lead him to seek treatment may be due to pressure of the growth upon some internal structure.

If one surveys the histories in cases of peripheral chondrosarcoma, one cannot fail to be impressed by the fact that antecedent *trauma* is mentioned much more commonly in connection with the emergence of the lesion in these cases than in cases of central chondrosarcoma. Since a peripheral chondrosarcoma may attain a fairly large size without producing significant clinical complaints, it may well be that the local trauma merely directed attention to a lesion which was already present. Probably the largest role that one can attribute to trauma is that of exacerbating the course of the lesion, and that only if the local trauma has been severe.

When palpable, the tumor mass is usually found to be firm, hard, and not very tender, and the overlying skin is never red or warm. If the mass abuts upon a joint, the latter is likely to be found swollen and its motion somewhat restricted. If the mass finally comes to compress a local nerve trunk or nerves, there will be corresponding neurological symptoms such as radiating pain, numbness, and/or paresthesia.

## ROENTGENOGRAPHIC AND PATHOLOGIC FINDINGS

**Roentgenographic Findings.**—In general, the peripheral chondrosarcomas are not difficult to single out roentgenographically. In connection with them, the *x*-ray findings relating to solitary or multiple exostosis are associated with the picture of a large, spottily and fuzzily opaque adjacent tumor mass. Peripherally, the mass may show radiopaque streaks extending out from the main area of radiopacity. The streaky areas are, of course, those in which the tumor cartilage is less heavily calcified than in the central part of the mass (see Fig. 104).

For comparison it should be remembered that even a solitary osteochondroma sometimes attains a fairly large size and may likewise appear rather heavily opaque, at least in part, although it has *not* undergone malignant transformation. However, the radiopacity, even if considerable, is confined within the delimiting shell of the lesion, and there is no streaky radiation of the opacity into the neighboring soft parts (Fig. 45, p. 149). Another problem of roentgenographic differential diagnosis relates to the juxtacortical osteogenic sarcoma. The radiopacity of that lesion is usually fairly uniform rather than spotty and fuzzy. Tufts of radiopacity may jut into the neighboring soft parts, but these tufts are usually just as dense as the rest of the radiopaque area (Fig. 85, p. 281).

**Gross Pathology.**—It is difficult to give a single account which will do justice to the gross picture presented by peripheral chondrosarcoma. Nevertheless, the findings from two pertinent cases may serve for illustrative purposes. In the case illustrated in Fig. 104-*B*, surgical exploration showed that the tumor was attached to and had apparently arisen from the surface of one side of the sacrum. The resected specimen (Fig. 104-*C*) consisted of the tumor mass *in toto* and the part of the sacrum from which it had sprung. The mass was more or less globular in shape, measured about 22 cm. in length, 15 cm. across, and 15 cm. in thickness, and had muscle adherent to its outer surface. In hemisection the cartilage composing the tumor was found firm and bluish white. It presented the appearance of small, faceted lobules of cartilage, some of which showed calcification about their periphery. Continuous with the main tumor mass was a portion of sacrum which presented exostotic outgrowths along its margin.

Two years after the resection of the original tumor mass in this case, a recurrent tumor was removed from the buttock. The recurrent tumor tissue consisted of a number of large nodular masses of cartilage buried in muscle, fat, and fascial tissue. Three years later there was another local recurrence, and 3 years after that, a third recurrent tumor was removed. Thus, in an interval of 8 years after the original tumor mass was resected, there were three local recurrences, and still the tumor had neither spread into the pelvis nor metastasized. This is all the more interesting in view of the fact that the cytologic appearance of the tumor tissue became increasingly ominous from recurrence to recurrence and the fact that in the original specimen the tumor cartilage hardly gave any cytologic indication of malignancy at all.

### *Figure 104*

*A*, Roentgenograph showing a peripheral chondrosarcoma which has developed on the basis of a solitary osteocartilaginous exostosis of a tibia. The patient was a man who was 46 years of age at the time when the affected limb was amputated. He had been aware for 24 years of a tumor mass in the upper part of the leg. Lately, the tumor had begun to enlarge rather rapidly.

*B*, Roentgenograph showing a large peripheral chondrosarcoma which had sprung from the sacrum in the case of a man affected with hereditary multiple exostosis. Note the fuzzy radiopacities in the tumor area. The patient was 37 years of age and had been aware for 2 years of a tumor mass in the left buttock. Though the mass was increasing in size, there was no pain connected with its presence.

*C*, Photograph showing the cut surface of the specimen resected in the case illustrated in *B*. Above, one notes part of the sacrum, attached to which is a large, faceted cartilaginous tumor. Excision was followed by 3 local recurrences in the course of 8 years, but the tumor has not yet spread into the pelvis or metastasized.

*D*, Roentgenograph showing a huge chondrosarcoma which has sprung from the surface of a femur in the case of a man 41 years of age affected with hereditary multiple exostosis. The patient stated that he had discovered a mass in the thigh only 5 weeks before entering the hospital. However, he had been aware of bony bumps on other bones since he was 8 years old (see also Fig. 105).

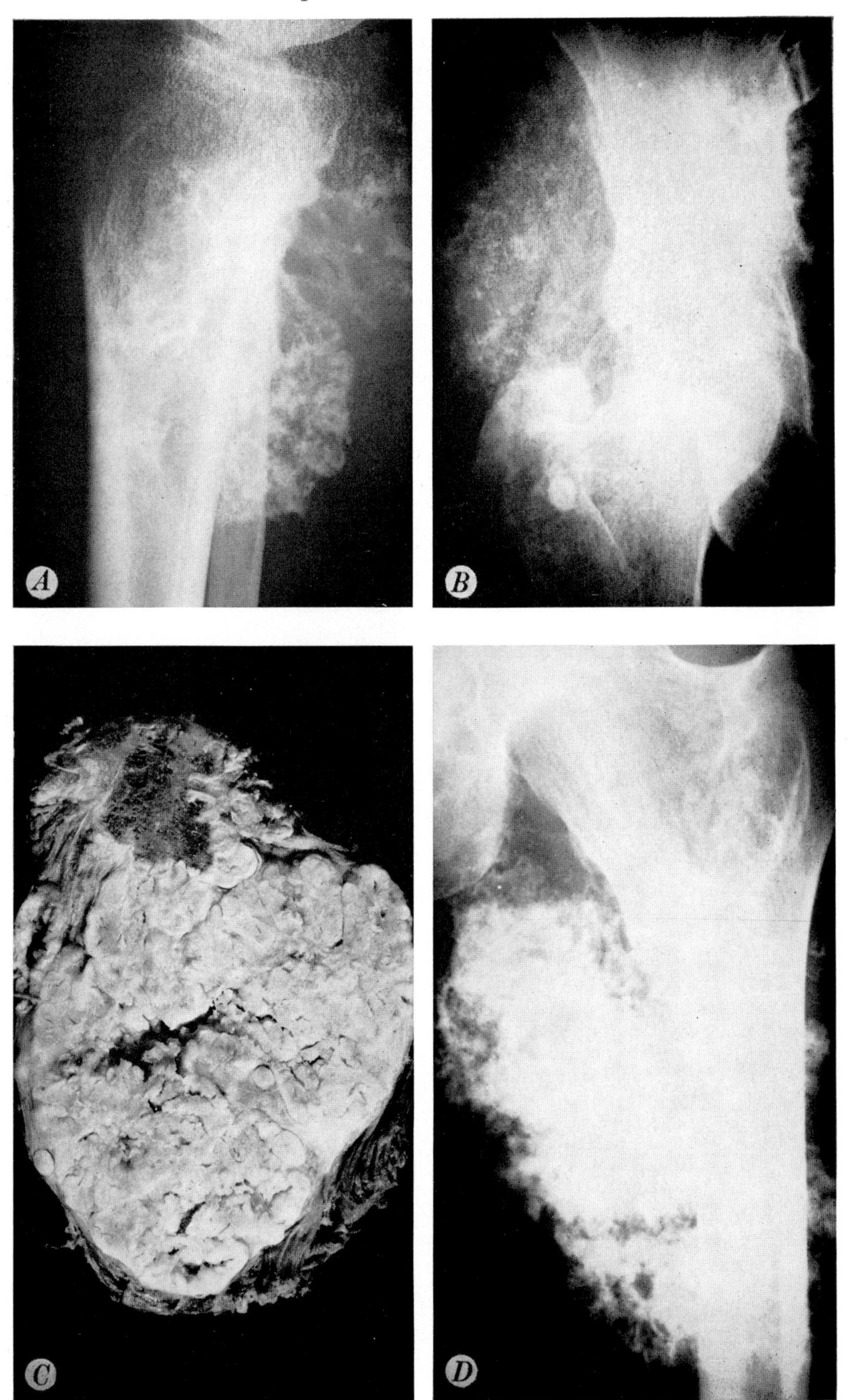


*Figure 104*

In the case illustrated in Fig. 104-*D*, the condition was treated by disarticulation at the hip joint. When the overlying soft parts had been removed from the affected part of the femur, a rather coarsely lobulated cartilaginous tumor was exposed and found to be partially enveloping the bone. The tumor mass as a whole measured approximately 20 cm. in length, 14 cm. across at its widest point, and up to 9 cm. in thickness. The tumor surrounded the neck of the femur and overlay the anterior and lateral and medial surfaces of the upper part of the femoral shaft. The posterior surface of the affected part of the shaft was free of tumor tissue. When the femur and engulfing tumor mass were hemisectioned, the cut surface again showed the faceted character of the tumor cartilage. In places this cartilage was rather heavily calcified, and in the area where the calcification was considerable one could see osseous tissue apparently representing metaplastic ossification of calcified tumor cartilage. Furthermore, the sectioned specimen showed that, although the cortex adjacent to the tumor tissue had been invaded in some places, the tumor had not broken through the cortex and invaded the medullary cavity (see Fig. 105).

Though the chondrosarcoma in this case was treated by disarticulation, this procedure did not prevent a recurrence, probably because it was not sufficiently radical in view of the location of the tumor. The first local recurrent mass of cartilage was removed 2 years after the disarticulation, and a second recurrent mass was removed 6 months later. In the subsequent 3½ years, no further recurrences have appeared, and the patient is in good health. However, one cannot say after so short an interval that the patient has certainly been cured.

**Microscopic Findings.**—What has been said about the cytologic stigmata of malignancy in connection with central chondrosarcoma applies in a general way to peripheral chondrosarcoma as well. However, in a particular peripheral chondrosarcoma, the cytologic stigmata of malignancy are often not obvious. In fact, unless tissue blocks from many different areas of such a lesion are taken for histologic examination, the evidences of malignancy may be missed. For instance, the lesional cartilage as a whole may not be very cellular, and many of the sections may show only an occasional cell with a double nucleus and no cells with bizarre nuclei—appearances which might lead to interpretation of the lesion as a benign cartilage growth. Nevertheless, sections prepared from other parts of the lesion will show plumping up of all the nuclei, quite a number of cells with double nuclei,

***Figure 105***

*A*, Photograph showing a large peripheral chondrosarcoma (see Fig. 104-*D*) which is oriented to the anterior surface of the upper part of the shaft of a femur. Note the lobulated appearance of the tumor cartilage.

*B*, Photograph showing the posterior view of the tumor in the femur shown in *A*. The bumpiness of the femoral neck and intertrochanteric area represents an exostotic outgrowth. Below and to the sides of the shaft one notes the tumor, which has not enveloped the posterior surface of the shaft.

*C*, Photograph showing the femur and adherent chondrosarcoma in longitudinal section. Note the faceted appearance of the tumor cartilage as a whole. Note also the speckled whitish areas representing calcification which are prominent in the lower part of the tumor. Although the tumor is intimately connected with the cortex of the femur and is invading it, especially in the region of the lesser trochanter, it has not broken into the medullary cavity of the bone (see *D* and *E*).

*D*, Roentgenograph of a transverse slice of the femur and chondrosarcoma, approximately at the level of the lesser trochanter. The tumor cartilage is not very heavily calcified in this region. Note that the medullary cavity has not been invaded by the tumor.

*E*, Roentgenograph of a transverse slice of the femur and chondrosarcoma somewhat below the level shown in *D*. At this lower level the tumor cartilage is heavily calcified.

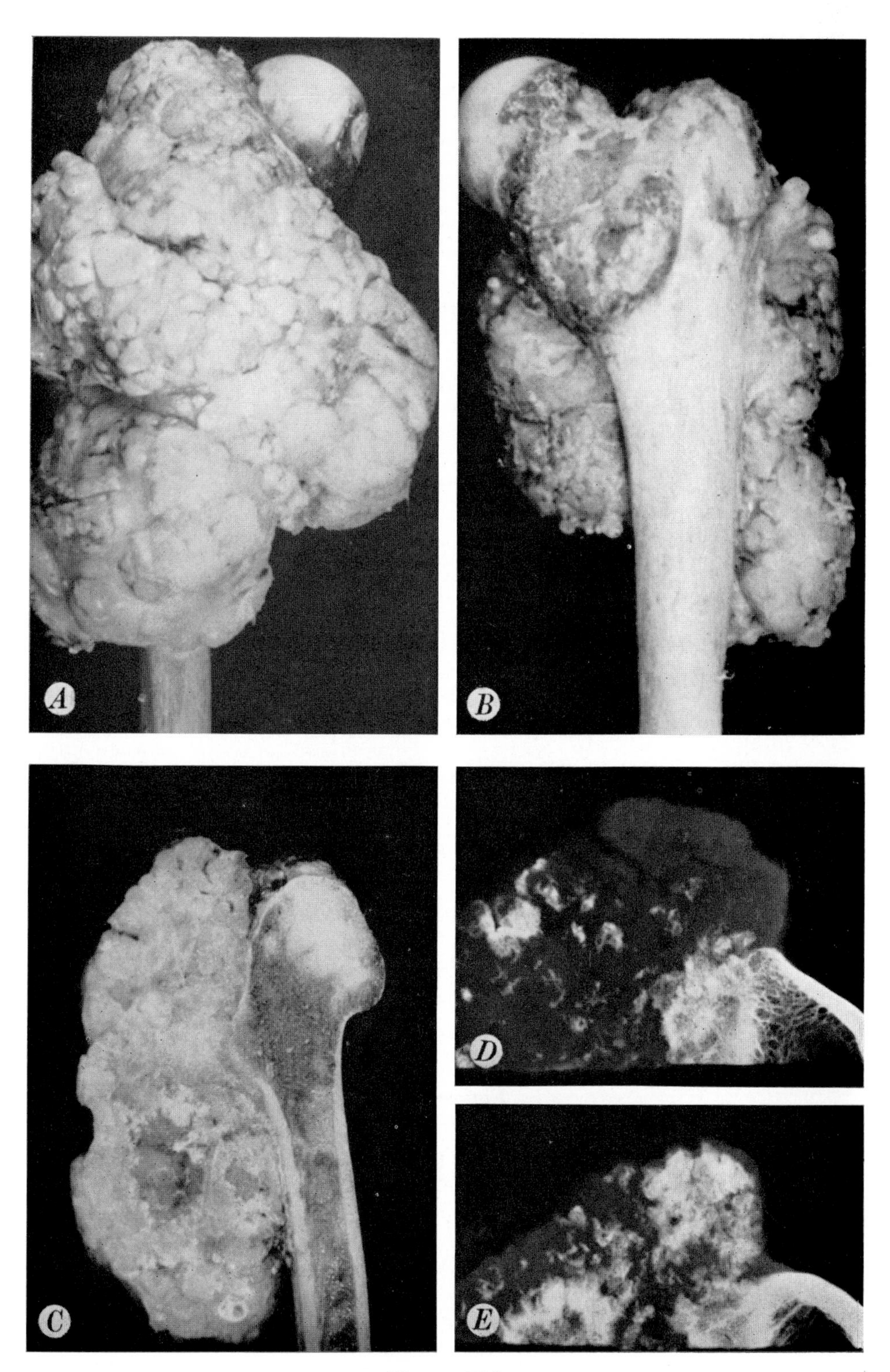


*Figure 105*

and an occasional bizarre giant nucleus—indubitable evidences of malignancy in a cartilage tumor.

In still other peripheral chondrosarcomas, tissue sections from all parts of the lesion will already show that the tumor cartilage is cellular, that all the nuclei are plump, and that many of them are double. In any case, no matter how subtle the histologic evidences of malignancy may be in the original lesion, they become increasingly clear-cut in any recurrences which may take place. Indeed, in a second or third recurrence the tumor cartilage may show numerous cells with giant bizarre nuclei and even some nuclei in mitotic division (see Fig. 106).

## TREATMENT

The principles of treatment for peripheral chondrosarcoma are the same as those outlined for central chondrosarcoma. Thus, in accordance with the location of the lesion and the degree of cytologic malignity presented by a biopsy specimen, the surgical indications are: wide excision, amputation, or fore- or-hindquarter ablation.

Many of the peripheral chondrosarcomas occur in the general region of the hip joint or shoulder joint, and the growths have often attained large size by the time the patient appears for treatment. Hence one is often faced with the practical problem of deciding how radical the surgery should be for peripheral chondrosarcoma affecting the upper part of a humerus or femur or part of a scapula or innominate bone.

In relation to such sites, complete local excision of the lesion such as would be necessary to prevent recurrence may be difficult and should not be undertaken unless the chances of success appear to be quite good. If such an excision is attempted, however, a recurrence does not necessarily preclude the possibility that a more radical intervention can still be undertaken in the expectation of a favorable outcome. Thus, while a forequarter or hindquarter amputation will usually produce a cure in such cases if undertaken as the initial intervention, the lesion is often still amenable to such surgery even after one or more recurrences. Altogether, cases of peripheral chondrosarcoma have to be evaluated individually in regard to the best surgical approach.

***Figure 106***

*A*, Photomicrograph (× 250) showing the cytologic appearance characteristic of the tumor tissue in the peripheral and uncalcified portions of the chondrosarcoma illustrated in Figure 105. Note that the nuclei of the tumor cells are not particularly prominent, that only an occasional cell shows a double nucleus, and that none of the cells show bizarre nuclei. Indeed, the roentgenographic and gross pathologic findings in this lesion at this stage speak more strongly in favor of chondrosarcoma than do the cytologic findings.

*B*, Photomicrograph (× 250) of tissue from the first recurrence of the lesion shown in *A*. Note that many of the cells now show plump nuclei and that the cytologic picture is becoming more clearly representative of chondrosarcoma.

*C*, Photomicrograph (× 250) of tissue from the second recurrence in this case. Note that most of the cell nuclei are plump, and that some cells have double or bizarre nuclei. The cytologic picture is now that of an indubitable chondrosarcoma.

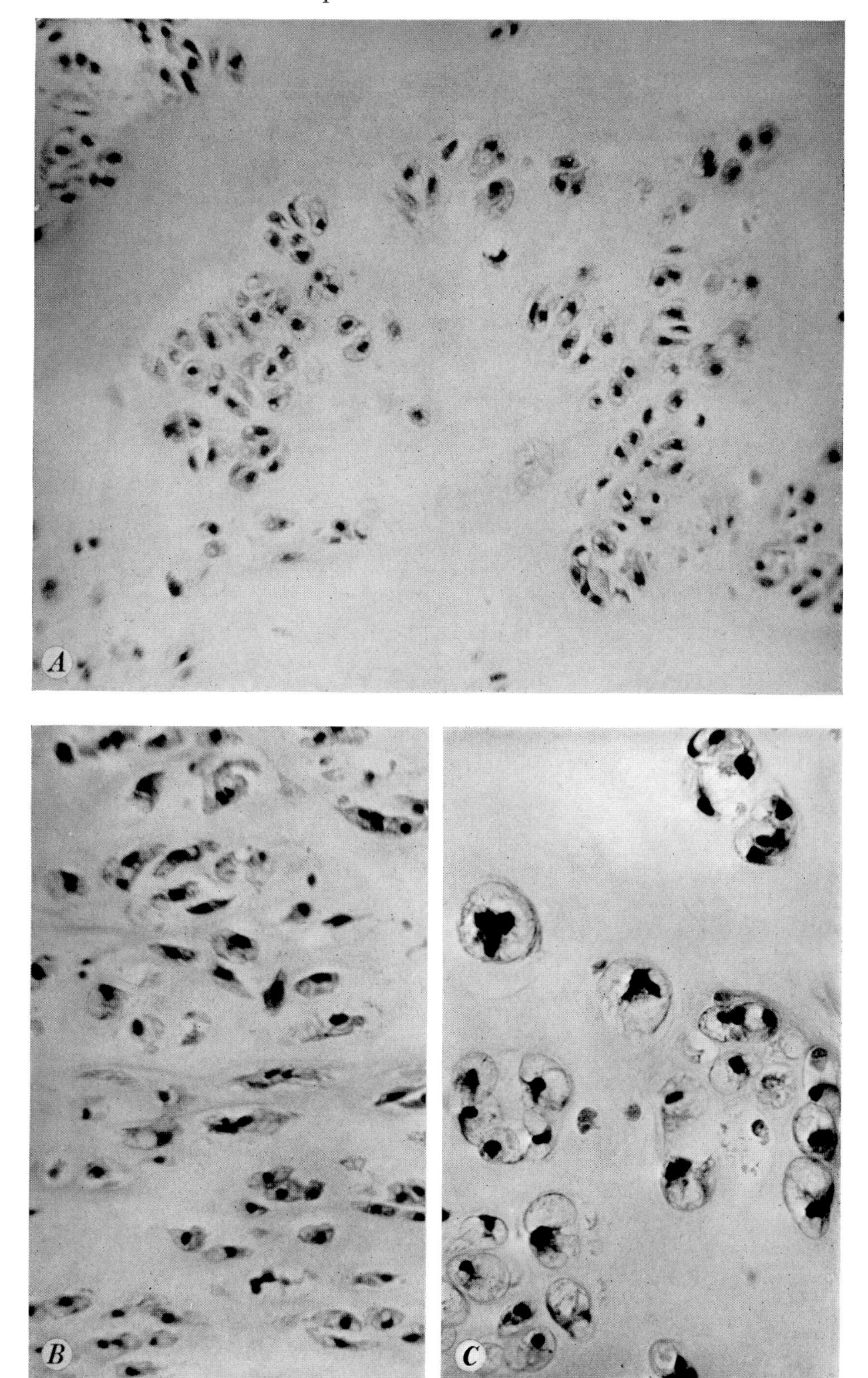


*Figure 106*

## REFERENCES


Bessler, W.: Das Beckenchondrom und Chondrosarkom, Virchows Arch. f. path. Anat., *323*, 72, 1953.

Calvi, N.: Contributo alla conoscenza radiologica dei condrosarcomi, Tumori, *39*, 308, 1953.

Coley, B. L., and Higinbotham, N. L.: Secondary Chondrosarcoma, Ann. Surg., *139*, 547, 1954.

Copeland, M. M.: Tumors of Cartilaginous Origin, Clinical Orthopaedics, *7*, 9, 1956.

Cruickshank, A. H.: Chondrosarcoma of a Phalanx with Cutaneous Metastases, J. Path. & Bact., *57*, 144, 1945.

Dahlin, D. C., and Henderson, E. D.: Chondrosarcoma, A Surgical and Pathological Problem, J. Bone & Joint Surg., *38-A*, 1025, 1956.

Ernst, P.: Ungewöhnliche Verbreitung einer Knorpelgeschwulst in der Blutbahn, Beitr. z. path. Anat. u. z. allg. Path., *28*, 255, 1900.

Fodden, J. H.: The Central Malignant Chondroma of Bone, Canad. M.A.J., *63*, 362, 1950.

Ghormley, R. K.: Chondromas and Chondrosarcomas of the Scapula and the Innominate Bone, Arch. Surg., *63*, 48, 1951.

Harrington, S. W.: Surgical Treatment of Intrathoracic Tumors and Tumors of the Chest Wall, Arch. Surg., *14*, 406, 1927.

Jaffe, H. L.: Hereditary Multiple Exostosis, Arch. Path., *36*, 335, 1943.

Jaffe, H. L., and Lichtenstein, L.: Solitary Benign Enchondroma of Bone, Arch. Surg., *46*, 480, 1943.

————: Chondromyxoid Fibroma of Bone, Arch. Path., *45*, 541, 1948.

Keiller, V. H.: Cartilaginous Tumors of Bone, Surg., Gynec. & Obst., *40*, 510, 1925.

Kósa, M.: Chondroblastom in der venösen Blutbahn, Virchows Arch. f. path. Anat., *272*, 166, 1929.

Lichtenstein, L., and Jaffe, H. L.: Chondrosarcoma of Bone, Am. J. Path., *19*, 553, 1943.

Monro, R. S., and Golding, J. S. R.: Chondrosarcoma of the Ilium Complicating Hereditary Multiple Exostoses, Brit. J. Surg., *39*, 73, 1951.

O'Neal, L. W., and Ackerman, L. V.: Chondrosarcoma of Bone, Cancer, *5*, 551, 1952.

Phemister, D. B.: Chondrosarcoma of Bone, Surg., Gynec. & Obst., *50*, 216, 1930.

————: Conservative Surgery in the Treatment of Bone Tumors, Surg., Gynec. & Obst., *70*, 355, 1940.

Sugarbaker, E. D., and Ackerman, L. V.: Disarticulation of the Innominate Bone for Malignant Tumors of the Pelvic Parietes and Upper Thigh, Surg., Gynec. & Obst., *81*, 36, 1945.

Warren, S.: Chondrosarcoma with Intravascular Growth and Tumor Emboli to Lungs, Am. J. Path., *7*, 161, 1931.

Chapter

# 21

# Malignant Vascular Tumors

A *malignant vascular tumor* may be broadly defined as a sarcoma which demonstrates vasoformative capacity as part of its intrinsic nature. There are a number of tumors which come under this general definition. In addition to hemangiosarcoma and lymphangiosarcoma, such lesions as malignant hemangiopericytoma and Kaposi's sarcoma are often included in this category. (See Stout, Stout and Murray, Nelson and Morfit, and Landing and Farber.) In the present chapter, however, we are concerned mainly with the *hemangiosarcoma*, often also denoted as the *malignant hemangioendothelioma* or *angiosarcoma*. This vasoformative sarcoma is distinguished by the fact that its basic tumor cells are endothelioblasts and, as such, tend strongly toward the formation of blood channels in the course of their proliferation. The other malignant vasoformative tumors mentioned above have little practical importance in relation to the skeleton, and it is even doubtful whether a lymphangiosarcoma occurs in bones at all.

The hemangiosarcoma is a rare tumor altogether, and it is highly unusual for it to appear in bone as a primary lesion. Indeed, when it is encountered in bone, it usually represents a metastasis from an extraskeletal hemangiosarcoma or direct extension to the bone by a hemangiosarcoma of the overlying soft parts. In any case, it should be borne in mind that a hemangiosarcoma almost never arises from a pre-existing benign hemangioma. Whether as a primary or as a metastatic lesion, the tumor is more likely to be encountered in the form of multiple foci in one or more bones than as a solitary lesion affecting a single bone area. In connection with multiple hemangiovascular lesions of bone, it seems likely that some cases of the rare so-called "benign metastasizing hemangioma" represent instances of "underdiagnosed" hemangiosarcoma metastatic from an extraskeletal hemangiosarcoma, or of hemangiosarcoma primary in multiple bone sites. On the other hand, those multiple vascular tumors of bone which are indubitably benign in their histologic appearance in the various sites must be regarded as benign hemangiomas primary in multiple bone sites. (For the discussion of the benign vascular tumors of bone, see p. 224.)

Whether present in solitary or in multiple form, the hemangiosarcomas encountered in bone (like those encountered elsewhere) fall into two general groups. In one group the lesion is of low malignancy and shows a histologic pattern characterized by the presence of numerous small blood channels lined by layers of endothelial cells. On the other hand, one encounters hemangiosarcomas which are frankly malignant and tend to metastasize rapidly. In such a case the histologic pattern of the lesion may be the one expected in a hemangiosarcoma or, on the other hand, it may be so anaplastic that the picture is dominated by undifferentiated sarcomatous stromal cells, few vascular clefts being present.

## CLINICAL CONSIDERATIONS

The clinical manifestations of hemangiosarcoma consist mainly of pain and swelling and present little that is distinctive. Also, because of the rarity of the condition, no significant statements are possible about its age distribution and sex incidence. However, insofar as one can judge, there is no predilection for either sex or any particular age group. When a hemangiosarcoma appears as a solitary lesion, the site is more likely to be a long bone than some other kind of bone. There are also cases in which multiple bone areas show involvement simultaneously. On the other hand, one may encounter a case in which the disorder first becomes clinically manifest in a single bone but in which additional lesions subsequently appear in other bone sites. Even in such a case these other lesions are not necessarily metastatic lesions and may again simply represent hemangiosarcoma in multiple sites.

The *roentgenographic findings* offer little to distinguish the hemangiosarcoma from other malignant bone tumors producing solitary or multiple areas of bone destruction. The lesional area or areas are likely to be strikingly radiolucent. The regional cortex is often found destroyed, and there may be bulging of the local bone contour. Be that as it may, one arrives at the diagnosis through tissue examination, and to avoid pitfalls it should be made from an adequate sample removed through an incisional biopsy. (See Fig. 107.)

## PATHOLOGIC FINDINGS

**Gross Pathology.**—A hemangiosarcoma is likely to reveal its vascular character grossly by its dark, brownish or bluish red color. Also, the tissue tends to be of soft consistency. If seen intact in its bone setting, the lesional tissue may not be sharply delimited from the neighboring tissue. However, if the hemangiosarcoma

### *Figure 107*

*A*, Roentgenograph showing an area of lytic destruction produced by a hemangiosarcoma involving the proximal end of the third metacarpal bone. There is nothing in the *x*-ray picture which gives much help toward establishing the diagnosis. (The microscopic appearance of the lesional tissue in this case is illustrated in Fig. 109-*A*.) The patient was a man who developed local pain and swelling after an injury to the hand. The affected bone began to present roentgenographic evidence of lytic destruction, and the *x*-ray picture illustrated shows the state of the bone destruction 2 months later. The lesion was treated by local resection, insertion of a bone graft, and postoperative radiation therapy. Almost 5 years later there was no evidence of recurrence.

*B*, Roentgenograph showing an area of lytic destruction produced by a hemangiosarcoma involving part of the lower end of the shaft of a femur. Again the *x*-ray picture is nondescript. (The microscopic appearance of the lesional tissue removed from the bone site in question is illustrated in Fig. 109-*B*.) The patient was a boy 14 years of age who was admitted to the M. D. Anderson Hospital of Houston, Texas, with a history of anemia, loss of weight, and a local swelling about the knee. At that time a skeletal survey showed merely the illustrated lesion in the femur. It was treated by curettage, and numerous fragments of firm, hemorrhagically discolored tumor tissue were removed from the lesional area. Several months later the boy was found to have developed very pronounced osteoporosis of many bones, and particularly of the vertebral column, which showed compression of several bodies. Lytic destructive lesions in bones other than the femur had not appeared as yet. The great likelihood is, however, that they will appear and that the boy is suffering from a generalized hemangiosarcomatosis of the skeleton and possibly of internal organs also.

*C*, Roentgenograph of a foot from a case of hemangiosarcoma involving multiple bone sites. Lesions are present in the proximal phalanx of the big toe, in the first metatarsal bone and in the navicular and cuboid bones. The patient was a man 25 years of age. The condition was treated by amputation above the ankle, and a 6-year follow-up finds the patient cured of his disease. Cytologically, the lesional tissue was that of a well differentiated hemangiosarcoma, resembling in its histologic pattern the lesion illustrated in Fig. 109-*A*.

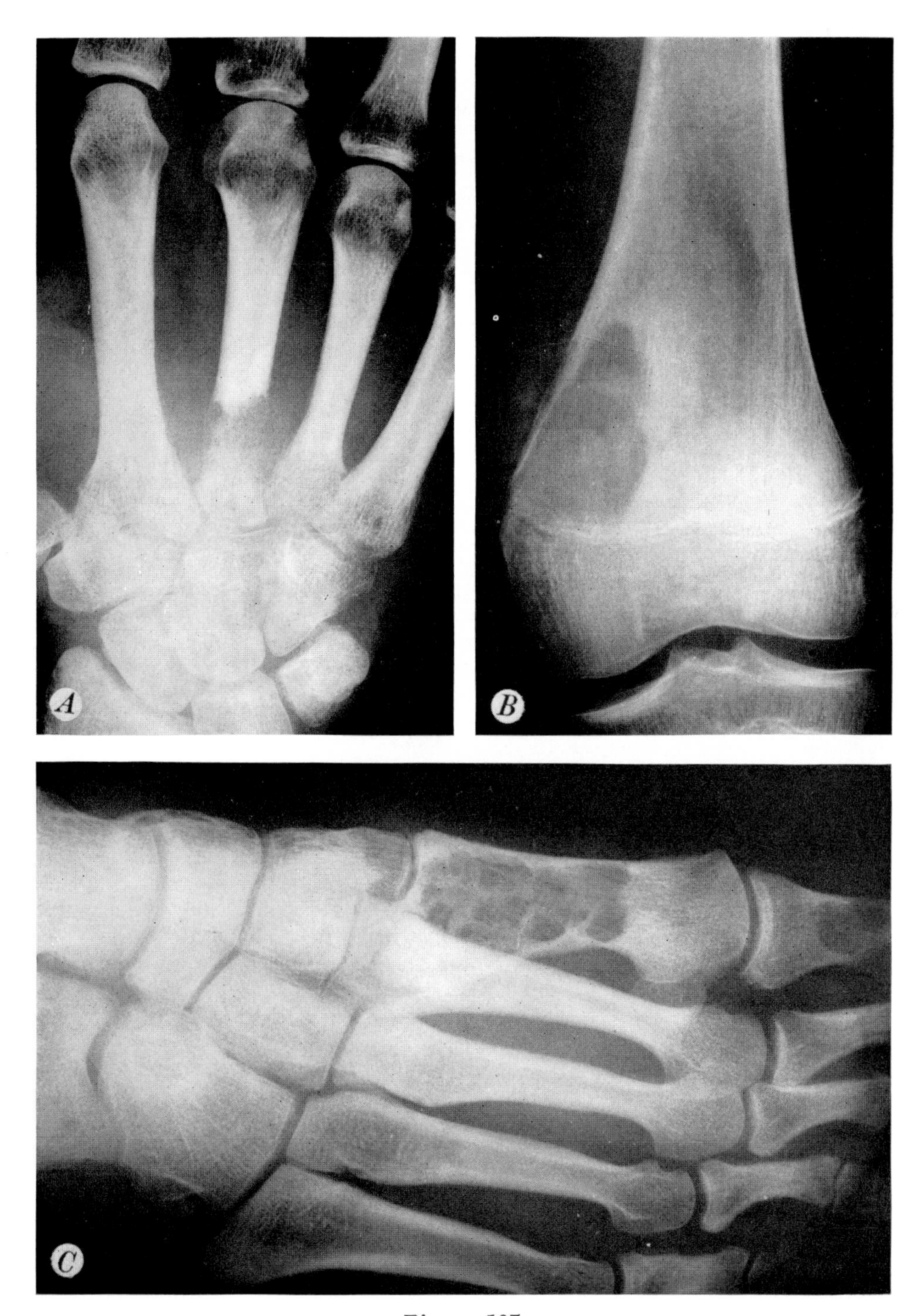


*Figure 107*

is one in which the blood channels have become obstructed by endothelial proliferation, the telltale characteristic reddish color may not be striking or may be absent altogether. Indeed, under these conditions the tumor tissue may even suggest an anaplastic fibrosarcoma in its gross appearance and texture. (See Fig. 108.)

**Microscopic Pathology.**—In the last analysis, as already indicated, the diagnosis of hemangiosarcoma of bone has to rest upon the histologic pattern presented by the lesional tissue. This pattern can vary in its detail from lesion to lesion and even within different areas of the same lesion. Its distinctive feature is the presence of aggregations of anastomosing vascular spaces which are lined by atypical endothelial cells. The stroma between the capillary spaces varies in amount but is largely composed of still undifferentiated endothelioblasts.

In some lesions the evidence of the formation of vascular spaces is striking throughout. Specifically, one notes numerous rounded or cleft-like capillaries which are lined by roundish or oval endothelial cells. Many of the vascular spaces may contain blood cells, though many may appear to have become partially obliterated by heaping up of the endothelial lining cells. Here and there one may also find nests of endothelial cells not surrounding a lumen at all. However, as Stout points out, whenever a lesion which is not forming vascular spaces is nevertheless suspected of being a hemangiosarcoma, its vascular character can be demonstrated by the use of silver stains to bring out the reticulin which will be found surrounding the cords of endothelial cells.

In these well differentiated hemangiosarcomas, the histologic pattern is more suggestive of the benign hemangioendothelioma often encountered in the skin in children than of those hemangiosarcomas (see below) in which the tendency of the basic endothelioblasts of the tumor toward vascular differentiation is less striking. Their behavior, too, is different from that of these poorly differentiated hemangiosarcomas. In particular, they grow more slowly, do not tend to metastasize readily, and, if present in solitary form, are on the whole responsive to local excision followed by radiation therapy. (See Fig. 109.)

A poorly differentiated hemangiosarcoma may still show, in many areas, considerable evidence of vasoformative capacity. In such areas the blood channels may be mere slits or large and cavernous, but in either case the lining endothelial cells are usually rather flattened and not piled up in the lumens. On the other hand, in areas where the proliferating tumor cells are not forming vascular spaces, they may be present in sheets or cords and may be rather spindle-shaped. Usually, however, a poorly differentiated hemangiosarcoma still contains, in one area or another, sufficient evidence of its vasoformative character to permit the correct

***Figure 108***

*A*, Photograph of a longitudinally sectioned tibia showing 3 foci of angiosarcoma represented by the dark areas. In addition to lesions in the tibia, there were also lesions in the fibula and in several bones of the corresponding foot. The histologic pattern of the lesional tissue in this case corresponded more or less closely to that illustrated in Fig. 110-*A*.

*B*, Photograph showing part of a longitudinally sectioned tibia which has been invaded by a hemangiosarcoma primary in the overlying soft parts. Note the dark lesional area standing out from the unaffected part of the bone. Some time before the amputation, an attempt had been made to cure the condition by local excision of the soft-tissue tumor, but recurrence of the tumor and invasion of the bone made amputation necessary.

*C*, Photograph (natural size) of a celloidin section showing the architectural tissue pattern of a hemangiosarcoma affecting the lower half of a femur. The blood channels are more obvious in the part of the lesion involving the bone shaft than in the tumor tissue in the end of the bone. (Doctor C. Howard Hatcher of the University of Chicago kindly supplied the section.)

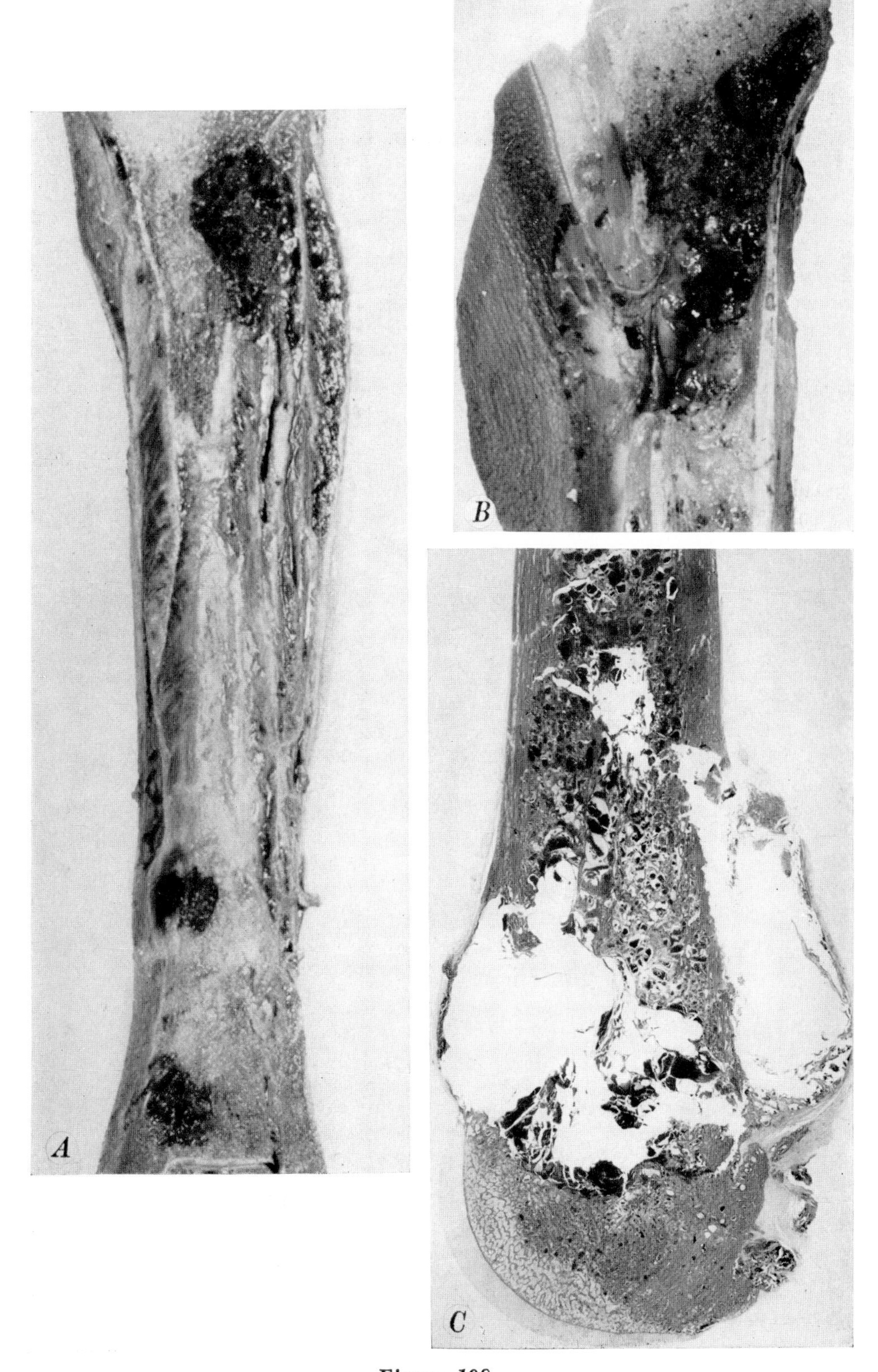


*Figure 108*

interpretation. Nevertheless, if the hemangiosarcoma is a highly anaplastic one, and in particular if spindle-shaped cells are numerous, the lesion might easily pass for a poorly differentiated fibrosarcoma. (See Fig. 110.)

In general, a hemangiosarcoma does not seem to be more prone to metastasis than various other sarcomas. Metastasis of a hemangiosarcoma usually takes place by way of the blood stream, though metastasis by way of the lymphatics to regional lymph nodes also occurs (see Bauer and Stanford).

**Differential Diagnosis.**—In view of the rarity of hemangiosarcoma, particularly in skeletal sites, the diagnosis of hemangiosarcoma of bone should be made with great caution. In this connection the question of the interpretation of cases reported, for instance by Thomas, under the heading of "angioendothelioma of bone" arises. It comes up because the interpretation of that lesion as a primary vascular tumor of bone seems to be inconsistent with the described cytologic pattern of the lesional tissue. The constituent cells of the tumor are stated to be large and polyhedral or cylindrical in shape, and to have a well defined cell membrane, clear cytoplasm, and a small, vesicular nucleus. Also, the cells are described as being arranged in cords or alveolar formation. It is further recorded in these reports that many of the alveolar lumens may be found filled with blood. It is probably this fact that has created the misleading impression that the lesion is a primary vascular tumor of bone. Actually, the bone lesion in these cases is a highly vascularized metastatic carcinoma and specifically, in most instances, a carcinoma metastatic from a hypernephroma. Altogether, if one does use the term "angioendothelioma" of bone, it should be kept for a sarcoma demonstrating vasoformative capacity, and in particular for a tumor in which clear-cut vascular spaces lined by endothelium are being delimited. That is, if used at all, the term should be employed only as a synonym for hemangiosarcoma.

Other metastatic carcinomas, if highly vascularized and undifferentiated, may also sometimes be misinterpreted as hemangiosarcomas. These others include thyroid carcinoma, choriocarcinoma, and even undifferentiated tumors metastatic from the lungs or stomach. It goes without saying that highly vascularized sarcomas of various types metastatic to a bone site are also subject to misinterpretation as hemangiosarcomas. Even a malignant synovioma might be so misinterpreted, on account of the fact that it forms cell-like clefts which may become filled with blood in consequence of surgical trauma. It has also been suggested that the so-called adamantinoma of limb bones actually represents a malignant vascular tumor (malignant angioblastoma) rather than an epithelial tumor. For further discussion of this particular question, see page 222.

***Figure 109***

*A*, Photomicrograph (× 125) showing the tissue pattern of a hemangiosarcoma which mimics the pattern of the so-called "benign hemangioendothelioma." (The tissue came from the lesion illustrated in Fig. 107-*A*.) Note the capillary spaces lined by hypertrophied endothelial cells. Note also that, in the upper left-hand part of the picture, the endothelial cells are present in clusters and not in orderly arrangement as the lining cells of vascular spaces.

*B*, Photomicrograph (× 125) showing the tissue pattern of a hemangiosarcoma in which the vascular spaces are present mainly as anastomosing clefts lined by endothelial cells. (This tissue came from the lesion illustrated in Fig. 107-*B*.)

*C*, Photomicrograph (× 250) showing in higher detail the histologic architecture of the vascular clefts and lining endothelial cells observed in *B*. The field illustrated comes from the lower central part of that picture.

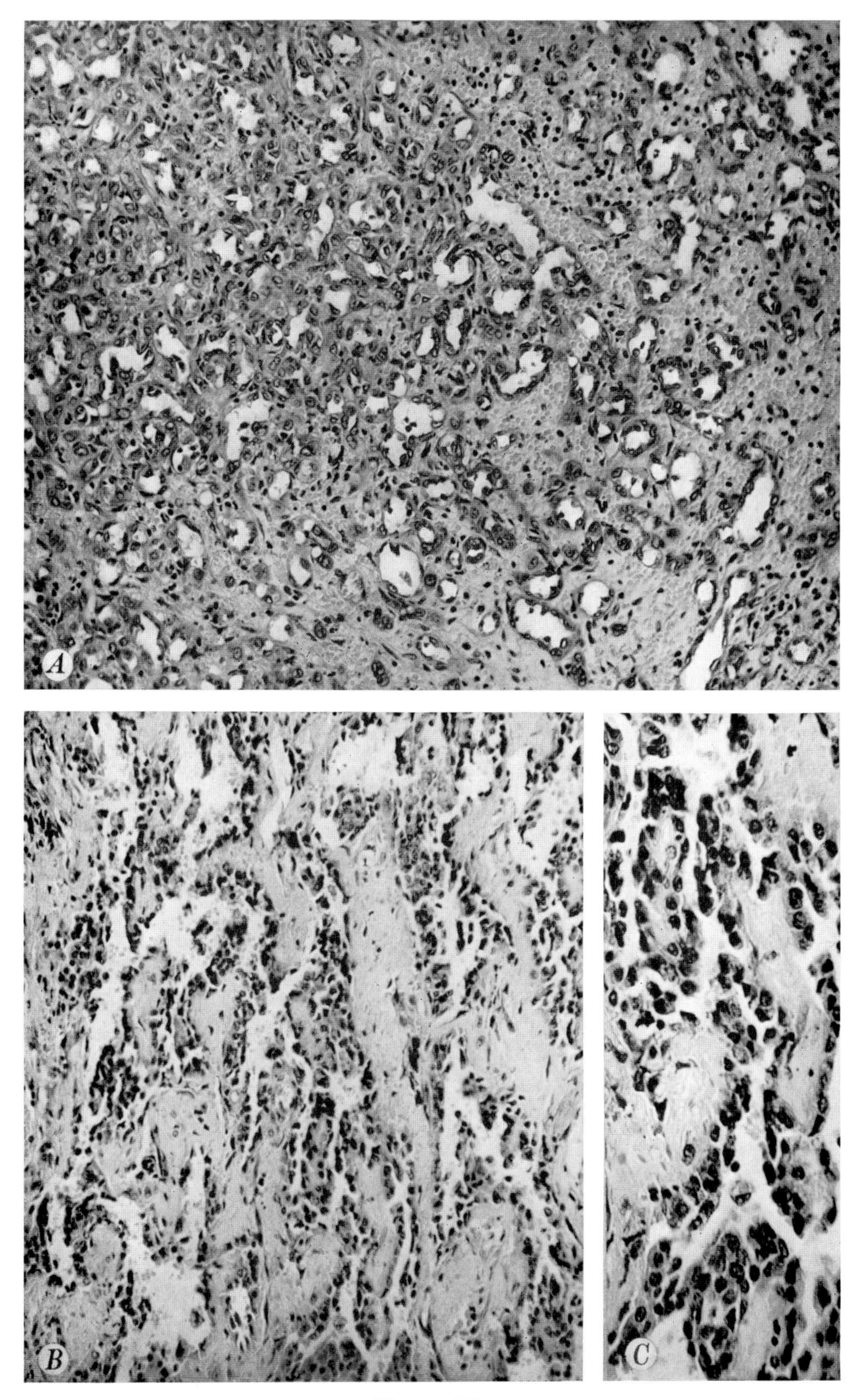


*Figure 109*

## TREATMENT

The treatment of a hemangiosarcoma of low malignancy in a solitary bone site may well consist of local resection and postoperative radiation therapy. If a tumor of this type is present in multiple sites in the bones of one limb, amputation is indicated. Hemangiosarcomas of high malignancy appearing in limb bones, in solitary or multiple form, are best treated by amputation. Whether of low or high malignancy, hemangiosarcomas appearing in sites inaccessible to surgery naturally call for treatment by radiation alone.

## REFERENCES

Aegerter, E. E., and Peale, A. R.: Kaposi's Sarcoma: A Critical Survey, Arch. Path., *34*, 413, 1942.

Bauer, D. deF., and Stanford, W. R.: Splenic Hemangiosarcoma: A Case with Lymphatic and Vascular Metastases, Arch. Path., *41*, 668, 1946.

Fienberg, R., and Baehr, F. H.: Hemangioendothelioma of Tibia with Metastasis to the Popliteal Artery, Arch. Path., *31*, 811, 1941.

Gloggengiesser, W.: Angiomartige Umwandlung des Gefässmesenchyms als Systemerkrankung, Beitr. z. path. Anat. u. z. allg. Path., *103*, 256, 1939.

Hirsch, E. F., and Ryerson, E. W.: Metastases of the Bone in Primary Carcinoma of the Lung: A Review of So-called Endotheliomas of the Bones, Arch. Surg., *16*, 1, 1928.

Köhlmeier, W.: Zur Kenntnis der Angiome des Knochens, Wien. klin. Wchnschr., *50*, 274, 1937.

Kolodny, A.: Angio-Endothelioma of Bone, Arch. Surg., *12*, 854, 1926.

Landing, B. H., and Farber, S.: Tumors of the Cardiovascular System, Atlas of Tumor Pathology, Section III, Fascicle 7, Armed Forces Institute of Pathology, Washington, D.C., 1956.

Lutz, J. F., and Pusch, L. C.: Angio-Endothelioma of Bone, J.A.M.A., *113*, 1009, 1939.

Nelson, W. R., and Morfit, H. M.: Lymphangiosarcoma in the Lymphedematous Arm after Radical Mastectomy, Cancer, *9*, 1189, 1956.

Pollak, A.: Angiosarcoma of the Sternum, Am. J. Surg., *77*, 522, 1949.

Rabson, S. M.: Multiple Mesenchymal Hemendothelioma, Arch. Path., *25*, 185, 1938.

Robinson, J. M., and Castleman, B.: Benign Metastasizing Hemangioma, Ann. Surg., *104*, 453, 1936.

Schlopsnies, W.: Über ein systematisiertes Angioplastisches Sarkom in Milz, Leber und Knochenmark, Virchows Arch. f. path. Anat., *274*, 85, 1929.

Stout, A. P.: Hemangio-endothelioma: A Tumor of Blood Vessels Featuring Vascular Endothelial Cells, Ann. Surg., *118*, 445, 1943.

Stout, A. P., and Murray, M. R.: Hemangiopericytoma: A Vascular Tumor Featuring Zimmermann's Pericytes, Ann. Surg., *116*, 26, 1942.

Thomas, A.: Vascular Tumors of Bone, Surg., Gynec. & Obst., *74*, 777, 1942.

Töpfer, D.: I. Über ein infiltrierend wachsendes Hämangiom der Haut und multiple Kapillarektasien der Haut und inneren Organe. II. Zur Kenntnis der Wirbelangiome, Frankfurt. Ztschr. f. Path., *36*, 337, 1928.

Wollstein, M.: Malignant Hemangioma of the Lung with Multiple Visceral Foci, Arch. Path., *12*, 562, 1931.

### *Figure 110*

*A*, Photomicrograph (× 125) showing the pattern of a hemangiosarcoma which is less differentiated than the hemangiosarcomas illustrated in Fig. 109. Note the numerous vascular spaces lined by flattened endothelial cells. Observe also that, in the area illustrated, the endothelial cells between the vascular spaces are also spindle-shaped.

*B*, Photomicrograph (× 125) illustrating the tissue pattern in another part of the section from which *A* was prepared. Note that the endothelial cells are spindle-shaped and that vasoformative activity is not conspicuous.

*C*, Photomicrograph (× 250) illustrating the pattern in still another part of the section from which *A* was prepared. Here, vasoformation is prominent and numerous small vascular spaces lined by hypertrophied endothelial cells are in evidence.

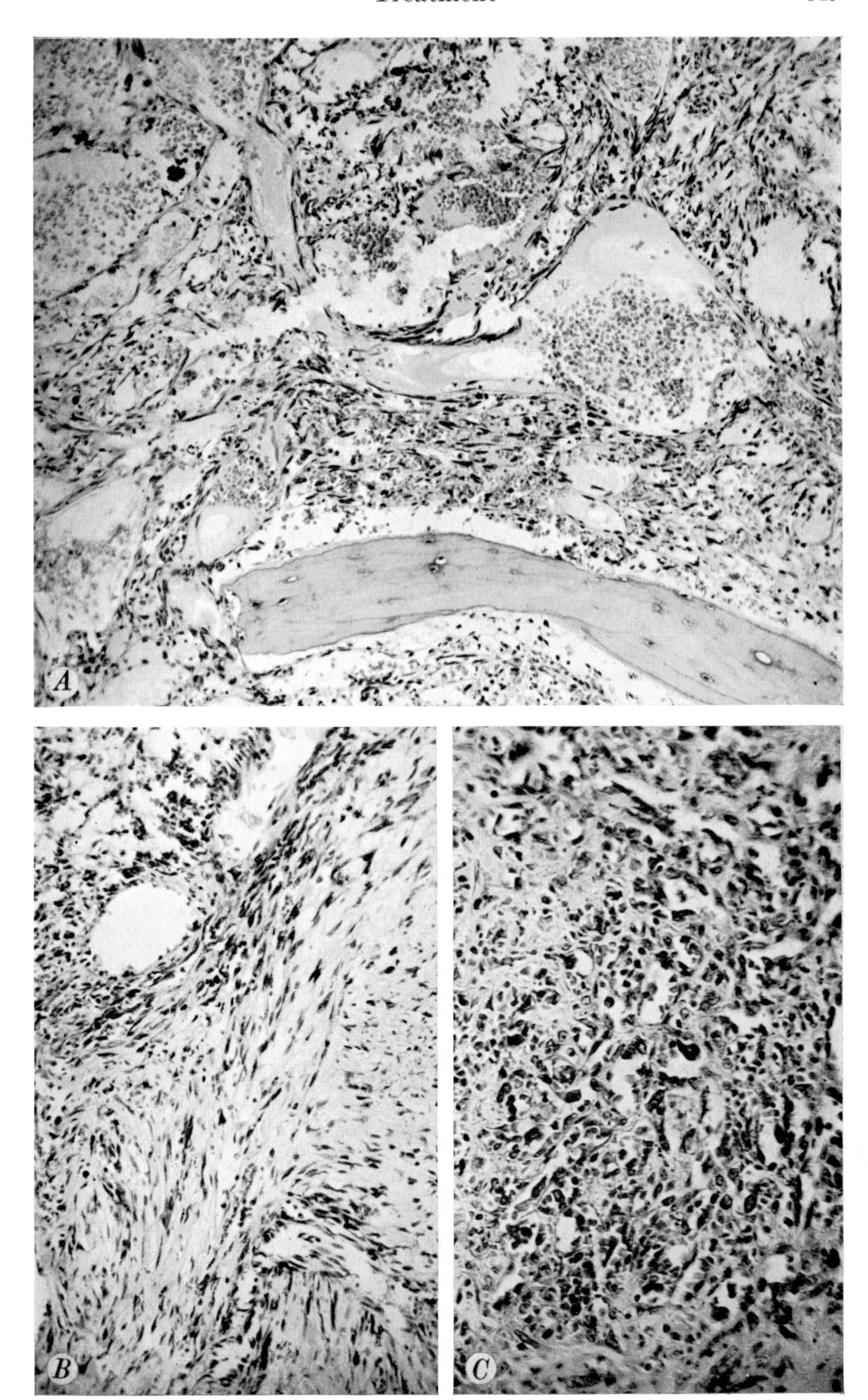


*Figure 110*

Chapter

# 22

# Ewing's Sarcoma

THE *Ewing sarcoma* is a specific primary malignant tumor of bone which Ewing singled out in the early 1920's as a clinicopathologic entity. Previously such cases had usually been relegated to the rather nondescript and general category of "round cell sarcoma" of bone. Though the Ewing sarcoma soon gained wide acceptance as an entity, it nevertheless became the focal point for much critical discussion. In consequence, much of what was embodied in the original descriptions of the lesion (relating to its histogenesis and histology and to certain clinical features) has been modified. (See Oberling, Stout, Jaffe, and Lichtenstein and Jaffe.) However, the doubt expressed by some that a bone tumor entity such as Ewing described exists at all (see Willis) has turned out to be unjustified.

A patient affected with Ewing's sarcoma is usually a young person. Most often, the presenting lesion is in a long bone of a lower limb or in a pelvic bone. Roentgenographically, in one case or another a Ewing sarcoma may be hard to distinguish, for instance, from an eosinophilic granuloma of bone, a focus of bone infection, or an osteogenic sarcoma. Histologically, in areas not modified by secondary change such as necrosis or hemorrhage, the lesional tumor tissue is characterized by the presence of cells which lack clearly delimited boundaries and whose nuclei are roundish and of fairly uniform appearance.

However, it must be borne in mind that this cytologic pattern may be simulated, for example, by tissue from a malignant lymphoma (especially a primary reticulum cell sarcoma of bone) or a focus of neuroblastoma metastatic to a bone. On the other hand, a pathologist studying a biopsy specimen from a suspected case of Ewing's sarcoma may also have considerable difficulty in making the correct diagnosis if the tissue submitted happens to be largely necrotic. In such a case the presence of many leukocytes in the necrotic tissue may even lead to misinterpretation of the condition as an infection.

Against this background it is evident why the diagnosis of Ewing's sarcoma often presents difficulties. Caution in making this diagnosis is all the more justified in view of the fact that the lesion is not a very common one. No matter how the condition is treated, it is nearly always ultimately fatal. In fatal cases, autopsy usually reveals tumor tissue widely disseminated through the skeleton and often also in visceral organs, especially the lungs.

**Nomenclature.**—Ewing called the lesion "diffuse endothelioma" or "endothelial myeloma" of bone. These names were based on the idea that the tumor was derived from vasoformative tissue, and that the tumor cells were, in the broadest sense, angioendothelial cells. Oberling, on the other hand, held that the tumor cells are derived from the immature reticular cells (the supporting mesenchymal cells) of the bone marrow. On this account, he suggested the name "reticulosarcoma of the bone marrow" for the lesion. Oberling's view of the histogenesis is the one which is generally favored at present. Nevertheless, it appears that designation of the lesion as a "reticulosarcoma" is open to considerable misunderstanding. This is so because of the confusingly varied interpretations existing as to the neoplastic potentialities of the mesenchymal reticular framework of the lymphoid and myeloid tissues. Hence the writer prefers the neutral name of Ewing's sarcoma, which has the additional advantage of signalizing Ewing's pioneer work in the delimitation of the entity.

## CLINICAL CONSIDERATIONS

**Incidence.**—As already indicated, the Ewing sarcoma is not a very common lesion. Indeed, it is much rarer than osteogenic sarcoma or chondrosarcoma. The *sex* difference in incidence is not striking. However, most though not all observers have found that the condition is somewhat more common in males than in females.

As to *age* incidence, our experience is in line with the general observation that a very large proportion of the cases in any series fall within the second decade of life. Most of the rest of the patients are slightly under 10 years or slightly over 20 years of age. In any event, it is unusual to see a Ewing sarcoma in a middle-aged or elderly person. Furthermore, the patients are not often below 5 years of age. The latter finding is useful in the clinical differential diagnosis between Ewing's sarcoma and sympathetic neuroblastoma metastatic to the skeleton, most cases of which are seen in patients under 5 years of age (see Wyatt and Farber).

**Localization.**—In connection with localization, let us consider first the presenting lesion—that is, the one giving rise to the complaints which brought the patient to the hospital. The two most common sites of the presenting lesion are some part of an innominate bone or a long tubular bone. Indeed, in about half of the cases in our experience, the presenting lesion was in some part of an innominate bone. Localization of the lesion in some trunk bone other than an innominate bone was also not unusual. However, the incidence reported in the literature for localization of the presenting lesion in a trunk bone tends to be somewhat lower than we found it in our own series. In most of our remaining cases the presenting lesion was in a femur, tibia, fibula, or humerus. In an occasional case, roentgenographic examination of the rest of the skeleton on admission already reveals one or more additional but clinically silent foci of bone involvement, or even pulmonary metastases.

**Clinical Complaints and Findings.**—Survey of the clinical histories in a representative group of cases will show that local and/or referred pain is the one consistent complaint. With few exceptions, the pain is of at least some months' standing, and sometimes it is found to have been present for at least a year before admission. Usually, also, the pain has become increasingly severe and persistent during the immediately preceding weeks or months. With the local pain there are often complaints related to spread of the tumor beyond the limits of the bone and varying with the location of the presenting lesion. Thus, for instance, from patients in whom some part of an innominate bone is involved, there are usually complaints of disability relating to the hip joint and sometimes also of radiating pain running down the lower limb. In connection with location of the lesion near the articular end of a long bone, there are sometimes complaints of lameness or stiffness of the joint in question, perhaps associated with effusion into it. In the cases in which the lesion is in a lumbar vertebra, there are, in addition to the local pain, complaints ascribable to implication of nerve trunks in the area. For instance, there may be pain radiating down the limbs, and tingling sensations and weakness in the latter. Location of the lesion in a rib may be found associated with pleural effusion, as it was in one of our cases. Naturally, other locations of the presenting lesion (for instance, in the skull) are associated with their own special clinical disabilities.

Just as local pain is the dominant clinical complaint, so the presence of a local tumor mass is the dominant clinical finding in the patients at the time of admission.

Indeed, at that time a more or less prominent tumor mass is usually palpable at the site of the lesion. This fact indicates the strong tendency of the Ewing sarcoma to break out through the cortex of the bone and to spread in the surrounding tissues. Notably large tumor masses are palpable in some of the cases in which the tumor is somewhere in an innominate bone. Spreading internally toward the pelvic cavity, the tumor beyond the limits of the bone can then sometimes be palpated as an elastic irregular globular mass, through the rectum if the tumor is low down, or in the lower quadrant of the abdomen if it is higher up. Spreading externally, a tumor springing from an innominate bone sometimes produces a large mass palpable in the groin or in the gluteal region. In one of our cases in which the presenting lesion was in the shaft of a humerus, there was likewise a very large extra-osseous tumor mass connected with the bone. When the presenting tumor is in a superficially located bone such as a clavicle or a rib, the mass produced by the extra-osseous spread of the tumor tissue can often, of course, be seen as well as palpated.

Tenderness to pressure at the site of the lesion can almost always be noted. Not infrequently the veins of the skin overlying the presenting lesion are found prominent. However, it is only exceptionally that increased local heat is noted in the course of the physical examination.

If one surveys the temperature charts and the laboratory findings, what appears to be significant information of clinical value often emerges. Even before a biopsy is done, many of the patients are found to run a slight fever, as indicated by daily rises in temperature to about 101° F. These same patients generally present a definite secondary anemia (with a red blood cell count of about 3,500,000), and sometimes also a definite leukocytosis. In addition, they usually show a high

***Figure 111***

*A*, Roentgenograph showing an area of mottled rarefaction in the neck and upper part of the shaft of a femur in a case of Ewing's sarcoma. Note on the left the small amount of periosteal new bone deposited on the cortex. The patient was a boy 7 years of age who was admitted to the hospital with a history of limping, and of pain in the hip for about 7 weeks. Since the child also had some fever, the clinical impression, before a diagnostic biopsy was done, was that the condition was osteomyelitis. After the diagnosis of Ewing's sarcoma had been made, the femoral lesion was treated with *x*-radiation. Nevertheless, the child died 10 weeks after admission to the hospital. Such a rapidly fatal course is not unusual in cases of Ewing's sarcoma in which the condition is associated with fever at the time when the diagnosis is first established.

*B*, Roentgenograph showing a fairly large area of lytic destruction in the upper part of an ilium in a case of Ewing's sarcoma. The patient was a boy 19 years of age who had been complaining of pain in the sacro-iliac region for almost 2 years. The pain was mild and intermittent at first, but had become quite severe and steady. The patient died with evidences of widespread metastases $1\frac{1}{2}$ years later.

*C*, Roentgenograph showing the appearance of a Ewing sarcoma in the ischium in which the picture is dominated by radiopacity. The patient was a young man 20 years of age who gave a history of pain in the thigh for about 3 months. In view of the *x*-ray picture, the diagnosis before biopsy was "sclerosing" osteogenic sarcoma. The patient died of spread of the Ewing sarcoma 5 months after admission to the hospital.

*D*, Roentgenograph showing a Ewing sarcoma in the shaft of a fibula, the picture again being dominated by radiopacity. The patient was a boy 18 years of age who complained of intermittent pain in the lower part of the leg in question for almost a year. The area affected also showed swelling and was tender. Biopsy established the diagnosis of Ewing's sarcoma. This case, like the other cases illustrated in the plate, was treated by radiation therapy. The patient died of pulmonary metastases about $2\frac{1}{2}$ years after the onset of his complaints.

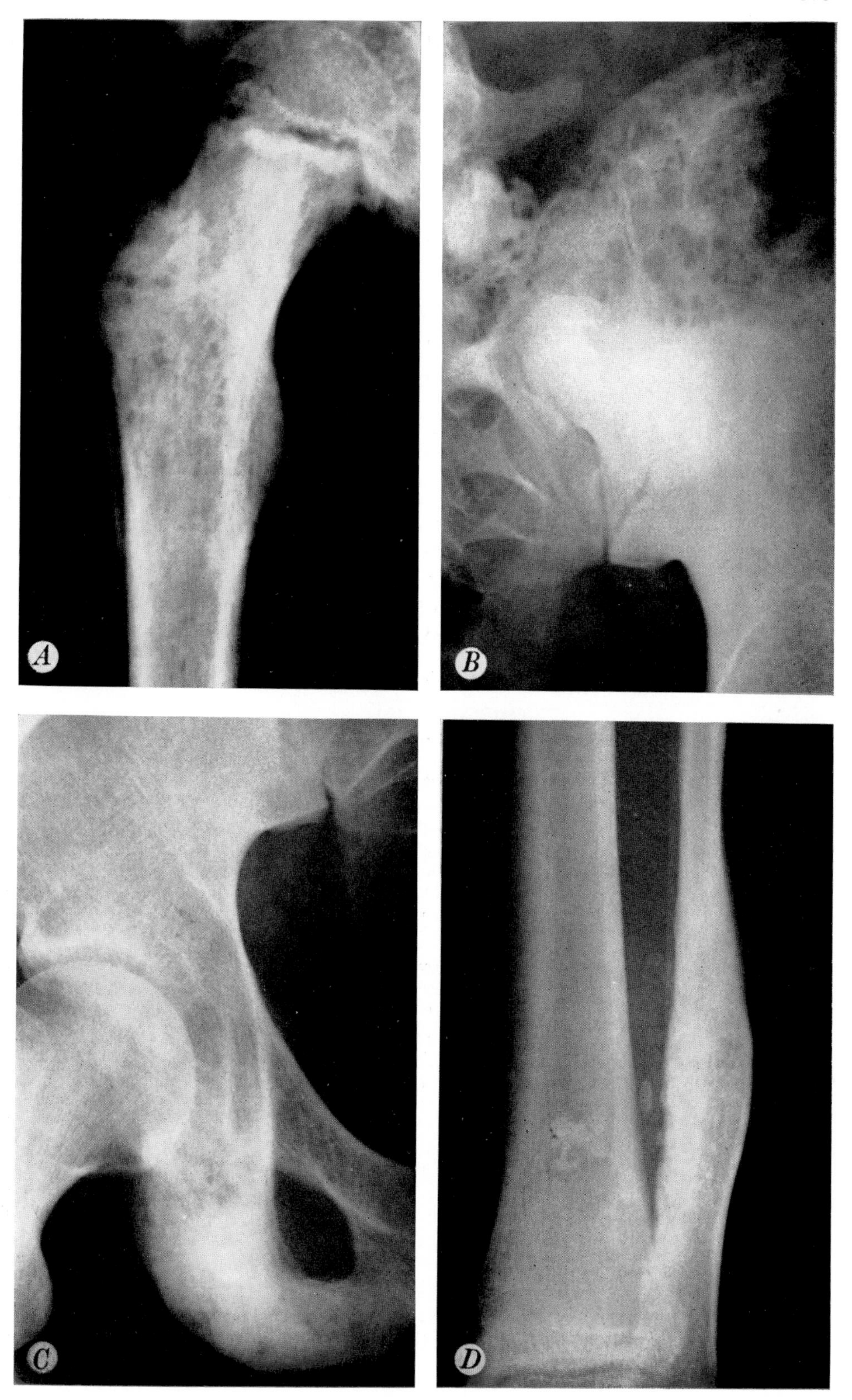


*Figure 111*

sedimentation rate of the blood. Taken together, slight fever, secondary anemia, and an increased sedimentation rate seem to be even more significant as to the immediate prognosis than the size of the presenting lesion. Specifically, the cases in which the presence of some fever and secondary anemia, even alone, were noted were found by the writer to be those which tended to run a fulminating course, usually ending in death within a few months after admission to the hospital. On the other hand, those patients who had no fever on admission, and no anemia or increased sedimentation rate, tended to survive for a year or more after admission, though in them too the disease was usually ultimately fatal.

## ROENTGENOGRAPHIC FINDINGS

A Ewing sarcoma, as it develops in a bone site, ordinarily induces bone lysis, not associated with much reactive new bone formation. Consequently, what one ordinarily sees in the early *x*-ray picture of the affected region is a smaller or larger area of mottled rarefaction. However, in an occasional presenting lesion, one will find that much of the lesional area is relatively radiopaque. The radiopacity is the result of new bone formation at the lesional site. It must be borne in mind, however, that this bone formation represents a local reactive osteosis, and that the Ewing sarcoma tissue itself has no osteogenic potentialities. (See Fig. 111.)

The mottled rarefaction shown by the lesion reflects destruction of the spongiosa and, to a lesser degree, of the overlying cortex. In the early stage the rarefaction is likely to be associated with a trace of periosteal new bone apposition, in reaction to the tumor tissue which has penetrated beyond the cortex. At first the picture may even suggest an inflammatory lesion (possibly a pyogenic or tuberculous osteomyelitis or an eosinophilic granuloma) rather than a tumor. However, al-

### *Figure 112*

*A*, Roentgenograph in a case of Ewing's sarcoma showing a faint area of rarefaction in the condylar part of a femur, associated with an indistinct soft-tissue mass overlying the cortex of the condyle. On the basis of the biopsy findings, the limb was ablated. The gross specimen is illustrated in Figs. 113-*A* and *B* and shows that, though only a small area of involvement was visible roentgenographically, tumor tissue was disseminated throughout the femur. The patient was a boy 19 years of age whose local complaints were of only 3 months' standing at the time of the disarticulation. He died with widespread dissemination of the disease $3\frac{1}{2}$ months after that.

*B*, Roentgenograph showing the appearance of a fibula altered by a Ewing sarcoma. This is one of the few instances in our case material in which significant parallel layers of periosteal new bone deposition were evident in the *x*-ray picture of a Ewing sarcoma. The patient was a boy 16 years of age who gave a history of some pain and swelling just below the knee, of 1 month's standing. On admission, he had anemia, fever, and an increased sedimentation rate. He died of widespread dissemination of the disease 7 months after the onset of his complaints.

*C*, Roentgenograph of a tibia involved by a Ewing sarcoma. From this picture it would be difficult to deduce anything more specific than that one was dealing with a tumor which had broken into the interosseous space and provoked some streaky new bone formation. The patient was a girl 10 years of age. Her complaints were of pain in the right leg for about 3 months, associated with the presence of a palpable tumor mass. She died of widespread pulmonary metastases $1\frac{1}{2}$ years after the onset of her complaints.

*D*, Roentgenograph of a humerus affected with a Ewing sarcoma. Note the large extraosseous tumor mass and the transverse radiopaque streaks in it. Clinically, on the basis of this picture, the tumor was interpreted as an "osteolytic" osteogenic sarcoma. The patient was a girl 8 years of age who died 7 months after the diagnosis of Ewing's sarcoma was established by biopsy. She died at home and no autopsy was performed

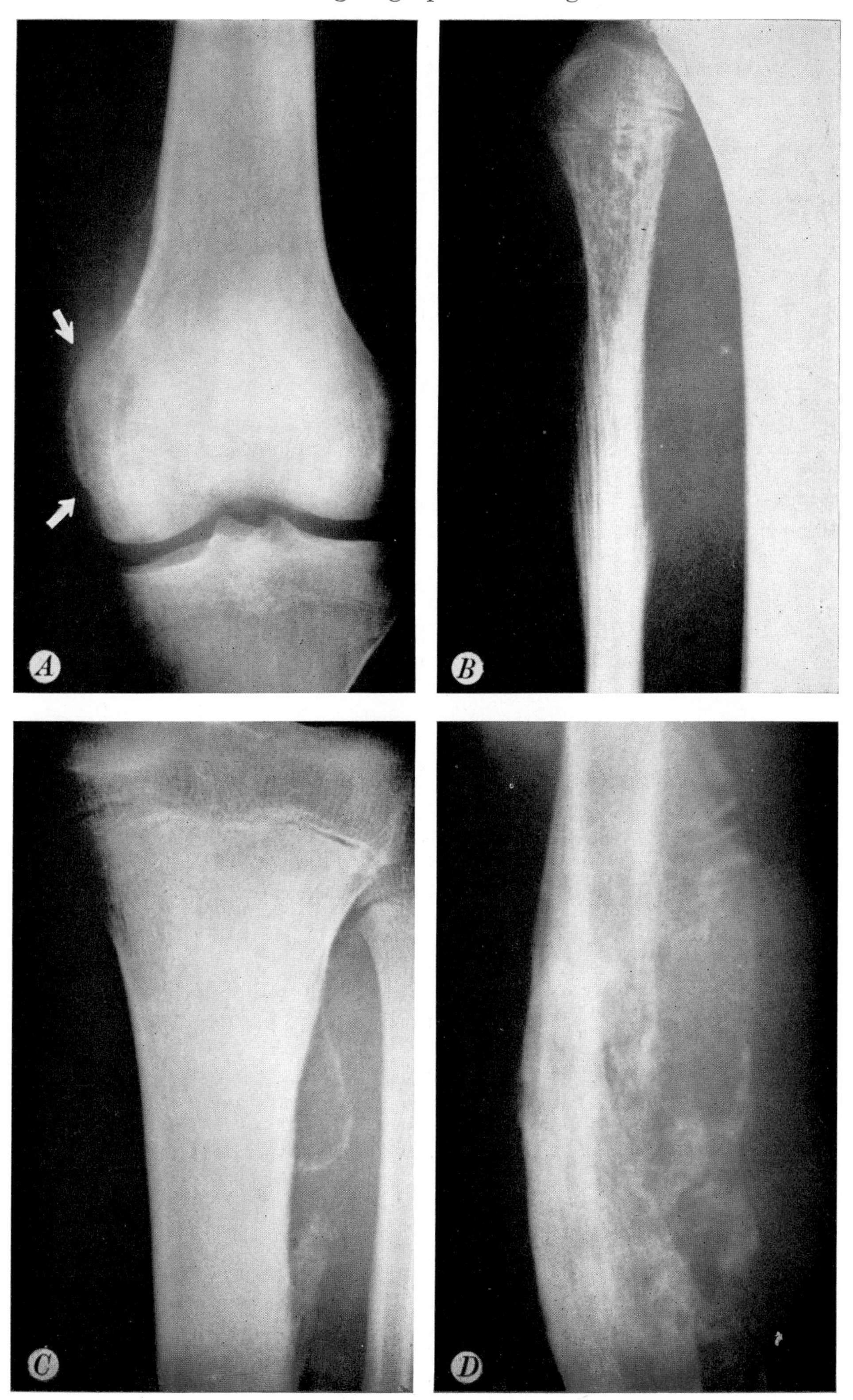


*Figure 112*

ready within a month or so, the roentgen picture in such a case presents evidence of rapid extension of the pathologic area within and beyond the bone, strongly supporting now a diagnosis of malignant tumor. At any rate, even if the roentgenograph still shows only a relatively small area of bone destruction, this should not be taken as indicating the actual extent of anatomic involvement of the affected bone. Indeed, the marrow spaces throughout the bone may already be riddled by tumor tissue, whose presence is not being reflected roentgenographically where it has not caused lytic resorption of osseous tissue.

In the cases in which the initial roentgenograph of the presenting lesion already shows rather clearly that one is dealing with a malignant tumor, one usually notes a large area of bone destruction, often along with a large overlying soft-tissue mass. The affected bone area may show distention of its outline, but if present this is not pronounced. However, the affected area appears irregularly rarefied and mottled from the presence of smaller or larger foci of relative radiolucency and shows disruption of the cortical outline over a smaller or larger region.

If one considers a whole series of cases of Ewing's sarcoma, one can also state that reactive new bone deposition by the periosteum where the tumor tissue is penetrating the cortex is certainly not conspicuous. When, as is commonly the case, Ewing's sarcoma involves bones other than long bones, evidence of periosteal new bone apposition is often demonstrable but rarely striking. It may even not be a striking finding in connection with involvement of long bones. Indeed, in a given case a substantial portion of the shaft may show irregular mottled rarefaction, perhaps in the complete absence of significant periosteal bone apposition. On the other hand, one may observe a case in which extensive involvement of the shaft is associated with onionskin-like periosteal new bone apposition, but the latter is not likely to be found extending completely around the circumference of the shaft. In still another instance, the *x*-ray picture may show the presence of more or less transverse streaks of radiopacity in the soft-tissue mass overlying the surface of the bone rather than concentric periosteal stratification. Thus, altogether, if the shaft of a long bone is the site of a Ewing sarcoma, one does not by any means commonly observe the concentric onionskin-like layers of periosteal new bone of a laminated pattern often held to be so characteristic of the *x*-ray picture of this tumor. (See Fig. 112.)

It cannot be too strongly emphasized that it is sometimes quite difficult to make a differential diagnosis, on a roentgenographic basis, between Ewing's sarcoma and other malignant tumors of bone. This problem may arise in relation to malignant lymphoma or metastatic malignancy (including metastatic neuroblastoma). Should the presenting lesion be heavily radiopaque, the picture may suggest a "sclerosing" osteogenic sarcoma. Should the tumor mass overlying the affected bone area present transverse radiopaque streaks, one might think that one was dealing with an "osteolytic" osteogenic sarcoma. Sometimes too, as already noted, a solitary eosinophilic granuloma or some other inflammatory lesion may be mistaken for a Ewing sarcoma, or vice versa. To make certain that a suspected tumor is a Ewing sarcoma, tissue examination is essential. However, one must stress the idea that a pathologist confronted by a biopsy specimen from a suspected case of Ewing's sarcoma may easily be mistaken in his opinion on this basis also. That is true especially if the tissue available is meager or substantially necrotic.

**"Metastatic" Bone Lesions.**—As noted, in a case of Ewing's sarcoma, lesions may already be manifest roentgenographically, on admission, in bones other than the one with the presenting lesion, or become manifest in them subsequently. Whether such lesions represent metastases from the presenting bone lesion or represent independent tumor growths in these bones does not precisely concern us at this point (but see p. 360). As to their roentgenographic appearance, these additional lesions, too, show up essentially as lytic ones. They appear first as rather faint, slightly mottled areas of rarefaction. As the resorption of the bone increases, the small multiple roundish foci of rarefaction become more distinct and may merge into larger, more clear-cut areas of radiolucency. In flat bones such as the skull bones or the ilium, multiple clear-cut punched out areas of rarefaction may appear in consequence of lytic destruction of the spongiosa and overlying cortex. Even a pathologic fracture of a long bone from destructive resorption of the spongiosa and cortex at a given site may become manifest. However, in any case, the actual extent of involvement of the skeleton as the case proceeds toward fatal termination is never adequately reflected roentgenographically.

## PATHOLOGIC FINDINGS

**Gross Pathology.**—Since cases of Ewing's sarcoma are now usually treated by irradiation rather than by amputation, there are few current opportunities for observing a presenting lesion intact in its setting within the affected bone. For such observations one has to go back to cases from former days. Let us consider the gross changes in an affected femur in which, at the time when the limb was amputated, the alterations visible roentgenographically involved only the medial condyle and the adjacent part of the shaft. The cortex of the shaft in this region was fuzzy and had a soft-tissue swelling about 2 cm. in thickness superposed upon it. However, when the femur was stripped of its surrounding muscles and cut in the frontal plane, practically the entire bone was found riddled with tumor tissue.

Inspection revealed tumor tissue not only in the medial condyle, but also in the lateral condyle and contiguous portions of the shaft, and indeed in the major marrow cavity and even in the marrow spaces of the spongiosa of the upper end of the femur. The tumor tissue in the region of the medial condyle and that which had penetrated beyond the cortex in this region was for the most part hemorrhagically discolored. It was also interspersed with yellowish areas reflecting necrosis of both the tumor tissue and spongiosa. Elsewhere for the most part the tumor tissue was not modified by hemorrhage or necrosis. Where it was not so modified, it was whitish, and, notably in the major marrow cavity, took the form of massed, soft, glistening tumor nodules. Thus the disease area visible in the preamputation *x*-ray of this femur was merely the area in which the changes were most destructive in regard to the osseous tissue. The discrepancy thus indicated between the extent of involvement revealed in the *x*-ray picture and that found anatomically brings out the importance of irradiating the entire bone if radiation therapy is given. (See Fig. 113.)

It is worth noting furthermore that in the course of dissection of the ablated limb in this case, neither the inguinal nor the popliteal lymph nodes were found enlarged or involved by tumor. Also, in spite of the extensive implication of the femur, no tumorous involvement was discernible in the tibia, fibula, or foot bones, all of which were opened and examined. These negative findings are of interest because, $3\frac{1}{2}$ months after the disarticulation of the limb, the patient died, and at autopsy presented widespread tumorous involvement of the rest of the skeleton, along with visceral metastases.

In contrast to the findings in the femoral lesion just described, let us now consider those noted in relation to an affected ilium showing a large tumor mass extending beyond the limits of the bone. The patient in this case was a young girl whose complaints (despite the large size of the presenting lesion) had been of only short duration at the time of admission to the hospital. At that time the patient already showed a tumor mass of the size of a neonate head, fixed to the ilium and palpable in the lower quadrant and groin. Though this patient appeared to be in good general health on admission, $x$-ray examination of the chest already showed pulmonary metastases too. No surgery was undertaken and the patient died 4 months later.

At autopsy, the huge tumor mass was found overlying the inner surface of the affected innominate bone. This mass had pushed the urinary bladder and the genital organs anteriorly and the sigmoid and rectum medially. Furthermore, on removing the innominate bone, it was found that posteriorly too the tumor had extended through the ilium and was bulging into the gluteal muscles and penetrating the capsule of the hip joint. The extra-osseous tumor tissue itself was soft, friable, extensively hemorrhagic, spongy and cystic on the whole, and in many places almost diffluent. The iliac portion of the bone was riddled through by tumor tissue which was cystic in many places, and the bone showed many defects in its cortex both on the inner and outer aspects.

In regard to the bones other than the one with the presenting lesion, autopsy regularly reveals that much of the rest of the skeleton is also involved by tumor. Indeed, the involvement is much more extensive than one would have suspected from the roentgenographs taken even just before death. Thus, the calvarium is likely to show tumor tissue permeating the diploic spaces and, in addition, areas in which the tumor tissue has eroded or completely destroyed the tables. In the latter case the calvarium will show actual defects, not infrequently several centimeters in diameter. These are filled with cellular, gray-white or even greenish yellow tumor tissue which may bulge or even penetrate the regional calvarial coverings. The marrow spaces of the ribs and sternum, too, are likely to be crowded with tumor tissue. Thinning and erosion of the cortex of these bones may be associated with the presence of focal masses of tumor tissue beneath the periosteum.

As to the vertebral column, if large segments are opened, the marrow spaces of the bodies, arches, and spinous processes will likewise be found extensively infiltrated by tumor tissue. In the cases which we autopsied, the vertebral column sometimes showed areas in which the tumor tissue in the marrow spaces and the supporting spongy bone appeared yellowish in consequence of necrosis. Where there was no necrosis, the tumor tissue was grayish, soft, and obviously cellular. Sometimes the tumor tissue is found extending through the bodies and beneath the anterior vertebral ligament in many places. It may also be found to have ex-

***Figure 113***

*A*, Photograph showing, in sagittal section, the lower half of a femur involved by a Ewing sarcoma. The tumor tissue in the condylar area and that overlying the cortex is hemorrhagic and was substantially necrotic. Note tumor tissue extending up through the major marrow cavity. Relatively little of this extensive involvement was manifest in the $x$-ray picture of the lower end of this femur as shown in Fig. 112-*A*.

*B*, Photograph of the upper half of the femur shown in *A*. Note the roundish nodules of tumor tissue in the upper part of the major marrow cavity. The tumor tissue also permeates the marrow spaces of the spongiosa of the neck and upper part of the shaft of the bone.

*C*, Photograph of the cut surface of an innominate bone heavily involved by Ewing's sarcoma. The iliac portion of the bone has been largely destroyed, and the tumor has broken through and extended widely beyond the limits of the bone. The patient was a girl 16 years of age whose complaints were of short duration but who already presented a large tumor mass on admission to the hospital. She, too, was treated by $x$-ray irradiation, but she died 4 months after admission. At autopsy, widespread skeletal and visceral dissemination of the Ewing sarcoma was found.

*D*, Photograph showing, in sagittal section, lower lumbar vertebræ and sacrum in a case of Ewing's sarcoma in a boy 17 years of age coming to autopsy. The bones removed at autopsy (a large segment of the vertebral column and many ribs) showed diffuse infiltration of the marrow spaces of the spongiosa by tumor tissue. Visceral metastases were also present.

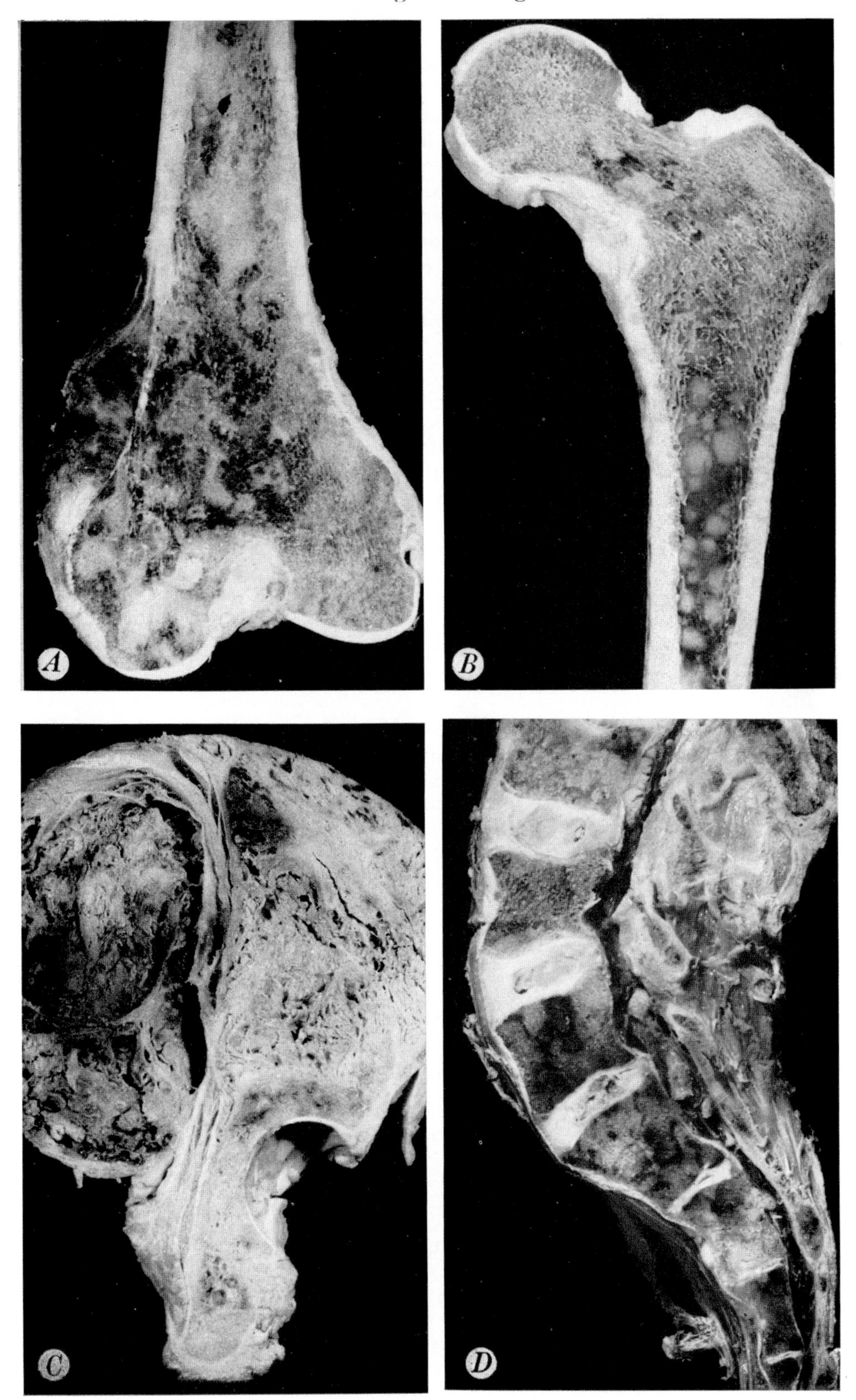


*Figure 113*

tended beneath the dura of the spinal canal. When this is so, it may have narrowed the spinal space and cuffed and compressed some part of the cord, causing degeneration of the latter.

The wide dissemination of the sarcoma in the bones which is observed at autopsy raises the question of whether one is dealing with metastatic spread or with independent multicentric development of the sarcoma. The writer leans toward the latter conception. That is, he tends toward the opinion that the same carcinogenic influence which provokes the mesenchymal supporting framework of the bone marrow to tumor formation at the site of the presenting lesion activates the mesenchymal framework of the marrow practically throughout the skeleton. No proof is yet available, however, for either conception. Indeed, a definite answer to the question of metastasis *vs.* independent development must be held in abeyance in regard to Ewing's sarcoma just as it must, for instance, in regard to myelomatosis (plasmacytoma).

In regard to the *visceral involvement* found at autopsy in cases of Ewing's sarcoma, it should be noted first that the lungs may be found free of tumor tissue or, on the contrary, riddled through with metastatic nodules. Under the latter conditions the parietal pleura, too, may be found studded with tumor masses, some of which are large and fungating. The liver may present numerous metastases, mainly in the form of nodules a few millimeters to somewhat more than a centimeter in diameter. In one case or another, metastases may be observed also in one or more of the following organs: heart, spleen, kidneys, pancreas, and thyroid. Finally, it should be noted that the lymph nodes, by and large, tend to be free of tumor tissue, though sometimes the paravertebral and pelvic lymph nodes do show, albeit only microscopically, some nests of tumor cells in the peripheral sinuses. These usually represent extensions of the tumor tissue from the underlying involved vertebræ.

**Microscopic Pathology.**—In his original descriptions, Ewing stated that the type cell of the tumor was a small polyhedral cell with pale cytoplasm, a small hyperchromatic nucleus, and a well defined cell border. He stated that, though tending to be arranged in compact broad sheets, the tumor cells, at least in some places in a given tumor, were often found lying around tiny or larger vascular spaces in "perithelial" arrangement or, still circularly but not around a vessel, in "rosette" formation. Enlarging experience has shown that this description of the cytology of the tumor is heavily slanted in the direction of what one sees in lesional tissue which is undergoing degeneration.

### *Figure 114*

*A*, Photomicrograph (× 500) showing the cytology of a cellular and relatively unmodified area of a Ewing sarcoma. Note that the tumor cells are enmeshed in a loose and more or less vacuolated cytoplasmic fabric. One can expect to see this characteristic histologic pattern only in areas of the lesion in which the tumor tissue is well preserved.

*B*, Photomicrograph (× 500) illustrating the cytology of the tumor tissue of a Ewing sarcoma not showing the characteristic pattern presented in *A*. This tissue came from an area adjacent to one which showed frank degeneration and necrosis. Note that the nuclei are, in general, smaller than in *A*, and that some are pyknotic.

*C*, Photomicrograph (× 250) showing so-called "perithelial" arrangement of tumor cells in a Ewing sarcoma. Note that tumor cells are collaring vascular spaces, but that the actual tumor cells are not an integral part of the walls of the vascular spaces. Cytologic appearances such as these are likely to be found in tumor areas which are grossly hemorrhagic.

*D*, Photomicrograph (× 500) showing the rosette-like formations sometimes encountered in a Ewing sarcoma. Note that these formations are constituted by rings of viable tumor cells surrounding cores of degenerating tumor cells, the shadows of which are still perceptible. Compare these spurious rosettes (or pseudorosettes) with the genuine rosettes encountered in neuroblastoma, as shown in Fig. 115-*C*.

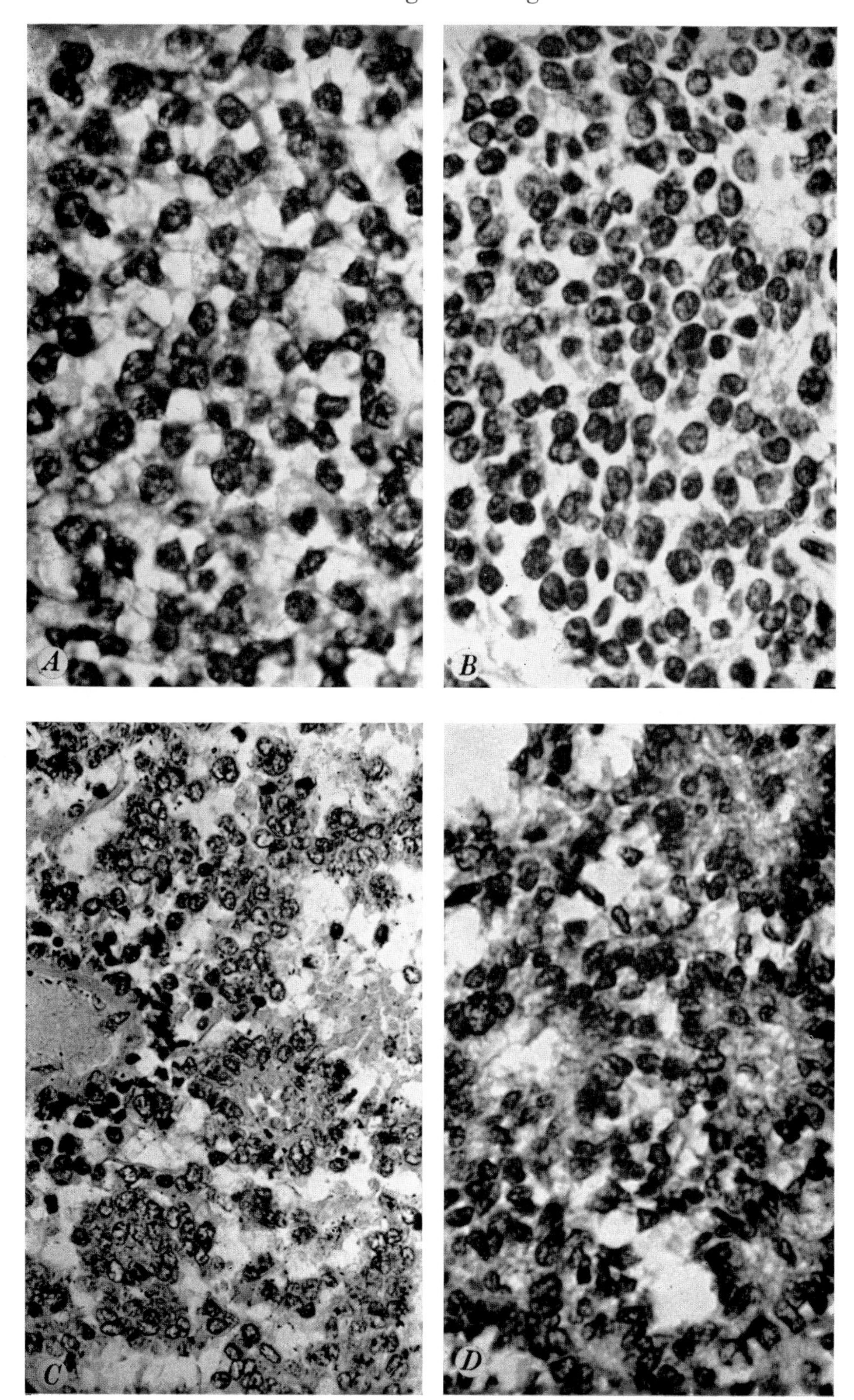


*Figure 114*

Characteristically, the cytology of the Ewing sarcoma is manifested through the presence of smaller or larger fields of tumor cells which lack clearly delimited cell boundaries and whose nuclei (which are sometimes crowded together) are of fairly uniform appearance. These nuclei are round or ovoid, are about twice as great in diameter (or, in the case of the ovoid ones, perhaps three times as great in widest axis) as the nucleus of a lymphocyte, and have finely divided or powdery chromatin and often one or more nucleoli. As a rule, the individual nuclei appear enmeshed in, and slightly separated by, a loose, more or less vacuolated cytoplasmic fabric. In some tumor fields, however, they may be found crowded together (perhaps to such an extent that many of them are even pressed into an oval shape). In such fields, of course, there is but little cytoplasm between them. It should also be noted that, in the fields presenting the general cytologic picture just described, vascularity is usually not at all a prominent feature of the tumor tissue. (See Fig. 114.)

In an individual case, areas showing the characteristic cytology as described above may have to be searched for in a biopsy specimen from the presenting bone lesion if the tumor tissue has undergone abundant secondary changes. Degeneration is indicated in the nuclei of the tumor cells by pyknosis and reduced size, and such nuclei are now likely to be surrounded by a narrow zone of cytoplasm with a delimiting cell border. It is such cells that, as indicated, approximate most closely the description given by Ewing for the type cell of the tumor. Intermingled with the fields in which the tumor cells are undergoing degeneration there are usually fields of various sizes in which the cells have undergone necrosis. Degenerating, but particularly necrotic, tumor tissue may, in some places, be heavily infiltrated by polymorphonuclear leukocytes. Thus a biopsy specimen may show large fields in which the appearance of the individual tumor cells has been altered by degeneration and necrosis, areas in which the tumor tissue as a whole has been modified by hemorrhage and reparative reaction to it, and even areas in which reactive inflammatory changes dominate the picture.

Free hemorrhage into smaller or larger tumor tissue fields, especially if it is extensive, comes to be associated with the ingrowth of many blood vessels into those fields. If the tumor tissue in these areas is not necrotic, one will note that many of these vessels are collared by tumor cells. However, the vessel spaces are not lined by the actual tumor cells, and between the latter and the lining cells there is tissue representing the wall of the vascular space. It is true that in such tumor fields one does see tumor cells about capillary spaces or around larger vascular spaces in so-called "perithelial" arrangement. However, one does not see this orientation of tumor cells to any pronounced extent except in connection with hemorrhage. It is on this account that no distinctive cytologic significance attaches to such findings. Indeed, perivascular orientation of tumor cells is observed also in connection with sarcomas of other kinds in which focal areas have undergone extensive hemorrhage.

We turn now to the question of the presence, in Ewing's sarcoma tissue, of rosette (or pseudorosette) formations. In connection with an occasional Ewing's sarcoma, some authors have reported finding, and have illustrated, formations in which cells are arranged circularly (though not around a vessel) in so-called rosette formation (see Foote and Anderson, and Gharpure). However, if one studies the illustrations in question, it can be seen that the centers of these formations represent degenerated cells whose shadows are still perceptible, rather than fibrillar or granular cores as in neuroblastoma. In our own material we too have occasionally encountered a tumor field in which viable tumor cells were disposed about cores of degenerating ones. In one case this was a rather prominent feature, but even then the formations were not clearly suggestive of the rosettes of neuroblastoma. (See p. 363.)

Finally, we come to the question of reticulum fibrils in Ewing's sarcoma tissue. It appears that these are not a consistent nor a prominent feature of the histologic picture. Indeed, there is considerable variability in regard to these fibrils, from lesion to lesion and even from part to part of the same tumor section. Some of the lesions, in part or throughout, have at most only a few stray argyrophil fibrils in a whole low power field. Other lesions show more numerous fibrils. Even in them, however, these are irregularly distributed and are seen only between smaller and larger groups of tumor cells. In no Ewing sarcoma did we regularly see large fields of tissue showing a lattice or meshwork of reticulum fibrils outlining not merely cell groups, but the individual tumor cells, as they do in reticulum cell sarcoma. In view of this variability, it is clear that there is no characteristic pattern for the Ewing tumor tissue insofar as these fibrils are concerned.

## DIFFERENTIAL DIAGNOSIS

Some mention has already been made of the problems relating to differentia diagnosis. On the one hand, we may be confronted by cases which seem to repre sent Ewing's sarcoma on clinical and roentgenographic grounds but which turn out to represent some other condition when a biopsy specimen from the lesion is studied. For instance, a solitary eosinophilic granuloma of bone not infrequently presents an *x*-ray picture suggesting a Ewing sarcoma. However, the distinctive histologic tissue pattern of the eosinophilic granuloma of bone is now clearly established, so that the differential diagnosis is not hard to make in these cases. Nevertheless, there can be no doubt that before the concept of eosinophilic granuloma of bone was clarified, some misdiagnosed cases of that condition which were cured by radiation therapy came to be regarded as instances of cured Ewing's sarcoma. Again, a focus of bone infection may simulate a Ewing sarcoma in the *x*-ray picture, but in these cases, too, tissue examination (and/or bacteriologic examination) readily clarifies the diagnosis.

On the other hand, one occasionally encounters a Ewing sarcoma whose *x*-ray picture may suggest an osteogenic sarcoma (either "osteolytic" or "sclerosing"). In such cases, too, the biopsy examination readily permits the proper distinction. Indeed, even if the affected bone area appears in the *x*-ray picture as a focus of dense radiopacity, one still finds fields of cells characteristic of the Ewing sarcoma interspersed through the large amount of osseous tissue which has been laid down in reaction to it.

Finally, one encounters cases in which, on histologic grounds, one might misinterpret the lesion as a Ewing sarcoma because the tumor cells in the biopsy specimen appear as "round cells." Such cases include neuroblastoma metastatic to bone, undifferentiated carcinoma metastatic to bone, and malignant lymphoma (particularly primary reticulum cell sarcoma) of bone.

**Neuroblastoma.**—The neuroblastoma (sympathicoblastoma) usually develops from the sympathetic tissue of the adrenal medulla, but may originate from sympathetic tissue elsewhere in the body. While the subjects are usually infants or young children (most often under 5 years of age), the tumor does occasionally appear in an adult.

What characterizes the tumor cytologically is the presence of tumor cells arranged in rosettes. Typically, the rosettes are ball-like aggregations of tumor cells enclosing a small central meshwork of filamentous neurofibrils, some of which can be shown to constitute processes of the cells making up the periphery of the rosette. However, because of degeneration, the fibrils may be difficult to demonstrate and the rosettes may appear as formations in which several rows of cells surround a finely granular eosin-staining core without a central lumen. In a particular case, rosettes may be fairly numerous in both the primary growth and any metastases developing, conspicuous in the primary growth and sparse or even absent in the metastases, or difficult to find in either. As to the type cell of the tumor, there are differences from lesion to lesion depending on the predominating level of maturation of the sympathicoblasts. In any event, the tumor cells are nearly always round cells, and frequently they have vesicular nuclei and even some cytoplasmic processes.

The neuroblastoma commonly metastasizes to bones, and the skeletal metastases are often already widespread when the bones are first roentgenographed. Indeed, one can anticipate finding, at least at autopsy, a malignant adrenal tumor as the primary lesion in infants and children who present clinically tumorous involvement of cranial bones, proptosis from tumorous involvement of the orbital region, and tumorous enlargement of the preauricular and other regional lymph nodes. However, in some cases the first clinical manifestation of a neuroblastoma comes from a focus of metastasis to a single bone (not infrequently a long bone) and roentgenographic examination of the rest of the skeleton fails to reveal any destructive bone lesions elsewhere. The tumor cells in the biopsy specimen from such a metastatic lesion are likely to be round cells with vesicular nuclei, and the tumor tissue in such a metastatic focus is not likely to show rosettes. Hence it is not surprising that such a bone lesion, especially if it occurs in a child, might be interpreted as a Ewing sarcoma. (See Fig. 115.)

Against this background we are in a position to understand the skepticism expressed by Willis about the validity of the concept of Ewing's sarcoma. This skepticism was based on experience with two cases in point. In both of these there was a

***Figure 115***

*A*, Roentgenograph showing a rarefying destructive lesion in the neck of a femur, caused by a metastasis from a neuroblastoma and representing the lesion which brought the patient to the hospital. The patient was a boy 3 years of age whose clinical complaints were of pain in the affected hip region and limping of 3 months' duration. A biopsy was done on the assumption that this lesion represented a focus of bone infection, but the tissue sections (see *B*) showed that the lesion was a malignant tumor. The fact that the femoral tumor represented a metastatic focus of neuroblastoma became evident only from the histologic findings relating to a cervical lymph node (see *C*) removed because the child had developed a generalized lymphadenopathy.

*B*, Photomicrograph (× 500) showing the histologic appearance of the tissue removed from the femoral focus of neuroblastoma illustrated in *A*. Note the roundish tumor cells and the absence of rosettes, which, indeed, were not found in any of the numerous tissue sections prepared from the curetted material.

*C*, Photomicrograph (× 500) showing the rosette formations presented by the lymph node removed from the cervical region in the case in question. The child died at home about 1 year after the onset of the pain in the hip region, and the primary site of the neuroblastoma never became known.

*D*, Photograph of part of a calvarium from another case of neuroblastoma. In this case, autopsy proved the primary lesion to be in an adrenal, and the calvarium shows metastatic involvement, as it so often does, at least terminally, in cases of neuroblastoma. The patient was a female child 21 months of age who was brought to the hospital because she had been vomiting after feeding. At the time of admission, there were already numerous metastatic osteolytic areas in various other bones. The child died 2 months after admission to the hospital, and widespread dissemination of the neuroblastoma throughout the skeleton was noted at autopsy.

*E*, Photograph of the calvarium shown in *D*, sectioned in the frontal plane through the tumorously involved area. The metastatic tumor mass is largely hemorrhagic and has destroyed portions of the frontal bone. Rosettes were observable in the viable tumor tissue in this calvarial focus of metastasis.

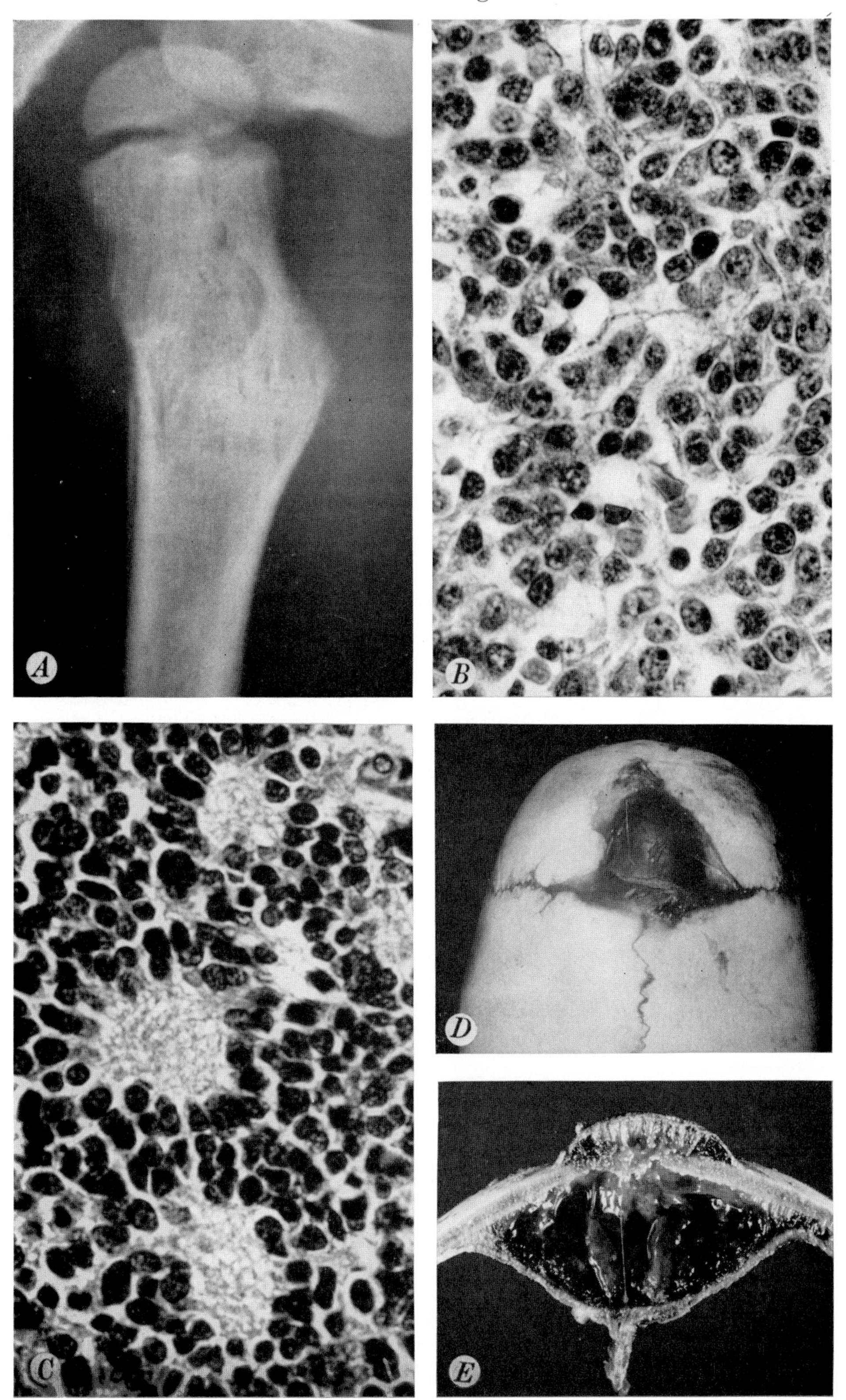


*Figure 115*

presenting tumor in a femur which had the usually accepted clinical and roentgenographic characteristics of the Ewing sarcoma. In these cases the clinical course, and in particular the susceptibility of the bone lesion to radiation therapy, seemed to support this diagnosis. In neither case were rosettes found in the material taken for biopsy from the femoral lesion, and the biopsy findings too seemed to support the diagnosis of Ewing's sarcoma. However, in both cases it was revealed at autopsy that the femoral tumor actually represented metastasis from a neuroblastoma, primary in an adrenal in one instance and in the left lumbar sympathetic chain in the other. Though rosettes were not found in the femoral metastases, they were found in the primary lesion in each case. These experiences emphasize the importance of paying careful attention to the adrenals and sympathetic chains at autopsy in any supposed case of Ewing's sarcoma, to rule out the possibility of neuroblastoma.

There can be no doubt that Willis was correct in holding that a presenting bone lesion which is in fact a metastasis from a neuroblastoma may not be recognized as such on the basis of a biopsy and may be misinterpreted as a Ewing sarcoma. However, with due allowance for the necessity of diagnostic caution, the weight of evidence has sustained the existence of a primary bone tumor entity such as Ewing singled out. That, on the other hand, a large proportion of cases of sympathetic neuroblastoma have certain distinctive clinical and roentgenographic features of their own can be gathered from the mass of material on which Wyatt and Farber have reported.

**Undifferentiated Metastatic Carcinoma.**—As already indicated, it is unusual for a Ewing sarcoma to appear in a mature or elderly adult. Thus, if a biopsy specimen from a solitary destructive bone lesion shows tumor tissue whose cytologic appearance seems consistent with that of a Ewing sarcoma, one should nevertheless hesitate in making that diagnosis if the patient is an adult. In such cases one may be dealing with a focus of metastasis so undifferentiated cytologically as to present a more or less uniform pattern of round cells, the primary growth still being clinically silent. The primary lesion may be in a bronchus, breast, testis, or the stomach, for instance. Thus, in any supposed case of Ewing's sarcoma in an adult, one is not justified in feeling sure that that diagnosis is correct unless at least the possibility that one is dealing with metastasis from a small cryptic cancer has been carefully ruled out by a searching autopsy (see Hirsch and Ryerson, and Sternberg).

**Primary Reticulum Cell Sarcoma.**—The concept of primary reticulum cell sarcoma of bone grew out of the dilemma created by cases supposedly representing Ewing's sarcoma but not running the baleful clinical course typical for that tumor (see Parker and Jackson). Indeed, the differential diagnosis between these two lesions is often a practical problem difficult to solve. On the one hand, a diagnosis of reticulum cell sarcoma cannot be made with any assurance on the basis of the *x*-ray picture. Also, the two lesions do not differ strikingly in their cytology, since both are composed of so-called round cells. However, the cell nuclei of the reticulum cell sarcoma are on the whole somewhat larger, and, while they are usually round to oval, many of them may be indented. If the lesional tissue is stained for reticulum, the latter is found to run in delicate threads and strands around groups of tumor cells and also between individual cells, which is not the case in a Ewing sarcoma.

Furthermore, the fact that the primary reticulum cell sarcoma of bone may remain essentially restricted to the affected bone site for a long time represents an important biological difference between it and the Ewing sarcoma. It is this fact that gives the former lesion a more favorable prognosis, and the latter, of course, has a bearing on treatment. Thus, if the cellular pattern of a given lesion favors a diagnosis of reticulum cell sarcoma of bone, and there is as yet no clinical evidence of distant spread of the tumor, one may even be justified (when the lesion is in a suitable site) in urging amputation of the affected part. (For further details concerning primary reticulum cell sarcoma of bone, see p. 416.)

## TREATMENT

The treatment of choice for Ewing's sarcoma is radiation therapy. Adequate irradiation directed against the presenting lesion usually has a remarkable local effect on the tumor. This effect is likely to be most striking if the presenting lesion is in a limb bone. The area treated should be large and should definitely extend beyond the lesional area as shown in the *x*-ray picture. As indicated in the discussion of the pathology, a Ewing sarcoma apparently involving only the condylar area of a femur in the *x*-ray picture may actually be found spread throughout the entire bone when examined anatomically. Hence, if possible, the entire bone in which the tumor is located should be irradiated.

A tumor dose of 4,000 to 5,000 r delivered through a number of portals and fractionated at the rate of 200 to 300 r per day seems usually to be sufficient to bring the primary lesion under control and to relieve the local complaints. Not infrequently, radiation therapy is supplemented by a course of nitrogen mustard and/or Coley's toxin. However, despite the fact that the presenting lesion may come to be substantially if not completely healed under such treatment, the patients usually develop, sooner or later, additional destructive bone lesions and pulmonary metastases. Radiation therapy may be used against these lesions, also, with temporary beneficial effect.

The published survival rates for Ewing's sarcoma are somewhat difficult to evaluate. In our experience, Ewing's sarcoma is almost regularly fatal, the great majority of the patients being dead within 3 years from the time of onset of the local clinical complaints. Indeed, it is to be suspected that reported 5-year survival rates exceeding 3 or 4 per cent should be regarded with some skepticism in respect to the correctness of the diagnoses. In fact, it can safely be assumed that survival rates of 10 per cent or more include many cases not actually representing Ewing's sarcoma.

## REFERENCES


BARDEN, R. P.: The Similarity of Clinical and Roentgen Findings in Children with Ewing's Sarcoma (Endothelial Myeloma) and Sympathetic Neuroblastoma, Am. J. Roentgenol., *50*, 575, 1943.

COHEN, J., BROWN, K. A., and GRICE, D. S.: Ewing's Tumor of the Talus (Astragalus) Simulating Aseptic Necrosis, J. Bone & Joint Surg., *35-A*, 1008, 1953.

EDWARDS, J. E.: Primary Reticulum Cell Sarcoma of the Spine. Report of a Case with Autopsy, Am. J. Path., *16*, 835, 1940.

EWING, J.: Diffuse Endothelioma of Bone, Proc. New York Path. Soc., *21*, 17, 1921; and: Further Report on Endothelial Myeloma of Bone, Proc. New York Path. Soc., *24*, 93, 1924.

FOOTE, F. W., JR., and ANDERSON, H. R.: Histogenesis of Ewing's Tumor, Am. J. Path., *17*, 497, 1941.

GARBER, C. Z.: Reactive Bone Formation in Ewing's Sarcoma, Cancer, *4*, 839, 1951.

GHARPURE, V. V.: Endothelial Myeloma (Ewing's Tumor of Bone), Am. J. Path., *17*, 503, 1941.

HIRSCH, E. F., and RYERSON, E. W.: Metastases of the Bone in Primary Carcinoma of the Lung: A Review of So-called Endotheliomas of the Bones, Arch. Surg., *16*, 1, 1928.

JAFFE, H. L.: The Problem of Ewing Sarcoma of Bone, Bull. Hosp. Joint Dis., *6*, 82, 1945.

LICHTENSTEIN, L., and JAFFE, H. L.: Ewing's Sarcoma of Bone, Am. J. Path., *23*, 43, 1947.

MCCORMACK, L. J., DOCKERTY, M. B., and GHORMLEY, R. K.: Ewing's Sarcoma, Cancer, *5*, 85, 1952.

MCKENZIE, A. H., and DAY, F. G.: Eosinophilic Granuloma of the Femoral Shaft Simulating Ewing's Sarcoma, J. Bone & Joint Surg., *39–A*, 408, 1957.

MCSWAIN, B., BYRD, B. F., JR., and INMAN, W. O., JR.: Ewing's Tumor, Surg., Gynec. & Obst. *89*, 209, 1949.

Melnick, P. J.: Histogenesis of Ewing's Sarcoma of Bone; With Post-Mortem Report of a Case Am. J. Cancer, *19*, 353, 1933.

Neely, J. M., and Rogers, F. T.: Roentgenological and Pathological Considerations of Ewing's Tumor of Bone, Am. J. Roentgenol., *43*, 204, 1940.

Oberling, C.: Les réticulosarcomes et les réticulo-endothéliosarcomes de la moelle osseuse (sarcomes d'Ewing), Bull. Assoc. franç. p. l'étude du cancer, *17*, 259, 1928; and: Oberling, C., and Raileanu, C.: Nouvelles recherches sur les réticulosarcomes de la moelle osseuse (sarcomes d'Ewing), Bull. Assoc. franç. p. l'étude du cancer, *21*, 333, 1932.

Parker, F., Jr., and Jackson, H., Jr.: Primary Reticulum Cell Sarcoma of Bone, Surg., Gynec. & Obst., *68*, 45, 1939.

Sternberg, C.: Zur Frage des sogenannten Ewings Tumor, Frankfurt. Ztschr. f. Path., *48*, 525, 1935.

Stout, A. P.: A Discussion of the Pathology and Histogenesis of Ewing's Tumor of Bone Marrow, Am. J. Roentgenol., *50*, 334, 1943.

Stowens, D.: Neuroblastoma and Related Tumors, Arch. Path., *63*, 451, 1957.

Swenson, P. C.: The Roentgenologic Aspects of Ewing's Tumor of Bone Marrow, Am. J. Roentgenol., *50*, 343, 1943.

Wang, C. C., and Schulz, M. D.: Ewing's Sarcoma: A Study of Fifty Cases Treated at the Massachusetts General Hospital, 1930–1952 Inclusive, New England J. Med., *248*, 571, 1953.

Willis, R. A.: Metastatic Neuroblastoma in Bone Presenting the Ewing Syndrome, with a Discussion of "Ewing's Sarcoma," Am. J. Path., *16*, 317, 1940; and: Colville, H. C., and Willis, R. A.: Neuroblastoma Metastases in Bones, with a Criticism of Ewing's Endothelioma, Am. J. Path., *9*, 421, 1933.

Wyatt, G. M., and Farber, S.: Neuroblastoma Sympatheticum; Roentgenological Appearances and Radiation Treatment, Am. J. Roentgenol., *46*, 485, 1941.

Chapter

# 23

# Myelomatosis (Multiple Myeloma)

One may define *myelomatosis* (*multiple myeloma*) as a cancerous disease which takes its origin in the bone marrow and which is further characterized by a tendency of the tumorous involvement to remain limited to the bones and by the fact that at least some of the cells of the lesional tissue resemble plasma cells. In addition, myelomatosis is very often associated with certain biochemical aberrations relating to the blood serum, and most distinctively with a rise in the serum globulin content, often due to the presence of abnormal globulins. Also, the disease is commonly associated with the appearance of proteinaceous plugs in the renal tubules, frequently leading to severe renal insufficiency due to the development of the so-called "myeloma kidney." In some instances of myelomatosis an amyloid-like substance comes to be deposited in the tumor tissue proper and/or the viscera, muscles, and other soft parts.

The tumor cells of myelomatosis apparently arise from the primitive marrow reticulum. In some cases, many (or even practically all) of the tumor cells of the lesional tissue are small round cells resembling the ordinary tissue plasma cells in their histologic details. For this reason the disease is often also denoted as "plasmacytoma" or "plasma cell myeloma" of bone. However, in other cases, most of the cells are larger than the ordinary plasma cell, though similar to the latter in a general way. Furthermore, in some tumors or tumor fields, many of the cells may be not only large but otherwise bizarre in appearance, though these are interspersed with smaller cells, some of which do appear like the common plasma cell. The indicated variations in the histologic appearance of the tumor cells in sections of the lesional tissue seem to represent merely different stages of development, degeneration, or differentiation of the basic tumor cell. It seems best, on the whole, to designate this cell in a neutral way as the "myeloma cell," and the condition as "myelomatosis" or "multiple myeloma." In any event, the disease is one which should be kept distinct from the other primary cancerous disorders involving the hematopoietic system (notably the lymphomas and leukemias).

Myelomatosis appears mainly in older people. Its clinical manifestations are likely to be vague for a long time. In the past, the presence of the disease was often not suspected in a clinical case unless *x*-ray examination revealed clear-cut foci of bone destruction in a number of skeletal sites. Currently, however, the disease is frequently discovered before obvious destructive bone lesions have appeared. This earlier detection has been made possible through the wide use of sternal marrow puncture smears for studying the cytology of the bone marrow in clinically ambiguous cases. If such a case is one of myelomatosis, the bone marrow smears may already show excessive numbers of myeloma (plasma) cells. Also, in these early cases, biochemical examination of the blood may already reveal aberrations in the serum globulin pattern.

General weakness and/or bone pain are the usual initial complaints. Not infrequently the bone pain leads to the detection of a destructive lesion in one or another skeletal site. Progress of the disease over the skeleton may be steady and rapid, sometimes from the beginning and sometimes after a static period. In any event, the tumor tissue usually comes to be spread widely through the marrow spaces of the bones, but, in addition, many large, discrete tumor foci are present. These foci are the sites of extensive lytic destruction of the local spongy bone and cortex. It is such areas that appear in the *x*-ray pictures as punched-out radiolucencies scattered over the skeleton, and it is to this picture that the name "multiple myeloma" is best suited. Occasionally the involvement of the marrow spaces remains diffuse, the case running its course without the development of discrete tumor foci in the bones, and hence without the appearance of punched-out lytic areas in the *x*-ray pictures. Nevertheless, in such cases the *x*-ray picture may reveal a generalized osteoporosis, sometimes mild but sometimes quite pronounced. To the pattern of the skeletal involvement in such cases, the term "diffuse myelomatosis" is often applied. On the other hand, there are cases in which the disease seems to flourish in a single bone site (often as a large, destructive lesion) for months before other bone sites become affected. Occasionally it remains so localized for years, and there seem even to be instances in which it does not spread at all. It is to these latter, rare cases of the disease that the term "solitary myeloma" or "solitary plasmacytoma" of bone has come to be applied.

### *Figure 116*

*A*, Roentgenograph showing a destructive myelomatous lesion of the body of the 10th thoracic vertebra in a case in which this was the presenting lesion that brought the patient to the hospital. The subject was a woman 35 years of age who had complained of progressively increasing pain in the back for 6 months. Since a skeletal survey failed to reveal involvement of other bones, the initial clinical impression was that the lesion represented a focus of carcinoma metastasis. Because of neurological findings referable to pressure on the spinal cord, a laminectomy was done and the diagnosis of myelomatosis was established through the examination of tissue from the lesional area. The patient died 7 months after the onset of her complaints, and Fig. 119-*C* shows the gross appearance of the vertebral lesional area after its removal at autopsy.

*B*, Roentgenograph from another case of myelomatosis in which the presenting lesion was in the vertebral column. Note the narrowing of the disk space between the 9th and 10th thoracic bodies and the partial collapse of these bodies, especially the 10th. The patient was a man 55 years of age who had complained of pain in the back for about 3 months, but whose pain had suddenly become acute after a misstep. Roentgenographic survey of the rest of the skeleton failed to reveal other bone lesions. Because of this fact, and in view of the *x*-ray picture presented by the affected part of the column, the initial clinical impression was that the lesion represented a focus of vertebral tuberculosis. The correct diagnosis was established when a sternal marrow puncture smear revealed the presence of abnormal numbers of myeloma cells and chemical analysis of the blood showed hyperglobulinemia.

*C*, Roentgenograph of an osteolytic femoral lesion which was the presenting lesion in another case of myelomatosis. The patient was a woman 53 years of age who gave a history of aching pain in the thigh of 4 months' duration. A skeletal survey, including examination of the calvarium, revealed no other obvious bone lesions. Because of this fact and because the femoral lesion was in a site commonly affected by metastatic cancer, the original clinical impression was that one was dealing with a focus of metastasis from a clinically occult carcinoma. The serum calcium, inorganic phosphate, and alkaline phosphatase values were within normal limits, but a sternal marrow puncture smear was not done. The patient was readmitted 1 year later, and very pronounced osteolytic changes were now found in many bones, including the humerus (see *D*) and calvarium (see Fig. 117-*A*). At this admission a sternal marrow puncture smear showed numerous myeloma cells, the serum calcium and globulin values were strikingly elevated, and the urine was found to contain Bence Jones proteins.

*D*, Roentgenograph of the humerus from the case described in *C*. One year earlier, this humerus had presented no apparent involvement roentgenographically.

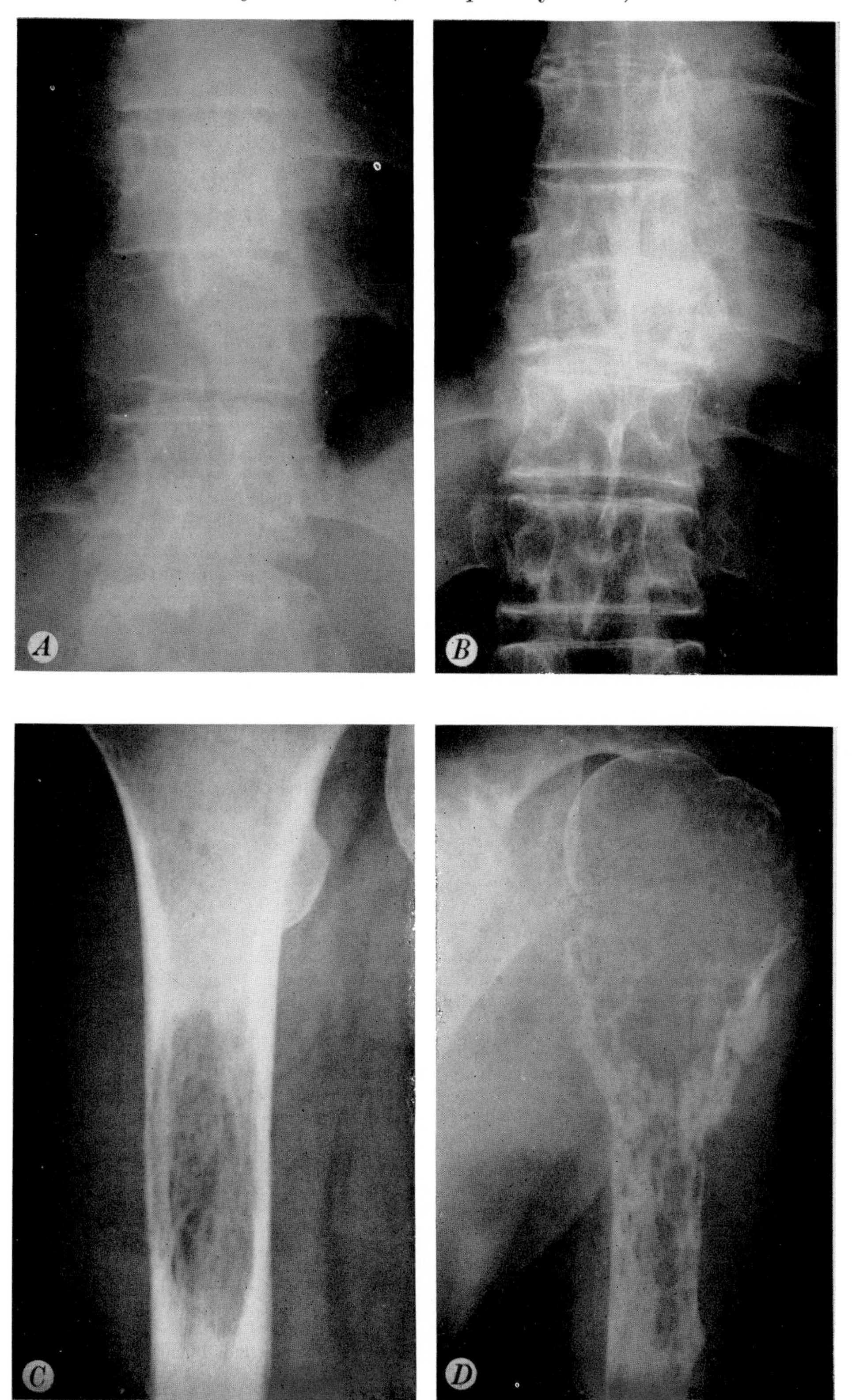


*Figure 116*

Though at autopsy the skeleton may be found riddled through with myelomatous tumor tissue, it is only infrequently that gross myelomatous foci are found in the viscera and other extraskeletal parts. Nevertheless, even in the absence of gross infiltrations, microscopic examination not infrequently reveals the presence of smaller or larger numbers of myeloma cells within the spleen, the liver or the lymph nodes, and occasionally in other organs as well. Also, in some cases, myeloma cells may invade the blood stream. Ordinarily under these circumstances, relatively few myeloma cells are found in the blood smears. Terminally in an occasional case they are so numerous as to create a leukemic blood picture—that of so-called plasma-cell leukemia. (Recent comprehensive and critical discussions of the disease include those by Lichtenstein and Jaffe, Meacham, and Carson, Ackerman, and Maltby.)

## CLINICAL CONSIDERATIONS

**Incidence.**—Myelomatosis is encountered fairly often, but its actual general incidence is difficult to estimate, since many cases still escape clinical detection. As to *sex incidence,* the disease is more common in males than in females. Indeed, one often finds the statement that it is at least twice as common in males.

As to *age incidence,* the patients are between 50 and 70 years of age in about three-quarters of any representative group of cases. Most of the rest are between 40 and 50 or else, though less often, between 30 and 40 years of age. In persons under 30 years of age, the disease is definitely uncommon. However, a few unequivocal cases of myelomatosis have even been observed in adolescents or children (see Gordon and Schneider, and Schmaus). In this connection, the writer has seen the case of a boy who presented the first manifestations of the disease at the age of 13 and died of it at the age of 18.

**Clinical Complaints and Course.**—For some weeks or months before the diagnosis is established, a patient affected with myelomatosis may have only vague, general complaints. There may be relatively mild aching pains referable to the bones,

***Figure 117***

*A,* Roentgenograph of the skull from the case of myelomatosis illustrated in Figs. 116-*C* and *D.* A picture taken 1 year previously had revealed nothing abnormal. Note the numerous punched-out roundish rarefactions. Identical roentgenographic appearances may be produced by osteolytic carcinoma metastases. Furthermore, in some cases of myelomatosis (see Fig. 121), involvement of the calvarium may be slight in comparison with that of the rest of the skeleton.

*B,* Roentgenograph showing extensive changes from myelomatosis in part of an innominate bone and a femur from a patient who, on admission for diagnosis, already presented devastatingly severe involvement of practically the entire skeleton. The patient was a man 45 years of age who had lost weight and complained of pain in both lower limbs for about 10 months. He had a severe anemia, and his urine contained Bence Jones protein. He died 4 months after admission, and an autopsy was done.

*C,* Roentgenograph showing, in the upper end of a femur, a large, trabeculated, osteolytic lesion which proved, on the basis of tissue examination, to be a myeloma. The patient was a woman 52 years of age who had had complaints relating to the hip region for about 3 years. She transferred to another institution, where she received radiation therapy, from which clinical improvement resulted. Four years later the case was reported from that institution as one of solitary myeloma, since no other skeletal lesions seemed to be present. However, almost 10 years after the onset of complaints, the patient died of myelomatosis, which had become disseminated over the skeleton. This case shows that even 3 or 4 years are not enough to establish a case firmly as one of solitary myeloma.

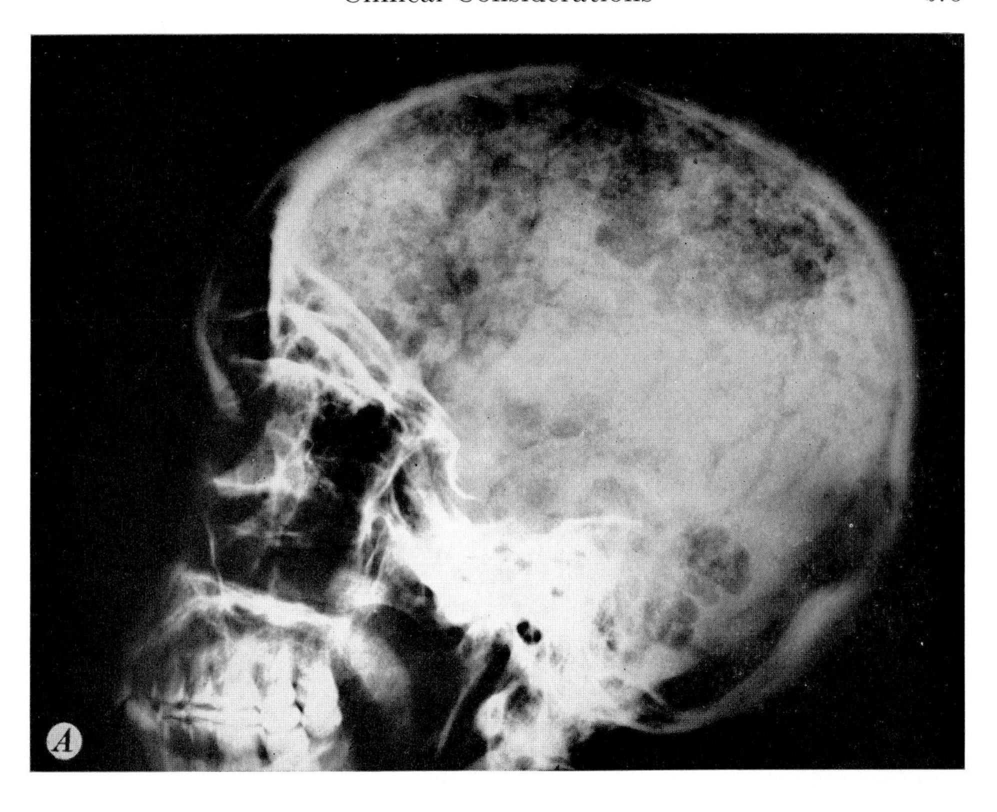


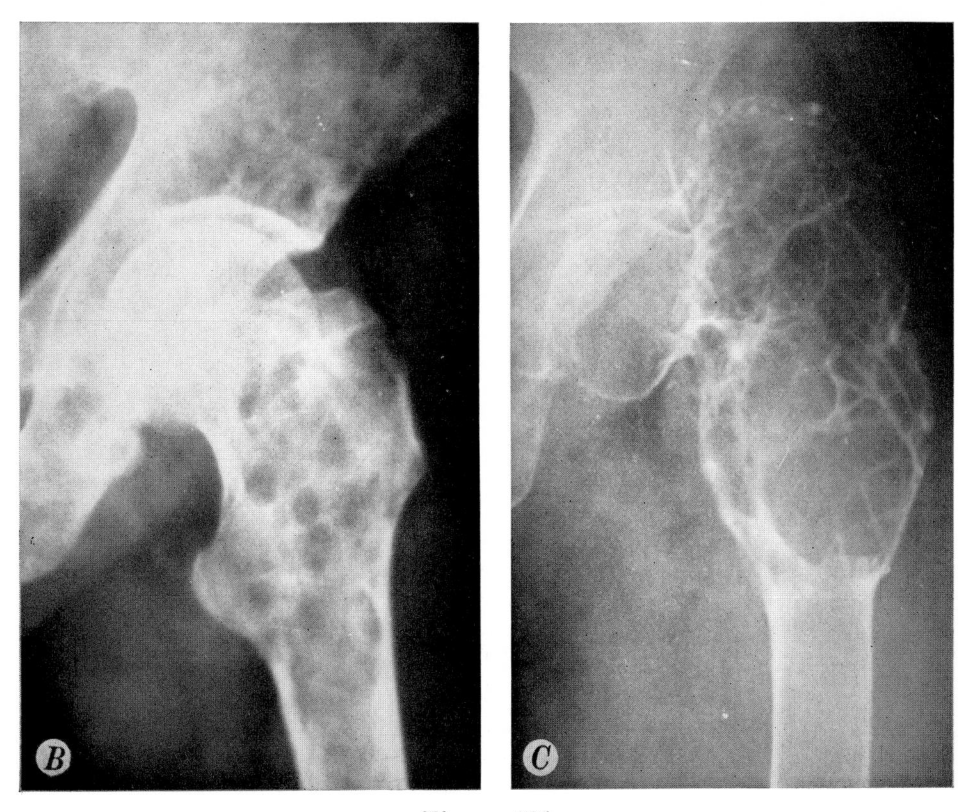


*Figure 117*

perhaps associated with some general weakness and possibly some weight loss and/or anemia. Indeed, such a clinical picture, when presented by an elderly person, warrants a sternal marrow puncture directed toward a search for myelomatosis. If it is not through the general complaints mentioned that the disease comes to light, it is nearly always pain relating to some particular skeletal part that focuses attention upon its presence. Most often this pain is referred to the back —more commonly the lower part of the back than the upper. In some of the cases starting with relatively mild pain in the back, a minor exertion or trauma is followed by the abrupt onset of severe back pain, associated with radiating pains and even paraplegia. Roentgenographic examination will then usually show areas of osteolytic destruction in one or more vertebral bodies, and some affected bodies may even be found more or less collapsed. When one or more lumbar bodies are affected, the patient may suffer not only from severe pain localized to the back, but also from sciatica, even if there is no compression of affected vertebræ. This is accounted for by the spread of myeloma tissue out of the bone, and its presence between the bone and the dura.

When not referable to the back, the local presenting complaint is quite likely to relate to a long bone. Roentgenographic examination will then show a large focus of lytic destruction which may be in the shaft or lie toward an end of the bone. The affected area may appear expanded and uniformly radiolucent or somewhat trabeculated, and be in imminent danger of fracture. Occasionally, when the presenting lesion is in a long bone, it may even be severe pain and disability from a fracture through the affected area that first makes the disease clinically conspicuous.

In a minority of the patients the presenting condition may relate to still another skeletal part. Thus, a rib or clavicle may have developed a palpable swelling or undergone fracture, or a palpable swelling may have appeared in the sternum or in relation to a skull bone, for instance.

The degree of involvement of the rest of the skeleton at the time when the presenting lesion is first noted varies widely. Sometimes the presenting lesion seems to be unaccompanied by any obvious changes detectable roentgenographically in the rest of the bones. Sooner or later, in most of these cases, the rest of the skeleton comes to show widespread demineralization and many areas of lytic destruction. In other cases, roentgenographic survey may show that the presenting lesion is already associated with destructive lesions in many other bones. (See Figs. 116 and 117.)

As more and more of the bone marrow becomes crowded out and replaced by the myelomatous tumor tissue, the patient becomes increasingly anemic. A severe cachexia may also eventually supervene. Another circumstance contributing to fatal termination of the case may be progressive renal insufficiency. This ensues from plugging of the renal tubules by proteinaceous material (already noted), and concomitant scarring of the renal parenchyma. Compression of the cord and consequent transverse myelitis may be associated with the development of an ascending infection of the urinary tract.

In a general way it can be stated that, apart from such or other intervening complications which may cut life short, patients affected with myelomatosis are likely to survive for 2 or 3 years from the time of onset of complaints. Some few survive much longer (8 or 10 years and occasionally even more), and in some of these patients the whole skeleton may long have been riddled with myeloma foci. In contrast, there are cases of myelomatosis in which the skeleton is by no means strikingly affected roentgenographically, but in which the patient succumbs within a few months to some intervening complication. These statements about survival do not, of course, apply to cases of so-called "solitary myeloma" (see p. 379).

## CLINICAL LABORATORY FINDINGS

**Marrow Puncture Smears.**—By study of sternal (or iliac) marrow puncture smears, it is often possible to establish the diagnosis of myelomatosis when the clinical and roentgenographic findings are still equivocal, and to confirm the diagnosis when it is already suspected on these grounds. A sternal marrow puncture smear in which plasma cells make up more than 3 per cent of the nucleated cells may be regarded as abnormal. If the plasma cells make up as much as 10 per cent, and if they are all of the so-called "typical" small variety, one may be dealing with myelomatosis, but one cannot be certain of it on this basis alone. This is so because small numbers of uniformly small plasma cells may be found also in smears from patients suffering from a variety of other diseases, including liver disease and carcinoma metastatic to the bones. In the latter instance, the smear showing an increased number of plasma cells comes from irritated marrow adjacent to a metastatic bone focus.

When the proportion of plasma cells is greater than 10 per cent, the diagnosis of myelomatosis from the smear rests on fairly firm ground. Indeed, in a representative group of cases of the disease, about 75 per cent of them are likely to show definitely excessive numbers of plasma (myeloma) cells at the time when the first sternal marrow puncture smear is taken. At this time, in accordance with the degree of infiltration of the sternal marrow by myeloma cells, the percentage of myeloma cells among the nucleated cells will be found to range up to 60 or 70 per cent and to average about 35. As the disease progresses, repeated smears will bring the incidence of positive sternal marrow puncture findings closer to 100 per cent (Fig. 118-*A*).

In a given case of myeloma, many or most of the myeloma cells in the smear may be of the small "typical" plasma cell variety. On the other hand, there are numerous cases in which the smears show relatively few small cells, but many cells which are large and otherwise bizarre, including some with multiple nuclei (see Bayrd). The large cells are held to represent myeloma cells of an anaplastic, immature type. Smears showing many large cells, giant multinuclear cells, and a definite lack of the typical small plasma cells sometimes raise problems of differential diagnosis. It should be noted that these variations from case to case in the cytologic detail of the myeloma cells in marrow smears are in line with what one also observes in the tissue sections made from open biopsy or autopsy material in different cases. Be that as it may, we have found that cases of myeloma in which many cells are of the large or giant type seem to be the cases most likely to run a fulminating clinical course.

**Other Hematologic Findings.**—Patients affected with progressing myelomatosis show an anemia which may become very severe. Indeed, as already pointed out, the presence of an unexplained anemia, particularly in an older person, should suggest the advisability of exploring the case for evidences of myeloma. Unless depressed by radiation or drug therapy, the white blood cell count in most cases of the disease tends to be within normal limits, and the differential formula is usually not much altered. Nevertheless, careful search of the blood smears in untreated cases is likely to reveal an occasional plasma cell, or at most a few plasma cells, in a fair proportion of them. However, now and then one encounters a case in which the white cell count is high and in which a large percentage of the white cells are plasma cells. In one such case studied by the writer, the white cell count rose steadily from 6,000 to 40,000, and 30 to 54 per cent of the cells were plasma cells. Such cases of myelomatosis, in which the tumor cells invade the blood stream, are well known and have been discussed under the heading of plasma-cell leukemia (see Muller and McNaughton, Patek and Castle, and Piney and Riach).

It is worth noting that cases of myelomatosis characterized by frank invasion of the blood stream apparently exhibit a strong tendency toward extraskeletal spread, manifest at autopsy in the form of diffuse and occasionally nodular infiltration of the spleen, liver, lymph nodes, and sometimes also of the kidney, pancreas, skin or other organs.

**Serum Calcium, Inorganic Phosphate, and Alkaline Phosphatase.**—Hypercalcemia is a common finding in cases of multiple myeloma. About half of the patients in any representative group of cases can be expected to show it. When elevated, the *serum calcium* value is likely to be around 13 to 15 mg. per 100 ml., though occasionally it may be around 18 mg. (normal value 9.5 to 10.0 ± 0.5). The hypercalcemia is best conceived as resulting mainly from the mobilization of calcium from the bones in the process of resorption of the osseous tissue by the growing myeloma tissue. Still, in one case of myelomatosis studied by the writer in which the skeleton was found devastated on roentgenographic examination and the marrow puncture smear yielded positive findings, the serum calcium value was, if anything, slightly below normal. Hypercalcemia may be observed, whether or not hyperproteinemia is also present in a given case. Indeed, the highest calcium levels noted by us were observed mainly in cases in which hyperproteinemia was not present. The presence of hypercalcemia in a patient should not make one think that one is necessarily dealing with a case of myelomatosis. Indeed, hypercalcemia occurs characteristically in association with primary hyperparathyroidism, and it also appears occasionally in connection with cancer which has produced widespread osteolytic metastases in the bones (see Jaffe and Bodansky).

The serum *inorganic phosphate* value is not elevated in the disease unless renal insufficiency develops. However, such insufficiency is a frequent terminal finding in connection with the disease. Concomitantly the serum nonprotein nitrogen also becomes elevated. The serum *alkaline phosphatase* activity is usually within the normal range. However, we have found that in an occasional case, as the disease advances and pathologic fractures occur, the alkaline phosphatase value may become moderately elevated. This elevation represents a healing response to the fractures and is not directly attributable to the myelomatosis.

***Figure 118***

*A*, Photomicrograph (× 450) showing the appearance of a sternal marrow puncture smear which is crowded with myeloma cells. Note that, characteristically, the myeloma cells present eccentrically placed nuclei. Note also that many of the nuclei are large and that some of the cells contain double nuclei.

*B*, Photograph showing the cut surface of several vertebral bodies from a case in which the clinical picture was dominated by widespread extraskeletal deposition of amyloid, but in which microscopic study of the bones removed at autopsy showed diffuse myelomatous involvement of the marrow. The patient was a woman 42 years of age in whom amyloid infiltration of the skin and subcutis had led to remarkable scleroderma-like thickening of these parts and the occurrence of verrucæ containing amyloid on the eyelids (see *C*), about the anus, on the oral mucous membranes, and along the margins of the tongue. At autopsy, extensive deposits of amyloid were noted also in the muscles, lungs, liver, spleen, stomach, intestines, and lymph nodes. Note that the vertebral bodies present no alteration in gross architecture. Furthermore, the bones did not cut with abnormal ease. The presence of myelomatosis in this case was established only by microscopic examination of the bones, which showed diffuse and substantial replacement of the bone marrow by myeloma cells. Had the bones not been examined microscopically, the presence of the myelomatosis could have been overlooked and the case considered merely one of primary idiopathic amyloidosis.

*C*, Photograph of the patient described in *B*. Note the verrucæ about the eyelids, the thickening of the mucous membrane of the lower lip, and the thickening of the fingers—all due to infiltration of amyloid.

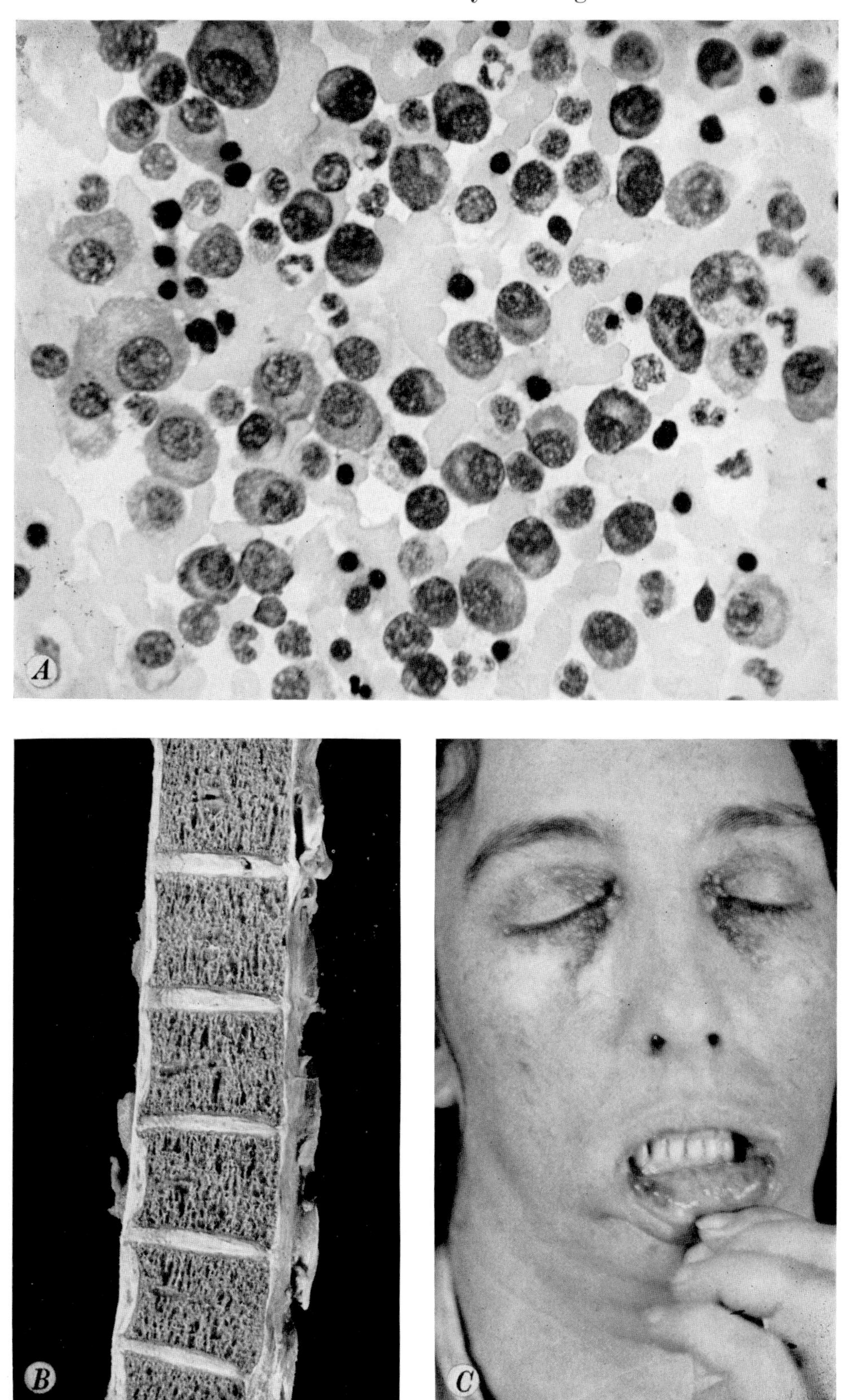

*Figure 118*

**Serum Proteins.**—In about 50 to 60 per cent of any representative group of cases, one is likely to encounter an elevation of the serum protein level. Indeed, in an occasional case the total serum protein value may come to be as high as 15 gm. per 100 ml. or even more (normal total protein value 6.5 to 7.5 gm. per 100 ml.). However, the albumin fraction of the serum protein (normal value 4 to 5 gm. per 100 ml.) is not elevated in multiple myeloma and indeed is often below normal. Thus, it is an increase in the globulin fraction (normal value 2 to 3 gm. per 100 ml.) that accounts for the hyperproteinemia when any is present. Indeed, in one case or another of myelomatosis with hyperproteinemia, we have obtained globulin fraction values of 10 gm. and even more. Briefly, then, if a case shows hyperproteinemia, one will find the albumin value normal or below normal, the globulin value elevated, and thus a reversal of the normal ratio (about 2 to 1) of albumin to globulin. The globulin aberrations are apparently contributed by the myeloma cells.

In recent years, much work has been done on the particulars of the globulin aberration. By the Howe fractionation procedure, Gutman has shown that the hyperglobulinemia is often due to an increase in both the euglobulin fraction and the pseudoglobulin fraction. However, a hyperglobulinemia associated with an increase in both of these globulin fractions is also to be observed in certain chronic infectious diseases. Nevertheless, if the hyperglobulinemia as a whole is very pronounced, the finding of an elevated euglobulin and pseudoglobulin speaks rather for myeloma than for chronic infectious disease. The presence of a pronounced hyperglobulinemia without any increase in the euglobulin value is an even more significant finding in favor of multiple myeloma. Furthermore, in some cases of myeloma the Howe fractionation method may reveal peculiarities in the salting-out behavior of the proteins. These peculiarities are known to be due to the presence of proteins of the Bence Jones type and other abnormal proteins. The finding of such proteins in the serum is virtually pathognomonic for multiple myeloma.

The serum proteins in cases of myeloma have also been studied by the ultracentrifuge technique and by the Tiselius electrophoretic technique. The former technique has yielded information about the molecular weights of the abnormal globulins present in the serum, thus helping to differentiate them. The Tiselius electrophoretic technique has revealed abnormal peak patterns for the globulins in almost all cases, the majority of peaks occurring in the gamma globulin and beta globulin areas. These peaks reflect either the presence of excessive amounts of normal gamma globulin and/or beta globulin, or the presence of abnormal globulins (including proteins of the Bence Jones type) having electrophoretic mobilities similar to those of the beta and gamma globulins normally present. For routine clinical investigation of the serum proteins, however, the method of filter paper electrophoresis has come into wide use. By the application of paper electrophoretic techniques, one observes increases in beta and/or gamma globulin fractions in those cases of myeloma in which a frank hyperglobulinemia is present. Even in cases in which hyperglobulinemia is minimal or absent, paper electrophoretic patterns often display evidence of small abnormal components in the beta and/or gamma globulin areas.

**Bence Jones Proteinuria.**—The term "Bence Jones protein" refers not to a single protein, but to a group of proteins with closely related properties. We have observed it in about 40 per cent of our cases. This incidence is in line with what has been noted by many others, though much higher and much lower incidences have also been reported. In explanation of variations in the incidence of Bence Jones proteinuria, it is to be noted that: (1) It may be undetectable in casual urine specimens but present in a 24-hour specimen; (2) it may be present at certain times but not at others (that is, its occurrence may be intermittent rather than continuous); (3) it may be absent from the urine early in the course of the disease and become evident later on; and (4) it may be searched for repeatedly in the course of the disease in a given case and never found at all. In this connection, it should be pointed out that if one employs the old standard method for the detection of Bence Jones urinary protein by heat coagulation and solution at temperatures above 60° C., the presence of this protein occasionally goes undetected. Therefore, in cases of suspected myelomatosis, routine screening of urine specimens for Bence Jones protein by paper electrophoresis is valuable because it permits the detection of trace amounts of this type of protein even in the presence of large amounts of albumin and other proteins, which interfere with the detection of the Bence Jones protein in the urine if the old method is used.

Bence Jones proteinuria is not a necessary concomitant of hyperglobulinemia. In fact, one is more likely to observe it in cases in which hyperglobulinemia is absent or slight than in cases in which it is pronounced. Furthermore, it is interesting to note that in the cases in which Bence Jones protein is observed in the urine, there is very likely to be at least a qualitative aberration in the serum globulin peaks, as evidenced by electrophoretic studies. It is stated, though not well corroborated, that Bence Jones proteinuria is occasionally found in conditions other than multiple myeloma, and particularly with leukemia and with carcinoma extensively metastatic to the bones. At any rate, for all practical purposes, the presence of Bence Jones proteinuria constitutes one of the most reliable clinical laboratory criteria for the presence of myelomatosis.

## ROENTGENOGRAPHIC AND GROSS PATHOLOGIC SKELETAL FINDINGS

**Solitary Myeloma of Bone.**—The problem of so-called "solitary myeloma" of bone has had a good deal of attention centered upon it. Cases are not at all unusual in which a patient seeks treatment because of a destructive lesion in some one bone, the lesion is established by biopsy as a plasma cell tumor, and roentgenographic examination of the skeleton fails to reveal clear-cut myelomatous involvement of any other bones at that time. However, within some months or at most a year or two, nearly all of these cases come to reveal destructive lesions in other bones, and also myeloma cells in the sternal marrow puncture smears. That is, sooner or later these cases show themselves as belonging in the category of multiple rather than solitary myeloma. Indeed, it is to be noted that many of the cases reported as instances of solitary myeloma had merely not been followed long enough to manifest their true nature as cases of myelomatosis (Fig. 117-*C*).

Multiple bone involvement in myelomatosis probably represents multifocal tumor growths rather than metastases to the various bones from a single primary bone lesion. If this is the fact, it is understandable: (1) that in some cases, myeloma foci may appear in many bones simultaneously; (2) that in other cases there may be an interval of months and possibly a year or two between the appearance of the presenting lesion and that of lesions in other bones; and finally (3) that, in very rare cases, no lesions in other bones appear at all, even in the course of a number of years. Of course, it is only to the last-named group of cases that the term "solitary myeloma" is strictly applicable.

In connection with the question of solitary myeloma, there are a few carefully followed cases in which, many years after the presenting bone lesion had been diagnosed as a myeloma (and treated in one way or another), the patient still did not show myelomatous involvement of other bones. A striking case in point was reported by Stewart and Taylor. The patient was a man 34 years of age who presented himself with a large osteolytic lesion in the upper half of a humerus, which had broken out into the neighboring soft parts. Biopsy showed the tumor to be composed essentially of cells resembling plasma cells, and a forequarter amputation was performed. A follow-up extending over 8 years failed to reveal any evidence either of local recurrence or of myelomatous involvement of other bones. In a personal communication, Stewart informed the writer that this was still true 18 years after publication of that report.

In the cases acceptable as instances of solitary myeloma, the plasma cells of the lesional tissue do not show the atypism which they often reveal in cases of disseminated myeloma. Furthermore, the biochemical findings relating to the blood serum are ordinarily within the normal range (see Christopherson and Miller, and Carson, Ackerman, and Maltby). Indeed, the solitary myeloma of bone has even been held to be a lesion closer to the relatively benign (or at least only locally malignant) solitary plasmacytoma (myeloma) of soft tissues than to myelomatosis of bones. These soft-tissue solitary plasmacytomas generally arise in relation to the nasopharynx or the conjunctiva, but occasionally in lymph nodes and, very rarely, elsewhere (see Hellwig).

The favorable response of most cases of plasmacytoma of soft parts to local surgical intervention and/or radiation therapy is much like that observed in some of the cases of solitary myeloma of bone so treated. However, there are also occasional instances of localized plasmacytoma primary in soft parts in which, after many years, the condition not only recurs but tends to spread widely over the skeleton as well as other tissues (see Jackson, Parker, and Bethea). In these cases, as in cases of myelomatosis primary in bones, no therapy is able any longer to check a fatal termination.

Cases of localized myeloma of bone have also been reported on the basis of autopsy findings, but in none of these cases was there a very long interval between

***Figure 119***

*A*, Photograph showing, in sagittal section, a severely altered vertebral column from a case of myelomatosis. The patient was a man 31 years of age whose presenting lesion was in the right clavicle. He had sustained a trauma to that region, the affected bone area subsequently became swollen, and a biopsy established the diagnosis of myelomatosis. The patient died $1\frac{1}{2}$ years after the onset of his difficulties. Note that many of the vertebral bodies have undergone compressional collapse, and that many of the intervertebral disks are expanded. The osseous tissue of the vertebral bodies has been substantially resorbed and replaced by myeloma tissue, which in some places takes the form of discrete tumor nodes. It is also noteworthy in this case that throughout the patient's hospitalization, which lasted for 1 year, numerous determinations of the serum calcium showed a striking hypercalcemia. On the other hand, neither the ordinary chemical methods nor electrophoretic methods revealed, at any time, abnormal serum proteins or even a hyperglobulinemia. Furthermore, repeated examination of the urine failed to reveal Bence Jones proteinuria. At autopsy, some of the internal organs showed metastatic calcification, which was most striking in the lungs (see Figs. 123-*B* and *C*).

*B*, Roentgenograph of part of a sagittally sectioned vertebral column from another case of myelomatosis in which the column was heavily involved. Some of the vertebral bodies have undergone compressional collapse. All show numerous radiolucencies, the large ones representing areas in which all the spongy bone has been destroyed.

*C*, Photograph of part of the sagittally sectioned spine removed at autopsy in the case described in connection with Fig. 116-*A*. Note the almost total destruction and collapse of the body of the 10th dorsal vertebra, and also the extradural encuffment of the cord at that level. The other vertebræ are not collapsed, but show miliary to small pea-sized grayish white areas of tumor tissue. The compression of the spinal cord was followed by transverse myelitis and ascending infection of the urinary tract. Terminally, the patient presented the blood picture of plasma-cell leukemia.

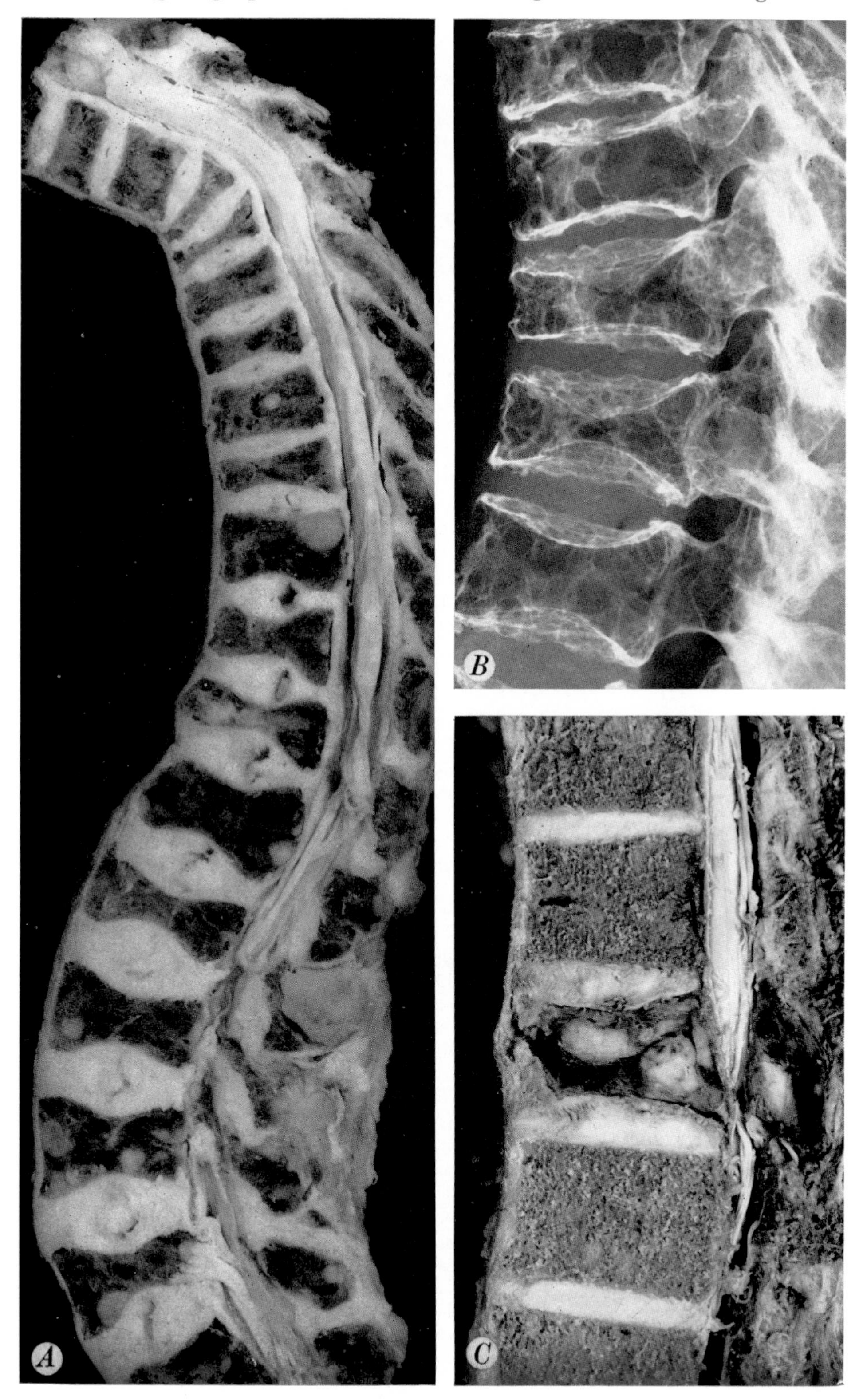


*Figure 119*

the clinical emergence of the solitary lesion and the autopsy. What these cases do prove is that the disease may persist in the form of a solitary lesion for some time before becoming disseminated over the skeleton. Thus, Rutishauser reports an instance of a woman who had a large, destructive lesion of the upper femoral shaft which proved at autopsy to be a plasma cell tumor, while the other bones failed to reveal evidence of myeloma. A fracture through the affected femur had occurred about 5 months before the patient's death, and she had given a history of local disability for some months before the occurrence of the fracture. Raven and Willis report the case of a man who suffered a paraplegia from collapse of the 5th and 6th cervical vertebræ, which, at autopsy some months later, were found to be the site of a plasma cell tumor. No evidences of myeloma were found in the many other bones examined grossly at autopsy and subsequently studied histologically.

Lumb reports the case of a man presenting a tumor which had destroyed practically the entire sacrum and had spread out into the iliac bones and adjacent soft parts. The patient survived for a year after the onset of his local complaints and died of uremia. In this case, too, there was no evidence of myeloma in the numerous bones examined at autopsy and subsequently studied microscopically. This case is further of interest in that: (1) during life, the patient presented Bence Jones proteinuria, and (2) the uremia from which he died could be related to renal tubular blockage by proteinaceous casts. Such findings are certainly unusual in a case of myeloma limited to a single skeletal area, and indeed their presence in a case apparently of this kind is usually regarded as ruling out the possibility that the myeloma in question is actually localized.

**Diffuse and/or Multiple Myeloma.**—No single description is generally applicable to the gross and roentgenographic findings in the bones in cases of widespread involvement by myeloma. At one extreme there is the occasional case in which such bones as are removed at autopsy present no obvious changes externally and do not seem particularly soft when being cut open. In the bones from one such case, the writer found that the spongy trabeculæ were still numerous and the bone

***Figure 120***

*A*, Photograph showing, in longitudinal section, the upper part of a femur in a case of myelomatosis. Note that the contour of the bone is not modified. Nevertheless, the marrow has been replaced by myeloma tissue which, here and there, takes the form of discrete whitish nodules. The patient was a man 45 years of age who complained of nosebleeds, weight loss, weakness, dizziness, and vague aches in the bones and joints, dating back to about 1 year before admission. On admission he was found to have a severe anemia and a pronounced hyperglobulinemia, and myeloma cells were demonstrated in the sternal marrow puncture smears. The roentgenographs showed numerous small roundish radiolucencies in many of the bones. However, no large lytic destructive lesions were observed. The patient died about 1½ years after the onset of his complaints.

*B*, Photograph showing, in longitudinal section, the upper part of a femur in another case of myelomatosis. In this case the femur is deformed and is the site of a pathologic fracture. The skeleton in general was devastated by the disease.

*C*, Photograph showing, as a macerated specimen, the lower lumbar vertebral bodies and the innominate bones and sacrum from a case of myelomatosis. Note the "moth-eaten" appearance created by the destruction of the osseous tissue and representing the radiolucencies which were observed in the clinical $x$-ray picture of the part. The patient was a man 59 years of age who was admitted to the hospital on account of pain in the lower part of the back of only 3 months' standing. Hypercalcemia was present and also Bence Jones proteinuria. The patient died 1 month after admission, and the autopsy revealed the wide dissemination of the destructive changes throughout the skeleton.

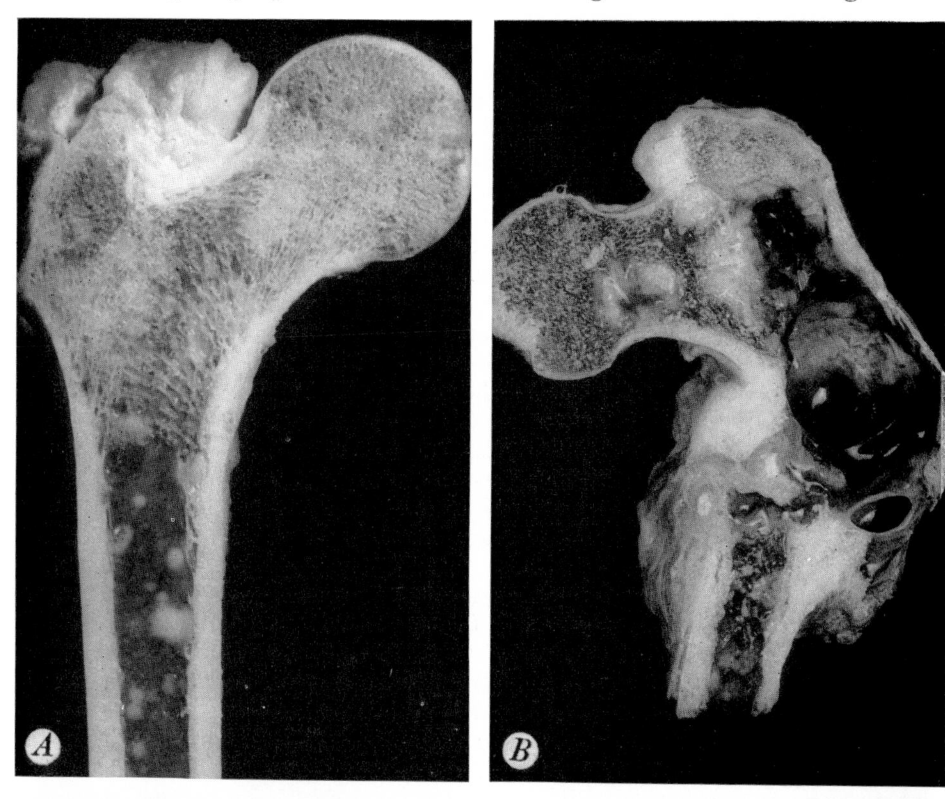


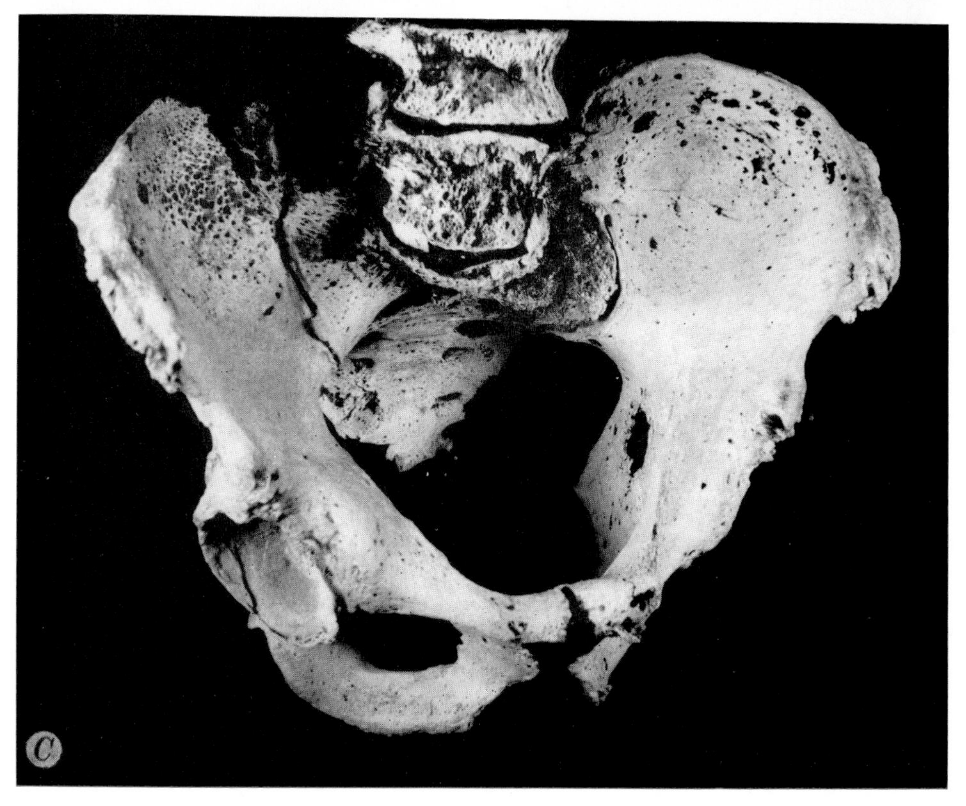


*Figure 120*

cortices not significantly thinned. However, on close inspection the marrow was found modified and, specifically, replaced more or less diffusely by grayish tissue which, on histologic examination, was found to consist mainly of myeloma cells. The mildness of the gross changes in this case of diffuse myelomatosis was in accord with the fact that, during life, roentgenographic study of the bones failed to reveal any significant general porosity or punched-out rarefactions (Fig. 118-*B* and *C*).

In a few other cases of diffuse myelomatosis which came to autopsy, though the bones removed still presented no obvious external changes, they did cut with abnormal ease. Furthermore, their cortices were found thinned from the medullary side, and the spongy trabeculæ reduced in number and thickness. In the vertebral column, some of the intervertebral disks were expanded and some of the bodies narrowed by compressional collapse. In the various bones studied from these cases, the marrow spaces were found filled by grayish white tumor tissue which, here and there, was even present in the form of small but discrete tumor nodules. Thus, there was not only tumor tissue in the marrow spaces, but actual widespread though slight reduction of the osseous tissue, from encroachment upon it by the myeloma tissue. In the bones presenting pathologic changes of this magnitude, the clinical roentgenographs had shown, as might be expected, thinning of the cortex and diffuse rarefaction of the spongiosa, associated with the presence of small but discrete mottled rarefactions in the spongiosa. This is likely to be most striking in the ends of the long bones. Cases of diffuse myelomatosis showing *x*-ray changes of this character might be mistaken for instances of pronounced generalized osteoporosis if one judged them by the *x*-ray findings alone.

However, the classical roentgenographic picture is that in which, in addition to widespread general porosity of the bones, one sees also numerous small or fairly large punched-out rarefactions. These punched-out areas of osteolysis show no evidence of osteoblastic reaction around them or within them. In a particular case, they may be widely distributed, being found in the calvarium, ribs, vertebræ, pelvic bones, and also some of the long bones. One or another of the latter bones may also show, either in the shaft or toward an end, a large expanded area which may be uniformly rarefied or somewhat trabeculated. Such a roentgenographic picture not infrequently raises the clinical problem of differential diagnosis between multiple myeloma and carcinoma which has produced widespread osteolytic metastases.

In cases of multiple myeloma in which the roentgenographic picture is of this character, autopsy reveals, of course, that the bones are more or less gravely altered. Specifically, some or even many of the ribs may show single or multiple distentions of contour. The vertebral column is likely to show deformity due to collapse of one or even a number of the bodies. Long bones, and especially one or both of the femora, are likely to manifest swellings, or deformity due to pathologic fracture.

***Figure 121***

*A*, Roentgenograph of the skull from a case of myelomatosis in a man 51 years of age who was known to have been suffering from the disease for 9 years. The interesting feature is the comparative lightness of the involvement of the calvarium, as observed shortly before death, in relation to the involvement of other skeletal areas as observed at autopsy ( see *C*). Note the relatively sparse, small, roundish rarefactions in the calvarium.

*B*, Roentgenograph of a number of segments from the calvarium removed at autopsy in the case illustrated in *A*.

*C*, Roentgenograph of several affected ribs in this case showing strikingly severe alterations due to the myelomatous involvement. The vertebral column and long bones were also devastated by the disease.

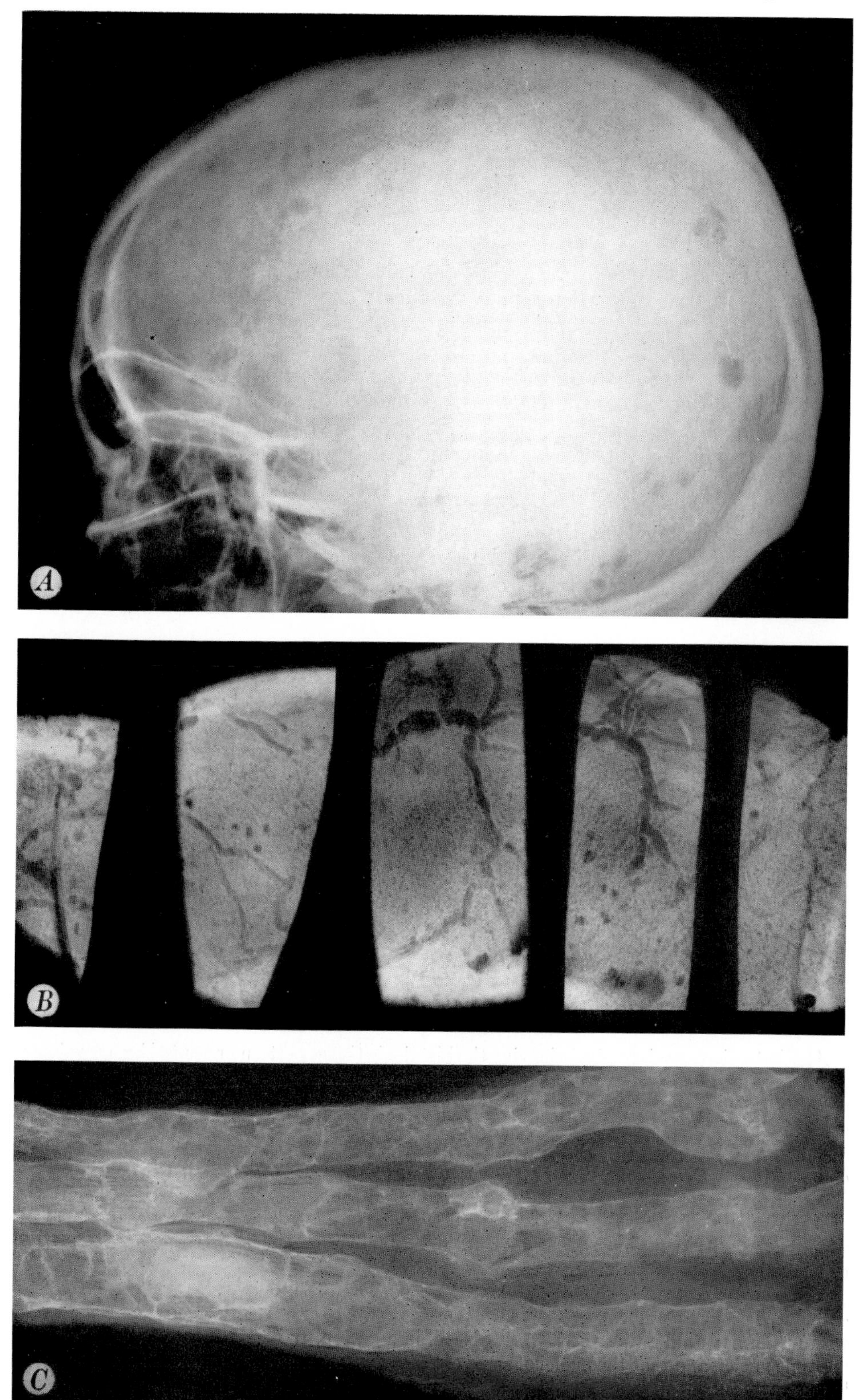


*Figure 121*

When cut open, such severely affected bones will show substantial thinning of the cortex. In some places the latter may have undergone complete lytic destruction, and tumor tissue will then be found distending the periosteum. The spongy bone also will be found substantially resorbed and, in many places, entirely lacking. Myeloma tissue not only diffusely fills the marrow spaces, but is also present in the form of large discrete tumor masses. The tumor tissue itself may, in many places, be hemorrhagically discolored and, in some places, softened and cystified in consequence of the hemorrhage into it (see Figs. 119 and 120).

Great emphasis is usually laid upon the diagnostic value of the presence of several or even many roundish, punched-out rarefactions in *x*-ray films of the calvarium. It is true that when *x*-rays show clear-cut and widespread involvement of the rest of the skeleton, in the form of numerous punched-out rarefactions, the calvarium, too, is quite likely to show these, though frequently it does not. However, precisely when one turns to the films of the calvarium because the films of the other bones do not show the conventional picture of multiple myeloma, the calvarium, too, fails to show it (see Jaffe). Whether or not the films of the calvarium present the punched-out areas, gross examination will reveal that the marrow of the diploic spaces, like that elsewhere, has been substantially replaced by the tumor tissue. At a site corresponding to a clear-cut, punched-out rarefaction, one will find that the myeloma tissue is present as a tumor nodule which has destroyed the diploic bone and usually also thinned the tables. However, one only seldom finds the inner and outer tables completely destroyed at a site of punched-out calvarial rarefaction (see Fig. 121).

## HISTOPATHOLOGY OF THE MYELOMA TISSUE

In areas not modified by hemorrhage and softening, the tumor tissue is found quite cellular, there being practically no supporting stroma between the tumor cells. In some cases, as noted, sections prepared from the tumor tissue show that the myeloma cells are rather uniform and predominantly small, and resemble the ordinary plasma cell. Such cells are rather roundish or oval, the nucleus tends to be eccentric and may contain a nucleolus, and there is relatively little cytoplasm. The chromatin particles of the nucleus are likely to be concentrated chiefly around the periphery, and the cytoplasm tends to stain pinkish with eosin. Sections treated with Pappenheim or iron-hematoxylin stain reveal that these cells have many of the staining peculiarities of ordinary inflammatory plasma cells. Interspersed

***Figure 122***

*A*, Photomicrograph (× 450) showing the histologic tissue pattern presented by a myeloma composed of predominantly small tumor cells of almost uniform size which resemble the ordinary tissue plasma cell. A myeloma presenting this cytologic appearance is commonly designated as a plasma cell myeloma or a plasmacytoma.

*B*, Photomicrograph (× 450) showing the pattern of a myeloma in which many of the cells are larger than in *A*. Note also that many of the cells present deep-staining hyperchromatic nuclei.

*C*, Photomicrograph (× 450) showing the histologic pattern presented by a myeloma in which many of the myeloma cells have multiple nuclei and in which, on the average, the nuclei are larger than those illustrated in *A* and *B*.

*D*, Photomicrograph (× 450) showing tissue from a myeloma whose cytologic pattern is dominated by comparatively large cells, though there is also a sprinkling of smaller cells with nuclei not unlike those seen in *A*. Note, in addition, that a number of the cells have multiple nuclei, and that the nuclei of some of these multinuclear myeloma cells are markedly hyperchromatic.

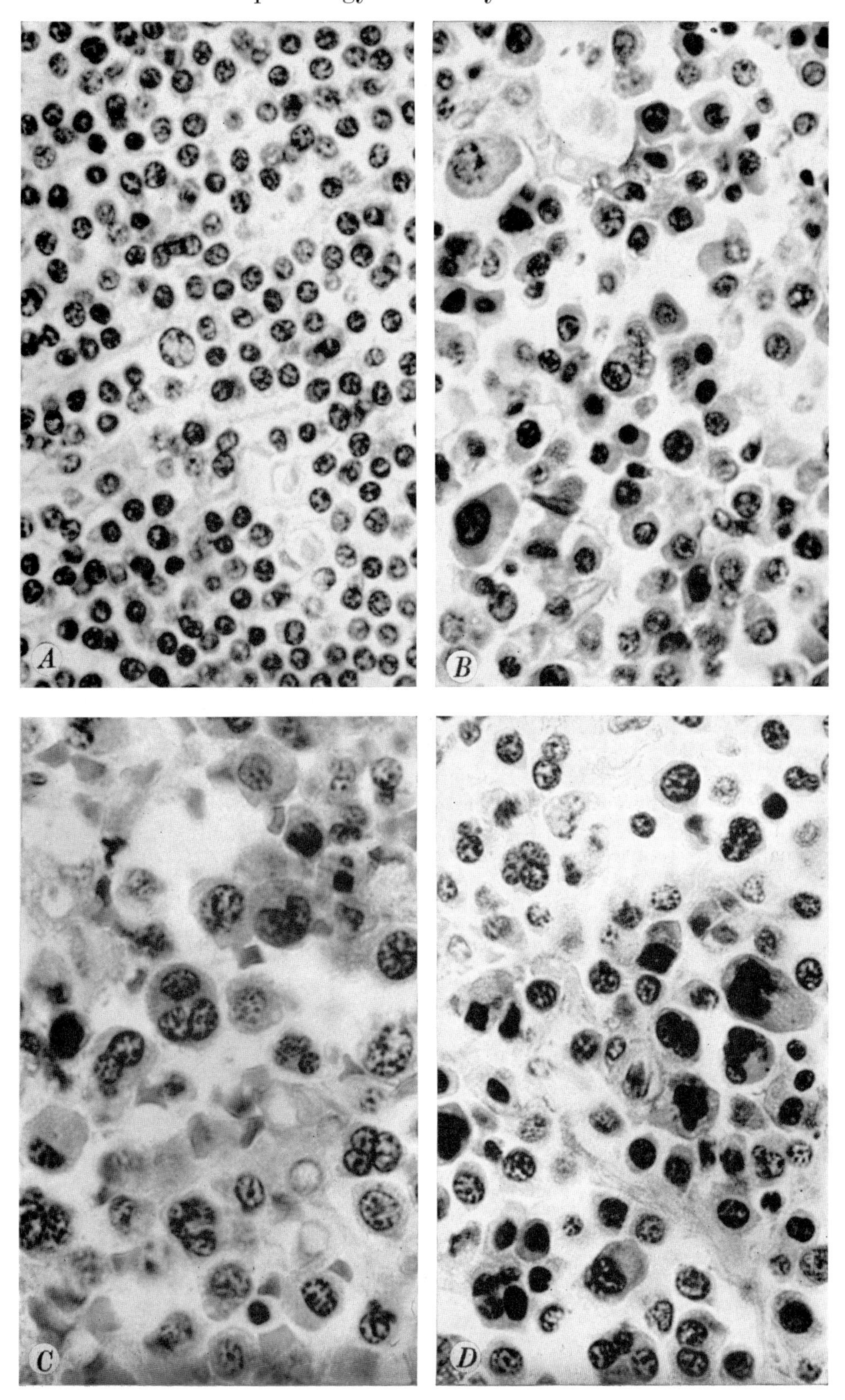


*Figure 122*

among the small myeloma cells there may be some myeloma cells which, though of the same general character, are larger in respect to both cytoplasm and nucleus. There may also be very occasional cells with double nuclei, but there is no tendency to cellular irregularity otherwise. As indicated, it is for the myelomas showing this cytology that the name "plasma cell myeloma" or "plasmacytoma" is most appropriate.

In other cases, sections will show that many of the myeloma cells are large, and indeed large cells sometimes dominate the cytologic picture in tissue taken from one area or another. However, variable numbers of small, typical myeloma cells will be found among the large ones in any case. The large myeloma cells generally exceed the myeloblast in size. Their cytoplasm is often abundant, and the nucleus, which may or may not be eccentrically placed, is fairly large, and round, oval, or even reniform. In some tumor fields, veritable tumor giant cells may also be found. These cells present large, hyperchromatic nuclei, giant nuclei of bizarre shape, and sometimes giant multiple nuclei. Then, again, some large cells in mitotic division may be encountered. Indeed, were it not for the fact that variable numbers of the more classic myeloma cells are found scattered among the large and bizarre giant cells, one might hesitate to interpret the cytologic findings in these cases as those of myeloma (see Fig. 122).

At any rate, the fact that one observes differences in regard to cytologic detail among the tumor cells as one passes from one area or one case of myelomatosis to another has led to much discussion. This has centered around the question of whether these differences express merely variations of one basic cell type or whether they indicate that various kinds of marrow cells may give rise to myelomatosis. Those who have favored the latter conception have held specifically that, in addition to the so-called plasma cell myeloma, there exist, for instance, myeloblastic, lymphoblastic, erythroblastic, and megakaryoblastic myelomas. At present there is a trend away from this idea. The opinion prevailing now is that all myelomas are made up of cells of the same fundamental type, and that the variations of cytologic detail observed in the tissue sections are, as already indicated, merely expressions of various stages of development, differentiation, anaplasia, or degeneration occurring in the basic cell (see Wallgren, and Lichtenstein and Jaffe). The results of sternal marrow puncture smear studies have tended to support this opinion (see Bayrd, and Wintrobe).

At one time the writer believed that correlation of the cytologic aspects of the myelomas with the pertinent biochemical data strongly suggested that it was the large cell myelomas particularly which are characterized by hyperglobulinemia and, rather often, by Bence Jones proteinuria. However, further experience with myeloma has led the writer to believe that there is actually no such correlation. This further experience does, however, support the idea that the myelomas in which many of the cells are large and anaplastic (as shown also by sternal marrow smears) are the ones which run a relatively rapid fatal course.

It should be noted that, despite large experience, a pathologist may occasionally misread a tissue section prepared from an open biopsy specimen in a case of myelomatosis. This may happen even in the absence of bizarre and atypical cells in the tissue sections. The misleading factor may be that, while the cells of the myeloma tissue are of uniformly small size, processing of the tissue had produced staining artifacts suggesting interpretation of the cells as lymphocytes, and hence of the lesion as a lymphosarcoma. Sometimes myeloma cells of larger size may be misinterpreted as reticulum cells, and the lesion be designated erroneously as a reticulum cell sarcoma. There are other pitfalls, also. For instance, on the basis of a biopsy section alone (that is, without knowledge of the clinical aspects of the case), a Ewing sarcoma or a focus of neuroblastoma may occasionally be miscalled a myeloma, or vice versa. It is for this reason that a diagnosis of myelomatosis based on tissue sections from a biopsy specimen should be confirmed, if possible, by findings from a sternal marrow puncture smear, or from direct smears from the specimen, stained with Wright stain.

## EXTRASKELETAL PATHOLOGIC FINDINGS

**Visceral Involvement in Myelomatosis.**—Of course, we are not referring here to the direct outgrowth of tumor tissue from affected bones into neighboring tissues, but rather to involvement due apparently to metastatic spread. In a few of our autopsied cases, we found one or more gross extraskeletal myeloma foci. These are most likely to be found in the liver, spleen, or lymph nodes, though occasionally they have been noted elsewhere. In our cases, such tumor foci were generally only a centimeter or two in diameter, though occasionally somewhat larger. In relation to the spleen in particular, a number of instances of more or less massive gross myelomatous involvement have been reported (see Churg and Gordon). On the other hand, the finding of microscopic infiltrations of myeloma cells, particularly in the liver, spleen, and lymph nodes, is more common. In fact, it is held that, if searched for carefully, microscopic infiltrations, particularly in these sites, will be found more often than not (see Lowenhaupt). In a given case coming to autopsy, one may find merely such microscopic infiltrations, or these may be associated with the presence of one or more gross tumor foci.

**Myeloma Kidney.**—As noted, in many cases of myelomatosis the kidneys show certain microscopic changes which have come to be regarded as characteristic of the disease; hence the term "myeloma kidney" (see Mallory, Oliver, and Newns and Edwards). Gross alterations may or may not be present, and are slight at most. The kidneys are likely to be of normal size, but occasionally are somewhat enlarged or somewhat contracted. The corticomedullary outline, though usually still discernible, may be blurred.

The glomeruli, as a rule, show no specific changes. The significant changes relate to the tubules. Many of these are found blocked by proteinaceous casts. These represent protein (Bence Jones protein or other abnormal proteins) precipitated in the tubules while the urine is undergoing concentration there by reabsorption of water. The obstructing casts are found particularly in the loops of Henle and in the collecting tubules. Many of the casts are surrounded by multinucleated giant cells. The latter are regarded by some as foreign-body giant cells, but it is more likely that they represent agglomerations of desquamated tubular epithelium cells. As a rule, many of the tubules above the region of blockage are dilated, though others are collapsed and atrophied. One may also find some interstitial fibrosis, and some round cell infiltration not related to infection (Fig. 123–*A*). As to the glomeruli, here and there in the kidneys, many of them may show thickening of the basement membranes of their capillaries (see Kobernick and Whiteside). However, the aberration in question is usually not striking, nor is it peculiar to multiple myeloma. These capillary changes are hardly ever as severe as those associated with chronic glomerulonephritis, arteriolar nephrosclerosis, and diabetic glomerulosclerosis. Be that as it may, the common occurrence of proteinuria in multiple myeloma is probably to be related to the glomerular changes.

It is thus tubular blockage and its consequences that constitute the myeloma kidney and are so often the cause of renal insufficiency in patients suffering from multiple myeloma. Indeed, the writer has seen a case in which the renal insufficiency led to death of the patient, and in which the presence of myelomatosis was not suspected clinically and was established only at autopsy. An occasional case has also been reported in which a patient has died of renal insufficiency from tubular blockage although the skeletal involvement by myeloma was of very limited scope (see Lumb).

Other renal changes are encountered in one case or another, with or without the specific changes. Thus, one often finds some arteriosclerotic renal changes, in accordance with the age of the patient. Also, a more or less pronounced pyelonephritis may be encountered, if vertebral collapse has resulted in damage to the spinal cord, and infection of the urinary tract has supervened.

**Metastatic Calcification.**—Some degree of metastatic calcification may be encountered if lytic destruction of the bones has been associated with a pronounced hypercalcemia, and particularly if severe renal insufficiency has also been present (Figs. 123-*B* and *C*). Among the most common sites are the kidneys, where the calcification usually takes the form of calcium granules in the tubular epithelium and interstitial connective tissue. However, in one of our cases coming to autopsy, the renal calcification was apparent even grossly. The kidneys in this case showed yellowish streaks within some of the pyramids, and fine yellowish calcific gravel was present in many of the calyces and also within the urinary bladder. Evidence of calcification may likewise be found in the lungs. Indeed, in one of our cases the calcification was so heavy that the lungs felt indurated and the cut surfaces showed numerous patchy areas which were yellowish and gritty. Microscopically, widespread deposits of calcium were noted in the interstitium of the pulmonary parenchyma. Calcium deposits have also been found in the gastric mucosa and even in still other tissues in cases of myelomatosis coming to autopsy (see Froboese).

**Amyloid Deposition.**—Amyloid deposition is not uncommon in connection with myelomatosis. The writer observed it in about 10 per cent of the cases which he studied. Its occurrence is very likely to be associated with the presence of hyperglobulinemia and/or Bence Jones proteinuria. When it is not found so associated, the likelihood is that the presence of abnormal globulins would be revealed by electrophoretic studies of the blood, even though the total blood protein value is not elevated. This fact affords grounds for speculation as to the relationship of circulating abnormal globulins to the formation of amyloid in these cases. There is the possibility that the organism becomes hypersensitive to these globulins, and that the amyloid deposition is the end product of an antigen-antibody mechanism (see Magnus-Levy, Lichtenstein and Jaffe, and Dahlin and Dockerty).

Anatomically, amyloid deposition in multiple myeloma may be manifest in any of several patterns. Most often, it is only the myelomatous bone lesions that show the amyloid. In some cases the latter is scattered and so small in amount as to be

***Figure 123***

*A*, Photomicrograph (× 125) showing dilated renal tubules which are obstructed by proteinaceous casts about which there are multinuclear giant cells. This is the characteristic picture observed in the so-called myeloma kidney, and indeed it is often possible to make a diagnosis of multiple myeloma from the appearance of the kidney sections alone.

*B*, Roentgenograph of a lung from the case of myelomatosis described in Fig. 119-*A*. In this case the skeleton was devastated by the disease and the patient presented a pronounced hypercalcemia of long standing. Terminally, there was a mounting renal insufficiency.

*C*, Photomicrograph (× 65) showing the histologic pattern presented by the tissue sections prepared from the lung illustrated in *B*. The dark-staining areas represent calcium which has been deposited in the pulmonary interstitial tissue.

*D*, Photomicrograph (× 65) showing amyloid infiltration of myelomatous tumor tissue. In this case the amyloid formed gross tumor masses in some places. However, there was no extraskeletal amyloid deposition, but many of the renal tubules were plugged by proteinaceous casts.

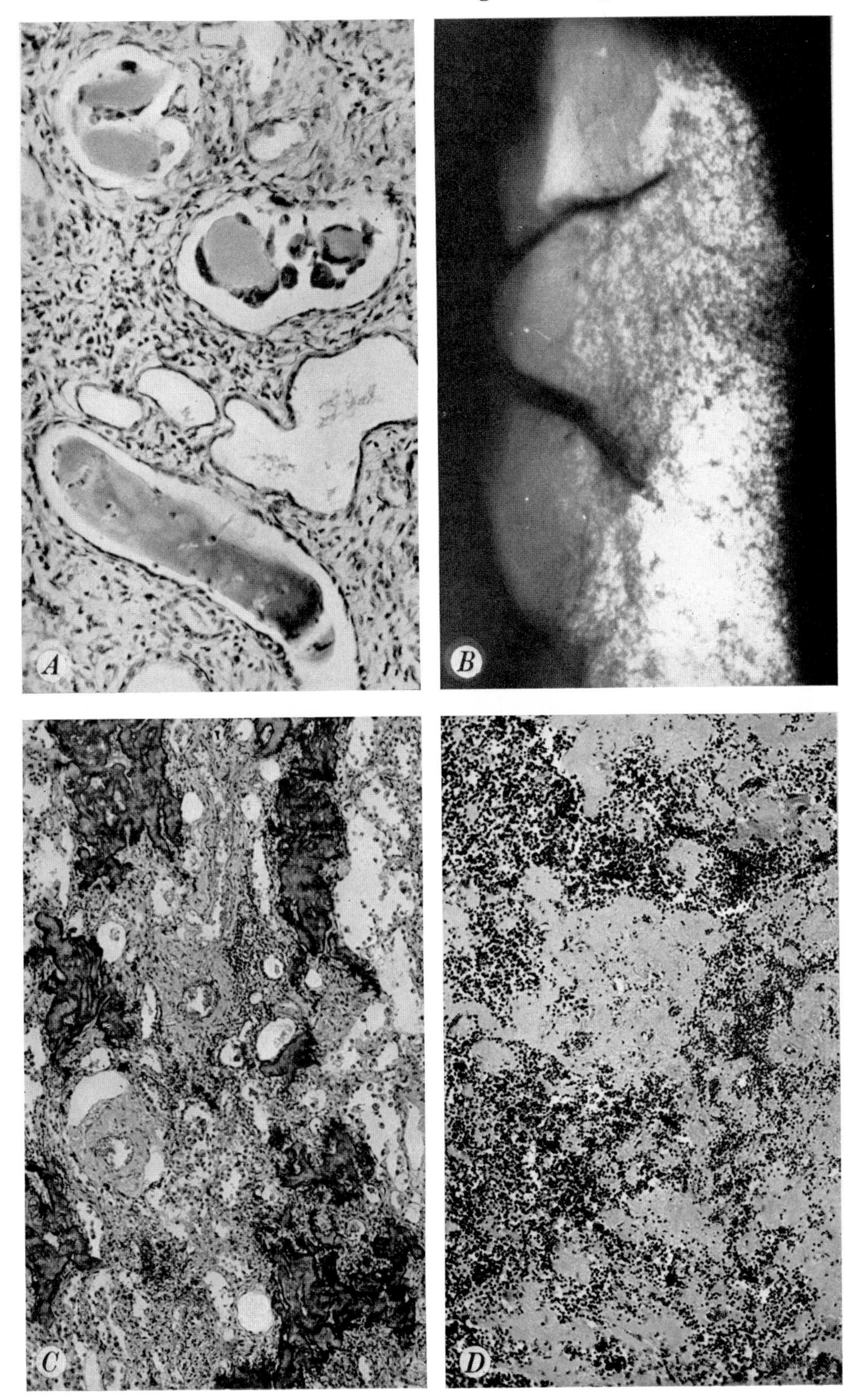


*Figure 123*

detectable only microscopically in the myelomatous tumor tissue. Indeed, in one autopsied case studied by the writer, the little amyloid present was still mainly confined within individual myeloma cells. Again, there are cases in which, in addition to a sprinkling of amyloid through the myelomatous tissue, one finds some grossly visible amyloid tumor masses in affected bones (Fig. 123-*D*). Freund described a case in point in which there were several large amyloid tumor masses, some of which had even broken out of the confines of the bone, so that amyloid and tumor tissue had spread to neighboring soft parts.

More rarely, one observes a case in which deposition of amyloid in relation to the myelomatous bone lesions is associated with large amyloid tumor masses in the soft parts. Some of these masses may be in the muscles and connective tissues overlying the bones and joints, and some may even be remote from the skeleton, perhaps appearing as large intra-abdominal masses. In one such case which the writer had an opportunity of reviewing, some of the extra-osseous amyloid tumor masses also contained myeloma tumor cells.

Finally there are the cases, again rare, in which the amyloid deposition is essentially extraskeletal and there is little or no amyloid in the myelomatous tumor tissue in the bones (see Paige, and Tarr and Ferris). The present writer has observed a case of this kind, also. In that case there was extensive amyloid infiltration of the tongue, mucous membranes, subcutaneous tissues, and muscles, and also of certain of the internal organs, including the lungs, but not of the myelomatous tissue in the bones. In fact, the presence of myelomatosis in this case was not suspected until certain of the bones had been subjected to gross and microscopic examination. Also, the spleen, liver, and kidneys were not at all affected. In some such cases, these organs do show a little amyloid. These cases of myelomatosis (multiple or diffuse) in which the amyloid deposition is essentially extraskeletal may raise the problem of differential diagnosis from so-called primary (or idiopathic) systemic amyloidosis (see Iverson and Morrison). In this connection, before accepting any supposed instance of the latter condition, one should take pains to rule out the presence of clinically occult myeloma.

The gross amyloid tumor masses seen in cases of myelomatosis are usually firm, and, when cut, have a grayish yellow or pinkish color, and the sheen and consistency of fish flesh. Microscopically, the amyloid appears as amorphous, poorly cellular, eosinophilic aggregates. Many of these may be found surrounded by smaller or larger numbers of foreign-body giant cells. Some of the amyloid material may even be somewhat calcified. It is noteworthy also that the amyloid shows some peculiarity in that it may fail to give the usual metachromatic staining reactions with one or another, or perhaps all, of the dyes commonly employed for the detection of amyloid appearing in cases of chronic infection. On this account, the term "paraamyloid" is sometimes used for the amyloid-like substance encountered in some cases of myelomatosis and in the cases of so-called primary (or idiopathic) systemic amyloidosis.

## DIFFERENTIAL DIAGNOSIS

The diagnosis of myelomatosis strongly suggests itself if, in an elderly person many bones, including those of the calvarium, are found to present osteolytic defects on *x*-ray examination. However, practically identical *x*-ray pictures may be seen in cases of carcinoma widely metastatic to the bones. In particular, the roentgenographic differential diagnosis creates a problem in those cases of osteolytic carcinoma metastasis in which the primary lesion is clinically occult.

Be that as it may, current cases of myelomatosis do not usually present numerous osteolytic defects at the time when they first come up for diagnosis. Indeed, one often observes merely some vaguely defined rarefactions in a few bones, or a large osteolytic defect in a single bone. Also, sometimes (when myelomatous infiltration of the bone marrow is diffuse) skeletal changes may not be apparent at all roentgenographically, in spite of general complaints referable to the bones. In such equivocal or initially obscure cases, the lead may come from the discovery of anemia, hypercalcemia, hyperglobulinemia, and/or evidence of renal insufficiency.

It must be recognized, however, that these pertinent findings are not all present in every case or necessarily present in the early stages of evolution in any given case; nor are they necessarily pathognomonic in themselves. Hypercalcemia occurs characteristically with hyperparathyroidism and occasionally with osteolytic (osteoclastic) carcinoma extensively metastatic to the skeleton. However, hypercalcemia associated with hyperglobulinemia and/or Bence Jones proteinuria is clearly indicative of myelomatosis. On the other hand, hyperglobulinemia *per se* (that is, in the absence of skeletal roentgenographic changes and/or hypercalcemia) is also not necessarily indicative of myelomatosis. It is known to occur with other conditions, too, and particularly with chronic infections (notably lymphogranuloma venereum and sarcoidosis) and occasionally with cirrhosis of the liver, chronic nephritis, rheumatoid arthritis, lupus erythematosus, and viral hepatitis.

The most reliable guide for the diagnosis of myelomatosis in any stage of the disease is the finding of myeloma cells in the sternal marrow puncture smears. Indeed, the use of sternal marrow puncture smears often leads to the discovery of the disease when the clinical findings are nondescript and when skeletal roentgenographic changes are either equivocal or absent. Certainly no large osteolytic bone lesion in an elderly person should be subjected to an open biopsy unless sternal marrow puncture smears have been found negative for myeloma cells and such cells could not be demonstrated from smears made from a needle biopsy of the lesion, if the latter is in an accessible site. It is true that if the myelomatous involvement is localized to one skeletal area, the results of the sternal marrow smear may be negative. However, the involvement of the marrow sooner or later becomes widespread, although this dissemination may not yet be represented by the presence of additional osteolytic areas in the *x*-ray picture.

Open biopsy is indicated when the results of the sternal marrow puncture smear are negative. Biopsy of some obviously affected and readily accessible bone site will usually resolve any possible doubt as to the diagnosis, since the histologic recognition of myeloma ordinarily entails no difficult problems in differential diagnosis. However, once in a while there is diagnostic difficulty even under these circumstances, because the myeloma cells fail to present their characteristic histologic appearance. This happens when the tissue submitted for examination has been traumatized or when processing of the tissue has produced shrinkage of the cells or introduced staining artifacts.

## TREATMENT

Treatment of myelomatosis consists mainly of general supportive measures, measures to relieve distressing bone pain, and the handling of such complications as fractures and pressure upon the spinal cord. Among the more important general supportive measures are the use of repeated transfusions to combat anemia, and encouragement of an ambulatory state (rather than bed rest) as much as possible.

The feeling about roentgen therapy for the disease is not so enthusiastic as it was at one time. Certainly the myelomatous tissue is not very radiosensitive, and the irradiated lesions do not tend to heal in. When the skeletal involvement is widespread, irradiation, even of multiple affected sites, does not seem to prolong life, and indeed may even shorten it if the treatment is too intense. However, it is worth trying for relief of pain when one is dealing with a destructive lesion in a strategic area (such as the vertebral column), or with a large painful lesion elsewhere. Irradiation is probably most useful when a single painful lesion is still the only one from which the patient is obviously suffering.

Drugs recently used in the treatment of myelomatosis include radioactive isotopes, nitrogen mustard, urethane, ACTH, and cortisone. These have been used singly or sometimes in various combinations. All of these agents have been found of value in the relief of pain in a certain percentage of the cases in which they have been given.

The drug currently most favored is urethane. Some workers have reported relief of pain in as many as half of the patients by this drug. The relief of pain is temporary, so that repeated courses of treatment are necessary. However, some patients do not tolerate urethane well, and some exhibit actual toxic reactions even if the drug is used in moderation. In a small percentage of cases, treatment with urethane has been found not only to relieve pain, but actually to be associated with a reduction in the serum globulin level and occasionally even with a reduction in the radiolucency of some of the bone lesions. While it seems likely that, in some cases, urethane delays the fatal outcome of the disease, at least for some months, there are other cases in which it seems even to have shortened life expectancy. Altogether, urethane and the other drugs mentioned have not shown themselves to be more than palliative in the management of the disease.

Fractures, especially of long bones, may, of course, call for surgical measures. These also have a place in the relief of neurological complaints arising from pressure against the spinal cord, for which laminectomy is indicated. It is advised that laminectomy be followed by roentgen therapy. In an occasional case of ostensibly solitary myeloma of a long bone, amputation has been carried out. (For further details relating to the problem of solitary myeloma, see p. 379.)

## REFERENCES

Adams, W. S., Alling, E. L., and Lawrence, J. S.: Multiple Myeloma: Its Clinical and Laboratory Diagnosis with Emphasis on Electrophoretic Abnormalities, Am. J. Med., *6*, 141, 1949,

Bayrd, E. D.: The Bone Marrow on Sternal Aspiration in Multiple Myeloma, Blood, *3*, 987. 1948.

Bell, E. T.: Renal Lesions Associated with Multiple Myeloma, Am. J. Path., *9*, 393, 1933.

Carson, C. P., Ackerman, L. V., and Maltby, J. D.: Plasma Cell Myeloma. A Clinical, Pathologic and Roentgenologic Review of 90 Cases, Am. J. Clin. Path., *25*, 849, 1955.

Christopherson, W. M., and Miller, A. J.: A Re-evaluation of Solitary Plasma-Cell Myeloma of Bone, Cancer, *3*, 240, 1950.

Churg, J., and Gordon, A. J.: Multiple Myeloma with Unusual Visceral Involvement, Arch. Path., *34*, 546, 1942.

Dahlin, D. C., and Dockerty, M. B.: Amyloid and Myeloma, Am. J. Path., *26*, 581, 1950.

Forbus, W. D., Perlzweig, W. A., Parfentjev, I. A., and Burwell, J. C., Jr.: Bence-Jones Protein Excretion and its Effects upon the Kidney, Bull. Johns Hopkins Hosp., *57*, 47, 1935.

Freund, E.: Über diffuses Myelom mit Amyloidtumoren, Frankfurt. Ztschr. f. Path., *40*, 400, 1930.

Froboese, C.: Ein neuer Fall von multiplem Myelom (Erythroblastom) mit Kalkmetastasen in Lungen, Nieren und der Uterusschleimhaut, Virchows Arch. f. path. Anat., *222*, 291, 1916.

Gordon, H., and Schneider, B.: Plasma-Cell Myeloma in a Child, Internat. Clin., *4*, 173, 1940.

Gutman, A. B.: Tumors of the Skeletal System: Medical Aspects, Bull. New York Acad. Med., *23*, 512, 1947.

Harrington, W. J., and Moloney, W. C.: The Treatment of Multiple Myeloma with Urethane, Cancer, *3*, 253, 1950.

Hellwig, C. A.: Extramedullary Plasma Cell Tumors as Observed in Various Locations, Arch. Path., *36*, 95, 1943.

Innes, J., and Rider, W. D.: Multiple Myelomatosis Treated with a Combination of Urethane and an Oral Nitrogen Mustard, Blood, *10*, 252, 1955.

Iverson, L., and Morrison, A. B.: Primary Systemic Amyloidosis, Arch. Path., *45*, 1, 1948.

Jackson, H., Jr., Parker, F., Jr., and Bethea, J. M.: Studies of Diseases of the Lymphoid and Myeloid Tissues. II. Plasmatocytomata and Their Relation to Multiple Myelomata, Am. J. M. Sc., *181*, 169, 1931.

Jaffe, H. L.: Tumors of the Skeletal System: Pathological Aspects, Bull. New York Acad. Med., *23*, 497, 1947. (See p. 507.)

Jaffe, H. L., and Bodansky, A.: Serum Calcium: Clinical and Biochemical Considerations, J. Mt. Sinai Hosp., *9*, 901, 1943; *and:* Diagnostic Significance of Serum Alkaline and Acid Phosphatase Values in Relation to Bone Disease, Bull. New York Acad. Med., *19*, 831, 1943.

Kobernick, S. D., and Whiteside, J. H.: Renal Glomeruli in Multiple Myeloma, Lab. Invest., *6*, 478, 1957.

Korngold, L., and Lipari, R.: Multiple-Myeloma Proteins. III. The Antigenic Relationship of Bence Jones Proteins to Normal Gamma-Globulin and Multiple-Myeloma Serum Proteins, Cancer, *9*, 262, 1956.

Lawrence, J. H., and Wasserman, L. R.: Multiple Myeloma: A Study of 24 Patients Treated with Radioactive Isotopes ($P^{32}$ and $SR^{89}$), Ann. Int. Med., *33*, 41, 1950.

Lichtenstein, L., and Jaffe, H. L.: Multiple Myeloma: A Survey Based on Thirty-five Cases, Eighteen of Which Came to Autopsy, Arch. Path., *44*, 207, 1947.

Loge, J. P., and Rundles, R. W.: Urethane (Ethyl Carbamate) Therapy in Multiple Myeloma, Blood, *4*, 201, 1949.

Löhlein, M.: Eiweisskristalle in den Harnkanälchen bei multiplem Myelom, Beitr. z. path. Anat. u. z. allg. Path., *69*, 295, 1921.

Lowenhaupt, E.: Proliferative Lesions in Multiple Myeloma with Special Reference to Those of the Spleen. The Origin of the Plasma Cell, Am. J. Path., *21*, 171, 1945.

Lumb, G.: Solitary Plasmocytoma of Bone with Renal Changes, Brit. J. Surg., *36*, 16, 1948.

Luttgens, W. F., and Bayrd, E. D.: Treatment of Multiple Myeloma with Urethan: Experience with Sixty-six Cases over a Two-and-a-half-year Period, J.A.M.A., *147*, 824, 1951.

Magnus-Levy, A.: Bence-Jones-Eiweiss und Amyloid, Ztschr. f. klin. Med., *116*, 510, 1931; *and:* Multiple Myelome: VII Euglobulinämie. Zur Klinik und Pathologie. Amyloidosis, Ztschr. f. klin. Med., *126*, 62, 1933.

Mallory, T. B.: Case Records of the Massachusetts General Hospital (Case 25511. Plasma-cell Myeloma, Diffuse; Myeloma Kidneys), New England J. Med., *221*, 983, 1939.

Meacham, G. C.: Plasma Cell Myeloma, Ann. Int. Med., *38*, 1035, 1953.

Muller, G. L., and McNaughton, E.: Multiple Myeloma (Plasmatocytomata) with Blood Picture of Plasma Cell Leukemia, Folia haemat., *46*, 17, 1931.

Nelson, M. G., and Lyons, A. R.: Plasmacytoma of Lymph Glands, Cancer, *10*, 1275, 1957.

Newns, G. R., and Edwards, J. L.: A Case of Plasma-cell Myelomatosis with a Large Renal Metastasis and Widespread Renal Tubular Obstruction, J. Path & Bact., *56*, 259, 1944.

von Numers, C.: Cytological Studies on Plasma Cell Myeloma, Acta path. et microbiol. scandinav., *33*, 240, 1953.

Oliver, J.: New Directions in Renal Morphology: A Method, Its Results and Its Future, Harvey Lect., *40*, 102, 1944–1945.

Osserman, E. F., and Lawlor, D. P.: Abnormal Serum and Urine Proteins in Thirty-five Cases of Multiple Myeloma, as Studied by Filter Paper Electrophoresis, Am. J. Med., *18*, 462, 1955.

Paige, B. H.: A Case of Myeloma with Unusual Amyloid Deposition, Am. J. Path., *7*, 691, 1931.

Patek, A. J., Jr., and Castle, W. B.: Plasma Cell Leukemia, Am. J. M. Sc., *191*, 788, 1936.

Perla, D., and Hutner, L.: Nephrosis in Multiple Myeloma, Am. J. Path., *6*, 285, 1930.

Piney, A., and Riach, J. S.: Multiple myeloma. Aleukaemic and Leukaemic, Folia haemat., *46*, 37, 1931.

Putnam, F. W., and Hardy, S.: Proteins in Multiple Myeloma. III. Origin of Bence-Jones Protein, J. Biol. Chem., *212*, 361, 1955.

Raven, R. W., and Willis, R. A.: Solitary Plasmocytoma of the Spine, J. Bone & Joint Surg., *31-B*, 369, 1949.

Rubinstein, M. A.: Multiple Myeloma as a Form of Leukemia, Blood, *4*, 1049, 1949.

Rundles, R. W., Dillon, M. L., and Dillon, E. S.: Multiple Myeloma. III. Effect of Urethane Therapy on Plasma Cell Growth, Abnormal Serum Protein Components and Bence Jones Proteinuria, J. Clin. Investigation, *29*, 1243, 1950.

Rutishauser, E.: Zur Frage der solitären Myelome, Centralbl. f. allg. Path. u. path. Anat., *58*, 355, 1933.

Schmaus, K. A.: Multiples Myelom (Plasmocytom) bei einem Jugendlichen, Chirurg, *21*, 48, 1950.

Stewart, M. J., and Taylor, A. L.: Observations on Solitary Plasmocytoma, J. Path. & Bact., *35*, 541, 1932.

Tarr, L., and Ferris, H. W.: Multiple Myeloma Associated with Nodular Deposits of Amyloid in the Muscles and Joints and with Bence Jones Proteinuria, Arch. Int. Med., *64*, 820, 1939.

Wallgren, A.: *Untersuchungen über die Myelomkrankheit*, Uppsala, Almqvist & Wiksells, 1920.

Wintrobe, M. M.: *Clinical Hematology*, 4th ed., Philadelphia, Lea & Febiger, 1956. (See p. 1072.)

# Chapter 24

# Leukemia and Lymphoma

THIS chapter is concerned mainly with the *skeletal manifestations* of the leukemias and the lymphomas. As to the *leukemias*, it is mainly in connection with acute leukemia in children that skeletal manifestations are prominent. The affected children often have complaints referable to the bones and/or joints, and conspicuous changes are often found in the *x*-ray pictures of the skeleton. Indeed, it is complaints due to skeletal changes that not infrequently lead to the discovery that the child is suffering from leukemia. In adults affected with leukemia, skeletal manifestations occur mainly in the chronic cases and are not very common even in these.

In connection with the *generalized malignant lymphomas*, it is not unusual for the patient to complain, in the course of his disease, of pain referable to one or another bone area and to present corresponding destructive skeletal changes visible roentgenographically. In fact, in an occasional case it may even be pain due to such a lesion that leads to the discovery of the basic lymph node involvement. Among the generalized lymphomas, it is in Hodgkin's disease that destructive skeletal changes are most commonly encountered. They are also fairly common in connection with lymphosarcoma, especially if the latter has become widely disseminated through the bone marrow and the clinical picture has gone over into that of a chronic lymphatic leukemia.

Finally, this chapter deals with the rather complex and by no means fully clarified subject of *lymphoma primary in bone*. In this connection the discussion centers mainly around the so-called "primary reticulum cell sarcoma of bone." Because of certain overlapping histologic appearances, the differentiation of primary reticulum cell sarcoma of bone from Ewing's sarcoma often presents a problem. However, accumulating experience with both conditions has tended to accentuate the differences between them. This experience is establishing more and more firmly the idea, first developed by Parker and Jackson, that primary reticulum cell sarcoma of bone does represent a distinct bone tumor entity which belongs among the lymphomas and should not be confused with Ewing's sarcoma (p. 350).

## LEUKEMIA

Leukemia is a cancerous disease which takes its departure in the bone marrow and runs a fatal course. It is characterized by tumorous proliferation of one or another type of the white blood cells. The leukemic tumor cells come to crowd out and substantially replace the red marrow and even the fatty marrow of the bones, and often appear in large numbers in the circulating blood. They also accumulate in the lymph nodes and notably in the spleen, liver, and kidneys, but, in one case or another, may also be found in almost any other body structure.

The recent increase in the incidence of leukemia in man has become a matter of medical concern. It has been estimated that the death rate from leukemia in the United States has risen from 14 to 61 per million population during the period from 1921 to 1951 (see Shimkin). It is true that most of the current cases represent instances of so-called "spontaneous" leukemia. On the other hand, it is well established that exposure to ionizing radiation can induce leukemia. Thus, an especially high incidence of the disease has been demonstrated in respect to radiologists, persons treated with *x*-rays for ankylosing spondylitis or thymic enlargement, and particularly among survivors of atomic bomb explosions. In regard to the radiation from natural "background" sources to which man is constantly exposed, it seems probable that this may even be a small factor in the incidence of so-called "spontaneous" leukemia. Furthermore, there seem to be indications that even small increases in the amount of "background" radiation, if persistent, will raise this incidence. In this connection, Lewis estimates that if, on account of increasing pollution of the air, the population were to reach and maintain a body level of strontium 90 amounting to one-tenth of the maximum permissible concentration, one could expect an increase of 5 to 10 per cent in the incidence of "spontaneous" leukemia. For an adult, the maximum permissible concentration of $Sr^{90}$ in the skeleton has been estimated at 1 microcurie.

Cytologically, the leukemias fall into two general groups—the myelogenous (myeloid) and the lymphatic. However, one encounters instances in which it is difficult to decide to which of these two categories the case belongs. In the myelogenous leukemias the tumor cells are related to the cells of the bone marrow, and in the lymphatic leukemias to the cells of the lymphoid tissue. The categories of myeloid and lymphatic leukemia are further subclassified into the myelocytic, myeloblastic, lymphocytic, lymphoblastic, and others on the basis of the particular type of cell predominating. The so-called monocytic leukemia probably represents a form of myeloid leukemia.

In any of the varieties of leukemia, the clinical course may be acute or chronic. On the whole, those myelogenous or lymphatic leukemias in which immature or "blast" cells dominate tend to run an acute course. The cases of leukemia which are considered acute are those in which the period of survival is a year or less from the time of onset of symptoms. However, without treatment, many patients with acute leukemia fail to survive for more than a few weeks, and a large proportion of patients are dead within a few months in any event.

As to the leukocyte count in the peripheral blood in cases of leukemia, it is to be noted that this may range from less than 5,000 per cu. mm. to more than 100,000. When the count is 5,000 or less, the case is usually classed as one of "aleukemic" leukemia.

Leukemia is observed somewhat more frequently in males than in females. The age range of the patients is wide, extending from early infancy into advanced age. Infants a few weeks old are sometimes already found affected, and there are even reports of cases of congenital leukemia. A large proportion of the patients are young children, and in them the leukemia usually runs an acute course and is more often of the lymphatic (and specifically the lymphoblastic) than of the myeloid type. Also, leukemia in children is not infrequently associated with an "aleukemic" peripheral blood picture. In subjects who have reached adult life, the leukemia is somewhat more likely to be of the myeloid than of the lymphatic variety, and the disease more often runs a chronic course. The latter is in accordance with the fact that, in adults, the leukemic cells are more frequently of the mature type, the leukemia being of the myelocytic or lymphocytic variety. However, among the oldest subjects taken by themselves, the lymphatic form of leukemia comes to predominate over the myeloid form.

Acute leukemia ordinarily sets in with manifestations simulating acute infection. Pallor, weakness, and other evidences of severe anemia may soon become apparent. Inflammatory or even gangrenous lesions may be noted in the oral mucosa. In addition, the latter may show evidence of hemorrhage, and this may also be manifested in the skin, in the form of a purpuric eruption. The spleen and superficial lymph nodes may be found enlarged but are by no means regularly so in the earlier stages of the disease. Study of the blood is likely to show thrombocytopenia, and the white cell count is rather likely to be between 15,000 and 30,000, though it may be much lower or much higher. The differential count is very often abnormal, and the smears tend strongly to show many "blast" cells of one kind or another. In the presence of such clinical and hematologic findings, the recognition that the patient is suffering from leukemia is easy.

On the other hand, in some cases of acute leukemia, especially in children, the nature of the underlying disease may not be apparent at first or perhaps for some time, because neither the clinical nor the hematologic manifestations are characteristic. In such cases the diagnostic difficulties may be enhanced by the fact that the child's presenting complaints relate mainly to the skeleton. There may be pains in various bones and in joints, and even swelling of joint regions. Such complaints may make one think, certainly at first, that one is dealing with a case of acute pyogenic osteomyelitis, scurvy, or even rheumatic fever rather than with leukemia. However, in adults suffering from acute leukemia, skeletal complaints are only rarely among the presenting manifestations.

Chronic leukemia is insidious in its onset. The clinical manifestations include weakness and other indications of anemia, and enlargement of lymph nodes and/or the spleen. Complaints referable to the skeleton are not common, and at any rate a relatively late manifestation. Patients with obvious chronic leukemia, whether of the lymphocytic or myelocytic type, have an average survival period of about 3 years. A shorter survival period is not unusual, and, on the other hand, a survival period extending beyond 5 years is not at all rare, especially with lymphocytic leukemia.

## SKELETAL MANIFESTATIONS OF LEUKEMIA IN CHILDREN

As noted, a child suffering from leukemia often complains of pain and tenderness in various long bones, and/or migratory pains in joints and even swelling of joint regions. Indeed, one may fail to think of leukemia in such a case if the leukemia is of the "aleukemic" type and if other characteristic clinical manifestations of leukemia are lacking. The finding of roentgenographic changes in the bones may put one on the track of the correct diagnosis in such a case. It will at least rule out rheumatic fever and rheumatoid arthritis of childhood (Still's disease), which are among the conditions sometimes simulated by leukemia in children when the presenting complaints relate to bones and joints. Furthermore, it may well lead to investigation of the sternal marrow with the aid of puncture smears, which will almost certainly disclose the presence of the leukemia. This procedure is, of course, of diagnostic value even if the spleen is not yet enlarged, lymph nodes are not palpable, and the peripheral blood findings are not decisive either.

In any representative group of leukemic children, at least 50 to 60 per cent can be expected to show bone changes of some kind roentgenographically (see Fig. 124). An aberration very often to be noted is the presence of a narrow transverse zone of increased radiolucency at the shaft ends of long bones. This is apparently the earliest and mildest change. It tends to appear first at those epiphysial-diaphysial junctions of long bones where endochondral bone growth is most active. Thus, if present at all, such zones, which may be only a few millimeters wide at first, are most likely to be found in the knee area. Sooner or later, however, the shaft ends of other long bones will probably reveal them too (see Baty and Vogt, Snelling and Brown, and Silverman).

These juxta-epiphysial radiolucent zones apparently have their pathologic basis:

(1) in a depression of endochondral bone formation at the sites in question, which is a natural accompaniment of the general illness of the child, and (2) in the fact that the resorptive pressure effect of the leukemic tumor tissue in the marrow spaces at these sites is being exerted upon particularly labile osseous trabeculæ (see Erb, and Follis and Park). These zones may disappear if the leukemia undergoes remission, either spontaneously or in consequence of therapy. At any rate, it is to be noted that juxta-epiphysial radiolucent zones are not pathognomonic for leukemia. Indeed, they are observed almost regularly in scurvy, where they represent, in terms of pathology, the scorbutic zone of detritus. Also, somewhat analogous zones are occasionally observed in children affected with severe illness of some other kind, where they again represent the effects of disturbed endochondral bone growth.

As the leukemic infiltration of the marrow becomes more pronounced, the metaphysial ends of many of the long bones are likely to appear rather strikingly rarefied as a whole, so that the original transverse radiolucent zones no longer stand out as such. Furthermore, in consequence of focal erosion of the cortex by tumor tissue, the ends of long bones in particular may show numerous small, roundish radiolucencies (see Fig. 125). In some cases the calvarium and even the bones of the hands and feet likewise come to show generalized rarefaction, along with small focal punched-out radiolucencies.

In other cases, however, the bones of a leukemic child may already show, even in the first roentgenographs, large areas of lytic destruction reminding one of those produced by skeletal metastases in cases of neuroblastoma in childhood. However, in neuroblastoma metastatic to bone (as in metastatic cancer in general), the roentgenographic evidence of skeletal involvement, even if widespread, is not likely to include involvement of bones below the knees and below the elbows. In leukemia, on the other hand, if there is such severe involvement of the skeleton, these more distal bones of the extremities are often also found affected. Furthermore, in a case in which the bones are severely involved, one or another long bone may be the site of a pathologic fracture, and one or several affected vertebræ may even undergo compressional collapse.

Another common skeletal manifestation of leukemia in children is periosteal new bone deposition. Occasionally a child may be admitted because of pain relating to a long bone, associated with some fever and with *x*-ray changes in the bone in question which are highly suggestive of an acute osteomyelitis. That is, much of the bone shaft may show mottled rarefaction, and much new bone may be found deposited on the bone cortex. The deposition represents a reaction of the periosteum to irritation and lifting of it by the leukemic tissue. The latter reaches the periosteum mainly by way of the haversian canals, many of which become widened and broken through as the tumor tissue spreads along them. In fact, while, during life, evidence of periosteal new bone deposition may have been noted only on one or a few long bone shafts, microscopic study of bones removed at autopsy is likely to show that ribs and even other bones which seemed unaffected clinically are also the site of various amounts of periosteal new bone deposition (see Jaffe).

Some children with leukemia show increased radiopacity of bones (osteosclerosis) without evidence of periosteal new bone deposition or radiolucent osteolytic lesions. In all probability, these are children whose primary illness is osteopetrosis (marble bone disease) and in whom leukemia has developed as a terminal phase of that disorder.

**Treatment.**—In connection with the treatment of acute leukemia in children, Farber has established the palliative value of the various folic acid antagonists. In cases of acute lymphatic (lymphoblastic) leukemia in children, remissions can also be induced by ACTH and/or cortisone. In fact, some workers attempt to induce the initial remission with ACTH or cortisone and then maintain the remission with subtoxic doses of the antifolic antagonists, alternating the latter if resistance develops to a given one. In a personal communication to the writer, Farber has stated that through the appropriate use of the various antimetabolites, sometimes in conjunction with ACTH, remissions are induced in 40 to 50 per cent of children

***Figure 124***

*A*, Roentgenograph showing narrow transverse zones of increased radiolucency at the shaft ends of the long bones in the knee region of a child suffering from acute lymphatic leukemia. Note that beyond the transverse zones the bone shafts show evidence of mottled porosity. The patient was a boy 3 years of age whose illness was of 3 months' standing at the time of admission to the hospital. At that time he presented a severe anemia, a low white blood cell count with "blast" cells in the smears, and evidence of leukemic infiltration of the bone marrow as revealed by sternal marrow puncture smears. Generalized lymphadenopathy and enlargement of the liver and spleen were also manifest. The child died 7 months after the onset of his illness and came to autopsy. (See also Fig. 125.)

*B*, Roentgenograph of the knee area of a child affected with acute lymphatic leukemia who had been under treatment with cortisone and the antifolic antagonists for about 4½ months at the time when this picture was taken. Note the zones of increased radiopacity where zones of increased radiolucency had been present before treatment. Note also that the osseous structure in general now shows no abnormalities. The child was a boy 6 years of age who was admitted because of pain in the left arm and fever. On account of these complaints and the roentgenographic appearance of the left humerus at that time (*C*), the child was thought to be suffering from an acute osteomyelitis. It soon became evident, however, that the lymph nodes, liver, and spleen were enlarged. Study of the peripheral blood and sternal marrow puncture smears helped to establish the diagnosis of acute leukemia.

*C*, Roentgenograph showing the appearance of the humerus on admission of the patient referred to in *B*. Note the mottled rarefaction of the bone and the evidence of periosteal new bone deposition—appearances which seemed to suggest an acute osteomyelitis. Note also the narrow zone of radiolucency at the upper end of the humeral shaft.

*D*, Roentgenograph indicating the appearance of the humerus illustrated in *C* about 1 month after the child had been treated with cortisone and antifolic antagonists. Observe that while the periosteal reaction is now more striking (actually on account of considerable deposition of new bone), the mottled rarefaction of the humerus as a whole has receded under the therapy, and the radiolucent zone has disappeared. Nevertheless, the child died of his leukemia about 3 months later.

*E*, Roentgenograph showing a large area of osteolysis in the upper end of the shaft of the right femur in a child suffering from lymphatic leukemia. Analogous osteolytic lesions were present at the time of admission in the opposite femur and in the upper ends of both tibial shafts (*F*), and there were numerous osteolytic lesions in the humeri and in the calvarium. The patient was a girl 6 years of age whose complaints were mainly of pain, of 1 month's standing, referred to the lower limbs. There was no obvious lymphadenopathy, and the peripheral blood smears failed to reveal the presence of abnormal cells. One of the tibial lesions was biopsied, and the tissue sections showed small tumor cells with hyperchromatic nuclei. Despite the absence of rosettes, it was thought that the bone lesions probably represented foci of metastasis from a neuroblastoma. The tumor cells were held to be of the sympathogonioma type—cells which are difficult to distinguish from lymphocytes. Five months later, however, the peripheral blood and bone marrow smears showed the presence of "blast" cells, and the diagnosis was revised to leukemia. The child died about 1 year after the onset of her illness, and the case came to autopsy. Widespread leukemic infiltration was found in the bone marrow, and leukemic infiltrations were also noted in the kidneys, spleen, liver, and various lymph nodes.

*F*, Roentgenograph of the upper end of a tibia as it appeared at the time of admission in the case illustrated in *E*.

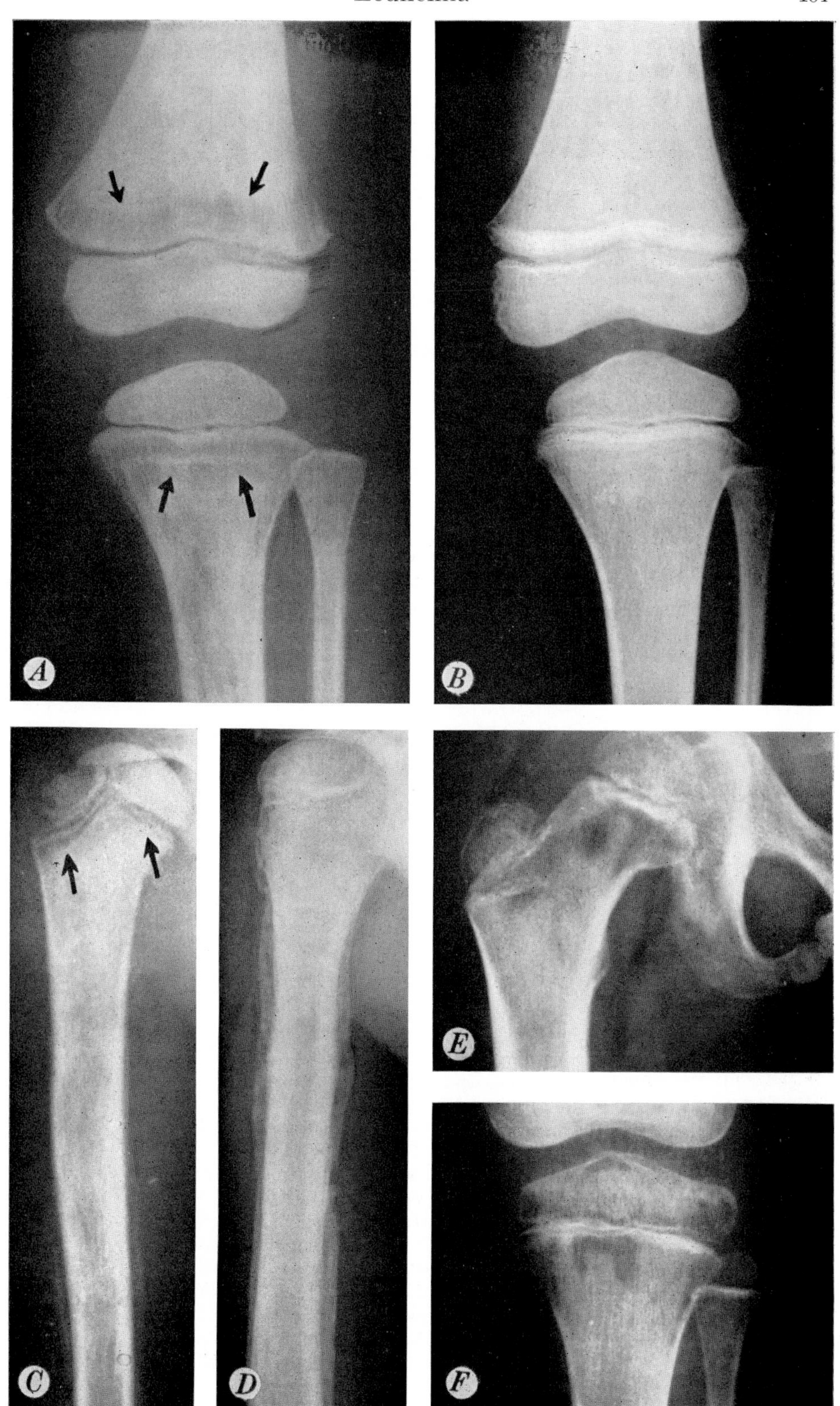

*Figure 124*

affected with acute leukemia. Furthermore, about 50 per cent of the children treated in this way survive for at least a year.

Children so benefited tend to show regression of their skeletal lesions, and the juxta-epiphysial radiolucent zones in particular usually disappear. As Silverman points out, one may now find, instead of them, zones of increased radiopacity. These resemble the radiopaque bands familiar in cases of poisoning of young children by heavy metals. Evidence of cortical destruction and concomitant periostitis may also substantially disappear. However, when the leukemic child becomes refractory to the treatment and enters the terminal phase of the disease, roentgenographs show the reappearance of skeletal lesions.

## SKELETAL MANIFESTATIONS OF LEUKEMIA IN ADULTS

In adults affected with leukemia, the occurrence of roentgenographically detectable skeletal changes is much less common than in children. Indeed, in adults affected with acute leukemia, such changes are nearly always absent, despite the widespread tumorous infiltration of the bone marrow found at autopsy. On the other hand, adults affected with chronic leukemia occasionally do show skeletal changes roentgenographically in the course of their disease (see Fig. 126). However, there can be no doubt that the often stated incidence of 8 to 10 per cent for skeletal changes in leukemia of adults includes many cases of lymphosarcoma in which, more or less terminally, the peripheral blood came to present the picture of lymphocytic leukemia.

Be that as it may, in one case or another of chronic leukemia in an adult, the bones may show rather generalized porosity, often not very pronounced. Also, one or more bones may present areas of discrete or confluent rarefaction, sometimes even alternating with small patches of radiopacity. Some bones may exhibit evidence of periosteal new bone deposition. Fractures, especially of ribs, can sometimes also be visualized.

Anatomic examination of a definitely porotic bone from a leukemic adult reveals that its spongiosa is wide-meshed, the trabeculæ being thin and even lacking in some places. The bone cortex will be found thinned from the medullary side, and its haversian canals enlarged. The leukemic marrow is gray-red on the whole. In places, however, it may be dark red from hemorrhage, or yellowish in consequence of necrosis. Wherever a large patch of the leukemic marrow is necrotic, the osseous

***Figure 125***

*A*, Roentgenograph showing the appearance presented 3 months later by the femur illustrated in Fig. 124-*A*. Note the general porosity of the end of the bone, and the numerous small, punched-out radiolucencies. The anatomic basis for this *x*-ray picture is made clear by *B*, which shows the external appearance of that femur after its removal at autopsy 1 month later.

*B*, Photograph illustrating the posterior surface of the femur shown in *A*. A number of small and discrete roundish defects of the cortex are visible. In addition, immediately above the condylar area of the bone, the cortex as a whole is spongified. Through the innumerable cortical defects, tumor tissue had extended beneath the periosteum.

*C*, Photograph of the femur shown in *B*, after it had been sectioned in the frontal plane. Note the modification of the cortex at the end of the shaft and the wide-meshed appearance of the spongiosa above the epiphysial cartilage plate area.

*D*, Photomicrograph (× 65) illustrating the histologic appearances at the plate area of the femur shown in *C*. Note the lack of active endochondral ossification and the wide spongy marrow spaces. The tumor cells in these enlarged spaces are lymphoblasts.

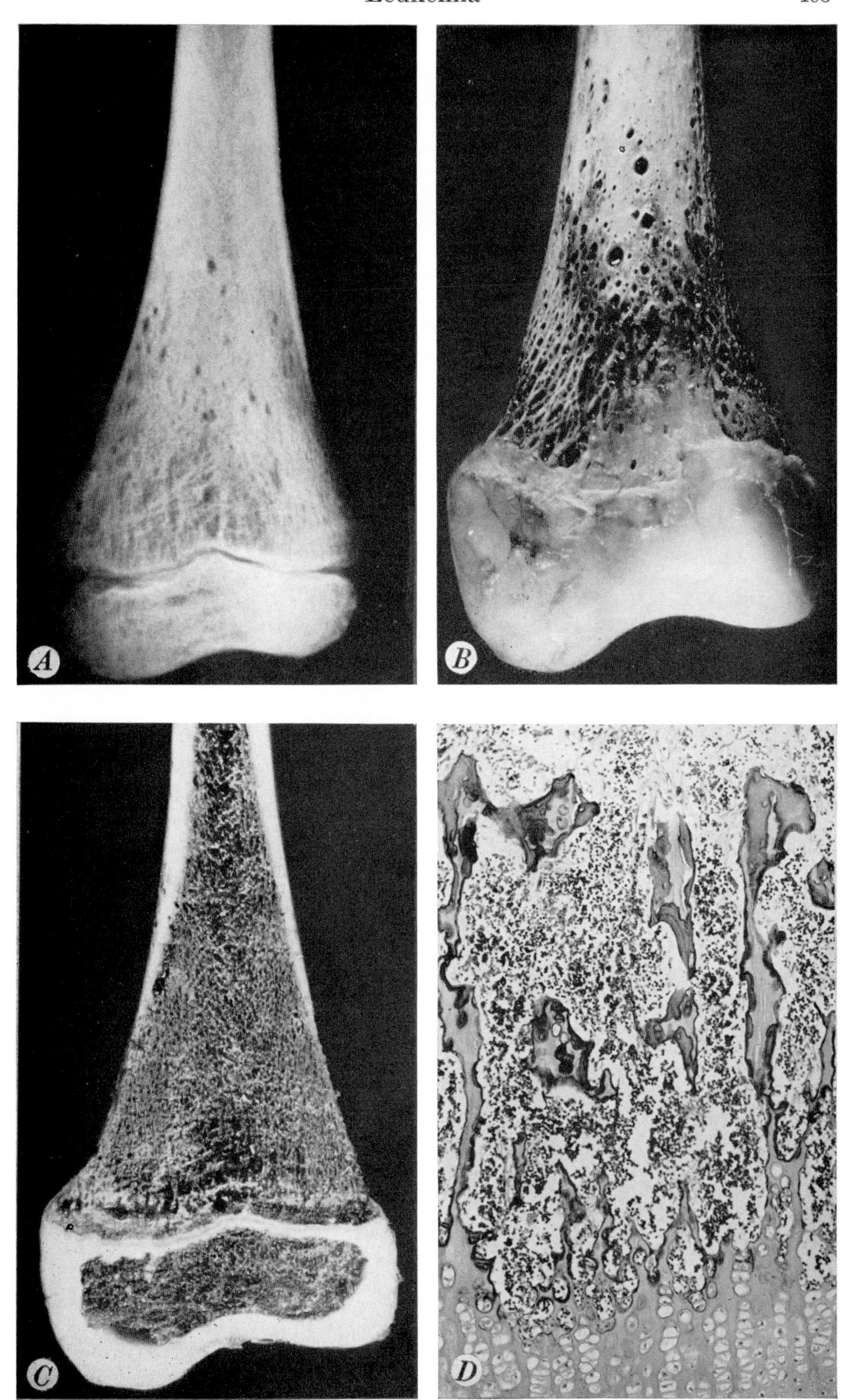


*Figure 125*

trabeculæ within the area will also be found to show necrosis, and the latter sometimes even extends to the overlying cortex (see Apitz).

Roentgenographic examination of the calvarium may have revealed many smaller or larger areas of increased radiolucency. If so, these will be found to correspond to areas in which the osseous tissue has largely disappeared and been replaced by grayish red foci of leukemic tissue. In other bone sites, too, if there has been roentgenographic evidence of osteolysis, the local cortex will be found substantially resorbed. If leukemic tissue has extended beneath the periosteum, new bone deposition is likely to be demonstrable. In sites of pronounced osteolysis, as in areas where the bone is merely uniformly porotic, the bone resorption is due mainly to pressure from the expanding leukemic tissue. In an occasional case, severely porotified vertebral bodies may show compressional collapse. If bones have undergone fracture (as ribs sometimes do), the fracture is more likely to be found in an area which has been the site of necrosis than in one which has been merely porotified. In older necrotic areas, furthermore, one may note evidence of connective-tissue repair and even many trabeculæ of new bone in the area of repair.

Diffuse increased radiopacity (osteosclerosis) of many of the bones is also said to occur in some cases of leukemia in adults. The development of a more or less

***Figure 126***

*A*, Roentgenograph showing collapse of the first and third lumbar vertebral bodies in a case of chronic myelogenous leukemia. The patient was a woman 52 years of age who was first admitted to the hospital on account of pain in the lower part of the back of 5 weeks' standing. Because of her complaints, a skeletal survey was done. The only positive finding at that time was a compression fracture of the fifth lumbar vertebra (not shown), but subsequently the vertebral bodies illustrated also collapsed. Further clinical study of the patient showed an anemia and a very much elevated white blood cell count, associated with the presence of numerous myelocytes in the blood smears. Also, the liver and spleen were found enlarged. Striking demineralization of the vertebral column and/or collapse of vertebral bodies is on the whole unusual in chronic myeloid leukemia of adults. The patient in this case died 2 years after this *x*-ray picture was taken. Autopsy revealed findings classical for chronic myelogenous leukemia insofar as the spleen, liver, and lymph nodes were concerned. In regard to the skeleton, it showed that, in addition to collapse of the first, third and fifth lumbar vertebræ (due to leukemic infiltration), there was widespread leukemic infiltration of the marrow of numerous other bones removed and opened.

*B*, Roentgenograph of the hip area in a woman 48 years of age who had been suffering from generalized lymphosarcoma and who eventually came to present the peripheral blood picture of chronic lymphocytic leukemia. Note the pathologic fracture through the large area of lytic destruction in the upper part of the femoral shaft. In chronic lymphatic leukemia, areas of lytic bone destruction appear most frequently when the leukemia develops as a terminal phase in the clinical evolution of a lymphosarcoma.

*C*, Photograph of the upper part of a femur, cut in the sagittal plane, from a case of chronic myeloid leukemia. The patient was a man 63 years of age who presented lymphadenopathy and splenomegaly, but a rather low peripheral white blood cell count. However, a small number of abnormal cells were present in the peripheral blood smears. None of the bones removed at autopsy showed any alteration in contour. Nevertheless, when cut open, all bones removed showed evidence of infiltration of the marrow by the tumor tissue. Note that in the femur illustrated, the major marrow cavity is occupied by the leukemic tumor tissue, as are the spongy marrow spaces in the trochanteric areas. The marrow spaces of the spongiosa of the head of the bone are not heavily infiltrated by tumor tissue.

*D*, Photomicrograph (× 65) showing, in cross section, an area of the cortex of the femur illustrated in *C*. Note that the haversian canals are somewhat enlarged and crowded with the tumor cells. The surface of the cortex shows a small deposit of subperiosteal new bone. This represents a reaction to the spread of the tumor cells beneath the periosteum by way of the haversian canals.

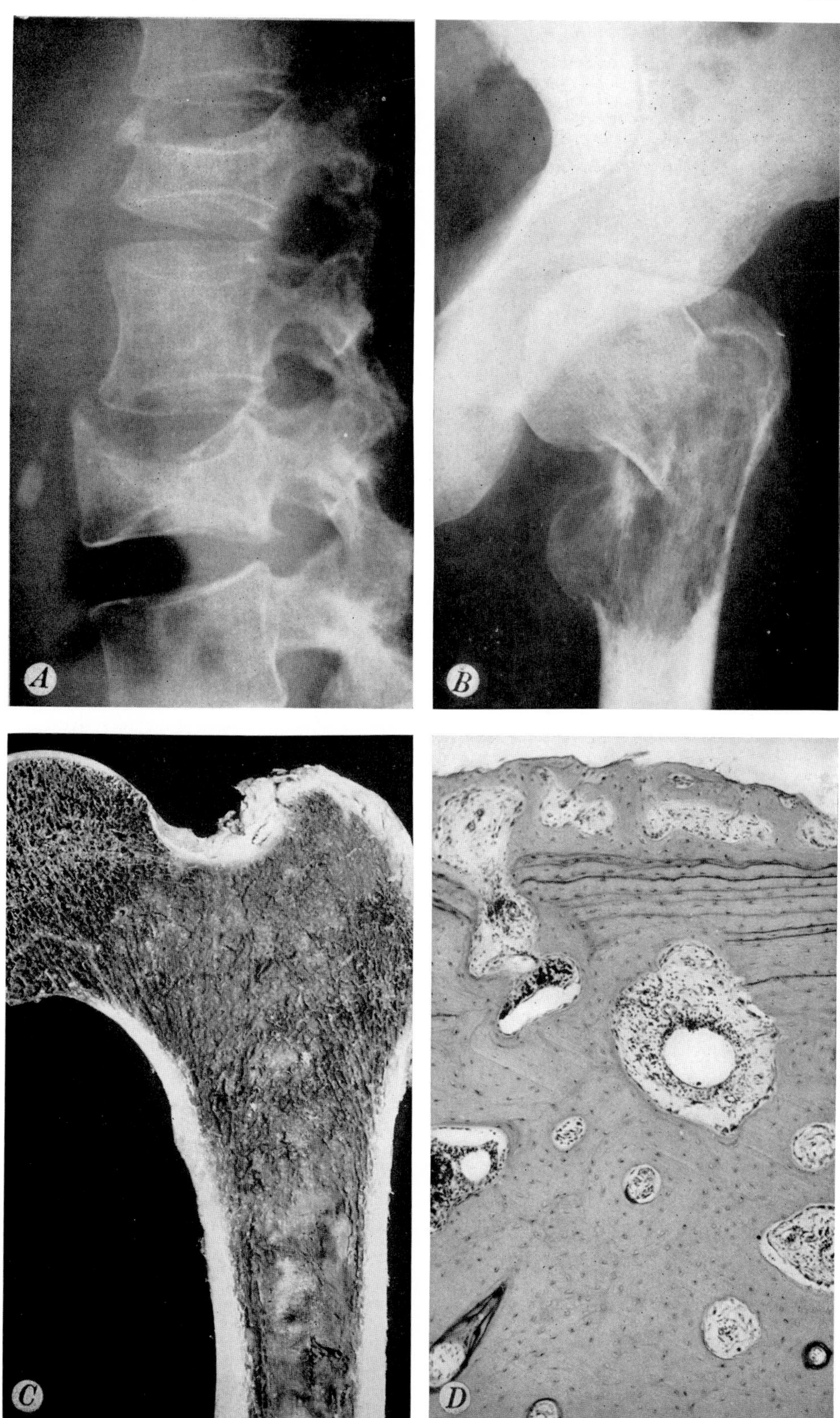


*Figure 126*

generalized osteosclerosis, not attributable to radiation, in a case starting as one of leukemia can safely be regarded as rare. Indeed, the likelihood is that most cases of widespread osteosclerosis in which the sclerosis is regarded as having been engrafted on a leukemia really represent instances of "myelosclerotic anemia" with a pronounced terminal leukemoid picture (see Sussman, and Wyatt and Sommers).

**Treatment.**—In the treatment of chronic leukemia, the antifolic antagonists now known seem to be contraindicated. The chemotherapeutic agents of value in chronic lymphocytic leukemia are the mustard congeners. For chronic myelocytic leukemia, myleran and urethane have been found useful. In both chronic lymphocytic and chronic myelocytic leukemia, radiation therapy is also indicated (see Wintrobe *et al.*).

## GENERALIZED MALIGNANT LYMPHOMA

The various primary cancerous conditions arising in lymph nodes or other lymphoid tissues are now commonly grouped together, as proposed by Gall and Mallory, as the malignant lymphomas. These include, in descending order of frequency, Hodgkin's disease, lymphosarcoma, reticulum cell sarcoma, and giant follicle (follicular) lymphoma. However, it must be recognized that: (1) Occasionally the assignment of a particular case of malignant lymphoma to one or another of these subgroups requires some forcing; and that (2) in some cases the lesional tissue changes its cytologic character in the course of further evolution of the disease, so that the case no longer fits into the subgroup to which it was originally assigned.

All of the malignant lymphomas are distinctly more prevalent among males than among females, in the proportion of about 2 to 1. As to age distribution, one can say in general that, with the exception of Hodgkin's disease, they are relatively uncommon below the age of 20. Hodgkin's disease predilects the age group between 20 and 40, while the other lymphomas predilect that between 40 and 65. The cases of giant follicle lymphoma in particular lie mainly toward the upper end of this age distribution.

By far the most common site of departure for the malignant lymphomas is the cervical lymph nodes. Other common sites of origin are the axillary, inguinal, mediastinal, and abdominal nodes, but almost any lymphoid aggregate in the body may constitute the point of departure in one case or another. Early in the clinical course of the malignant lymphomas, smears of the peripheral blood fail to reveal aberrations in the white blood cell count. Later, in consequence of involvement of the bone marrow, large numbers of tumor cells may appear in the peripheral blood. This is particularly true in regard to lymphosarcoma, which, in many cases, comes to show great numbers of lymphocytes in the peripheral blood, giving the case in question the aspect of a lymphocytic leukemia. In connection with Hodgkin's disease, on the other hand, even though the bone marrow eventually becomes heavily infiltrated, the peripheral blood apparently never presents a corresponding leukemic picture.

Irrespective of the particular lymph nodes originally implicated, the involvement of the lymphatic tissues is likely to be found quite striking and generalized when a case has run its course and come to autopsy. The affected lymph nodes are found enlarged, are often matted together into packets, and, when cut, reveal obvious alteration of gross architecture. Furthermore, there are usually some foci of lymphoma in various other organs and tissues. If bones are removed and opened, they not uncommonly reveal a greater or lesser amount of tumorous infiltration of the marrow. Some bones, also, may be the site of localized destructive lesions which have been the source of clinical complaints.

## SKELETAL CHANGES OF GENERALIZED MALIGNANT LYMPHOMA

The bones usually become involved either by direct extension of the disease from affected neighboring lymph nodes, or by metastatic spread by way of the vascular and/or lymphatic channels. However, one cannot rule out the possibility that, in a case of lymphoma, some foci of skeletal involvement may develop independently of extension or metastasis, as expressions of the general disease. The development of a destructive lesion in one or another skeletal area may occur even relatively early in the course of a malignant lymphoma. Indeed, sometimes attention is first called to the presence of malignant lymphoma by complaints arising from a skeletal lesion. As a rule, in such cases the skeletal complaint merely happens to occupy the foreground of the clinical picture, and study of the patient reveals indubitable involvement of lymph nodes. In cases of Hodgkin's disease, this skeletal emphasis is not at all unusual. Those rarer cases of malignant lymphoma which apparently start in a bone site and tend to remain restricted to that site and its regional lymph nodes are ordinarily referred to as "lymphoma primary in bone" (p. 415).

Direct invasion of bones is most likely to affect those skeletal areas which stand in closest proximity to affected chains of lymph nodes. These areas, of course, are particularly vertebral bodies, the vertebral ends of ribs, the sternum, and the ilium along its crest and near the sacro-iliac joint. In addition to being the principal sites of direct extension, these areas may share in metastatic involvement, which may be widespread over the skeleton. Metastasis by way of the blood stream results in scattered miliary seeding of the marrow of various bones with lesional tissue. Such miliary metastatic lesions are clinically silent, as a rule, and are also not likely to be detectable roentgenographically. In some skeletal areas they, too, may grow into rather large foci of the disease, become recognizable in the *x*-ray picture because of local destruction of osseous tissue, and also give rise to clinical manifestations.

In any event, in considering the question of skeletal implication in malignant lymphoma, one should distinguish between: (1) the incidence as ascertained clinically (and roentgenographically) and (2) the incidence as ascertained on the basis of autopsy findings in cases in which many of the bones have been examined for gross and microscopic evidence of the disease. Naturally, the frequency with which one finds skeletal involvement is much higher among carefully autopsied cases than among those evaluated only clinically. This higher incidence is due to the fact that, along with any large, obvious foci in one or more bones, whose presence may have been known clinically, autopsy reveals that in many other bones there is, as noted, at least miliary seeding of the marrow spaces with lesional tissue peculiar to the disease. Indeed, it seems likely that some evidence of bone involvement, amounting at least to miliary seeding of the marrow of some bones, would probably be found at autopsy in practically all cases of malignant lymphoma in which the disease had been free to run its full clinical course.

**Hodgkin's Disease.**—Hodgkin's disease is distinguished from the other lymphomas by the cytologic peculiarities of the lesional tissue. Foremost among these is the presence of Reed-Sternberg cells. These are large cells with a large single nucleus which is often multilobed, or they are actual giant cells with multiple nuclei. They are apparently derived from the locally proliferating reticulum cells. Sooner or later, other cells, including lymphocytes, eosinophilic leukocytes, neutrophilic leukocytes, plasma cells, and fibroblasts, appear in varying proportions in the lesional tissue. Areas of focal necrosis usually become apparent also. Furthermore, a reactive fibrosis sets in, and this is sometimes so intense that the basic cellular pattern of the lesion becomes obliterated. In some cases, sooner or later, the lesional tissue pattern changes to an indubitable sarcomatous one. That pattern is dominated by great numbers of Reed-Sternberg cells, variable in size and nuclear configuration, and is often referred to as *Hodgkin's sarcoma.* In some cases, furthermore, the affected lymph nodes apparently show the cytologic pattern of Hodgkin's sarcoma from the beginning.

The incidence of *skeletal involvement* in Hodgkin's disease as observed on a clinical basis is usually reported as being around 10 to 20 per cent. On the other hand, when established on the basis of autopsy findings, the incidence has been variously reported, for example, as 34 per cent (see Uehlinger), 61 per cent (see Jackson and Parker), and 78 per cent (see Steiner).

Not uncommonly, it is study of biopsy material from a bone lesion that first establishes the fact that a patient is suffering from Hodgkin's disease (see Fig. 127). By far the most common site for clinically manifest bone involvement is, as noted, the vertebral column (particularly the lower thoracic and upper lumbar portion). The involvement of vertebræ relates mainly to the vertebral bodies, clinical complaints arising from destructive lesions in the processes and spines being much less common. Probably next in frequency as a source of clinical complaint is the innominate bone (especially its iliac portion). The appearance of a clinical lesion in the sternum, a scapula, or one or another rib is also not rare. Occasionally a clinically manifest lesion develops in a long bone. Now and then, some other bone is the site of a lesion giving rise to clinical complaints.

Attention is usually directed to a bone lesion by pain. However, roentgenographic examination of the skeleton in a case of Hodgkin's disease may reveal, along with the painful lesion, one or more other areas of bone involvement which are clinically silent. On the other hand, pain is sometimes localized to a bone site perhaps for months before any bone lesion becomes apparent roentgenographically. Particularly if there is involvement of the sacro-iliac area, the local pain may be associated with radiating pains, and if appropriate vertebræ are affected there may even be neurologic signs of pressure upon the cord. Rather rarely, a lesion in a rib, or a rather extensive one in a long bone, leads to pathologic fracture of the bone.

### *Figure 127*

*A*, Roentgenograph showing a destructive lesion in the left half of the third lumbar vertebra, which was proved by biopsy to be the site of Hodgkin's disease. The patient was a man 39 years of age whose presenting complaint was pain relating to the vertebral lesion in question. There was no clear-cut evidence of lymphadenopathy on admission. Indeed, a generalized lymphadenopathy did not become apparent until 15 months after the onset of the patient's pain. At that time, biopsy of an enlarged axillary node also revealed evidence of Hodgkin's disease, and the presence of widespread Hodgkin's disease was confirmed at autopsy not long thereafter.

*B*, Photomicrograph (× 250) illustrating the general histologic pattern of the tissue removed at biopsy from the lesion illustrated in *A*. Among the smaller cells, many of which are eosinophilic leukocytes, one notes some large cells which represent the Reed-Sternberg cells characteristic of Hodgkin's disease.

*C*, Roentgenograph of the upper end of the right femur in a case of Hodgkin's disease showing a destructive lesion in the region of the greater trochanter. Pain from this femoral lesion was the presenting complaint. In this case, too, the concomitant involvement of lymph nodes was inconspicuous at the time. The patient was a young man 19 years of age who died 3 years after the onset of his complaints. Autopsy revealed widely disseminated Hodgkin's disease heavily involving the skeleton. (See also *D*, and Fig. 128.)

*D*, Photograph showing, for comparison with *C*, the gross anatomic appearance of the right hip joint area, which was removed at the autopsy in this case. In addition to the involvement of the bones by the Hodgkin's disease, one can note massive tumorous involvement of the soft tissues about the joint.

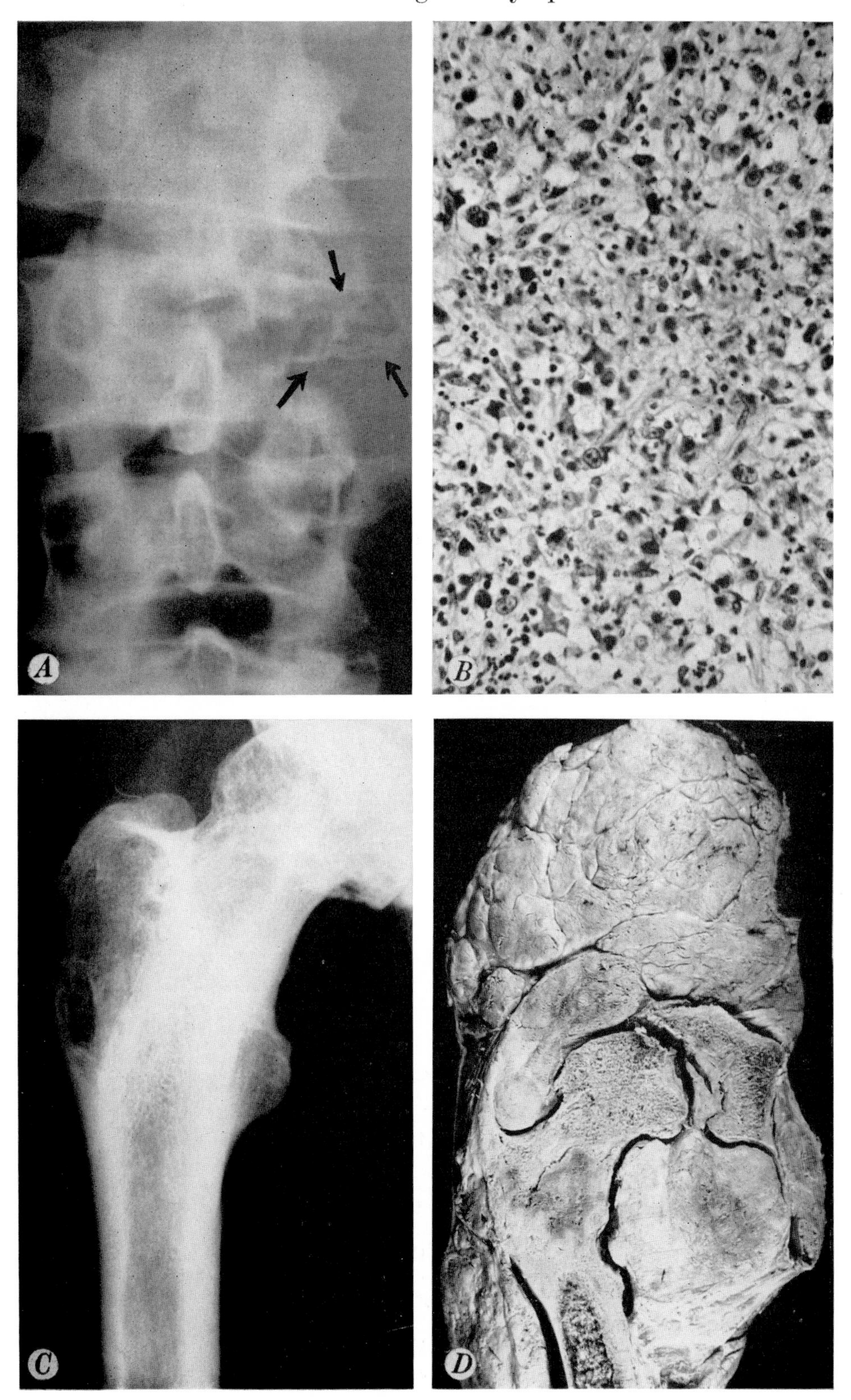


*Figure 127*

There is no characteristic roentgenographic picture for areas of bone involvement in Hodgkin's disease. Osteolytic destruction of one or more vertebral bodies may have caused their collapse. In relation to affected flat bones, one may find multiple punched-out areas of radiolucency or one or more large radiolucent areas. If an area of bone destruction is in a long bone, the local cortex may be found invaded and broken through in places. Extension of the lesional tissue beyond the bone may have provoked the deposition of new bone by the periosteum. At a site of bone involvement, one often finds that the relatively radiolucent osteolytic areas are intermingled with areas of relative radiopacity. The latter is due to an osteoplastic reaction in some parts of the lesional area, apparently following in the wake of necrosis. Occasionally an affected bone area is predominantly radiopaque, in consequence of a particularly strong osteoplastic reaction in the lesion. Rather rarely, in relation to affected vertebræ, the osteoplastic reaction has been so pronounced that one sees the picture of a so-called "ivory vertebra" (see Hultén).

When bones are removed at autopsy in a case of Hodgkin's disease and cut open, one will find that any small, scattered foci of disease in the bone marrow are grayish or yellowish and stand out strikingly against the unaffected marrow. In some areas one may find somewhat larger foci of marrow involvement, while the local trabeculæ are still intact. As the foci increase in size, their presence is increasingly likely to be associated with destruction of the regional osseous tissue. Ultimately a large focus of bone involvement starting in the marrow may extend to the cortex and even destroy it at some point. A vertebral body so affected may be completely replaced by soft, rubbery, yellowish tissue which, in places, may be extending beneath the ligaments or against the dura. A lesion in which osteoplastic reaction has occurred will, on the other hand, be firm on account of the deposition of new bone in the tumor tissue. (See Fig. 128.)

As to cytologic detail, the pattern of the lesions is not essentially different in the bones from what it is in other organs affected by the disease, some lesions being more cellular and others more scirrhous. However, occasionally a Hodgkin's bone lesion, if considered apart from the case as a whole, may present a cytologic problem of differential diagnosis from eosinophilic granuloma of bone. This problem arises notably if the Hodgkin's tissue is quite cellular and contains numerous eosinophiles and if the Reed-Sternberg cells are few and have been overlooked. However, in eosinophilic granuloma the histiocytes, in some places at least, tend to show a meshy arrangement, and any areas of necrosis present are not ringed by connective tissue as they are likely to be in Hodgkin's disease.

**Lymphosarcoma.**—In lymph nodes or nodal areas affected with lymphosarcoma, microscopic examination shows that the germinal centers have disappeared, the sinuses have become filled with lymphoid cells, and the capsule and trabeculæ

***Figure 128***

*A*, Photograph showing the cut surface of the upper end of the left femur, for comparison with Fig. 127-*D* from the same case. Note the small, discrete patches and a number of larger patches of tumor tissue representing Hodgkin's disease. About the hip joint on this side, however, there were no large extra-osseous tumor masses.

*B*, Photograph showing the cut surface of the lower half of the femur illustrated in *A*. Note the widespread distribution of tumor tissue through the interior of the bone.

*C*, Photograph showing the cut surface of the 3 lower lumbar vertebræ and the sacrum from the same case of Hodgkin's disease. The body of the fourth lumbar vertebra has been almost completely replaced by tumor tissue. The latter is also grossly evident to some degree in all the other bones illustrated.

*D*, Photomicrograph (× 450) showing the histologic pattern characteristic of the tumor tissue wherever encountered at autopsy in this case of Hodgkin's disease.

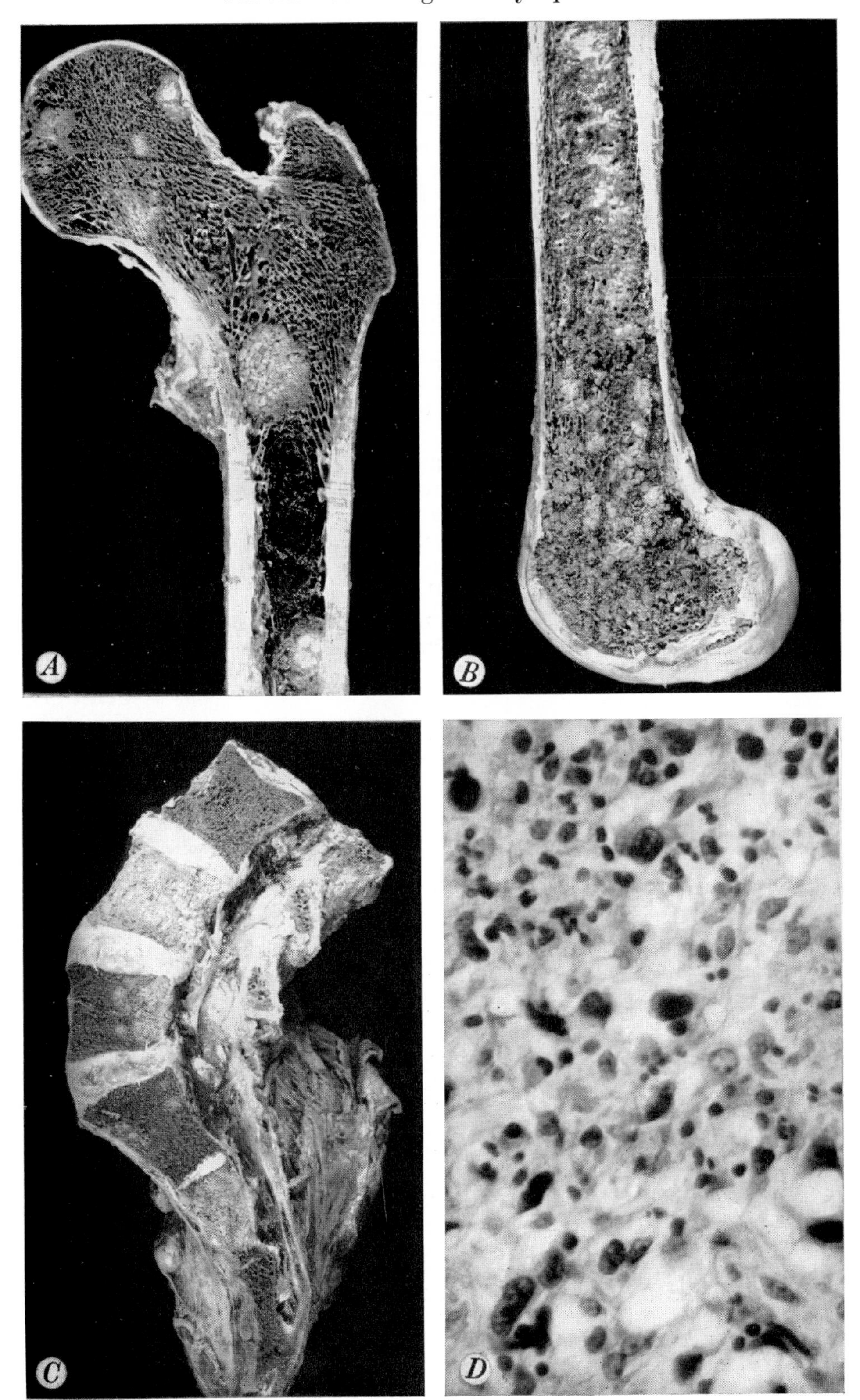


*Figure 128*

have undergone more or less infiltration with such cells. In most cases of lymphosarcoma the general histologic pattern presented by the enlarged and otherwise altered nodes becomes one composed, almost throughout, of small, adult lymphocytes. In other cases of lymphosarcoma the histologic pattern is one in which lymphoblasts (more primitive, larger lymphocytes) pervade the lesional tissue. Many of these lymphoblasts may present mitotic division figures.

In some cases of lymphosarcoma (about 20 per cent), lymphoid cells eventually enter the blood stream, sometimes in large numbers, and create the peripheral blood picture of lymphatic leukemia. It is especially in these cases that autopsy reveals lymphoid infiltrations of smaller or larger size, widely distributed not only in the viscera but also through the bone marrow. In which of the cases of lymphosarcoma a terminal change to lymphatic leukemia will occur cannot be anticipated on the basis of study of affected lymph nodes removed for diagnostic biopsy at the time of the initial study of the case. Cases of lymphosarcoma presenting the terminal picture of lymphatic leukemia are often referred to as instances of lymphosarcomatosis.

As to *skeletal involvement,* we are not especially concerned here with dissemination of the lymphosarcoma through the marrow of the bones, such as is likely to be found at autopsy, especially in those cases in which the disease terminates as a lymphatic leukemia. The findings in such cases correspond to what has already been described in connection with the bone changes of leukemia in adults (p. 402). We are interested rather in the localized destructive bone lesions which are the source of clinical complaints. Clinically manifest localized bone lesions are to be observed in about 10 per cent of the cases of lymphosarcoma (see Sugarbaker and Craver, and Coles and Schulz). Though one or more such lesions may appear relatively early in the course of a given case, it is only exceptionally that attention is first directed to the presence of lymphosarcoma by complaints arising from skeletal involvement. In this respect, there is somewhat of a contrast with Hodgkin's disease.

In a particular instance, only a single skeletal site, or several such sites, may be affected. As in Hodgkin's disease, so also in lymphosarcoma, the vertebral column is predilected. The skull, the pelvis, the ribs, and long bones are the other common sites, but taken together they do not greatly exceed the vertebral column in frequency of involvement.

***Figure 129***

*A*, Roentgenograph showing a large osteolytic lesion in the acetabular area of an innominate bone in a case of lymphosarcoma. The patient was a woman, 65 years of age on admission, who was known to have been suffering from lymphosarcoma for 3 years. For 3 months before admission she had been complaining of severe local pain. The destructive bone lesion illustrated was the only one found in the skeletal survey.

*B*, Roentgenograph showing a large, mottled area of lytic destruction in the shaft of a femur in a case of lymphosarcoma. The patient was a woman 68 years of age who had developed cervical and axillary lymphadenopathy 5 years before admission. The original lymph node biopsy revealed the histologic pattern of a giant follicle lymphoma. A lymph node biopsy 3 years later showed that the pattern had changed to that of lymphosarcoma. The destructive lesion in the femur illustrated developed in the course of 4 months. A skeletal survey showed an analogous destructive lesion in a humerus. The histologic pattern of the punch biopsy specimen from the femoral lesion is shown in *C*.

*C*, Photomicrograph (× 450) illustrating the histologic pattern of the biopsy specimen removed from the lesion shown in *B*. Note the domination of the picture by small lymphocytes, warranting a diagnosis of lymphosarcoma.

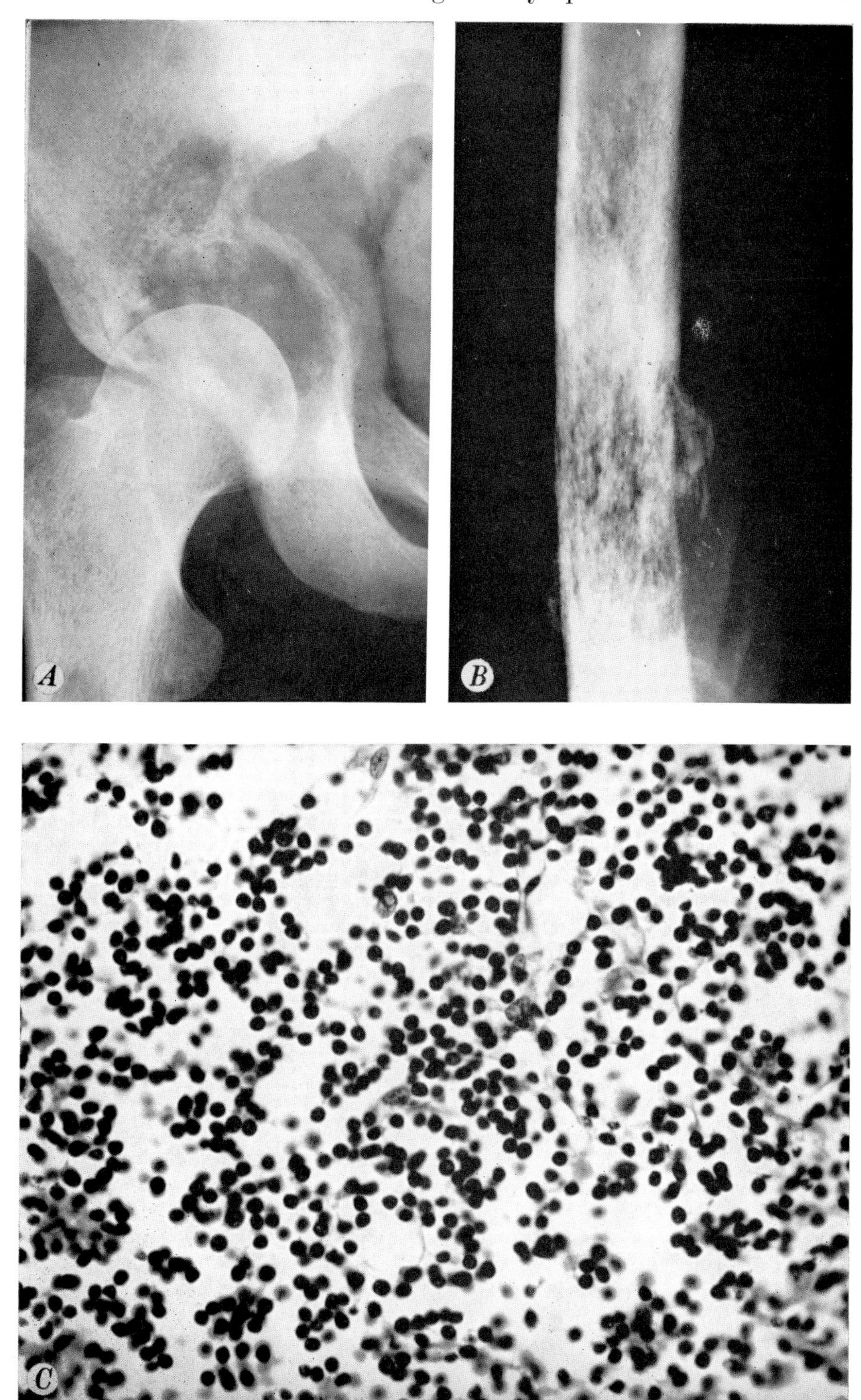


*Figure 129*

Boring pain localized to the affected skeletal area is the usual complaint, and if the affected site is superficially located there may be a palpable swelling. Usually, roentgenographic examination will then already show a focus of essentially osteolytic alteration of the bone (see Fig. 129). However, as in Hodgkin's disease, the patient may complain of local bone pain before the local bone destruction has become sufficiently extensive to be detectable roentgenographically.

**Giant Follicle Lymphoma.**—Since we are concerned with the lymphomas largely insofar as they affect the bones, we need give but little attention to giant follicle lymphoma. This is the lymphoma which has an early, relatively benign stage, characterized by enlarged nodes showing numerous large follicles or germinal centers. The giant follicle lymphoma as such seems not to be associated with skeletal involvement. When, in the later stage, the condition becomes frankly malignant, the striking follicular structure of the nodes is lost and the character of the disease usually becomes that of lymphosarcoma. When it changes into a lymphosarcoma, it may come to involve bones, but the skeletal manifestations then are not different from what they would be if the disorder had started as a lymphosarcoma.

**Reticulum Cell Sarcoma.**—Reticulum cell sarcoma tends to follow the general pattern of the other malignant lymphomas, starting in a chain of lymph nodes, spreading to other chains, and eventually metastasizing widely to various organs and tissues. The basic tumor cell is held to be derived from primitive mesenchyme and to be different from the lymphocyte. The reticulum cell is distinctly larger than the lymphocyte, has abundant cytoplasm, and often shows cytoplasmic processes. The nucleus is often eccentric in position and not infrequently indented. Occasionally, in areas in which sheets of such cells predominate, one may see a few very large cells with multiple nuclei. Tissue sections of a reticulum cell sarcoma which have been impregnated with silver show reticulum fibers scattered diffusely among the cells.

However, pathologists are by no means in accord as to the cytologic criteria which justify a diagnosis of reticulum cell sarcoma in a particular case. Indeed, what one person may call a reticulum cell sarcoma another may want to designate as a Hodgkin's sarcoma, and vice versa. Furthermore, it should be noted that it is sometimes difficult to decide, on the basis of the cytologic pattern presented by tissue from a biopsy specimen, whether one is dealing with a reticulum cell sarcoma or with a completely undifferentiated metastatic carcinoma.

In reticulum cell sarcoma, clinical manifestations resulting from the occurrence of *localized bone destruction* in one or more skeletal areas are not at all uncommon, appearing in perhaps 10 or 15 per cent of the cases. In regard to predilected sites, clinical complaints, and the roentgenographic appearance of the affected bones, the skeletal lesions found in connection with generalized reticulum cell sarcoma follow, on the whole, the pattern of those occurring with lymphosarcoma. Hence they require no further discussion.

It should be noted, however, that in contrast to the other malignant lymphomas, reticulum cell sarcoma in particular not infrequently starts in a bone site and fails to spread except locally, perhaps even for some years (see below).

**Treatment.**—In the general treatment of the malignant lymphomas, radiation therapy still remains the most valuable procedure. Of the chemotherapeutic agents, nitrogen mustard is also of value and can be alternated with radiation therapy, especially in cases of Hodgkin's disease. On the other hand, the folic acid antagonists are contraindicated, and cortisone and ACTH are of dubious usefulness.

In any event, we are concerned here mainly with the treatment of the localized destructive bone lesions appearing in connection with these disorders. For these lesions the local application of radiation therapy is clearly the most valuable procedure known at present. Pain referable to a bone site in a case of generalized lymphoma may be an indication for local treatment even though no lesion can, as yet, be visualized in the *x*-ray picture. Irradiation therapy with 600 to 1,500 r can be expected to relieve the pain at the site of a clinically manifest bone lesion. It can also be expected to relieve neurologic complaints due to pressure on the cord and issuing nerves from a lesion in the vertebral column, to the extent to which the neurologic damage is still reversible. However, irradiation therapy to a particular bone site usually has to be repeated, since, if the patient continues to survive, the lesion is almost sure to become active again.

## LYMPHOMA PRIMARY IN BONE

As already indicated, attention is sometimes first called to the presence of a *generalized* malignant lymphoma by complaints arising from a skeletal lesion. This happens most often in connection with Hodgkin's disease. Indeed, it is not unusual for a case of Hodgkin's disease to be identified through biopsy of a painful bone lesion, the lymph node involvement which antedated the bone involvement having been overlooked, most probably because of inconspicuous location. Occasionally in a case of Hodgkin's disease, skeletal involvement may even dominate the clinical picture, thrusting the associated involvement of lymph nodes and viscera into the background. However, such cases again do not represent instances of lymphoma primary in bone, since the skeletal involvement is secondary to that of the lymphoid tissues.

The term *lymphoma primary in bone* is meant to refer to cases in which a lymphoma starts in a bone or skeletal area. In some cases the lymphoma may even remain restricted to the skeletal area originally affected. In others, lymph nodes regional to the affected skeletal area sooner or later become involved. In still other cases (a small minority), a number of skeletal sites come to present lymphoma lesions either simultaneously or successively. In these cases, too, any lymph gland involvement appearing early in the course of the disease tends to affect only nodes regional to the areas of skeletal involvement. Eventually, in any of these cases, the lymphoma may become generalized, but this generalization does not alter the fact that, at least at first, the lymphomatous involvement was restricted to a skeletal part or parts.

While it may be true that any of the various lymphomas may appear in the form of lymphoma primary in bone, it is only in connection with reticulum cell sarcoma that this occurrence has been established by abundant experience. Nevertheless, the writer has recently had the opportunity of studying a case of Hodgkin's disease which took this form. The patient was a man 30 years of age whose presenting lesion was an area of lytic destruction in the neck and intertrochanteric region of a femur. A biopsy specimen from the femoral lesion showed tissue presenting the histologic pattern of Hodgkin's disease. The lesion in question was treated by irradiation, healed in rapidly, and has remained healed.

About 16 months after study of the femoral lesion, the patient developed pain in the back and showed roentgenographic evidence of lytic destruction of 2 midthoracic vertebræ. This, too, yielded to radiation therapy. About 6 months later, several ribs on one side of the chest became painful and showed focal areas of lytic destruction, and these lesions, too, were successfully treated by irradiation. The latest skeletal episode (2½ years after biopsy of the femoral lesion) has been a recurrence of the lesion in the midthoracic part of the column, associated with the development of a paraplegia.

During the entire clinical course so far, the patient has been examined repeatedly for evidence of superficial lymphadenopathy, but none has been noted. Also, *x*-ray films of the chest have failed to reveal any mediastinal lymphadenopathy. When this patient will come to show widespread involvement of lymph nodes, such as is ordinarily found in Hodgkin's disease, one cannot tell. At any rate, the case seems to be a convincing example of lymphoma primary in bone in which the lymphoma represents Hodgkin's disease and not reticulum cell sarcoma. Such cases are rare, and we turn now to the more common "primary reticulum cell sarcoma of bone."

## PRIMARY RETICULUM CELL SARCOMA OF BONE

It was Parker and Jackson who first called attention to the lesion now known as "primary reticulum cell sarcoma of bone." As a clinicopathologic entity, the con-

### *Figure 130*

*A*, Roentgenograph illustrating the appearance of a primary reticulum cell sarcoma of bone in the lower end of a femur. The patient was a man 50 years of age who had had difficulty relating to the knee for the previous $3\frac{1}{2}$ years. Specifically, he complained of intermittent bouts of pain, and there was also slight swelling of the affected bone area. The nature of the lesion was not suspected from the *x*-ray picture, and a biopsy was done. This revealed the pattern of a reticulum cell sarcoma (Fig. 131-*A*), and a high thigh amputation was carried out. A 2-year follow-up revealed that the patient is in good general health and shows no other bone lesions and no lymphadenopathy. However, the ultimate prognosis in the case must still be guarded.

*B*, Roentgenograph showing the appearance of a primary reticulum cell sarcoma of bone located in the midshaft area of a femur. The patient was a man 38 years of age who had had pain relating to the thigh for about $1\frac{1}{2}$ years prior to admission. He was in good general health and presented no lymphadenopathy. The femoral lesion was interpreted as a focus of chronic osteomyelitis on the basis of the *x*-ray picture. At the surgical intervention, the lesional tissue was found extensively necrotic. On the basis of microscopic examination, one could not be certain that the lesion was not a focus of infection. However, the presence of some small nests of reticulum cells did indicate the possibility of a tumor. The patient returned 2 months later because a pathologic fracture through the lesional area had occurred. Examination again failed to reveal any lymphadenopathy or additional bone lesion. Tissue removed for histologic study at the time of this admission did present the pattern of a reticulum cell sarcoma, and the patient received radiation therapy. The patient died about $1\frac{1}{2}$ years later, showing what seemed to be pulmonary dissemination of the disease, but no autopsy was done.

*C*, Roentgenograph showing the appearance of a primary reticulum cell sarcoma in a tibia which again suggests a focus of infection more strongly than a tumor. The patient was a man 37 years of age who had been complaining over a period of 5 months of pain referred to the leg. There was no lymphadenopathy at the time of admission, and findings from the sternal marrow puncture smears were negative. The diagnosis was established through study of a biopsy specimen from the lesion, and radiation therapy was instituted. About 3 months later, the inguinal glands on the same side as the bone lesion showed slight enlargement, and these too were irradiated. The patient was lost to follow-up after about $2\frac{1}{2}$ years, but, before that, showed substantial healing of the tibial lesion and good general health.

*D*, Roentgenograph showing a lytic lesion above the acetabulum of the right ilium, established by tissue examination as a reticulum cell sarcoma. Seven years earlier, the patient (a woman then 49 years of age) presented a reticulum cell sarcoma of the right humerus. This was irradiated and has remained healed. During the entire interim of 7 years, the patient was free of lymphadenopathy. However, about 5 months after the appearance of the iliac lesion, she returned to the hospital with an enlarged lymph node in the region of the second rib. This was apparently the first evidence that the case was no longer one of reticulum cell sarcoma restricted to the skeleton. The condition now proceeded to run a steadily downhill course, and the patient died about a year later. Autopsy revealed widespread involvement of the lymph nodes (particularly the mediastinal and mesenteric nodes), the liver and spleen, and the marrow of all the bones removed and examined.

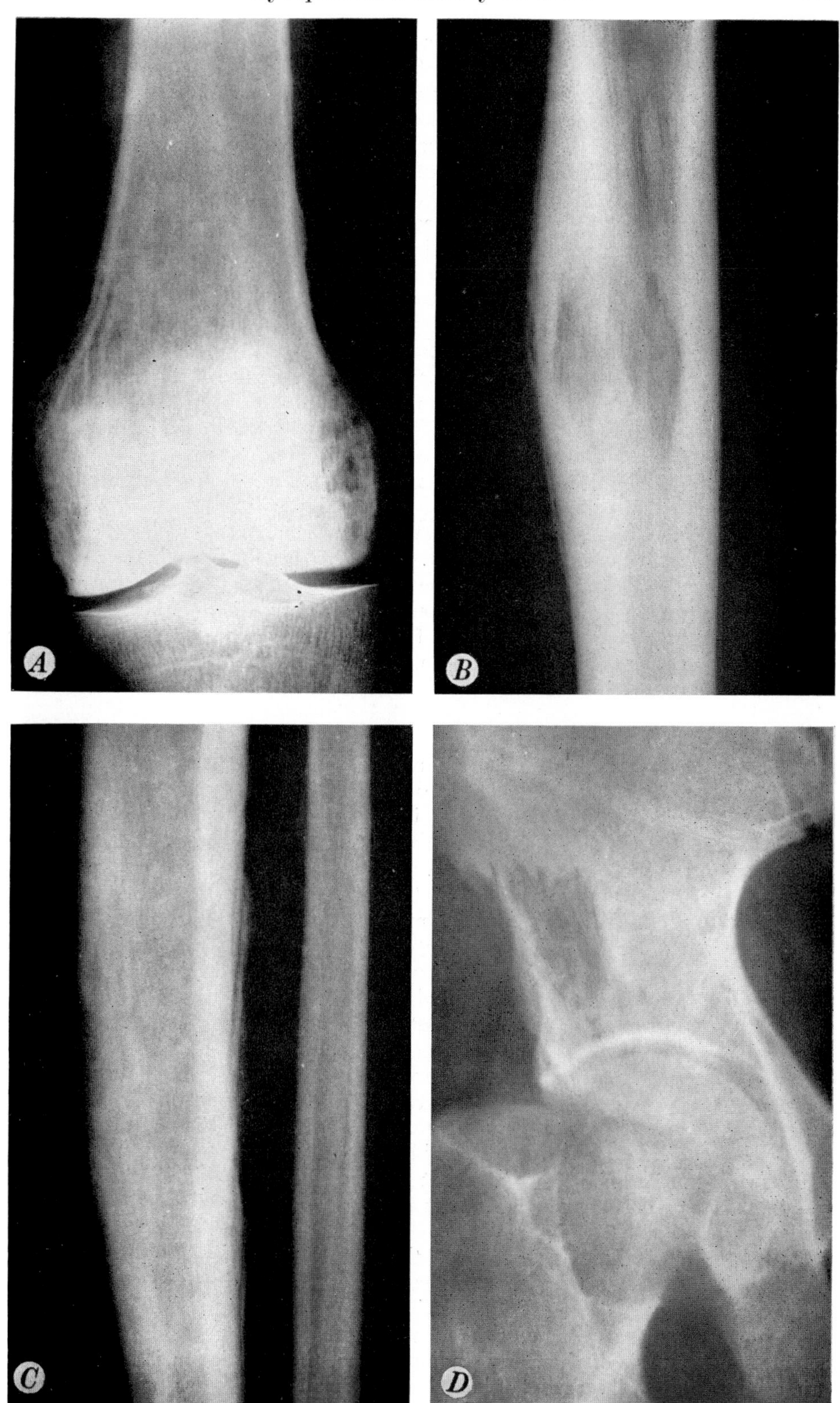


*Figure 130*

dition is being more and more definitely established in a growing body of literature (see also McCormack *et al.*, Fripp and Sissons, and Francis, Higinbotham, and Coley). The concept of this lesion grew out of the dilemma created by cases supposedly representing Ewing's sarcoma but not running the baleful clinical course typical of that sarcoma. The cells of the primary reticulum cell sarcoma of bone are apparently derived from the primitive mesenchyme in the marrow of the affected bone.

In the group of cases originally reported, there had been repeated surgical interventions and recurrences, and the bone lesion usually came to present as a bulky tumor mass. Now that the concept has become better clarified, cases of primary reticulum cell sarcoma of bone are often diagnosed and treated before a large destructive lesion has developed. In fact, many cases are now recognized at a stage in which there is only a slight thickening of the bone, and the *x*-ray picture of the lesion may not even indicate clearly that one is dealing with a tumor at all. As indicated in the general discussion of lymphoma primary in bone, there seem to be occasional cases of primary reticulum cell sarcoma of bone in which, successively or simultaneously, a number of skeletal areas are affected. However, the present discussion will concentrate on the much more common cases in which the clinical picture at the time of admission is dominated by a single bone lesion.

**Clinical Considerations.**—The condition is more common in males than in females, in the proportion of at least 2 to 1. As to *age* distribution, about half of the patients are below the age of 40. However, it is exceptional to see the condition in a person under 10 years of age, although a fair proportion of the patients are between 11 and 20 years of age. Most of the rest are between 40 and 60 years of age. Thus, in respect to age distribution, primary reticulum cell sarcoma of bone contrasts with generalized reticulum cell sarcoma, nearly all of whose victims are above the age of 40. It contrasts also with Ewing's sarcoma, whose victims are preponderantly below 25 years of age.

As to the *bone site* affected, long tubular bones, and in particular the femur, tibia, and humerus are predilected. Localization to an innominate bone, scapula, rib, or some part of the vertebral column is not exceptional, but other localizations are definitely rare. Within a long bone the lesion may be located in the middle of the shaft or near one end of the bone.

The *clinical complaints* are usually not striking and only rarely related to an antecedent trauma. The presenting complaint is generally pain, often described as being of an aching character. Along with the pain there is likely to be some swelling at the affected bone site, perhaps associated with local tenderness. In occasional instances the pain is quite mild and intermittent at first, leaving periods of weeks or months during which the patient is free from it. Indeed, the writer has seen several cases in teen-age subjects in which, on account of the mild and intermittent character of the complaints and the absence of significant changes in the *x*-ray picture, several years elapsed before the true nature of the condition was unmasked. On the other hand, in a case in which the lesion involves a vertebral body, the complaints may be severe and dominated by neurologic manifestations. Furthermore, in one case or another, it may be the occurrence of a pathologic fracture through the affected bone that first brings the patient under definitive medical care.

**Roentgenographic Findings.**—Though the *x*-ray picture presented by a primary reticulum cell sarcoma of bone sometimes suggests an inflammatory bone lesion, it more often suggests that one is actually dealing with a tumor. (See Fig. 130.) Even when the picture does favor the idea of a tumor, however, one usually cannot be sure. on the basis of the *x*-ray findings alone, that the lesion is specifically a primary reticulum cell sarcoma of bone (see Sherman and Snyder, and Wilson and

Pugh). In the last analysis, the diagnosis depends upon the histologic examination of tissue from the lesion. However, even after study of a biopsy specimen, problems of histologic differential diagnosis may still remain.

The leading feature of the *x*-ray picture is the presence of irregular patchy areas of radiolucency representing osteolysis in the interior of the affected bone part. The foci of radiolucency are not infrequently found intermingled with patchy areas of radiopacity which reflect reactive new bone formation at the site of the tumor. If the tumor tissue has invaded the regional cortex of the bone, as it is very likely to do, smaller or larger areas of cortical destruction can be noted. Concomitantly, part of the regional cortex may be found thickened. In any event, however, the contour of the affected part of the bone is usually only slightly distended, at most. Whether or not the original cortex is found thickened, it frequently shows some periosteal new bone apposition on its outer surface, but this too is usually not striking. When the lesion has broken the bounds of the cortex and extended into the surrounding soft parts, an extra-osseous tumor mass of variable size will be apparent, but there is usually no evidence of ossification within this mass.

**Pathologic Findings.**—Gross specimens showing a primary reticulum cell sarcoma of bone intact in its setting and unmodified by previous treatment are now rarely available for study. This is so because irradiation rather than amputation is now the usual initial (and often the only) therapeutic procedure used against the condition. On the basis of earlier specimens, the tumor tissue can be described as being usually firm but sometimes rather soft and friable. In a case in which the tumor tissue is rather firm, it is likely to appear whitish or grayish white, while the tumor tissue of softer consistency is likely to be pinkish gray in color. In a lesion in which the tumor tissue has extensively destroyed the local osseous tissue and penetrated the cortex so as to produce a large extra-osseous mass, areas of necrosis and cystification may also be seen here and there in the tumor tissue. All in all, on the basis of gross appearance, it is hard to tell the difference between a primary reticulum cell sarcoma and a Ewing sarcoma or a fibrosarcoma of bone, or even to differentiate it from an extremely "osteolytic" osteogenic sarcoma.

In regard to the microscopic appearance of the lesion in question, one notes that the tumor tissue is pervaded by cells which usually contain a fairly large single nucleus which is roundish or oval in general, but may be indented or lobulated. The chromatin may be finely divided and scattered, or, on the other hand, it may be coarser and nucleoli may be present. The cytoplasm stains palely with eosin and may be sparse. Some few cells may contain large double nuclei, but true tumor giant cells are not seen. Mitotic figures are sometimes prominent. Scattered foci of smaller cells (lymphocytes) are frequently also present among the tumor cells. There is a variable amount of intercellular stroma, which, in some lesions or areas, is represented merely by delicate strands of collagen and in others by dense collagen bundles. When the neoplastic tissue is stained in order to bring out the reticulum, the latter is found to run in delicate threads and strands around groups of tumor cells and also between individual tumor cells. (See Fig. 131.)

**Differential Diagnosis.**—In respect to differential diagnosis, the lesion raises some complex problems. If one examined an abnormal lymph node (from the neck or some other site) and found it presenting the cytologic pattern described above, one would hardly hesitate in making a diagnosis of reticulum cell sarcoma. However, if one studies a biopsy specimen from a solitary destructive bone lesion which presents that cytologic pattern, one must consider a number of diagnostic possibilities before calling the lesion a primary reticulum cell sarcoma of bone. For instance, under certain conditions there may be difficulty in distinguishing, on cytologic grounds, between primary reticulum cell sarcoma of bone and a focus of cancer metastatic to a bone. This is so when biopsy of the cancerous lesion shows the tumor tissue to be highly undifferentiated, when the primary cancer is clinically silent, and when the focus of bone metastasis is the presenting lesion and seems to be the only one.

However, the condition creating the greatest problem of differential diagnosis is Ewing's sarcoma. In fact, certain workers even maintain that there is no essential difference between the two conditions, and that the distinctions which have been drawn between them are artificial (see Magnus and Wood). It is true that in both conditions the tumor cells are so-called round cells, and that on this account it is sometimes difficult to decide, on a cytologic basis, whether to place a given tumor in one category or the other. However, in general, the cell nuclei of the primary reticulum cell sarcoma of bone are somewhat larger than those of the Ewing sarcoma. Also, in the former lesion the individual nuclei are usually surrounded by a delimited zone of cytoplasm, while in a Ewing sarcoma the cell nuclei often appear enmeshed in a loose and more or less vacuolated cytoplasmic fabric. Furthermore, as noted, when a primary reticulum cell sarcoma of bone is appropriately stained, one usually observes a lattice or meshwork of reticulum fibers outlining groups and individual cells. For the Ewing sarcoma, on the other hand, there is no characteristic pattern so far as these fibrils are concerned.

On the clinical side, a large majority of subjects affected with reticulum cell sarcoma of bone are above 20 years of age, while the large majority of those affected with Ewing's sarcoma are below this age. Furthermore, in cases of the reticulum cell sarcoma, the clinical course is often a torpid one, not only in respect to the local lesion, but also in respect to the general condition of the patient. Thus the local lesion is often slow in evolving and the relevant complaints tend to be quite mild. Also, the lesion frequently remains localized to the affected bone area for a long time or permanently, or involves only the regional lymph nodes in spreading. These various aspects of the condition account for the fact that primary reticulum cell sarcoma of bone is fairly often curable by radiation therapy and/or amputation. All these features are in sharp contrast to those of Ewing's sarcoma. The latter is usually already disseminated through the marrow of the bones at the time when the nature of the presenting bone lesion is first recognized, and is almost always fatal within 2 or 3 years.

In spite of the differences which have been outlined, one might still wish to maintain that primary reticulum cell sarcoma of bone represents merely a relatively banal form of Ewing's sarcoma. In support of this idea one might point out that in both of these conditions the tumor cells are probably derived from the immature reticular cells (the supporting mesenchymal cells) of the bone marrow. In addition, one might say that if one surveys the literature relating to primary reticulum cell sarcoma of bone, one finds that many of the cases had originally been held to represent Ewing's sarcoma. That is, in many of the cases included in reported series, the diagnosis of reticulum cell sarcoma represents a revised diagnosis, made in retrospect on the basis of re-evaluation of the tissue sections in the light of the clinical course pursued by the case. Despite all the obscurities, the writer is among those who hold that primary reticulum cell sarcoma of bone and Ewing's sarcoma represent distinct entities. However, even if one regards them as representing

***Figure 131***

*A*, Photomicrograph (× 450) showing the characteristic cytologic pattern presented by tissue from a reticulum cell sarcoma. The tissue illustrated came from the femoral lesion shown in Fig. 130-*A*.

*B*, Photomicrograph (× 450) illustrating the arrangement of the reticulum fibers which is characteristic for reticulum cell sarcoma.

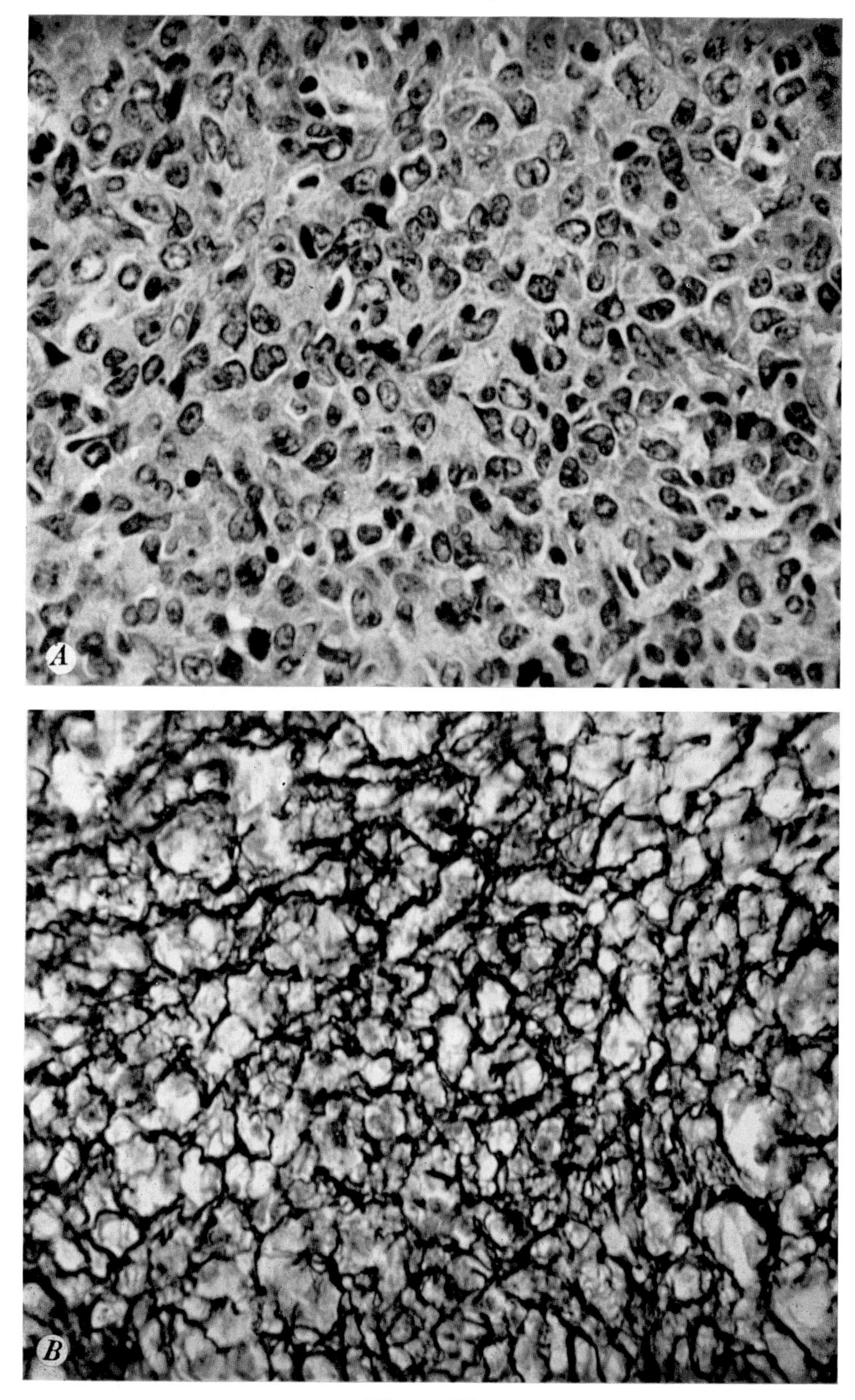


***Figure 131***

merely variants of the same basic tumor, it is important to keep them apart for clinical purposes.

**Course.**—As indicated, the course pursued by cases of primary reticulum cell sarcoma of bone is variable. There can be no doubt that in some cases the lesion may remain localized to the affected bone part without involving even the regional lymph nodes. In other cases the disease may still show a tendency to remain localized, but does spread to the extent of involving the regional lymph nodes. It is the cases showing such restricted involvement that are most subject to cure by irradiation and/or amputation if the lesion is in an accessible site. In such cases of restricted involvement and favorable location of the presenting lesion, cures are not infrequently effected even though the disease has been in existence for a number of years.

When the location is unfavorable, the patient may succumb to complications due to local involvement even though the disease has not become disseminated. Thus Edwards reports the case of a woman 59 years of age in whom a reticulum cell sarcoma apparently originated in the first lumbar vertebra and was the source of clinical complaints for 3 years before death. Autopsy revealed that, though the tumor had spread out somewhat locally, distant lymph nodes were not involved, nor was the spleen, and there were no visceral metastases.

In still other cases, a reticulum cell sarcoma in a bone site may heal in under radiation therapy, but some years later the patient may come to show one or more similar lesions in other bone sites. Even then, though some lymph nodes may also be involved, the disease remains one which centers in the skeleton. In a pertinent case studied by the writer, the patient, a woman 49 years of age, presented a destructive lesion in the upper end of the right humerus. There was no evidence of lymphadenopathy. The bone lesion was treated by irradiation and healed in. Seven years later the patient returned with a lytic lesion in the right ilium, just above the acetabulum. This lesion, too, was treated by irradiation, after biopsy had confirmed the presence of a reticulum cell sarcoma. About 5 months later the patient returned with an enlarged lymph node in the costochondral area of the second rib. No generalized lymphadenopathy was evident. Special interest attaches to the fact that the enlarged lymph node removed showed the histologic pattern of a giant follicle lymphoma. (Details regarding the subsequent course in this case are given in the legend for Figure 130–*D*.)

In another case the site of the presenting reticulum cell sarcoma was the right innominate bone. The patient was a man 60 years of age whose complaints were of about 1 year's standing. Originally he complained of pain referred to the right thigh, but shortly before admission he noted enlargement of the right hip and groin area. The lymph nodes in the right inguinal region were found enlarged, but there was no generalized lymphadenopathy. An *x*-ray picture of the pelvis revealed a large destructive lesion affecting practically the entire right innominate bone. A number of enlarged lymph nodes were removed from the right groin, and they showed the pattern of reticulum cell sarcoma. Before death, lesions appeared in several other bone sites. Autopsy failed to reveal involvement of any lymph nodes except those adjacent to the lesion in the ilium, and neither the spleen nor the liver was found involved. Indeed, the only visceral metastasis found was a focus only 1 cm. in diameter in a kidney. Thus in this case, too, the course was one in which the disease centered in the skeleton, while distant lymphatic involvement was absent and visceral involvement was negligible.

Finally, one encounters cases in which a reticulum cell sarcoma presents as a primary lesion in a single bone site and even yields to radiation therapy, but in which the disease eventually becomes generalized. That is, the terminal picture in such cases is one of conventional reticulum cell sarcoma showing widespread involvement of lymph nodes and also involvement of the spleen, liver, and lungs, along with the marrow of many bones. Such dissemination may appear within a year or two after the presenting bone lesion has been discovered, or may occur even years later.

**Treatment.**—As to methods of treatment, the question of the relative merits of irradiation alone and of surgery followed by irradiation is still not settled. If irradiation is used, 3,000 to 4,000 r is the dose usually delivered to the tumor. Often this destroys the tumor permanently. On the other hand, it is not unusual for the latter to reappear in the original irradiated site, perhaps years later. In other cases, as noted, a focus of reticulum cell sarcoma appears in one or more other bone sites, or the disease finally becomes generalized. Those who favor surgical treatment for the presenting lesion propose amputation (or wide excision) if the lesion is in a site permitting this. The supplementary use of local irradiation therapy as soon as possible after the surgical intervention is usually recommended.

It appears that irradiation and/or amputation can be expected to produce cures in about 25 per cent of the cases of primary reticulum cell sarcoma of bone. However, in view of the wide variation in the course pursued by the disease, it is clear that one must be cautious about the ultimate prognosis in any given case. Indeed, a treated case may seemingly be cured for as long as 5 years and still come to show a local recurrence, or the development of lesions in other bone sites, or even widespread dissemination of the disease. In any event, the ultimate prognosis is better for primary reticulum cell sarcoma of bone than for most bone sarcomas, and very much better than for Ewing's sarcoma. In fact, any case interpreted as one of Ewing's sarcoma in which the patient survives beyond a 2- or 3-year period must be carefully re-evaluated in the light of the idea that the case may be one of primary reticulum cell sarcoma instead.

## REFERENCES


Apitz, K.: Über Knochenveränderungen bei Leukämie, Virchows Arch. f path. Anat., *302*, 301, 1938.

Baty, J. M., and Vogt, E. C.: Bone Changes of Leukemia in Children, Am. J. Roentgenol., *34*, 310, 1935.

Coles, W. C., and Schulz, M. D.: Bone Involvement in Malignant Lymphoma, Radiology, *50*, 458, 1948.

Coley, B. L., Higinbotham, N. L., and Groesbeck, H. P.: Primary Reticulum-Cell Sarcoma of Bone, Radiology, *55*, 641, 1950.

Craver, L. F.: Lymphomas and Leukemias, Bull. New York Acad. Med., *23*, 79, 1947.

Dresner, E.: The Bone and Joint Lesions in Acute Leukaemia and their Response to Folic Acid Antagonists, Quart. J. Med., *19*, 339, 1950.

Edwards, J. E.: Primary Reticulum Cell Sarcoma of the Spine, Am. J. Path., *16*, 835, 1940.

Erb, I. H.: Bone Changes in Leukaemia. Part II. Pathology, Arch. Dis. Childhood, *9*, 319, 1934.

Farber, S.: Some Observations on the Effect of Folic Acid Antagonists on Acute Leukemia and Other Forms of Incurable Cancer, Blood, *4*, 160, 1949.

Follis, R. H., Jr., and Park, E. A.: Some Observations on the Morphologic Basis for the Roentgenographic Changes in Childhood Leukemia, Bull. Hosp. Joint Dis., *12*, 67, 1951.

Francis, K. C., Higinbotham, N. L., and Coley, B. L.: Primary Reticulum Cell Sarcoma of Bone, Surg., Gynec. & Obst., *99*, 142, 1954.

Fripp, A. T., and Sissons, H. A.: A Case of Reticulosarcoma (Reticulum-Cell Sarcoma) of Bone, Brit. J. Surg., *42*, 103, 1954.

Gall, E. A., and Mallory, T. B.: Malignant Lymphoma. A Clinico-Pathologic Survey of 618 Cases, Am. J. Path., *18*, 381, 1942.

Hultén, O.: Ein Fall von "Elfenbeinwirbel" bei Lymphogranulomatose, Acta radiol., *8*, 245, 1927.

Ivins, J. C., and Dahlin, D. C.: Reticulum-Cell Sarcoma of Bone, J. Bone & Joint Surg., *35-A*, 835, 1953.

Jackson, H., Jr., and Parker, F., Jr.: Hodgkin's Disease. II. Pathology, New England J. Med.. *231*, 35, 1944; and IV. Involvement of Certain Organs, New England J. Med., *232*, 547, 1945.

Jaffe, H. L.: Skeletal Manifestations of Leukemia and Malignant Lymphoma, Bull. Hosp. Joint Dis., *13*, 217, 1952.

KHANOLKAR, V. R.: Reticulum Cell Sarcoma of Bone, Arch. Path., *46*, 467, 1948.
LEWIS, E. B.: Leukemia and Ionizing Radiation, Science, *125*, 965, 1957.
LUMB, G.: *Tumours of Lymphoid Tissue*, Edinburgh and London, E. & S. Livingstone, Ltd., 1954.
MAGNUS, H. A., and WOOD, H. L.-C.: Primary Reticulo-sarcoma of Bone, J. Bone & Joint Surg., *38-B*, 258, 1956.
McCORMACK, L. J., IVINS, J. C., DAHLIN, D. C., and JOHNSON, E. W., JR.: Primary Reticulum-Cell Sarcoma of Bone, Cancer, *5*, 1182, 1952.
PARKER, F., JR., and JACKSON, H., JR.: Primary Reticulum Cell Sarcoma of Bone, Surg., Gynec. & Obst., *68*, 45, 1939.
PATRASSI, G.: Zerstörungsvorgänge am Skelett im Verlauf leukämischer Erkrankungen, Beitr. z path. Anat. u. z. allg. Path., *86*, 643, 1931.
POYNTON, F. J., and LIGHTWOOD, R.: Lymphatic Leukaemia, with Infiltration of Periosteum Simulating Acute Rheumatism, Lancet, *1*, 1192, 1932.
RODGERS C. L., DONOHUE, W. L., and SNELLING, C. E.: Leukaemia in Children, Canad. M.A.J., *65*, 548, 1951.
ROSENTHAL, N.: The Lymphomas and Leukemias, Bull. New York Acad. Med., *30*, 583, 1954.
SHERMAN, R. S., and SNYDER, R. E.: The Roentgen Appearance of Primary Reticulum Cell Sarcoma of Bone, Am. J. Roentgenol., *58*, 291, 1947.
SHIMKIN, M. B.: Hodgkin's Disease. Mortality in the United States, 1921–1951; Race, Sex and Age Distribution; Comparison with Leukemia, Blood, *10*, 1214, 1955.
SILVERMAN, F. N.: The Skeletal Lesions in Leukemia, Am. J. Roentgenol., *59*, 819, 1948; and: Treatment of Leukemia and Allied Disorders with Folic Acid Antagonists; Effect of Aminopterin on Skeletal Lesions, Radiology, *54*, 665, 1950.
SNELLING, C. E., and BROWN, A.: Bone Changes in Leukaemia. Part I. Clinical and Roentgenological, Arch. Dis. Childhood, *9*, 315, 1934.
SOUTHAM, C. M., CRAVER, L. F., DARGEON, H. W., and BURCHENAL, J. H.: A Study of the Natural History of Acute Leukemia with Special Reference to the Duration of the Disease and the Occurrence of Remissions, Cancer, *4*, 39, 1951.
STEINER, P. E.: Hodgkin's Disease: The Incidence, Distribution, Nature and Possible Significance of the Lymphogranulomatous Lesions in the Bone Marrow; A Review with Original Data, Arch. Path., *36*, 627, 1943.
STRANGE, V. M., and DE LORIMIER, A. A.: Reticulum Cell Sarcoma Primary in the Skull, Am. J. Roentgenol., *71*, 40, 1954.
SUGARBAKER, E. D., and CRAVER, L. F.: Lymphosarcoma, J.A.M.A., *115*, 17, 1940.
SUSSMAN, M. L.: Skeletal Changes Associated with Diseases of the Blood, Bull. New York Acad. Med., *26*, 763, 1950.
UEHLINGER, E.: Über Knochen-Lymphogranulomatose, Virchows Arch. f. path. Anat , *288*, 36, 1933.
UEHLINGER, E., BOTSZTEJN, C., and SCHINZ, H. R.: Ewingsarkom und Knochenretikulosarkom. Klinik, Diagnose und Differentialdiagnose, Oncologia, *1*, 193, 1948.
VALLS, J., MUSCOLO, D., and SCHAJOWICZ, F.: Reticulum-cell Sarcoma of Bone, J. Bone & Joint Surg., *34-B*, 588, 1952.
VIETA, J. O., FRIEDELL, H. L., and CRAVER, L. F.: A Survey of Hodgkin's Disease and Lymphosarcoma in Bone, Radiology, *39*, 1, 1942.
WILSON, T. W., and PUGH, D. G.: Primary Reticulum-Cell Sarcoma of Bone, with Emphasis on Roentgen Aspects, Radiology, *65*, 343, 1955.
WINTROBE, M. M., CARTWRIGHT, G. E., FESSAS, P., HAUT, A., and ALTMAN, S. J.: Chemotherapy of Leukemia, Hodgkin's Disease and Related Disorders, Ann. Int. Med. ,*41*, 447, 1954.
WYATT, J. P., and SOMMERS, S. C.: Chronic Marrow Failure, Myelosclerosis and Extramedullary Hematopoiesis, Blood, *5*, 329, 1950.

Chapter

# 25

# Lesions Peculiar to the Jawbones

In this chapter we are concerned mainly with various cysts and tumorous lesions which are indigenous to the jawbones. That is, we shall concentrate on lesions which are distinctive for the jawbones and which do not represent merely jawbone localizations of lesions usually occurring elsewhere in the skeleton.

Among the cysts in question we have the so-called *odontogenic cysts.* These are epithelial-lined structures, some of which (the *periodontal cysts*) develop in consequence of dental infection, while others (the *follicular cysts*) result from aberrations in dental development. However, there is another group of jawbone cysts—the *nonodontogenic cysts*—so called because the teeth play no direct role in their development. Most of the nonodontogenic cysts are lined by epithelium, and these are of developmental origin. Some of them (the *fissural cysts*) apparently form in the wake of entrapment of epithelium along the fissural fusion lines of the developing jawbones. Others (the *vestigial cysts*) form from vestiges of the nasopalatine duct.

One usually also reckons among the nonodontogenic jawbone cysts those uncommon mandibular cysts whose walls are not epithelialized. These are commonly denoted as *traumatic cysts* of jawbones, but their traumatic origin may be questioned. Their inclusion among lesions peculiar to the jawbones may not seem justified, since they apparently represent the jawbone equivalent of the solitary bone cyst familiar in relation to long tubular bones (p. 63). Nevertheless, it seems useful to discuss them in the present chapter because of the problems of differential diagnosis which they present.

Under the heading of *odontogenic tumors* we shall discuss a number of more or less solid lesions whose tissue presents histologic patterns suggestive of one or another stage in the evolution and differentiation of the odontogenic mesoderm, odontogenic ectoderm, or combinations of the two. In particular, we shall take up the myxoma, cementoma, ameloblastoma, and odontoma. The *myxoma* is a growth composed mainly of loose-meshed stellate cells and devoid of any calcified intercellular elements such as cementum or dentin. The *cementoma* is composed of more differentiated connective tissue, containing cementum in particular, sometimes even in considerable amounts. The *ameloblastoma* (formerly called adamantinoma) represents the odontogenic tumor composed essentially of epithelium. The term *odontoma* embraces a considerable variety of odontogenic tumors. It includes lesions containing mesodermal and ectodermal tissue elements alone, lesions composed of these tissues along with some of their calcified derivatives (cementum, dentin, and/or enamel), and also lesions containing even more highly differentiated dental elements in the form of organized tooth structures.

Various benign and malignant tumorous lesions not peculiar to the jawbones are also encountered in these bones. Thus, while a focus of fibrous dysplasia may occur in a jawbone alone, it is quite common to find that one or both jawbones are affected (often along with other parts of the skull) in cases in which the disease heavily involves the extracranial skeleton. Another fibro-osseous lesion encountered in jawbones is the so-called "fibrous osteoma." The roentgenographic and pathologic features of that lesion are more or less interchangeable with those observed in connection with a focus of fibrous dysplasia affecting a jawbone. Since the writer holds that the fibrous osteoma is basically of the same nature as fibrous dysplasia of bone, the various fibro-osseous lesions of jawbones are considered in the chapter on Fibrous Dysplasia (p. 136).

Once in a while, also, a jawbone is the site of a tumor such as is commonly encountered as a solitary primary lesion in a long tubular bone. Thus one occasionally observes in a jawbone such lesions as: a desmoplastic fibroma, a fibrosarcoma, chondroma, chondrosarcoma, or even an osteogenic sarcoma. Since the morphology and clinical behavior of these lesions present nothing special in relation to jawbones, the reader is referred to the appropriate chapters for the pertinent facts about these tumors. A jawbone may also become involved, for instance, in a case of Ewing's sarcoma, myeloma, or lymphoma, or even present a focus of metastatic malignancy. The jawbone localizations of these various conditions need not particularly concern us here either. However, when they involve jawbones, all these various conditions are likely to raise problems of differential diagnosis in relation to tumors peculiar to jawbones.

Finally, it is important to note that the giant-cell tumor of bone as it is known in relation to extracranial skeletal parts is rarely encountered in jawbones. Those jawbone lesions which do contain multinuclear giant cells develop as expressions of hyperparathyroidism (*"brown tumor" of hyperparathyroidism*) or represent a reparative lesion containing giant cells and developing on some other basis (*giant-cell reparative granuloma of jawbones*). In relation to the gums, the common "giant-cell epulis" is now frequently denoted as the *peripheral giant-cell reparative granuloma*, again with the aim of delimiting it from the conventional giant-cell tumor (see Bernier and Cahn).

## ODONTOGENIC CYSTS

As already indicated, the odontogenic cysts are those epithelial-lined cysts of jawbones whose occurrence is connected in some way with the teeth. The odontogenic cyst representing a sequela of dental infection is oriented to the root or roots of the infected tooth and is usually denoted in particular as a *periodontal* (or *radicular*) *cyst*. Those odontic cysts which have their origin in aberrations of dental development are referred to as *follicular cysts*. The latter are further subclassified into the *primordial* and the *dentigerous* cysts. A primordial follicular cyst is one which

### *Figure 132*

*A*, Roentgenograph showing a periodontal cyst of the residual type in the upper jaw. The patient was a man 43 years of age who had had many teeth extracted in both the upper and lower jaws because of dental infection, and the cyst illustrated is one which has developed or persisted after the extraction of infected teeth.

*B*, Roentgenograph showing a small periodontal cyst oriented to the apex of a tooth. Note the area of radiolucency beyond the root and the demarcation of the area peripherally by a narrow margin of radiopacity. The patient was a woman 37 years of age who gave a history of intermittent toothache of long standing. On extraction of the tooth, the cyst remained attached to the root (see *C*), as is often the case with such periapical radicular cysts.

*C*, Photomicrograph (× 35) illustrating the general architecture of the cyst attached to the root of the tooth shown in *B*. When opened, the cyst was found to contain some brownish flaky material. Note that the cyst merges with the periodontal membrane. That the wall of the cyst is heavily inflamed is also apparent, even under the low magnification shown.

*D*, Photomicrograph (× 125) showing the epithelial lining of the cyst wall removed in the case illustrated in *A*.

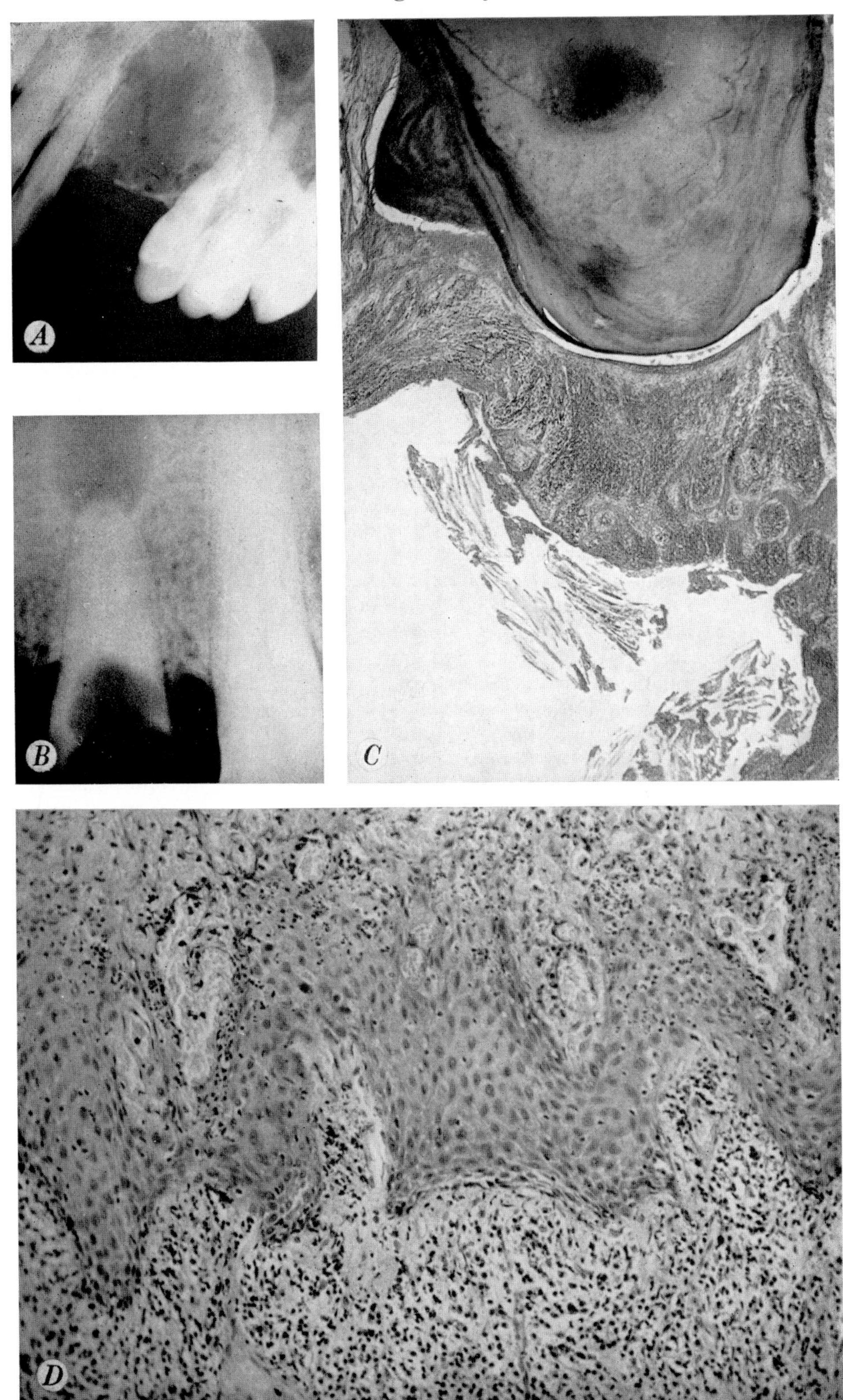


*Figure 132*

begins its development before the odontogenic epithelium of the evolving tooth germ has begun to lay down enamel. A dentigerous follicular cyst is one which begins its development from the enamel organ after the crown of the tooth has formed. (See Robinson, and Stafne and Millhon.)

## PERIODONTAL (RADICULAR) CYSTS

The periodontal cyst is a very common lesion. Practically always, it develops in the wake of a pulp infection associated with the formation of inflammatory granulation tissue about the root or roots of a nonvital tooth. The lesion is found more often in the maxilla than in the mandible, and a majority of the subjects are middle-aged. In the maxilla the cyst is usually located in the anterior part of the bone, while in the mandible it tends to have a posterior location.

When a periodontal cyst is oriented to the apex of the tooth, as it usually is, it is also called a *periapical* cyst. If the cyst is one which has developed or persists after extraction of an infected tooth, it is sometimes also denoted as a *residual* cyst. A periodontal cyst which is found oriented along the sides of the root is often referred to as a *lateral* cyst. The lateral periodontal cysts are rare and are not necessarily of infectious-inflammatory origin.

In the evolution of a periodontal cyst, the infection spreads from the dental pulp through a foramen or a perforation into the periodontal membrane and beyond it. A focus of inflammatory granulation tissue forms about the root of the affected tooth. Sooner or later the granulation tissue becomes enveloped by a layer of epithelium. This is derived from the epithelial cells which are very likely to be lying dormant in the periapical tissues. In the further evolution of the cyst, fluid transudates into the area, the granulation tissue liquefies, and the epithelial lining coat comes to be enveloped by a coat of fibrous connective tissue. As the cyst enlarges, it destroys the neighboring osseous tissue of the jawbone. If the cyst grows to considerable size, it may even thin the cortex and expand the bone contour in the part of the bone where it is located. A periodontal cyst spreading in a lateral direction may even push unaffected teeth aside.

When the presence of a periodontal cyst is associated with clinical complaints, these are likely to consist of localized pain and swelling, and if there is drainage from the cyst into the oral cavity, there may be a "bad taste" in the mouth. Roentgenographically, the cyst shows up as a smaller or larger area of "nonloculated" radiolucency oriented to the root of a tooth. (See Fig. 132.) Fairly often, it is demarcated peripherally by a narrow margin of radiopacity, but this may be absent if the cyst is heavily infected. As to treatment, a periodontal cyst is ordinarily managed by extracting the affected tooth and excising the related cyst wall *in toto* (see Thoma, and Nathan).

When opened, the cyst is often found to contain purulent fluid. On microscopic examination of the cyst wall, one finds that its lining epithelium consists of a thin layer of squamous epithelial cells. The lining cells may be ulcerated in some places, while in other places the epithelium may present evidences of reparative proliferation. The cyst wall itself is likely to be permeated by leukocytes, lymphocytes, and other inflammatory cells. Occasionally a mandible containing a large periodontal cyst becomes so weakened that a pathologic fracture occurs through the cystic area. A large cyst located in a maxilla may break into the maxillary sinus.

As to differential diagnosis, it is usually hard to distinguish histologically between the wall of a periodontal cyst and the wall of an infected follicular cyst. The differentiation has to be made on the basis of the clinical and *x*-ray findings. Specifically, one has to ask whether the cyst was oriented to the root of the tooth, indicating that one was dealing with a periodontal cyst, or to the crown of an unerupted tooth, as it is in connection with the common or dentigerous type of follicular cyst. However, it is often difficult to distinguish even roentgenographically between a residual periodontal cyst and a primordial follicular cyst (see below).

## FOLLICULAR CYSTS

As already pointed out, those epithelial-lined odontogenic cysts which result from an aberration in dental development are known as follicular cysts. They are much less common than the periodontal cysts. Follicular cysts may begin their development early or late in the course of evolution of the implicated tooth, and are subclassified accordingly as *primordial* and *dentigerous* cysts. Multiple (multilocular) follicular cysts are occasionally encountered. They may be of the primordial or the dentigerous type alone, or may represent a combination of the two types. Occasionally the epithelial lining of a follicular cyst undergoes tumorous proliferation, resulting in the formation of an ameloblastoma or, very rarely, an epidermoid carcinoma.

**Dentigerous Cyst.**—This is the more common type of follicular cyst. It is encountered somewhat more often in the mandible than in the maxilla. It starts its development after the crown of the tooth has already been formed. The tooth implicated is nearly always a permanent or a supernumerary tooth. The cyst is often symptomless and therefore may not be discovered until years after it has developed. In the treatment of dentigerous cysts (as of follicular cysts in general) it is important to remove the cyst wall completely, in view of its malignant potentialities (see Cahn, and Sonesson).

The development of a dentigerous cyst seems to be instigated by the occurrence of regressive changes in the stellate reticulum of the enamel organ. Fluid accumulates within the latter, and it becomes detached from the crown. As more and more fluid gathers, the neighboring connective tissue becomes compressed to form the fibrous coat of the cyst. The lining epithelium of the cyst wall is apparently derived from the external epithelial layer of the enamel organ. The cyst formation hinders the eruption of the implicated tooth. As the lesion grows larger, it destroys the local spongiosa of the jawbone. If it grows very large, it may even thin the cortex and expand the contour of the implicated area of the bone. In the $x$-ray picture the cyst shows up as a focus of radiolucency which is usually surrounded by a zone of margination. The tooth around which it has developed can be visualized unless, of course, the tooth has been extracted in a previous surgical intervention against the cyst. (See Fig. 133.)

When the lesion is entered in the course of its surgical removal, the fluid it contains may be found to be either amber colored and clear, or much darker and cloudy. If the cyst has become infected, it may even contain pus. The tooth within the cyst is generally of normal structure, although its roots may be stunted.

The cyst wall is composed of fibrous connective tissue and is usually attached to the periodontal membrane at the neck of the tooth. Evidence of inflammation of the wall is lacking unless the cyst has become infected. The inner lining of the cyst wall is a layer of stratified squamous epithelium. This lining layer may be intact throughout, or may be ulcerated in places. Cholesterol crystals surrounded by foreign-body giant cells may be seen on the surface and even within the wall of the cyst. In some cysts the epithelial lining cells may be found keratinized in places and/or undergoing hypertrophy. In the latter connection one may note papillary projections of epithelium into the lumen and/or proliferation of epithelial buds from the basal layer of the epithelial lining. It is because the epithelial lining of a dentigerous cyst is derived from the enamel organ that this lining (like the lining of follicular cysts in general) has the potentiality of forming an ameloblastoma. This happens only rarely, but if it does occur, the cyst space may come to be substantially occupied by a more or less solid tumor of this type.

**Primordial Cyst.**—As already implied, a primordial cyst develops through cystification of odontogenic epithelium before the latter has differentiated to secrete enamel and before the mesenchymal papilla of the evolving tooth has formed dentin and pulp. Thus it is distinguished from the dentigerous cyst by its earlier appearance and by the fact that it does not contain the crown of a tooth, the development of a tooth having been arrested. However, in the histopathology of its sac, it is entirely similar to the dentigerous cyst.

A primordial cyst is located most often in the third molar region of the mandible. Thus it usually involves the angle of that bone and frequently extends into the ascending ramus. Indeed, any cyst, whether unilocular or multilocular, which is located in the ramus and which is not obviously associated with a tooth is usually a primordial cyst. The cyst is most often discovered while the subject is still young, but sometimes not until adult life has been reached. In whatever part of a jawbone the primordial cyst is noted, a tooth will be missing from the dental arch, unless the cyst has arisen from the germ of a supernumerary tooth.

In the *x*-ray picture the lesion shows up as a focus of radiolucency surrounded by a narrow zone of radiopacity. If the lesional area appears multilocular, as it not infrequently does, clinical differentiation from ameloblastoma (p. 442) may be difficult. Furthermore, in connection with an edentulous jaw, the differentiation between a primordial cyst and a residual periodontal cyst is also not very readily made on the basis of the *x*-ray picture.

## NONODONTOGENIC CYSTS

The nonodontogenic cysts—those cysts whose occurrence is not connected with dental infection or maldevelopment—fall into two main categories (see Fig. 134). One group comprises those which are lined by epithelium. These *epithelialized cysts* are usually subclassified on the basis of pathogenesis into the *fissural cysts* and the *vestigial cysts*. The fissural cysts are, in a sense, epithelial inclusion cysts.

***Figure 133***

*A*, Roentgenograph showing a follicular cyst containing the crown of a molar and located in a mandible. This dentigerous follicular cyst expanded the contour of the affected part of the mandible, and it was the resulting facial asymmetry that led to discovery of the lesion. The cyst was extirpated *in toto*, and the topography of the lining of the cyst wall is shown in *C*.

*B*, Roentgenograph showing a somewhat larger dentigerous follicular cyst which has developed in relation to the crown of the second lower molar.

*C*, Photomicrograph (× 165) showing a thick layer of stratified epithelium which lined the inner surface of the dentigerous cyst removed from the lesion illustrated in *A*. Note the absence of evidences of infection, in contrast to what one regularly encounters on microscopic examination of the wall of a periodontal cyst.

*D*, Roentgenograph showing a very large follicular cyst in a mandible. In this case the cyst wall showed evidence of ameloblastomatous transformation (see *E*). The patient was a man 63 years of age, and, though the cyst had undoubtedly been present for many years, the complaints (swelling of the jaw, later associated with some pain) were of only a few months' standing at the time of his admission to the hospital.

*E*, Photomicrograph (× 65) showing the histologic pattern presented in some places by the wall of the follicular cyst illustrated in *D*. Note that epithelial cells in cord and follicle formation lie deep in the connective-tissue wall of the cyst, constituting the evidence of ameloblastic transformation.

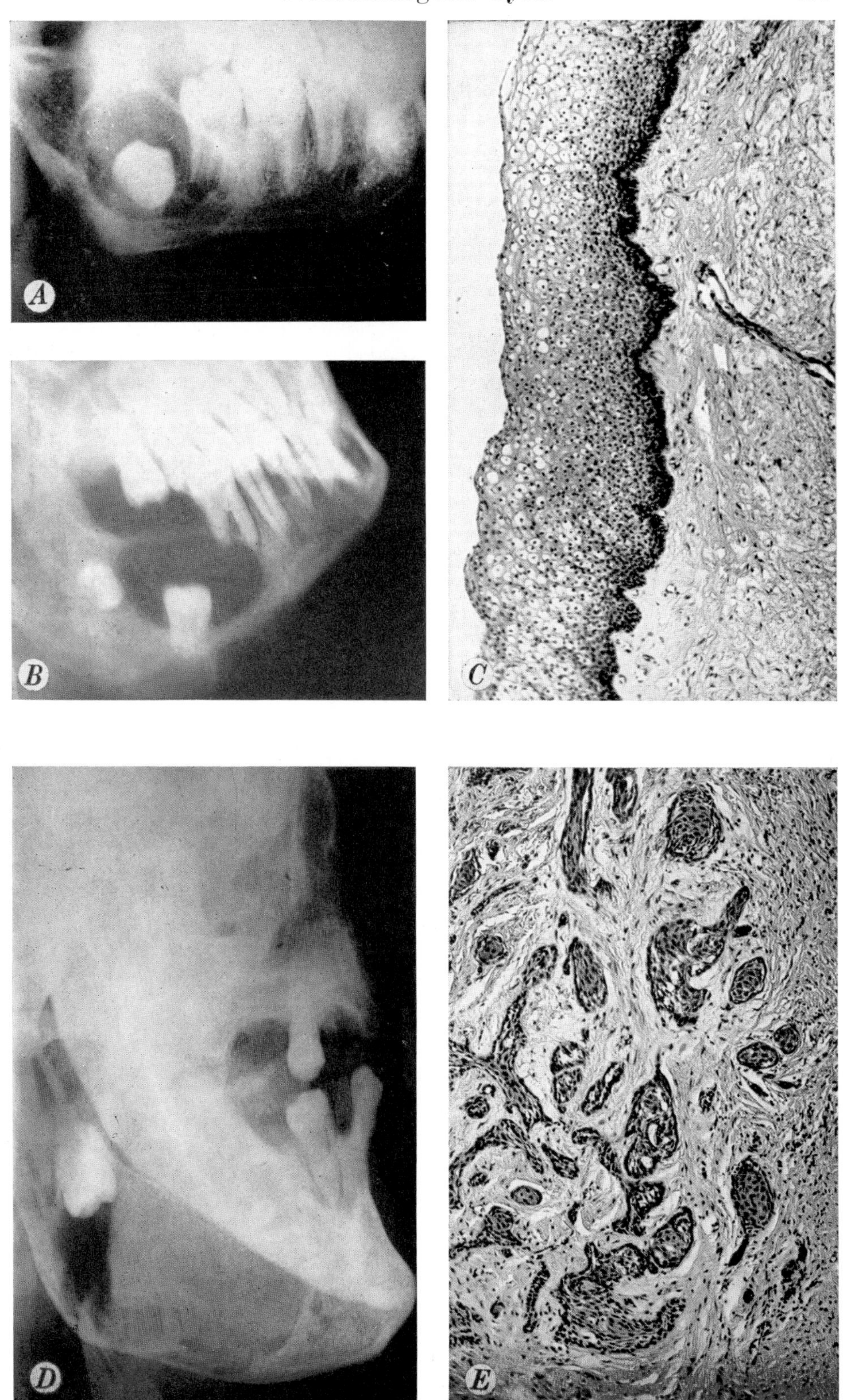


*Figure 133*

Their epithelium is apparently derived from epithelium which has become entrapped somewhere along the fissural (fusion) lines of the various component parts of the developing jawbones during early embryonic life. The vestigial cysts develop from vestiges of the nasopalatine duct. The other category of nonodontogenic cyst—the *nonepithelialized cyst*—is represented by a bone cavity usually filled with fluid and lined at most by an attenuated connective-tissue membrane. In the pathogenesis of this type of cyst, trauma has usually been inculpated, but actually its connection with trauma is doubtful, as will be brought out later.

## FISSURAL AND VESTIGIAL CYSTS

As already indicated, epithelial cells may become trapped, early in embryonic life, in the fissures between still unfused component parts of the maxillæ and the mandible and eventually give rise to cysts. The fissural inclusion cysts are uncommon. They are usually subclassified as follows, in accordance with their locations: the *median* cyst, the *globulomaxillary* cyst, and the *naso-alveolar* cyst. A cyst derived from vestiges of the embryonic nasopalatine duct is referred to as a *nasopalatine* cyst. It is encountered even more rarely than the fissural cysts.

**Median Cysts.**—These develop in the median fissure between the two parts of the mandible or the median fissure between the maxillæ. In relation to the upper jaw, a median cyst may be located between the roots of the central incisors, in which case it is denoted as an "alveolar median cyst." Or it may be located in the posterior part of the palate, in which case it is denoted as a "palatine median cyst." In any case, when entered, a median cyst is usually found to contain some fluid. Its wall is a thick layer of fibrous connective tissue whose inner surface is lined by stratified squamous epithelium.

**Globulomaxillary Cyst.**—This type of fissural cyst forms at the site of fusion of the globular and maxillary processes of the upper jaw. It develops in the alveolar bone between the roots of the lateral incisor and canine and pushes these roots apart. If it is still rather small, the cyst usually appears in the *x*-ray picture as a unilocular radiolucent area of teardrop shape which occupies the alveolar bone be-

### *Figure 134*

*A*, Roentgenograph illustrating a median fissural cyst in the upper jaw between the roots of the central incisors. The patient was a man 30 years of age who had no complaints referable to the condition, the lesion being discovered incidentally in the course of routine *x*-ray examination of the teeth.

*B*, Roentgenograph showing a globulomaxillary cyst of the upper jaw. Note that the roots of the lateral incisor and canine are pushed apart in the manner characteristic of this lesion. The patient was a man 19 years of age who presented merely a slight swelling of the gum.

*C*, Photomicrograph (× 65) illustrating the histologic pattern of the wall of a nasopalatine cyst. Note that the lining cells are columnar rather than squamous cells and that many of the cells are goblet cells.

*D*, Roentgenograph showing a nonepithelialized cyst (so-called traumatic cyst) in a mandible. Note the loculated appearance of the cyst and the scalloping between the roots of the teeth in its vicinity. The patient was a boy 17 years of age, and the lesion was discovered incidentally in the course of routine *x*-ray examination of the teeth. The histologic appearance of the cyst wall in this case is shown in *E*.

*E*, Photomicrograph (× 25) illustrating the attenuated cortex of the mandible. Applied to the inner surface of the cortex (top) is an extremely attenuated connective-tissue membrane.

(The writer is indebted to Doctor Theodor Blum and the New York Institute of Clinical Oral Pathology for the material illustrated.)

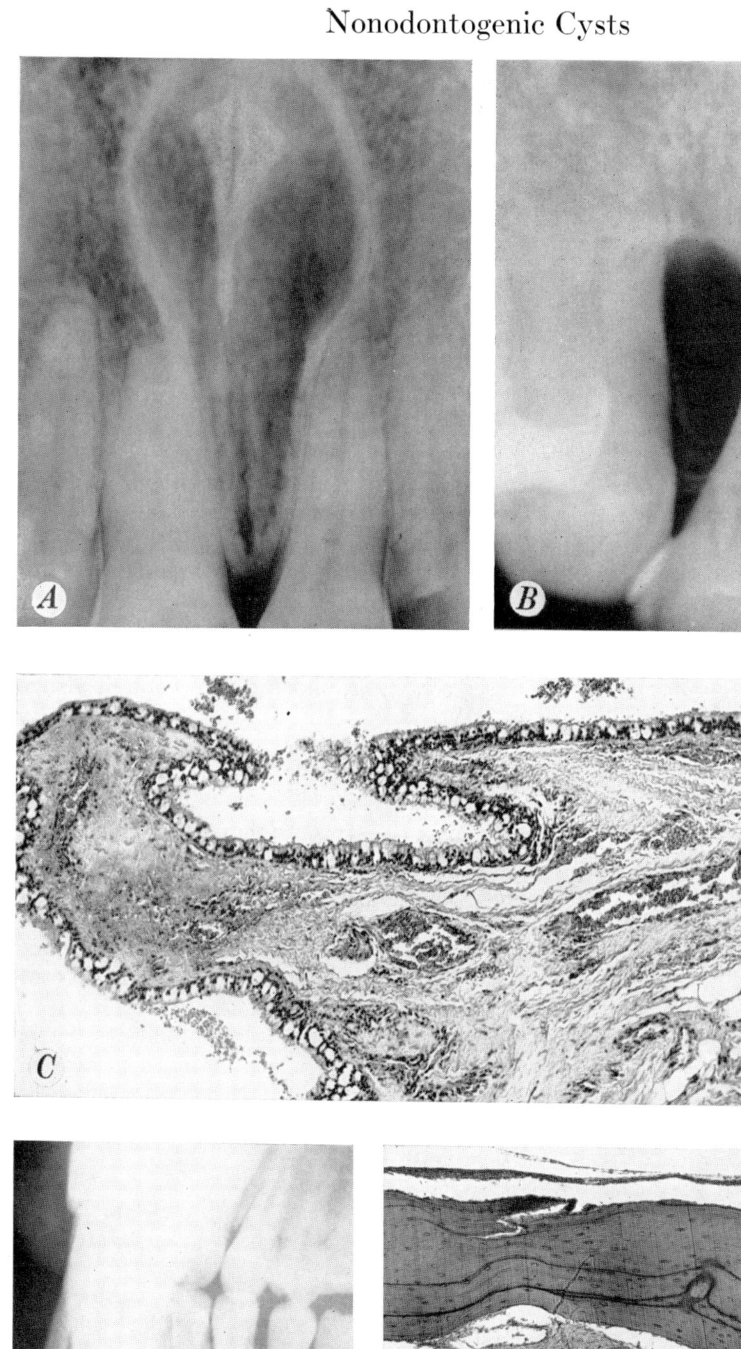


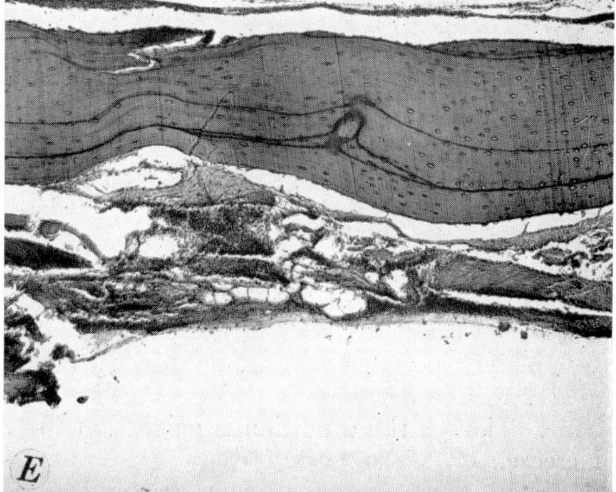


*Figure 134*

tween the teeth in question. As it grows larger, the cyst extends beyond the apices of the teeth and may cause destruction of at least the premaxillary portion of the palate. Because this cyst is oriented to the apices of the teeth, it may easily be mistaken for a periodontal radicular cyst, especially if it reaches a large size. The cyst wall is composed of a thick, firm membrane of connective tissue whose inner surface is lined by epithelium. The latter is usually a layer of stratified squamous cells, but in some places the lining cells may be ciliated columnar cells.

**Naso-alveolar Cyst.**—This cyst forms where the globular, lateral, nasal, and maxillary processes meet, and gives rise to a swelling at the site of attachment of the wing of the nose. Such a cyst tends to be located on or near the surface of the bone rather than within it (see Schroff). As it grows, the cyst encroaches on the nasal cavity, causing a bulging inside the nostril. The fluid content of the cyst is usually of a mucous consistency and brownish color. The inner lining of its tissue sac is composed of cylindrical epithelial cells interspersed with goblet cells.

**Nasopalatine Cyst.**—As noted, this type of cyst has its origin in epithelial vestiges of the nasopalatine ducts. It may develop in one of the incisive canals or in both simultaneously. As it enlarges, it produces a swelling on one or both sides along the midline of the anterior portion of the hard palate, or in the floor of the nares. If the cyst has become infected, as it frequently does, it may be tender and painful and there may be an intermittent discharge from it. The fibrous coat of the cyst is likely to be quite thick, especially if the cyst has become inflamed. The epithelial lining cells may be squamous or columnar, and the fluid content accordingly serous or mucoid.

## NONEPITHELIALIZED CYSTS

This type of cyst is of rather rare occurrence. It represents a jawbone cavity usually filled with fluid and ordinarily lined by an extremely attenuated connective-tissue membrane. Indeed, it resembles the so-called solitary bone cyst familiar particularly in relation to the humerus and other long tubular bones (p. 63).

Blum, who was among the first to describe this type of cyst, held that it develops in the wake of trauma and hence denoted it as the "traumatic bone cyst." Most other workers, too, favor the idea of a traumatic origin for this lesion, and accordingly it has also been called the "hemorrhagic extravasation cyst" and the "solitary (hemorrhagic) cyst" (see Rushton and Cantab, and Waldron). In giving consideration to the possible causative role of trauma, it is to be noted that the patient does not usually inculpate a trauma spontaneously, and that the traumatic incident elicited on questioning often occurred years before the cyst was discovered. In view of the frequency with which trauma is suffered by jawbones (particularly the mandible) and the rarity of solitary jawbone cysts, it seems justifiable to doubt the causal role of trauma in this connection (see Jaffe). In discussing the pathogenesis of the solitary cyst of long tubular bones, the writer critically reviewed and rejected the role of trauma which had been proposed as the underlying cause for these cysts, too. An alternative explanation (and a much more plausible one in the writer's opinion) is that the cysts in both these locations represent the consequence of an aberration in the development and growth of the local osseous tissue.

The nonepithelialized jawbone cyst nearly always occurs in the mandible. In relation to this bone it is most often found in the subapical region, on the right or left side of the body of the bone, and most often in the posterior part of it. It is seen mainly in young persons, most of the patients being between 10 and 20 years of age. Clinically, there is likely to be some enlargement of the affected part of the bone. Though the condition is painless at first, pain may develop and gradually increase.

Roentgenographically, the cyst presents as a more or less circumscribed uniform or somewhat trabeculated rarefaction shadow usually having no sharply delimited radiopaque border. The periodontal lamella about the roots of the teeth in the vicinity of the cyst is ordinarily intact. Scalloping of the bone between the teeth is often to be seen.

When the cyst is entered surgically, it is generally found to contain serous fluid if there has been no presurgical hemorrhage into the cyst. Under these circumstances the latter is found lined, as already noted, merely by a very attenuated connective-tissue membrane. If there has been hemorrhage, the surface of the lining membrane may have adherent to it, in some places, organizing blood clot and some multinuclear giant cells. The cortex of the mandible in the neighborhood of the cyst is likely to be found attenuated through resorption, in consequence of the pressure exerted upon it. Treatment of the condition consists of surgical evacuation of the fluid content, followed by curettage.

## ODONTOGENIC TUMORS

The odontogenic tumors are those jawbone tumors whose constituent tissue suggests in its cytologic pattern one or another of the patterns produced by the odontogenic mesoderm and/or odontogenic ectoderm in the course of the evolution of teeth. The odontogenic *myxoma* is composed throughout of a loose primitive connective tissue suggestive of the mesenchymal elements encountered in the tooth germ. The *cementoma* represents a somewhat more differentiated odontogenic connective-tissue tumor characterized by the presence of various amounts of cementum in the lesional tissue. A jawbone tumor showing a considerable amount of dentin in its connective-tissue substratum could be denoted as a *dentinoma,* but this type of lesion is rare, and it is probably not important to separate it from the odontomas (see below).

The *ameloblastoma* is composed essentially of epithelium, and it derives its name from the fact that the arrangement of its epithelial cells runs the gamut of the patterns observed in the developing and/or differentiating enamel organ of the tooth. The ameloblastomas do not lay down enamel. However, the existence of the small, clinically unimportant malformation known as the *enameloma* should at least be mentioned. This consists of a pearl-like deposit of enamel which is apparently formed from remnants of the enamel organ and usually appears at the base of the tooth root.

Finally, the odontogenic tumors include the *odontomas.* The odontoma is a tumor-like malformation containing both mesodermal and epithelial odontogenic tissues, alone or in association with their calcified derivatives (enamel, dentin, and cementum). In its most highly differentiated form an odontoma consists of organized tooth structures or even actual teeth.

### MYXOMA

The so-called myxoma of jawbones is a benign tumor of rather rare occurrence. It may appear in either jaw, and the subject is usually a young person. As will be indicated, the clinical and anatomic peculiarities of the myxoma of jawbones are such as to make it highly probable that that lesion is a tumor indigenous to the jawbones, despite the fact that myxomas also occur in soft parts. The tumor usually develops insidiously and may have come to occupy a large part of the affected bone before its presence is discovered. The presenting complaint may be merely local swelling of the involved jawbone.

In the $x$-ray picture the lesional area presents as a rather large focus of radiolucency which may show coarse or delicate trabeculation (see Fig. 135). Since these findings may be associated with the absence of a tooth, or the presence of a partly erupted or an unerupted tooth, they may suggest the possibility of an ameloblastoma or a follicular cyst. Thus, as is so often the case with jawbone tumors, definitive treatment must await study of a biopsy specimen. The treatment for these cases is radical local excision of the tumor area, but not necessarily block resection of the affected part of the bone.

Grossly, the cut surface of the lesional tissue has a slimy, mucoid appearance. Microscopically, the tissue presents the pattern of rather sparse stellate or somewhat elongated cells set in a basophilic mucoid intercellular material in which variable amounts of reticulin and collagen fibers may also be imbedded. Some lesions may be more collagenous than others, but there is hardly enough difference to justify a subcategory of "fibromyxoma of jawbones." On the whole, the myxoma of jawbones resembles the myxoma of soft tissues anatomically. However, its clinical behavior is unlike that of the latter lesion.

As indicated, the myxoma of jawbones is an essentially benign lesion and does not exhibit aggressive qualities. In contrast, the myxoma of soft tissues, while it does not tend to metastasize, is an aggressive lesion which is likely to recur again and again unless the first surgical intervention consists of radical local excision. Another point tending to confirm the odontogenic nature of the myxoma of jawbones is the fact that the lesion does not seem to have any exact counterpart among the tumorous lesions of the bones of the limbs or thorax. The lesion which it comes nearest to resembling is the chondromyxoid fibroma of bone (p. 203), and even here the histologic similarity is not very close.

## CEMENTOMA

A cementoma is a tumorous lesion of jawbones which is apparently derived from odontogenic connective tissue and which is further characterized by the formation of cementum in the lesional tissue (see Stafne, and Bernier and Thompson). In some cementomas the basic spindle cell stroma overshadows the cement material. Such a cementoma may be designated as a *fibrocementoma*, but is sometimes also denoted as a "cementoblastoma" or as an "odontogenic fibroma." In a fibrocemen-

***Figure 135***

*A*, Roentgenograph of a myxoma in the maxilla. Note the delicate trabeculation of the lesional area, which on the whole is radiolucent. The patient was a woman 23 years of age who complained merely of swelling of the upper jaw. Local resection of the lesional area resulted in cure. (The $x$-ray picture in this case was supplied by Doctor Theodor Blum and the New York Institute of Clinical Oral Pathology.)

*B*, Roentgenograph showing a large radiolucent area resulting from the presence of a myxoma in the mandible. In this case the rather characteristic delicate trabeculation was absent.

*C*, Photomicrograph (× 250) illustrating the histologic appearance typical for the tissue of a myxoma of a jawbone. Note the sparse, somewhat elongated stellate cells, set in a loose intercellular substance. Though a myxoma may have some collagen fibers, these are never so abundant as in the lesion shown in *D*.

*D*, Photomicrograph (× 125) illustrating the appearance of a highly collagenized desmoplastic fibroma. This type of connective-tissue growth is not an odontogenic tumor. While occasionally observed in a jawbone, it is more often seen in extracranial skeletal areas. The desmoplastic fibroma (p. 298) is a benign lesion, apparently never metastasizing although it shows a tendency to recur.

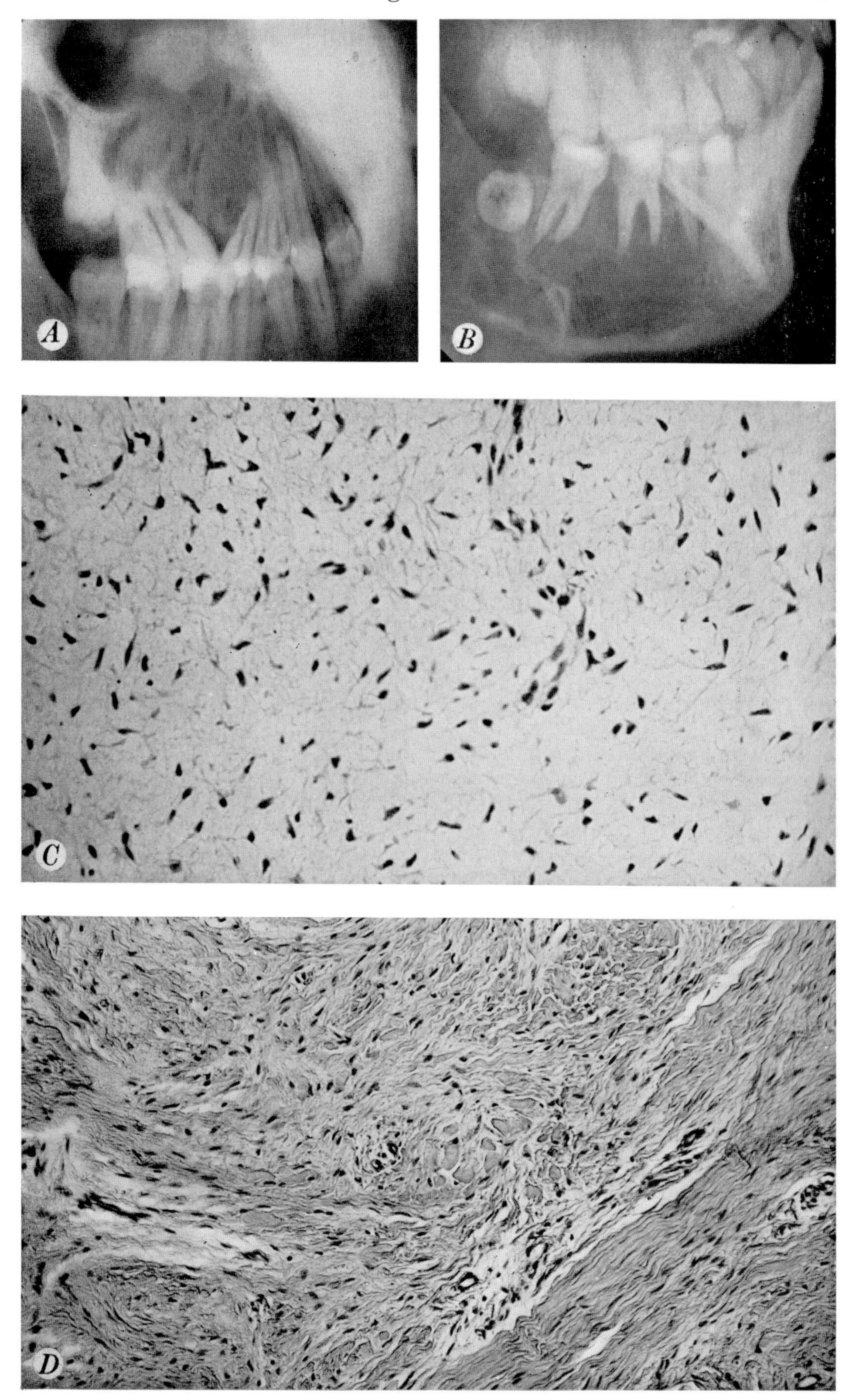


***Figure 135***

toma the cement material consists largely of cementicles and/or spherites of cementum, which may be rather sparse in some lesions and even fairly abundant in others. Much more commonly, however, the cementum in a cementoma is so abundant that the fibrous tissue substratum of the lesion may be completely submerged, perhaps throughout the lesion. Such a cementoma may be designated as a *sclerosing cementoma,* since it often consists to a large extent of compacted and highly calcified masses of cementum. (See Figs. 136 and 137.)

**Fibrocementoma.**—The fibrocementoma is a rather rare lesion. It may affect either jawbone, though it is more commonly encountered in the mandible. In a mandible it generally presents as a fairly large expansile lesion which shows up in the *x*-ray picture as a more or less delimited focus of radiolucency within which some radiopacities are observed, especially in the subapical part of the lesional area. On the other hand, the involved part of the bone may cast an almost uniformly radiolucent shadow or, if such cementum as is present is evenly distributed through the lesional tissue, the shadow may be faintly cloudy. The lesion may grow to such size that the contour of the bone becomes very much bulged, and the cortex may even be destroyed in some places, though the periosteum is not likely to be violated.

On microscopic examination one notes that the stromal cells are numerous and oval or slightly more elongated. Cementicle formation is inaugurated by spotty deposition of intercellular substance between the stromal cells. The intercellular substance becomes calcified. The cementicles emerge as small roundish bodies which, in sections stained with hematoxylin and eosin, show a dark, granular interior having a more or less lamellated configuration, and a light, pink periphery.

It is commonly held that the lesion we are calling the sclerosing cementoma represents the terminal evolutionary stage of the fibrocementoma. However, though the two varieties of cementoma apparently have a common histogenic basis, they seem to develop along different lines, the sclerosing cementoma usually laying down large amounts of cementum from the start. Nevertheless, the question arises of whether an occasional fibrocementoma may lay down so much cementum in the course of its evolution that one would be justified in calling the ultimate lesion a sclerosing cementoma. In the writer's opinion, this possibility does exist, but the problem of nomenclature would arise only in connection with an occasional exceptionally large sclerosing lesion which has bulged the contour of the bone.

### *Figure 136*

*A,* Roentgenograph showing a fibrocementoma located in a mandible of a young girl who had complained only of a local swelling and some tenderness. When the lesion was curetted, the tissue corresponding to the radiolucent part of it was found to be essentially spindle cell connective tissue, containing but little cementum (see Fig. 137-*A*).

*B,* Roentgenograph of a molar tooth which has a very condensed and sclerotic mass of cementum attached to its roots. The patient was a woman 40 years of age, and the sclerosing cementoma in question was localized to the mandible in the region of that tooth.

*C,* Roentgenograph showing a sclerosing cementoma in a mandible. The patient was a woman 36 years of age, and the lesion in the mandible was found in the course of routine *x*-ray examination of the teeth. The histologic pattern of the lesional tissue in this case is shown in Figure 137-*B*.

*D,* Roentgenograph showing involvement of the lower and also the upper jaw by a sclerosing cementoma. The patient was a woman 57 years of age who was aware of progressive swelling of the jaws for a period of 5 years before this roentgenograph was taken. Clinical examination showed that the gum over the front part of the enlarged mandible was ulcerated. The pattern of the tissue removed from the front part of the mandible is shown in Fig. 137-*C*.

*E,* Roentgenograph showing a very extensive sclerosing cementoma affecting the upper jaw. The patient in this case, too, was a woman.

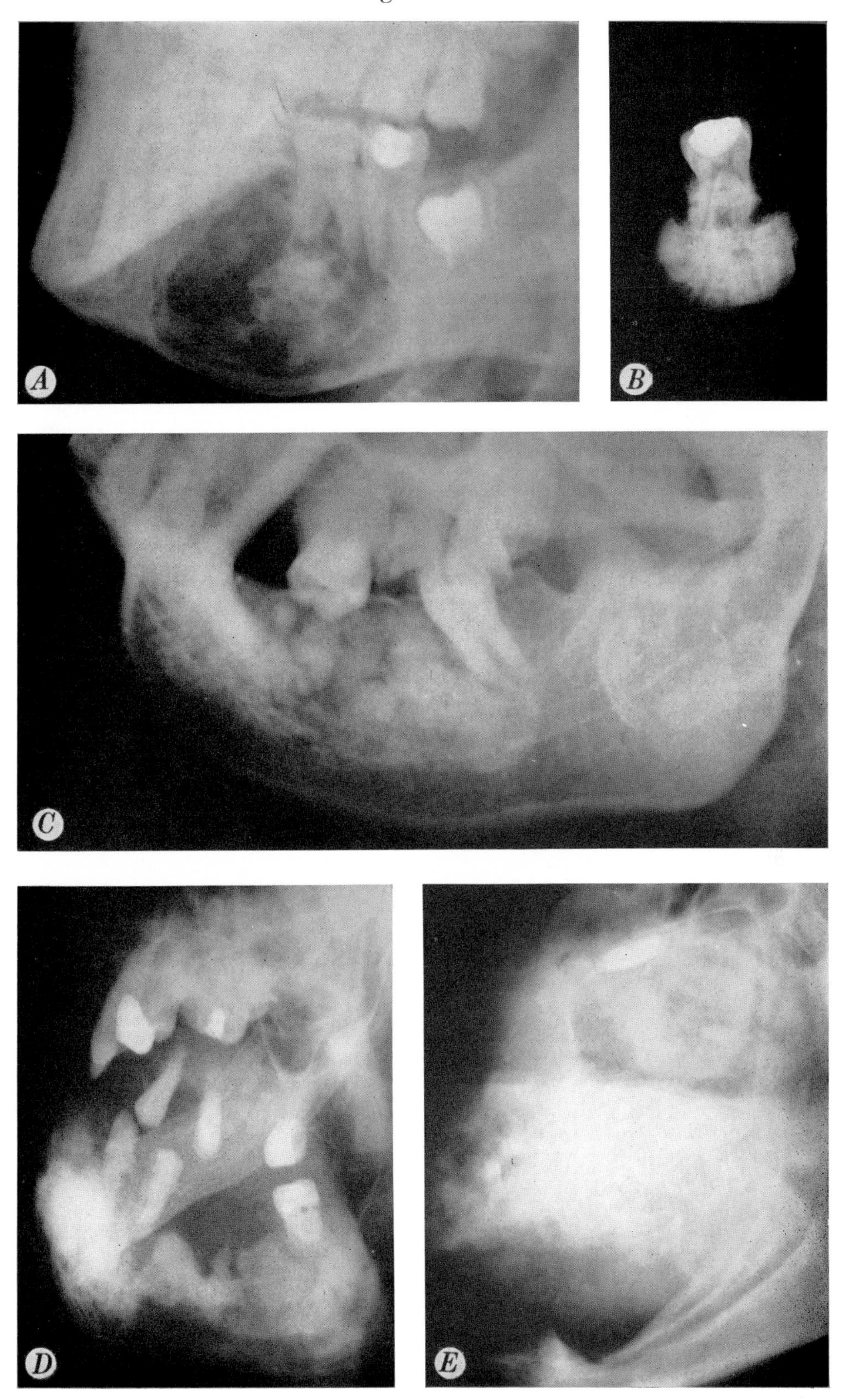


*Figure 136*

The problem of nomenclature and differential diagnosis of fibrocementoma has to be considered also in relation to fibrous osteoma (ossifying fibroma) and fibrous dysplasia of jawbones. There can be no doubt that occasionally a case of fibrocementoma is misinterpreted as a case of fibrous osteoma of a jawbone. The latter jawbone lesion is composed of intermingled fibrous connective tissue and osseous tissue (not cementum) in various proportions. Furthermore, the fibrous tissue substratum in this lesion is not odontogenic but osteogenic connective tissue. Thus, the fibrocementoma should be kept distinct from the fibrous osteoma or ossifying fibroma of jawbones (p. 136).

On the same basis, fibrocementoma of jawbones should be delimited from fibrous dysplasia of jawbones. It is true that the writer has stated in another connection that the fibrocementoma may be regarded as the odontogenic counterpart of fibrous (fibro-osseous) dysplasia appearing in a jawbone (see Jaffe). However, he believes that the two lesions should nevertheless be held apart. Certainly a considerable amount of confusion is introduced in regard to both cementoma and fibrous dysplasia if they are not. This confusion is compounded if, as some have done, one counts even small sclerosing cementomas as belonging in the category of fibrous dysplasia.

**Sclerosing Cementoma.**—This lesion is not at all uncommon. It is far more likely to be located in the lower than in the upper jaw, and in the anterior part of these bones than on the sides. It is seen much more often in females than in males, and the subjects are nearly always adults. The lesion develops within the jawbone and is usually oriented to the apex of one or more teeth. As a rule, the lesion is not a large one, and often it is not found to have increased in size even if it has been followed for years after it was first discovered. A small sclerosing cementoma often comes to light by chance in the course of *x*-ray examination of the teeth, the lesion not having given rise to any clinical complaints. On the other hand, an occasional sclerosing cementoma may involve the periapical region of many teeth, even causing expansion of the affected part of the jawbone, and also pain and other clinical complaints. Once in a while, also, an instance of sclerosing cementoma is encountered in which the condition is present on both sides of a jawbone or in both jawbones. In cases of multiple involvement, the extent of implication of the mandible is likely to be striking.

On microscopic examination a sclerosing cementoma is found to be composed essentially of cementicles which in many places have become matted and fused together into large concretions of cementum. In some areas where the cementum has become compacted, cement material may be apposed in layers upon the concretions. The resultant highly compacted and calcified masses then present a histologic appearance suggestive of condensed atypical osseous tissue rather than cementum. The amount of fibrous tissue present in a sclerosing cementoma is likely to vary considerably. In areas in which the cementicles are scattered, the

***Figure 137***

*A*, Photomicrograph (× 25) illustrating the histologic pattern of the fibrocementoma shown in Fig. 136-*A*. Note the spindle connective-tissue cells and the sparse cementicles.

*B*, Photomicrograph (× 25) showing the pattern of a moderately sclerosed cementoma. There is a considerable amount of cementum set in a fibrous stroma. The tissue in question came from the case illustrated in Fig. 136–*C*.

*C*, Photomicrograph (× 25) illustrating the histologic appearance of a highly sclerotic cementoma. Note the compacted cementicles. The tissue shown comes from the case illustrated in Fig. 136-*D*.

*D*, Photomicrograph (× 100) bringing out the histologic details of the compacted cementum shown in *C*.

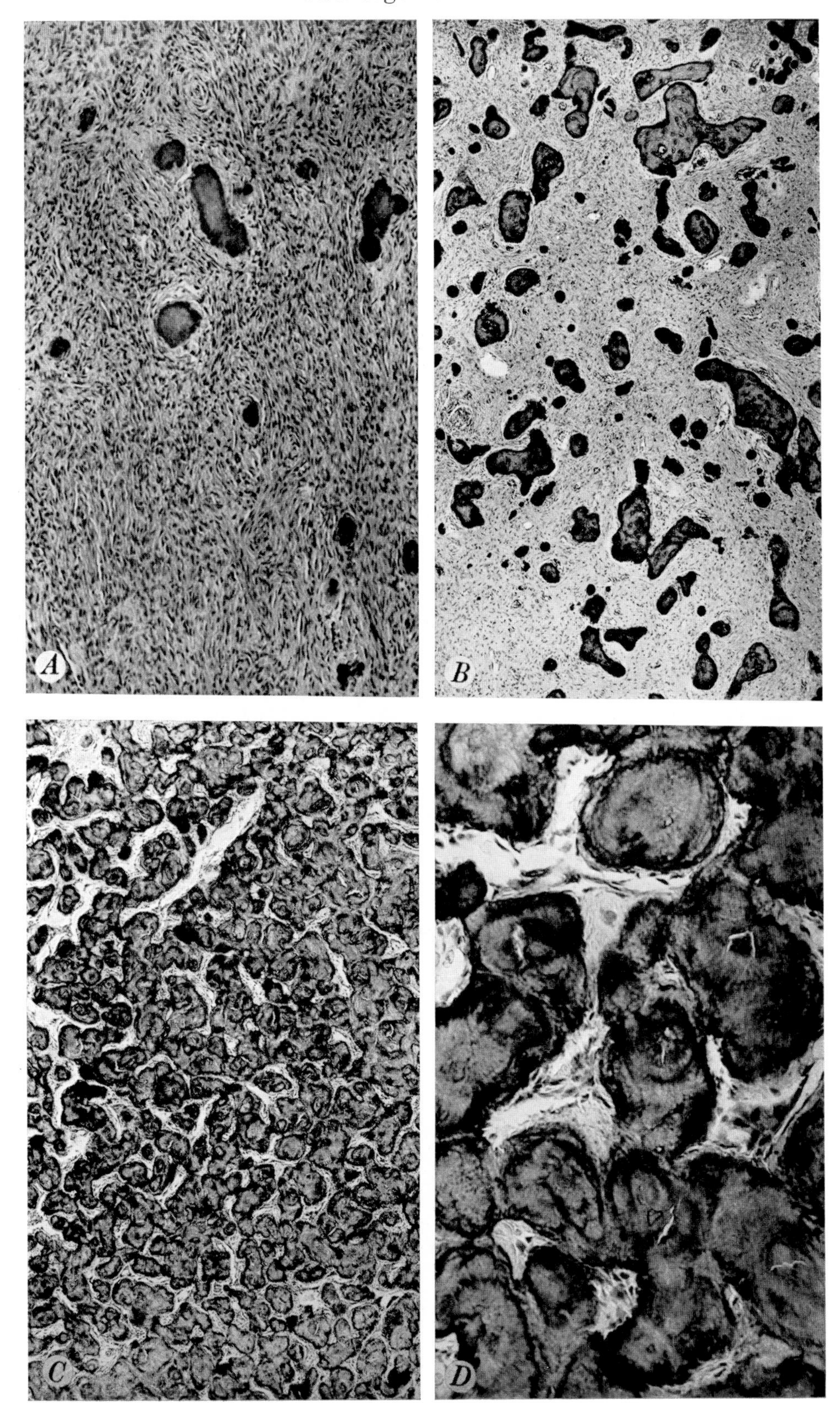


*Figure 137*

latter are usually found set in a rather cellular fibroblastic tissue. Between the large concretions of cementum the connective tissue is more sparse and somewhat collagenous. Indeed, in some fields there is very little connective tissue between the aggregations of cementum.

The anatomic composition of the cementoma is reflected in its roentgenographic appearances. Of course, the more cementum the lesion contains and the more densely it is compacted, the more radiopaque the lesion will appear. Areas in which the lesional tissue is essentially fibrous will appear radiolucent. Thus, in some cases the lesion shows up in the *x*-ray picture as a more or less uniformly radiopaque single roundish shadow. In other cases one sees smaller multiple juxtaposed roundish radiopacities separated by areas of radiolucency representing stromal tissue which has not yet become heavily calcified. It is conceivable that a small evolving lesion may present an essentially radiolucent shadow and hence be mistaken for a periodontal radicular cyst. This possibility of confusion results from the subapical location of the lesion, in association with its still meager cementum content.

## AMELOBLASTOMA

The ameloblastoma is a slowly growing epithelial tumor affecting the jawbones. Its name is derived from the fact that the cytologic tissue patterns produced by the proliferating tumor cells resemble those presented by the developing and/or differentiating enamel organ. However, in contrast to the epithelial cells of the enamel organ (ameloblasts), the tumor cells of the so-called ameloblastoma do not form enamel. The tumor is basically a benign lesion, but it tends to recur again and again if not radically extirpated. Eventually it may change its character and become a locally invasive malignant tumor which occasionally even metastasizes (see Sharp, Bullock, and Binkley).

It is more or less generally held that an ameloblastoma may take its origin from the epithelium which gives rise to the enamel organ, or from the evolved enamel organ or persisting cell rests of it. On the other hand, it is known that an ameloblastoma may develop from the epithelial lining of an odontogenic cyst. Furthermore, some hold that it may also form from the deep layer of the surface epithelium covering the jawbones. A point of special interest in connection with the ameloblastoma of jawbones is the fact that once in a great while one encounters in a long

### *Figure 138*

*A*, Roentgenograph showing an ameloblastoma involving the maxilla of a man 32 years of age. The diagnosis was established by examination of a biopsy specimen (see *E*), since it could not be made from the *x*-ray picture.

*B*, Roentgenograph showing an ameloblastoma involving the mandible. The patient was a boy 17 years of age who gave a history of local swelling of the mandible of 1 month's standing. On removal, the tumor was found to be a solid, firm tissue mass whose histologic pattern is illustrated in Fig. 139-*C*.

*C*, Roentgenograph showing an ameloblastoma in its typical location in a mandible. Note the multilocular appearance of the lesional area. The patient was a woman 52 years of age who had complained of pain and swelling in the lesional area over a period of 5 years. The histologic pattern of the lesional tissue removed in this case is illustrated in Fig. 139-*D*.

*D*, Roentgenograph showing the appearance of an ameloblastoma in an edentulous mandible. The patient was a woman 44 years of age who was admitted because of a slight swelling on the right side of the mandible. Note the multilocular appearance of the involved area.

*E*, Photomicrograph (× 65) showing the histologic tissue pattern of the ameloblastoma of the maxilla illustrated in *A*.

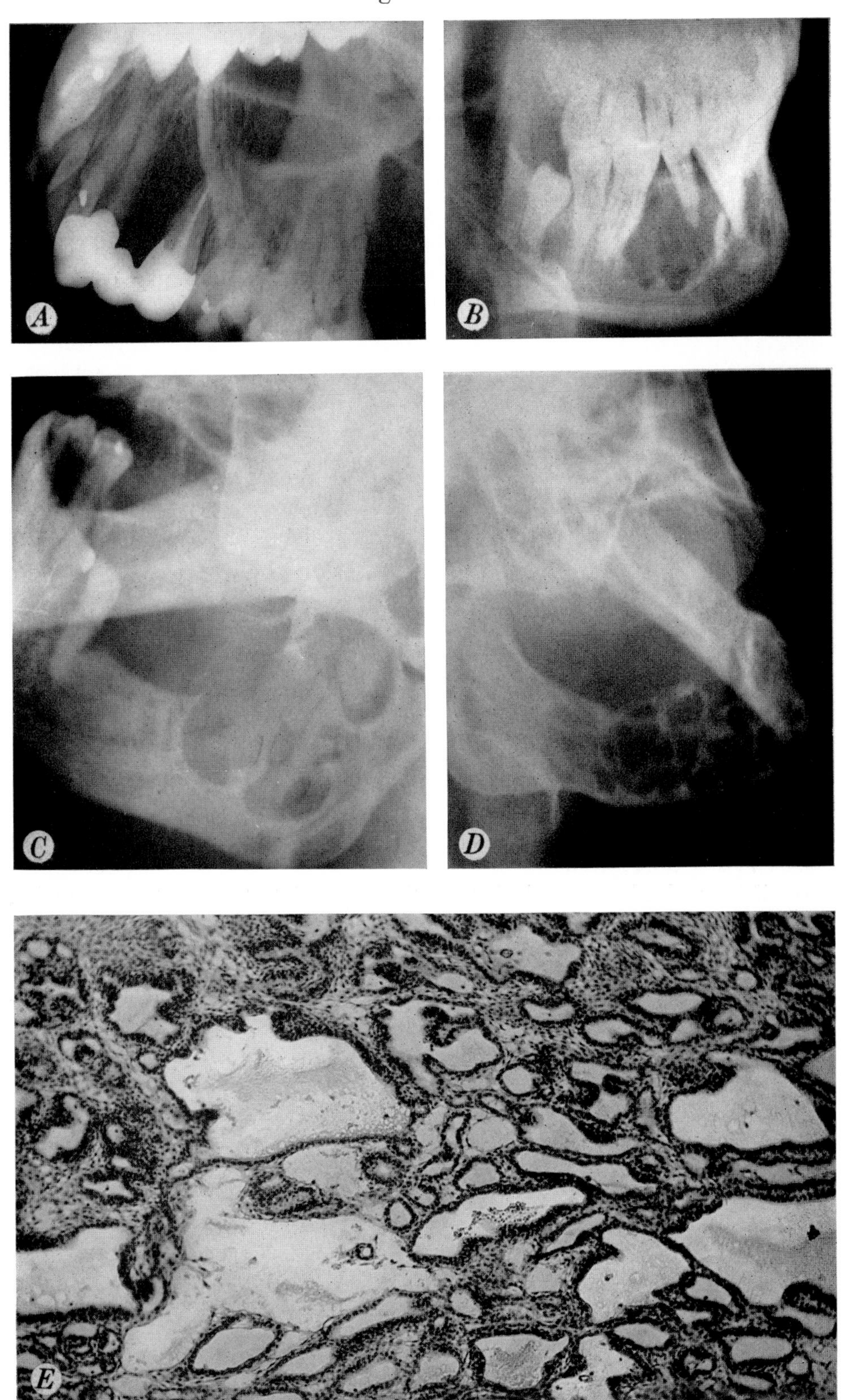


*Figure 138*

bone (usually a tibia) a tumor whose cytologic pattern simulates that of the jawbone lesion. The extracranial lesion in question, whose pathogenesis is obscure, is commonly denoted as the adamantinoma of limb bones (see p. 213).

The mandible is much more often the site for an ameloblastoma than the maxilla (see Fig. 138). The lesion is observed somewhat more commonly in males than in females. The subject is frequently a young adult when the lesion is discovered, but may even be a child or an old person.

There is nothing distinctive about the complaints and clinical findings. The tumor may be present without giving rise to complaints and be discovered in the course of routine *x*-ray examination of the teeth. On the other hand, it may be a painless swelling of the jaw that leads to detection of the lesion. Sooner or later, however, there are complaints of pain, and this is likely to be noted earlier when the tumor is in the upper jaw than when it is in the lower.

In the *x*-ray picture the lesion frequently presents as a rather large, multilocular, radiolucent shadow in the affected part of the bone, associated with local expansion of its contour. Less commonly, it presents as a unilocular rarefaction shadow. If the lesional area contains a tooth, one might think, from the picture, that one was dealing with a dentigerous cyst. Indeed, the roentgenographic differential diagnosis between ameloblastoma and other cystic and solid lesions of the jaws is often difficult. In any case, the definitive diagnosis must usually await histologic examination of a biopsy specimen from the lesion.

**Pathology.**—In respect to gross appearance, an ameloblastoma may present as a solid encapsulated tumor mass whose cut surface appears whitish in color and granular rather than smooth in texture. On the other hand, the tumor may be more or less cystified, being permeated by smaller or larger smooth-walled spaces containing yellow fluid which may even be of a viscid consistency. Should the ameloblastoma be one which is developing in the wall of an odontogenic cyst, the tumor is likely to be represented by a more or less irregular mass of tissue protruding into the cavity of the cyst. In its growth, the tumor of course erodes the osseous tissue neighboring upon it, often causes expansion of the contour of the affected bone part, but does not tend to violate the covering periosteum even if part of the bone cortex is destroyed. This tendency of the untreated tumor to remain confined to the affected jawbone, taken in conjunction with the fact that it tends to recur if incompletely removed, dictates the appropriate treatment. Specifically, as early as possible, the original lesion should be subjected to wide surgical resection including a margin of normal bone around the tumor.

In respect to histologic pattern, ameloblastomas reveal a good deal of variety from lesion to lesion. (See Figs. 138-*E* and 139.) In a given one, a particular pattern tends to predominate, but in certain parts of it other patterns are also to be found. Thus in some lesions the picture is characterized particularly by strands

***Figure 139***

*A*, Photomicrograph (× 65) illustrating the histologic pattern of an ameloblastoma in which the picture is dominated by ramifying and interconnected cords of epithelial cells.

*B*, Photomicrograph (× 65) of an ameloblastoma in which the histologic pattern is dominated by follicle formation. In the left upper part of the picture, degeneration of the cells in the interior of a follicle has resulted in its cystification.

*C*, Photomicrograph (× 65) showing the pattern of an ameloblastoma in which the cells in the interior of some of the follicles show a tendency to form epithelial pearls.

*D*, Photomicrograph (× 125) showing the epithelial cells of an ameloblastoma arranged in acinar and duct-like formations. The tissue in question came from the case illustrated in Fig. 138-*C*.

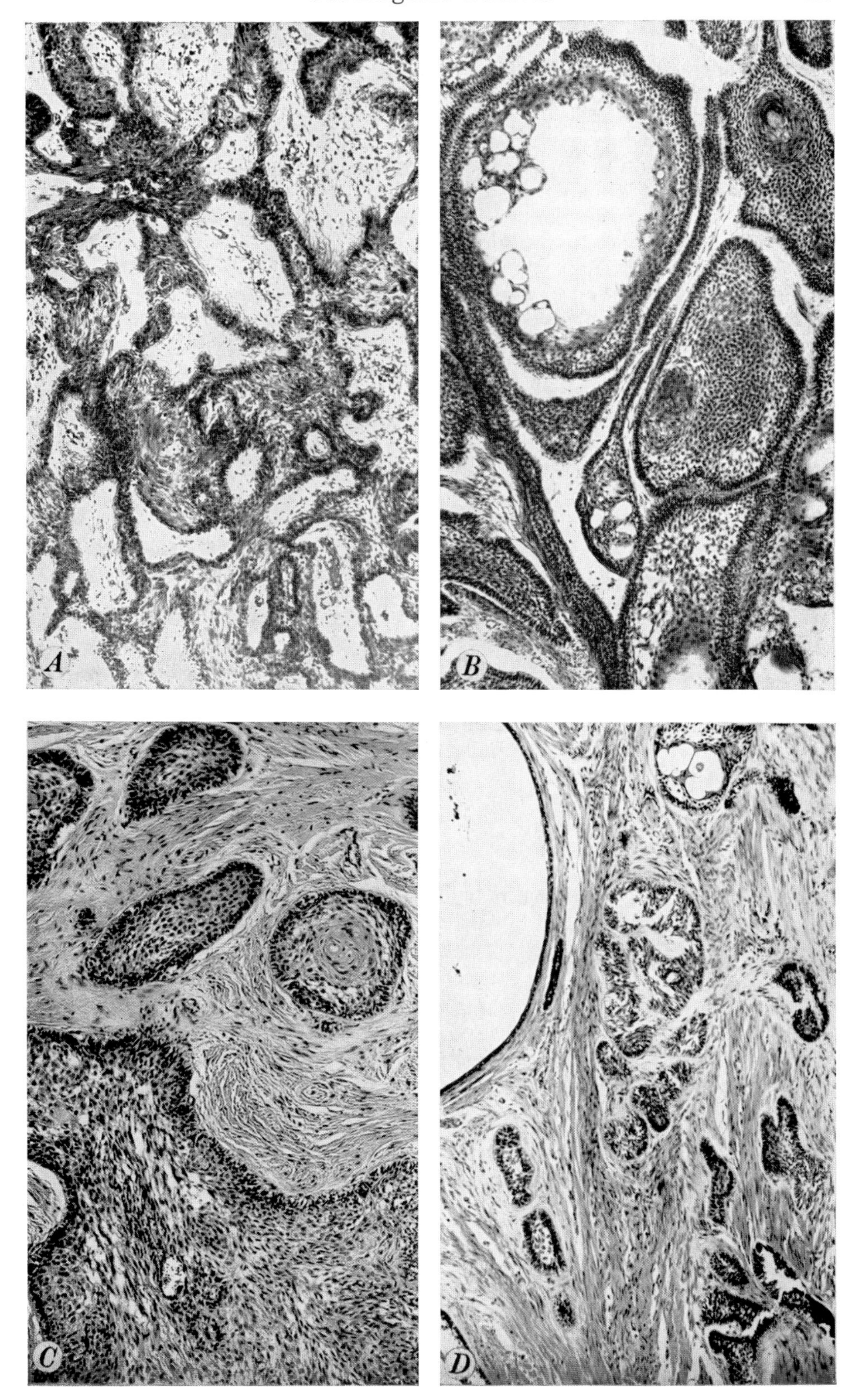


*Figure 139*

or cords of epithelial cells set in variable amounts of a loose fibrous stroma. In others, one sees a striking picture produced by ramifying and interconnected cords of epithelial cells which, along the margins of the cords, are cuboidal or cylindrical in shape. Again, the lesional tissue may be dominated by sheets of stellate cells bordered by cuboidal cells.

Somewhere in most of the lesions, and predominantly in some, one sees follicle formation. The follicles are composed of central cores of stellate cells bordered by columnar cells. In the interior of some of the follicles, one may even note squamous cells showing a tendency to "pearling." In other follicles, degeneration of the stellate cells results in cystification. Cystified neighboring follicles may fuse to form larger or even very large cysts, which are again lined by cylindrical cells. In another variation of the general histologic pattern, the tissue shows mainly follicle-like structures whose cells within the interior present a good deal of squamous differentiation and a pronounced tendency to form epithelial pearls. It should also be noted that some ameloblastomas may show areas in which the tumor cells are arranged in acinar and duct-like formations. Finally, in rare instances one encounters an ameloblastoma in which at least some of the epithelial cells contain melanin pigment (see Battle, Hovell, and Spencer). In connection with the histologic differential diagnosis of ameloblastoma, it should be emphasized that a jawbone may be the site of a primary or metastatic carcinoma. Indeed, unless special care is exercised, such a carcinoma may be misinterpreted as an ameloblastoma on account of its epithelial nature and its superficial resemblance to the latter tumor.

As indicated, an ameloblastoma is basically a benign tumor, but its locally aggressive character explains its strong tendency to recur if inadequately removed. However, the recurrence may be slow to manifest itself, years sometimes elapsing between the surgical intervention and the recurrence. In time, especially if recurrences have followed repeated unsuccessful attempts at removal, an occasional lesion has been known to metastasize to regional lymph nodes. Several instances have been reported in which the tumor spread to the lungs, but this occurrence is probably due to implantation of tumor tissue aspirated during surgery. Once in a

***Figure 140***

*A*, Roentgenograph showing a partially mature odontoma (odontoblastoma) in a mandible. The patient was a boy 11 years of age whose chief complaint was local swelling of the face, which had been noted for about 5 months. The odontoma is one in which only part of the lesional tissue has evolved into mature tooth structure. Note that in the vicinity of the well formed tooth there are small, roundish radiopacities representing such mature tooth substance. However, to either side there is a considerable amount of lesional tissue casting a ground glass shadow. The latter reflects the presence of enamel, cementum, and dentin, representing calcified derivatives of the still active and proliferating odontogenic ectoderm and mesoderm (see *C*).

*B*, Roentgenograph showing a completely evolved, mature odontoma in the maxilla. The patient was a girl 17 years of age who had been aware of some pain and a local swelling for about 10 months. Note the compacted, radiopaque appearance of the lesion, reflecting the fact that it is composed throughout of organized tooth substance (see *D*).

*C*, Photomicrograph (× 65) illustrating the histologic pattern to be observed in parts of an odontoma containing hard and soft elements. Note the presence of connective tissue and epithelial cells intermingled with calcified elements representing dentin and cementum.

*D*, Photomicrograph (× 12) illustrating the histologic pattern observed in the mature odontoma shown in *B*. Note the presence of compacted agglomerations of well differentiated and organized tooth structures surrounded merely by a fibrous capsule.

(The writer is indebted to Doctor Theodor Blum and the New York Institute of Clinical Oral Pathology for the material illustrated.)

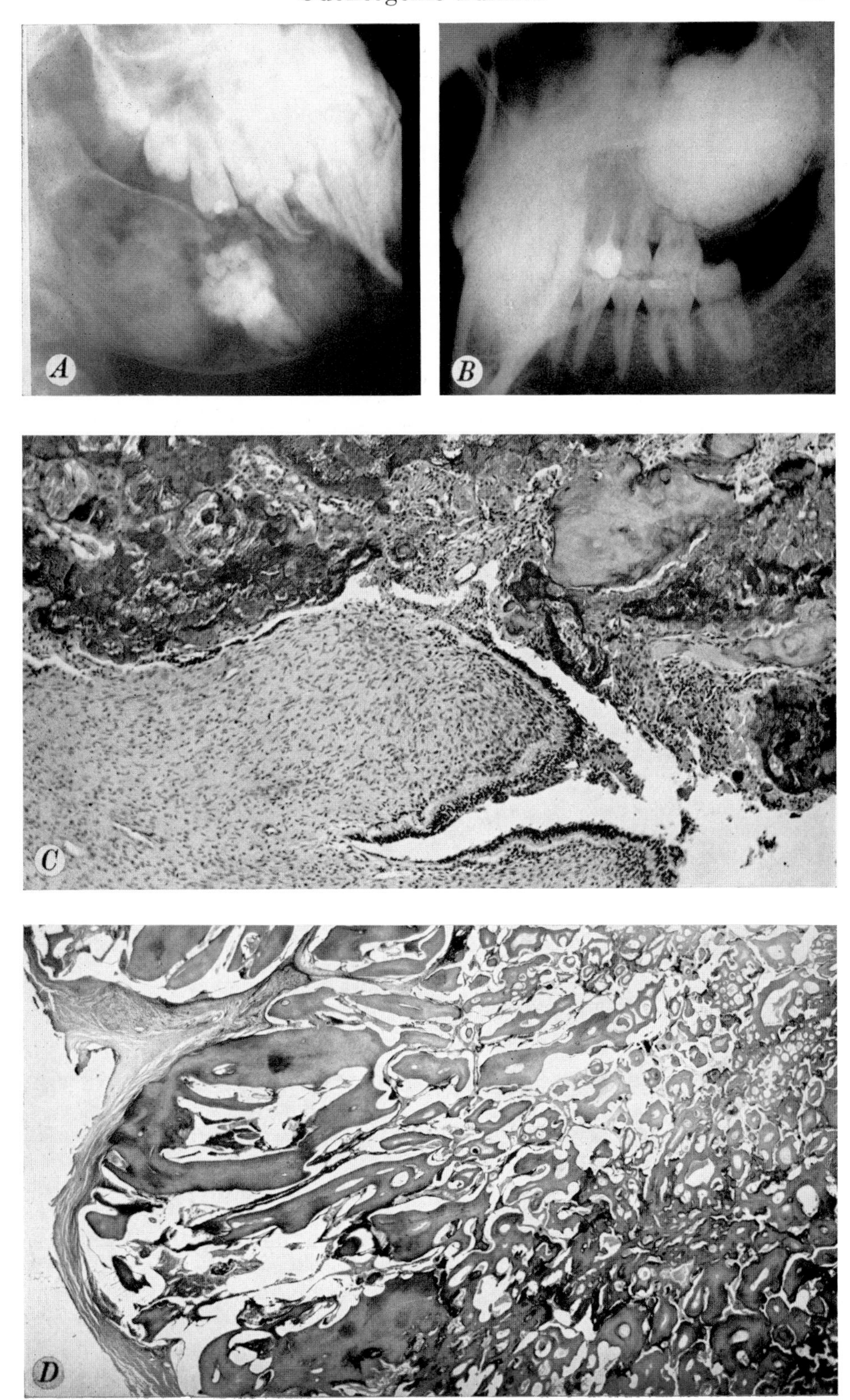


*Figure 140*

while, too, an ameloblastoma undergoes frank malignant transformation, usually into an epidermoid carcinoma but sometimes (through malignant transformation of its stroma) into a sarcoma.

### ODONTOMA

Under the general heading of odontoma one may group together the various mixed odontogenic tumors. (See Fig. 140.) Some are composed solely of odontogenic epithelium and odontogenic mesenchyme, and these are often denoted as the *soft odontomas.* In these lesions the epithelial cells are lined up in the form of drawn-out cords and/or small compact buds, but do not tend to form the clear-cut follicular structures characteristic of the ameloblastoma. Interspersed between the epithelial elements is a rather abundant amount of connective tissue. This may be poor in cells and rather collagenous or composed instead of a loose meshwork of stellate cells. In accordance with the histologic tissue pattern of the soft odontoma, it is sometimes also called an "ameloblastic fibroma" (see Thoma). The lesional area appears radiolucent in the *x*-ray picture, and it is difficult to differentiate it from one or another form of cyst or from a conventional ameloblastoma. If not adequately excised, a soft odontoma is prone to recurrence.

Another variety of mixed odontogenic tumor is that in which the presence of odontogenic epithelium and mesenchyme is associated with the presence of various amounts of their calcified derivatives (enamel, cementum, and dentin) and even some more highly organized tooth tissue. Such tumors (in which hard and soft elements are intermingled) are often also referred to as *odontoblastomas* (see Thoma and Goldman). In the *x*-ray picture the lesional area may be more or less radiolucent, but if calcified material is relatively prominent, the area will show radiopacities of various size and density. These lesions, too, often recur if not thoroughly excised.

Complete evolution of an odontoblastoma results in what is known as a hard or *mature odontoma.* That lesion contains little if any of the basic formative cellular tissue. Instead, it is composed mainly of rather well differentiated and organized tooth structures appearing as agglomerations of abortive and/or even fairly completely formed teeth, surrounded by a fibrous capsule. In the *x*-ray picture the mature odontoma often appears as an irregularly lobulated, dense focus of radiopacity, in accordance with its composition of compact tooth tissue. The lesion is usually clinically dormant, but it may eventually produce expansion of the affected part of the bone. However, it is an entirely innocuous lesion and can often be pried out of its bed intact after having been decompressed and loosened from the surrounding tissues. It has no tendency toward recurrence.

## LESIONS CONTAINING MULTINUCLEAR GIANT CELLS

Lesions located in or about the jawbones and containing multinuclear giant cells are often uncritically interpreted as giant-cell tumors. However, it is only rarely that a lesion in such a site fully corresponds in its cytologic pattern and clinical behavior to the indubitable giant-cell tumor whose familiar site is the end of one or another long bone of a limb (p. 18). Indeed, the writer has seen only one example of a genuine giant-cell tumor in a jawbone, the lesion having been located in the mandible. Histologically, most of the constituent tissue of an unquestionable giant-cell tumor shows great numbers of large, multinuclear giant cells distributed more or less evenly through the tissue, and these cells are set in a rather cellular stroma of spindle-shaped or polyhedral cells. This tissue pattern contrasts with the patterns presented by the various other lesions, now to be considered, which also contain giant cells but which do not represent the giant-cell tumor.

**"Brown Tumor" Focus of Hyperparathyroidism.**—A jawbone is not an uncommon site of such a focus. The lesion produces one or more areas of lytic destruction in the affected jawbone area. The contour of the bone in that area may be expanded, and the lesion may even erupt from the bone and produce an epulis-like swelling under the gum.

The pathogenesis of the "brown tumor" can be reasonably conceived as follows: The hyperparathyroidism leads to active bone resorption and fibrous scarring; in a bone area which has undergone considerable resorption and extensive replacement by fibrous tissue, hemorrhage into the replacement tissue may occur; multinuclear giant cells appear in the wake of the hemorrhage, and organization of the lesional area continues with the formation of delicate trabeculæ of osteoid and osseous tissue. Altogether, then, such a "brown tumor" focus apparently represents a reparative scarring reaction associated with the presence of giant cells in an area heavily damaged by the local effects of hyperparathyroidism.

Details which help in the histologic identification of a "brown tumor" include the following: The giant cells are small and often clumped or bunched, sometimes in nodular arrangement, especially about areas of hemorrhage; the stromal cells are delicate and there is often evidence of osseous metaplasia of the stroma. The fact that a "brown tumor" might be misinterpreted histologically as a giant-cell tumor has already been considered in connection with the differential diagnosis of giant-cell tumor (p. 34), and the lesion is illustrated in Figure 7 (p. 37). In establishing hyperparathyroidism as the basis for a lesion thought to be a "brown tumor," the finding of an elevated serum calcium level is of primary importance.

**Giant-cell Reparative Granuloma of Jawbones.**—Independently of hyperparathyroidism, one occasionally encounters a jawbone lesion which likewise raises the problem of differentiation from giant-cell tumor. This is the so-called "giant-cell reparative granuloma of jawbones" (see Jaffe). The name is intended to convey the idea that the lesion is not a neoplasm in the true sense, but represents instead a local reparative reaction. The giant cells observed in the lesional tissue apparently do not constitute elements in a tumorous proliferation, as they do in a genuine giant-cell tumor of bone, but instead seem to be connected with the occurrence of hemorrhage into the interior of the bone.

The lesion is not a common one. It occurs more often in the mandible than in the maxilla. Most often, the patients are between 10 and 25 years of age. Roentgenographically, the lesion appears as a roundish or oval area of radiolucency which is sometimes faintly trabeculated. It thins and expands but does not perforate the cortex of the affected jawbone. In general, the roentgenographic appearance of the lesion is thus rather nondescript and not such as to permit a definitive preoperative diagnosis.

When the lesional area is entered, one finds that it contains a variable amount of soft, spongy, reddish, friable tissue. The histologic pattern presented by the lesional tissue is a rather characteristic one. In a fairly loose, vascular stroma composed of small spindle-shaped cells, one notes a good deal of hemorrhagic extravasation. The multinuclear giant cells are sparse, small, and unevenly distributed, and often clumped in areas of hemorrhage. One will note also some microscopic fields of edema and even cystification. Between the microscopic lobules of this lesional tissue one may see, here and there, some delicate trabeculæ of newly formed osteoid and bone. The lesion is illustrated in Figure 8 (p. 39), and the description given above follows closely the previous remarks on the lesion made in connection with its differential diagnosis from giant-cell tumor (p. 36).

The giant-cell reparative granuloma of jawbones is a benign lesion which yields readily to therapy. The therapeutic procedure of choice is curettage, after which the lesion usually heals in. Occasionally the curettage has to be repeated, but if a lesion which is thought to represent a giant-cell reparative granuloma has recurred, one must make sure that the patient is not suffering from hyperparathyroidism, and that the jaw lesion in question does not represent an expression of that disease. The lesion has also been found to yield to radiation therapy after the diagnosis has been established by biopsy (see Berger). However, the results obtained through curettage of the lesion are usually so satisfactory that, in view of its benignity, it seems unnecessary to run such risks as radiation therapy, even in small doses, may entail.

## REFERENCES


Battle, R. J. V., Hovell, J. H., and Spencer, H.: Pigmented Adamantinomata, Brit. J. Surg., *39*, 368, 1952.

Bennett, I. B., and Chilton, N. W.: Traumatic Cysts of Mandible, J. Am. Dent. A., *32*, 51, 1945.

Berger, A.: Solitary Central Giant-cell Tumor of the Jaw Bones, J. Oral Surg., *5*, 154, 1947.

Berger, A., and Jaffe, H. L.: Fibrous (Fibro-osseous) Dysplasia of Jaw Bones, J. Oral Surg., *11*, 3, 1953.

Bernier, J. L., and Cahn, L. R.: The Peripheral Giant Cell Reparative Granuloma, J. Am. Dent. A., *49*, 141, 1954.

Bernier, J. L., and Thompson, H. C.: The Histogenesis of the Cementoma, Am. J. Orthodontics (Oral Surg. Sect.), *32*, 543, 1946.

Blum, T.: Unusual Bone Cavities in the Mandible: Traumatic Bone Cysts, J. Am. Dent. A., *19*, 281, 1932.

Cahn, L. R.: The Dentigerous Cyst as a Potential Adamantinoma, Dent. Cosmos, *75*, 889, 1933.

Hertz, J.: Adamantinoma. Histo-Pathologic and Prognostic Studies, Acta chir. scandinav., *102*, 405, 1952.

Holdsworth, W. G., and Rowe, N. L.: Adamantinoma, Brit. J. Surg., *43*, 255, 1955.

Jaffe, H. L.: Giant-cell Reparative Granuloma, Traumatic Bone Cyst, and Fibrous (Fibro-osseous) Dysplasia of the Jawbones, Oral Surg., *6*, 159, 1953.

Lucas, R. B., and Thackray, A. C.: Histology of Adamantinoma, Brit. J. Cancer, *5*, 289, 1951.

Manley, E. B.: Adamantinoma in Relation to Tooth Development, Australian J. Dent., *58*, 137, 1954.

Nathan, A. S.: Unilocular Cysts of the Jaw Bones, Bull. Hosp. Joint Dis., *17*, 197, 1956.

Rankow, R. M., and Hickey, M. J.: Adamantinoma of the Mandible: Analysis of Surgical Treatment, Surgery, *36*, 713, 1954.

Robinson, H. B. G.: Classification of Cysts of the Jaws, Am. J. Orthodontics (Oral Surg. Sect.), *31*, 370, 1945.

Rushton, M. A., and Cantab, B. C.: Solitary Bone Cysts in the Mandible, Brit. Dent. J., *81*, 37, 1946.

Schroff, J.: Unusual Cysts of the Maxilla: Cyst of Naso-Palatine Duct. Cyst of Facial Cleft Area (Fissural Cyst), Dent. Items Interest, *51*, 107, 1929.

Sharp, G. S., Bullock, W. K., and Binkley, F. C.: Ameloblastoma of the Jaws, Oral Surg., *8*, 1013, 1955.

Sonesson, A.: Odontogenic Cysts and Cystic Tumours of the Jaws, Acta radiol. (Supp. 81), 1950.

Stafne, E. C.: Periapical Fibroma: Roentgenologic Observations, J. Am. Dent. A., *30*, 688, 1943.

———: Value of Roentgenograms in Diagnosis of Tumors of the Jaws, Oral Surg., *6*, 82, 1953.

Stafne, E. C., and Millhon, J. A.: Periodontal Cysts, J. Oral Surg., *3*, 102, 1945.

Stoll, H. C., Marchetta, F. C., and Schobinger, R.: Malignant Epithelial Tumors of the Mandible and Maxilla, Arch. Path., *64*, 239, 1957.

Thoma, K. H.: Diagnosis and Treatment of Odontogenic and Fissural Cysts, Oral Surg., *3*, 961, 1950.

———: *Oral Pathology*, 4th ed., St. Louis, The C. V. Mosby Co., 1954.

Thoma, K. H., and Goldman, H. M.: Odontogenic Tumors: A Classification Based on Observations of the Epithelial, Mesenchymal, and Mixed Varieties, Am. J. Path., *22*, 433, 1946.

———: Central Myxoma of the Jaw, Am. J. Orthodontics (Oral Surg. Sect.), *33*, 532, 1947.

Tratman, E. K.: The Classification of Odontomes, Brit. Dent. J., *91*, 167, 1951.

Umiker, W., and Gerry, R. G.: Pseudo Giant Cell Tumor (Reparative Granuloma) of the Jaw, Oral Surg., *7*, 113, 1954.

Waldron, C. A.: Solitary (Hemorrhagic) Cyst of the Mandible, Oral Surg., *7*, 88, 1954.

Chapter

# 26

# Chordoma

The *chordoma* is a malignant tumor which apparently takes its origin from a persisting ectopic remnant of the notochord.* It is a locally infiltrative and destructive tumor which grows slowly and does not readily metastasize. The sites of predilection for the chordoma are the base of the skull in the region of the spheno-occipital synchondrosis and the sacrococcygeal region of the vertebral column. A chordoma which develops at the base of the skull never reaches the large size frequently attained by a chordoma in the sacrococcygeal region.

Histologically, the tissue of a chordoma characteristically shows, in part or throughout, vacuolated cells, some of which are so tremendously distended by vacuoles that they are denoted as "physaliphorous cells." Furthermore, there is likely to be a good deal of mucin between the smaller or larger characteristically vacuolated cells. Indeed, unless a lesion suspected of being a chordoma presents these histologic features at least in some areas of the tumor, its identification as a chordoma remains in doubt.

It is the clinical and pathologic peculiarities of these malignant tumors of notochordal tissue that will mainly concern us in this chapter. However, mention must be made of the fact that, especially in the region of the spheno-occipital synchondrosis, one occasionally encounters a small, innocuous nodule of tissue representing a proliferated rest of heterotopic notochordal tissue. The existence of such nodules in the clival region was familiar to pathologists long before the chordoma was identified as a tumor entity.

*The notochord is formed by a proliferation of cells from the cephalic end of the primitive streak. It first appears as a midsagittal rod of cells lying ventral to the neural tube, with which its dorsal surface is in contact, and forming the roof of the archenteron in the midline. It then closes off ventrally to form an elongated cylinder, but it temporarily retains its contact with the neural tube and gut. Thus, at a very early stage in the development of the human embryo (about the third week), the formed notochord is present as a longitudinal, nonsegmented rod of cells extending along the midaxis from the region of Rathke's pouch (future sphenoidal region) to the most caudal segment.

The notochord (along with the adjacent neural tube) soon becomes surrounded by a sheath of mesoderm. This sheath becomes chondrified and later ossified, forming, at the anterior extremity, the basiocciput and basisphenoid, and elsewhere the vertebral column. In the course of this chondrification and ossification of the mesodermal sheath around the notochord, the latter begins to disappear. Indeed, this disappearance is already well under way during the second month of fetal life.

Specifically, in relation to the vertebral column, the notochordal tissue within the developing vertebral bodies becomes obliterated, but the notochordal tissue in the intervertebral disks persists in the nucleus pulposus. At its cranial end, likewise, the notochord becomes substantially obliterated in the course of the development of the base of the skull in the vicinity of the foramen magnum. However, remnants of notochordal tissue not infrequently persist in relation to the pharyngeal surface of the base of the skull and on the cranial aspect of the base (or possibly even within the bone) in the vicinity of the spheno-occipital synchondrosis. In the sacrococcygeal region the notochord is continued into the tail end of the embryo. In this region, too, the notochord undergoes regression and involution, but it is not unusual for notochordal remnants to persist, especially in and about the end of the coccyx.

When originally noted, these nodules were mistakenly held to represent rests of degenerated cartilage and were denoted accordingly by the name of "*ecchondrosis* physaliphora spheno-occipitalis." However, when their relationship to notochordal remnants was surmised, this relationship was expressed in the name "*ecchordosis* physaliphora spheno-occipitalis." In occasional instances, small, proliferated rests of heterotopic notochordal tissue are also found elsewhere along the path of the original notochord than in the clival region. Currently, the name "*benign chordoma*" is often used to denote such small proliferated notochordal rests, irrespective of their site. However, since the term "chordoma" has acquired the connotation of a malignant tumor, the term "benign chordoma" should perhaps be avoided in any connection.

There is a strong possibility that most of the malignant chordal tumors evolve out of proliferated rests of heterotopic notochordal tissue. This evolution cannot be proved, since, unless they undergo malignant transformation, such rests are completely innocuous and clinically silent. However, indirect evidence of such an evolutionary course is afforded by the fact that, at the base of the skull, the true chordomas occur precisely in the site where the benign proliferated rests of notochordal tissue (the ecchordoses) have most often been noted. On the other hand, a chordoma in this area may possibly develop out of a notochordal vestige in the region of the spheno-occipital synchondrosis without having passed through the stage of being an ecchordosis.

The other common site of the true chordoma is the sacrococcygeal region. This is a site in which one could expect to encounter persisting ectopic notochordal tissue, in view of what is known about the development and regression of the caudal end of the notochord (see Horwitz) and the postnatal development of the sacrum and coccyx. There is a strong possibility that careful study of the sacrococcygeal area of the vertebral column in a large series of autopsies will show that proliferated notochordal rests are not rare in this site, either. Congdon, in fact, encountered a "benign chordoma" as a chance finding in a coccyx which had been resected surgically in connection with operative intervention against a carcinoid of the rectum.

## CLINICAL CONSIDERATIONS

**Incidence.**—The malignant tumors of chordal tissue (the chordomas) are of relatively rare occurrence. However, since the condition is a striking one, individual instances are frequently recorded, and many reviews based on collected cases are also to be found in the literature. As to *sex* incidence, the condition is apparently more common in males than in females. As to *age* incidence, it does not seem to predilect any particular decade of life. In occasional instances the lesion has been observed even in the first decade of life, and all the succeeding decades through the seventh are well represented in the case reports. However, one notes that in any large collected series of cases, a definite majority of the spheno-occipital chordomas fall within the age group 30 to 60 years, and a definite majority of the sacrococcygeal chordomas within the age group 40 to 70 years.

**Localization.**—As already indicated, the chordomas are observed mainly in the cranial and caudal regions. Indeed, approximately 35 per cent occur in the cranial region (predominantly in the spheno-occipital area), 55 per cent in the caudal region (mainly in the sacrococcygeal area), and only about 10 per cent elsewhere along the vertebral axis (the thoracic area being a less common site of the lesion than the cervical or lumbar areas). The relatively infrequent occurrence of chordomas in the cervical, thoracic, and lumbar parts of the column is probably to be related to the lower incidence of notochordal ectopia in those parts of the column. It is true that, after birth, notochordal remnants are retained, sometimes even into adult life, within the nucleus pulposus of the intervertebral disks of this region. However, a vertebral chordoma appearing in one of these parts of the column seems to arise not in an intervertebral disk, but in the vertebral body, and hence, here as elsewhere, to have its origin in an ectopic chordal rest.

**Clinical Complaints and Findings.**—In any site, pain is usually the initial complaint. It is attributable to destruction of bone at the site of the lesion's growth, and/or involvement of some part of the brain or spinal cord, or nerves issuing from them. However, the details of the complaints will, of course, vary with the location of the tumor.

Thus the clinical picture produced by a chordoma in the region of the spheno-occipital synchondrosis is likely to be dominated early by neurologic aberrations, since the lesion may erode and invade the sella and also involve the brain stem and regional cranial nerves, at least through pressure. Once in a while, the tumor even erodes through the base of the skull and extends into the roof of the pharynx. Usually, however, a chordoma found in the nasopharyngeal region is one which has begun there. A sacrococcygeal chordoma frequently produces a palpable tumor mass, though this finding, too, is usually preceded by complaints of pain. The mass grows steadily, though often slowly, and may become very large and visible externally. The bulk of the tumor mass may present anteriorly or posteriorly. Bladder and bowel function may be disturbed, and neurological complaints appear because the pelvic nerves tend to become surrounded and infiltrated by the tumor tissue. In connection with chordomas involving the cervical or lumbar parts of the column, neurological complaints and findings are again noted early. In these locations the tumor is usually related to the posterior aspect of the affected vertebral body or bodies, and soon produces compression of the spinal cord or cauda equina. Neurological complaints will also be prominent if the chordoma arises in the thoracic part of the column, but, as already noted, it is unusual for the lesion to develop there.

Since the clinical manifestations of a cranial chordoma are similar to those produced by other cranial neoplasms growing in the region of the clivus, its clinical diagnosis is very difficult. When the lesion is in the sacrococcygeal region, the idea that one may be dealing with a chordoma is much more likely to come to mind on the basis of the clinical findings. However, irrespective of the site of the lesion, the definitive diagnosis of a chordoma must depend upon microscopic examination of the lesional tissue.

The clinical course pursued by a chordoma varies with its site, but is baleful in the vast majority of cases. It is particularly bad for the spheno-occipital chordomas, because of their unfavorable location. Chordomas in this site nearly always lead to death within 2 or 3 years after the onset of complaints, whether or not attempts at surgical removal of the lesion have been made. On the other hand, patients affected with chordomas in the sacrococcygeal region not infrequently survive for 5 to 10 years, especially under repeated palliative surgical therapy.

**The Possible Role of Trauma.**—In occasional case reports, a severe local trauma is mentioned as a factor in the causation of a sacrococcygeal chordoma. The factor of trauma is supposed to act by liberating chordal tissue from the injured bone site and thus permitting proliferation of the extruded tissue. This concept probably had its basis in an experimental study by Ribbert in which he showed that puncturing intervertebral disks of young rabbits and liberating nucleus pulposus tissue results in the formation of small, innocuous nodules of proliferated chordal tissue. However, Congdon, who confirmed these findings in rabbits, noted that these nodules eventually underwent involution.

The idea that trauma is important in the causation of chordoma does not stand up under critical consideration. In the first place, the lower part of the back is a site often severely traumatized, but even sacrococcygeal chordomas are of relatively rare occurrence. Furthermore, the wide practice of surgical curettage of one or more lumbar intervertebral disks in the treatment of patients presenting the sciatic syndrome has not increased the incidence of lumbar chordomas. Finally, any explanation offered for the sacrococcygeal chordomas ought also to be applicable to the cranial chordomas, but trauma can hardly be inculpated in regard to the latter.

## ROENTGENOGRAPHIC FINDINGS

On *x*-ray examination, a chordoma in the region of the clivus is usually found limited to the area of the midline at first, but it may eventually spread widely in all directions. The tumor tends to cause erosive destruction of the sphenoid and may be found to have extended into the sphenoidal sinuses and even beyond them, giving rise to additional local osteolytic changes. The tumor mass itself frequently shows scattered radiopacities, representing calcification going on in the lesional tissue. Air injection studies are likely to indicate also upward displacement of the third ventricle, while the cerebral aqueduct and the fourth ventricle are likewise displaced, often backward. Such roentgenographic findings, taken together with the clinical findings (especially multiple cranial nerve palsies) are indeed of considerable diagnostic value. However, they are not conclusive, since other tumors involving the region in question may likewise produce them (see Wood and Himadi).

In the sacrococcygeal area, an early finding is expansion of the affected part of the bone, associated with obliteration of the normal markings. The tumor tissue in the involved area is likely to cast a more or less ground glass shadow. Smaller or larger areas of radiolucency appear sooner or later, in consequence of complete lytic destruction of parts of the bone and perforation of the cortex. Extension of tumor tissue into the pelvis or posteriorly toward the buttock is manifested by the presence of a rather well defined soft-tissue mass which may likewise show scattered radiopacities. (See Fig. 141.)

### *Figure 141*

*A*, Roentgenograph from a case of chordoma involving the sacrococcygeal region. Note that the sacrum is somewhat expanded and that it lacks, through most of its extent, the normal trabecular markings. In the lateral projection, it was apparent that the shadow cast by the coccyx was also abnormal. The patient was a man 52 years of age who gave a history of progressively worsening bouts of pain, of 2 years' standing, in the lower part of the back. Of late, the pain had been radiating down both lower extremities, and physical examination showed diminution of ankle jerks and the presence of sensory changes in the lower limbs. At the surgical intervention, tumor tissue was found to have broken out of the sacrum in all directions, and tissue submitted for anatomic study established the diagnosis of chordoma. Postoperatively, over an interval of 4 months, the patient received about 13,000 r of irradiation to the entire sacrococcygeal region. However, this apparently produced at most only slight shrinkage of the residual tumor mass.

*B*, Photograph showing, at three different levels, the cut surface of one of two large masses of chordoma tissue removed in the course of surgical intervention against the second recurrence of a sacrococcygeal chordoma. Where the tissue was not hemorrhagic, it appeared bluish white to grayish white in color and was soft and mucoid. The characteristic lobular pattern of the tumor tissue is also evident. The patient was a man 46 years of age whose complaints were of 9 years' standing at the time of the surgical procedure against the second recurrence. The original complaint was of pain in the lower back. Later the pain began to radiate down both lower extremities. Within 2 years after the onset of the patient's complaints, difficulties relating to the bladder and bowel appeared. A biopsy at this time established the diagnosis of chordoma. In addition to the two partial surgical resections, the patient was given four courses of very intensive radiation over a period of 5 years. The total dosage was approximately 25,000 r, but this treatment did not prevent the development of the recurrences.

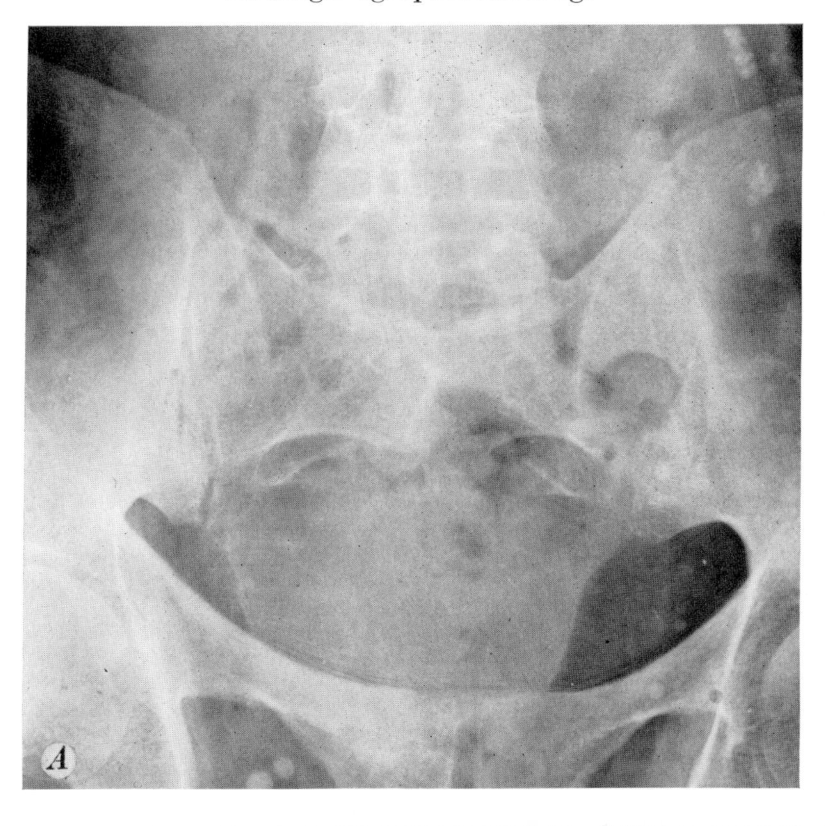


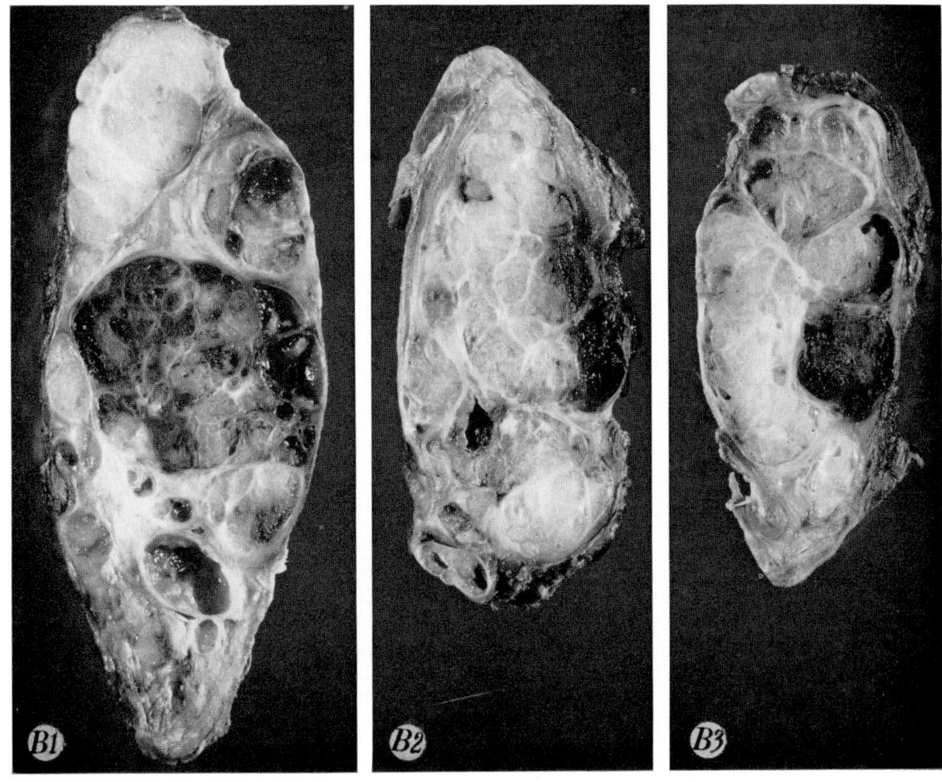


*Figure 141*

Vertebral chordomas characteristically produce foci of osteolysis, usually in two or more adjacent vertebræ. The intervertebral disk between affected adjoining vertebræ may or may not be found destroyed. Affected vertebræ may also show areas of increased radiopacity. Thus, in some cases the picture is that of a lesion which has produced both osteolytic and osteoblastic changes. In addition, one may note a soft-tissue tumor mass in the area of the bone involvement. However, all these *x*-ray findings are so common with various other lesions affecting vertebral areas that they offer little help in establishing the diagnosis of chordoma. Indeed, in regard to vertebral sites, the diagnosis of chordoma is not likely to be made without the aid of tissue examination. As already noted, it is also often not until a biopsy is done that the diagnosis is established even when the lesion is in one of its more common sites.

## PATHOLOGIC FINDINGS

It was the early pathologico-anatomic studies of Müller and of Ribbert that laid the foundation for our knowledge of the chordoma. The histogenetic aspects of the tumor were first worked out in detail by Alezais and Peyron. The contributions of Stewart and of Cappell (alone and with their co-workers) are likewise still basic to our understanding of the subject. Numerous reports on individual cases, and review articles summarizing experience with this intriguing lesion have since appeared (see Montgomery and Wolman, Mabrey, and Congdon).

As already implied, our knowledge of the malignant chordal tumors has grown out of the observations relating to the so-called *ecchordosis physaliphora spheno-occipitalis.* This represents merely a proliferated mass of heterotopic notochordal tissue occurring at the base of the skull, in the general region of the clivus. It presents as a soft, transparent jelly-like nodular structure usually not more than a few millimeters in diameter. The lesion can be seen to project through an aperture in the dura, and a more or less slender pedicle attaches it to the middle of the dorsum sellæ. The lesional tissue may also be loosely adherent to the pia arachnoid, over the pons. Microscopically, the nodule shows few cells, and those present are highly vacuolated and contain mucin. Here and there one sees large intercellular collections of homogeneous material which in places gives the staining reaction of mucin.

An ecchordosis does not tend to produce pressure or tissue destruction at the site of its growth and hence does not give rise to clinical complaints. Thus its presence is ordinarily discovered as an incidental finding at autopsy and often only when a special search is made for it. Making such a search, Ribbert found ecchordoses in the region of the clivus in 2 per cent of a large series of autopsies, and Stewart and Burrow found them in 1.5 per cent. There is a strong possibility that

***Figure 142***

*A*, Photomicrograph (× 125) illustrating the histologic pattern observed in a case of chordoma of the first lumbar vertebra in a girl 14 years of age. Intracellular vacuolation is not prominent, but could be demonstrated here and there within the lesional tissue (see *B*). Note that the tissue is highly cellular, and that the cells are small, roundish, and closely compacted, so that one may have difficulty in deducing that the lesion is a chordoma.

*B*, Photomicrograph (× 450) showing, in detail, the character of the chordoma cells in an area of the tissue illustrated in *A*. Some of the cells show vacuolation of their cytoplasm.

*C*, Photomicrograph (× 125) presenting a histologic pattern more characteristic of a chordoma. There is considerable mucin between the cells. The latter are distended, and many of them show vacuolation of their cytoplasm.

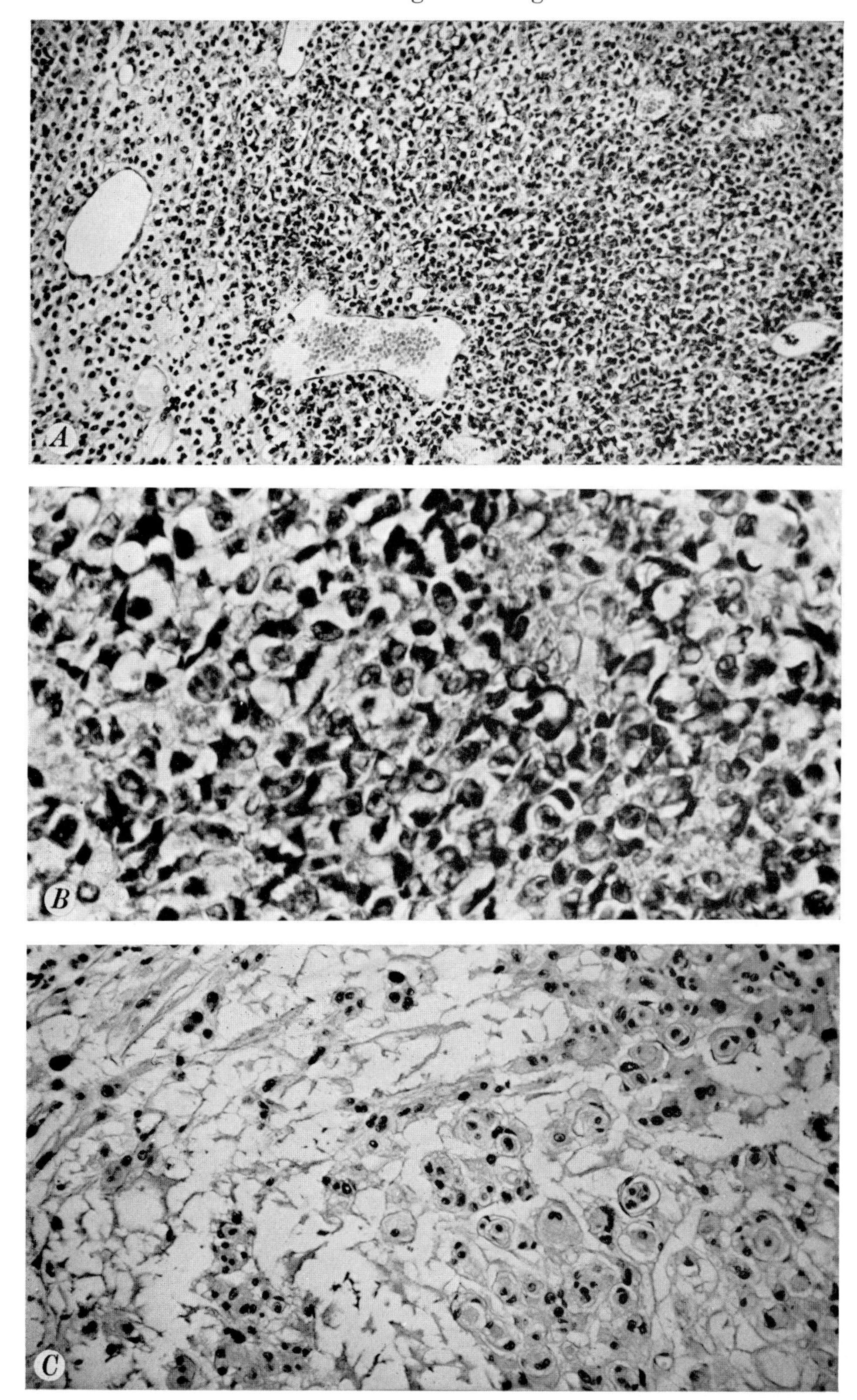


*Figure 142*

the chordomas developing in the region of the clivus usually originate from such ecchordoses.

**Gross Pathology.**—Chordomas located at the base of the skull (or in the cervical region) are relatively small in comparison with those encountered in the sacrococcygeal region. This difference is ascribable to the fact that tumors in the former areas involve vital structures and hence lead to death before they have been able to attain great size. A chordoma in the region of the clivus is only infrequently more than 7 cm. in its largest dimension. It presents as a nodulated mass covered by the dura, which in places may be extremely attenuated or even penetrated by the tumor tissue. If the tumor has broken through the dura, tumor tissue may be found adherent to the adjacent part of the brain or actually invading it. It is likely also to surround and compress regional cranial nerves. On the deep surface of the chordoma, there is often evidence of destruction of the central portion of the base of the skull, and tumor tissue may even be found extending into the nasopharynx, orbits, and/or nasal sinuses.

The lesional tissue itself is soft, and its cut surface presents a lobular pattern in which the lobules are delimited by septa of fibrous tissue. While some areas of the tumor tissue may be grayish in color, others are likely to be glistening and semitranslucent, on account of their mucin content. Furthermore, the cut surface of the tumor is likely to show larger or smaller areas of discoloration from recent or old hemorrhage (Fig. 141-*B*).

In relation to the vertebral column, a chordoma seen at autopsy is usually found already involving more than a single vertebral body. The body in which the tumor took its origin is likely to be found more or less completely replaced by tumor tissue. On breaking out of the body posteriorly, the tumor tends to spread beneath the posterior longitudinal ligament, and it may be found to have invaded one or more adjacent vertebræ. In one case or another, the regional intervertebral disks may be spared. In other cases, however, they too are invaded and may be found substantially or completely destroyed. In consequence of posterior extension of the tumor, the spinal canal is likely to be narrowed and the cord compressed locally. However, the dura is usually not penetrated, though local spinal nerves are usually found surrounded by, or imbedded in, the tumor tissue. Anteriorly, the tumor tissue is likely to extend out of the vertebral body principally affected and to invade the local prevertebral muscles and fascia. In consequence, a fairly large tumor mass may also be present in front and/or to the sides of the column. In respect to the gross appearance of the actual tumor tissue, a vertebral chordoma does not differ essentially from a cranial chordoma as already described.

The sacrococcygeal chordomas have so much latitude for expansion that, although their rate of growth tends to be slow, they may ultimately attain tremendous size. Growing in front of the sacrum, the tumor may substantially fill the pelvis, while at the same time it often extends behind the sacrum and even gains exit from the pelvis into one or both buttocks. Within the pelvis the tumor mass, generally lobulated, is usually covered by peritoneum on its anterior aspect. Naturally, the

***Figure 143***

*A*, Photomicrograph (× 125) showing an area of a chordoma in which the tissue pattern is dominated by pools of mucin between and around the chordoma cells, many of which present vacuolation of their cytoplasm.

B, Photomicrograph (× 450) illustrating a group of typical physaliphorous cells surrounded by a considerable amount of intercellular mucin.

*C*, Photomicrograph (× 450) showing cells arranged in concentric spherical formations. This is another cytologic appearance sometimes observed in a chordoma.

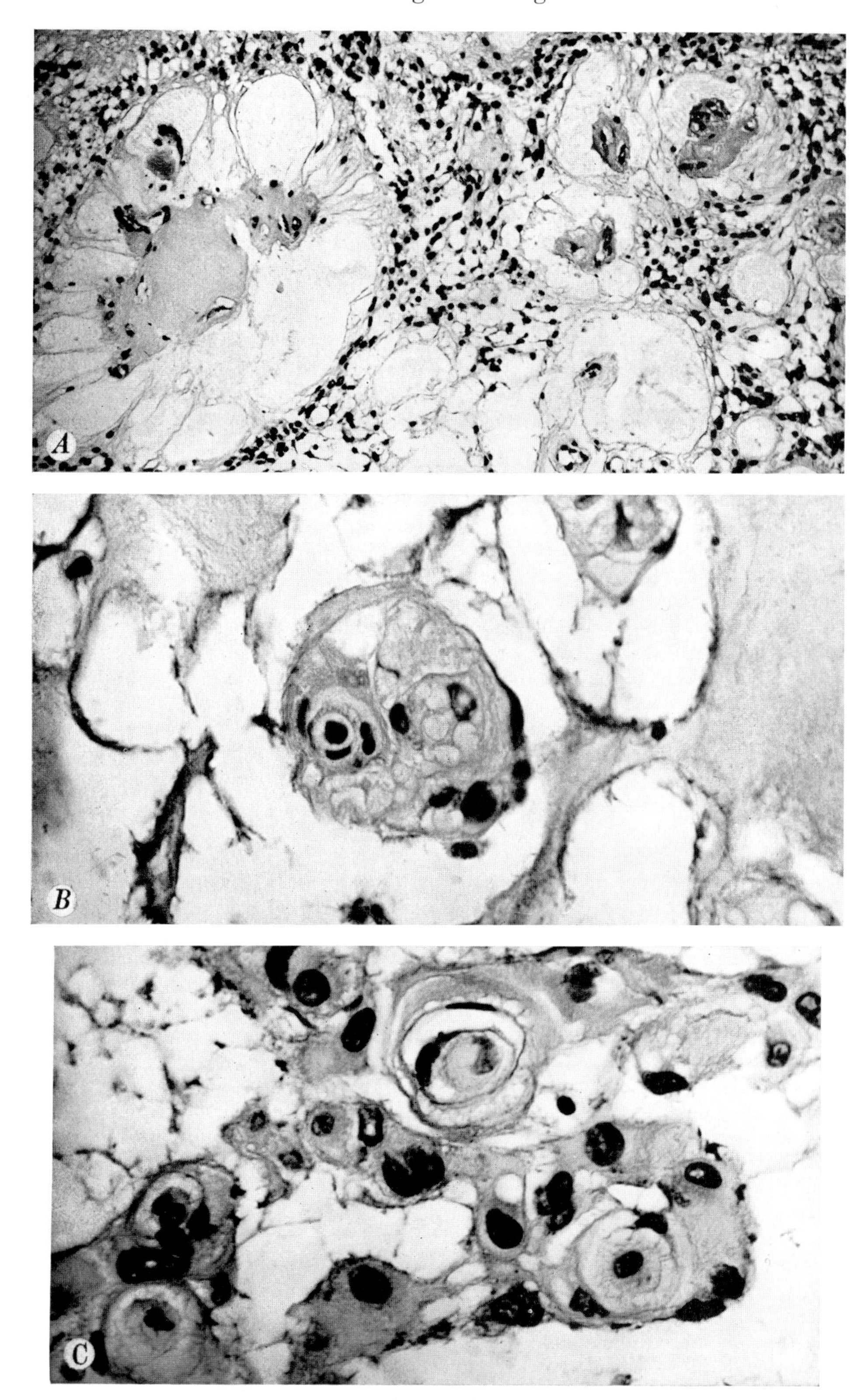


*Figure 143*

rectum, bladder, and, in the female, the uterus and its adnexa are likely to be compressed, displaced, and even partially encased by the growth. The tumor tissue may be found to have spread retroperitoneally into the abdominal cavity, in the direction of the kidneys. The sacrum and coccyx are likely to be substantially destroyed and replaced by the lesional tissue, which may also be found extending in the postsacral direction. Further examination may reveal that tumor tissue has also spread through one or both ischial notches into the buttocks. Having persisted for a long time and grown to large size, the tumor tissue of a sacrococcygeal chordoma usually shows extensive hemorrhage, necrosis, and cystification. However, a substantial part of the tumor is nevertheless likely to consist of rather characteristic gelatinous tissue.

**Microscopic Pathology.**—In histologic detail, the chordomas may show considerable variety from lesion to lesion and even within different areas of the same lesion. Some tumors, in part or throughout, are highly cellular, and the cytoplasm of the cells in these areas may show little or none of the vacuolation which one looks for in a chordoma. Other tumors show, in part or throughout, distended and strikingly vacuolated cells and also considerable intercellular mucin. The presence of intracellular vacuolation and intercellular mucin is held to indicate maturation of the lesional tissue and is most striking in the most mature tumor tissue areas. (See Figs. 142 and 143.)

In tumors or tumor fields in which the tissue is relatively immature, it is highly cellular. Furthermore, the cells are closely compacted, small, roundish, and well defined, and their cytoplasm shows little if any vacuolation. Indeed, if the lesion has to be evaluated only from tissue areas presenting such histologic appearances, one cannot be sure that it is a chordoma. In areas in which the tumor tissue is more mature, many of the tumor cells show pronounced distention from the accumulation of vacuoles within them, constituting the so-called physaliphorous cells. The lesional tissue may even show very pronounced vacuolation of practically all the cells and, in places, demarcation between individual cells may be lost. Finally, in some lesions or lesional fields, the histologic tissue pattern is that of smaller or larger pools of mucin, in and between which only sparse and strikingly vacuolated cells remain.

The large physaliphorous cells usually consist of a nucleus enveloped by a narrow ring of cytoplasm encircled in turn by a larger or smaller zone of well defined vacuoles. Sometimes even the nucleus of the physaliphorous cell is vacuolated. Under appropriate staining, some of the vacuoles show a mucin content. Apparently the discharge of mucin from the intracellular vacuoles leads to the accumulation of mucin between the tumor cells. In highly mucinous areas of the tumor one may also observe small spherical formations apparently resulting from the concentric layering of several cells. Cells in mitotic division are rarely seen, but may be observed, especially if the chordoma is an anaplastic one. In such a lesion, tumor fields suggesting the appearance of an undifferentiated fibrosarcoma are to be noted, intermingled with fields presenting the characteristic histologic appearance.

Once in a while, one may be faced with the problem of deciding histologically whether a tumor represents a chordoma or a chondrosarcoma. It is true that one sometimes observes in a chondrosarcoma (whether or not the latter has undergone myxomatous degeneration) some cells with vacuolated cytoplasm or even an occasional cell with a vacuolated nucleus. However, if one's observation covers many blocks of tissue from various parts of the lesion in question, the diagnostic dilemma can usually be readily resolved. If the chordoma is one in which, more or less throughout, the cells are small and not strikingly vacuolated, it still will not show the type of intercellular matrix which is characteristic of a cartilage tumor. On the other hand, a chondrosarcoma never shows large physaliphorous cells with vacuoles honeycombing the cytoplasm, such as most chordomas are likely to show somewhere. Furthermore, in a chordoma the intercellular material consists predominantly of mucin, and one finds no chondroid matrix such as a chondrosarcoma is sure to show somewhere in its lesional tissue, even if it has undergone myxomatous degeneration in many parts.

**Metastasis.**—When chordomas in all locations are considered, the over-all incidence of metastasis is not very high. Chordomas at the base of the skull rarely metastasize, while those in the sacrococcygeal area not infrequently do so. Furthermore, metastasis seems usually to have occurred only after the tumor had been present for at least some years. Invasion of local venous channels by the growing chordoma has been noted repeatedly, but this invasion is not regularly associated with the appearance of remote metastases.

Willis describes a case of sacral chordoma in which the tumor was found to have invaded the main iliac and femoral veins and metastasized widely to the lungs. In addition, metastases were found in the skin and many of the internal organs, but lymph node involvement was limited to some of the bronchial nodes. Widespread metastasis such as was observed in this case is exceptional. Usually the metastatic foci noted have been small and sparse, and sometimes it was only the liver and/or some lymph nodes that were involved.

## TREATMENT

Since chordomas grow slowly and do not readily metastasize, total excision of the tumor is, in theory, the procedure of choice. Unfortunately, this procedure is impractical, whatever the location of the lesion. The difficulty is that radical surgery would bring disastrous effects, because of inevitable damage to some part of the nervous system. Nevertheless, partial surgical removal is usually of definite palliative value, whatever the site of the tumor. When the lesion is in the sacrococcygeal region, repeated partial excisions often help to maintain the patient in fair condition for many years. It should be noted, however, that when the lesion is in this area, the patient often survives for some years without any treatment at all. The palliative value of postsurgical irradiation of chordomas is debatable. In any event, a chordoma oriented to some part of the skeleton is always ultimately fatal, irrespective of any treatment given.

## REFERENCES


Alezais, and Peyron: Contribution à l'étude des chordomes: Chordome de la région occipitale, Bull. Assoc. franç. p. l'étude du cancer, *7*, 194, 1914.

Bérard, L., Dunet, C., and Peyron, A.: Les Chordomes de la région sacro-coccygienne et leur Histogénèse, Bull. Assoc. franç. p. l'étude du cancer, *11*, 28, 1922.

Bruce, J., and Mekie, E.: Chordoma, Surg., Gynec. & Obst., *65*, 40, 1937.

Burrow, J. le F., and Stewart, M. J.: Malignant Spheno-Occipital Chordoma, J. Neurol. & Psychopath., *4*, 205, 1923.

Cappell, D. F.: Chordoma of the Vertebral Column with Three New Cases, J. Path. & Bact., *31*, 797, 1928.

Coenen, H.: Das Chordom, Beitr. z. klin. Chir., *133*, 1, 1925.

Congdon, C. C.: Benign and Malignant Chordomas. A Clinico-Anatomical Study of Twenty-Two Cases, Am. J. Path., *28*, 793, 1952.

————: Proliferative Lesions Resembling Chordoma Following Puncture of the Nucleus Pulposus in Rabbits, J. Nat. Cancer Inst., *12*, 893, 1952.

Horwitz, T.: Chordal Ectopia and Its Possible Relation to Chordoma, Arch. Path., *31*, 354, 1941.

Mabrey, R. E.: Chordoma: A Study of 150 Cases, Am. J. Cancer, *25*, 501, 1935.

Montgomery, A. H., and Wolman, I. J.: Sacrococcygeal Chordomas in Children, Am. J. Dis. Child., *46*, 1263, 1933.

MÜLLER, H.: Ueber das Vorkommen von Resten der Chorda dorsalis bei Menschen nach der Geburt und über ihr Verhältniss zu den Gallertgeschwülsten am Clivus, Ztschr. f. rat. Med., *2*, 202, 1858.

RIBBERT: Ueber die Ecchondrosis physalifora sphenooccipitalis, Zentralbl. f. allg. Path. u. path. Anat., *5*, 457, 1894.

————: Ueber die experimentelle Erzeugung einer Ecchondrosis physalifora, Verhandl. d. Kong. f. inn. Med., *13*, 455, 1895.

SENSENIG, E. C.: Adhesions of Notochord and Neural Tube in the Formation of Chordomas, Am. J. Anat., *98*, 357, 1956.

STEWART, M. J., and BURROW, J. LE F.: Ecchordosis Physaliphora Spheno-Occipitalis, J. Neurol. & Psychopath., *4*, 218, 1923.

STEWART, M. J., and MORIN, J. E.: Chordoma: A Review, with Report of a New Sacrococcygeal Case, J. Path. & Bact., *29*, 41, 1926.

UHR, N., and CHURG, J.: Hypertrophic Osteoarthropathy; Report of a Case Associated with a Chordoma of the Base of the Skull and Lymphangitic Pulmonary Metastases, Ann. Int. Med., *31*, 681, 1949.

WILLIS, R. A.: Sacral Chordoma with Widespread Metastases, J. Path. & Bact., *33*, 1035, 1930.

WOOD, E. H., JR., and HIMADI, G. M.: Chordomas: A Roentgenologic Study of Sixteen Cases Previously Unreported, Radiology, *54*, 706, 1950.

Chapter

# 27

# Tumors Developing at Sites of Pre-existing Bone Disease

THE present chapter deals mainly with the occurrence of tumors in bones affected with *Paget's disease*. Some consideration is also given to tumors developing in relation to bones affected with *chronic osteomyelitis*. Though apparently appropriate to this chapter, the matter of malignant transformation of pre-existing benign tumorous lesions need not be discussed here. It is sufficiently considered in the discussions of the various individual types of the benign lesions which sometimes undergo such transformation. In that connection, it seems sufficient to mention, for instance, that in an occasional case of fibrous dysplasia, a sarcoma becomes engrafted upon an affected bone (p. 134). The high incidence of malignant transformation of benign cartilaginous tumors is generally recognized, and this has been given attention in the discussions relating to solitary and multiple enchondroma (pp. 180 and 194) and solitary and multiple osteocartilaginous exostosis (pp. 150 and 164). Furthermore, the occurrence of malignant transformation of giant-cell tumor has been considered in the chapter dealing with that lesion (p. 30).

On the other hand, it may be worth noting here that a solitary bone cyst seems never to undergo spontaneous sarcomatous transformation. Nor are such benign lesions as the fibrous cortical defect or the non-ossifying fibroma subject to this change. Even in hyperparathyroidism, in which the bones may become severely altered through resorption, fibrous replacement, and the deposition of new osseous tissue, the affected bones never become the site of unquestionable sarcoma. It is true that in cases of hyperparathyroidism in which the skeleton has become severely altered, one frequently observes, in one or another affected bone, the so-called giant-cell or "brown" tumors, even large ones. However, these again have never been known to undergo malignant transformation. Thus, the absence of sarcomatous transformation in hyperparathyroidism stands out in contrast to what is observed in connection with Paget's disease. Indeed, the tendency toward sarcomatous transformation sets off Paget's disease sharply from all the other metabolic bone diseases.

## SARCOMA COMPLICATING PAGET'S DISEASE

Paget's disease of bone is a fairly common disorder, and the appearance of a sarcoma in connection with it is not at all unusual. As to Paget's disease itself, this may be found involving a single bone, several bones, or even many bones in a given case (see Schmorl, and Jaffe). However, in most of the cases coming under clinical observation, the skeletal involvement is more or less limited rather than very widespread. In fact, not infrequently only a single bone or bone part is found affected when the subject first comes under clinical observation. Indeed, cases such as Paget originally described, in which the skeletal involvement is very extensive, actually represent only a small proportion of the total cases of the disorder. In regard to the distribution of the skeletal changes in general, it is also worth noting that this shows no regularity or symmetry even in the cases in which much of the skeleton is involved. As to sarcoma complicating the disease, it is of special interest that this may develop in an affected bone (or even several affected bones) whether the total skeletal involvement is limited or extensive. A sarcoma may even develop in an affected bone in a case in which the Paget's disease appears to be limited to that bone.

**Incidence.**—As already indicated, the engraftment of a sarcoma upon a bone affected with Paget's disease is by no means uncommon. However, it is difficult to state the over-all incidence of this complication with any precision. Among those cases in which the skeleton is heavily involved by the disease, the incidence seems to approach 10 per cent. Among cases of Paget's disease in which the number of bones affected is not large, the incidence is certainly lower than 10 per cent, and perhaps as low as 2 or 3 per cent. Indeed, if the numerous cases of nonclinical Paget's disease of limited extent are taken into account in the statistics on malignant transformation, the over-all incidence can safely be said to be much lower than even 2 or 3 per cent. How very numerous these mild cases really are is shown by the

***Figure 144***

*A*, Roentgenograph showing a large osteolytic lesion produced by a sarcoma involving the upper third of the shaft and part of the head of a humerus. The tumor has broken out of the bone, especially medially, and the bone shaft is also the site of a pathologic fracture (see *B*). The patient was a man 65 years of age who had been complaining for 1 month of increasingly severe pain relating to the right shoulder. From the *x*-ray picture illustrated (which was taken at the time of admission), one could not be certain that the sarcoma had been engrafted upon a bone affected with Paget's disease. However, an *x*-ray picture taken elsewhere, 9 months earlier, was available for comparison because the part in question had been injured in the course of a brawl. That picture showed that the humerus was clearly the site of Paget's disease, and that the sarcoma was apparently already evolving. A skeletal survey at the time of admission revealed that Paget's disease was also present in the lower end of the right radius and in the pelvic bones. The affected upper limb was disarticulated.

*B*, Photograph of the humerus shown in *A*, sectioned in the sagittal plane. Note that the central part of the tumor is hemorrhagic and cystified. Microscopic examination revealed that the tumor was essentially a highly anaplastic polymorphocellular sarcoma very rich in sarcoma giant cells. There was no evidence of osteogenesis anywhere in the tumor tissue. Histologic study of the nonsarcomatous part of the humerus showed it to be the site of Paget's disease, as was the lower end of the radius. Roentgenographic examination of the chest 1 year after the disarticulation revealed a large focus of pulmonary metastasis.

*C*, Roentgenograph showing the lower part of a sectioned femur altered by Paget's disease and presenting a large focus of osteolysis produced by a sarcoma in one of the condylar areas. The patient was a man 60 years of age whose only difficulty relating to his Paget's disease prior to the clinical emergence of the sarcoma was a slight bowing deformity of both tibiæ. A skeletal survey made at the time of admission showed that the Paget's disease involved not only the femur in question, but also the calvarium, the pelvic bones, both tibiæ, and the left fibula. The complaints referable to the sarcoma were that the knee region had been painful for 3 months and that the pain was growing worse. The lower end of the femur was tender to palpation and was the site of a local swelling. The affected lower extremity was amputated, but no follow-up information is available in this case.

*D*, Photograph of the femur shown in *C*. The Paget's disease is indicated by the thickening and altered architecture of the cortex and the thickening and abnormal compaction of the spongy bone. The sarcoma on the right appears as a focus of firm fibrous tissue which manifested no grittiness on palpation. Microscopic examination of numerous tumor areas revealed that the tissue pattern was the same throughout. The pattern was that of a lattice of sarcomatous spindle-shaped cells, interspersed with large numbers of round cells, many of which were apparently lymphocytes and reticulum cells. Osteogenesis was not in evidence anywhere in the tumor tissue.

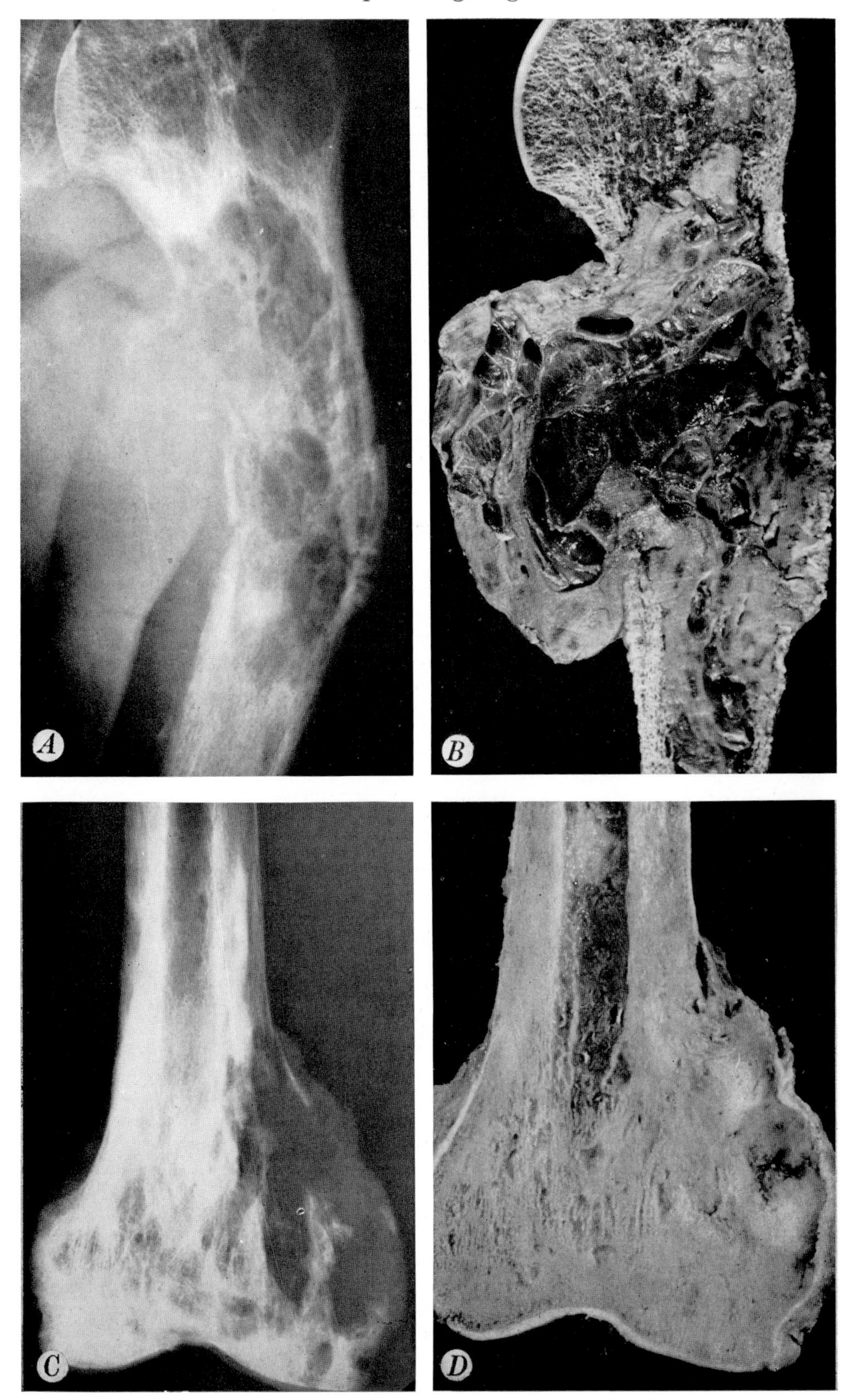


***Figure 144***

fact that in about 3 per cent of persons over 40 years of age coming to autopsy, some degree of Paget's disease (frequently involving only part of a single vertebral body) can be found in the vertebral column if this is removed and examined. Thus, in evaluating any report giving data on the incidence of the complication, one must give due consideration to the range of severity of the Paget's disease in the cases included in the report.

**Clinical Emergence of the Sarcoma.**—It is not unusual, in the milder cases of Paget's disease, first to discover the presence of the disease only because a sarcoma has become engrafted upon one or another of the affected bones. Thus a sarcoma appearing in a bone of a middle-aged or older person may well instigate a roentgenographic search for Paget's disease in that bone and in the rest of the skeleton, for frequently in these age groups, a bone sarcoma has its foundation in Paget's disease. (See Fig. 144.)

How limited the Paget's disease may be and still be the basis for sarcoma is illustrated by the following experiences of the writer, to which he could add others. He has observed 2 cases of Paget's disease limited to the cranium, in both of which a sarcoma appeared in the occiput; a case in which the disease was limited to the 6th thoracic vertebra, insofar as one could judge from the skeletal survey pictures,

***Figure 145***

*A*, Photograph showing the cut surface of a sarcomatously transformed innominate bone (along with part of the sacrum and femur) removed in a case of Paget's disease which came to autopsy. The patient was a woman 72 years of age in whom Paget's disease was widely distributed over the skeleton and had been known to be present for at least 10 years. However, her complaints relating to the sarcoma were of only 3 months' standing. In particular, the region of the left hip became the site of increasingly severe pain, and a rapidly enlarging tumor mass appeared there. *X*-ray examination of the affected ilium showed it to be riddled with large areas of osteolysis, intermingled with blotchy areas of radiopacity. Death occurred 4 months after the onset of the acute complaints. At autopsy, the left innominate bone was found largely replaced by a tumor which was also extending into the neighboring musculature, the local tumor mass measuring 20 × 17 × 13 cm. Both femora were also removed, and these too were found to be the site of cancer, presenting multiple foci of tumor tissue involving both the spongiosa and the cortex. Furthermore, metastases to the lungs and heart were noted. On microscopic examination, the histologic pattern of the tumor in the innominate bone was found to vary in detail from place to place. In some tissue fields it was that of an osteogenic sarcoma, in others it was that of a fibrosarcoma which was highly anaplastic here and there, and in still other areas the pattern resembled that of a malignant giant-cell tumor.

*B*, Roentgenograph showing the lower half of a femur altered by Paget's disease and also presenting a sarcoma whose shadow is largely radiopaque. In conformity with this finding, the tumor tissue in the gross specimen (see *C*) showed considerable grittiness. The patient was a woman 48 years of age. The presence of the Paget's disease had been discovered fortuitously a year or so before admission, in connection with *x*-ray study of the kidneys for renal colic. The complaints relating to the sarcoma in the femur were of only 2 months' standing and consisted of increasing local pain and swelling. There was no history of injury. A skeletal survey on admission showed Paget's disease in the calvarium, vertebral column, pelvic bones, and femora. *X*-ray examination of the chest revealed no evidence of metastasis, and the limb presenting the sarcoma in the femur was amputated. However, re-examination of the chest 3 months later revealed innumerable smaller and larger radiopaque foci of metastasis in the lungs.

*C*, Photograph of the femur shown in *A*, cut in the frontal plane. The tumor tissue felt gritty more or less throughout, and a pathologic fracture extending transversely across the bone can be seen. Microscopic study of various areas of the tumor revealed everywhere the pattern of an osteogenic sarcoma—that is, a spindle cell sarcoma showing the formation of considerable tumor osteoid and tumor bone.

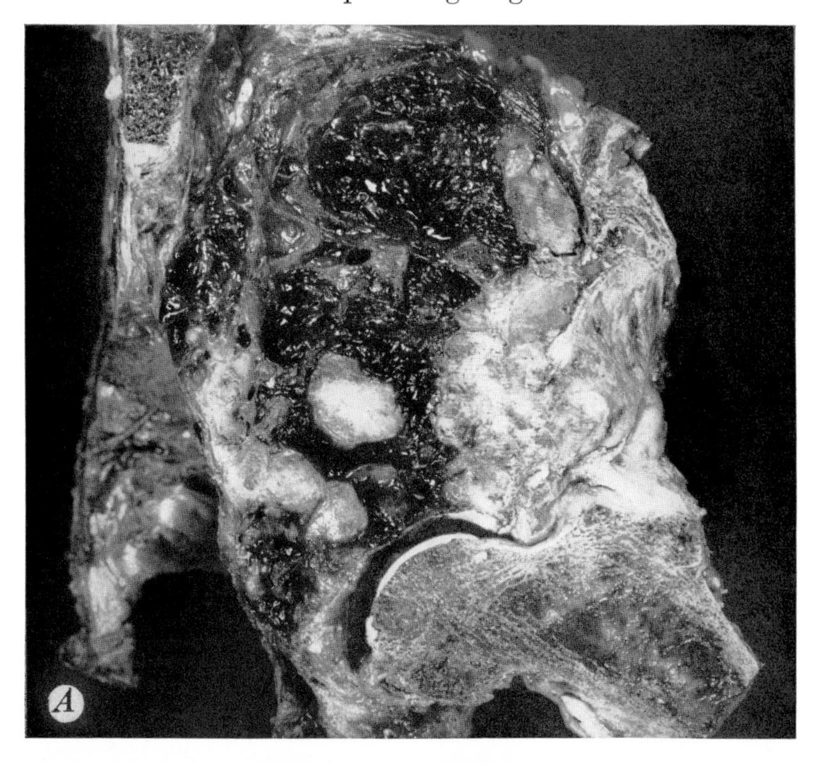

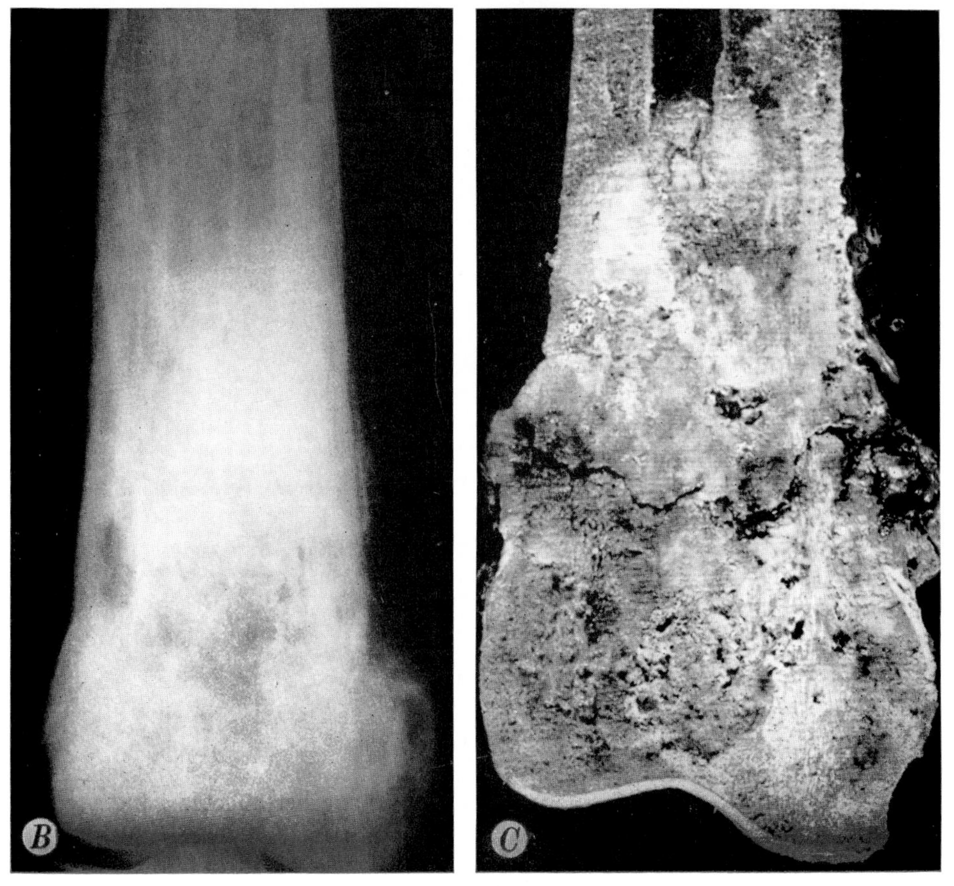

***Figure 145***

and that vertebra became the site of a sarcoma; a case in which the disease was limited to the pelvic bones and 5th lumbar vertebra and a sarcoma appeared in one of the ischia; a case in which the disease was limited to the left innominate bone and the upper end of the right femur and the latter was the site of a sarcoma; a case of sarcoma appearing in an affected scapula, in which subsequent study also revealed Paget's disease in the pelvic bones; a case in which a sarcoma appeared in an affected humerus and in which a subsequent skeletal survey also revealed Paget's disease in the lower end of the homolateral radius and in the pelvis; and a case in which a sarcoma appeared in a tibia known for 13 years to be affected with Paget's disease and in which it turned out that that disease was also present in the lower lumbar vertebræ and in the pelvic bones.

In a case of widespread Paget's disease, when a sarcoma appears in one affected bone or bone part, other foci of sarcoma are usually already present or soon become apparent in other affected parts. The question naturally arises whether these other foci of sarcoma represent metastatic or independent sarcomas. Autopsy findings in such cases point strongly to independent (multicentric) origin of these other sarcomas. This conception is also supported by those cases in which the Paget's disease is of limited extent, but in which, some months after the appearance of the sarcoma in one bone, a focus of sarcoma appears in one or several of the few other bones affected by the disease. A point indirectly favoring the multicentric origin of the sarcomas in these various cases of Paget's disease is the fact that, in cases of osteogenic sarcoma occurring in children, skeletal metastases are definitely uncommon.

Not infrequently, in a case of sarcoma complicating Paget's disease, a *trauma* is inculpated in relation to the onset of the difficulty. In other cases, however, there is no history of antecedent trauma, and this fact already casts some doubt upon the importance of trauma as an instigating factor. Even greater weight in this connection belongs to the finding, already noted, that, in cases of very widespread Paget's disease, sarcoma may appear in various bone sites simultaneously. Obviously, in such a case, a trauma at a single bone site cannot account for the development of sarcomas at sites remote from the traumatized area. At most, then, a trauma seems merely to attract attention to a sarcoma already present. If the trauma should be so severe as to induce a fracture through the tumor site or otherwise disrupt the tumor, local acceleration of the sarcoma's growth would, of course, be favored. In any event, the occurrence of a trauma has no bearing on the ultimate outcome of the case, since sarcoma complicating Paget's disease is invariably fatal, even in cases in which there has been no trauma.

**Clinical and Roentgenographic Findings.**—When a sarcoma is evolving in a site of Paget's disease, the patient comes to complain of more or less continuous aching and gnawing pain referred to that area. Concomitantly, a tumorous swelling usually appears at the painful site. Often the tumor mass grows rather rapidly. These complaints and findings are in contrast to the conditions prevailing in cases of Paget's disease not complicated by sarcoma. A person affected with uncomplicated Paget's disease is often unaware of its presence. In such a case the disease may be discovered quite fortuitously in the course of roentgenographic examination of some visceral part which has been the source of complaint. In other cases the Paget's disease comes to light when a region such as a lower limb or the lower part of the back is roentgenographed merely because of discomfort or relatively mild pain. Indeed, these may be the sole complaints even when the disease has already spread widely over the skeleton. In still other cases the patients may be aware, in addition, of increasing curvature of the lower limbs, increasing size of the head, and/or progressive deafness. Thus, when a patient with Paget's disease begins to complain of definite and increasing pain at one or another affected bone site, one should immediately be alert to the possibility that a sarcoma is developing there. (See Fig. 145.)

That the serum *alkaline phosphatase value* is elevated in cases of Paget's disease is well known. When the disease is of limited extent, the alkaline phosphatase values may range between 5 and about 25 Bodansky units, in accordance with the number of bones affected and the severity of the involvement. When the disease is very widespread and still progressing, it is not unusual to find alkaline phosphatase values of 50 to 125 units. When sarcomatous changes occur in connection with the disease, the phosphatase value tends to become higher than it was before the complication appeared. Should the sarcoma be of a type which lays down large amounts of tumor osteoid and osseous tissue, and should many bones be sites of sarcomatous transformation, the serum alkaline phosphatase value may rise to extremely high levels, such as 200 Bodansky units, or even higher (see Jaffe and Bodansky).

On *roentgenographic examination*, a sarcoma appearing in connection with Paget's disease often stands out as a smaller or larger irregular area of radiolucency (representing osteolysis) against a background of bone altered by the disease. The presence of streaky radiopacities within the osteolytic area or in the tumor tissue which has gained exit from the bone reflects ossification going on in the tumor tissue. On the whole, however, the sarcomas of Paget's disease do not show striking radiopacity. Indeed, one only infrequently sees the dense, eburnated radiopaque shadows representing heavy ossification of the tumor tissue, which are so commonly observed in connection with osteogenic sarcoma occurring *de novo*—that is, the osteogenic sarcoma predilecting adolescents and young adults. This is true irrespective of whether only one bone affected with Paget's disease shows a sarcoma or multiple sarcomas are present in the skeleton.

**Pathologic Findings.**—In respect to *gross appearance*, some of the sarcomas encountered are essentially fibrous tumors and manifest little or no grittiness of the tumor tissue. In others, the lesional tissue may feel quite gritty, at least in some areas. It is unusual, however, for the tumor to be so heavily ossified that large areas of it are hard and eburnated. If the sarcoma is a bulky one, much of the lesional tissue may, in fact, be hemorrhagic and cystified, although the hemorrhagic and cystic areas are usually found interspersed with areas in which the tumor tissue is still firm and, in places, even somewhat gritty. In view of this range of the gross findings, it is not surprising that there is also a good deal of variety in regard to histologic detail among the individual lesions and even between different areas of the same lesion.

In accordance with the gross findings, the *microscopic pattern* is occasionally that of a collagenized fibrosarcoma more or less throughout. In other lesions it is that of a highly cellular and, on the whole, anaplastic fibrosarcoma rich in sarcoma giant cells. In still others, areas in which the tumor tissue presents the pattern of an anaplastic fibrosarcoma rich in sarcoma giant cells are interspersed with areas in which numerous multinuclear giant cells resembling those seen in giant-cell tumor are set against a background of plump spindle cells. Thus, the sarcoma in such an instance manifests the pattern of an anaplastic and indeed polymorphocellular fibrosarcoma in some tissue fields and that of a malignant giant-cell tumor in other fields. Furthermore, in most of the tumors the sarcomatous stroma also expresses osteogenic potentialities, in part or throughout. Consequently, one may encounter a sarcoma in which the pattern is that of a fibrosarcoma in some areas, a malignant giant-cell tumor in others, and an osteogenic sarcoma in still others. In those of the sarcomas whose histologic pattern comes to be dominated by osteogenesis, the large amount of tumor osteoid and osseous tissue formed may even create the pattern of a so-called "sclerosing" osteogenic sarcoma.

Even this variety, however, does not express the full range of the cytologic possibilities. In one case studied by the writer, not only was tumor osteoid and bone being formed, but in many places (even in areas in which ossification was going on) the sarcomatous stromal tissue seemed to be composed of cells resembling malignant myeloid elements. Just as arresting as this case was one in which the tumor showed the pattern of a chondrosarcoma throughout.

It is difficult to explain this complexity of cytologic expression manifested by the sarcomas appearing in connection with Paget's disease. All we know is that the basic tissue from which they arise reveals, even within the same tumor, manifold potentialities for differentiation along mesenchymal lines. Hence it is important to recognize that a random sample of the tumor tissue from a given sarcoma often does not represent the pattern of the tumor tissue throughout the lesion. Thus it is probably best in all cases to denote the tumor simply as a sarcoma complicating Paget's disease, rather than to try to narrow its designation down to some specific variety of bone sarcoma.

**Prognosis and Treatment.**—The occurrence of sarcoma in a case of Paget's disease is very ominous. The patients developing multiple sarcomas, of course, all die soon. (See Fig. 146.) Specifically, most of them succumb with metastases in the lungs (and usually also elsewhere) in the course of about 6 months. Those who do not succumb within this time live only a little longer. If the sarcomatous involvement seems to be limited to one bone (particularly of a limb), amputation may constitute good palliative treatment. In the writer's experience, however, the patients in such cases, too, have succumbed to pulmonary metastases.

## GIANT-CELL TUMOR COMPLICATING PAGET'S DISEASE

Once in a great while, a bone part affected with Paget's disease shows a tumor or even multiple tumors presenting the tissue pattern of a conventional giant-cell tumor throughout. That is, in these lesions the tumor tissue is completely devoid of ominous histologic features. So far as the writer's experience goes, this occurrence has been observed only in relation to the skull. In a particularly illuminating case which he followed, 12 giant-cell tumor lesions appeared successively in the course of 8 years in relation to the frontal, parietal, temporal, occipital, and upper facial region. As to the Paget's disease itself, this involved not only the skull, but also the vertebral column, the innominate bones and the femora. In none of

***Figure 146***

*A*, Roentgenograph of a femur in a case of widespread Paget's disease in which innumerable foci of sarcoma appeared practically simultaneously in many of the affected bones (see also *B*). The patient was a woman 65 years of age who had been unaware that she had any skeletal disease until difficulties due to the complicating sarcoma began to appear. Her presenting complaint was pain and swelling in the left elbow, due to the development of a sarcoma at the lower end of the left humerus, which was a site of Paget's disease. Soon thereafter, small, nodular swellings appeared on other affected bones. Note the densely radiopaque foci in the femur, representing areas of sarcoma in which the formation of tumor osteoid and tumor bone was found conspicuous on microscopic examination. The patient died with extensive pulmonary metastases about 6 months after the onset of her complaints.

*B*, Roentgenograph of a tibia from the case illustrated in *A*. Note that in this bone, too, there are multiple areas of radiopacity representing multiple foci of osteogenic sarcoma.

*C*, Photomicrograph (× 4) illustrating a cross section through a femur affected with Paget's disease and representing 2 independent foci of osteogenic sarcoma oriented to the cortex of the bone at that level.

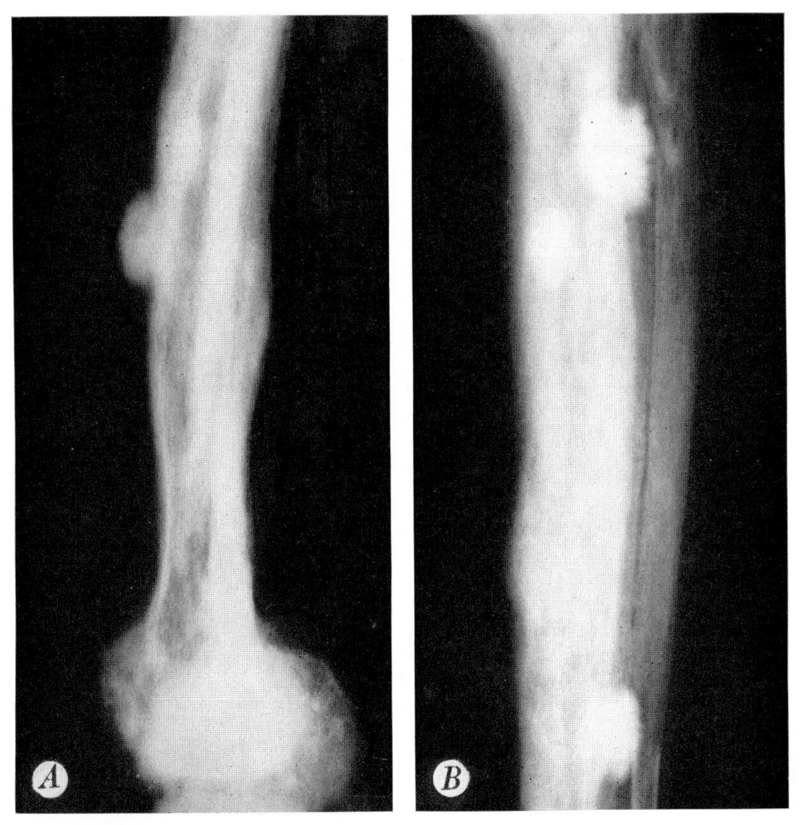


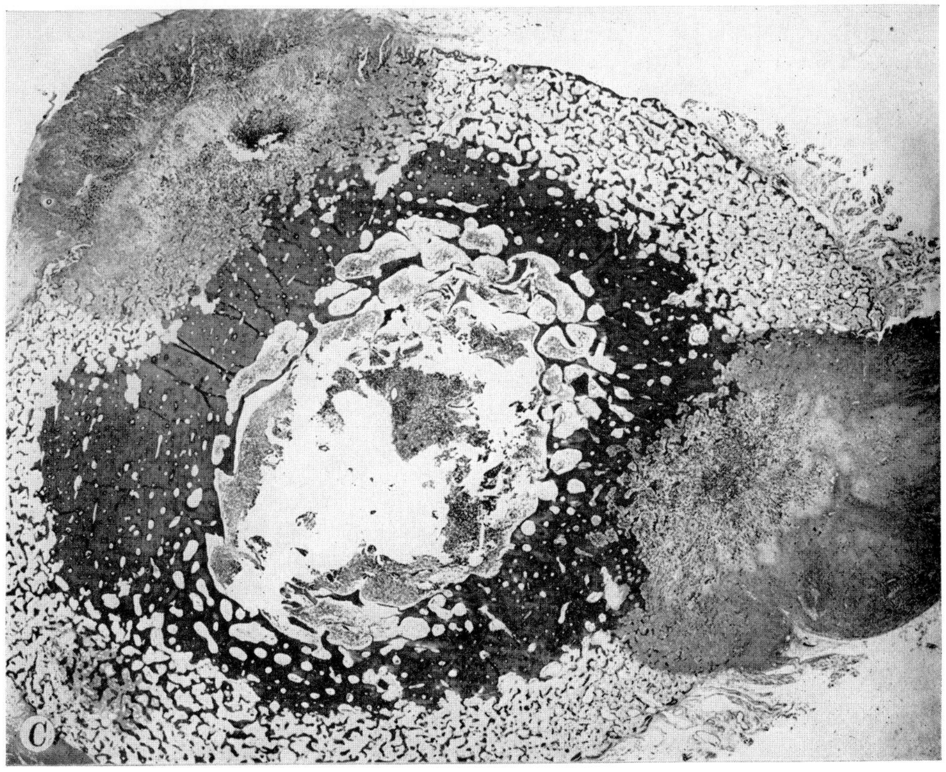


***Figure 146***

these other skeletal parts has any type of tumor developed to complicate the Paget's disease.

All of the tumors were manifest externally as local swellings. A number of them were as large as 6 × 6 cm. in diameter and projected as much as 3 cm. on the surface. None of the lesions gave rise to much pain, and some caused no pain at all. Roentgenographically, wherever a tumor had appeared, one could note an irregular area of radiolucency representing osteolysis. In the course of the 8-year period, tissue was removed from 3 of the tumors for histologic study. In each instance the tissue presented the pattern of numerous large, multinuclear giant cells set in a rather meager stroma of spindle-shaped cells. Accordingly, the pattern presented by each of the 3 lesions examined histologically was interpreted as that of a conventional giant-cell tumor.

The individual tumors were treated with irradiation, some lesions receiving roentgen rays and others gamma radium rays. The total dosage given to the 12 lesions together in the course of the 8 years amounted to 62,000 r (48,000 r of $x$-rays and 14,000 r of gamma rays). Most of the lesions shrank perceptibly under this treatment. That these tumors were multicentric is indicated by the fact that while a given lesion was shrinking under treatment, another was developing at a clearly different though not necessarily remote site. (See Fig. 147.)

From the experience relating to this case, and from what one can gather from an occasional other case which has been reported in the literature, it appears that the outlook for continued survival when Paget's disease is complicated by giant-cell tumor (as contrasted with sarcoma) is not bad. Just what the ultimate outcome will be in the particular case detailed above cannot be predicted. Other tumors are likely to develop, or some of the original ones may recur, and eventually there may be serious damage to vital tissues, either from direct extension of tumor tissue or from hemorrhage. Furthermore, so much irradiation has already been given in the attempt to check the growth of the various tumors that there is a possibility of the eventual development of a postirradiation sarcoma in one or another of the treated areas.

## TUMORS COMPLICATING CHRONIC OSTEOMYELITIS

The possibility that a malignant tumor may evolve at a site of chronic osteomyelitis associated with sinus formation is generally recognized. The bone infection may have followed upon a war wound, developed in consequence of a compound fracture from an accident, or been caused by hematogenous spread of the bacterial agent (see Benedict, and McAnally and Dockerty, Marks and Turner, Gillis and Lee). Nearly always, the tumor is a squamous cell carcinoma, but in very rare instances it is a sarcoma. As to localization, it is of interest that when a cancer does

***Figure 147***

*A*, Roentgenograph of a calvarium affected with Paget's disease and showing, in the fronto-parietal region, areas of radiolucency resulting from the development of foci of giant-cell tumor. As indicated in the text, 12 independent foci of giant-cell tumor appeared in various parts of the skull in the course of 8 years in this case. The patient was a woman who was 46 years of age at the time when the first giant-cell tumor lesion appeared, and she also presented evidences of Paget's disease in other parts of the skeleton.

*B*, Photomicrograph (×125) showing the pattern, typical of a conventional giant-cell tumor, which was demonstrated by the tissue removed from the presenting lesion in the case illustrated in *A*. Two other tumor foci were also biopsied and presented the identical histologic tissue pattern.

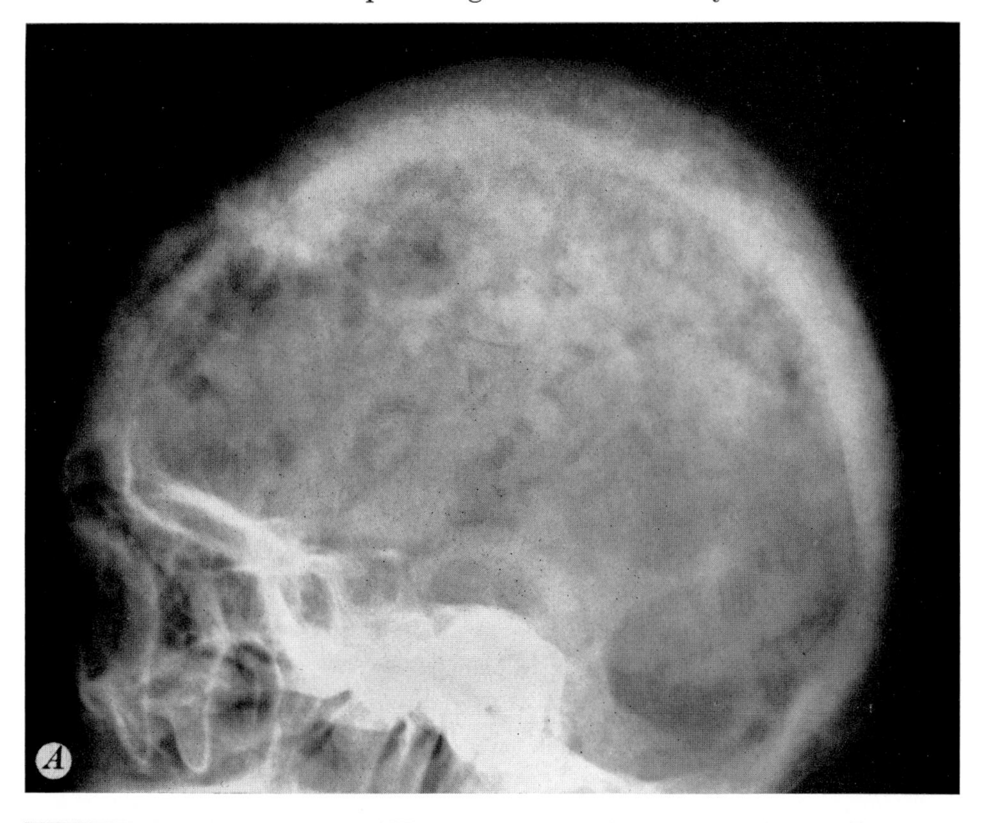


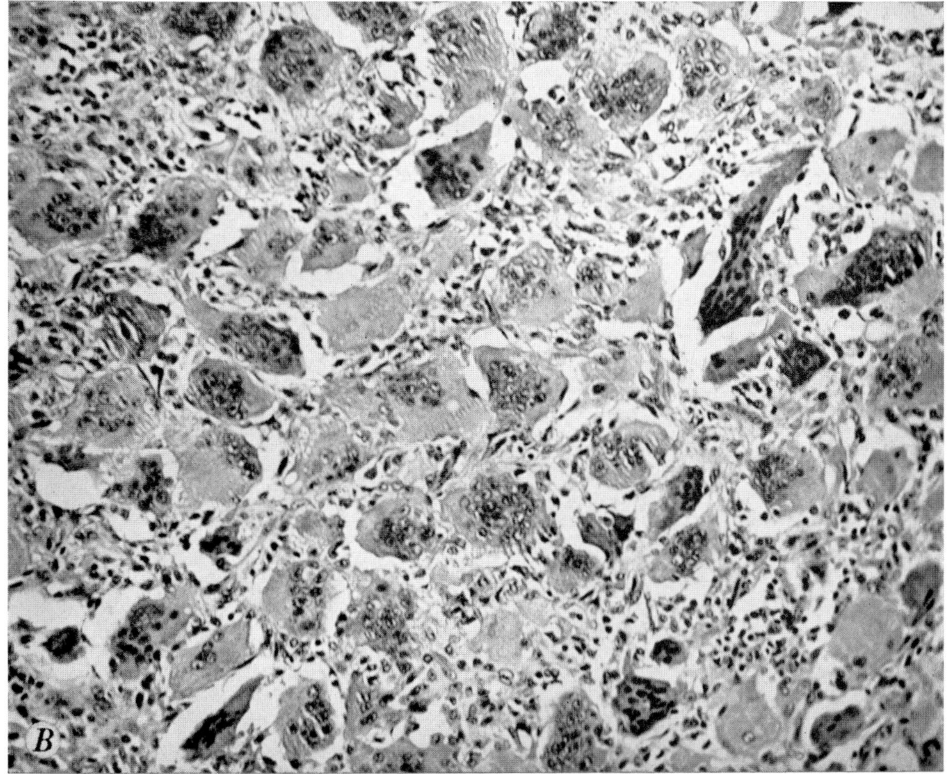


*Figure 147*

appear in connection with chronic osteomyelitis, the bone involved is almost always a bone of a lower extremity or of the pelvis. Most often it is a tibia or a femur.

A complicating cancer has been found in only about 0.25 to 0.5 per cent of cases of protracted chronic osteomyelitis. One of the factors favoring the higher incidence is the predominance, in a given series, of cases in which the osteomyelitis has been present for a particularly long time. Indeed, it is usually only among cases in which the osteomyelitis has persisted for at least 20 or 30 years and in which sinuses are still present that one begins to see instances of this complication. The writer's experience embraces 10 cases, representing an incidence of about 0.5 per cent of the cases of chronic osteomyelitis treated at the Hospital for Joint Diseases in the course of the past 30 years. However, in the future, cancer complicating chronic osteomyelitis is likely to be observed even less frequently, because of the modern management of chronic osteomyelitis by aggressive surgery and antibiotic therapy.

**Squamous Cell Carcinoma.**—The carcinoma may arise in the epithelialized lining of a bone cavity (such as often forms in stubborn cases of osteomyelitis) and invade the neighboring bone before extending along the sinus tract toward the surface of the limb. More often, however, the carcinoma begins in the region of the superficial mouth of the sinus and extends down along the sinus tract and eventually into the bone. In the latter cases, the fact that one is dealing with a carcinoma is often obvious clinically from the appearances at the mouth of the sinus and the adjacent skin. Thus the sinus may be rimmed by a large fleshy area of ulceration with hard, rolled edges, or a fungating tumor mass may be present at and around the mouth of the sinus.

Even in the absence of such indications of local cancerous transformation, one should be alert to the possibility that a cancer is evolving deep in the bone if there is increased pain and increased foul discharge and/or bleeding from the sinus. In an occasional case the growth of the cancer tissue within the osteomyelitic bone may so have weakened the latter that a pathologic fracture supervened. In any suspected case of carcinoma evolving at the site of a chronic osteomyelitis, a biopsy should also be done to establish or rule out the diagnosis. (See Fig. 148.)

The cancer tissue usually presents, in rather clear-cut fashion, the microscopic pattern of a squamous cell carcinoma. Indeed, the lesional tissue may reveal, in part or throughout, the intercellular bridges and central keratinous nests or "epithelial pearls" which easily identify the tumor as one originating from squamous epithelium.

### *Figure 148*

*A*, Roentgenograph showing a focus of chronic osteomyelitis in the lower part of a tibia, at which site a squamous cell carcinoma appeared (see *C*). The patient was a man 66 years of age whose osteomyelitis dated back to late childhood. The lower part of the leg had been the site of several sinuses which had been draining more or less constantly for 26 years before the affected limb was amputated on account of the complicating cancer.

*B*, Photograph showing a tibia which has been invaded by a squamous cell carcinoma in a case of chronic osteomyelitis associated with the presence of a draining sinus at the site of the subsequence cancer. The patient was a man 64 years of age who had suffered a shrapnel wound of the leg 38 years prior to admission. He developed a focus of osteomyelitis in the tibia, associated with the presence of a draining sinus. The carcinoma began to evolve about 1 year prior to amputation of the affected limb. At the time of the amputation, the regional inguinal lymph nodes were found enlarged. A subsequent radical lymph node resection revealed that the enlarged nodes were the site of metastases. The patient died of massive pulmonary embolism subsequent to the lymph node dissection. At autopsy, metastases were *not* found in the lungs or elsewhere.

*C*, Photomicrograph (× 75) illustrating the cytologic pattern of the squamous cell carcinoma from the case illustrated in *A*.

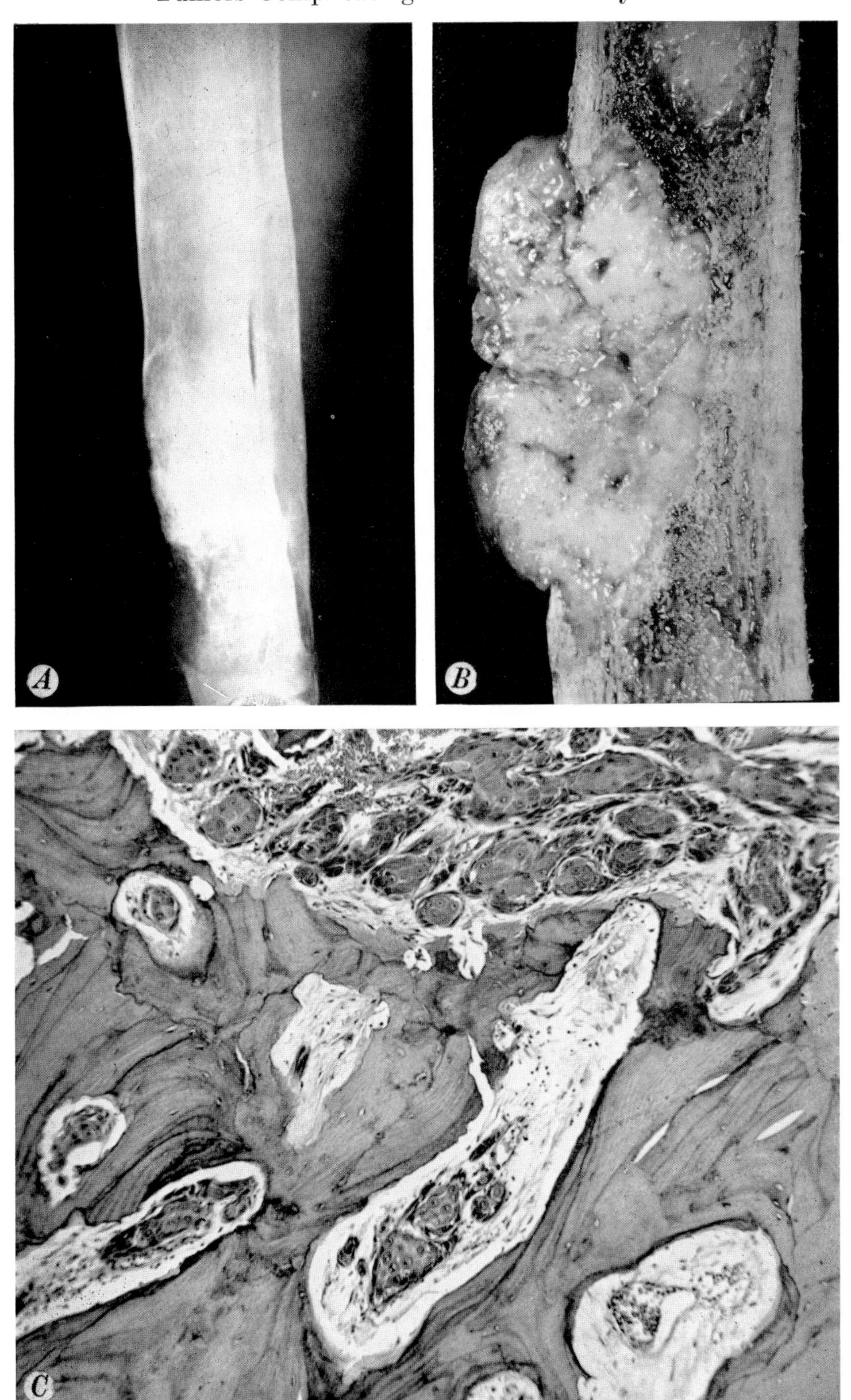


*Figure 148*

On the other hand, one may encounter a case in which, in part or throughout, the lesional tissue is not well differentiated and fails to show these elements. In an occasional instance the anaplasia may even be so extreme that the tissue pattern may suggest a spindle cell sarcoma rather than a carcinoma. The literature contains several reports of cases in which, on this account, the complicating cancer was first thought to represent a sarcoma, but in which subsequent histologic findings established it as a carcinoma.

Another histologic diagnostic problem which sometimes arises is the differentiation between a squamous cell carcinoma and pseudoepitheliomatous hyperplasia going on in the epithelialized sinus wall or adjacent skin. Actually, if sufficient tissue sections are studied, the problem is usually readily resolved. The cells in the isolated epithelial nests from an area of pseudoepitheliomatous hyperplasia turn out to be quite well differentiated and to resemble very closely the epithelial cells of the neighboring benign epidermis and epidermal "pegs."

Clinically, when one is confronted with a case of osteomyelitis of very long standing, associated with persistent sinus formation, one must be guided by the fact that there is some danger of the development of a squamous cell carcinoma. If repeated attempts by modern therapy have failed to obliterate the sinus, amputation may well be considered as a preventive measure. For a case in which a squamous cell carcinoma has already appeared, amputation is clearly indicated. As to the regional lymph nodes, it should be pointed out that they are likely to show enlargement in these cases. However, when they have been examined histologically, their enlargement has been found attributable, much more often than not, to chronic lymphadenitis rather than metastasis. Occasionally, however, the regional lymph nodes are already metastatically invaded, and this involvement, too, must be considered in the surgical approach and prognosis. In such cases, if amputation (and resection of affected regional lymph nodes) is much delayed, pulmonary and other visceral metastases, and consequently death, can be expected in about 50 per cent of the pertinent cases. If the regional lymph nodes are not involved at the time of the amputation, and especially if the carcinoma has not yet invaded the medullary cavity of the osteomyelitic bone, the ultimate prognosis is very much better.

**Sarcoma.**—As already noted, it is only very rarely that a sarcoma develops at the site of a chronic osteomyelitis. In a suspected instance, care must be taken to rule out the possibility that one is dealing with a highly anaplastic carcinoma which is mimicking the histologic pattern of a sarcoma, rather than with an actual sarcoma. An acceptable example of a sarcoma complicating an osteomyelitis was reported by Waugh. For 48 years prior to the appearance of the tumor, the patient had had a focus of chronic osteomyelitis and abscess formation, associated with the presence of a discharging sinus, at the lower end of a femur. The tumor was a fibrosarcoma which grew to large size in the course of 3 months. It bled easily and was heavily

### *Figure 149*

*A*, Roentgenograph showing a tibia in a case of chronic osteomyelitis complicated by the appearance of a sarcoma. The radiolucent areas in the tibia represent foci of sarcoma destroying the bone (see *B*). The patient was a woman 37 years of age whose osteomyelitis was of 26 years' standing. For about 12 years before the appearance of the sarcoma, draining sinuses were present. The development of the sarcoma was associated with an increase in the drainage and the occurrence of local bleeding.

*B*, Photograph of the sectioned tibia from the case illustrated in *A*. The osseous tissue throughout the affected tibia is modified, and 2 large foci of sarcoma are to be noted in the midportion of the bone.

*C*, Photomicrograph (× 250) illustrating the cytologic pattern of the sarcoma in this case. The tumor is a spindle cell sarcoma and is heavily infected.

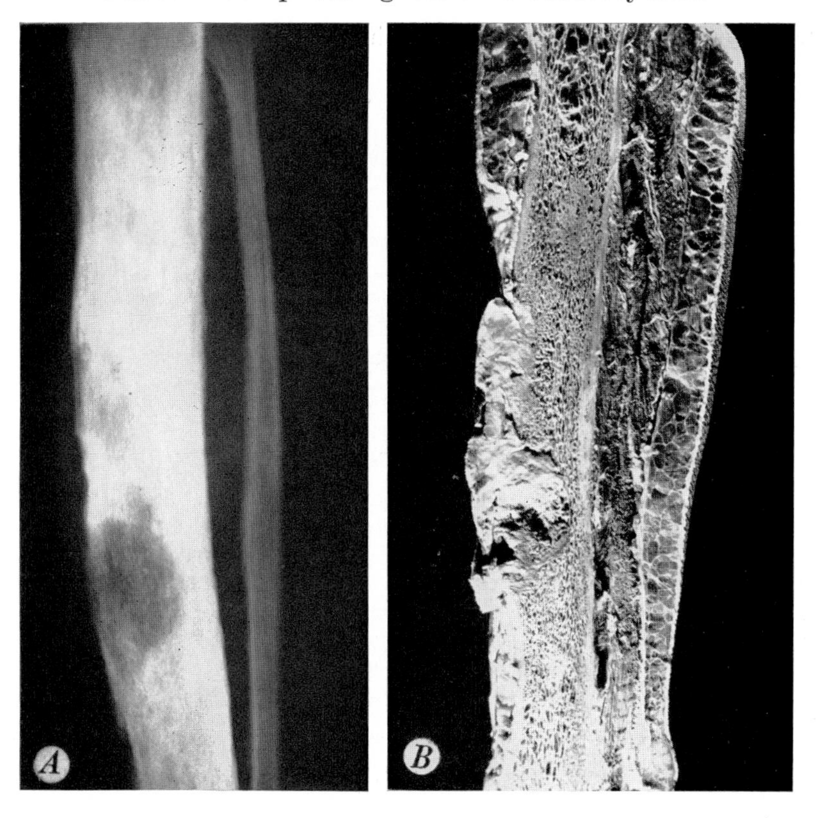


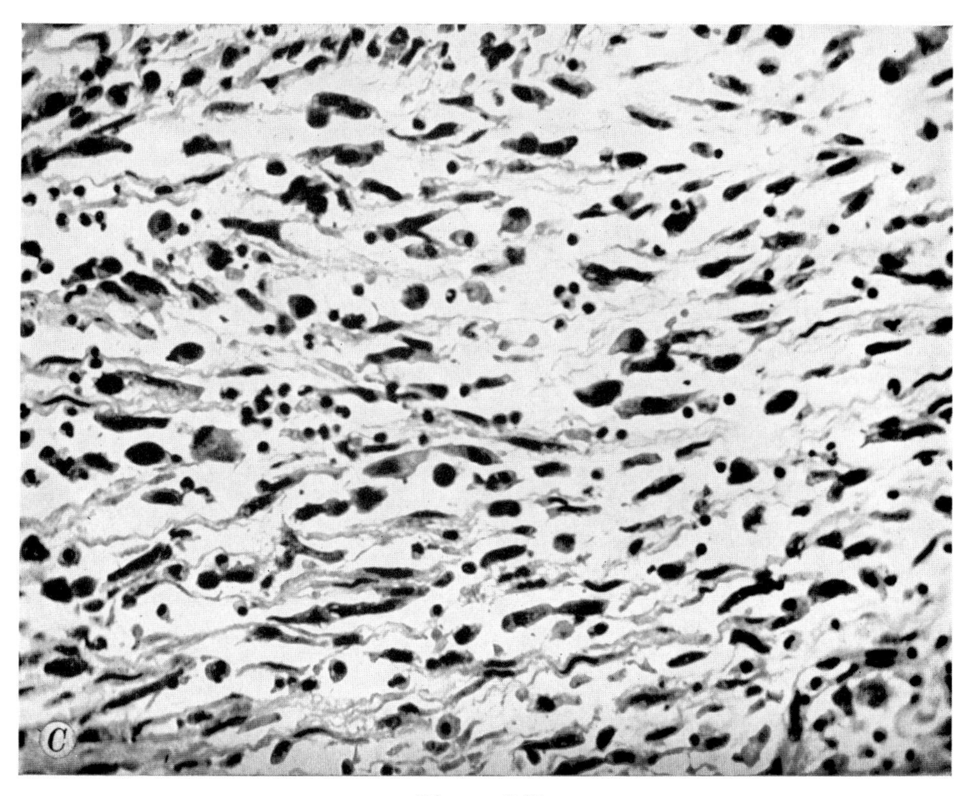


*Figure 149*

infected. It had apparently arisen from the granulation tissue of the sinus wall, and not only fungated externally but was invading the interior of the femur.

The writer, too, has observed a case of sarcoma complicating osteomyelitis. (See Fig. 149.) In this case a tibia had been the site of a draining chronic osteomyelitis for 26 years, but the sarcoma was again only of several months' standing. In the course of this short time, a large, fungating, rather vascular, foul-smelling and discharging tumor mass had appeared on the surface of the leg. On anatomic study of the amputated affected limb, the sarcoma was found also to be invading the interior of the osteomyelitic tibia. Tissue sections showed the histologic pattern of the tumor to be that of an infected, vascular, and edematous fibrosarcoma. Ten years after the amputation, the patient was still free from both local recurrence and metastasis. It may well be that the sarcoma in such cases corresponds to what the older pathologists were denoting as the granulation tissue sarcoma.

## REFERENCES


VON ALBERTINI, A.: Über Sarkombildung auf dem Boden der Ostitis deformans Paget. (Kasuistischer Beitrag), Virchows Arch. f. path. Anat., *268*, 259, 1928.

BENEDICT, E. B.: Carcinoma in Osteomyelitis, Surg., Gynec. & Obst., *53*, 1, 1931.

COLEY, B. L. and SHARP, G. S.: Paget's Disease: A Predisposing Factor to Osteogenic Sarcoma, Arch. Surg., *23*, 918, 1931.

DERMAN, H., PIZZOLATO, P., and ZISKIND, J.: Multicentric Osteogenic Sarcoma in Paget's Disease with Cerebral Extension, Am. J. Roentgenol., *65*, 221, 1951.

DEVAS, M. B.: Malignant Change in Chronic Osteomyelitis, Brit. J. Surg., *40*, 140, 1952.

GILLIS, L., and LEE, S.: Cancer as a Sequel to War Wounds, J. Bone & Joint Surg., *33-B*, 167, 1951.

HILTON, G.: Osteoclastoma Associated with Generalised Bone Disease, Brit. J. Radiol., *23*, 437, 1950.

JAFFE, H. L.: Paget's Disease of Bone, Arch. Path., *15*, 83, 1933.

JAFFE, H. L., and BODANSKY, A.: Diagnostic Significance of Serum Alkaline and Acid Phosphatase Values in Relation to Bone Disease, Bull. New York Acad. Med., *19*, 831, 1943.

MANEY, A. W.: Lymphatic Dissemination of a Sarcoma Superimposed on Paget's Disease of the Os Calcis, Brit. J. Surg., *40*, 84, 1952.

MARKS, K. L., and TURNER, W. L.: Carcinoma Occurring in the Sinuses of Chronic Osteomyelitis, Brit. J. Surg., *38*, 206, 1950.

MCANALLY, A. K., and DOCKERTY, M. B.: Carcinoma Developing in Chronic Draining Cutaneous Sinuses and Fistulas, Surg., Gynec. & Obst., *88*, 87, 1949.

NIEBAUER, J. J.: Development of Squamous-Cell Carcinomata in the Sinus Tracts of Chronic Osteomyelitis, J. Bone & Joint Surg., *28*, 280, 1946.

NOLI, G., and ZINCONE, P.: Osteodistrofia pagetica e degenerazione sarcomatosa, Rass. ital. chir. med., *4*, 397, 1955.

PLATT, H.: Sarcoma in Abnormal Bones, Brit. J. Surg., *34*, 232, 1947.

RUSSELL, D. S.: Malignant Osteoclastoma and the Association of Malignant Osteoclastoma with Paget's Osteitis Deformans, J. Bone & Joint Surg., *31-B*, 281, 1949.

SCHMORL, G.: Über Ostitis deformans Paget, Virchows Arch. f. path. Anat., *283*, 694, 1932.

SUMMEY, T. J., and PRESSLY, C. L.: Sarcoma Complicating Paget's Disease of Bone, Ann. Surg., *123*, 135, 1946.

DE VULPIAN, P., and KIRSCH, J.: Sur la transformation de la maladie osseuse de Paget en tumeur maligne, Paris méd., *40*, 622, 1950.

WAUGH, W.: Fibrosarcoma Occurring in a Chronic Bone Sinus, J. Bone & Joint Surg., *34-B*, 642, 1952.

Chapter

# 28

# Radiation Injury and Postradiation Sarcoma of Bones

It is well known that *ionizing radiation* (from any source) is capable of producing serious damage to the various tissues of the body. In regard to *external radiation*, it became evident early that persons whose work involved the use of roentgen rays or radium and who had failed to protect themselves adequately often developed an extremely stubborn dermatitis of the exposed parts. Furthermore, it was found that, not infrequently, an epidermoid carcinoma eventually evolved somewhere in the affected skin. It also soon became established that other tissues, too, may be damaged by excessive exposure of the surface of the body to roentgen and radium rays. In respect to the blood-forming tissues, it became known that this may lead to the development of a fatal anemia and even leukemia, resulting from damage to the bone marrow (see Ledoux-Lebard, Rolleston, and Colwell and Russ). Aside from its effects on the bone marrow, external radiation was found capable of causing injury to the osseous tissue proper and (in growing subjects) to the cartilage at sites of endochondral ossification.

The growth-inhibiting effects of injury to epiphysial cartilage plates by external radiation were already demonstrated on an experimental basis by Perthes in 1903, and additional experimental and clinical reports on these effects have been accumulating since then. In regard to the osseous tissue proper, external radiation was shown to have a necrotizing action, and the special vulnerability of the osteocytes (the bone cells encased in the bone matrix) came to be emphasized. The complex of changes which may appear in bone more or less devitalized by external radiation was denoted by Ewing as "radiation osteitis" (see also Nageotte, and Phemister). Bones so affected were found to be brittle and highly susceptible to fracture, as well as to supervening infection, especially if the damaged bone was a jawbone (see Regaud). Furthermore, it has since come to be recognized that a bone area injured by radiation sometimes becomes the site of a sarcoma. However, the eventual development of a postradiation sarcoma is less likely to occur after external than after internal radiation.

In regard to the damaging effects of *internal radiation* on human beings, great historic interest attaches to the work of Martland. In 1925, the latter began to call attention to various pathologic conditions (notably anemia, focal bone necrosis, osteomyelitis, pathologic fracture, and bone sarcoma) which were appearing as late sequelae of the ingestion and/or inhalation of radioactive substances. The victims (mainly young women) were watch dial painters who had been repeatedly ingesting small amounts of radium, mesothorium, and/or radiothorium in the course of their work. This happened because they had formed the habit of pointing with their lips the brushes which they used in applying to the dials the luminous paint containing these substances. The experiences with this industrial hazard focused attention upon another group of cases, presenting more or less analogous late effects of internal radiation. These were cases in which salts of radium and/or mesothorium had been misguidedly administered for therapeutic purposes to subjects affected with various medical disorders. A great wealth of clinical and radiobiological information based on follow-up studies on cases of both these types can be found in the recent publications by Looney, and Aub *et al.*

The early experimental studies of the effects of internally deposited radioactive substances were largely instigated by the desire to elucidate the problems presented by such clinical cases. These experimental studies have not only confirmed the pathologic findings in the clinical cases, but have yielded valuable information about bone metabolism in general and skeletal mineral metabolism in particular. The various radioactive elements show up well in the bones because they have a selective affinity for the skeletal tissues, and practically all ingested, inhaled, or injected radioactive material which is not excreted is ultimately stored in the bones.

Interest in the whole problem of radiation injury has recently been strongly reactivated by awareness of the medical dangers connected with the production and utilization of atomic energy. In consequence, many of the "bone-seeking" radioactive isotopes have become the object of intensive experimental study often centering about their early and late effects upon the skeleton (see Heller, Vaughan *et al.*, Hamilton, and Fink *et al.*). This group includes radiostrontium ($Sr^{89}$ and $Sr^{90}$), which is of special practical interest because it is a fall-out product of atomic explosion. Indeed, the potential late effects on human beings of the cumulative storage of radioactive strontium following contamination of air and soil have come to be a matter of concern. There can be little doubt that increasing contamination can be expected to produce a further rise in the already increasing incidence of leukemia (see Lewis). There is also the possibility that a very late effect of contamination of the air and soil by radioactive isotopes may be a rise in the incidence of bone sarcoma among subjects in whom the isotopes have become lodged in the bones in amounts exceeding the maximum permissible concentration. For an adult, the maximum permissible concentration of $strontium^{90}$ in the skeleton has been estimated at 1 microcurie. Langham and Anderson, and Eckelmann *et al.* present data demonstrating the slight but definite recent increase in concentration of $strontium^{90}$

***Figure 150***

*A*, Roentgenograph showing the upper end of a femur 3 years after the area had received 6,200 r of *x*-radiation on account of a giant-cell tumor. The patient was a woman 42 years of age who was free of complaints from the giant-cell tumor at the time when this picture was taken, the treatment apparently having destroyed the tumor. Note that the irradiated site appears vaguely loculated and that there is a margin of sclerosis delimiting the site of the treated lesion. However, 4 years later the appearance of the area was dominated by osteolysis, a fibrosarcoma having developed at the site of the previous giant-cell tumor.

B, Roentgenograph showing the upper end of a tibia which had been treated by *x*-radiation 4 years previously on account of the presence of Paget's disease. The patient was a man 48 years of age, and the fracture visible was of several years' standing when this picture was taken. Note the presence of areas of blotchy radiopacity, especially in the immediate vicinity of the fracture. The amount of *x*-radiation given is not known, but must have been large. Because of nonunion, extensive radiation dermatitis of the leg, and a large area of ulceration and sloughing of the skin at the level of the fracture, the limb was ablated. The sectioned tibia showed not only the gross changes of Paget's disease, but also numerous whitish calcareous foci surrounded by fibrous tissue in the immediate vicinity of the fracture line and beyond it.

*C*, Photomicrograph (× 65) illustrating the pattern of radiation osteitis found almost everywhere in the tibia shown in *B*. Note that the necrotic osseous tissue shows evidence of disintegration, and that the interosseous tissue is poor in cells, fibrillar and, in some areas, calcified.

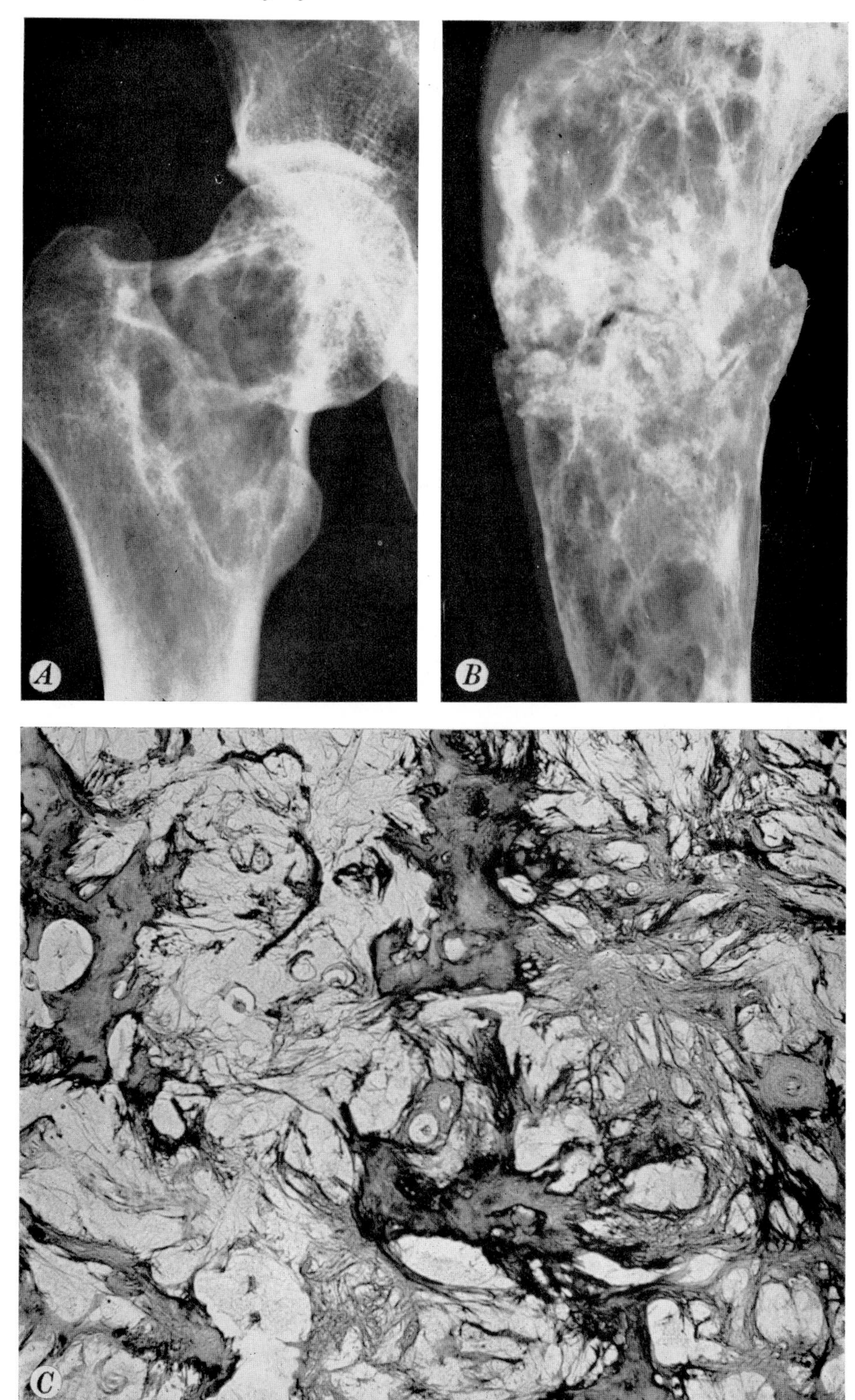


*Figure 150*

in human bones which is resulting from radioactive fall-out due to the current testing of nuclear weapons.

In addition, the question of the genetic effects of ionizing radiation has again come to the fore. In this connection, it has been known for some time that external radiation of pregnant animals may induce in the offspring such congenital malformations as dwarfing, clubbing of the feet, absence of digits, etc. Also, descendants of female animals whose gonads had been irradiated before pregnancy may be similarly affected, although sometimes not until generations later (see Bagg, and Murphy and de Renyi). Instances have also been reported in which analogous abnormalities appeared in the offspring of women whose ovaries had undergone radiation in the course of therapeutic use of the rays in the treatment of some medical disorder (see Fick). The genetic effects of atomic radiation have not as yet been fully assessed. To what degree the results of the work showing genetic mutations in lower forms are applicable to man remains to be established. At any rate, it is already clear from work with such forms (fruit flies, etc.) that *x*-radiation causes mutations by profoundly disturbing the chromosomes and/or their genes (see Muller). A review of the general problem of the genetic hazards of nuclear radiations is presented by Glass, and the question of the health hazards in the diagnostic use of *x*-rays has also been recently surveyed by Hodges.

## RADIATION OSTEITIS

The term "radiation osteitis" serves a useful purpose, despite its connotation of inflammation, to which there has been some objection. As noted, it was employed by Ewing to denote in particular the incidental damaging effects which came to be manifested in bones when *x*-rays and radium packs had been used in the treatment of various bone lesions. However, the term may reasonably be extended to include the damage produced in bones by internal radiation. Indeed, the direct harmful effects of radiation on bones are fundamentally the same, whether the source of the

***Figure 151***

*A*, Roentgenograph showing radiopacity in the hip joint area and partial collapse of the femoral head in the case of a woman whose work had involved the application of paint containing radium to watch dials. Analogous changes were present in the bones of the opposite hip joint area. (This illustration was supplied by Dr. Robert S. Sherman of the Memorial Hospital, New York City.)

*B*, Roetgenograph showing a tibia and fibula altered in consequence of the internal deposition of radioactive material. Note the numerous oval cortical radiolucencies, particularly prominent in relation to the fibula. The patient was a woman 47 years of age who had worked for 20 years as a radium dial painter. At the time of admission, she also presented a large, destructive lesion in the right ischium, which had become the site of a fibrosarcoma (Fig. 157). The estimated body content of radium at this time was 2.6 micrograms. (The clinical information and illustrative material in this case were kindly supplied by Dr. C. Howard Hatcher of the University of Chicago.)

*C*, Roentgenograph (enlarged) showing the changes produced by the internal deposition of radium in the upper end of a tibia removed at autopsy in another case of chronic radium poisoning. Note the irregular radiopacities in the spongiosa. The patient was a woman 82 years of age who had received radium chloride in connection with the treatment of "arthritis" of the spine 34 years before her death. In the interim, she had developed a severe anemia, suffered pathologic fractures of various bones, and came to show a destructive arthritis of the right hip. About 12 years before her death, the radium content of her body was estimated at 10 micrograms. (The clinical information and illustrative material in this case [see also Figs. 152 and 153] were again kindly supplied by Dr. Hatcher.)

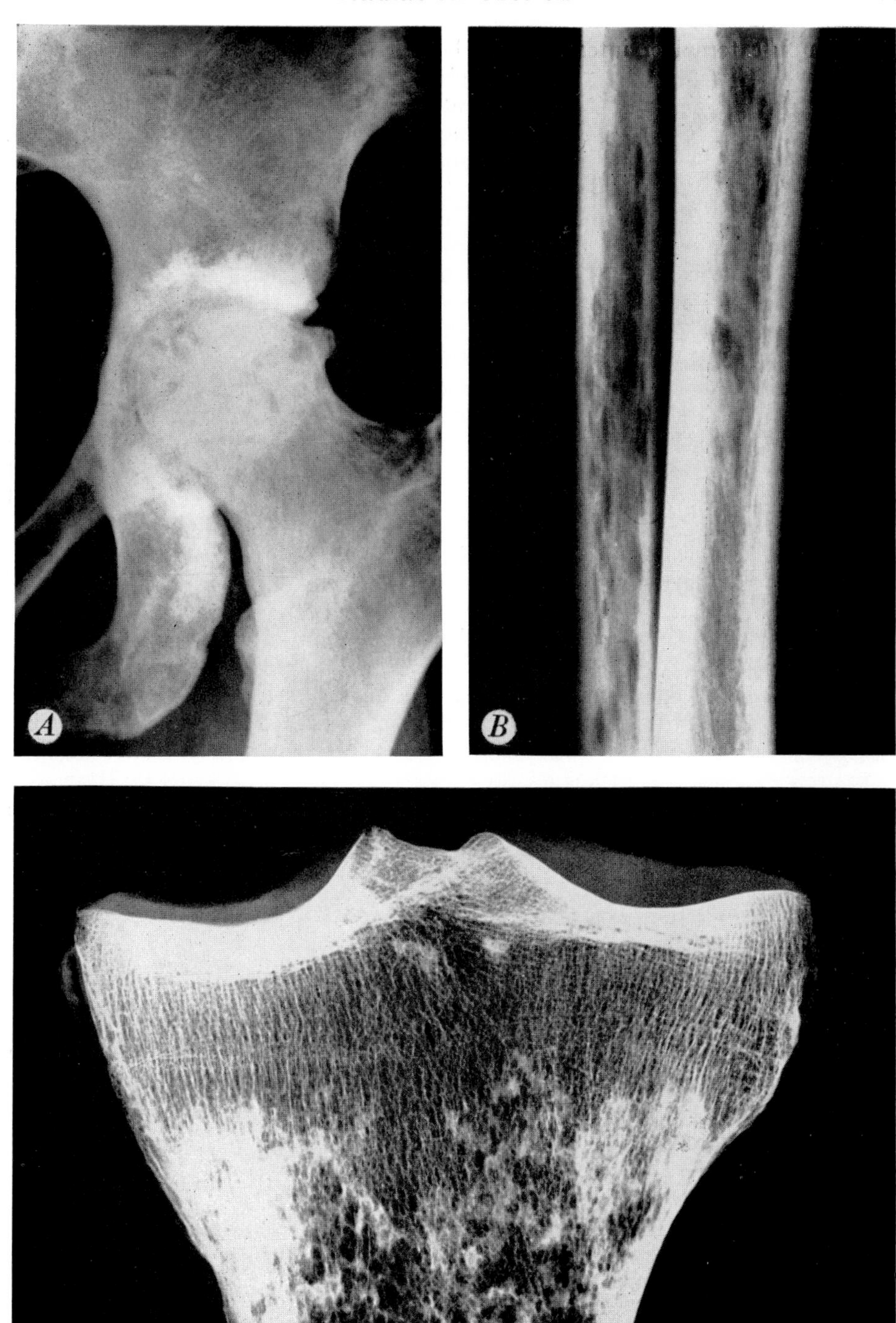


*Figure 151*

radiation is external or internal and whether the subjects are human beings or experimental animals. The histologic picture to be observed in connection with damage from ionizing radiation represents, in various combinations, aseptic bone necrosis, disintegration of necrotic bone, and the compensating reparative reaction.

The extent of the bone damage depends, of course, upon the intensity of the radiation. To a greater or lesser degree, the latter injures and/or destroys not only the cellular elements of the bone marrow, but also the cells involved in the formation, maintenance, and reconstruction of the osseous tissue proper—that is, osteoblasts, osteocytes, and osteoclasts. Since normally functioning osteocytes are essential to the maintenance of the organic matrix of the osseous tissue (collagen fibers and cement substance), degenerative changes in the collagen are likewise a feature of radiation damage. If the bones are still growing, the cartilage cells at the epiphysial cartilage plates are also damaged. Indeed, these cells are particularly vulnerable to radiation injury, and bone growth is consequently disturbed. The injury to the various cellular constituents of the bone seems to be a direct effect of the radiation upon them, and not an indirect effect resulting from radiation damage to the blood vessels supplying the affected bones. However, if the radiation does injure the blood vessels, the resultant disturbance of the blood supply will contribute to the cellular damage produced directly by the radiation.

The damaging effects of *external radiation* on bones have been the subject of numerous experimental studies on animals. In man, they have been noted when such radiation has been directed for therapeutic purposes to some part of the skeleton itself or even to the soft tissues adjacent to that skeletal part. Of course, when *x*-radiation has been applied to only a part of a bone, the direct damage from it may eventually be largely or completely repaired. However, if the radiation has been given on account of a local tumor and has been completely effective against it, the radiated site may still show up roentgenographically, even years later, as a multiloculated area of sclerosis (see Fig. 150). The osseous tissue in the sclerotic area is likely to show at least some degree of residual necrosis and postnecrotic disintegration. Lining the interior of the sclerotic area of bone one will find a thick layer of deteriorated connective tissue which may contain some bizarre cell nuclei. It is possible that the sarcoma which occasionally appears as a sequela of *x*-radiation may have its origin from such cells (see below).

As to *internal radiation*, it is well known that when radioactive substances such as radium or mesothorium gain entry to the body (through ingestion, inhalation, or injection), most of what is taken in at a given time is fairly rapidly excreted. It has also been established that such small amounts of the radioactive material as are retained in the body are stored almost exclusively in the bones, and specifically in the osseous tissue proper. More recent studies have indicated that the retained radioactive material is most probably incorporated in the lattice of the apatite complex constituting the mineral substance of the osseous tissue. However, some hold that it is bound to the protein matrix of the osseous tissue.

The radioactive material tends to concentrate especially at sites where osseous tissue is being laid down in the course of bone growth or maintenance, or being

***Figure 152***

*A*, Roentgenograph (enlarged) showing the upper end of the right femur (except for the head) from the case described in Figure 151-*C*. Note the extensive radiopacity in the neck and subtrochanteric region of the bone. The changes observed in the *x*-ray picture reflect the presence of a pronounced radiation osteitis in the area shown (see *B*).

*B*, Photomicrograph ($\times$ $1\frac{1}{2}$) illustrating the topography of the radiation osteitis in the upper end of the femur shown in *A*. See Figure 153-*A* for histologic details.

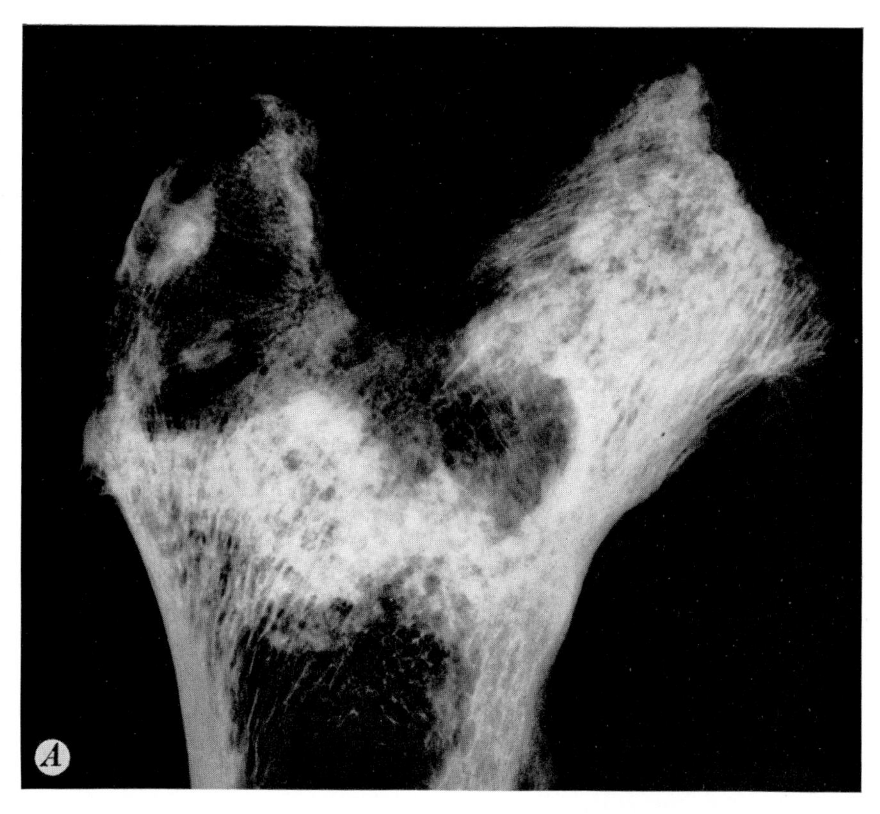


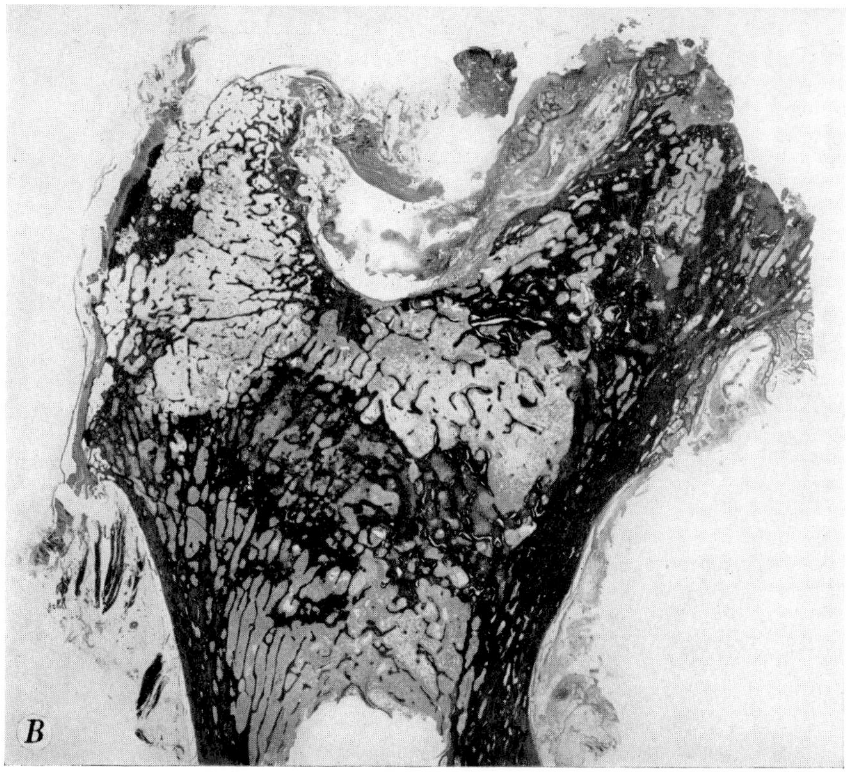


*Figure 152*

reconstructed in the course of metabolic wear and tear. At any rate, it is not uniformly dispersed through the osseous tissue in a particular bone, but has a rather patchy distribution. Furthermore, the radioactive material which accumulates at a given site does not necessarily remain fixed there. That is, some or even all of what has been deposited at any one site may be mobilized in the course of time, and what is not excreted may be redeposited at a new site of bone deposition or reconstruction.

This is the general pattern of deposition, retention, and redistribution of radium or mesothorium in the skeleton, irrespective of whether, for instance, the radioactive material has been given by injection in a single and relatively large dose to an animal, or ingested in repeated small amounts over a long period by a human being. Furthermore, this pattern is essentially the same for the large group of so-called "bone-seeking" radioactive isotopes, many of which have also been studied experimentally in regard to their localization and retention in the skeleton. Also, since the radioactive substances or the products of their decay have very long half-lives, they continue indefinitely to bombard and injure the cellular elements of the bone at the site of their lodgment. Thus radioactive elements entering the skeleton are not only widely disseminated through it, but persist in the focal damage they create. It is for this reason that striking examples of radiation osteitis have been observed in the clinical cases in which radium and/or mesothorium have accumulated gradually in the bones over a long period of time. On the other hand, the rapid accumulation of radium, mesothorium, or one or another of the radioactive isotopes in the body of an animal or human being not infrequently induces a fatal blood dyscrasia even before the bones come to show the changes of radiation osteitis.

The *x-ray pictures* of bones which have been subjected for a long time to the damaging action of internally deposited radioactive substances present various abnormalities (see Fig. 151). A conspicuous finding is the presence of streaky, patchy, or even large blotchy areas of radiopacity. In relation to the ends of long bones, the extent of the radiopacity is sometimes considerable, and it may even reach to the articular cartilage. In an area in which the radiopacity is not very pronounced, the individual spongy trabeculae may still be clearly apparent, but where the radiopacity is intense, the trabecular markings may be more or less obliterated. The radiopacity reflects the presence of bone necrosis and its consequences, and if the articular end of a long bone is substantially necrotic, it may even show collapse.

Another common *x*-ray finding is the presence of scattered areas of radiolucency. For instance, some small, roundish radiolucencies, perhaps surrounded by sclerotic borders, may be observed in the calvarium. One may likewise note them at the ends of long bones, either by themselves or in alternation with areas of radiopacity.

**_Figure 153_**

*A*, Photomicrograph (× 65) illustrating the histologic details of the radiation osteitis in the intertrochanteric spongiosa of the femur shown in Figure 152-*B*. Note that the osseous tissue is necrotic, the bone cell lacunæ being devoid of osteocytes. Between the necrotic osseous trabeculæ there is a poorly cellular fibrillar tissue which shows streaky calcification. Apposed on the surface of the trabecula to the right there is a layer of dark-staining material possibly representing newly deposited atypical osseous tissue.

*B*, Photomicrograph (× 65) illustrating the histologic appearance presented by an area of altered femoral cortex in this case. Note the absence of osteocytes in the lacunæ, again indicating that the osseous tissue is necrotic. Many of the haversian canals are widened, and coalescence of adjacent modified canals has resulted in the appearance of large cavities in the cortex. It is the fusion of such cavities that produces the radiolucencies observed roentgenographically in the cortices of bones altered by chronic radium poisoning.

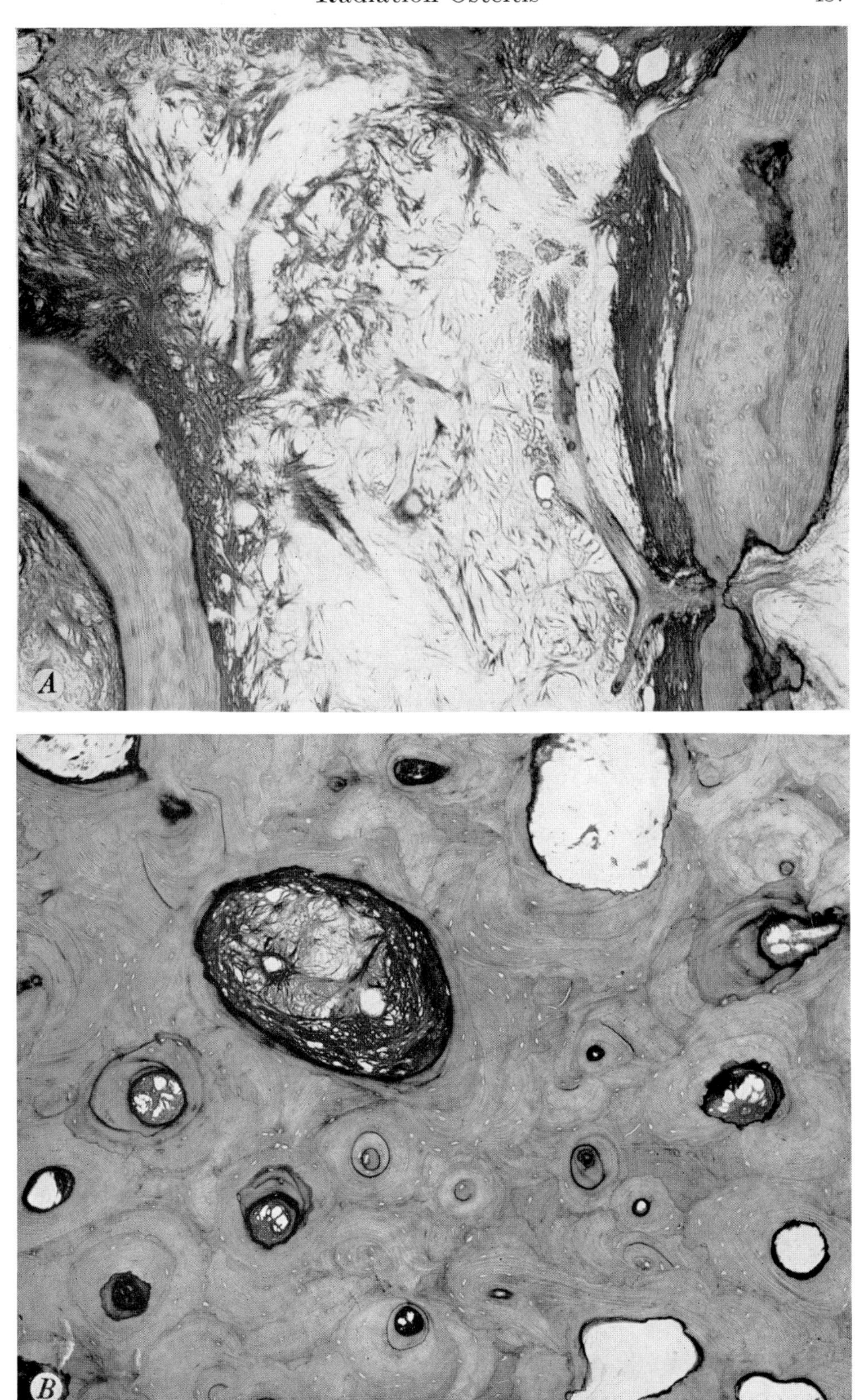


*Figure 153*

However, it is when the radiolucencies are present in the shaft cortex of long bones that they create the most striking picture. Here they usually have a drawn-out, oval form, and the long axis of the radiolucencies generally corresponds to the long axis of the bone. In some areas, furthermore, adjacent radiolucencies merge to produce a relatively large longitudinal focus of radiolucency.

On *microscopic examination*, a bone area which has undergone severe damage from internal radiation shows extensive necrosis of the osseous tissue, associated with necrosis and/or substantial scarring of the bone marrow. At most, only a few osteocytes are observed in the bone cell lacunae of the necrotic osseous tissue. That is, practically all the bone cell lacunae in the damaged area are likely to be found empty. Signs of repair of the bone necrosis by the process of creeping replacement are few or completely lacking. In particular, there is little evidence of osteoclasts eroding the margins of the necrotic bone, or of osteoblasts depositing new bone along these marginal surfaces.

Still, the osseous tissue does give way in places. Indeed, many of the haversian canals in the injured cortex are found much enlarged and many of the spongy trabeculae are thin. These changes represent the consequences of disintegration of the necrotic tissue along the margins both of the altered haversian canals and of the spongy trabeculae. The intertrabecular spaces and the enlarged haversian canals come to be filled with fibrillar connective tissue extremely poor in cells. This connective tissue is likely to be found heavily impregnated with calcium, particularly along the edges of the necrotic and disintegrating osseous tissue (see Figs. 152 and 153).

These microscopic details are reflected in the findings described above in relation to the *x*-ray picture. Thus, enlargement of the haversian canals and particularly fusion of several adjacent enlarged canals result in the radiolucencies observed in the shaft cortex of the affected bones. The small, roundish radiolucencies in the spongy bone are the result of thinning and disappearance of the local bony trabeculæ, and their replacement by fibrillar connective tissue. The patchy radiopacities

***Figure 154***

*A*, Roentgenograph showing an impacted fracture through the neck of a femur, apparently attributable to the effects of *x*-radiation. The patient was a woman 35 years of age who had been treated surgically 7 years previously for a carcinoma of the ovary. Postoperatively, she was given 4,000 r of *x*-radiation. She was free of complaints until about 2 months prior to the time when this picture was taken. At that time she began to complain of pain in the hip, but an *x*-ray picture did not reveal a fracture or other local abnormalities. A biopsy specimen from the fracture area showed that the fracture was not conditioned by a focus of metastasis.

*B*, Roentgenograph of a resected femoral head and neck presenting a postradiation fracture. The patient was a woman 60 years of age who had been treated surgically for a carcinoma of the vulva. Subsequently, over a period of about a month, she received a total of 20,000 r of *x*-radiation. Ten months after the end of the treatment, she complained of pain in the hip, and an *x*-ray picture taken at that time revealed a linear fracture line at the femoral neck. Despite some mild difficulties, the patient continued to be ambulatory. An *x*-ray picture taken about 4 months later showed that there had been displacement of the femoral head and impaction of the fracture fragments. On gross examination of the resected specimen, the fragments were found to be firmly held together by callus, there being no mobility between them. When sectioned, the specimen showed bony union between the fragments in some places. Furthermore, inspection of the cut surface failed to reveal gross evidence of aseptic necrosis in the femoral head.

*C*, Photomicrograph (× 65) showing the status of the head-neck junction in a place where the fracture fragments had not yet united. Note the necrotic, fragmented, and disintegrating osseous trabeculæ. This histologic appearance is quite similar to what one observes along the line of a so-called "fatigue fracture."

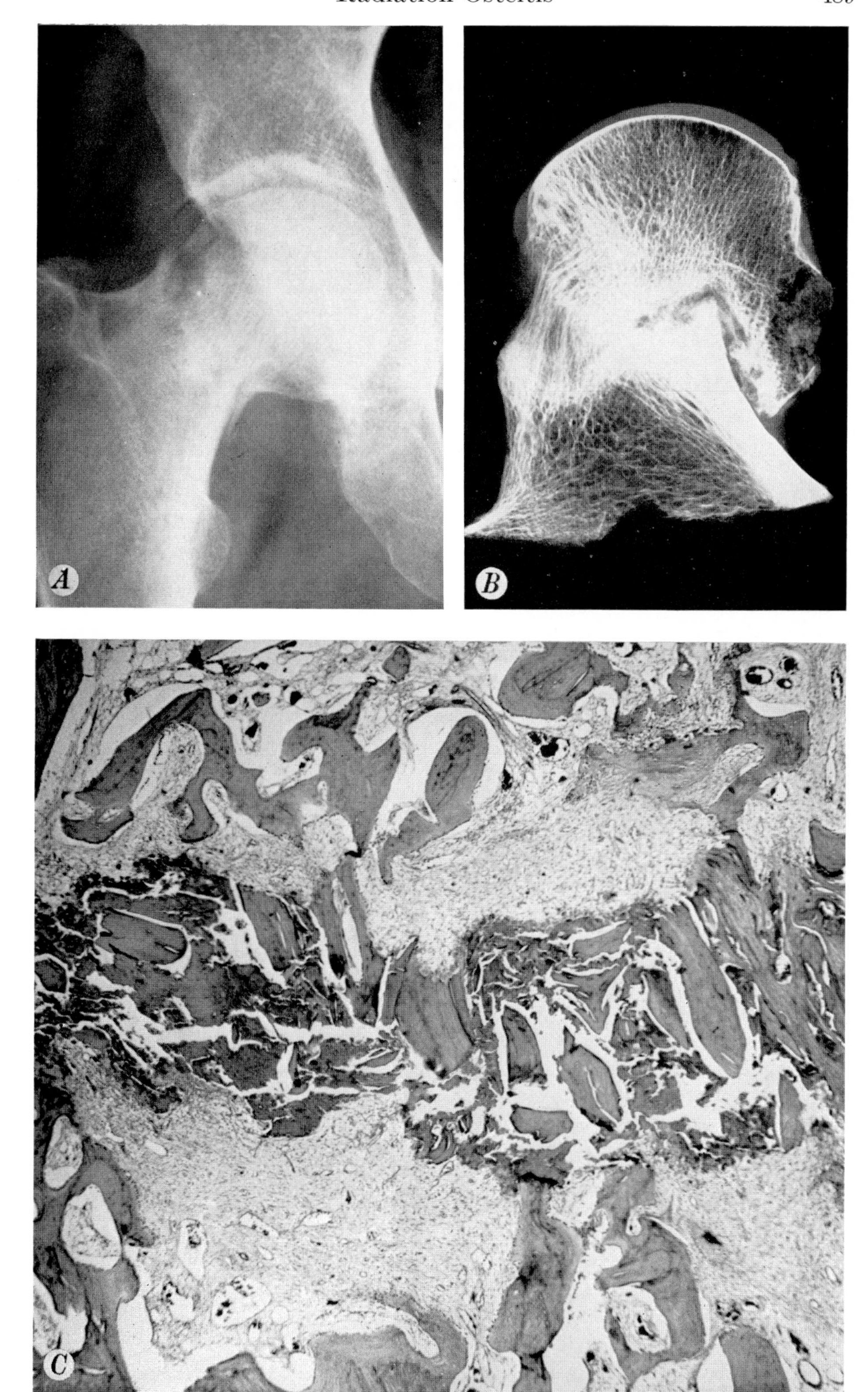


*Figure 154*

in the ends of the long bones represent large areas in which the intertrabecular marrow is scarred and heavily calcified. From all this it is also apparent why the necrotic end of a long bone severely damaged by radiation sometimes collapses, and why a pathologic fracture through an affected bone shaft may also occur.

**Retardation of Bone Growth.**—Numerous experimental studies on a variety of young animals have demonstrated the inhibiting effects of both external and internal radiation upon bone growth, and in particular upon longitudinal bone growth. The early studies in this field were largely confined to the effects of external radiation with $x$-rays. In the more recent experimental studies relating to bone growth in particular, it is again mainly $x$-rays that have been utilized (see Regen and Wilkins, Gall *et al.*, and Barr *et al.*). However, the growth-inhibiting effects of internal radiation (through the agency of radium salts and radioactive isotopes) have also received considerable attention (see Heller). In regard to experimental $x$-radiation, it appears that a dose of 600 r directed to the growth zone of a long bone retards its longitudinal growth, but that the latter is resumed at a normal rate after an interval of some weeks. A dose of 1,800 to 2,600 r given at one session can completely and permanently arrest longitudinal bone growth, though it is not until several weeks after the irradiation that its full effect is observed. The effects of ionizing radiation produced by the administration of radium or radioactive isotopes are similar to, but tend to be more drastic than, those of external radiation. However, when the isotopes are used in very low doses, growth may likewise eventually be resumed. After a short time, this may stop again, on account of premature closure of the epiphysial cartilage plates.

As already pointed out, the inhibiting effects of radiation on bone growth result from damage to the cells in the cartilage plate area. Specifically, it has been observed that after an effective dose of $x$-radiation, the cells of the plate cease to divide and lose their columnar arrangement. Also, many of the cartilage cells swell and degenerate. Consequently, there are no new columns of calcified cartilage matrix moving toward the metaphysis, and, since the osteoblasts have also been damaged, these are no longer depositing new bone in the zone of endochondral bone growth. Later, the plates appear swollen, but if the damage is severe, they may also present signs of premature closure. Eventually the stunted bones may also show abnormal curvatures. Entirely analogous but much more severe and extensive changes are observed at the growth zones after damage from internally deposited radioactive material.

These experimental findings have important clinical implications. If, for therapeutic purposes, one or more bones of a young child have received too large a dose of $x$-radiation (given at one session or at close intervals), their growth will be stunted. In fact, such an effect has been known to follow upon too vigorous radiation even of the soft parts or skin surrounding the bone or bones in question. The severity of the stunting of a long bone, for instance, and any curvature that may develop varies in accordance with the youthfulness of the subject at the time of radiation, the amount of radiation given, and the time which has elapsed since the radiation was applied. Certainly, in a child, any skeletal part which is exposed to $x$-radiation in excess of 2,000 r is likely to show disturbance in growth, and even smaller doses have been known to produce this effect (see Frantz, Neuhauser *et al.*, and Whitehouse and Lampe).

**Complicating Osteomyelitis.**—As already mentioned, this is particularly likely to occur when the site of the radiation osteitis is a jawbone. Indeed, the frequent occurrence of osteomyelitis in jawbones which have been damaged in the course of treatment of intra-oral cancer by external radiation was already discussed by Regaud in 1922. Furthermore, necrosis and engrafted infection of jawbones were not infrequently the first manifestations of chronic poisoning by radium and/or mesothorium suffered by the radium dial painters (see Blum, and Castle). In any of these cases a large part of the infected jawbone may eventually be sequestrated, and stubborn fistulae may appear. In the cases of the radium dial workers, there was little tendency toward healing through the formation of involucrum, and in some instances the osteomyelitis was complicated in turn by a septicemia. The source of the bone infection is usually bacteria from abscesses developing about the roots of teeth in the area which have likewise been damaged by the radiation. Sometimes the osteomyelitis becomes manifest only years after the jawbone has been injured by radiation. In any event, it is frequently precipitated by mechanical factors such as extraction of one or more infected teeth.

**Complicating Fracture.**—As has long been known, bones which have been severely damaged by radiation (whether external or internal) tend to become brittle and to fracture more easily than normal bones, and fracture healing tends to be slow. However, the literature relating specifically to fracture following radiation has centered mainly around cases of pathologic fracture of the neck of one or both femora in women who had received external radiation for cancer of the uterus or other pelvic organs. In cases of bilateral femoral neck fracture, the fractures have occasionally been more or less simultaneous, but more often some time has elapsed between them. Calculations of the incidence of the complication have ranged from as little as 0.1 per cent to about 3 per cent (see McCrorie, Gratzek *et al.*, Dalby *et al.*, and Kok). At any rate, even the lowest estimate is considerably higher than that for the incidence (about 0.03 per cent) of fracture of the femoral neck among women of comparable age who have not received radiation and in whom the area was not diseased. It is of interest in this connection that, in men who have received radiation for cancer of the prostate or bladder, postradiation fracture of the femoral neck seems not to occur.

Fracture of the femoral neck has been reported as appearing as early as a few months after radiation. However, when the interval is so short, and especially if the woman is over 60 years of age, the burden of proof falls upon those who would interpret the fracture as a consequence of the radiation damage. In many of the cases there is an interval of a year or two between the completion of the radiation therapy and the appearance of the complication, and in some cases the interval has been as long as 5 years or even longer. It is to be doubted that the interference with the blood supply to the hip area, through damage by radiation to the smaller or larger blood vessels in the area, is a factor in the production of the fracture (see Stephenson and Cohen).

Clinically, it is to be noted that the hip has usually been painful for several months before the fracture makes its appearance. In some cases, however, there is no antecedent pain. Roentgenographic examination of the hip area prior to the fracture may or may not have revealed abnormalities in the region of the femoral head and neck. In cases in which such aberrations have been observed, these have sometimes been merely small, scattered, circumscribed areas of increased radiolucency in the neck. The site of the impending fracture may be marked by an irregular transverse line of increased radiolucency. If the fracture has already occurred but is still incomplete, it will be noted that the fracture line is clearest in the lateral part of the neck. In general, these postradiation fractures of the femoral neck seem to have much in common, both clinically and anatomically, with the so-called "fatigue fractures." Healing of the fracture is usually slow, and sometimes only fibrous union takes place (see Fig. 154).

## BONE SARCOMA FOLLOWING EXTERNAL RADIATION

There is increasing awareness that a skeletal part which had been irradiated by roentgen rays or radium may eventually become the site of a sarcoma. Instances in which this effect of radiation has been produced in animals have been recorded. Postradiation sarcoma has also been observed in clinical cases, though it is by no means a common occurrence in this connection (see Jaffe *et al.*, Hatcher, Cahan *et al.*, Sabanas *et al.*, and Cruz *et al.*). For example, a sarcoma has been known to develop in a bone or bone part which had been irradiated in the course of treatment of an infection (articular tuberculosis), a nonmalignant tumorous bone lesion (giant-cell tumor, bone cyst, *etc.*), and even in an originally sound bone which merely happened to be within the field of the radiation.

In those clinical cases of postradiation sarcoma in which the dosage could be calculated with fair accuracy, the amount of radiation given has usually ranged from about 4,000 to about 6,000 r. In an occasional case the stated dosage has been as low as 1,500 r, and at the other extreme there are cases in which it has been 10,000 r or even more. The time interval over which the total dosage has been spread varies considerably. In the older cases it often amounted to a number of years, but in the more recent cases the total dosage was more often delivered within a period of a few months. In the reported cases, the interval between the end of the radiation treatment and the development of the sarcoma (the latent period) ranges from 3 to 20 years, more or less. However, in about half of the cases the latent period has been somewhere between 5 and 10 years. The sarcoma which evolves may present, almost throughout, the pattern of a polymorphocellular fibrosarcoma or that of an osteogenic sarcoma. In other cases the histologic pattern is rather complex, so that one cannot categorize the sarcoma precisely. In any event, it is noteworthy that, when once a postradiation sarcoma has appeared, death from pulmonary metastases usually ensues, even if the affected part is promptly amputated.

Taken by itself, the relative rarity of sarcoma following external radiation in clinical cases might lead one to question whether the radiation is really to be inculpated in the development of the sarcoma. What is probably the strongest evidence of a causal relation between external radiation and the development of a sarcoma in human bones is offered by its occurrence in cases of skeletal tuberculosis dating from the period when that condition was sometimes treated by radiation. Specifically, the older literature records a small number of cases in which sarcoma developed years after therapeutic irradiation of the knee region, in particular, for tuberculous gonitis (see Küttner). In this connection, it is known that sarcoma does not develop spontaneously in tuberculous bones and joints. Furthermore, now that radiation is no longer used in the treatment of skeletal tuberculosis, there have been no further reports of sarcoma complicating that condition.

On the other hand, when one comes to the question of sarcoma developing at the site of an irradiated nonmalignant tumorous bone lesion, one must give consideration to the possibility that the sarcoma might have developed even without radiation. This consideration arises particularly in connection with cases of giant-cell

***Figure 155***

*A*, Roentgenograph showing the upper end of a tibia 14 years after the area had been treated with *x*-radiation on account of a giant-cell tumor. Note the vaguely trabeculated appearance of the radiated site and the characteristic peripheral margin of sclerosis.

*B*, Roentgenograph illustrating the appearance, 9 years later, of the irradiated tibial site shown in *A*. The osteolysis present is the expression of a sarcoma which has developed there. Thus, a malignant tumor appeared 23 years after the treatment of the giant-cell tumor by *x*-radiation.

*C*, Photomicrograph (× 65) showing evidences of persisting radiation osteitis beyond the limits of the tumor. The tissue in question came from the sclerotic subchondral zone at the upper end of the tibia. Note the necrotic and disintegrated osseous tissue, below which there is a zone of fibrillar connective tissue poor in cells.

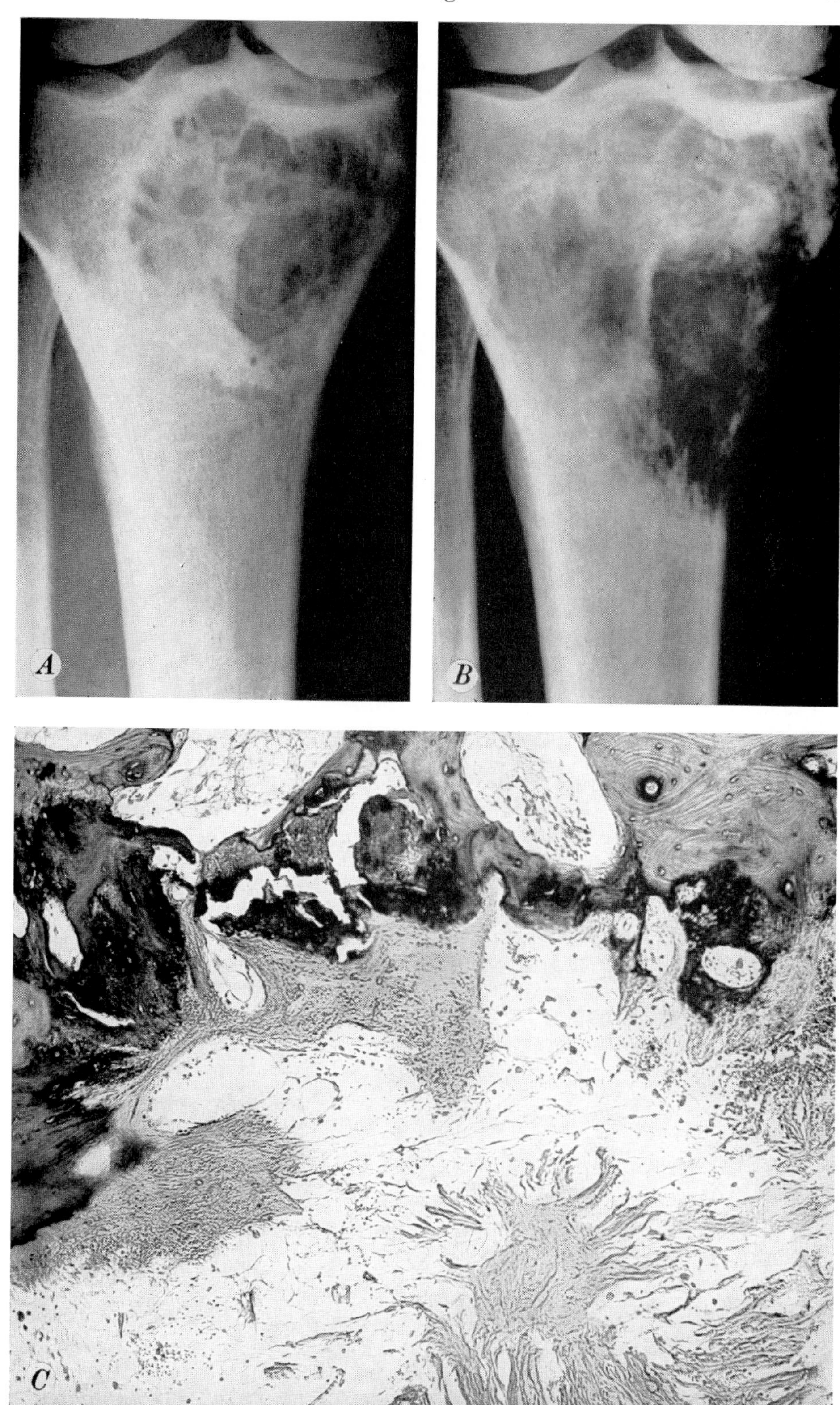


*Figure 155*

tumor, since it is not unusual for a giant-cell tumor to undergo malignant transformation spontaneously. However, it is to be noted that in the cases of giant-cell tumor in which a sarcoma appears after irradiation, the giant-cell tumor *per se* has apparently been destroyed by the radiation, since the patient becomes free of complaints relating to it. Indeed, the patient remains free of complaints during a latent period usually lasting for several years, at least, before the sarcoma appears. However, the bone area which has been the site of the giant-cell tumor will show sclerosis roentgenographically and, if examined anatomically, evidences of radiation damage. This being the case, the sarcoma can justifiably be held to have developed out of the local tissue damaged by the radiation, rather than out of residual giant-cell tumor tissue reactivated by the radiation. In contrast, those giant-cell tumors which undergo malignant transformation spontaneously do so progressively. That is, they are lesions which have not been contained or abolished by the local surgical measures undertaken against them and have simply become malignant in the course of time.

Though sarcomas have been known to appear in sound bones which have merely been within the field of external radiation, this occurrence is surprisingly rare in view of the general frequency with which radiation is given. Hatcher does report an instance of a sarcoma developing in a rib 11 years after a radical mastectomy in a woman who had received postoperative radiation therapy. He and others have also described instances in which a sarcoma developed in a sound bone lying in the path of radiation of an adjacent bone which was the site of a benign lesion.

## POSTRADIATION SARCOMA AT SITES OF GIANT-CELL TUMOR

The writer has personally studied 3 cases in which a sarcoma appeared at the site of a giant-cell tumor which had been given *x*-ray therapy. The giant-cell tumor was located in the upper end of a femur in one case, in the upper end of a tibia in another, and in the lower end of a tibia in the third. The subjects (2 men and 1 woman) were all middle-aged at the time when the sarcoma appeared. In each instance the original diagnosis of giant-cell tumor was already suggested by the roentgenographic appearance of the lesion and was confirmed histologically by examination of a biopsy specimen. In all 3 cases, surgical intervention was limited to removal of the biopsy specimen, and the only treatment given was *x*-ray therapy. In regard to 2 of the cases, accurate information about the total amount of radiation given is not available; in the third, the total amount was 6,200 r. In each of the cases, radiation was followed by abatement of the clinical complaints from the giant-cell tumor and by evidence of a local radiation effect in the form of a sclerosing reaction in the bone at the site of the original tumor. The latent period (that is, the interval of clinical

***Figure 156***

*A*, Roentgenograph showing the characteristic appearance of a large solitary bone cyst in a humerus. A pathologic fracture through the cyst has occurred.

*B*, Roentgenograph illustrating the appearance of the cyst shown in *A*, 3 months after the initiation of *x*-ray therapy. Note that the fracture has healed and that the lesional area is beginning to manifest sclerotization.

*C*, Roentgenograph showing the lesional area 2 years later. Observe that, as happens so often in connection with a bone cyst, the latter has moved away from the epiphysial cartilage plate. The residual lesional area appears sclerotized and multiloculated.

*D*, Roentgenograph revealing how the lesional area appeared approximately 4 years after the picture presented in *C* was made. The radiated bone region is now osteolytic, and a fibrosarcoma has developed in it.

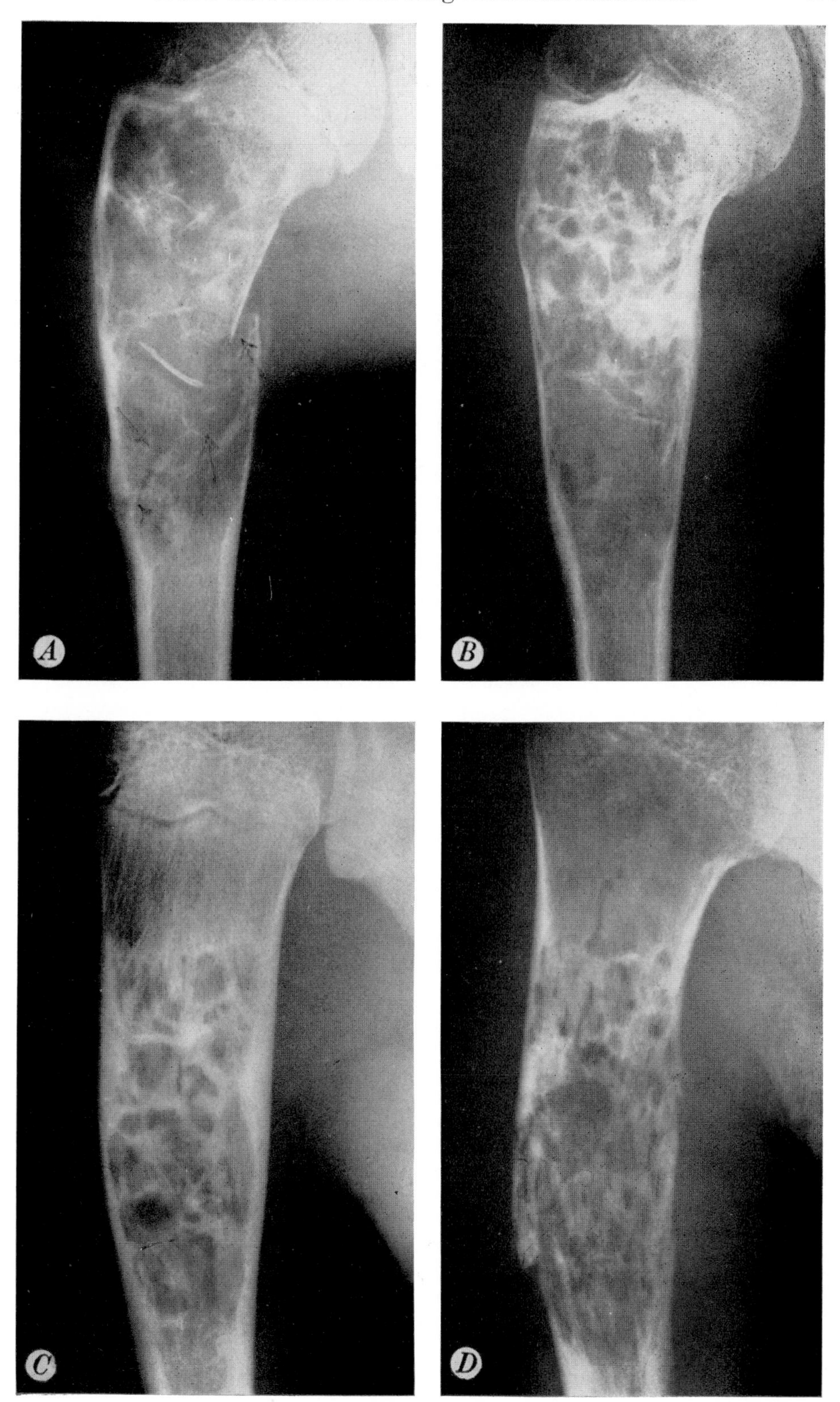


*Figure 156*

improvement before the appearance of clinical manifestation of the sarcoma) was 5 years in one case, 6 years in another, and 23 years in the third.

In this third case, which may serve as an example, the patient was a man who was 28 years of age in 1928, when he was found to have a giant-cell tumor in the upper end of the left tibia. He received *x*-ray therapy for this, and some months later his complaints had abated sufficiently to permit him to return to full duty as a policeman. In 1942 (that is, 14 years after his return to duty) he fell and injured the knee, and a roentgenograph of the upper end of the tibia showed a rather heavily sclerotic and trabeculated area marking the site of the irradiated tumor. He recovered quickly from the effects of the fall and was free from any complaints referable to that fall for the ensuing 9 years—that is, until 1951. In September of that year he began to complain of pain in the knee area, and, when he was admitted to our hospital in December, he presented a tense swelling in the region of the tibia. The affected area was tender and pulsating, and an *x*-ray picture showed evidence of extensive bone destruction at the sclerotic site of the previous giant-cell tumor. A midthigh amputation was done, but the patient succumbed to metastasis about 1 year later. Thus, a period of 23 years had elapsed in this case between the appearance and radiation treatment of a giant-cell tumor in the tibia and the development of a sarcoma at its site (see Fig. 155).

Anatomic study of the tibia in question showed that the site of the original giant-cell tumor was now occupied by a large and obviously malignant tumor which had thinned the cortex anteriorly and medially and to some extent laterally, and which had perforated it posteriorly to extend into the overlying soft parts. The sectioned specimen showed that the tumor tissue reached almost to the articular cartilage and was protruding distally quite far into the major marrow cavity. Blocks of tissue taken from various parts of the lesion showed that the microscopic pattern of the tumor tissue varied from place to place. In many areas the pattern was that of a conventional osteogenic sarcoma. In others, the tumor tissue showed no evidences of osteogenesis, the pattern being that of a fibrosarcoma. In still other areas one could note fields presenting the pattern of malignant giant-cell tumor.

However, what was most interesting in connection with the microscopic study of this specimen was the fact that one could still find evidence of radiation osteitis in the bone beyond the limits of the sarcoma. Between the sarcoma and the surrounding osseous tissue proper there was a thick layer of rather hyalinized and almost acellular connective tissue. Beyond this degenerated layer the residual osseous tissue showed evidence of aseptic necrosis and granular disintegration such as is commonly associated with radiation damage.

## POSTRADIATION SARCOMA AT SITES OF OTHER BENIGN BONE LESIONS

**Solitary Bone Cyst.**—A conventional bone cyst apparently never undergoes malignant transformation spontaneously. In the light of this fact, the occurrence of a sarcoma at the site of a cyst which has been radiated would seem to indicate that the radiation played a causal role. A case in point is that of a boy who, at the age of 12 years, suffered a pathologic fracture through the upper part of the shaft of the right humerus. An *x*-ray picture taken at that time (January 1937) revealed a large lesion whose location and *x*-ray appearance were so characteristic of the solitary bone cyst as to leave little doubt about the nature of the lesion. The latter was treated with repeated small doses of *x*-ray therapy extending over a period of 18 months, but information about the precise total amount of radiation given is not available. Within 3 months after the institution of the radiation therapy, an *x*-ray picture showed that the therapy had already induced a slight degree of sclerosis in the lesional area. An *x*-ray picture taken 2 years later (April 1939) revealed that the proximal part of the cyst had filled in, but that the persisting lesional area was loculated and sclerotic.

At this time the patient was entirely free of complaints, and he remained free of complaints referable to the humerus until July 1943. At the latter time he suffered a minor trauma to the arm, and shortly thereafter he began to complain of pain. An *x*-ray picture taken then showed that the lesional area which had previously been sclerotic was strikingly radiolucent and had obviously undergone extensive osteolysis. Shortly thereafter, a pathologic fracture occurred through the osteolytic area (see Fig. 156). Tissue from that area revealed the presence of an anaplastic fibrosarcoma and evidence that the bone region in which the sarcoma had developed was also the site of radiation osteitis. Thus, in this case the sarcoma developed $6\frac{1}{2}$ years after the institution of radiation therapy for a bone cyst of the humerus, and 5 years after the completion of the treatment (see Jaffe).

**Benign Chondroblastoma.**—Hatcher and Campbell report an instance of a benign chondroblastoma at whose site a chondrosarcoma was found about 4 years after the original lesion had been treated by curettage and 3,600 r of *x*-radiation. In associating the radiation with the appearance of the sarcoma in this case, it is significant that after the original lesion had been curetted and irradiated, the presenting clinical complaints rapidly subsided and the patient was free of any difficulties for the ensuing $3\frac{1}{2}$ years. Furthermore, the benign chondroblastoma (p. 44) is readily amenable to cure by curettage alone. Indeed, the writer has never seen a case in which the lesion underwent spontaneous malignant transformation.

**Fibrous Dysplasia.**—Several instances of sarcoma appearing at the site of a focus of fibrous dysplasia which had been treated with *x*-radiation are on record (see Cahan *et al.* and Sabanas *et al.*). In a case reported by the latter authors, the patient, a girl, showed a swelling of the right maxilla at the age of 6 years. That the lesion was benign was attested not only by the findings from 2 biopsies, but by the fact that it underwent but little change in the course of the next 9 years. When the patient was 15 years of age, the lesion was heavily irradiated. The precise dose of radiation given is not known, but it is recorded that the patient showed persisting severe radiation damage to the local soft tissues. Nine years after the completion of the *x*-ray therapy, the lesion in the maxilla underwent enlargement and local extension. At this time, tissue removed from it revealed the pattern of a fibrous dysplasia in some areas and an osteogenic sarcoma in others. The patient died 4 months later from the effects of intracranial extension of the complicating sarcoma.

It is true that, once in a while, a focus of fibrous dysplasia undergoes spontaneous malignant transformation (p. 134). However, when this happens, the case is usually one in which many bones are involved. On the other hand, the writer has never seen a case of fibrous dysplasia limited to a jawbone in which the lesion underwent spontaneous malignant transformation. Therefore, the case detailed above seems acceptable as one of sarcomatous transformation induced by radiation in a focus of fibrous dysplasia, as are the relevant cases reported by Cahan *et al.*

## BONE SARCOMA FOLLOWING INTERNAL RADIATION

Numerous studies on experimental animals (notably rabbits, rats, and mice) have shown that one or more bones of the animal may become the site of a sarcoma in consequence of the lodgment of one or another radioactive substance in the bones. These studies have indicated further that the incidence of sarcoma formation rises with the amount of radioactive material administered, provided that the dosage is not in itself inconsistent with survival of the animal. Under conditions of relatively high dosage and continued survival, there is usually an abrupt rise in the incidence of bone sarcoma among those animals in a given experiment who are surviving longest. It is worth noting also that radium is one of the most effective inducers of experimental bone sarcoma among the isotopes emitting alpha rays, and that strontium is one of the most effective among those emitting beta rays. Indeed, all other things being equal, radioactive strontium is outstandingly effective in the experimental induction of bone tumors (see Brues, and Owen *et. al.*).

In relation to human bones, our knowledge concerning bone sarcoma appearing in consequence of the deposition of radioactive substances comes, as already noted, mainly from two groups of cases. One group consists of those in which radium salts had been given either orally or intravenously for therapeutic purposes against a variety of nontumorous medical disorders. The other group comprises the cases in which radioactive salts (radium and/or mesothorium) had been ingested in the course of work involving the use of self-luminous paints. On the basis of findings in some of the cases of the luminous dial workers, the National Bureau of Standards, in 1949, set 0.1 microgram of fixed radium as the maximum permissible internal deposit—that is, the amount of radium that can safely be retained by the body. However, it now appears that in the cases on which this estimate was based, the patients had ingested mesothorium along with the radium. For this reason, Aub *et al.* hold that the maximum permissible level for radium is probably higher, since mesothorium is apparently more noxious to the body than radium.

As already indicated, Martland was the first to focus attention upon the fact that bone sarcomas were appearing among watch dial workers who had long been showing various other clinical manifestations of chronic radium (and mesothorium) poisoning. Since that time, more and more of the survivors of this industrial hazard have come to develop bone sarcomas. It was these experiences that also stimulated the studies of the occurrence of sarcoma among the persons who had been given radium for therapeutic purposes. In the cases from either source in which tumors appeared, the estimated burden of more or less fixed radioactive material (as estimated for radium) was always at least 0.5 microgram. However, even patients who have stored many times this amount of radium do not necessarily develop sarcomas (see Aub *et al.*, and Looney). When sarcomas have appeared, they have nearly always been associated with the changes of radiation osteitis (p. 482) distributed over the skeleton (see Fig. 157).

The incidence of complicating bone sarcoma in these two groups of cases taken together is about 20 per cent. In any event, since some of the subjects in question are still surviving, not all the returns have yet come in, and the incidence of the complication may finally come to be still higher. The latent period (that is, the time between the end of the intake of the radioactive material and the time of appearance of the sarcoma) in these various cases has a rather wide range. It is rarely less than 8 or 10 years, not infrequently 20 to 25 years, and sometimes much longer. Indeed, Woodard has recently commented on a case in which the latent period was about

***Figure 157***

*A*, Roentgenograph showing a sarcoma which has appeared in an ischium of a radium dial worker. The patient was a woman 47 years of age who had been subjected for 20 years to the industrial hazard in question (see also Fig. 151-*B*). Note that there is also patchy sclerosis in the ilium and in the neck of the femur, representing radiation osteitis in these areas.

*B*, Photomicrograph (× 1) showing the sarcoma illustrated in *A*. The tumor was specifically a fibrosarcoma. The osseous tissue about the acetabulum is the site of radiation osteitis (see *C*).

*C*, Photomicrograph (× 65) showing the radiation osteitis present in the acetabular area. The osseous tissue beneath the articular cartilage lacks osteocytes and is disintegrating in places. The intertrabecular marrow, too, has undergone necrosis.

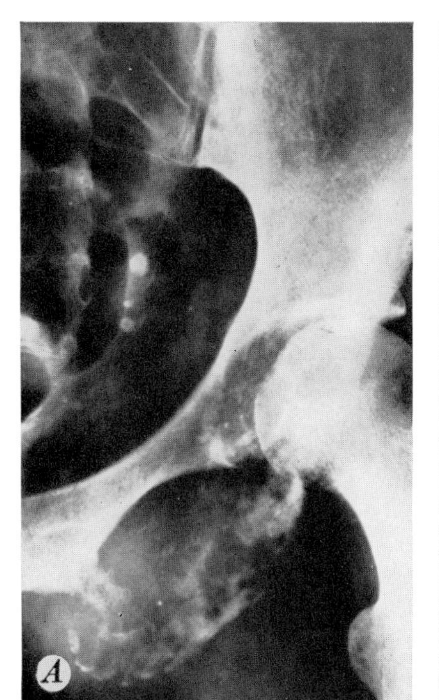


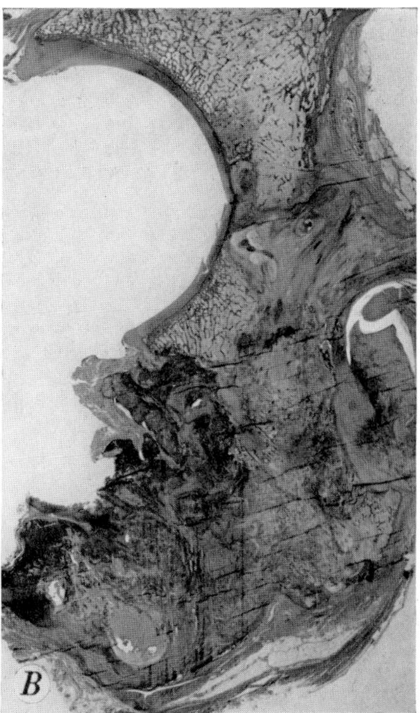


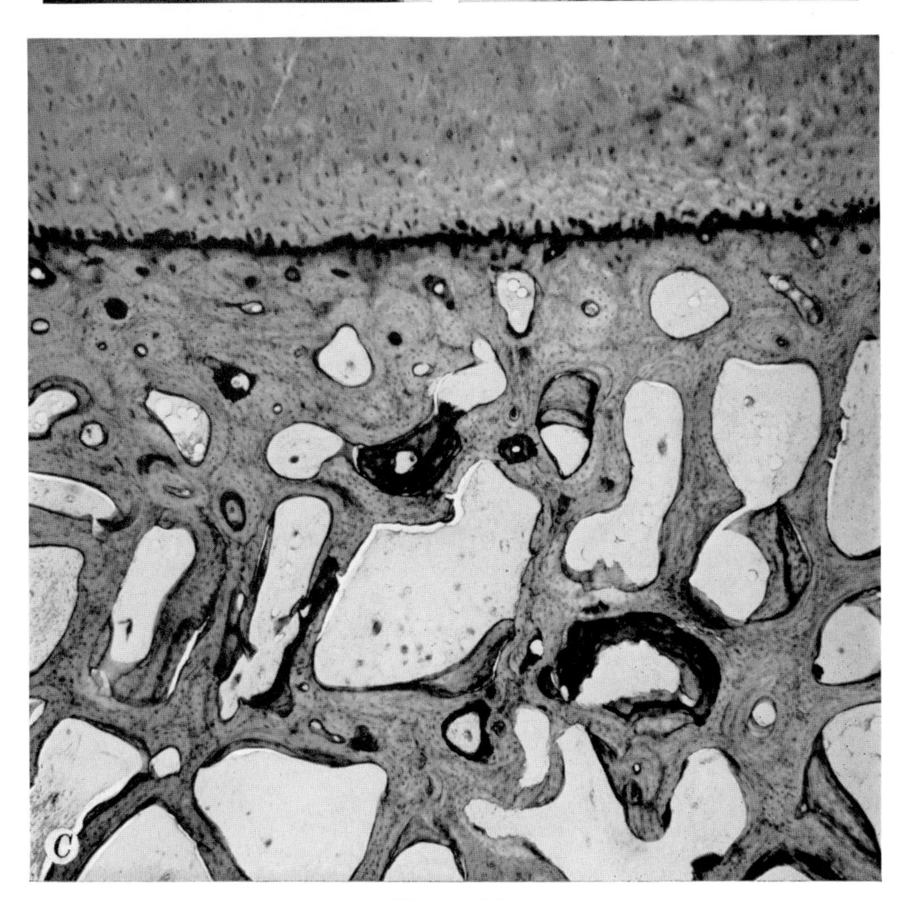


*Figure 157*

37 years. Be that as it may, the latent period for postradiation sarcoma following damage from internal radiation is generally much longer than that following external radiation.

The sarcoma may develop in almost any damaged bone site. However, like primary bone tumors in general, most of the tumors arising in connection with internal radiation have appeared in bones of the knee or hip region. Though the sarcoma formation has usually been limited to a single site, some cases have been reported in which sarcomas developed in several bone sites, apparently independently. Microscopically, the tumors have generally presented the histologic pattern either of an osteogenic sarcoma or of a fibrosarcoma (that is, a connective-tissue sarcoma devoid of evidences of osteogenesis). In any event, the occurrence of complicating sarcoma is followed within a year or so by death of the patient, usually from pulmonary metastases.

## REFERENCES


AUB, J. C., EVANS, R. D., HEMPELMANN, L. H., and MARTLAND, H. S.: The Late Effects of Internally-Deposited Radioactive Materials in Man, Medicine, *31*, 221, 1952.

BAGG, H. J.: Disturbances in Mammalian Development Produced by Radium Emanation, Am. J. Anat., *30*, 133, 1922.

BARR, J. S., LINGLEY, J. R., and GALL, E. A.: The Effect of Roentgen Irradiation on Epiphyseal Growth. I. Experimental Studies upon the Albino Rat, Am. J. Roentgenol., *49*, 104, 1943.

BLUM, T.: Osteomyelitis of the Mandible and Maxilla, J. Am. Dent. A., *11*, 802, 1924.

BRUES, A. M.: Symposium on Radioactive Isotopes: Biological Hazards and Toxicity of Radioactive Isotopes, J. Clin. Investigation, *28*, 1286, 1949.

CAHAN, W. G., WOODARD, H. Q., HIGINBOTHAM, N. L., STEWART, F. W., and COLEY, B. L.: Sarcoma Arising in Irradiated Bone. Report of eleven cases, Cancer, *1*, 3, 1948.

CASTLE, W. B., DRINKER, K. R., and DRINKER, C. K.: Necrosis of the Jaw in Workers Employed in Applying a Luminous Paint Containing Radium, J. Indust. Hyg., *7*, 371, 1925.

COLWELL, H. A., and RUSS, S.: *X-ray and Radium Injuries: Prevention and Treatment*, London, Oxford Univ. Press, Humphrey Milford, 1934.

CRUZ, M., COLEY, B. L., and STEWART, F. W.: Postradiation Bone Sarcoma: Report of eleven cases, Cancer, *10*, 72, 1957.

DALBY, R. G., JACOX, H. W., and MILLER, N. F.: Fracture of the Femoral Neck Following Irradiation, Am. J. Obst. & Gynec., *32*, 50, 1936.

ECKELMANN, W. R., KULP, J. L., and SCHULERT, A. R.: Strontium-90 in Man, II, Science, *127*, 266, 1958.

EWING, J.: Radiation Osteitis, Acta radiol., *6*, 399, 1926.

FICK, K. A.: Zur Frage der Erbschädigung durch Strahlen, München. med. Wchnschr., *91*, 312, 1944.

FINK, R. M. *et al.*: in *Biological Studies with Polonium, Radium, and Plutonium*, edited by R. M. Fink, New York, McGraw-Hill Book Co., Inc., 1950.

FRANTZ, C. H.: Extreme Retardation of Epiphyseal Growth from Roentgen Irradiation, Radiology, *55*, 720, 1950.

GALL, E. A., LINGLEY, J. R., and HILCKEN, J. A.: Comparative Experimental Studies of 200 Kilovolt and 1000 Kilovolt Roentgen Rays: I. The Biological Effects on the Epiphysis of the Albino Rat, Am. J. Path., *16*, 605, 1940.

GLASS, B.: The Genetic Hazards of Nuclear Radiations, Science, *126*, 241, 1957.

GRATZEK, F. R., HOLMSTROM, E. G., and RIGLER, L. G.: Post-irradiation Bone Changes, Am. J. Roentgenol., *53*, 62, 1945.

HAMILTON, J. G.: The Metabolism of the Fission Products and the Heaviest Elements, Radiology, *49*, 325, 1947.

HATCHER, C. H.: The Development of Sarcoma in Bone Subjected to Roentgen or Radium Irradiation, J. Bone & Joint Surg., *27*, 179, 1945.

HATCHER, C. H., and CAMPBELL, J. C.: Benign Chondroblastoma of Bone: Its Histologic Variations and a Report of Late Sarcoma in the Site of One, Bull. Hosp. Joint Dis., *12*, 411, 1951.

HELLER, M.: Bone. Chapt. V in *Histopathology of Irradiation from External and Internal Sources*, edited by W. Bloom, New York, McGraw-Hill Book Co., Inc., 1948.

HODGES, P. C.: Health Hazards in the Diagnostic Use of *X*-Ray, J.A.M.A., *166*, 577, 1958.

JAFFE, H. L.: Giant Cell Tumor of Bone: Problems of Differential Diagnosis, Bull. Hosp. Joint Dis., *5*, 84, 1944.

JAFFE, H. L., LICHTENSTEIN, L., and PORTIS, R. B.: Giant Cell Tumor of Bone: Its Pathologic Appearance, Grading, Supposed Variants and Treatment, Arch. Path., *30*, 993, 1940.

KOK, G.: Spontaneous Fractures of the Femoral Neck after the Intensive Irradiation of Carcinoma of the Uterus, Acta radiol., *40*, 511, 1953.

KÜTTNER, H.: Zur Frage der Geschwulstentstehung nach Röntgenbestrahlung von Gelenk- und Knochentuberkulosen, Arch. f. klin. Chir., *164*, 5, 1931.

LANGHAM, W. H., and ANDERSON, E. C.: Strontium-90 and Skeletal Formation, Science, *126*, 205, 1957.

LEDOUX-LEBARD, R.: Le cancer des radiologistes, Paris méd., *12*, 299, 1922.

LEWIS, E. B.: Leukemia and Ionizing Radiation, Science, *125*, 965, 1957.

LOONEY, W. B.: Late Effects (Twenty-Five to Forty Years) of the Early Medical and Industrial Use of Radioactive Materials. Their Relation to the More Accurate Establishment of Maximum Permissible Amounts of Radioactive Elements in the Body, J. Bone & Joint Surg., *37–A*, 1169, 1955; *38–A*, 175, 1956; and *38–A*, 392, 1956.

MARTLAND, H. S.: Histopathology of Certain Anemias due to Radioactivity, Proc. New York Path. Soc., *26*, 65, 1926.

————: Occupational Poisoning in Manufacture of Luminous Watch Dials, J.A.M.A., *92*, 466, 1929.

————: The Occurrence of Malignancy in Radio-active Persons, Am. J. Cancer, *15*, 2435, 1931.

MARTLAND, H. S., CONLON, P., and KNEF, J. P.: Some Unrecognized Dangers in the Use and Handling of Radioactive Substances: with Especial Reference to the Storage of Insoluble Products of Radium and Mesothorium in the Reticulo-endothelial System, J.A.M.A., *85*, 1769, 1925.

McCRORIE, W. D. C.: Fractures of the Femoral Neck following Pelvic Irradiation, Brit. J. Radiol., *23*, 587, 1950.

MULLER, H. J.: Our Load of Mutations, Am. J. Human Genet., *2*, 111, 1950.

MURPHY, D. P., and DE RENYI, M.: Postconception Pelvic Irradiation of the Albino Rat (Mus norvegicus): Its Effect upon the Offspring, Surg., Gynec. & Obst., *50*, 861, 1930.

NAGEOTTE, J.: Remarques sur l'ostéo-radio-nécrose de Cl. Regaud, Compt. rend. Soc. de Biol., *87*, 913, 1922.

NEUHAUSER, E. B. D., WITTENBORG, M. H., BERMAN, C. Z., and COHEN, J.: Irradiation Effects of Roentgen Therapy on the Growing Spine, Radiology, *59*, 637, 1952.

OWEN, M., SISSONS, H. A., and VAUGHAN, J.: The Effect of a Single Injection of High Dose of $^{90}$Sr in Rabbits, Brit. J. Cancer, *11*, 229, 1957.

PERTHES, G.: Ueber den Einfluss der Röntgenstrahlen auf epitheliale Gewebe, insbesondere auf das Carcinom, Arch. f. klin. Chir., *71*, 955, 1903.

PHEMISTER, D. B.: Radium Necrosis of Bone, Am. J. Roentgenol., *16*, 340, 1926.

REGAUD, C.: Sur la sensibilité du tissu osseux normal vis-a-vis des radiations X et Y et sur le mécanisme de l'ostéo-radio-nécrose, Compt. rend. Soc. de Biol., *87*, 629, 1922.

REGEN, E. M., and WILKINS, W. E.: The Effect of Large Doses of X-Rays on the Growth of Young Bone, J. Bone & Joint Surg., *18*, 61, 1936.

ROLLESTON, H.: Critical Review: The Harmful Effects of Irradiation (X-rays and Radium), Quart. J. Med., *24*, 101, 1930–31.

SABANAS, A. O., DAHLIN, D. C., CHILDS, D. S., JR., and IVINS, J. C.: Postradiation Sarcoma of Bone, Cancer, *9*, 528, 1956.

SCHWARTZ, L., KNOWLES, F. L., BRITTEN, R. H., and THOMPSON, L. R.: Health Aspects of Radium Dial Painting. I. Scope and Findings, J. Indust. Hyg., *15*, 362, 1933.

STEPHENSON, W. H., and COHEN, B.: Post-irradiation Fractures of the Neck of the Femur, J. Bone & Joint Surg., *38–B*, 830, 1956.

VAUGHAN, J. M.: The Effects of Radiation on Bone. Chapt. XXIII in *The Biochemistry and Physiology of Bone*, edited by G. H. Bourne, New York, Academic Press, Inc., 1956.

VAUGHAN, J. M., TUTT, M., and KIDMAN, B.: The Biological Hazards of Radioactive Strontium. In *Biological Hazards of Atomic Energy*, edited by A. Haddow, New York, Oxford Univ. Press, 1952.

WHITEH OUSE, W. M., and LAMPE, I: Osseous Damage in Irradiation of Renal Tumors in Infancy andChildhood, Am. J. Roentgenol., *70*, 721, 1953.

WOODARD, H. Q.: The Story of the Radium-dial Painters is not yet Finished, Cancer, *10*, opp. page 1, 1957.

Chapter

# 29

# Tumors Invading Bones from Overlying Soft Parts

THE soft parts overlying the bones and their periosteal coverings may be the point of departure for various tumors, both benign and malignant. Most of these tumors are to be related to the differentiated tissue constituents of the part: skin and its adnexa, supporting connective tissue, adipose tissue, muscle, and lymphoid tissue. Soft-tissue tumors composed of vascular or neural elements apparently also belong in this category. Although cartilage and osseous tissue are not normally present in soft parts, one occasionally encounters there a benign or malignant primary tumor containing one or both of these tissue elements. Furthermore, one may find a tumor (the so-called myxoma) whose tissue suggests primitive mesenchyme—a tissue likewise not normally present in mature soft parts.

In addition to tumors composed of tissue related to some single mesodermal element, one may encounter mixed soft-tissue tumors composed of a variety of mesodermal derivatives, and these tumors likewise may be either benign or malignant. To these mixed tumors Stout has given the name of "mesenchymoma." In any particular case, the mixed tumor is composed of a number of different tissues of mesodermal origin in various proportions—cartilage and/or osseous tissue, fibrous, adipose, lymphoid, or muscle tissue, for instance. However, in evaluating a soft-tissue tumor as a possible mixed mesodermal tumor, cartilage, osseous tissue, and even fibrous connective tissue should be considered together as a single tissue element. That is, when a lesion contains even all three of these tissues, the presence of some other mesodermal derivative in addition is needed to justify the diagnosis of a mixed mesodermal tumor. Indeed, altogether, a diagnosis of mesenchymoma has to be made with considerable discrimination. Otherwise, "mesenchymoma" becomes a sort of "wastebasket" category for soft-tissue tumors showing even minor aberrations from their basic histologic pattern.

This schematization of the soft-tissue tumors should not lead to the conclusion that these tumors always lend themselves easily to identification and placement in one category or another. It is true that, much more often than not, the classification of the lesion is relatively simple. This is so when the lesional tissue is dominated by some one type of cell and the nature of this cell (fibroblast, lipoblast, rhabdomyoblast, *etc.*) is clear.

Diagnostic difficulties arise when, as often happens, there has been extensive dedifferentiation and/or metaplasia of the tumor cells. Under these conditions, much of the tissue of a liposarcoma, for instance, may suggest histologically the pattern of a fibrosarcoma. Or a fibrosarcoma, for example, may have been so altered by dedifferentiation that it appears histologically as a polymorphocellular tumor which one cannot identify more precisely than as a sarcoma. In fact, if one reviews a large series of malignant soft-tissue tumors, many of them will be found not to lend themselves to any more specific diagnosis than "poorly differentiated sarcoma." Be that as it may, many of the complexities inherent in the diagnosis and differential diagnosis of the soft-tissue tumors have been resolved by Stout in his numerous publications in this field.

We are not concerned in this chapter with the soft-tissue tumors *per se*, but rather with the direct effects of their growth upon the regional bone or bones. As a matter of fact, it is not very often that such tumors actually invade or even deform the contour of bones in their vicinity. Indeed, a soft-tissue tumor (for example, a fibrosarcoma, liposarcoma, or chondrosarcoma) which has developed in a very fleshy part of an extremity may attain large size without encroaching upon bone. Even if a malignant soft-tissue tumor develops in an area which is not very fleshy, it is still likely that its main direction of growth will be outward (that is, away from the neighboring bone) rather than toward and into the bone.

Under certain conditions, however, soft-tissue tumors, even when they arise in the fleshy part of an extremity, do eventually invade bone. This happens notably when the tumor is deep-seated and originates near the periosteum, comes to involve the latter, and thus reaches and erodes the regional bone cortex. Also, irrespective of whether the tumor starts parosteally, if its site provides but little space for expansion, it tends rather strongly at least to deform the neighboring bone or bones and may actually erode and invade them. This is especially likely to occur in connection with tumors which arise in an interosseous space or in the soft tissues of the foot, the hand, or the wrist or ankle region. Indeed, in these latter sites, even nontumorous proliferative lesions of soft parts not infrequently come to deform and/or invade bone, as is well exemplified by the so-called pigmented villonodular lesions (p. 533).

Though the soft-tissue tumors do not frequently deform or invade neighboring bone or bones, they are, on the whole, more likely to do so if the tumor is malignant than if it is benign. Among the benign tumors, the hemangioma tends to constitute an exception to this general trend, especially if the soft tissues in which it has developed lie close to the bone. However, in any case, it is not the writer's intention to discuss the many individual soft-tissue tumors as such, but merely to give enough detail about certain ones to show the setting in which the bone involvement occurs.

## FIBROSARCOMA

Among the malignant soft-tissue tumors, the *fibrosarcoma* is the most common and the one most likely to be associated with invasion of regional bone. As to the benign fibrous lesions, even the diffusely proliferating fibroblastic growth of the palmar fascia (*palmar fibromatosis*) and its analogue in the plantar fascia apparently never come to involve neighboring bone.

In respect to *clinical findings*, most patients affected with fibrosarcoma are young or middle-aged adults, and it seems to show no sex predilection. The tumor is observed most often in the soft parts of the limbs or limb roots. It presents as a firm tissue mass and may be adherent to the skin if located superficially or, on the other hand, to bone if it is large and located in the deeper tissues. The tumor tends to grow slowly, and it is not unusual for it to have been present for several years before a spurt of growth led the patient to seek medical care. Pain is usually not a prominent complaint.

The history and clinical findings often do not contribute toward the definitive diagnosis of the tumor as a fibrosarcoma. *X*-ray examination of the part is also not specifically helpful, since it will show merely the presence of a somewhat lobulated soft-tissue mass—a type of shadow which might also be produced by a liposarcoma, for instance. If the presence of the tumor is associated with changes in the local bone or bones, the *x*-ray picture (comprising several different views) rarely leaves any doubt that the soft-tissue mass observed represents a tumor which is growing into the bone, rather than one which has started in the interior of the bone and broken out of it. In particular, one can usually see evidence of reaction of the bone to the tumor invasion, in the form of a zone of sclerosis at the site of the penetration. This is usually still true to some degree even if the tumor has penetrated widely into the bone and is growing freely within the medullary cavity. (See Fig. 158.)

As to the *pathologic findings,* a fibrosarcoma removed from the soft parts of an extremity appears grossly as a tumor mass often measuring 10 to 15 cm. in its

### *Figure 158*

*A*, Roentgenograph showing a globular soft-tissue tumor found on microscopic examination to be a well differentiated fibrosarcoma. The tumor has deformed the lower end of the fibula and is also eroding into the tibia and astragalus. The patient was a woman 34 years of age who had been aware of a somewhat painful swelling in the back of the left ankle for about 2 years. During the 6 months before her admission to the hospital, a definite tumor mass became palpable, and this was increasing in size. The extirpated tumor measured approximately 7 × 5 × 5 cm. and was of firm consistency. Its external surface was covered by a thin and closely adherent fibrous tunic which could not be peeled from the specimen. The cut surface was firm and varied in color from yellow to grayish white. It presented dense, coarse, irregularly directed bands of fibrous tissue which were set against a background of grayish white and more homogeneous fibrous tissue. For the histologic pattern of the lesional tissue, see *C*. The affected regional bone was not removed, and the capsule of the tibio-astragalar joint, to which the tumor was also attached, was not extirpated either. On this account, it is not surprising that the patient appeared 3 years later at another hospital with a local recurrence. The recurrent tumor was much larger than the original lesion, and a midleg amputation was then carried out. Histologic examination of the recurrent tumor showed that it was much more cellular than it had been in the original specimen. In a follow-up examination 3 years later, the stump showed a recurrent tumor mass which extended to the popliteal fossa, and a midthigh amputation was then done. The patient was found free of recurrence 2 years later, though one cannot be certain that she is cured. If the original intervention had consisted of a midleg amputation rather than an incomplete excision, the prolonged morbidity would have been avoided and one could feel much more secure about the ultimate prognosis.

*B*, Roentgenograph showing a large soft-tissue tumor found on microscopic examination to be a poorly differentiated fibrosarcoma. The tumor has extensively invaded and destroyed the lower part of the femur. The patient was a woman 47 years of age who, for about 7 years, had suffered from pain associated with a swelling in the back of the right knee. The *x*-ray picture in question was taken shortly before her admission to the hospital. The condition was treated by midthigh amputation. Dissection of the thigh area revealed a large tumor mass situated mainly posteriorly and laterally. The bone and the encuffing tumor mass were cut in the frontal plane. In the midportion of the amputated part of the femur, the major marrow cavity was found to contain a focus of tumor tissue about 2 inches in longitudinal extent. Below, in the region of the condyles, the destruction of the bone by the invading tumor was even more extensive, as one can observe in the *x*-ray picture. Within the femur the tumor tissue was demarcated everywhere by a zone of sclerotic osseous tissue. For the histologic pattern of the fibrosarcoma in this case, see *D*. A follow-up examination 7 years after the amputation revealed no evidence of local recurrence or metastasis.

*C*, Photomicrograph (× 225) showing the histologic pattern of the well differentiated fibrosarcoma illustrated in *A*. Note that the tumor fibroblasts appear as drawn-out spindle cells and that the cells are separated by abundant connective-tissue fibers.

*D*, Photomicrograph (× 225) showing the histologic pattern of the poorly differentiated fibrosarcoma illustrated in *B*. Note the great cellularity of the tumor tissue and the sparsity of intercellular fibers. Note also that the tumor fibroblasts are much larger and plumper than those shown in *C*. Sarcoma giant cells such as are to be observed in a poorly differentiated but frankly anaplastic fibrosarcoma were not present anywhere in the lesional tissue in this case.

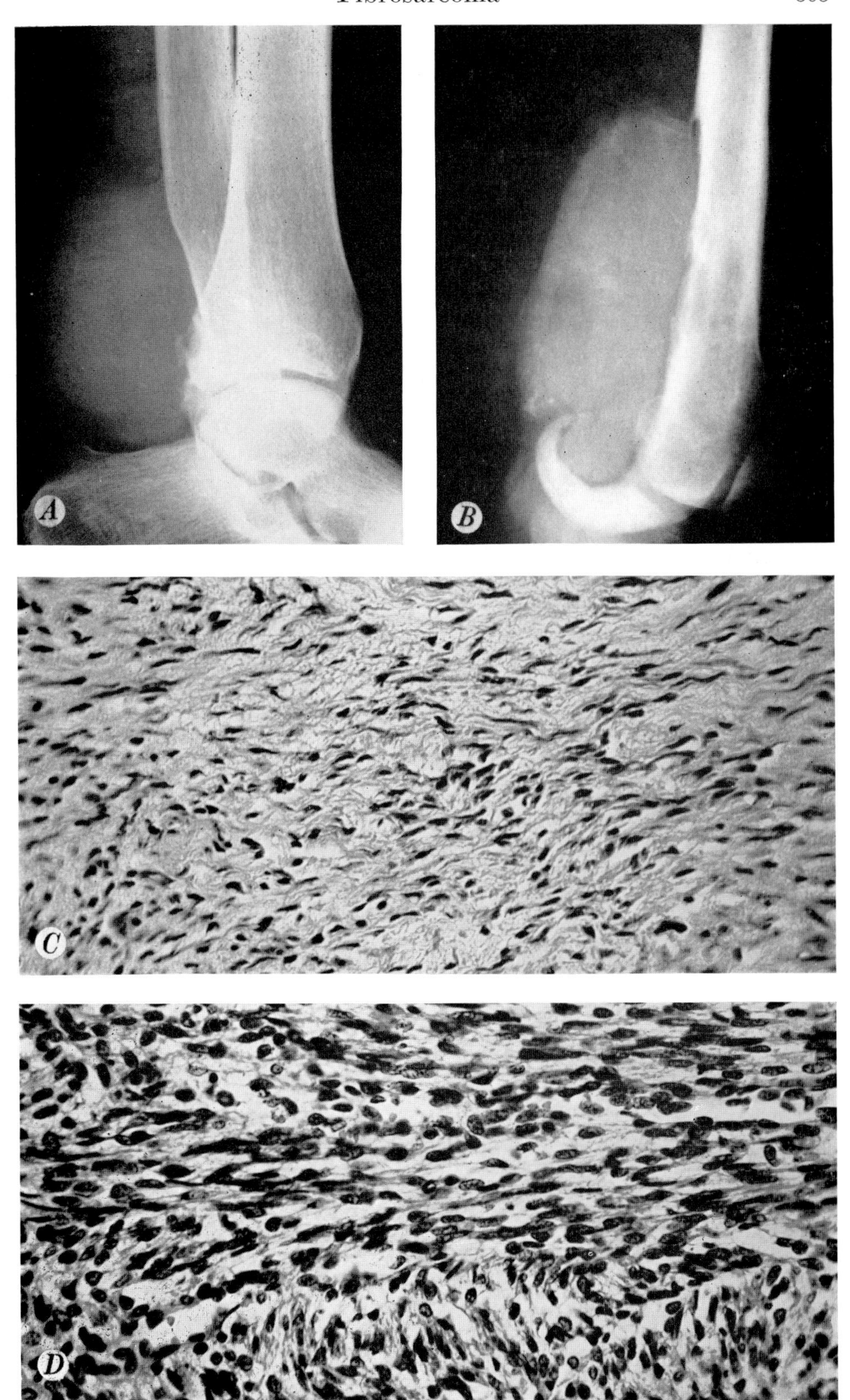


*Figure 158*

greatest dimension. It is usually quite firm and ordinarily has some muscle and/or fat adherent to its outer surface. When the specimen is sectioned, the cut surface usually appears whitish and often presents the pattern characteristic of a fibrous growth, as demonstrated by the presence of whorled tissue bundles. Some fibrosarcomas are less characteristic in this respect, in that the cut surface appears rather fleshy. Particularly in such lesions, one may also observe secondary changes represented by focal areas of hemorrhagic discoloration, edema, or even frank softening. The cut specimen usually also reveals that the tumor has no clearly defined capsule, and in fact one may observe irregular extensions of the tumor tissue here and there into the adherent muscle and/or fat. If the case is one in which the fibrosarcoma has involved the bone and an amputation has been done, detailed study will reveal just how and where the tumor is encroaching on the bone and perhaps even invading the marrow cavity.

In respect to the microscopic findings, what has already been said in regard to the cytology of the fibrosarcomas which start in bone (p. 304) is applicable to the fibrosarcomas primary in the soft tissues. Thus the latter, too, fall roughly into two histologic groups. In the category comprising the *well differentiated* lesions, the tumor cells are clearly larger and more drawn out than the ordinary adult fibroblasts, but few if any mitotic figures are seen. Though the tissue pattern as a whole does have a sarcomatous aura, little or no cellular anaplasia is observed. Furthermore, intercellular connective tissue fibers may be present in considerable amounts, and in some lesions or lesional areas, broad collagen bundles may even be prominent.

If one is dealing with a *poorly differentiated* lesion, the histologic picture of frank malignancy is much more clear-cut. The tumor tissue is likely to be highly cellular, and there is often but little fibrillar intercellular material between the crowded cells. The cells are usually still recognizable as fibroblasts, but are quite large and show variations in size, some nuclear hyperchromatism, and more than an occasional mitotic figure. In a poorly differentiated tumor, furthermore, some areas of frank anaplasia are commonly observed, and occasionally even the entire tumor is rather anaplastic. Under these conditions, the lesion shows a good deal of pleomorphism of the tumor cells (including the presence of sarcoma giant cells) and numerous mitotic figures. Since the fibroblastic nature of the tumor cells is no longer clear-cut, a highly anaplastic lesion is sometimes not readily identifiable as representing a fibrosarcoma at all. Indeed, this is not a problem relating to the fibrosarcomas alone. As already noted, the various other soft-tissue sarcomas sometimes also become so undifferentiated that there is difficulty in identifying the lesion in a given case in any more precise way than as a malignant soft-tissue tumor.

In respect to *treatment*, whether the fibrosarcoma is well or poorly differentiated, recurrence is almost certain unless the tumor is subjected to very radical excision. If the tumor has invaded the neighboring bone, the condition is probably best treated by amputation. This is the preferable initial approach unless one can include the entire affected bone area in the excision and is confident of being able to avoid contamination of the surgical field in the course of the intervention. In connection with treatment, it is also useful to know that many of the deep-seated fibrosarcomas of extremities are of the poorly differentiated variety. These tumors have a particularly high rate of recurrence and a particularly strong tendency to metastasize. However, metastasis is not likely to take place early, so that if the tumor is adequately treated at the first intervention the ultimate prognosis is not too unfavorable.

As a matter of fact, the first intervention is usually not adequate. Hence it is not surprising to find statements in the literature to the effect that 60 per cent or more of the patients treated for poorly differentiated fibrosarcomas have recurrences and that as many as 40 per cent or more ultimately succumb to metastasis. This nearly always occurs by way of the blood stream, and the lungs are the main site of the metastatic growths. On the other hand, though the recurrence rate for the well differentiated fibrosarcomas is also high if they are not adequately treated, very few of these lesions metastasize unless they change their histologic character.

# TUMORS OF ADIPOSE TISSUE

The various benign and malignant tumors of adipose tissue rarely deform or invade bone. Of course, the great majority of the benign tumors of adipose tissue (the *lipomas*) develop in subcutaneous sites and fail to attain great size. Even when a lipoma evolves in proximity to a bone (in a limb, for example) and even if it grows to fairly large size, the fact that the tumor has no infiltrative qualities and that it is also soft and yielding precludes its affecting neighboring bone. Indeed, one occasionally observes a very large and deep-seated intermuscular lipoma which is adherent to the periosteum and which nevertheless has not altered the bone.

Of interest in connection with the clinical diagnosis of deep-seated lipomas is the fact that they are more permeable to $x$-rays than are the soft tissues or, for that matter, any of the other soft-tissue tumors. Therefore, a deep-seated lipoma tends to show up as a definite circumscribed area of radiolucency. Should the lipoma become the site of fat necrosis (associated with calcification of necrotic areas), or should a meager encapsulating shell of osseous tissue develop about the lipoma, the diagnostic cue of radiolucency may, of course, be largely obliterated.

## LIPOSARCOMA

The *liposarcoma* is probably the second most common of the malignant soft-tissue tumors.* The subjects are usually older adults and more often males than females. The most common sites of the tumor are the thigh (usually the upper part), the back of the knee, the gluteal region, and the retroperitoneal area. In relation to limbs and limb roots, the tumor usually arises in the deep tissues rather than subcutaneously. As to the $x$-ray picture presented by a liposarcoma, it is to be noted that the latter casts a shadow which is denser than that of the neighboring soft tissues, in contrast to what is commonly observed in connection with the lipomas. (See Fig. 159.)

There is quite general agreement that it is exceptional for a liposarcoma to develop out of a pre-existing lipoma, and that the tumor is thus nearly always a malignant lipoblastic growth from the beginning. Liposarcomas tend on the whole to grow slowly for years and to attain large size if left to themselves. However, some grow very rapidly, becoming very large tumors even within a year, and these lesions have a rather strong tendency toward metastasis. In the course of its growth, or in consequence of recurrence, a liposarcoma occasionally comes to invade a neighboring bone (see Martin and Colson).

* Since adipose tissue is such an important constituent of bone marrow, one would expect to encounter, at least occasionally, a liposarcoma which has started in the interior of a bone. Actually, however, if primary liposarcoma of bone occurs at all, it is certainly extremely rare. On this account, before deciding on a diagnosis of primary liposarcoma of bone, one should be convinced that the liposarcoma was not one which had broken into the bone from the neighboring soft parts. Stewart, recognizing the problems inherent in the diagnosis of primary liposarcoma of bone, nevertheless reported three cases which he interpreted, largely by the process of elimination, as examples of the condition. His paper has been the point of departure for reports of other supposed instances (see Duffy and Stewart, Rehbock and Hauser, and Dawson). As to his own experience, the writer has not yet seen a case which he regarded as certainly representing primary liposarcoma of bone, though he does not wish to rule out entirely the possibility that such a tumor does exist.

In respect to the *pathologic findings,* a liposarcoma which has been sectioned presents grossly as a more or less encapsulated, somewhat nodular tissue mass which is often yellowish orange in color, though it may also show areas which are hemorrhagically discolored. The tumor tissue is much firmer than that of a simple lipoma, and it may be somewhat slimy in part or throughout. Here and there one may also note some areas of fibrous consistency, as well as areas in which the tumor tissue has undergone necrosis, but frank softening and cystification are usually not observed.

The microscopic appearance presented by the liposarcomas is quite variable, reflecting the differences in their malignant potentialities. As Stout points out, however, they have in common the fact that they reproduce cytologically the appearance of embryonal fat—either the ordinary myxoid variety or the less common brown fat.

Those of the tumors which are only locally malignant are now commonly denoted as the *well differentiated* liposarcomas. They are composed of an admixture of mature fat cells and myxoid tissue containing lipoblasts. Most of the lipoblasts are stellate or spindle-shaped, and their cytoplasm shows small vacuoles representing lipid, but some of the lipoblasts appear as "signet ring" cells because the cytoplasm is represented by a single large vacuole. However, the liposarcomas in question do not contain any bizarre lipoblasts, and, though they recur if not adequately extirpated, they do not tend to metastasize.

On the other hand, the liposarcomas which are fully malignant (the *poorly differentiated* liposarcomas) not only have a high recurrence rate but frequently metastasize. They contain few if any mature fat cells, are rich in lipoblasts, and may vary widely (from lesion to lesion and area to area) in respect to the amount of myxoid material they contain. In those tumors or tumor fields containing an abundance of myxoid, many of the lipoblasts appear as bizarre multinucleated giant cells whose cytoplasm is vacuolated. The uninuclear lipoblasts in myxoid areas may also be quite anaplastic and show many mitoses. In those tumors or tumor fields which are free of myxoid material, the lipoblasts are likely to appear as rounded, vacuolated cells suggesting the cells composing so-called "brown fat."

**Figure 159**

*A*, Roentgenograph illustrating extensive destruction of the lower part of a radius and ulna, induced by a fully malignant liposarcoma which had eroded into these bones. The patient was a man 58 years of age whose left forearm had been painful and swollen for the past 3 years. The tumor was treated by radical resection. It was removed intact, together with the first row of carpal bones and the radius and ulna to within 3 inches of the elbow joint. When the tumor mass was transected, the lesional tissue was found to be somewhat nodular and, on the whole, whitish yellow in color. Furthermore, the tissue was semimucoid in some areas, though in others it was firmer and cream yellow in color. The patient died with pulmonary metastases about one year after the surgical intervention.

*B*, Roentgenograph showing for comparison the appearance characteristic for a simple lipoma. Since the tissue of a simple lipoma is more readily permeable to *x*-rays than are the neighboring soft tissues, this benign lesion of adipose tissue stands out roentgenographically as an area of greater radiolucency.

*C*, Photomicrograph (× 225) showing the histologic pattern presented by tissue from a myxoid area in the poorly differentiated liposarcoma illustrated in *A*. Note that some of the lipoblasts appear as bizarre multinucleated giant cells and that many of the smaller lipoblasts are stellate.

*D*, Photomicrograph (× 225) from a firmer, non-myxoid tissue area of the lesion shown in *A*. On the whole, the lipoblasts appear as rounded, vacuolated cells, and the microscopic pattern of the tissue suggests in general that of brown fat.

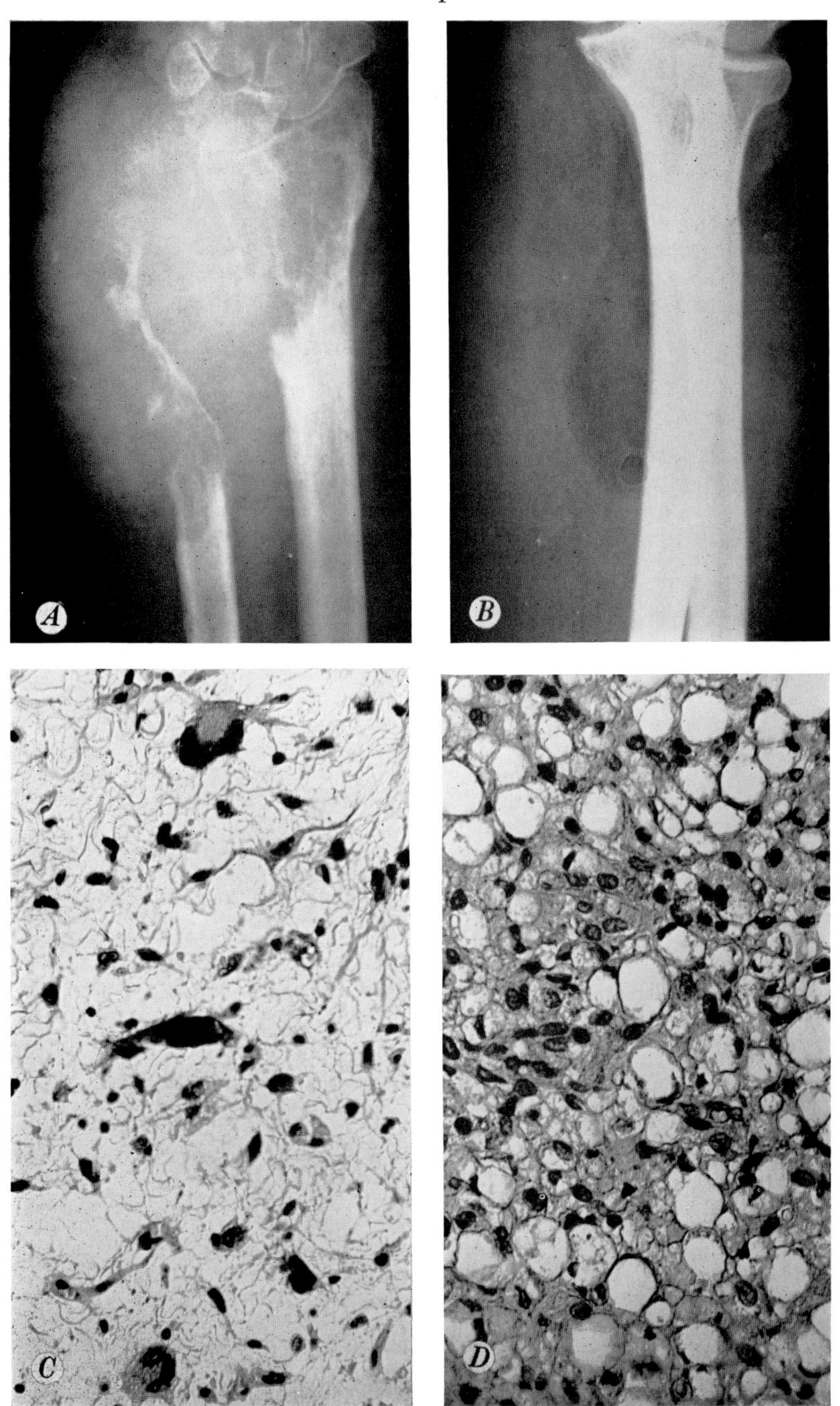


*Figure 159*

Though many of the poorly differentiated liposarcomas are essentially of the myxoid variety and some essentially of the "brown fat" variety, tumors containing lipoblasts of both these types of embryonal fat are also often observed. Furthermore, all fully malignant liposarcomas may show tissue areas in which the lipoblasts have become elongated and spindle-shaped, and in such places the cytologic pattern may even suggest fibrosarcoma.

The *treatment* appropriate for liposarcoma is surgical excision, and the tumor should be given a very wide berth. That is, it should not merely be shelled out of its bed, but removed intact in its setting with the adjacent soft tissues. As is true for malignant soft-tissue tumors in general, the surgical intervention should be undertaken only after histologic examination of a tissue specimen removed by incisional biopsy. If it is not feasible to extirpate the lesion intact in its setting and the tumor is in a limb, amputation is indicated to forestall recurrence and metastasis. On the other hand, radiation therapy is at best of only palliative value in the treatment of deep-seated liposarcoma.

## MALIGNANT TUMORS OF MUSCLE

The benign and malignant tumors of muscle fall into three categories: those derived from cells with granular cytoplasm which are apparently peculiar muscle cells (benign and malignant granular cell myoblastoma); those related to smooth muscle (leiomyoma and leiomyosarcoma); and those related to striated muscle (rhabdomyoma and rhabdomyosarcoma).

### *Figure 160*

*A*, Roentgenograph showing erosive destruction of the condylar region and adjacent portion of the shaft of a femur by a deep-seated soft-tissue tumor which proved to be a malignant granular cell myoblastoma. The patient was a man 64 years of age who, for at least 2 years, had complained of some pain and presented a palpable swelling in the popliteal region of the limb in question. The diagnosis was established by biopsy, and a midthigh amputation was done. Dissection of the specimen showed that the tumor mass outside of the bone was composed of rather soft tissue which was gray-yellow in color. When the amputated femur was sawed through in its long axis, one could note that, within the condylar region, the tumor extended to the articular cartilage and that proximally it was invading the medullary cavity of the local part of the shaft. In a follow-up examination made 2 years after the amputation, the patient showed neither local recurrence nor metastasis. Several months after this follow-up the patient succumbed to an acute myocardial infarction, but no autopsy was performed.

*B*, Photomicrograph (× 125) showing the cytologic architecture of the tumor in an area where some of the tissue (upper half of the picture) still presents the pattern of a granular cell tumor, while in the adjacent part (lower half of the picture) the cells have lost that pattern and are spindling out. The cytologic details pertaining to these two patterns are shown in *C* and *D*. Though some tissue samples taken from widely separated parts of the tumor showed this combination of cell types, others presented the granular cell pattern alone and still others the spindle cell pattern alone. However, the tumor tissue within the bone was almost entirely of the spindle cell type.

*C*, Photomicrograph (× 250) showing the cytologic details in an area in which the tumor tissue is still predominantly of the granular cell type. Note the suggestively alveolar or cord-like arrangement of the tumor cells. The cells are polyhedral, the cell outlines are distinct, and their cytoplasm presents a finely granular appearance. The cell nuclei are larger, on the whole, than those of the benign granular cell myoblastoma.

*D*, Photomicrograph (× 250) showing the pattern in an area in which the cells have spindled out. The presence of drawn-out cells with nuclei showing a tandem arrangement makes the picture suggest the familiar or usual form of rhabdomyosarcoma.

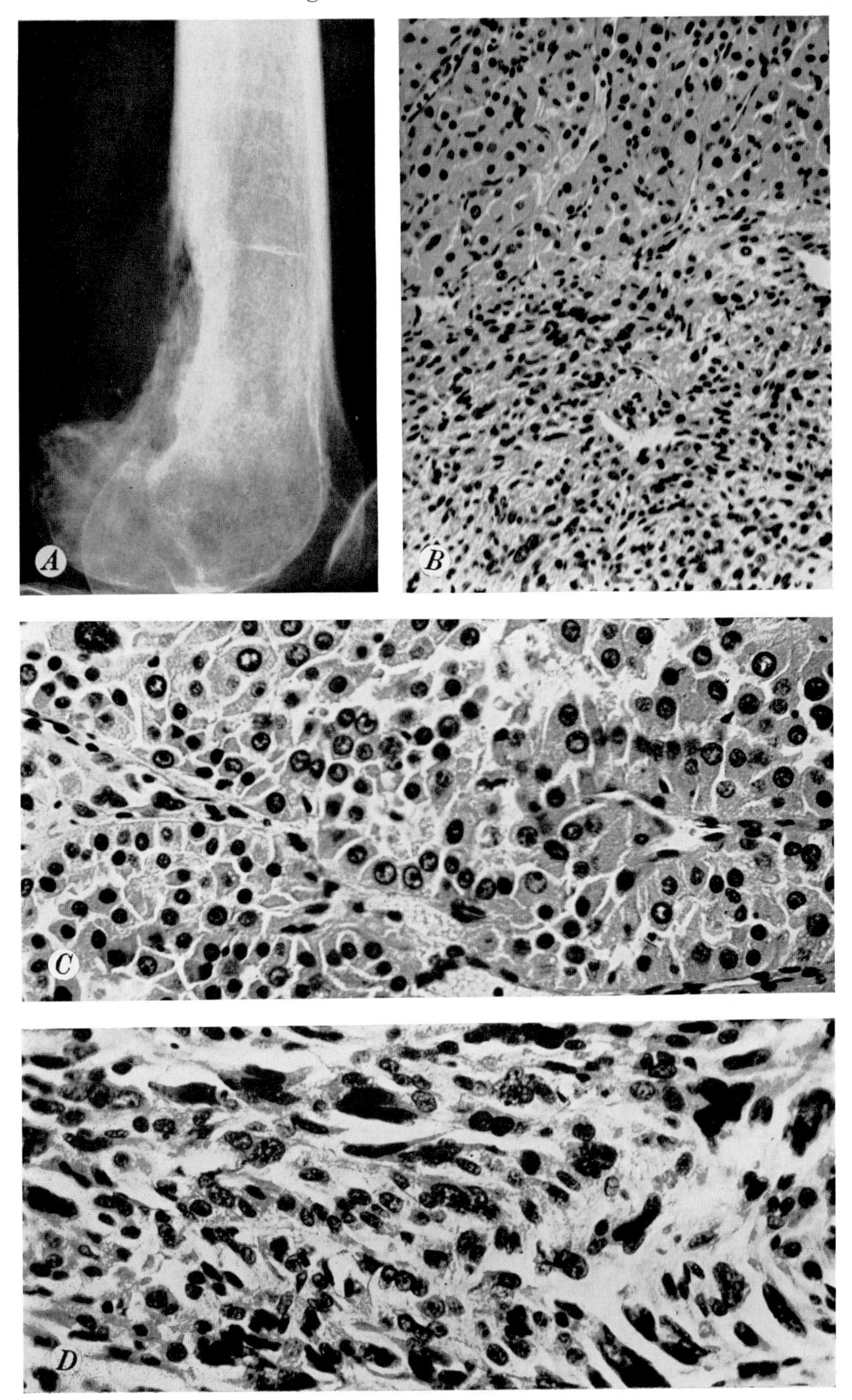


*Figure 160*

In connection with the muscle tumors, it is again almost solely the malignant varieties that come into question insofar as involvement of regional bone is concerned. However, even the rhabdomyosarcoma and the granular myoblastoma (benign or malignant) only infrequently involve neighboring bone, although they often occur in proximity to bone. The leiomyoma, though a fairly common tumor, is found mainly in the uterus and gastrointestinal tract, and this is likewise true in regard to the leiomyosarcoma. Thus involvement of regional bone by smooth muscle tumors is naturally exceptional. As to the rhabdomyoma (rare in any event), it is doubtful whether this is encountered elsewhere than in the heart.

## MALIGNANT GRANULAR CELL MYOBLASTOMA

The so-called granular cell muscle tumors are very peculiar lesions. Though there are those who doubt that they should be included among the muscle tumors at all, the writer nevertheless accepts them as such, in conformity with the interpretation given them by Stout and by Murray. In comparison with the *benign granular cell myoblastoma*, the corresponding malignant lesion is of rather rare occurrence. In any event, both forms of the lesion are prone to occur in the musculature of the extremities, though they also appear in many other sites.

The granular cell myoblastoma does not usually attain very large size, and the great majority of the benign lesions will not recur if completely excised. Even when located in the vicinity of a bone, the lesion rarely invades it. However, the writer has studied one example of a *malignant granular cell myoblastoma* which developed in the deep tissues behind the knee and did break into the neighboring bone. Specifically, this tumor appeared in the lower part of the thigh posteriorly and invaded the condylar region and the adjacent part of the shaft of the femur. (See Fig. 160.)

In respect to *histologic appearance*, the benign granular cell myoblastoma is composed of sheets of closely compacted, well defined polyhedral cells. The cell cytoplasm is abundant and shows many fine acidophilic granules, and the cell nuclei are small and stain deeply. Some of the malignant granular cell myoblastomas present the same general cytologic pattern as the benign ones, except for greater size of the cells and especially of the nuclei. In other malignant granular cell myoblastomas, however, the pattern is that of aggregates of cells in alveolar formation, the alveoli being outlined by delicate fibrous septa. In these lesions the cell nuclei are rather hyperchromatic, and the cytoplasm, while granular, may be somewhat vacuolated. It should be pointed out, however, that some workers do not accept the soft-tissue tumors showing this alveolar pattern as representing a so-called malignant granular cell myoblastoma (see Smetana and Scott, and Christopherson *et al.*). In any event, the malignant granular cell myoblastomas in general are not only locally malignant but are capable of metastasizing.

## LEIOMYOSARCOMA

As noted, the deep soft tissues of the extremities and torso are rarely the site of benign or malignant smooth muscle tumors. Already on this account alone, involvement of regional bone is even more unusual in connection with these tumors than with the tumors of fibrous tissue or adipose tissue. However, the writer has seen one case of a *leiomyosarcoma* which developed in the subcutaneous tissues of the lower part of a leg (on its anteromedial aspect) and grew large enough to produce a pressure deformity in the contour of the regional tibial cortex. The tumor, which appeared to be encapsulated, measured approximately 5 × 5 × 2 cm. and was intimately attached to the periosteum in the area where the tibia was deformed. Its cut surface appeared grayish and presented areas of hemorrhagic necrosis.

The *microscopic pattern* of the tumor tissue in this case was that conventional for leiomyosarcoma. In particular, the tumor cells were quite drawn out and spindle- or strap-shaped. In many places the cells were found arranged in whorled interlacing bundles. Between the cells there was a variable amount of connective tissue fibrils. The tumor cells were more or less uniform in size, but were larger than simple smooth muscle cells. Their nuclei were elongated, but less tapered than the cell as a whole. Intracellular myofibrils were not observed, but this is not infrequently the case with leiomyosarcomas in general. Mitotic division figures were also not apparent, and the absence of such figures is again not uncommon with these tumors. In this case, excision of the tumor, including the local periosteum and the modified tibial cortex, was not followed by recurrence or metastasis.

## RHABDOMYOSARCOMA

The malignant tumors of the skeletal musculature are relatively uncommon and constitute a very complex group of lesions. Within this group, four types have been singled out: the pleomorphic, alveolar, embryonal, and botryoid (see Horn and Enterline). The category of pleomorphic rhabdomyosarcoma represents the familiar form of the lesion. The rhabdomyosarcomas in the other categories are less well understood, and in fact many of the lesions placed in these categories have only recently been recognized as rhabdomyosarcomas (see Stobbe and Dargeon, Riopelle and Thériault, Mostofi and Morse, and Ober and Edgcomb).

The histologic hallmark of the rhabdomyosarcoma is the presence of tumor cells showing cross striations. Such cells are most often encountered in the familiar (so-called pleomorphic) type of rhabdomyosarcoma. However, in some instances even of this type it may be difficult to find cells with cross striations. In the other types of rhabdomyosarcoma (alveolar, embryonal, and botryoid), it is likewise often difficult to demonstrate cells with striations.

On the whole, the rhabdomyosarcomas do not often deform or invade neighboring bone. Apparently the embryonal rhabdomyosarcomas are more likely to do so than the other types. Furthermore, in the course of metastatic spread of these rhabdomyosarcomas, involvement of bones is also a common occurrence. (See Fig. 161.)

**Pleomorphic Rhabdomyosarcoma.**—This form of rhabdomyosarcoma predilects males, and the patients are usually middle-aged or older adults. The most common site of the tumor is a limb—most often a lower limb. The tumor usually grows rapidly, the common history being that the patient had been aware of its presence for a year or less. The size of the tumor may vary considerably from case to case, but it is usually deep-seated and not very firm under palpation.

On *histologic examination*, the tumor is found to be rich in cells, and many of these are elongated and drawn out, being ribbon-like or strap-shaped. The nuclei in these cells are often multiple and arranged in tandem. Also, one may note some very large cells with multiple nuclei and abundant intensely eosinophilic cytoplasm. Tumor cells showing longitudinal striations and, more importantly, cross striations may have to be searched for. If such tumor cells are found, identification of the lesion as a rhabdomyosarcoma is clear. If, as so often happens, they are not found, one may have to rely on the general pattern of the lesional tissue (great cellularity, drawn-out cells, tandem arrangement of the nuclei) in arriving at the diagnosis. In such cases the differential diagnosis usually rests between pleomorphic rhabdomyosarcoma and poorly differentiated fibrosarcoma.

These rhabdomyosarcomas tend strongly toward metastasis. This may take place even without being preceded by local recurrence following excision of the tumor. Such an occurrence indicates that the tumor had probably already metastasized before it was excised locally. If the excision has not been adequate, recurrence is almost certain to take place, and the incidence of metastasis is even higher.

**Alveolar, Embryonal, and Botryoid Rhabdomyosarcoma.**—The patients showing these morphologic forms of rhabdomyosarcoma are considerably younger, on the average, than those presenting the familiar pleomorphic form of the tumor. Indeed, patients affected with embryonal and botryoid rhabdomyosarcoma are often young children. None of these forms are as likely to occur in the limbs as is the pleomorphic rhabdomyosarcoma. The head and neck region, and in particular the orbit, is a common site for the embryonal variety of the tumor. The genitourinary tract is a common site for the botryoid, though the latter is also encountered in the cavities of the head region.

In respect to *gross appearance,* it is only the botryoid type that is at all distinctive. In particular, this form of rhabdomyosarcoma is found to consist of clustered masses of edematous polypoid tissue. In respect to the *microscopic findings,* the pattern characteristic of the alveolar rhabdomyosarcoma is one in which clusters of tumor cells are delimited by connective tissue trabeculæ, so that the appearance of the fields in question suggests the alveolar formations of adenocarcinoma. In these clusters, those cells which are not oriented to the trabeculæ tend to lie rather loosely. Most of these cells are small, round, and uninuclear. Some, however, are very large and multinucleated, and these giant cells are either roundish or strap-shaped. An occasional large and drawn-out cell, in particular, may show longitudinal and/or cross striations. In addition to tumor fields showing the characteristic alveolar

***Figure 161***

*A*, Roentgenograph showing a depression in the contour of the lower end of a tibia, caused by the growth of a soft-tissue tumor which proved to be a leiomyosarcoma. The patient was a woman 46 years of age. The history was that she had been aware for 4 years of a slowly growing but painless mass on the inner aspect of her right leg. At the surgical intervention, it was found that the tumor was adherent to the periosteum in the region where the tibia was deformed, but that it was otherwise well delineated and was apparently encapsulated. Excision of the tumor, including the local periosteum and modified tibial cortex, was not followed by local recurrence or metastasis.

*B*, Roentgenograph illustrating deformity and sclerosis of the right second metatarsal bone, produced by an embryonal rhabdomyosarcoma which had developed in the local soft tissues. The patient was a boy 9 years of age whose difficulty was of 6 weeks' standing. It related to a slowly enlarging though painless local swelling which presented on the dorsum of the foot. After the nature of the tumor had been established by biopsy, a low leg amputation was done. Nine months after the amputation, widespread skeletal metastases and also pulmonary metastases became apparent. (The clinical information and roentgenograph in this case were kindly supplied by Doctor John Caffey of the Babies Hospital, New York City.)

*C*, Photomicrograph (× 250) showing the histologic pattern commonly presented by the familiar (so-called pleomorphic) variety of rhabdomyosarcoma. Note the great cellularity of the tissue and the presence of large, drawn-out rhabdomyoblasts containing multiple nuclei. The section was prepared from a lesion representing a recurrence of the original tumor, which was situated in the deep tissues of the upper part of the right thigh. The patient was a man 59 years of age, and, because the lesion was a recurrent one, the limb was ablated. Three years later, however, the patient died, and autopsy revealed pulmonary metastases.

*D*, Photomicrograph (× 1100) showing a rhabdomyoblast with characteristic cross striations. The section was prepared from tissue of the primary lesion in a case of botryoid rhabdomyosarcoma. (I am indebted to Doctor William B. Ober of the Knickerbocker Hospital, New York City, for this illustration.)

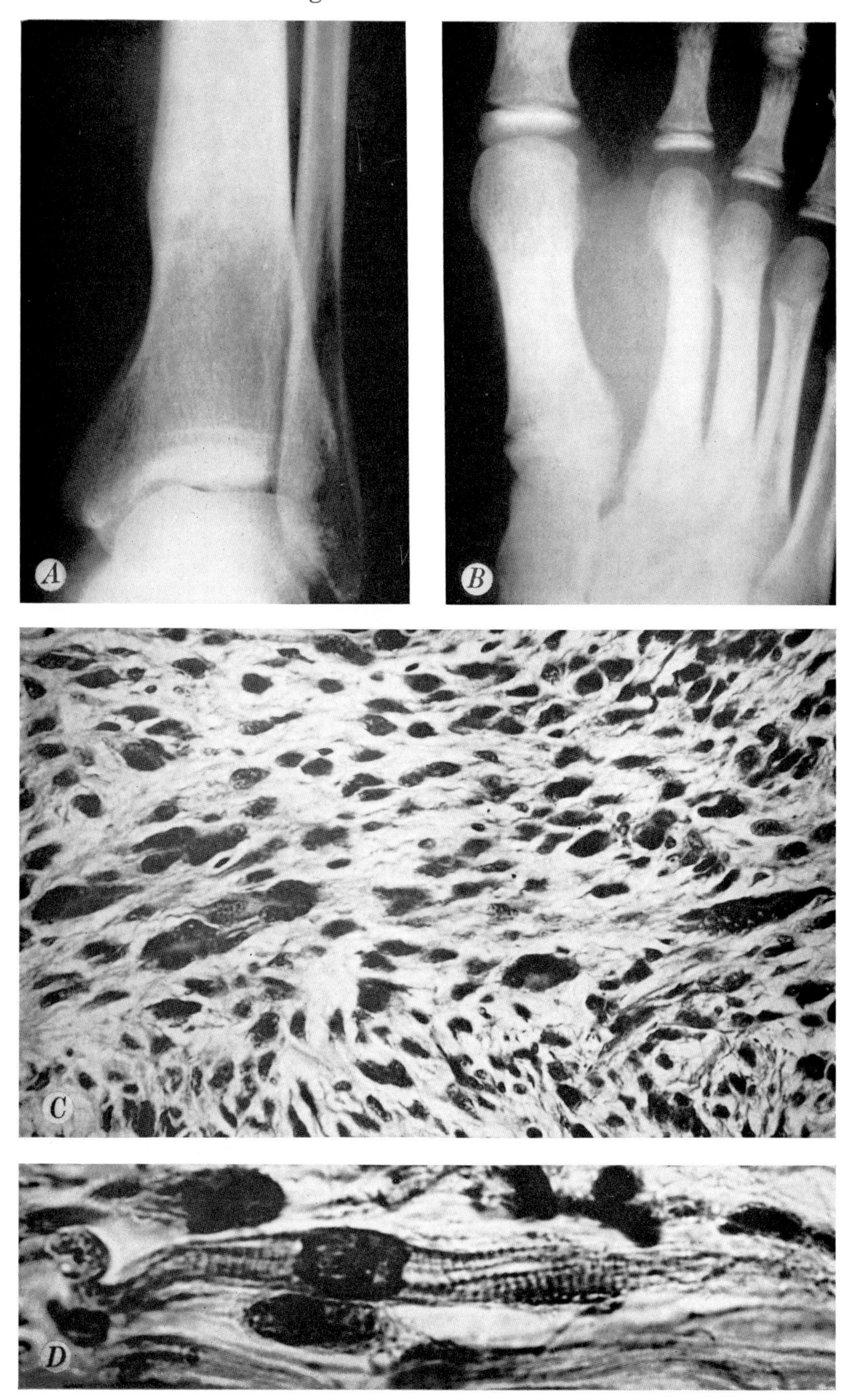

*Figure 161*

pattern, one may encounter fields in which the cells are essentially spindle-shaped or roundish and in which the alveolar pattern is lacking. Such fields may create the impression that the lesion in question represents an embryonal or a pleomorphic type of rhabdomyosarcoma.

In an embryonal rhabdomyosarcoma, too, there may be considerable variation in cytologic detail from part to part of the lesion. The basic cell is a long, tapering spindle cell with abundant eosinophilic cytoplasm and a single nucleus. Some of the drawn-out cells are enlarged about the nucleus, and in others the nucleus may be located at one end, so that the shape of the cell suggests a tadpole. The elongated cells sometimes show cross striations. In other fields, round cells may be numerous, and in still other fields one may find a mixture of round cells and drawn-out cells. Most of the round cells are small and poor in cytoplasm, but some are fairly large. In these, the nuclei are relatively small and the cytoplasm is strikingly eosinophilic.

As already indicated, the botryoid rhabdomyosarcoma, as a primary lesion, presents a distinctive gross appearance. The edematous, polypoid tumor tissue masses are covered by essentially normal mucous membrane of the site of origin, and their interiors tend to be very poor in cells. However, a multilayered band of tumor cells is to be found just beneath the mucous membrane. These are short spindle cells which show little cytoplasm, and many of their nuclei present evidence of mitotic activity. If the tissue comes from a focus of metastasis or from an area in which the tumor has invaded neighboring parts, the histologic pattern is likely to resemble that of an embryonal rhabdomyosarcoma.

All three of these forms of rhabdomyosarcoma tend strongly toward recurrence and metastasis (with or without involvement of regional lymph nodes) and are usually rapidly fatal if they have not been promptly and completely excised. For an embryonal sarcoma which has recurred, radiation therapy is sometimes of more than palliative value.

**Figure 162**

*A*, Roentgenograph showing a calcifying benign cartilage tumor (chondroma) which had developed in the palmar soft tissues overlying the midshaft of the right fourth metacarpal bone. The patient was a woman 32 years of age who had been aware for $1\frac{1}{2}$ years of a small but gradually enlarging mass in the region in question. The lesion was a source of pain, but only when the fingers were used. In the course of removal of the tumor it was noted that the latter was not attached to the bone. The specimen (see *B*) was a somewhat lobulated mass of cartilage measuring about 3 cm. across and 2 cm. in thickness. When it was transected, examination revealed that the lesional tissue was indeed heavily calcified, as had already been indicated by the *x*-ray picture.

*B*, Photograph of the specimen removed from the lesion illustrated in *A*. The lobulated character of the cartilage stands out clearly.

*C*, Roentgenograph illustrating the appearance of a juxtacortical chondrosarcoma which has developed beneath the periosteum of a humerus, near the upper end of the shaft. (The gross anatomy of the lesion is illustrated in *D*.) The patient was a woman 61 years of age whose complaint was that for 7 months she had had pain and limitation of motion in the right shoulder. The tumor has eroded the cortex, and a spur-like buttress of new bone has been formed by the irritated periosteum at the distal end of the lesion. Since the lesional cartilage has not undergone focal calcification, one does not see spotty radiopacity such as is often manifested by both benign and malignant cartilage growths in general.

*D*, Photograph showing the gross appearance of the chondrosarcoma whose roentgenographic appearance is illustrated in *C*. The lesion stands out in its setting, and the fact that it is eroding the cortex is plain, but the tumor tissue has not penetrated into the marrow cavity. The lesion in this case was treated by resection of the upper third of the affected humerus.

*E*, Photomicrograph (× 125) of tumor cartilage from the lesion shown in *D*. Cartilage cells with double nuclei can be seen, and also some cells with plump single nuclei. Such findings are sufficient to indicate that one is dealing with a malignant rather than with a benign lesion.

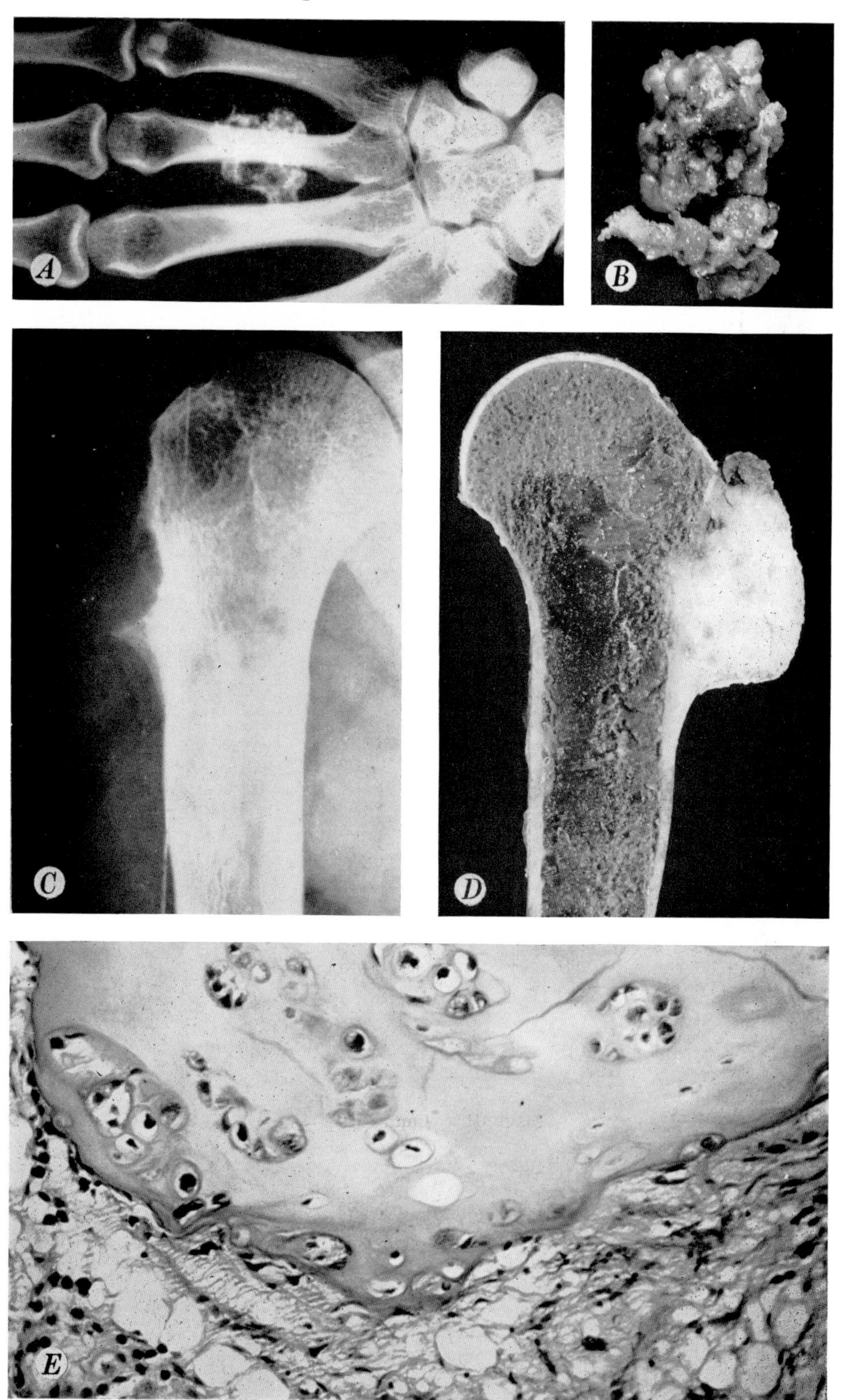

***Figure 162***

## TUMORS OF CARTILAGE

In the chapter on *juxtacortical chondroma* (p. 196), consideration is given to those benign cartilage tumors which develop in relation to the periosteal coverings of bones. These tumors (which thus do not represent cartilage tumors developing in actual soft parts) tend to be of small size, and though they erode the regional bone cortex, they usually do not break through the cortex into the medullary cavity. In accordance with the benignity of these lesions, the cartilage cells are nearly always uninuclear, the nuclei are not particularly plump, and they show no atypism even in those cells which are binuclear.

Occasionally one also observes a lesion which represents the malignant counterpart of the juxtacortical chondroma. The *juxtacortical chondrosarcoma*, while likewise developing in relation to the periosteum, not only erodes the local cortex but may break into the medullary cavity of the bone. (See Fig. 162.) In the juxtacortical chondrosarcoma the cytologic findings are analogous to those encountered in central chondrosarcoma (p. 326). Thus, as histologic examination reveals, the tumor cartilage in these cases is highly cellular, the cell nuclei are plump, many cells contain double nuclei, and there is at least an occasional cell with a large bizarre nucleus. The juxtacortical chondrosarcoma offers a relatively good prognosis even if the lesion is treated by local resection, provided that the latter completely removes the tumor intact in its regional setting of bone.

As noted, the juxtacortical chondrosarcoma represents the malignant counterpart of the juxtacortical chondroma. It is also the cartilage analogue of the *juxtacortical osteogenic sarcoma*. The latter lesion (see p. 279) is a malignant bone-forming

***Figure 163***

*A*, Roentgenograph of a foot in which a soft-tissue chondrosarcoma has partly destroyed the third metatarsal bone and also altered the second and fourth metatarsals. The patient was a woman 21 years of age who had been aware for 2 years of a painful and gradually enlarging swelling of the left foot. Clinically, a firm, nodular tumor mass was palpable, but the overlying skin was not adherent to the growth. The radiopacities in the lesional area are an indication of the fact that calcification is going on within the tumor cartilage. An amputation through the lower part of the leg was done, and part of the transected foot is illustrated in *B*. When the patient was last seen ($2\frac{1}{2}$ years after the amputation) there were no evidences of local recurrence or of metastasis.

*B*, Photograph of a longitudinal section through the foot shown in *A*. Note the lobular, faceted pattern of the tumor cartilage. Further dissection of the specimen revealed that, while the tumor had partly destroyed the third metatarsal bone, it had merely eroded the cortex of the second and fourth metatarsals and deformed the bones.

*C*, Roentgenograph showing a very large soft-tissue chondrosarcoma in the general region of a knee. Note the small blurry radiopacities which permeate the lesional area and which represent calcification going on within the tumor cartilage. Observe also that such radiopacities are likewise present in the articular space on the right. The patient was a man 54 years of age who had been aware for 2 years of an enlarging mass behind the left knee. The condition had come on insidiously and was associated with increasing pain. The tumor mass was of very firm consistency and was adherent to the tibia, but, as the *x*-ray picture shows, it had not caused any gross destruction of the regional bones.

*D*, Photograph showing, in posterior view, the knee region and the chondrosarcoma in the case illustrated in *A*, as they appeared after the overlying soft tissues had been cleaned away. The bulk of the chondrosarcoma is oriented to the tibia, and the tumor tissue appears whitish and nodular. The capsule of the joint is studded with small whitish nodules which likewise represent tumor tissue. Indeed, as was revealed by further dissection of the amputation specimen, the tumor had invaded the joint space and seeded itself on the synovial membrane.

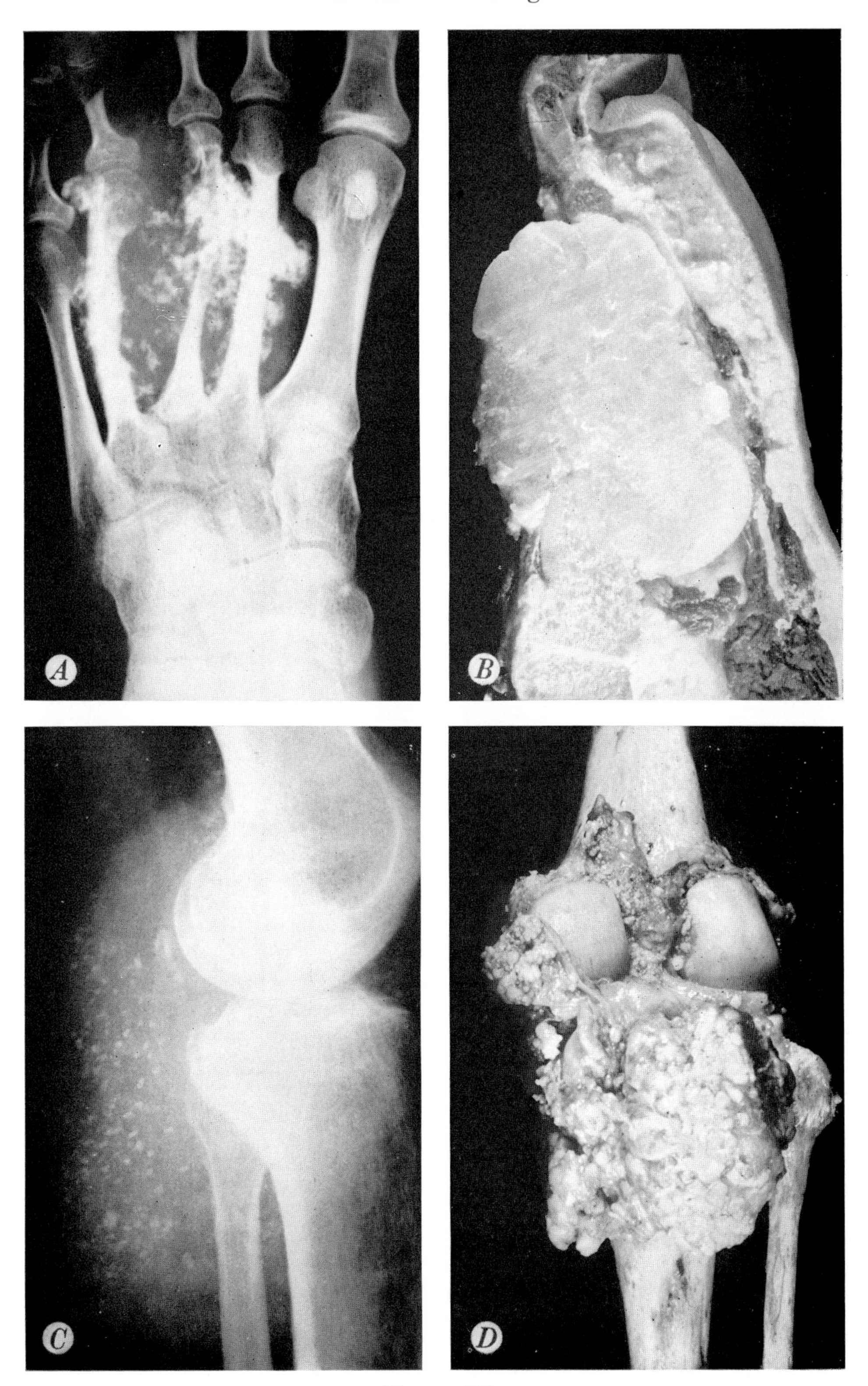

*Figure 163*

connective-tissue tumor which develops in relation to the periosteum of a bone. In accordance with its peripheral orientation, it too offers a relatively good prognosis, and certainly a far better one than the osteogenic sarcoma which starts in the interior of the bone (that is, the conventional osteogenic sarcoma).

## SOFT-TISSUE CHONDROMA

Benign cartilage tumors appearing in the somatic soft tissues but not oriented to the periosteum of bones are of infrequent occurrence (Fig. 162-*A* and *B*). The *soft-tissue chondromas* tend to grow very slowly and are usually still of small size when they first come under treatment. They usually do not deform or invade the neighboring bone. The focus of cartilage often appears spottily opaque in the *x*-ray picture. This opacity represents calcification of the cartilage matrix, and this calcification may be rather intense in some areas. In conformity with the fact that the lesion is a focus of growing cartilage, microscopic examination will show that the lesional tissue is moderately cellular in some places. In viable areas, however, the cells do not show bizarre or otherwise atypical nuclei, such as are often revealed by a malignant cartilage tumor. In the heavily calcified areas the cells are likely to have undergone necrosis, and the necrotic nuclei may appear swollen. When removed completely, these cartilage growths do not recur.

Cartilage growths oriented primarily to the capsules of joints are likewise encountered. With few exceptions, these growths are benign. The benign para-articular cartilage growths (*para-articular chondromas*) are also usually of small size. They are discussed in Chapter 31, which deals with synovial chondromatosis and other benign articular tumors.

## SOFT-TISSUE CHONDROSARCOMA

The *soft-tissue chondrosarcoma* is definitely rare. When such a tumor is encountered, it is quite likely to be in a lower limb. Just where in the soft parts the tumor begins may not be clear, but apparently it sometimes starts in muscle. A chondrosarcoma may also develop in the soft tissues about a joint. Indeed, sometimes it even penetrates the articular capsule and becomes seeded in the synovial membrane of the joint.

The patients are usually young or middle-aged adults. The tumor grows rather rapidly and may be fairly large by the time the condition is diagnosed. The roentgenographic picture may suggest the diagnosis. The helpful finding is the presence of spotty radiopacity in the soft-tissue mass representing the tumor. This is a reflection of calcification going on within the lesional cartilage. Indeed, some degree of spotty radiopacity is quite likely to be observed in connection with a soft-tissue chondrosarcoma. Occasionally, however, even a very large lesion fails to show any radiopacity, and the roentgenographic picture consequently does not point to the cartilaginous nature of the tumor. Furthermore, should a soft-tissue chondrosarcoma develop in the vicinity of a joint, and should it show only sparse radiopacities in its *x*-ray picture, one may be confronted with the problem of differentiating that picture from the one sometimes presented by synovioma (p. 582).

Be that all as it may, a soft-tissue chondrosarcoma does not often invade the regional bone or bones. It may do so if it is growing in a site where it has relatively little room for expansion—for instance, in the soft tissues of a foot. Indeed, in such a site the tumor may affect the local bones even before it has become very large. A chondrosarcoma which has developed deep in the groin may eventually invade the adjacent innominate bone and/or even the femur. This is particularly likely to happen if the tumor has attained large size. (See Fig. 163.)

The gross and microscopic *pathologic findings* in cases of soft-tissue chondrosarcoma (whether or not the tumor has invaded regional bone) are essentially the same as those described in connection with chondrosarcoma primary in bone (p. 314). The tumor ordinarily consists of a mass of rather firm and nodular cartilage. Its cut surface appears whitish and shows the lobular and faceted pattern characteristic of a cartilage growth. If the tumor is very large, it may show some edematous or mucoid areas or even some in which the tissue has undergone cystic degeneration. On microscopic examination the lesional tissue is found rather cellular on the whole. Most of the cartilage cell nuclei are plump, many cells have double nuclei, and some cells with large and bizarre nuclei are also to be seen.

The appropriate *treatment* for soft-tissue chondrosarcoma is surgery, and the procedure of choice depends on the site of the chondrosarcoma. If the lesion is accessible to complete radical local excision (that is, removal of the lesion intact in its setting of surrounding soft tissue), that procedure is preferable to amputation. This is so because (in conformity with chondrosarcoma in general) the tumor is not one which is likely to have metastasized by the time the patient comes under treatment. Even if the lesion recurs after an attempted local excision, distant metastases may still not be present. For a lesion in a site not lending itself to radical local excision, amputation should be done. This is particularly indicated if the tumor has invaded the regional bone. The over-all prognosis for soft-tissue chondrosarcoma is not too bad if the condition is adequately treated, and is certainly much better than for soft-tissue osteogenic sarcoma, now to be discussed.

## SOFT-TISSUE OSTEOGENIC SARCOMA

A *soft-tissue osteogenic sarcoma* (like an osteogenic sarcoma primary in bone) represents a malignant connective-tissue tumor which possesses, as an inherent feature, the capacity to form neoplastic osteoid and osseous tissue. The lesion is of rare occurrence, and the soft parts of limbs (especially the lower limbs) are its most common site. Only exceptionally does the tumor come to invade neighboring bone. The subjects are usually adults and occasionally even old adults. Commonly the lesion has been of only short duration (weeks or months) at the time when the patient comes under surgical care.

However, cases have been reported in which the tumor was of many years' standing. It seems probable that in most of these cases the lesion was not a fully malignant growth at the start. The likelihood is that at first it represented a bone-forming connective-tissue growth such as Fine and Stout denote by the name of "pseudomalignant osseous tumor of soft tissues." These lesions are in fact potentially malignant tumors, and indeed it may be very difficult to differentiate them histologically from the fully malignant soft-tissue osteogenic sarcoma. Apparently, in consequence of malignant transformation of the connective-tissue substratum of such an ossifying lesion, a fully malignant soft-tissue osteogenic sarcoma comes to replace it.

On the other hand, the writer is skeptical about references in the literature to the effect that a focus of conventional myositis ossificans sometimes undergoes malignant transformation into a soft-tissue osteogenic sarcoma. Indeed, a focus of post-traumatic myositis ossificans rapidly goes through a maturation process. If not removed, it comes to be represented merely by an encapsulated mass of well differentiated bone which is most condensed at its periphery. Thus the great likelihood is that, in the cases reported as representing malignant transformation of such a lesion, the nature of the basic condition had been misinterpreted.

A soft-tissue osteogenic sarcoma is not infrequently a large growth 10 cm. or more in its greatest diameter. In conformity with the fact that osteogenesis is going on in the lesional tissue, the $x$-ray picture of the tumor area shows radiopacity. This may vary in degree and extent from lesion to lesion, just as it does in connection with osteogenic sarcoma of bone. Even if the radiopacity is considerable, it is usually streaky in character. In the exceptional case in which a deep-seated soft-tissue osteogenic sarcoma invades neighboring bone, the fact that the tumor is extending into the bone (rather than coming out of it) is also usually apparent from the $x$-ray picture. Specifically, one notes that where the bone is being invaded the cortex is being hollowed out, and the border of the saucerized area may appear sclerotic. (See Fig. 164.)

In respect to the diagnostic value of the $x$-ray picture, it should also be borne in mind that a large soft-tissue tumor is not necessarily an osteogenic sarcoma even if it shows some streaky radiopacity. It might be a fibrosarcoma, a liposarcoma, or even a lipoma in which some tissue areas have undergone necrosis and in which the necrotic area has become the site of calcium deposition. Finally, it is to be

***Figure 164***

*A*, Roentgenograph showing the appearance of the lower end of a femur which is surrounded by a large tumor mass casting a faintly and fuzzily radiopaque shadow that proved to represent a soft-tissue osteogenic sarcoma. The patient was a girl 18 years of age who, for about 7 months, had been aware of a steadily enlarging and increasingly painful mass in the region of the left knee. The bulk of the tumor was located posteriorly, though that is not apparent from this projection. However, the picture does indicate that the tumor has guttered the cortex on both sides. What favors most strongly the interpretation of the lesion as a soft-tissue osteogenic sarcoma which has penetrated into the bone is the presence of the trough-like cortical defects, with their rather sharply delimited margins. Gross anatomic examination of the bone after amputation showed that some tumor tissue was present in the marrow cavity, but that the bulk of the tumor was extra-osseous and of a fibro-gritty consistency (see *C*). Follow-up one year after the amputation revealed that the patient was well and free of metastases.

*B*, Roentgenograph showing a large, roundish, rather radiopaque soft-tissue mass oriented to the upper end of an ulna and likewise representing a soft-tissue osteogenic sarcoma. In this case, too, the picture indicates that the tumor is eroding the cortex and extending into the bone. The histologic pattern of the biopsy specimen is illustrated in *D*. The diagnostic problem raised by this $x$-ray picture is whether the lesion should be interpreted as a soft-tissue osteogenic sarcoma which is extending into the bone or as a particularly aggressive juxtacortical osteogenic sarcoma. Since the lesion illustrated had not yet been subjected to any intervention, the general fuzziness of the radiopacity and the absence of clear delimitation of the tumor mass at its periphery speak strongly in favor of a soft-tissue osteogenic sarcoma which has become adherent to the bone. (For comparison with juxtacortical osteogenic sarcoma, see Fig. 85.)

*C*, Photomicrograph (× 65) showing the histologic features presented by the tissue of the lesion illustrated in *A*. The stroma of this tissue consists of spindle cells whose pattern suggests that of a well differentiated fibrosarcoma. Furthermore, one can see that trabeculæ of osseous tissue have been formed in the lesional stroma. In other words, since the stromal cells have demonstrated osteogenic capacity, the lesion is to be interpreted as a bone-forming connective-tissue sarcoma—that is, as an osteogenic sarcoma. Though the sarcomatous stromal cells are well differentiated, it should not be assumed that a lesion presenting this pattern cannot metastasize. In the case described by Umiker and Jaffe, the primary lesion in the soft parts also presented this type of histologic pattern. In that case, metastases eventually appeared, and in many of them the tumor tissue was clearly characteristic of an osteogenic sarcoma.

*D*, Photomicrograph (× 65) showing the histologic features of the biopsy specimen from the lesion illustrated in *B*. The pattern is clearly that of a fully malignant sarcoma forming osteoid and bone. Note the presence of several sarcoma giant cells in the lower part of the field.

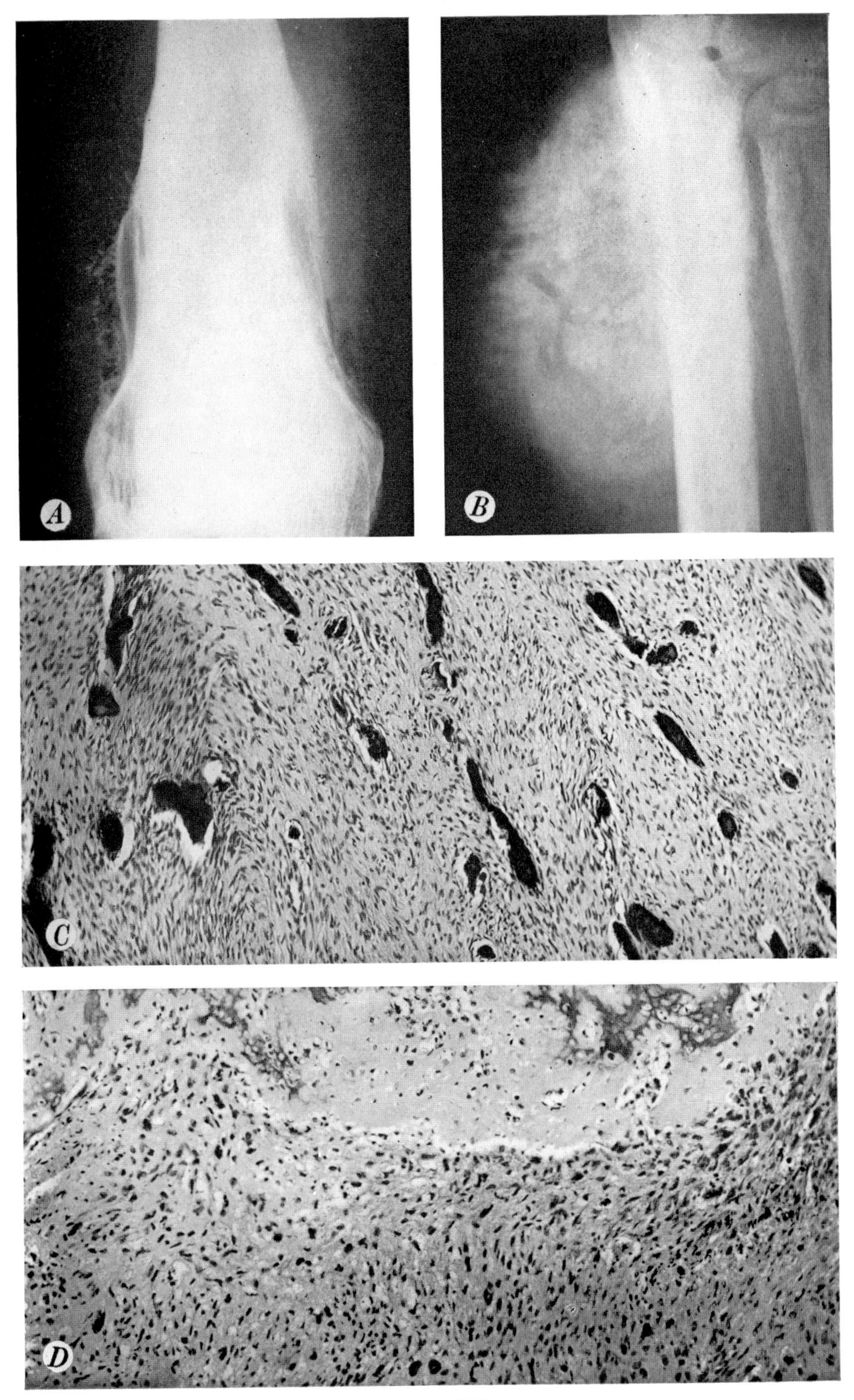


*Figure 164*

noted that the streaky radiopacity presented by a soft-tissue osteogenic sarcoma contrasts with the more or less discrete spotty radiopacity usually shown by a chondrosarcoma in which the lesional cartilage has undergone considerable calcification.

As to the *pathologic findings*, a soft-tissue osteogenic sarcoma which has been cut open is usually found to be whitish and somewhat gritty. In respect to cytologic detail, there may be a good deal of variety among the individual lesions. On the one hand, the sarcomatous connective-tissue stroma of the tumor may be found quite anaplastic and may show numerous sarcoma giant cells. In addition, one sees that tumor osteoid and tumor bone have been laid down in the sarcomatous stroma, and here and there even cartilage may have been formed. These appearances are precisely what one sees at the periphery of a very rapidly growing osteogenic sarcoma of bone.

On the other hand, there are lesions in which the basic stromal cells are likely to show relatively little anaplasia and to present as drawn-out spindle cells recalling the pattern of a fibrosarcoma. However, intermingled with the stromal cells, more or less throughout the lesion, one finds trabeculæ of osseous tissue. It is on this account that the designation of soft-tissue osteogenic sarcoma is still appropriate for such a lesion. In contrast, one should not designate as an osteogenic sarcoma a soft-tissue tumor which suggests a fibrosarcoma in its general cytologic pattern and shows only focal and sparse evidence of osteogenesis.

Irrespective of whether the lesion is one in which the basic stromal cells are anaplastic or one in which they are well differentiated, study of tissue from the periphery of the tumor fails to show a delimiting shell of osseous tissue. Indeed,

### *Figure 165*

*A*, Roentgenograph of a wrist area showing a lesion which proved on histologic examination to be an instance of the so-called pseudomalignant osseous tumors of soft tissues. The lesion presents as a small, roundish, soft-tissue shadow just sufficiently radiopaque at its periphery to stand out faintly. The patient was a girl 21 years of age who had been aware for 2 or 3 years of a small mass on the palmar surface of the wrist. The cut surface of the excised lesional mass appeared whitish and was somewhat gritty.

*B*, Photomicrograph (× 125) showing the tissue pattern seen in the interior of the excised lesion illustrated in *A*. Against a background of spindle-shaped cells (present on the left) one could see osteoid (present on the right) and trabeculæ of osseous tissue. However, nowhere in the lesional tissue could one observe evidences of anaplasia in the form of atypism of the stromal cells or the presence of sarcoma giant cells. Unfortunately, follow-up information is not available in this case.

*C*, Roentgenograph showing a focus of post-traumatic myositis ossificans which had developed deep in the muscles of a flank, between the lower lumbar vertebræ and the ilium. The patient was a girl 16 years of age who had suffered a severe fall and injured her back 19 days before this picture was taken. Note that most of the lesional area is already rather clearly delimited peripherally. The delimitation became much more striking in the course of the succeeding weeks, and the lesion as a whole came to stand out much more clearly.

*D*, Photograph (slightly reduced from natural size) of the sectioned focus of myositis ossificans from the case illustrated in *C*. The lesion was excised 3 months after the original traumatic incident. Note that it is very clearly delimited and that much of it is composed of osseous tissue. The whitish areas on the right represent those portions of the lesional tissue which have not yet matured and undergone replacement by trabeculæ of well formed osseous tissue.

*E*, Photomicrograph (× 20) showing the histologic pattern of the tissue at the periphery of the lesion shown in *D*. From above down, one notes, successively, compressed muscle, a capsule of fibrous tissue, and well formed osseous tissue set in loose fibrillar connective tissue.

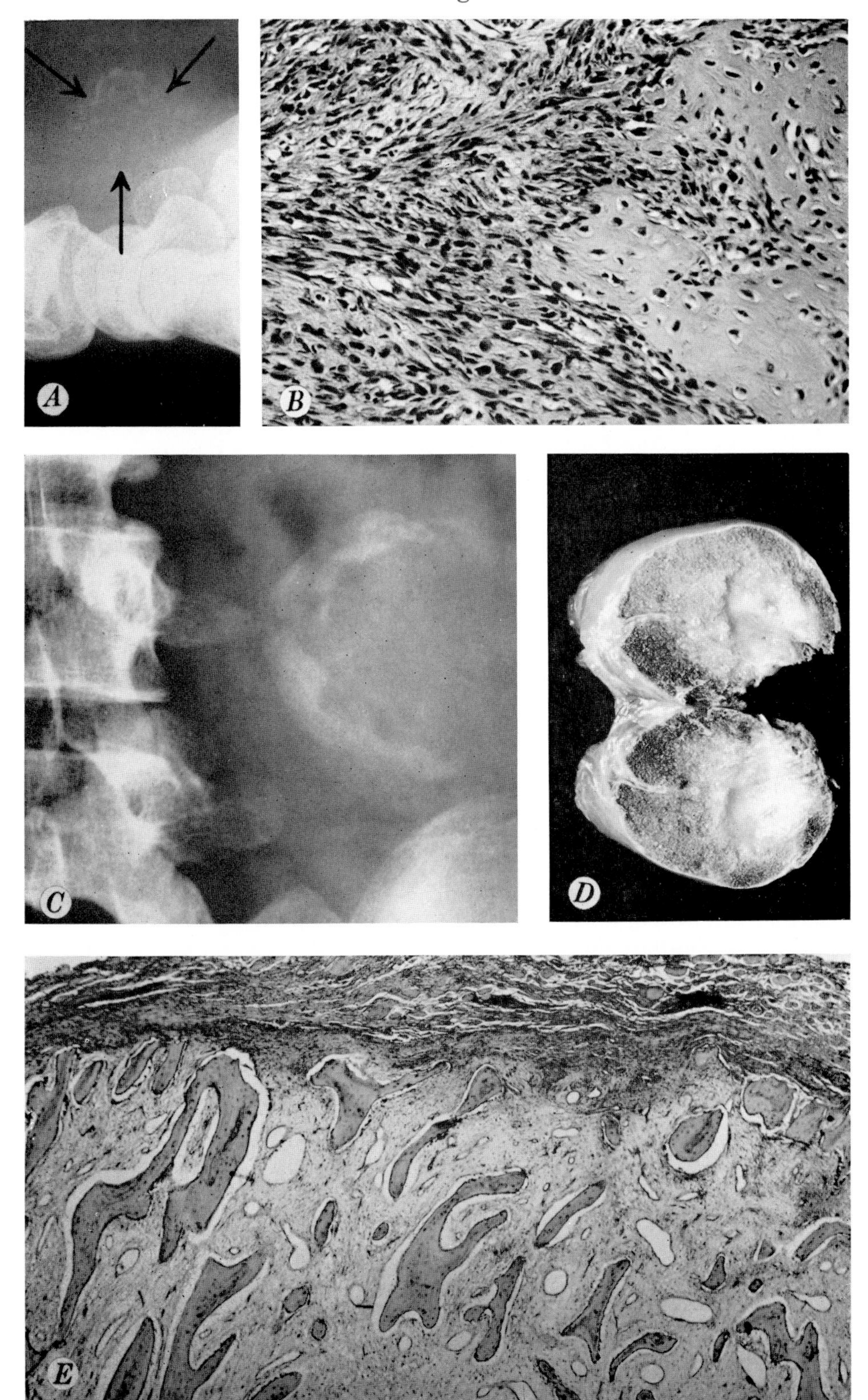

*Figure 165*

if a bone-forming connective-tissue lesion of soft parts shows encapsulation by a rim of well organized osseous tissue, one can practically rule out the possibility that it represents a true (that is, fully malignant) soft-tissue osteogenic sarcoma. This is so, despite the ominous impression which may be created by the cytologic appearance of tissue from the interior of the lesion.

Altogether, the diagnostic difficulty connected with soft-tissue osteogenic sarcoma is not that it is hard to recognize that lesion when it is present, but that one may misinterpret lesions of other kinds as instances of it. The principal lesions to be considered in this connection are: (1) bone-forming connective-tissue tumors of low malignancy (so-called pseudomalignant osseous tumors of soft tissues) and (2) post-traumatic myositis ossificans.

**Pseudomalignant Osseous Tumor of Soft Tissues.**—The so-called pseudomalignant osseous tumor of soft tissues is encountered only occasionally; its subjects are nearly always adolescents or young adults; and it seems to predilect females. Its usual site is in the soft tissues of a limb—most often a lower limb. The lesion does not ordinarily attain a size of more than 2 or 3 cm. by the time it is removed. In accordance with the presence of osseous tissue in it, the growth shows some radiopacity in its *x*-ray picture. As its name implies, the clinical behavior of the lesion is that of a benign growth, but its cytologic pattern might lead one to misinterpret it as a malignant tumor (see Figs. 165-*A* and *B*).

The lesion is to be distinguished not only from the clearly malignant soft-tissue osteogenic sarcoma, but also from conventional post-traumatic myositis ossificans. However, the development of the lesion is not associated with the occurrence of an acute local trauma and concomitant hemorrhage into the soft parts, such as are basic to the evolution of a focus of myositis ossificans. On the other hand, the absence of such a history of trauma does not exclude the possibility that one may be dealing with a clearly malignant osteogenic sarcoma of soft parts. Indeed, the latter lesion, too, apparently develops spontaneously and seems not to be connected with trauma.

On the basis of the *histologic findings*, it may be difficult to decide in a given case whether a spontaneously evolving bone-forming lesion of the soft parts represents a pseudomalignant or a fully malignant tumor. One of the most reliable microscopic indications that the growth is not really malignant is the presence of trabeculæ of well formed osseous tissue here and there at its periphery. An occasional lesion may even demonstrate the presence of an actual thin encapsulating shell of bone. In the interior of the lesion the tissue may be quite cellular, and here the basic stromal cells are spindle-shaped. Also, variable amounts of osteoid and osseous tissue are being formed in the stroma. However, a pseudomalignant lesion does not show atypism of its stromal cells or the presence of sarcoma giant cells, though variable numbers of small multinuclear giant cells are to be observed. While thus differing from a frankly malignant soft-tissue osteogenic sarcoma, the pseudomalignant lesion shows many of the same histologic features to be observed in a focus of post-traumatic myositis ossificans which is still in an early stage of its evolution.

The pseudomalignant tumor grows rather slowly. However, in contrast to a focus of post-traumatic myositis ossificans, it does not reach maturity and stop growing. It is true that the lesion does not metastasize and will not recur if completely excised. However, the writer is inclined to think that if it is not excised and continues to grow it may eventually undergo malignant transformation. Indeed, it seems probable that cases of clearly malignant soft-tissue osteogenic sarcoma in which the history indicates that the tumor has been present for many years represent instances of such transformation.

**Post-traumatic Myositis Ossificans.**—As already indicated, there is nearly always a definite history of a severe local trauma to the part in which a focus of myositis ossificans develops. If the part is easily accessible to palpation, a local painful soft-tissue swelling is to be felt soon after the trauma. Furthermore, the skin over the traumatized area usually shows, within a few days, discoloration due to diffusion of blood pigment. None of these features constitute essential parts of the clinical picture of soft-tissue osteogenic sarcoma.

An *x*-ray picture of the part, taken within about a week after the trauma, may not yet show a radiopaque shadow in the soft parts. However, within another week or so, such a shadow does appear, and in the course of the following weeks it enlarges somewhat and becomes more and more sharply delineated. Indeed, a focus of myositis ossificans usually reaches its maximum size and definitive outline in about two months or so from the time of the trauma. Also, it should be noted that a focus of so-called myositis ossificans is often not very densely radiopaque. Furthermore, it is rather clearly set off peripherally from the neighboring soft parts—a feature which again tends to contrast it with soft-tissue osteogenic sarcoma.

As to the *pathologic findings,* these too reveal the clear-cut peripheral delimitation of a focus of myositis ossificans. In fact, the osseous tissue at the periphery is usually the most mature part of the lesion and the part in which its innocent character stands out most plainly. Any muscle about the bony shell of the lesional area is found compressed and otherwise altered. However, it shows no invasion by tracts of connective tissue extending into it from the ossifying focus, such as commonly occurs in connection with a soft-tissue osteogenic sarcoma (see Figs. 165-*C*, *D* and *E*).

In the interior of a focus of myositis ossificans which has not reached full maturity, one may still see large fields of proliferating spindle cells in which osteoid, osseous tissue, and even cartilage are being laid down, and one may also note residual degenerating muscle fibers. However, any ominous-looking cytologic fields encountered in the interior of a myositis ossificans focus which might suggest that one was dealing with an osteogenic sarcoma can safely be discounted in view of the fact that the lesion has evolved rapidly and after a trauma, that it is well circumscribed, and that it presents no ominous cytologic features peripherally and is most mature there.

## VASCULAR TUMORS

Deep-seated, *localized hemangiomas* of the soft parts (muscle and/or fascia) are fairly common. Not infrequently, they affect the bone or bones in their immediate vicinity. A hemangioma may merely deform the bone contour by exerting a molding action through pressure as it enlarges. Again, through traction on the regional periosteum, it may provoke the latter to new bone deposition (traction periostitis) without altering the general shape of the bone. On the other hand, a relatively localized soft-tissue hemangioma may not only deform the regional bone and induce a traction periostitis, but may actually penetrate the periosteum and invade the bone. Indeed, when a bone of an extremity is the site of hemangiomatous involvement, the condition is much more likely to be the consequence of invasion of the bone from the overlying soft parts than to represent a lesion primary in the bone (see p. 236).

In addition to more or less localized hemangiomas of the deep soft parts of limbs, one encounters cases of *diffuse hemangiomatosis* of the soft parts, and in these cases the regional bones are quite likely to be found affected. Thus, without being deformed or otherwise modified, the long bones of the limb in question may show longitudinal overgrowth. This may amount to several inches and is due to excessive endochondral growth at their epiphysial cartilage plates, apparently stimulated by the increased vascularity of the part. In other cases the presence of widespread soft-tissue hemangiomatosis will be found associated with various specific alterations in the bones. In particular, one may note deformity of at least several of the bones, evidences of traction periostitis on several of them, and even the presence of circumscribed areas of radiolucency representing sites where the hemangioma has established itself within the bone.

The benign vascular tumors seem to appear more often in upper than in lower extremities and to predilect females. Most of the subjects who present hemangiomas of the soft tissues of limbs are children or young adults. Many of the adults likewise date their condition back to childhood. Indeed, in cases of diffuse hemangiomatosis, the abnormality may already be apparent at birth or shortly thereafter. The affected part of the limb is very likely to be visibly and palpably enlarged and is often tender to the touch. Discoloration of the overlying skin is more likely to be present if the hemangioma is diffuse than if it is of limited extent. Local pain is a frequent complaint. In fact, a deep-seated but small hemangioma is sometimes the cause of persistent and almost intractable pain.

*X*-ray examination is often of great value in the clinical diagnosis of the condition. (See Fig. 166.) In particular, it may reveal the presence of several or even many scattered radiopacities in the soft-tissue mass. These represent phleboliths—that is, organized and calcified thrombi in vascular channels of the tumor tissue. The

### *Figure 166*

*A*, Roentgenograph of a thumb whose proximal phalanx had become altered in contour (but not invaded) by a hemangioma of the soft tissues. Note the clearly outlined radiopacities representing phleboliths. The patient was a woman 30 years of age who gave a history of local pain and swelling of 3 years' standing. The overlying skin was not discolored.

*B*, Roentgenograph illustrating a bowing deformity of the lower part of the ulna which has resulted from the development of a hemangioma in the local musculature. The diagnosis is strongly suggested by the small, rounded, well defined radiopacities representing phleboliths. The patient was a girl 13 years of age who gave a history of a painless swelling of the right forearm of only 3 months' duration. No local heat, bruit or pulsation was present. Surgical intervention showed that the tumor had arisen from the pronator quadratus, and the entire lesion was excised without further incident. (Figure 72-*C*, p. 235, illustrates a very large hemangioma in the soft tissues of the calf, but that lesion had not affected the local bones at all.)

*C*, Roentgenograph showing several faint radiopacities in the interosseous region between the tibia and fibula and periosteal new bone deposition on the fibula as manifestations of a deep-seated hemangioma. The patient was a woman 37 years of age who had been suffering from intractable pain in the right leg for $4\frac{1}{2}$ years. Surgical exploration showed that the hemangioma had arisen in the region of origin of the tibialis posticus muscle. Excision of the hemangioma along with the portion of the fibula showing the traction periostitis brought prompt and lasting relief. (Figure 72-*B* illustrates a large hemangioma which developed in the soft tissues of a leg and did invade the fibula over a wide extent.)

*D*, Photograph illustrating hemangiomatosis with striking involvement of the left upper extremity and shoulder region. Small scattered hemangiomata are visible in the skin on the left side of the face and on the trunk. The patient was a woman 58 years of age in whom evidences of hemangiomatosis of the upper extremity in question were already present at birth. The left lower extremity also showed hemangiomatous involvement of the soft tissues. There was never any pain connected with the abnormality.

*E*, Roentgenograph showing part of the left hand and forearm in the case illustrated in *D*. Note the soft-tissue swelling representing the hemangiomatous involvement and the scattered roundish radiopacities representing phleboliths. The radius and ulna are somewhat deformed and otherwise altered, as were several of the phalanges not included in the picture.

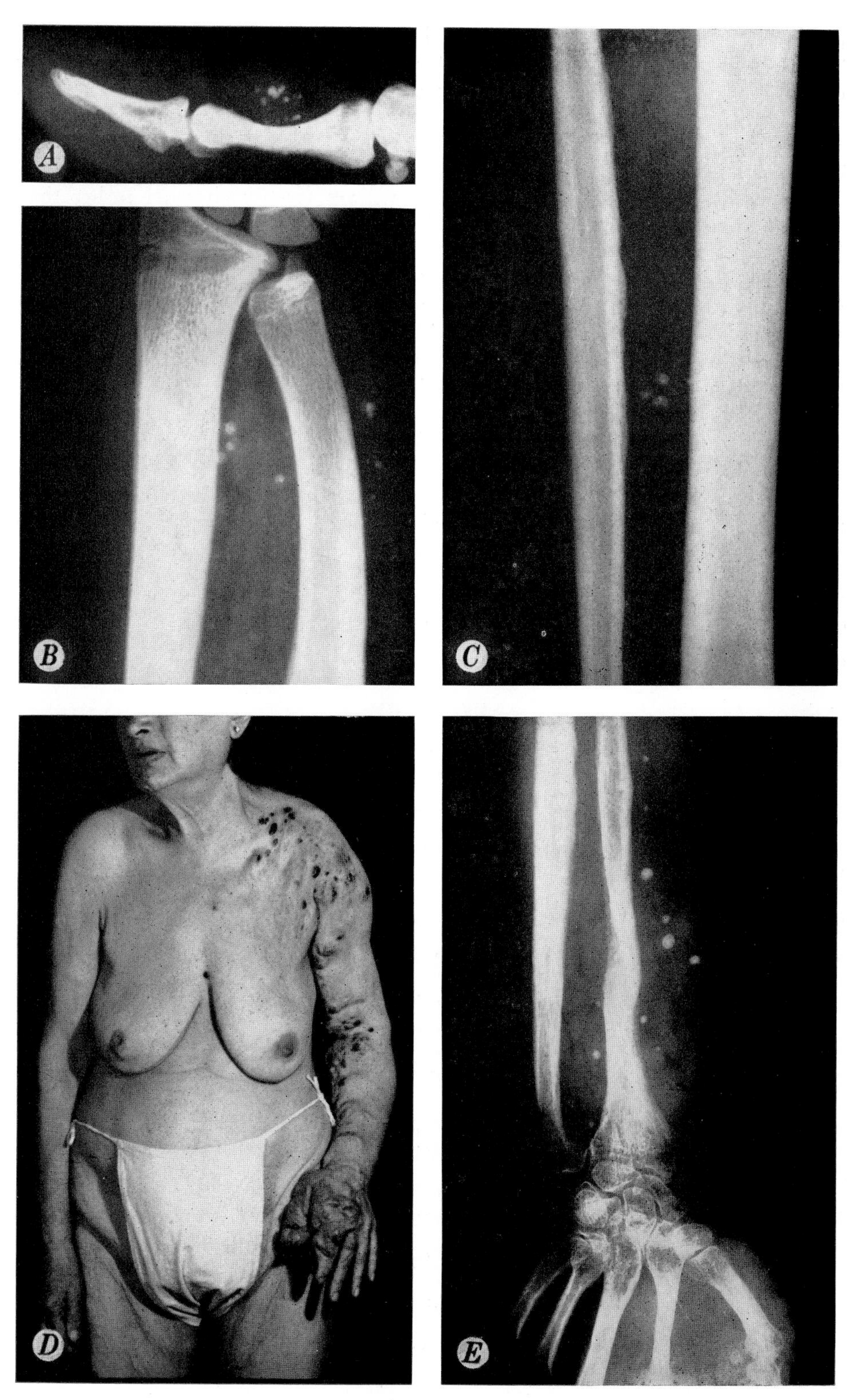


*Figure 166*

phleboliths show up as discrete, rounded radiopacities ranging in size from 1 or 2 mm. to as much as 5 mm. in diameter. Those phleboliths which are heavily calcified are likely to be very radiopaque. Those which are not completely calcified may show a relatively radiolucent center. For purposes of differential diagnosis it should be noted that radiopacities may also be seen in a soft-tissue tumor of cartilage in which the lesional tissue is undergoing calcification. In such a case, however, the radiopacities, even if numerous, are usually clumped rather than scattered, and they are also more blurred than those representing phleboliths (see Fig. 163-*C*).

On histologic examination it is apparent that the muscle, intermuscular connective tissue, and even fat of the lesional area are permeated by vascular channels. In some areas these will be found to consist of small, thin-walled capillaries. However, if one looks from area to area, the pattern of the vascular growth can usually be seen to be dominated by cavernously dilated capillaries, intermingled with which one can also find numerous sinuous vascular spaces. Here and there a lesion may also show one or more organizing and calcifying thrombi, which, as noted, produce the radiopacities to be seen in the *x*-ray picture in some cases.

Hemangiomas are benign growths, and it is doubtful whether the lesion ever undergoes transformation into a hemangiosarcoma. Treatment can therefore be guided by immediate practical and cosmetic considerations.

The *glomus tumor* represents a specialized vascular growth nearly always located beneath a nail. In rare instances it causes pressure erosion of the underlying phalanx. The question of involvement of bone by the glomus tumor is considered more fully elsewhere (see p. 254).

REFERENCES

Batts, M., Jr.: Periosteal Fibrosarcoma, Arch. Surg., *42*, 566, 1941.

Cappell, D. F., and Montgomery, G. L.: On Rhabdomyoma and Myoblastoma, J. Path. & Bact., *44*, 517, 1937.

Childs, P.: Rhabdomyosarcoma of Skeletal Muscle, Brit. J. Surg., *37*, 230, 1949.

Christopherson, W. M., Foote, F. W., Jr., and Stewart, F. W.: Alveolar Soft-Part Sarcomas. Structurally Characteristic Tumors of Uncertain Histogenesis, Cancer, *5*, 100, 1952.

Dawson, E. K.: Liposarcoma of Bone, J. Path. & Bact., *70*, 513, 1955.

Duffy, J., and Stewart, F. W.: Primary Liposarcoma of Bone, Am. J. Path., *14*, 621, 1938.

Fine, G., and Stout, A. P.: Osteogenic Sarcoma of the Extraskeletal Soft Tissues, Cancer, *9*, 1027, 1956.

Fulton, M. N., and Sosman, M. C.: Venous Angiomas of Skeletal Muscle, J.A.M.A., *119*, 319, 1942.

Golden, T., and Stout, A. P.: Smooth Muscle Tumors of the Gastrointestinal Tract and Retroperitoneal Tissues, Surg., Gynec. & Obst., *73*, 784, 1941.

Horn, R. C., Jr., and Enterline, H. T.: Rhabdomyosarcoma: A Clinicopathological Study and Classification of 39 Cases, Cancer, *11*, 181, 1958.

Johnson, E. W., Jr., Ghormley, R. K., and Dockerty, M. B.: Hemangiomas of the Extremities, Surg., Gynec. & Obst., *102*, 531, 1956.

Martin, M. E., and Colson, P.: Tumeur conjonctive de la cuisse avec atteinte de l'articulation de la hanche, Ann. d'anat. path., *13*, 534, 1936.

Mostofi, F. K., and Morse, W. H.: Polypoid Rhabdomyosarcoma (Sarcoma Botryoides) of Bladder in Children, J. Urol., *67*, 681, 1952.

Murray, M. R.: Cultural Characteristics of Three Granular-Cell Myoblastomas, Cancer, *4*, 857, 1951.

Ober, W. B., and Edgcomb, J. H.: Sarcoma Botryoides in the Female Urogenital Tract, Cancer, *7*, 75, 1954.

Ober, W. B., Smith, J. A., and Rouillard, F. C.: Congenital Sarcoma Botryoides of the Vagina, Cancer, *11*, 620, 1958.

Rehbock, D. J., and Hauser, H.: Liposarcoma of Bone, Am. J. Cancer, *27*, 37, 1936.

Riopelle, J. L., and Thériault, J. P.: Sur une forme méconnue de sarcome des parties molles; Le rhabdomyosarcome alvéolaire, Ann. d'anat. path., *1*, 88, 1956.

SMETANA, H. F., and SCOTT, W. F., JR.: Malignant Tumors of Nonchromaffin Paraganglia, Mil. Surgeon, *109*, 330, 1951.
STEWART, F. W.: Primary Liposarcoma of Bone, Am. J. Path., *7*, 87, 1931.
STOBBE, G. D., and DARGEON, H. W.: Embryonal Rhabdomyosarcoma of the Head and Neck in Children and Adolescents, Cancer, *3*, 826, 1950.
STOUT, A. P.: Fibrosarcoma: The Malignant Tumor of Fibroblasts, Cancer, *1*, 30, 1948.
——————: Liposarcoma—The Malignant Tumor of Lipoblasts, Ann. Surg., *119*, 86, 1944.
——————: Rhabdomyosarcoma of the Skeletal Muscles, Ann. Surg., *123*, 447, 1946.
——————: Tumors of the Soft Tissues; Atlas of Tumor Pathology, Section II, Fascicle 5, Armed Forces Institute of Pathology, Washington, D. C., 1953.
STOUT, A. P., and VERNER, E. W.: Chondrosarcoma of the Extraskeletal Soft Tissues, Cancer, *6*, 581, 1953.
UMIKER, W., and JAFFE, H. L.: Ossifying Fibrosarcoma (Extraskeletal Osteogenic Sarcoma) of Thigh Muscle, Ann. Surg., *138*, 795, 1953.

Chapter

# 30

# Pigmented Villonodular Synovitis, Bursitis and Tenosynovitis

UNDER the comprehensive name of *pigmented villonodular synovitis, bursitis* and *tenosynovitis*, we shall consider a group of interrelated benign lesions which develop in connection with the linings of: joints, bursæ, fibrous sheaths of tendons, and/or the fascial and ligamentous tissues adjacent to tendons. These lesions all seem to start as villous and nodular proliferations of the lining tissues in question. The pigmentation (brown or yellow-brown) is due to the presence of variable amounts of hemosiderin and lipid (of the nature of cholesterol) in the lesional tissue. At one stage or another, because of intergrowth and fusion of the villous and nodular proliferations, the lesional tissue may show cleft-like spaces bordered by synovial lining cells. Also to be observed are large numbers of roundish or polyhedral stromal cells which possess phagocytic capacity and take up the hemosiderin and lipid. Another cytologic feature common to the various lesions, especially in their nodular portions, is the presence of multinuclear giant cells.

Though recognizing that proliferative processes underlie the evolution of these lesions, the writer holds that the latter represent an inflammatory reaction (in the broadest sense of the term) rather than a true neoplastic condition. It was to express the combination of pigmentation, villous and/or nodular proliferation, and the inflammatory character of the lesional process that the designation "pigmented villonodular synovitis, bursitis and tenosynovitis" was coined to denote the condition in its various sites (see Jaffe *et al.*). There are various other interpretations of the nature of these lesions, and accordingly other names have also been applied to them (see "Nomenclature" and "Pathogenesis" below).

Wherever it occurs, the condition may appear in either a *localized* or a *diffuse* form. In cases in which it involves the synovial membrane of a large joint, it is nearly always the knee that is affected, and the involvement is about as likely to be localized as to be diffuse. In the localized form (*localized nodular synovitis*), the synovial membrane shows one or more sessile or stalked yellow-brown nodular outgrowths. In the diffuse form (*pigmented villonodular synovitis*), much or all of the synovial membrane appears brownishly pigmented and covered by villous and coarse nodular outgrowths, though either villi or nodules may predominate in a given case. In consequence of fusion, intergrowth, and compaction of the villous and nodular proliferations, the lesional tissue may present a spongy appearance in some areas. Indeed, the histologic pattern of such areas may lead to misinterpretation of the lesion as a malignant tumor if one is not familiar with the full range of the microscopic appearances which these diffuse synovial lesions may present.

Location of the lesion in the lining of a bursa is rare, and no particular bursa is predilected. In the few instances of bursal involvement which the writer has seen, the bursal lining was diffusely affected (*pigmented villonodular bursitis*). The lesional tissue was brown and the bursal surface covered by villous and nodular proliferations.

On the other hand, the occurrence of the condition in relation to tendon sheaths and/or the fascial and ligamentous tissues adjacent to them is very common. In this connection, the lesion is encountered very frequently in fingers and not infrequently in toes. Occasionally it develops in the palm of the hand, in the sole of the foot, or about the ankle or wrist. When it occurs in a finger, for instance, the lesion usually presents as a rather small, grayish yellow or yellow-brown tissue mass of firm consistency which is usually at least somewhat lobulated and sometimes strikingly so (*localized nodular tenosynovitis*). Instances of diffuse tenosynovial involvement (*pigmented villonodular tenosynovitis*) are rare. In the hand, one may occasionally observe diffuse involvement of the common flexor and/or extensor sheaths (the so-called ulnar and radial bursæ). Diffuse forms of involvement are also occasionally observed at the ankle and in the foot. In respect to these latter locations, it is often difficult to decide whether the lesion had actually developed in relation to tendon sheaths or in relation to the lining sheaths of the local fascial or ligamentous tissues.

In connection with the various lesions discussed in this chapter, it is of special interest that they sometimes erode the regional bone or bones in the course of their expansion (see Breimer and Freiberger). Indeed, the tenosynovial (or fascial or ligamentous) lesions, especially those developing in toes, in other parts of the foot, or at the ankle, not infrequently do this. Sometimes a diffuse articular synovial lesion likewise produces erosion of one or more bones entering into the formation of the joint. Cases in which regional bone destruction has occurred often raise problems of clinical differential diagnosis and even of treatment.

**Nomenclature.**—The writer has already outlined the reasons for the terminology which he uses in connection with the lesions under consideration. However, before it was recognized that the various lesions are interrelated, and before the comprehensive name "pigmented villonodular synovitis, bursitis and tenosynovitis" was accordingly introduced, the lesions were denoted in many different ways.

A localized nodular tenosynovial lesion which contained a good many lipid-bearing foam cells was often called a "xanthoma" of the tendon sheath, and if the lesional tissue had become heavily sclerotized, as it often does, it was frequently denoted as a "xanthogranuloma." Correspondingly, localized or diffuse articular synovial lesions containing considerable numbers of foam cells were likewise often designated as xanthomas. In general, however, such terms as "xanthoma," "xanthogranuloma," and "xanthomatous tumor" are no longer used for the lesion in any of its sites.

Because of the common finding of multinuclear giant cells in the tissue of these lesions, the condition was even more commonly referred to as a "giant-cell tumor" of a tendon sheath, synovial membrane, *etc.* However, reference to the lesion as a giant-cell tumor is definitely on the wane, though it has not yet completely disappeared from the current literature. To express the presence of giant cells and foam cells, the term "xanthomatous giant-cell tumor" was also frequently employed.

The name "benign giant-cell synovioma" has recently been introduced. The use of a name which includes the term "synovioma," even with the qualification "benign," is unfortunate. Actually, the term "synovioma" is now restricted to a highly malignant synovial tumor which often rapidly metastasizes. In this connection, it should be borne in mind that a diffuse pigmented villonodular synovial lesion (particularly a recurrent one) can come to present a highly complex histologic pattern suggestive of malignancy, despite the well-established fact that these lesions never metastasize. Indeed, this confusion can be found incorporated in the older literature, in which cases of this kind have been misdiagnosed and reported under such names as "fibrohemosideric sarcoma," "sarcoma fusogigantocellulare," and "malignant polymorphocellular tumor of the synovial membrane." Thus any name which includes the term "synovioma" may open the way afresh to misinterpretation of such benign but cytologically complex synovial lesions as sarcomas.

## PIGMENTED VILLONODULAR SYNOVITIS

The term *pigmented villonodular synovitis* refers, as already indicated, to a condition in which much or all of the synovial membrane of a joint is brownishly discolored, and in which its surface presents villous proliferations, usually intermingled with at least some nodular outgrowths, which may be sessile or stalked. However, tangling and intergrowth of the villous and nodular proliferations may result in a much more complex gross picture than the basic one just outlined. Histologically, too, there may be a good deal of variety from lesion to lesion. In the majority of cases the histologic diagnosis presents no problem. On the other hand, in a case in which the lesional tissue has become complexly matted, its histologic pattern may be misinterpreted as that of a synovial sarcoma. At any rate, the condition has been discussed in a large body of literature. The older references to the condition are cited by DeSanto and Wilson, Galloway *et al.* and Jaffe *et al.*

### CLINICAL CONSIDERATIONS

The diffuse form of pigmented villonodular synovitis is not a very common condition. The writer's experience with it covers 25 cases. Most of the subjects were young adults, though a few were middle-aged. The condition seems to show some predilection for males. As others have likewise found, the knee joint is by far the most common site for the condition. Among the cases studied by the writer, all but 4 involved that joint. In 2 of these it was a hip joint that was affected, and

***Figure 167***

*A*, Roentgenograph of a knee joint affected with pigmented villonodular synovitis and showing the alteration of articular soft tissues and erosion of bone which are sometimes encountered in this condition. Note the lobulated soft-tissue shadow, which represents thickened and otherwise modified synovial membrane. Note also the erosion of the femur (in the region of the condyles) and of the upper end of the tibia (in the region of the tibiofibular joint). The patella, too, is extensively eroded and is the site of a pathologic fracture, but the details of the changes in that bone are somewhat obscure because the reproduction of the roentgenograph was intended to bring out mainly the changes in the synovial membrane. The patient was a man 53 years of age whose difficulty relating to the knee was of 7 years' standing and was stated to have followed upon trauma to the knee. At the time of admission for treatment, there was no tenderness or loss of mobility in the affected knee, and aspiration of it yielded hemorrhagically discolored fluid.

*B*, Photograph of a diffusely affected synovium in a case of pigmented villonodular synovitis involving a knee. Observe that the thickened synovium is studded with nodules, which are most prominent in the lower part of the picture. The upper part of the specimen is pigmented and dominated by the presence of matted villous tissue in which a few nodules are also incorporated. The details relating to the middle portion of the specimen are somewhat obscured by the presence of a thin coating of fibrin. The patient was a woman 31 years of age whose difficulty relating to the affected knee joint was of 5 years' standing when the synovectomy was done. The condition set in abruptly with pain and swelling, and there was no history of possibly relevant trauma. The patient stated that she had had innumerable periodic attacks of pain and swelling of the knee. Repeated aspiration of the joint yielded serosanguineous fluid, but the latter promptly re-accumulated. A synovectomy was done, but this clearly did not cure the condition, since, 3 years after the surgery, the patient sought treatment elsewhere for what was apparently the same condition in the same knee.

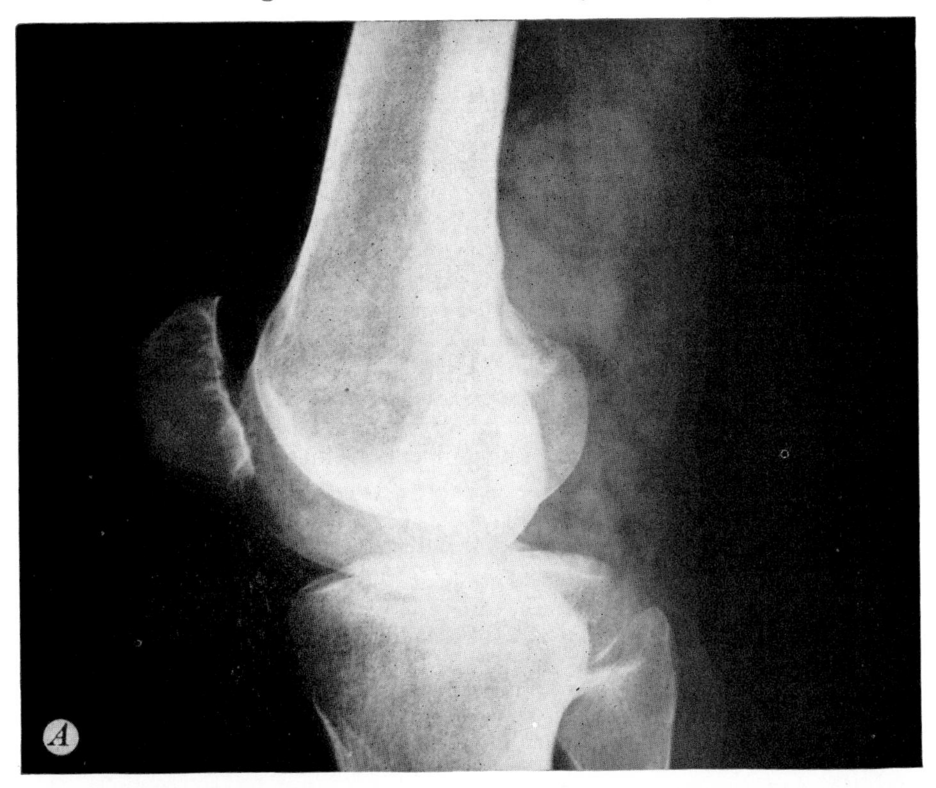


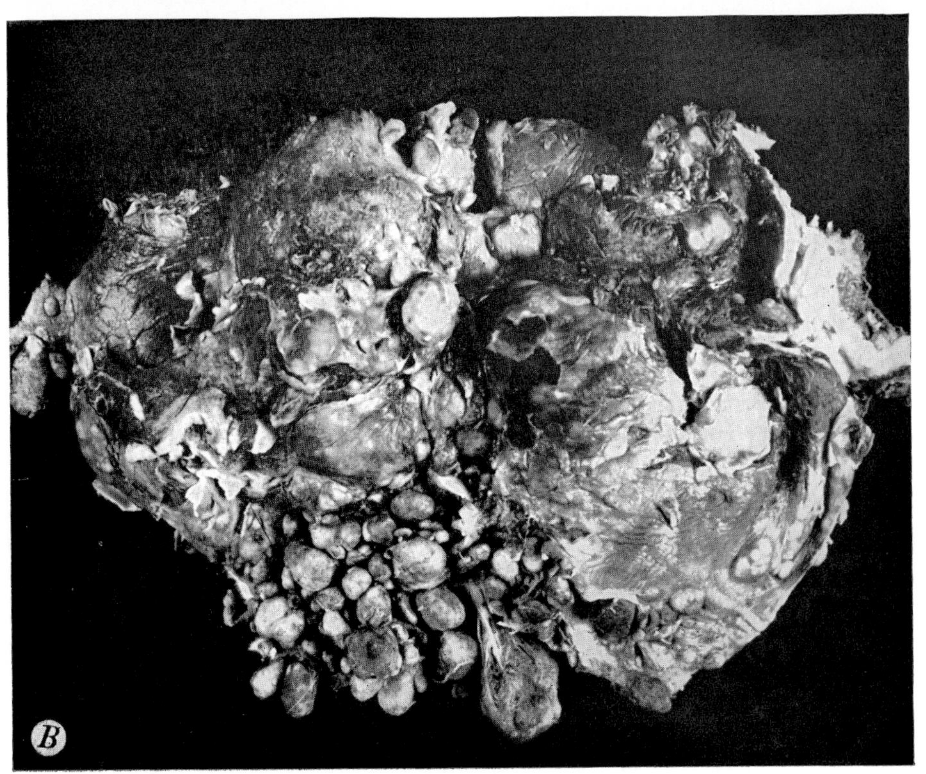


***Figure 167***

instances in which that joint was involved have also been reported in the literature (see Case Records of the Massachusetts General Hospital). In 1 of our remaining 2 cases the lesion was in an ankle joint, and in the other, in the calcaneocuboid joint. In respect to lesions in the latter locations, it is often difficult to decide whether the condition actually started in the synovium of the joint and then broke out of the joint, or whether it took the opposite course, starting in the periarticular area and breaking into the joint.

The principal *complaints* relating to the affected joint, as exemplified in the knee, are pain and swelling. These complaints are usually mild and intermittent, at least at first. Indeed, 2 or 3 years often elapse between the onset of the complaints and diagnosis and treatment of the condition. In the interim, there may have been some bouts of acute pain and locking of the joint, due to the crushing of altered synovium between the articular bone ends. These acute episodes are likely to be followed by an increase in the swelling of the affected joint, in consequence of additional effusion. Trauma is sometimes inculpated in the onset of the condition.

### *Figure 168*

*A*, Photograph of the synovium of a knee joint which shows the lesion in an essentially villous stage. The surface of the membrane is brownishly discolored and presents, over most of its extent, long tangled villi giving the membrane the general appearance of a scraggly beard. In the lower right-hand part of the picture (where the specimen has been incised), the surface presents a smoother appearance, due to fusion and matting down of the villi, and in this area the lesional tissue has a spongy texture. The patient was a man 22 years of age, and the complaints were of 2 years' standing. The principal difficulty was swelling of the joint, due to effusion, which always recurred promptly after each of many tappings. The fluid withdrawn was serosanguineous.

*B*, Photograph of the synovium of a knee which shows the lesion in an essentially nodular stage. The surface of the synovium is studded by numerous nodules, some of which are pedicled and others flat. These nodules, which vary in size, also varied in color, some being brown and others mainly gray, though speckled with brown and yellow. The nodules also differed in consistency, some being rather soft while others were firm and indurated on account of fibrosis and collagenization, as revealed on microscopic examination. The cut surface of the nodules, especially the larger ones, presented a vaguely lobulated appearance. The patient was a woman 21 years of age whose complaints were of 2 years' standing and had come on insidiously. They were mild at first, consisting of slight swelling of the joint and some loss of mobility, but subsequently the patient had episodes of locking of the knee. The aspirated fluid was serosanguineous. The treatment was synovectomy, the excision was apparently not complete, and the patient was subjected to a new intervention 18 months later, on account of recurrence of the lesion. After the second intervention she received 2 courses of radiation therapy at 6-month intervals, a total tissue dose of 4,480 r being given in 21 days. Follow-up examination 9 months after the second course of radiation showed that, while there was no recurrence, the functioning of the knee was still not quite normal.

*C*, Photograph illustrating the appearance of a recurrent lesion in a case of pigmented villonodular synovitis of a knee. On the left, the picture shows, laid open, the part of the lesion which occupied the quadriceps pouch. This lesional tissue is mainly brown in color, and matting of the villous proliferations has given it a finely porous texture. The right third of the specimen represents the intra-articular portion of the lesion, and its pigmented villous character is still apparent in some places. The patient was a young man 18 years of age whose difficulty relating to the knee was of $5\frac{1}{2}$ years' standing at the time of his admission to the hospital. He gave no history of trauma. At the original surgical intervention, the affected synovial membrane was found more or less uniformly villous, though the villi tended to be matted together. The synovectomy was followed by recurrence, and the specimen illustrated (the recurrent lesion) had been removed $2\frac{1}{2}$ years after the original lntervention. The subsequent treatment was radiation therapy, and when the patient was iast seen (almost 11 years after the second operation) there was every indication that the disease had been completely eradicated.

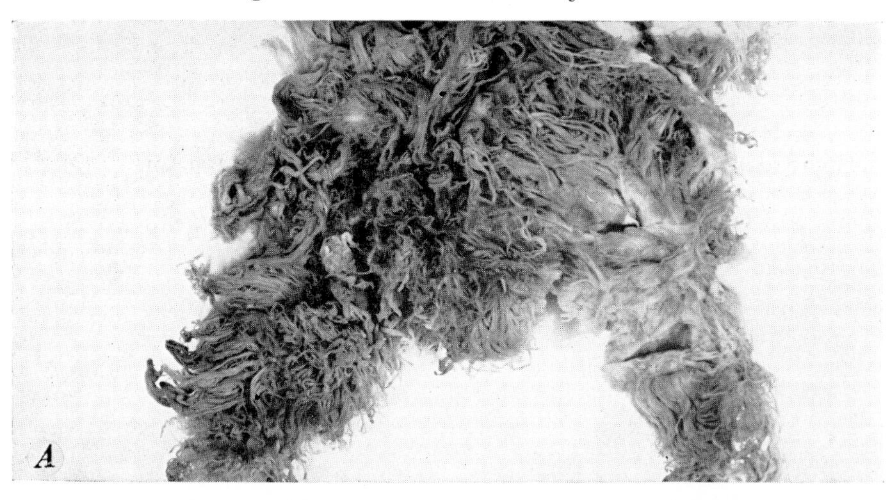

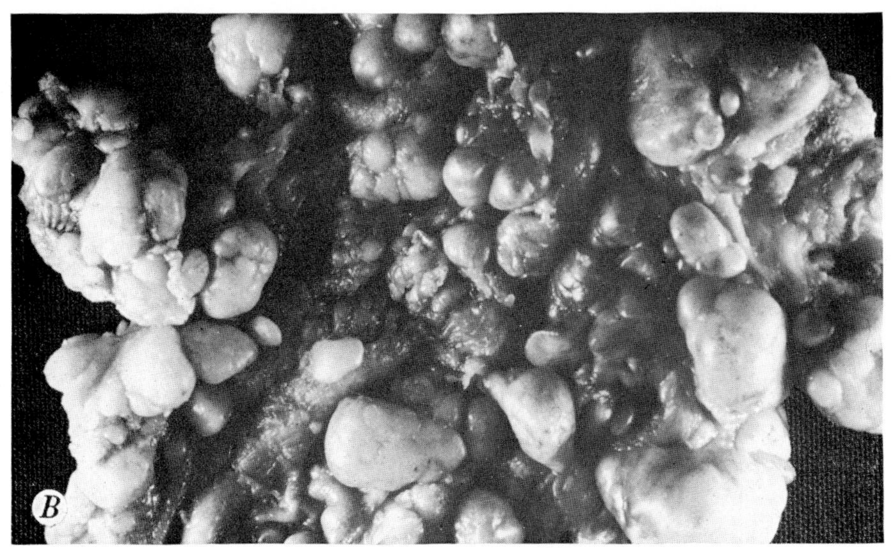

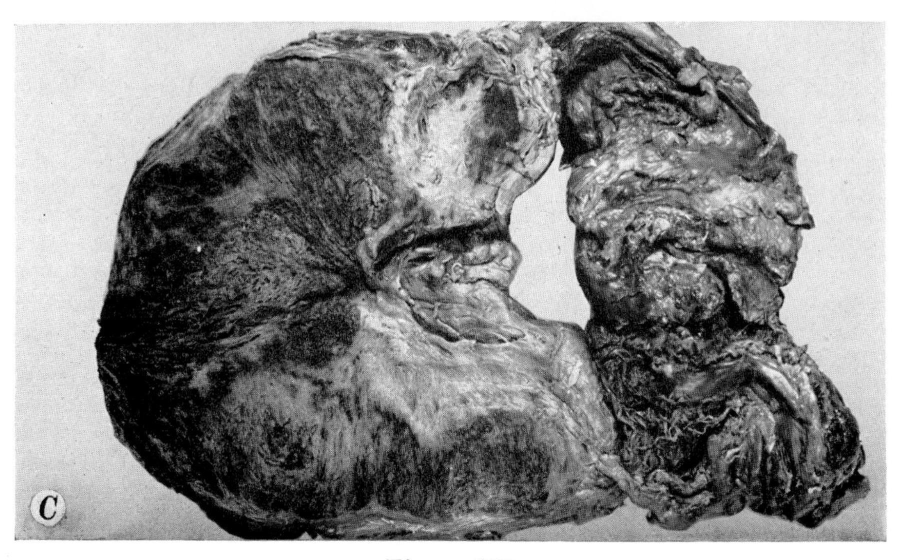

*Figure 168*

It is to be doubted, however, that it ever actually causes the condition, though when the latter is already present an acute trauma might aggravate it.

Aspiration of the swollen joint will yield dark brown or frankly serosanguineous fluid. This finding has diagnostic significance in a case in which the diagnosis of pigmented villonodular synovitis is already plausible on other grounds. In particular, it is significant: if the patient is a young adult; if the complaints have been mild and are of long standing; if there is no history of recent severe trauma to the joint; and if the patient is known not to be a hemophiliac. Indeed, the repeated aspiration of dark brown or serosanguineous fluid from a joint is strongly suggestive in itself of the presence of pigmented villonodular synovitis.

The *roentgenographic appearance* of the affected joint may also be helpful in arriving at a clinical diagnosis. This picture commonly reveals the presence of fluid in the joint. More significantly, the affected joint sometimes also reveals the presence of a large, often lobulated area of density representing the thickened and otherwise altered synovium (see Lewis, and Greenfield and Wallace). In an occasional instance there is also roentgenographic evidence of erosion of one or more of the bones entering into the formation of the joint. (See Fig. 167.) However, destructive erosion of bone is not so likely to occur with involvement of a knee joint as with involvement of a joint in which the articular space is more limited. An instance of retroperitoneal extension of the lesional tissue in consequence of bone destruction in an affected hip has been described (see Carr *et al.*).

## PATHOLOGIC FINDINGS

**Gross Pathology.**—A synovial membrane showing the condition in a predominantly villous form is of a rather uniform reddish brown color, usually shading down in some places to yellowish brown. For the most part, the villi are long, delicate, tangled and more or less matted together, but an occasional stubby villus, rather resembling a nodule, can also be noted. When the picture is dominated by tangled villi, the general appearance of the altered synovial membrane may suggest a scraggly brownish beard. However, even in such a lesion there will be thick, padlike areas which have resulted from compaction of the villi. When incised at right angles to the surface, such areas will be found to present the appearance of a coarse-meshed sponge.

### *Figure 169*

*A*, Photomicrograph (× 25) illustrating the histologic pattern of a tissue field in which villous proliferations (some of which have become fused) are projecting from the surface of a synovial membrane. (The section represents tissue obtained from the bearded villous portion of the specimen shown in Fig. 168-*A*.) The villi are rather vascular and contain a good deal of hemosiderin pigment both within the stromal cells and between the cells, but these details cannot be seen under this low magnification. It is the heavy pigmentation of the villi that accounts for their deep staining.

*B*, Photomicrograph (× 20) showing the pattern of a tissue field in which fusion and matting down of merged and swollen villi have occurred. (The section represents tissue obtained from the smoother, spongy part of the specimen shown in Fig. 168-*A*.) In some places the matted pigmented villi are separated only by narrow clefts, while elsewhere the spaces between them are much larger.

*C*, Photomicrograph (× 25) showing the pattern of a tissue field in which the fusion and matting down of the proliferations are even greater than in *B*. (The section represents tissue taken from the meshy and porous part of the specimen shown in Fig. 168-*C*.) The spaces are outlined by synovial lining cells, and between the spaces, some of the tissue is so heavily pigmented that all details are blurred. (For additional details, see Figs. 171-*A* and *B*.)

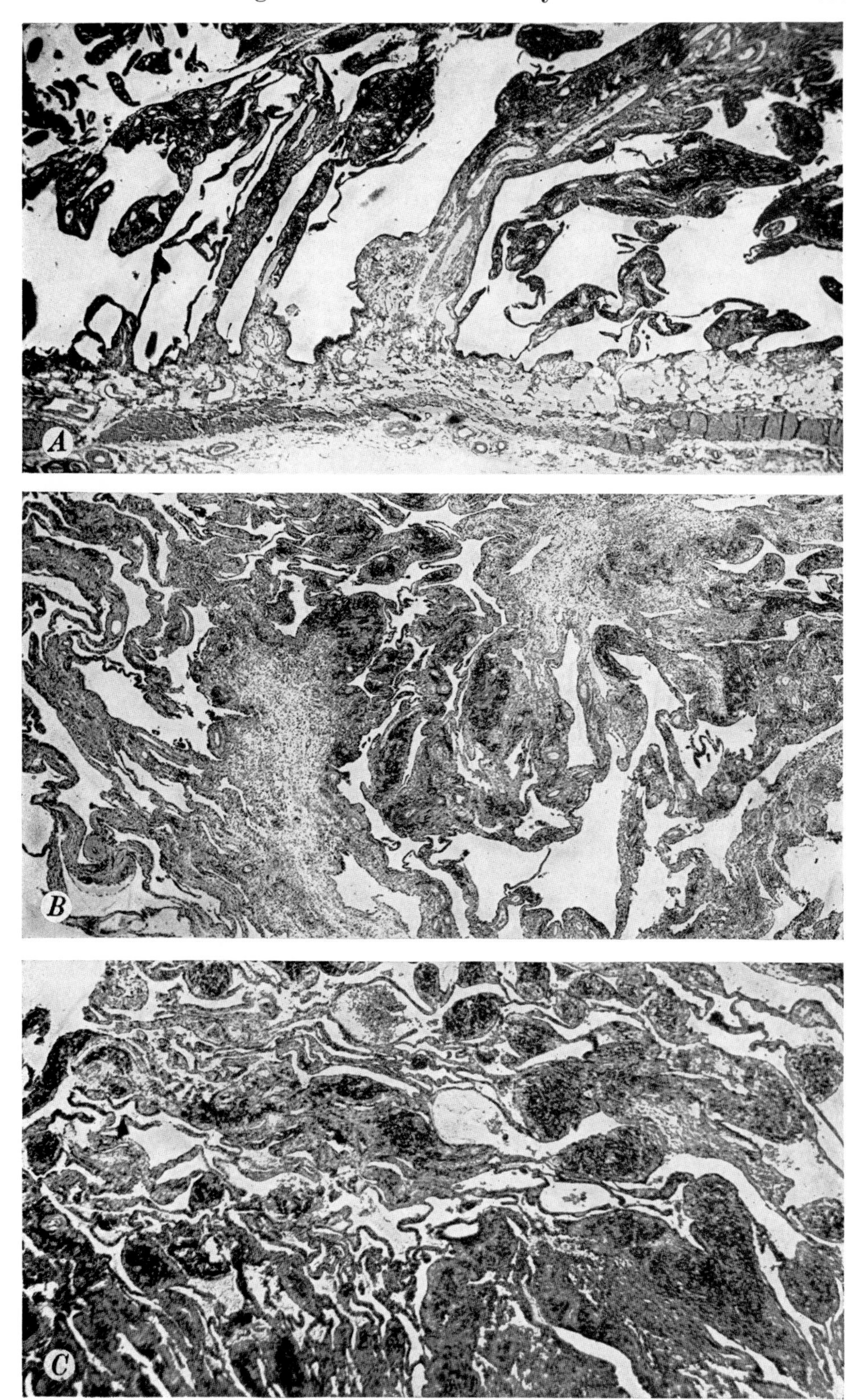


*Figure 169*

In a lesion in which villi and nodules are intermingled, the synovial membrane appears brownishly discolored and studded more or less patchily with individual and clustered nodules varying rather widely in size. Here and there on the surface of the membrane one may also find filmlike deposits of fibrin under which there are usually other residua of hemorrhage. Among the clumps of nodules and elsewhere on the synovial surface one may also see some pigmented villous areas. Some of the nodules are sessile, but most are pedicled, although the pedicle is quite short as a rule. The nodules tend to range between 0.5 and 1 cm. in diameter, but some may even be as large as 2 cm. When sectioned, the larger nodules usually reveal a smooth surface which is yellow-brown as a whole.

Then again, one may encounter a villonodular lesion whose gross picture has become very complex on account of lively intergrowth, fusion and compaction of the villi and nodules. Indeed, in an occasional instance these processes taking place in the lesion may result in the formation of a mass of brownish spongy tissue so large that it practically obliterates the articular cavity, as happened in connection with a recurrent lesion of a knee joint seen by the writer. (See Fig. 168.)

**Microscopic Pathology.**—Microscopic examination of an area covered by a beard of thin villi shows that the latter have a coating of synovial lining cells. Their supporting stroma of loose-meshed connective tissue contains a considerable number of thin-walled blood vessels and a variable number of roundish or polyhedral cells. Brownish pigment (consisting of hemosiderin granules) is to be noted in the cytoplasm not only of the lining cells, but also of the polyhedral cells, and some pigment is also present between the various cells. An area which had presented grossly a loose-meshed spongy appearance shows larger or smaller spaces lined by synovial cells between partitions representing thickened and agglutinated villi. In such an area the pigmentation is likely to be even heavier, both in the cells lining the spaces and in the numerous polyhedral cells present in the stroma of the fused partitioning villi.

In an essentially villonodular lesion, the villi present the same microscopic appearance (except for greater plumpness) as they do in an essentially villous lesion. As for the nodules, their histologic pattern is basically the same, whether they are small or large, sessile or stalked. The nodules are lined by one or more layers of more or less pigmented synovial lining cells. Some of the nodules are found to consist to a large extent of closely compacted roundish cells. Especially about the periphery of the nodules, many of these cells may be crowded with granules of

***Figure 170***

*A*, Photomicrograph (× 4) illustrating the histologic pattern of a tissue field in which rather plump stalked nodules protrude from the surface of the affected membrane. (The section represents tissue obtained from the highly nodular area shown in Fig. 167-*B*.) As higher magnification would reveal, the nodules are, for the most part, crowded with roundish stromal cells, and some of these contain pigment. Where this is the case, the nodules stain deeply. Those portions of the nodules which stain more lightly are areas in which a good deal of fibrosis and collagenization have occurred. Multinuclear giant cells are almost completely lacking in the various nodules shown.

*B*, Photomicrograph (× 20) illustrating the histologic pattern of a tissue field in which the surface of the membrane presents not only villous but also nodular proliferations. These nodules contain large numbers of multinuclear giant cells which show up merely as the scattered dark dots under this magnification. (See also Fig. 171-*C*.)

*C*, Photomicrograph (× 25) showing the pattern presented by a tissue field from an affected synovium in which a pigmented matted and villous area is present (upper left) in juxtaposition to nodular formations (lower middle and right). It is apparent even under this relatively low magnification that the nodules contain multinuclear giant cells.

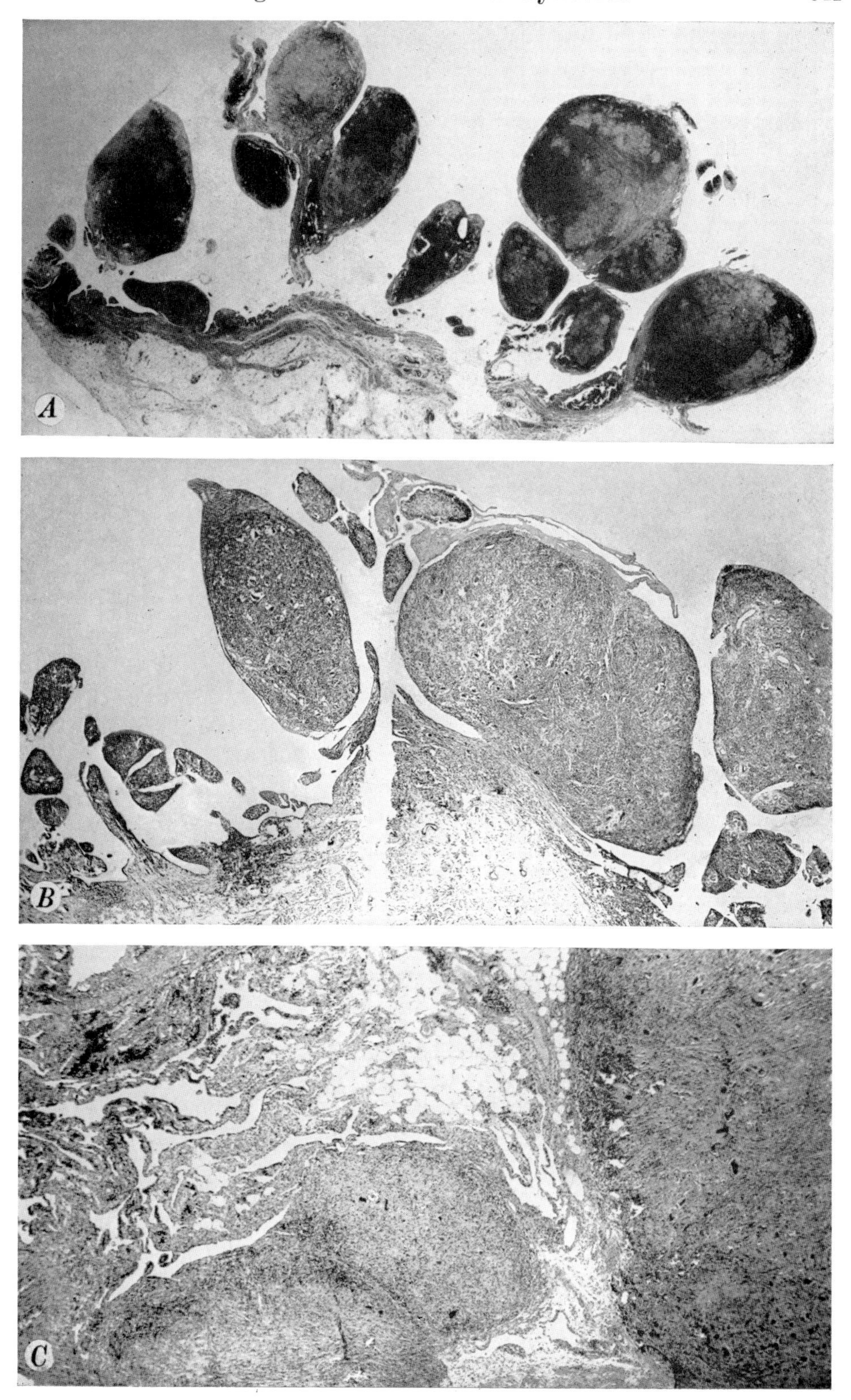


*Figure 170*

brown pigment. Cells containing lipid, with or without pigment, may also be observed. Multinuclear giant cells are likewise encountered, some nodules containing a few and others many of them. Ordinarily, these giant cells are of the so-called osteoclast type, the nuclei tending to congregate toward the middle of the cell. On the other hand, one may encounter a few, and in some lesions many, giant cells in which the nuclei are dispersed about the periphery of the cell. Such giant cells usually contain considerable lipid and sometimes also pigment.

In almost any villonodular lesion, many of the nodules show some evidence of fibrosis and collagenization. In some of the larger nodules this may be quite pronounced, and in an occasional one it is so extensive that the nodule is actually poor in cells, the latter apparently having been crowded out. It is noteworthy that, on a histologic basis alone, one cannot usually distinguish between the pattern presented by a large nodule from a pigmented villonodular articular synovial lesion and the pattern of a localized nodular tenosynovial lesion.

The histologic appearances presented by an exuberant spongy and matted synovial lesion are quite complex and may even be bewildering at first sight. In areas whose gross appearance is that of a close-meshed sponge, the spaces between the agglutinated villi are represented by mere clefts which are very narrow but still bordered by synovial lining cells. Between the clefts the tissue is likely to present a highly variegated pattern. In some places one finds large numbers of closely compacted roundish cells free or almost free of hemosiderin pigment. In other places these roundish cells may contain a considerable amount of pigment, and some or many of them may also have taken up lipid. A variable number of multinuclear giant cells may also be present. In tissue areas resulting from agglutination and intergrowth of nodules and villi, one likewise finds clefts lined by synovial lining cells and bordered by wide stretches of cellular tissue composed in the main of roundish cells which have phagocytosed pigment and/or lipid. In places the roundish cells are present in nodular agglomerations and interspersed with multinuclear giant cells.

In these exuberant lesions, an appreciable number of mitotic figures may also be seen. It is this fact and the great cellularity of these lesions that might lead one to think that the condition represents a malignant tumor. However, despite the suggestion of sarcoma conveyed by such histologic pictures, the writer's own experience includes no case in which such a lesion has metastasized. (See Figs. 169, 170 and 171.)

**Pathogenesis.**—Any explanation of the nature and genesis of diffuse pigmented villonodular synovitis must likewise be applicable to the diffuse villonodular tenosynovial and bursal lesions and to the localized nodular synovial and tenosynovial

***Figure 171***

*A*, Photomicrograph (× 125) showing in detail the histologic pattern presented by the area near the upper edge and about at the center of Fig. 169-*C*. Note the cleft-like spaces lined by flattened cells on the left, and the small richly cellular nodules on the right. The stromal cells of the nodules stain darkly on account of their high hemosiderin content.

*B*, Photomicrograph (× 65) showing in detail the histologic pattern presented by an area near the lower edge and to the right of the center of Fig. 169-*C*. In this area, where the lesional tissue is more condensed, lined cleft-like spaces are likewise prominent, but broad cords of tissue rich in stromal cells are present between the clefts.

*C*, Photomicrograph (× 125) showing the histologic pattern to be observed in a nodular area of a diffuse pigmented synovial lesion where the tissue contains multinuclear giant cells and foam cells.

*D*, Photomicrograph (× 125) showing the histologic pattern to be observed in a nodular area of a diffuse pigmented synovial lesion where the tissue is undergoing collagenization.

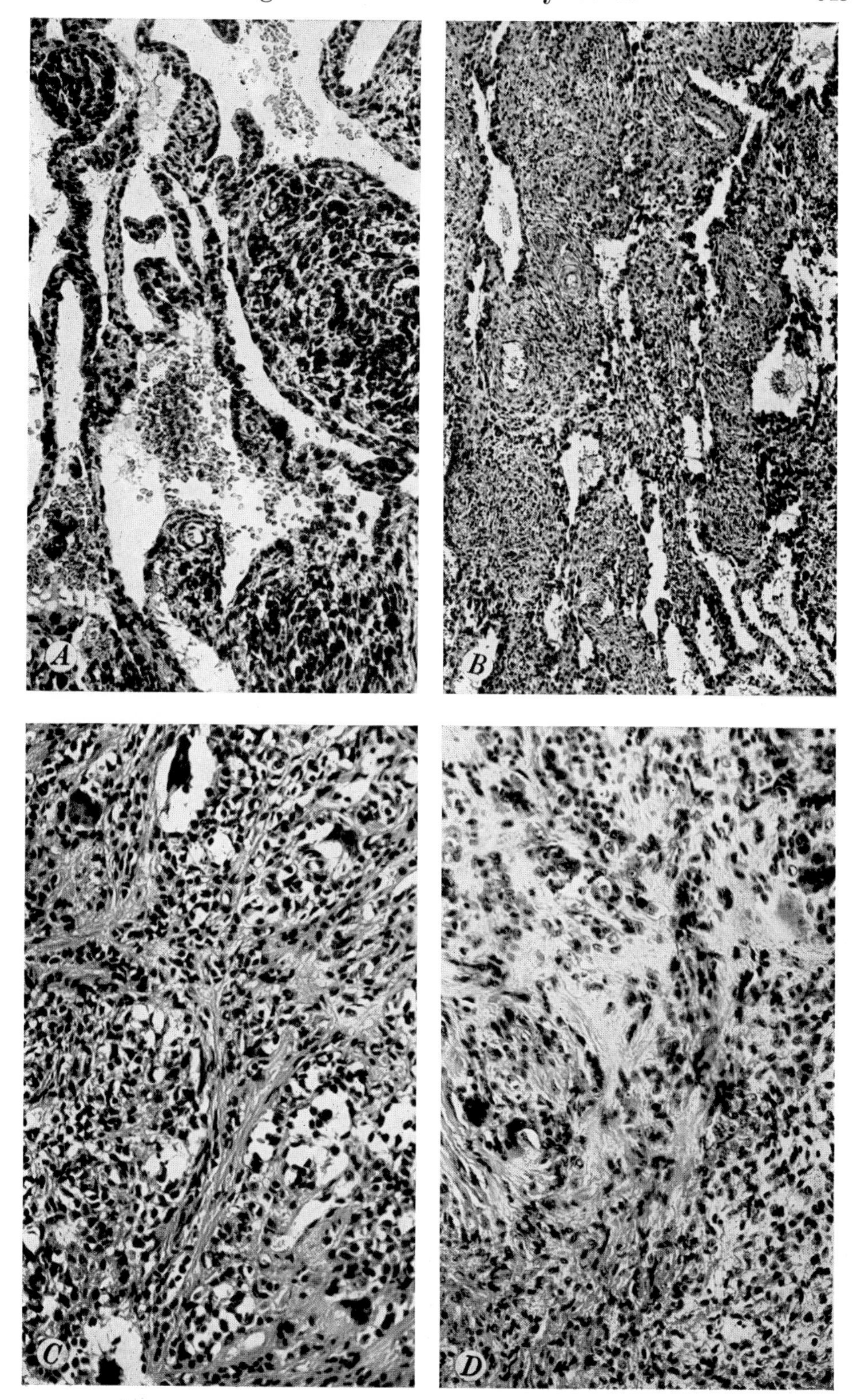


*Figure 171*

lesions. This is so because there can be no doubt that all these lesions are interrelated and thus represent merely different expressions of the same basic disorder.

The idea that the conditions under discussion arise as an inflammatory response to an imbalance (mainly local) of cholesterol metabolism has gone out of favor and no longer seems to require consideration. On the other hand, the idea that the lesion in its various sites and forms represents a true tumor in an oncological sense cannot be lightly discarded. Indeed, that concept has been held to be supported by the origin of the lesion from the linings of joints, bursæ, tendon sheaths and/or fascial and ligamentous tissues, and by the presence in the lesional tissue, at one time or another, of spaces bordered by synovial lining cells. Because the lesion is benign, contains giant cells and arises in synovial lining tissues, its supposed tumorous nature has been expressed in the name "benign giant-cell synovioma" (see Wright). The idea that the lesion is a true tumor is held to receive additional support from its behavior, in that it sometimes attains considerable size, that it sometimes erodes adjacent bones, and that it often recurs if not completed extirpated.

All this appears like formidable evidence in favor of the tumorous nature of the condition. There are other factors, however, which suggest an inflammatory process rather than neoplasia. Indeed, the whole cellular response activating the evolution of the lesions suggests an inflammatory reaction as the basis for the condition. This response centers around the accumulation of macrophages (the basic roundish cells) in the sublining layers of the affected structures. The assumption of phagocytic activity by these cells results in the appearance of multinuclear giant cells and of cells laden with hemosiderin and lipid. The spaces and clefts bordered by synovial lining cells in these lesions are due to the entrapment (following infolding and fusion) of villous proliferations, and are not formed within the lesional tissue by the proliferation of synovioblasts, as they are in the true synoviomas. Furthermore, these spaces are devoid of mucoid secretion, which is commonly present in the spaces of the indubitable tumors of synovial origin (see p. 586).

Finally, the whole natural course of the lesions under consideration tends in the direction of fibrosis, collagenization, and encapsulation. It is true that an occasional lesion does acquire an exuberant character and even becomes locally destructive, but this occurrence represents merely an aggravation of the original proliferative process, usually by irritation from intralesional bleeding.

Though the writer favors the idea that these lesions are of an inflammatory nature, there is still very little light on the question of what might provoke the inflammatory process. In view of the presence of hemosiderin pigment in the lesional tissue, it is natural to find that the condition (notably as it appears in joints) has been ascribed to the irritating effects of repeated intra-articular hemorrhage. Indeed, Young and Hudacek report having produced the changes of pigmented villonodular synovitis experimentally in the knee joints of dogs by the repeated intra-articular injection of autogenous blood.

However, even if the hemosiderosis in the clinical cases is due to absorption of blood into the synovial membrane, following on compression and laceration of vascular villi in the course of articular function, repeated intra-articular hemorrhage cannot account for the other cytologic features of the fully developed lesion. In this connection, the findings in affected joints in a case of hemophilia which the writer had the opportunity of studying are illuminating. In this case, repeated intra-articular hemorrhage had produced pronounced hemosideric pigmentation of the affected synovial membranes, which also became thoroughly villous, matted, and hypervascular. In addition, some of the joints showed disorganization of their bone ends. However, even in the severely affected joints, the synovial membrane did not present the other cytologic features of pigmented villonodular synovitis—foam cells and multinuclear giant cells among nodular collections or diffuse sheets of polyhedral stromal cells. In cases of hemophilia in which the bone ends of the joints are not severely altered, the cytologic picture presented by the synovial membrane is again not that of classic pigmented villonodular synovitis. In such joints one observes only that the synovium is heavily discolored and that the hemosiderin is confined to the synovial lining cells and the cells immediately below the lining (see Collins).

While functional trauma and hemorrhage are thus apparently not to be directly inculpated in the causation of a pigmented villonodular synovitis (for instance, in a knee joint), it cannot be denied that they could act as exacerbating factors. However, in connection with the localized tenosynovial lesions, it is hard to see how hemorrhage could be inculpated even as an exacerbating factor in the evolution of the lesion. Altogether, while the condition in its various sites is probably best interpreted as the expression of an inflammatory reaction, it must be conceded that we can offer no cue as to what the underlying cause of this reaction might be.

### TREATMENT

In a case of diffuse pigmented villonodular synovitis, total synovectomy (including meniscectomy) is indicated as the original therapeutic procedure. If extirpation of the lesional tissue has not been complete, there is considerable likelihood of recurrence. The latter is sometimes already evident within a few weeks. The recurrent lesion tends to become more florid than the original lesion, and on this account a new intervention should be undertaken as soon as evidence of recurrence appears. Should the second surgical intervention fail to lead to a cure, one might consider giving radiation therapy. Indeed, the writer has observed several cases in which *x*-ray therapy, given on account of recurrence, was followed by rather prompt amelioration and apparent cure of the condition. The appropriate total tissue dosage ranges between 1,500 and 2,500 r, given in divided doses of about 150 r daily.

## LOCALIZED NODULAR SYNOVITIS

As already indicated, the term *localized nodular synovitis* refers to that form of the condition under consideration in which only a limited area of the synovium of a joint is affected. The synovium shows merely a single sessile or stalked yellow-brown nodular outgrowth or at most a fused cluster of such outgrowths. The joint involved is again nearly always the knee.

### CLINICAL CONSIDERATIONS

Instances of the localized type of synovial involvement are perhaps slightly more common than those of the diffuse type. Also, the patients are older, on the average, more of them being mature adults. As to sex incidence, there seems to be no predilection for one sex over the other.

The duration of clinical complaints to the time when the patients come under definitive treatment varies from a few months to several years. On the whole, the clinical difficulties are mild. Not infrequently the history (as it relates to the knee) is that of swelling of the joint, relatively slight in amount and intermittent in character. The swelling is usually due to effusion, but the latter is rarely abundant enough to require aspiration. However, when this is done, it is likely to yield a straw-colored fluid rather than a hemorrhagically discolored fluid such as is encountered in the diffuse form of synovial involvement. Pain, often intermittent like the swelling, is also not infrequently reported and is probably to be related to catching of the lesional tissue between the articular bone ends. Under these circumstances there may also be episodes of locking and some limitation of motion (particularly of extension). Though a local trauma is sometimes inculpated in connection with onset of the difficulty in these cases, a history of such trauma is more often lacking, and trauma apparently bears no causal relation to the condition.

Physical examination may confirm the impression of slight swelling or enlargement of the joint. Furthermore, the examiner not infrequently senses that the joint contains a movable body. This, taken in conjunction with the clinical complaints, helps to explain why the trend of the preoperative diagnoses in these cases is toward internal derangement of the knee. Roentgenography is of no particular help in the diagnosis. In fact, the latter is usually not made until the joint is opened and the lesion exposed and examined. The appropriate *treatment* is excision of the affected part of the synovial membrane, and such treatment is not followed by recurrence of the lesion.

## PATHOLOGIC FINDINGS

**Gross Pathology.**—More often than not, the lesion consists of a single nodule issuing from some place in the synovial membrane. In the knee, the nodule is frequently found issuing from the membrane at a meniscocapsular junction. Occasionally, however, it is located at the intercondyloid fossa or eminence, near the patella, or even elsewhere. The knob of the nodule may measure from less than 1 cm. to several centimeters in its greatest diameter. It may be roundish or discoid, smooth or lobulated. If it is stalked, the stalk may be quite short or as much as several centimeters in length. The basic color of the knob, and often of the stalk too, is yellow or yellow-brown. In consistency, the nodule is firm and elastic on the whole. The synovial membrane immediately beyond the lesion is likely to be but little altered, but it may show slight brownish pigmentation and

***Figure 172***

*A*, Photograph showing a focus of localized nodular synovitis which had developed in the synovium of a knee at the meniscocapsular junction. The lesion appears as a stalked globular appendage and is faintly lobulated. It measured $2 \times 1\frac{1}{2} \times 1$ cm. and its color was yellow-brown. The patient was a man 28 years of age, and his complaints were of 3 years' standing. His principal difficulty was the occurrence of several episodes of acute pain, associated with the accumulation of fluid in the knee.

*B*, Photomicrograph ($\times$ 3) illustrating the general histologic pattern of the tissue from the lesion shown in *A*. Note the constituent lobules and the presence of several small clefts between them. The darkly stained areas represent viable tissue, and in these areas, multinuclear giant cells are present though not apparent at this magnification. In the more lightly stained areas, the lesional tissue is collagenized and also substantially necrotic, apparently in consequence of periodic crushing of the lesion between the articular bone ends.

*C*, Photograph showing a pigmented villonodular bursitis involving the bursa anserina. Note the numerous nodules in the wall of the bursa. In the central part of the picture the bursal lining is heavily pigmented and also villously transformed. The patient was a man 28 years of age who had been aware for 3 years of a slowly enlarging mass on the medial aspect of the upper part of a leg. For most of this time the lesion was not painful, but shortly before admission it had become so.

*D*, Photomicrograph ($\times$ 6) illustrating the histologic pattern of the affected bursal wall. The details of the histologic findings cannot be observed under such low magnification. However, the villi were heavily pigmented by hemosiderin, and in particular the large nodule on the right was composed of smaller fused nodules which contained many multinuclear giant cells and also showed evidences of collagenization.

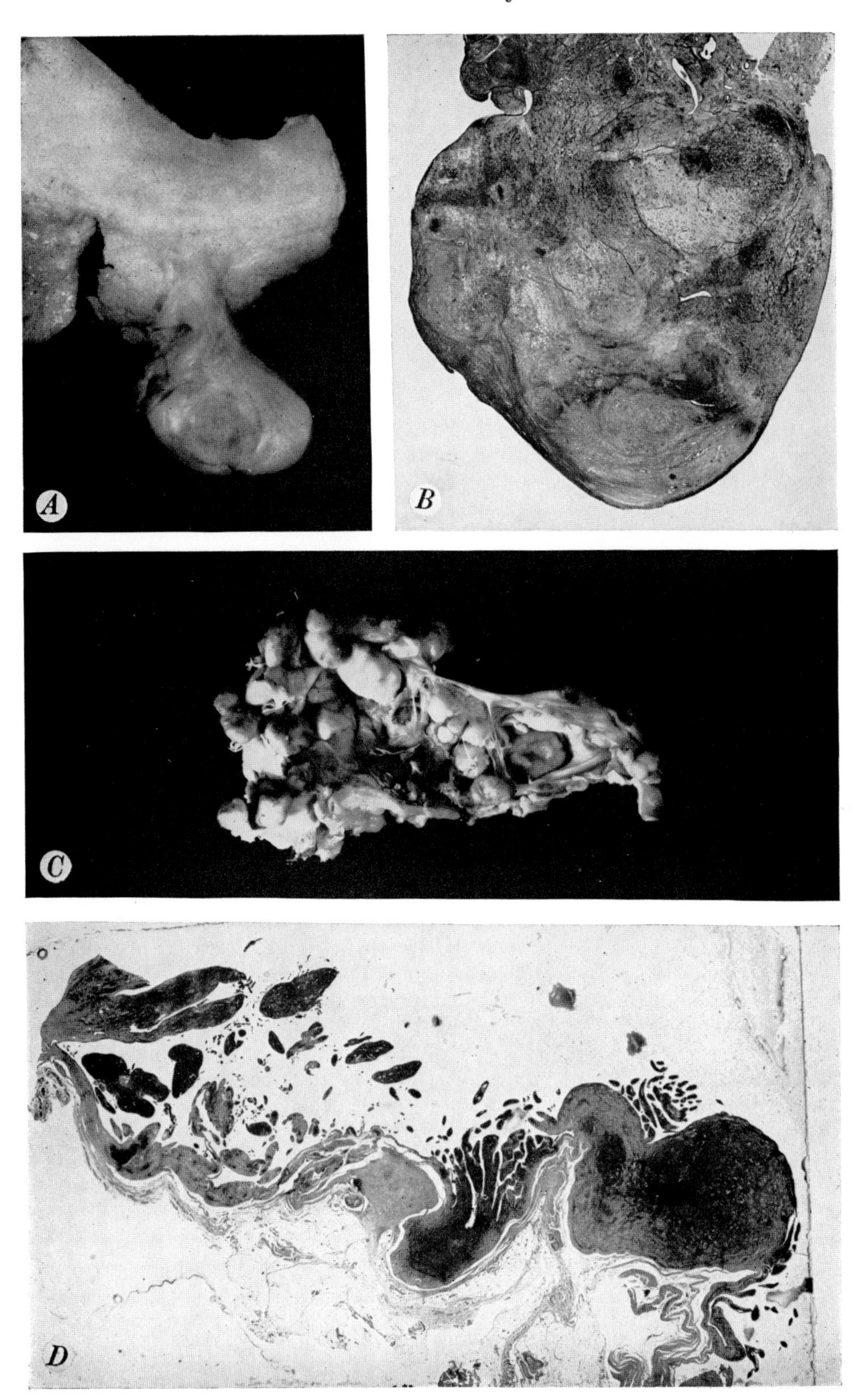


*Figure 172*

even slight villous transformation. The cut surface of the nodule or nodules may present a vaguely lobulated pattern and have a mottled yellow-brown color.

**Microscopic Pathology.**—The external surface of the nodule or nodules is covered by one or more layers of synovial lining cells, and many of the latter may be filled with granules of hemosiderin. If the cut surface of a nodule appeared lobulated, cleft-like spaces may be noted here and there between some of the more clear-cut lobules. In some specimens, the lesion as a whole still shows considerable cellularity. Under these conditions, one notes large numbers of roundish cells diffusely distributed or collected in large aggregates. An appreciable number of these cells may be rich in hemosiderin pigment. Others may be found to have taken up lipid, sometimes to such an extent that they appear as foam cells. Scattered among the roundish stromal cells are variable numbers of multinuclear giant cells. Furthermore, some degree of collagenization is almost regularly seen in the nodule as a whole or in its component lobules. In an occasional instance this may be so pronounced that the entire nodule is found poor in cells. Altogether, then, the histologic pattern presented by a nodule from a case of solitary nodular synovitis usually corresponds to what is likely to be observed in one or another of the larger nodules from the lesion in a case of diffuse pigmented villonodular synovitis (see Figs. 172-*A* and *B*).

Finally, it should be pointed out that one sometimes encounters in a joint a solitary stalked synovial nodule which is more or less fibrotic and necrotic and whose center may even be rich in cholesterol crystals. Such a nodule is apparently one which has become crushed in the course of articular function and then undergone further modification on account of interference with its blood supply.

## PIGMENTED VILLONODULAR BURSITIS

As noted, *pigmented villonodular bursitis* is encountered only infrequently. The sites in which the writer has seen it include the popliteal bursa (without concomitant involvement of the synovium of the knee joint) and the bursa anserina. An instance of involvement of the iliopectineal bursa has been reported by Weisser and Robinson. Occasionally a diffuse villonodular lesion is observed in the ankle region, and in such a case it may be difficult to decide whether the condition actually represents a pigmented villonodular bursitis or tenosynovitis. Furthermore, a diffuse pigmented villonodular lesion is sometimes encountered in the so-called radial and/or ulnar bursa of the wrist and hand. In view of the tenosynovial nature of these bursæ, it seems more appropriate to discuss these lesions as instances of diffuse pigmented villonodular tenosynovitis (p. 554).

In the cases of pigmented villonodular bursitis studied by the writer, the patients had been aware for some time of a slowly enlarging and somewhat painful mass at the affected site. In none of these cases had the bursal involvement interfered significantly with articular function.

On anatomic examination, the cavity of the affected bursa may be found still intact or largely obliterated. A bursa which has retained its cavity shows a lining of brownishly discolored villous fringes interspersed with nodular polypoid projections. A bursa whose cavity has been more or less obliterated (through fusion and intergrowth of the villous and nodular proliferations) appears as a brownishly discolored spongy tissue mass. In a lesion presenting this appearance, it is sometimes even difficult to be sure that the structure in which the condition developed was actually a bursa. In any event, what has already been said about the gross and microscopic findings relating to pigmented villonodular synovitis at the various stages of its evolution applies equally well to pigmented villonodular bursitis (see Figs. 172-*C* and *D*).

# LOCALIZED NODULAR TENOSYNOVITIS

The so-called *localized nodular tenosynovitis* (still often denoted as the giant-cell tumor of tendon sheaths) represents the most common and familiar expression of the conditions under consideration. Its sites of predilection are the fingers. Most often it is observed as a firm, somewhat lobulated, compact tissue mass not more than a few centimeters in greatest diameter, and its basic grayish color is mottled with yellow and brown. When it is present in this form, its relation to the diffuse pigmented and villonodular lesions discussed in this chapter is no longer obvious. This is so because the appearances representing the early villous and nodular stages of its evolution may have become completely obliterated. However, in the course of study of a large series of the tenosynovial lesions in question, an occasional one will be found which is still loose-meshed or spongy, at least in part. One of this kind not only sheds light upon the manner of evolution of the tenosynovial lesions in question, but helps to show that they are related to the obviously villonodular synovial and bursal lesions we have considered.

## CLINICAL CONSIDERATIONS

The writer has studied at least 200 examples of localized nodular tenosynovitis. As noted, in the great majority of the cases, the lesion is to be observed in the fingers. It shows no particular predilection for any one digit. The lesion may be located on the flexor or the extensor surface, or even on the lateral aspect of the digit, and occasionally it even more or less encircles the latter. When present elsewhere in the hand, it tends to be located in the region of a metacarpophalangeal joint, usually on the palmar surface. Sometimes the lesion is found at the wrist or the ankle, or in one or another toe. Only rarely does it appear in multiple sites—that is, in more than one finger, for instance. Indeed, any supposed case in which one finds multiple involvement should arouse the suspicion that one may actually be dealing with "xanthoma tuberosum multiplex" having its basis in familial hypercholesterinemia.

The condition seems to show a predilection for females. The great majority of the patients are young or middle-aged adults, and most of the rest are older people rather than children. The subjects often report merely that they have a nodule (on a finger or toe or at a wrist or ankle) which, after enlarging slowly for some years, has lately begun to enlarge more rapidly. Only occasionally do they complain of pain or interference with motion. The latter complaints arise when the lesion is impinging on a nerve or on the adjacent tendon or has merely become particularly large. Furthermore, the lesion sometimes erodes the neighboring bone, and may cause pain in this way also. The correct diagnosis can frequently be established preoperatively if one bears in mind that a small nodular mass of fibrous consistency, situated on a finger, represents, in all probability, a localized nodular tenosynovitis.

## PATHOLOGIC FINDINGS

**Gross Pathology.**—The precise site of origin of the so-called tenosynovial lesions is by no means always clear. There can be no doubt that many of them arise from the lining of the fibrous sheath of tendons. Certainly at the time of removal of the lesion, some of them also involve the fascial and ligamentous tissue adjacent to tendons, and these lesions may even have arisen from the linings of these structures. In connection with those lesions which develop on the extensor surface of the ends of the fingers, it is held by Wright, for instance, that they actually issue from the dorsal prolongations of the synovial membrane of the distal interphalangeal joints.

The extirpated lesion is usually oval or globular in shape and of rather firm consistency. It often measures between 1 and 3 cm. in its greatest dimension but may be smaller or larger. It appears faintly or definitely lobulated, and an occasional lesion may even show striking lobulation. Indeed, it may be possible to tease a distinctly lobulated lesion apart into a number of individual though connected smaller lobules. On the other hand, if gross lobulation is no longer distinct on the outer surface of the lesion, the cut surface may still reveal the lines which separated the individual lesions before they all became fused into a single mass. (See Fig. 173.)

### *Figure 173*

*A*, Photograph (enlarged by $\frac{1}{3}$) showing a localized nodular tenosynovial lesion which was removed from the region of the distal interphalangeal joint of a thumb. The lesion was of rather firm consistency and yellow-brown in color. It appears only faintly lobulated, its component nodular proliferations having undergone substantial agglomeration and fusion. The patient was a man 40 years of age who had been aware for 3 years of a slowly enlarging mass on the volar surface of the thumb. The lesion gave him no difficulty, and *x*-ray examination of the thumb revealed no changes in the bones. At the surgical intervention the lesion was found adherent to the sheath of the flexor tendon, but it did not penetrate the latter. There has been no recurrence.

*B*, Photograph (enlarged $2\frac{1}{2} \times$) of a strikingly nodular localized tenosynovial lesion which was removed from a finger. The lesion was located on the volar aspect in the vicinity of the interphalangeal joint. At the surgical intervention it was found that the lesion lay between the flexor tendon and the underlying bones and that it was producing pressure erosion of the cortex of the proximal phalanx. It was yellowish in color, and the cut surface also showed that the lesional tissue was composed of smaller nodules which were undergoing fusion (see Fig. 174-*A*). The patient was a man 40 years of age who had been aware of a swelling of the affected finger for 4 years. The lesion caused no clinical difficulty, and its growth was apparently so slow that he hardly noticed that the finger was enlarging.

*C*, Photograph (enlarged $2 \times$) showing the cut surface of a localized nodular tenosynovial lesion which was oriented to the volar surface of the distal half of an index finger. Note that, for the most part, the lesional tissue presents a nodular pattern and that its color is mottled. The lighter area represents that portion of the lesion which has undergone collagenization, while the darker area still contains considerable pigment. The patient was a woman 69 years of age who complained that for 2 years the finger had become increasingly painful and was enlarging. *X*-ray examination showed that the local bones were not affected.

*D*, Roentgenograph showing bone destruction produced by a localized nodular tenosynovial lesion affecting a large toe. The radiolucent defect in the distal end of the proximal phalanx is the result of actual penetration of lesional tissue into the bone, and the soft-tissue shadow represents this tissue. The patient was a woman 36 years of age who gave a history of gradual enlargement and intermittent pain in the toe of 3 years' standing. At the surgical intervention it was found that the lesion had apparently developed in relation to the extensor tendon sheath of the toe in question.

*E*, Photomicrograph ($\times$ 2) showing a localized pigmented villonodular lesion which is penetrating into the distal end of the middle phalanx of the fifth toe and is also involving the synovial membrane of the terminal interphalangeal joint. The lesion in question is a recurrent one. The patient, a woman 50 years of age, had had a nodule removed from the toe in question 5 years earlier at another institution. It is difficult to decide whether the recurrent lesion issued from the synovial membrane of the joint and then invaded the bone or whether it represents a tenosynovial lesion which had extended into both the regional joint and the phalanx.

*F*, Photograph showing a surgically exposed diffuse villonodular tenosynovial lesion affecting the so-called ulnar bursa. The lesion extends from the upper end of the carpal sheath to the tip of the fifth finger. Note the string of confluent nodules in the finger and the swelling which the lesional tissue has produced in the palm. Surgical dissection revealed that there was no involvement of the neighboring tendons. The patient was a woman 50 years of age who stated that for 2 years she had been aware of a progressively enlarging nontender growth in the area in question.

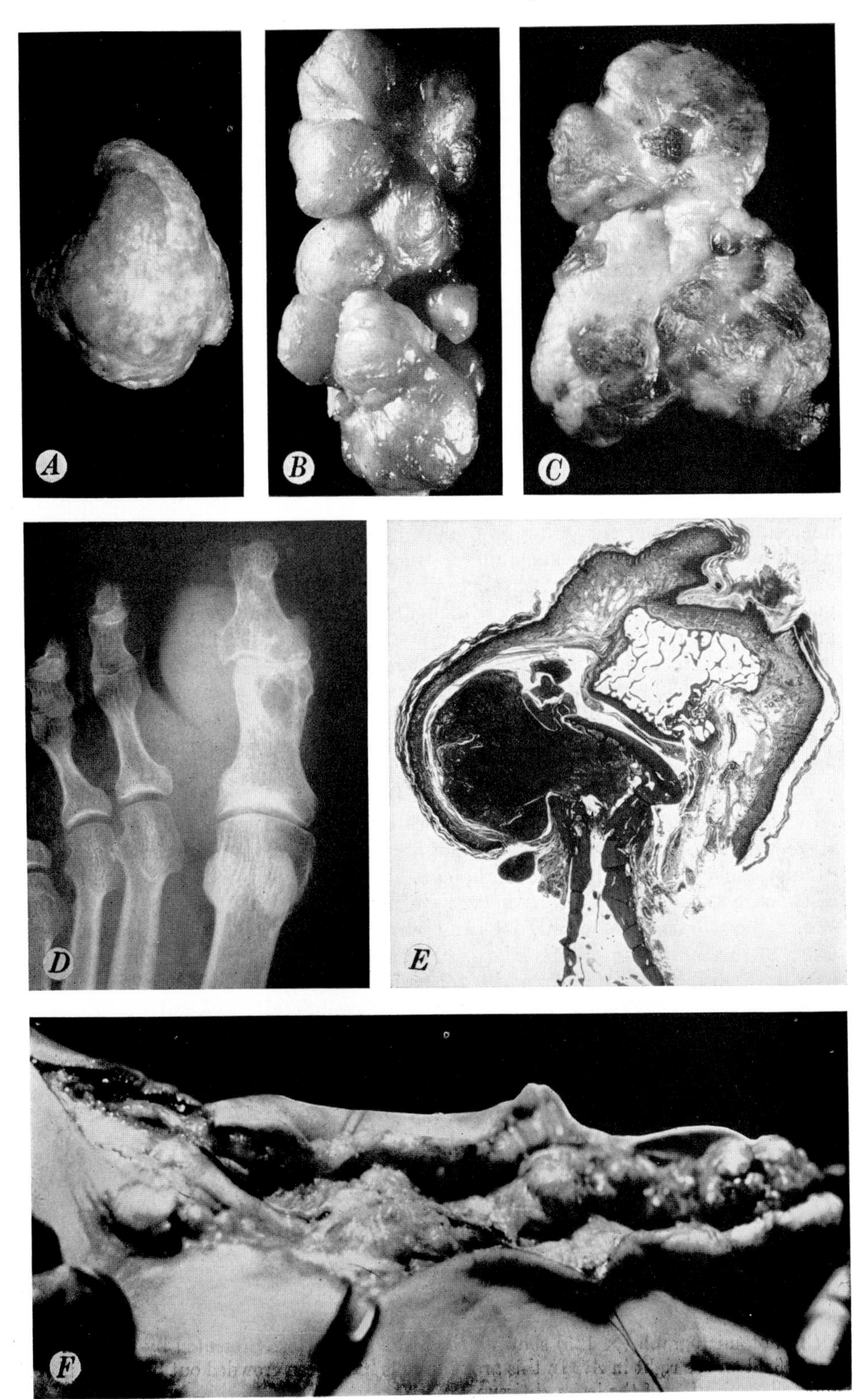


***Figure 173***

The lesional tissue ranges in color from gray to yellowish or reddish brown. In a particular specimen, the color is usually mottled rather than uniform throughout. The intensity of the yellow and brown discoloration reflects in a general way the abundance of lipid and hemosiderin respectively. Lesions which are especially firm are likely to be grayish in color, and microscopic examination shows them to be rich in collagen and relatively poor in cells, lipid, and hemosiderin. On the other hand, lesions which are rather soft are usually quite brown on account of the presence of a good deal of hemosiderin, and microscopic examination usually also shows them to be quite rich in cells.

**Microscopic Pathology.**—The details of the microscopic findings may vary considerably from lesion to lesion and even from part to part of the same lesion. Nevertheless, there is a basic finding which emerges from microscopic study of large numbers of the lesions in question. This is the fact that the lesion as a whole is the result of agglomeration and fusion of individual smaller nodular proliferations. Indeed, even if the lesion has presented grossly as a compact single nodule of tissue, some microscopic evidence that it originally consisted of multiple nodules can usually still be observed.

The basic cell of the nodule is a round cell. These roundish cells may be admixed with variable numbers of multinuclear giant cells and cells containing lipid and/or hemosiderin. The cells bearing lipid and hemosiderin are merely basic round cells which have taken up these substances. In the multinuclear giant cells, the nuclei are usually found distributed throughout the cell. However, one sometimes finds giant cells in which the nuclei are distributed about the periphery of the cell, and such giant cells show a good deal of lipid in their cytoplasm. In an occasional lesion, giant cells of this "foreign-body" type may even be quite prominent. Various degrees of collagenization and fibrosis are also to be observed. The heavier the collagenization of individual areas, the poorer they are in cells.

Occasionally a lesion shows not only the usual histologic pattern of more or less cellular lobules undergoing collagenization and fusion, but patterns representing even earlier phases in the development of the lesion. In particular, such specimens indicate that the lesion actually progresses by way of an initial villous pigmented stage through an intermediate nodular and cellular stage to a rather meagerly cellular, collagenous and fibrous end stage. Where the lesional tissue is still villous in character, the villi contain hemosiderin pigment and may be matted together. Where the villi have coalesced, one can observe cleft-like spaces and also the beginnings of small nodular proliferations. Furthermore, small nodules can be seen to have merged into larger ones, and where adjacent large nodules have formed, one notes that the clefts have become partly or completely obliterated. In places

***Figure 174***

*A*, Photomicrograph (× 4) illustrating the pattern presented by a localized nodular tenosynovial lesion whose constituent small nodules are merging into larger ones. The larger nodules are still discrete, and that is why the lesion appeared strikingly nodular in the gross (see Fig. 173-*B*). If they too had become agglomerated, the lesion would probably have appeared as a compact tissue mass, perhaps still faintly lobulated.

*B*, Photomicrograph (× 50) showing the histologic pattern presented by the boxed-out tissue field on the left in *A*. Note the two slits between fusing lobules and the presence of numerous multinuclear cells against a background of smaller cells representing the basic stromal cells.

*C*, Photomicrograph (× 125) showing the histologic pattern presented by the boxed-out tissue field on the right in *A*. In this area the cells have been crowded out by heavy fibrosis and collagenization of the lesional tissue.

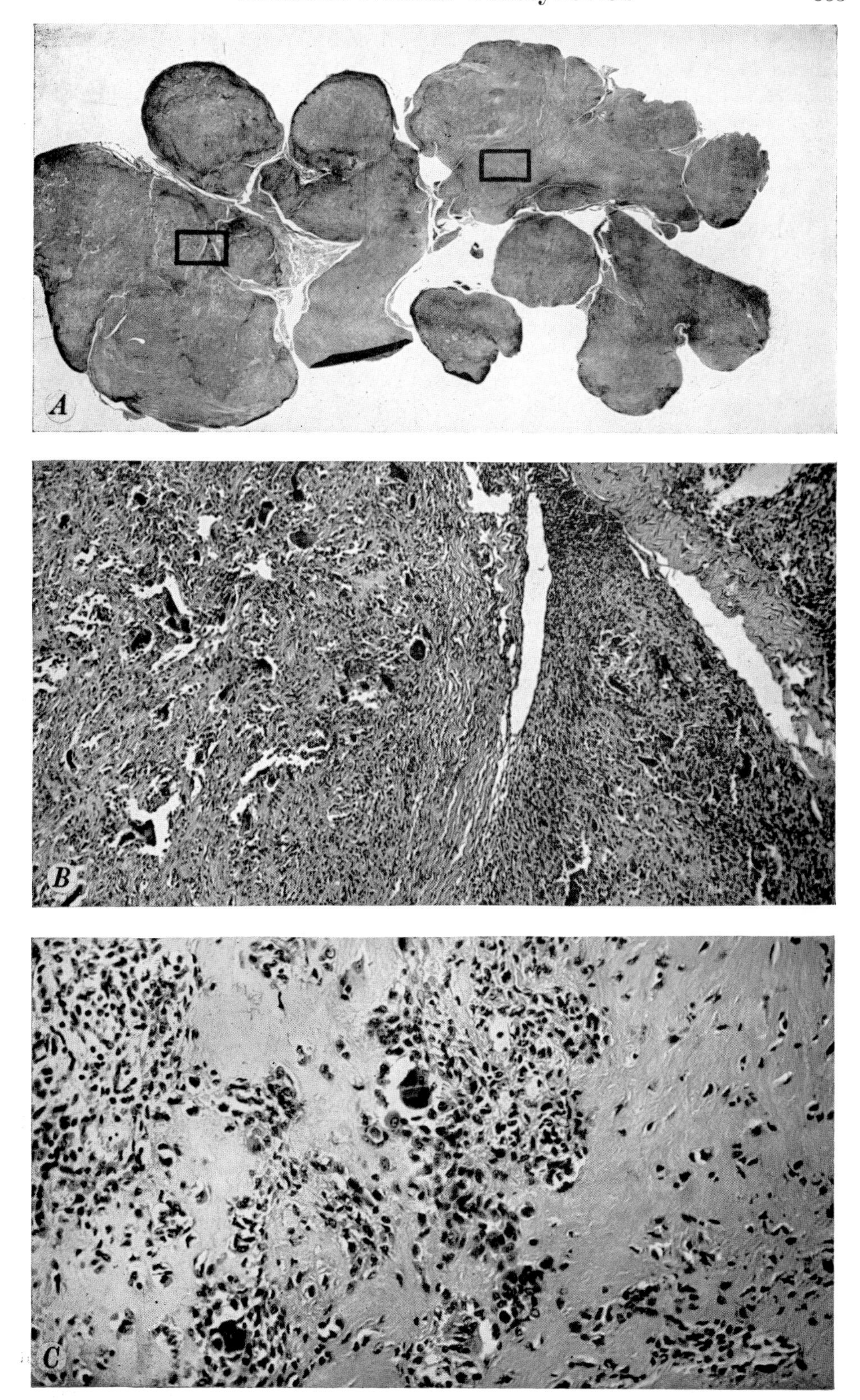


***Figure 174***

where the lesional tissue has reached its final mature stage, one finds that clefts are no longer present and that the tissue pattern is that of fused collagenized nodules which, however, may still contain variable numbers of roundish stromal cells, multinuclear giant cells, and cells bearing lipid and hemosiderin. (See Figs. 174 and 175.)

### TREATMENT

The treatment of choice for these lesions is local excision. In this connection, careful attention must be given to all extensions or ramifications of the lesional tissue, since recurrence is likely if any of it is left behind. In a case in which the lesion has recurred, a second surgical intervention is indicated. If the local bone has been invaded and removal of most of the lesional tissue is still feasible, any residual lesional tissue in the bone can usually be destroyed by radiation therapy (see p. 545), so that amputation of the digit so affected can usually be avoided. At any rate, it should be borne in mind that these lesions have no malignant potentialities, no matter how cellular or locally destructive they may be.

## PIGMENTED VILLONODULAR TENOSYNOVITIS

In addition to the common localized nodular tenosynovial lesions described in the previous section, one occasionally encounters an instance of diffuse and widespread involvement of synovial sheaths of the hand or foot. It is this *diffuse* type of tenosynovial involvement that is covered by the term *pigmented villonodular tenosynovitis*. Such lesions often attain large size, since they are not restricted to a single sheath. Indeed, particularly when present in the ankle and/or foot, the condition is very likely to involve also the local fascial and ligamentous tissues. Under these circumstances, the neighboring bones may be implicated through pressure erosion or actual penetration of the lesional tissue into these bones.

A striking instance of diffuse involvement of the synovial sheaths of the hand was described by Mason. In that case the lesion implicated the so-called ulnar and radial bursæ, had eroded the carpal bones at the base of the thumb, and passed between the second and third metacarpals to the dorsum, where it involved all the dorsal tendon sheaths. The lesional tissue was composed of innumerable con-

***Figure 175***

*A*, Photomicrograph (× 6) showing the pattern of a localized tenosynovial lesion which still presents evidence of its development through villous proliferation, infolding, and matting of the tissue. At the extreme left, one can still see villi which, under higher magnification, are found to be crowded with cells bearing hemosiderin. Somewhat to the right of this area there are sinuously winding channels between villi which have become thickened and invaginated and are undergoing agglutination. At the right, one can see a large nodule which represents the most evolved portion of the lesion. In this area the lesional tissue has undergone almost total fusion and compaction and become fibrosed and collagenized. The specimen came from the sheath of the flexor pollicis longus, and specifically from a site near the first metacarpophalangeal joint. The patient, a woman 35 years of age, stated that she had noted the presence of a "tumor" on her thumb for only 2 weeks prior to her admission to the hospital. She had not related its appearance to a trauma.

*B*, Photomicrograph (× 65) showing an invaginated villous fold from the tissue illustrated in *A*. Note the multinuclear giant cells set in a cellular stroma which, in places, is undergoing collagenization.

*C*, Photomicrograph (× 100) representing an area from another localized nodular tenosynovial lesion which still showed its early evolutionary phases. Note that several adjacent small nodular proliferations are fusing and undergoing collagenization.

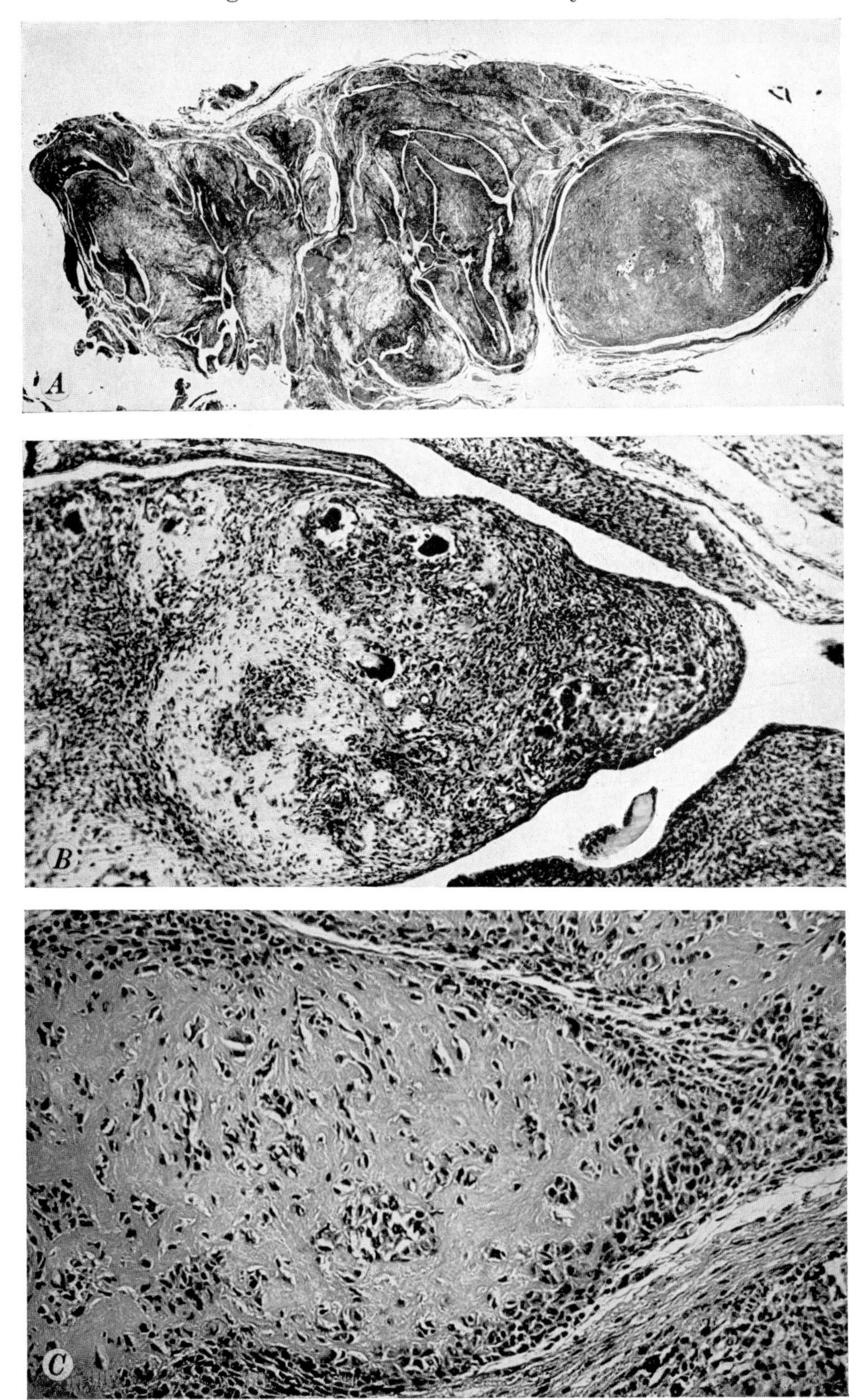

***Figure 175***

fluent nodular masses varying in color from gray through yellow to deep brown.

In a case studied by the writer in which the lesion was again in the hand, it was largely confined to the so-called ulnar bursa. The lesion, which was of 2 years' standing, extended from the tip of the fifth finger, involved the palm, and terminated near the upper end of the carpal sheath (see Fig. 173-*F*). The tendons themselves were unaffected. The resected specimen was found composed of confluent nodules of yellow-brown tissue. In the portion which had been located in the palm, a tendon sheath lumen was still identifiable, and one could recognize that the nodules had developed in the wall of the synovial sheath in that region. Some of the nodules in that area of the lesion had pedicles and were extending into the lumen of the bursa. In any event, practically all of the nodules, whether stalked or fused, were found on microscopic examination to be composed of roundish stromal cells interspersed with multinuclear giant cells and cells containing pigment and lipid. Here and there in some of the larger nodules there was evidence of collagenization of the lesional tissue.

In an instance of diffuse pigmented villonodular synovitis involving a foot, the patient had been aware for many years of a gradually increasing, relatively asymptomatic swelling on its lateral aspect. In this case the lesion apparently took its departure from the synovial sheaths of the peroneal tendons. The lesion had grown diffusely and had extended into the fascial and ligamentous tissues of the sole of the foot. Furthermore, it had eroded to some extent into the calcaneus, astragalus, cuboid, and scaphoid bones. The resected tissue was brownish in color and appeared villous and nodular. On microscopic examination, it presented the histologic pattern already described in regard to diffuse villonodular lesions in the hand and in other sites.

In another case in which a foot was affected, the lesion took its departure deep in the sole, involved the metatarsophalangeal joint of the second toe, and destroyed the bone ends of this joint. Actually, one could not be certain whether it had developed from the plantar aponeurosis or from the fibrous flexor sheath. In any event, the lesion presented as a large, firm, nodular mass of tissue in which the eroded bones were imbedded. On microscopic examination, the lesional tissue again showed the characteristic pattern of agglomerated nodules which were highly collagenized in some places but still presented, in other areas, multinuclear giant cells, foam cells, and even some cells bearing hemosiderin.

## REFERENCES


BREIMER, C. W., and FREIBERGER, R. H.: Bone Lesions Associated with Villonodular Synovitis, Am. J. Roentgenol., *79*, 618, 1958.

CARR, C. R., BERLEY, F. V., and DAVIS, W. C.: Pigmented Villonodular Synovitis of the Hip Joint, J. Bone & Joint Surg., *36-A*, 1007, 1954.

Case Records of the Massachusetts General Hospital (Case 37292), New England J. Med., *245*, 112, 1951.

COLLINS, D. H.: Haemosiderosis and Haemochromatosis of Synovial Tissues, J. Bone & Joint Surg., *33-B*, 436, 1951.

DESANTO, D. A., and WILSON, P. D.: Xanthomatous Tumors of Joints, J. Bone & Joint Surg., *21*, 531, 1939.

FLETCHER, A. G., JR., and HORN, R. C., JR.: Giant Cell Tumors of Tendon Sheath Origin, Ann. Surg., *133*, 374, 1951.

GALLOWAY, J. D. B., BRODERS, A. C., and GHORMLEY, R. K.: Xanthoma of Tendon Sheaths and Synov ial Membranes, Arch. Surg., *40*, 485, 1940.

GREENFIELD, M. M., and WALLACE, K. M.: Pigmented Villonodular Synovitis, Radiology, *54*, 350, 1950.

JAFFE, H. L., LICHTENSTEIN, L., and SUTRO, C. J.: Pigmented Villonodular Synovitis, Bursitis and Tenosynovitis, Arch. Path., *31*, 731, 1941.

LEWIS, R. W.: Roentgen Diagnosis of Pigmented Villonodular Synovitis and Synovial Sarcoma of the Knee Joint, Radiology, *49*, 26, 1947.
MASON, M. L.: Tumors of the Hand, Surg., Gynec. & Obst., *64*, 129, 1937.
MORTON, J. J.: Tumors of the Tendon Sheaths, Surg., Gynec. & Obst., *59*, 441, 1934.
RAGINS, A. B.: Benign Tumors of the Tendon Sheaths of Unusual Size, Ann. Surg., *93*, 683, 1931.
SHAFER, S. J., and LARMON, W. A.: Pigmented Villonodular Synovitis, Surg., Gynec. & Obst., *92*, 574, 1951.
SHERRY, J. B., and ANDERSON, W.: The Natural History of Pigmented Villonodular Synovitis of Tendon Sheaths, J. Bone & Joint Surg., *37-A*, 1005, 1955.
WEISSER, J. R., and ROBINSON, D. W.: Pigmented Villonodular Synovitis of Iliopectineal Bursa, J. Bone & Joint Surg., *33-A*, 988, 1951.
WRIGHT, C. J. E.: Benign Giant-Cell Synovioma, Brit. J. Surg., *38*, 257, 1951.
YOUNG, J. M., and HUDACEK, A. G.: Experimental Production of Pigmented Villonodular Synovitis in Dogs, Am. J. Path., *30*, 799, 1954.

Chapter

# 31

# Synovial Chondromatosis and Other Benign Articular Tumors

THE conditions to which attention is mainly devoted in this chapter are *synovial chondromatosis* and *hemangioma of joints*. Analogous lesions sometimes develop in relation to tendon sheaths and bursae mucosae, and some consideration is given to them also. However, neither synovial chondromatosis nor hemangioma of joints is seen very often, and their counterparts in tendon sheaths and bursae mucosae are of even rarer occurrence. Once in a while, a so-called *intracapsular* and/or *para-articular chondroma* is encountered. In such cases, a more or less circumscribed focus of cartilage develops in relation to the capsular apparatus of the joint, but by the time it is removed and studied anatomically, the lesional cartilage is usually found to have become substantially ossified. Instances of *lipoma* and *fibroma*, too, have been described as occurring in relation to articular capsules. However, it is mainly in the older literature that one finds reports of such cases, and it is often difficult to tell from the descriptions whether the lesions in question actually represented these conditions.

## SYNOVIAL CHONDROMATOSIS

As used here, the term *synovial chondromatosis* denotes the condition in which foci of cartilage develop in the synovial membrane of a joint, apparently through metaplasia of the sublining connective tissue of the membrane. Cartilage which has become detached from the affected membrane and entered the joint cavity may even increase in amount, since it is nourished by the synovial fluid. Furthermore, many of the cartilage foci (both in the synovial membrane and in the joint space) become calcified, and some may even become ossified. Because of the occurrence of calcification and ossification in the lesional cartilage, the name *synovial osteochondromatosis* is sometimes also used for the disorder.

### CLINICAL CONSIDERATIONS

Though many cases held to represent synovial chondromatosis (or synovial osteochondromatosis) have been reported in the literature, only a small number of them are acceptable as genuine instances of the condition, on the basis of the definition given above. Indeed, indubitable cases of synovial chondromatosis are not encountered very often. The writer's own experience covers 6 cases. One or more acceptable instances are also to be found in the reports by Beckman and Ivarsson, Jones, Rixford, Freund, and Leydig and Odell, among others.

Synovial chondromatosis is more likely to occur in males than in females, and the subjects are usually young or middle-aged adults. While the condition is also seen in older people, its occurrence below the age of puberty is certainly rare. As to localization, the knee joint is predilected, this being the site of the disorder in the great majority of the cases. Involvements of other large joints account for almost all the rest. Indeed, it is highly exceptional to encounter the lesion in one of the small diarthrodial joints. The condition is usually monarticular. In the rare cases in which it is polyarticular, it is usually both knees that are affected, though it may be other pairs of large joints or even two unpaired large joints.

Clinical difficulties are usually present for months or several years before the subject comes under definitive treatment. The amount of disability is generally greater when a hip or elbow is affected than when a knee or shoulder is involved. It is likely to be reported that the affected joint has been intermittently painful. In some cases, questioning elicits a history of possibly significant antecedent trauma, but more often it does not. The affected joint is usually found more or less enlarged and somewhat limited in range of motion, and it may even reveal clicking, grating or jamming. The examiner may sense the presence of fluid or of a mass or movable bodies in the joint.

The value of the *roentgenographic findings* in establishing the diagnosis depends in large measure upon the extent to which calcification and ossification have taken place, both in the cartilage present in the synovium and in the cartilage bodies within the articular cavity. In this connection, several cases are on record in which the affected joint contained considerable amounts of cartilage, but the condition could not be diagnosed as chondromatosis on a roentgenographic basis because the cartilage was neither calcified nor ossified. However, such cases represent the exception rather than the rule, and the *x*-ray findings usually do permit one to identify the condition clinically or at least to suspect its presence.

An affected knee joint, for instance, will show thickening of the synovium of the quadriceps pouch and of the anterior and posterior compartments of the joint. In addition, one will note at least some fuzzy and also some more distinctly spotty radiopacities in the region of the joint. It should be emphasized that in an unequivocal case of synovial chondromatosis one does not often encounter many large and very radiopaque bodies. Furthermore, the contour of the articular bone ends is usually not grossly altered. (See Fig. 176.)

Indeed, should a knee joint show many deeply radiopaque bodies and also present marginal exostoses and/or general irregularity in the contour of the articular bone ends, or one or more clear-cut defects at these ends, the condition is not likely to represent synovial chondromatosis. However, the possibility of misinterpreting some other condition as synovial chondromatosis is less likely to arise in connection with a knee joint than in connection with a hip or shoulder joint, for instance. Thus, if a hip joint is found even crowded with closely set, deeply radiopaque bodies, there is no justification for a diagnosis of synovial chondromatosis unless the synovial membrane shows evidence of cartilaginous metaplasia. In relation to the shoulder joint, too, the presence of numerous rather large, deeply radiopaque bodies should raise the suspicion that one may be dealing with something else than synovial chondromatosis.

Thus, in arriving at the diagnosis on the basis of the *x*-ray findings, one must bear in mind that conditions other than synovial chondromatosis may be associated with the presence of joint bodies. These conditions include osteochondritis dissecans, osteoarthritis, and neuropathic arthropathies. In these disorders, cartilaginous or osteocartilaginous fragments may be sheared off or broken off from the articular bone ends, may lie free in the joint or become implanted in the synovium, and may even continue to grow. Furthermore, in these and other conditions, joint bodies may also be formed through the calcification and chondrification of fibrin coagula that have accumulated in the articular space in consequence of a synovitis. Altogether, irrespective of the presence of cartilaginous or osteocartilaginous bodies in the joint space, there must be anatomic evidence that the synovial membrane is a site of formation of such bodies if a case is to be counted as one of synovial chondromatosis.

## PATHOLOGIC FINDINGS

**Gross Pathology.**—The affected synovium is found more or less thickened, and close inspection of it demonstrates that the cartilage tends to develop immediately

***Figure 176***

*A*, Roentgenograph of a knee joint affected with synovial chondromatosis. Note the thickening of the tissues in the region of the quadriceps pouch and in the posterior and anterior compartments of the joint. The speckled and fuzzy radiopacity in the articular soft tissues represents calcification and ossification of the lesional cartilage. The patient was a man 33 years of age who complained of pain, swelling, and stiffness of the joint. The difficulties were of 2 years' standing and were not related to an antecedent trauma. Surgical exploration of the joint revealed the presence of hundreds of small cartilaginous bodies (rice bodies), some of which were gritty. The resected synovial membrane showed numerous small cartilaginous bodies within its substance, and microscopic examination revealed that some of these, too, were undergoing calcification and ossification.

*B*, Roentgenograph of another knee joint affected with synovial chondromatosis, again showing thickening and fuzzy radiopacity of the soft tissues of the joint. The patient was a man 32 years of age whose complaints relating to the knee were pain, swelling, and stiffness. He stated that the difficulties had set in after an acute injury to the part. About 2 years after the onset of his complaints, a synovectomy was done, and the resected specimen is illustrated in Figure 177-*C*.

*C*, Roentgenograph showing a shoulder joint which contains numerous discrete rounded radiopaque bodies. These are also present in the various recesses of the joint. The patient was a woman 32 years of age whose complaints were of 6 years' standing and consisted mainly of repeated intermittent attacks of local pain, of short duration. At the surgical intervention, the joint bodies were removed, along with a good deal of synovial membrane. Both grossly and microscopically, the membrane failed to reveal cartilaginous metaplasia, though it did show a moderate degree of villous hypertrophy. When sectioned, many of the bodies were found to be entirely cartilaginous (though their cores were calcified), while other bodies had cores of osseous tissue. Since the synovial membrane failed to show any evidence of cartilage formation, this case should not be interpreted as a true example of synovial chondromatosis. Indeed, it is one of those cases, not uncommon, in which it is difficult to find an adequate explanation for the formation of joint bodies.

*D*, Roentgenograph of a hip joint whose distended articular capsule is crowded with closely set radiopaque bodies representing so-called joint mice. The patient was a man 29 years of age whose lower limbs had been paralyzed since early childhood in consequence of poliomyelitis. His recent complaints relating to the hip were of 2 years' standing and consisted mainly of repeated attacks of pain, associated with increased limitation of motion. When the joint was explored, it revealed not only hundreds of cartilaginous bodies, but also extensive fibrillization and roughening of its articular cartilages. The synovial membrane was thickened and congested and somewhat villously hypertrophied, but presented no gross or microscopic evidence of intramembranous cartilage formation. Microscopic examination of the articular cartilage removed from the joint revealed that innumerable fragments of cartilage had been separating off from its articular surface. The joint bodies had undoubtedly formed out of the bits of sheared off cartilage, which had continued to grow in the joint space, being nourished by the synovial fluid. Thus, this case again should not be interpreted as an example of synovial chondromatosis. Instead, it represents an instance of the development of joint bodies in consequence of degenerative changes occurring in the articular cartilages. These changes may have been initiated by the numerous manipulations and surgical interventions to which the hip had been subjected. These were carried out at various times before the patient was 9 years old, presumably as palliative procedures in connection with the postpoliomyelitic paralysis.

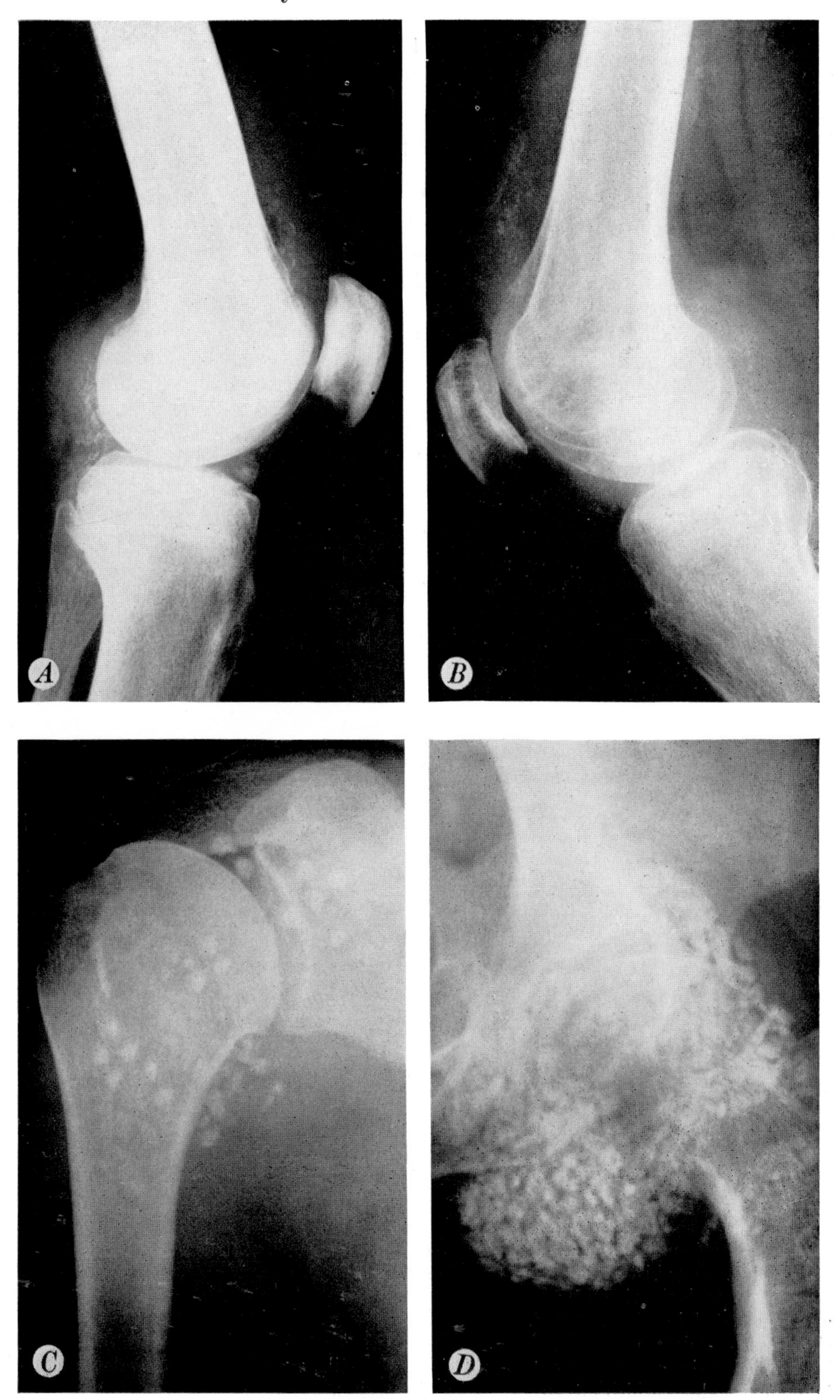


*Figure 176*

beneath its thin lining layer. The amount and distribution of the lesional cartilage are likely to vary among the specimens. For instance, in one lesion the gross picture may be dominated by large clusters of cartilaginous nodules protruding here and there from the surface of the membrane or even hanging from it by stalks. Other parts of the same specimen may show the lesional cartilage in the form of discrete flat nodules 3 or 4 mm. in diameter, and many very minute nodules may be found scattered over the surface of the rest of the membrane. In another lesion the conspicuous feature may be the presence of discrete but closely set cartilage nodules measuring up to 4 or 5 mm. in diameter and studding almost the entire synovium. However, these may be so numerous and so closely agglomerated in some places that they produce locally the effect of an almost solid, broadly based mass of cartilage rising from the surface of the synovium. On the other hand, in a case in which the involvement of the synovial membrane is less extensive, one may observe only a few cartilage nodules imbedded in the synovium or pendent from it.

Be that as it may, the lesional cartilage feels firm and appears hyaline on the whole. However, if the cartilage is cut through in various places, it is likely to show areas in which the tissue is whitish and gritty on account of calcification. Here and there one may also find spotty and even fairly large areas in which the lesional cartilage has apparently been undergoing replacement by osseous tissue. The extent to which calcification and ossification are going on in the lesional tissue is, of course, best demonstrated if one roentgenographs the specimen and also submits portions of it to histologic examination. (See Fig. 177.)

As noted, variable amounts of cartilage are also found in the articular cavity of the affected joint. In one case or another, the major joint space and its recesses may contain hundreds of small molded cartilage bodies. Or one may find relatively few of such small cartilage fragments, along with some larger cartilage masses composed of clustered nodules which likewise had their origin in the membrane. In still other instances, the joint cavity may show, in addition or even alone, one or several ossified cartilaginous bodies which may measure as much as 1 or 2 cm. in greatest dimension.

**Microscopic Pathology.**—It is generally held that the cartilage which develops in the synovial membrane in a case of synovial chondromatosis results from metaplasia of the sublining connective tissue of the membrane. In support of this idea it should be recalled that the synovial membrane is derived from the same portion

***Figure 177***

*A*, Photograph illustrating the gross appearance of the resected synovial membrane of a knee joint which was the site of synovial chondromatosis. Note the large clusters of cartilage nodules protruding and hanging from the synovial membrane. In addition, one can see numerous tiny and somewhat larger flat nodules of cartilage in the sublining layer of the membrane. The patient was a woman 37 years of age whose complaints were of 4 years' standing and consisted principally of pain and recurrent attacks of locking of the joint.

*B*, Roentgenograph (enlarged 2 ×) of a thin slice of tissue cut from the specimen of synovial chondromatosis illustrated in *C*. The tissue slice was roentgenographed on end, so that the upper margin of the picture represents the superficial aspect of the thickened membrane. In addition to the densely radiopaque foci (representing lesional cartilage which is undergoing calcification and ossification), one can see fainter roundish cartilage foci which are not so modified. (For histologic details, see Figure 178.)

*C*, Photograph showing the gross appearance of the resected synovial membrane from the case illustrated in Figure 176-*B*. The surface of the synovium shows numerous small, closely set nodules on both the right- and left-hand sides of the picture. The central area is occupied mainly by a crescent-shaped ridge of cartilage made up of a great number of individual nodules which are compressed and merging.

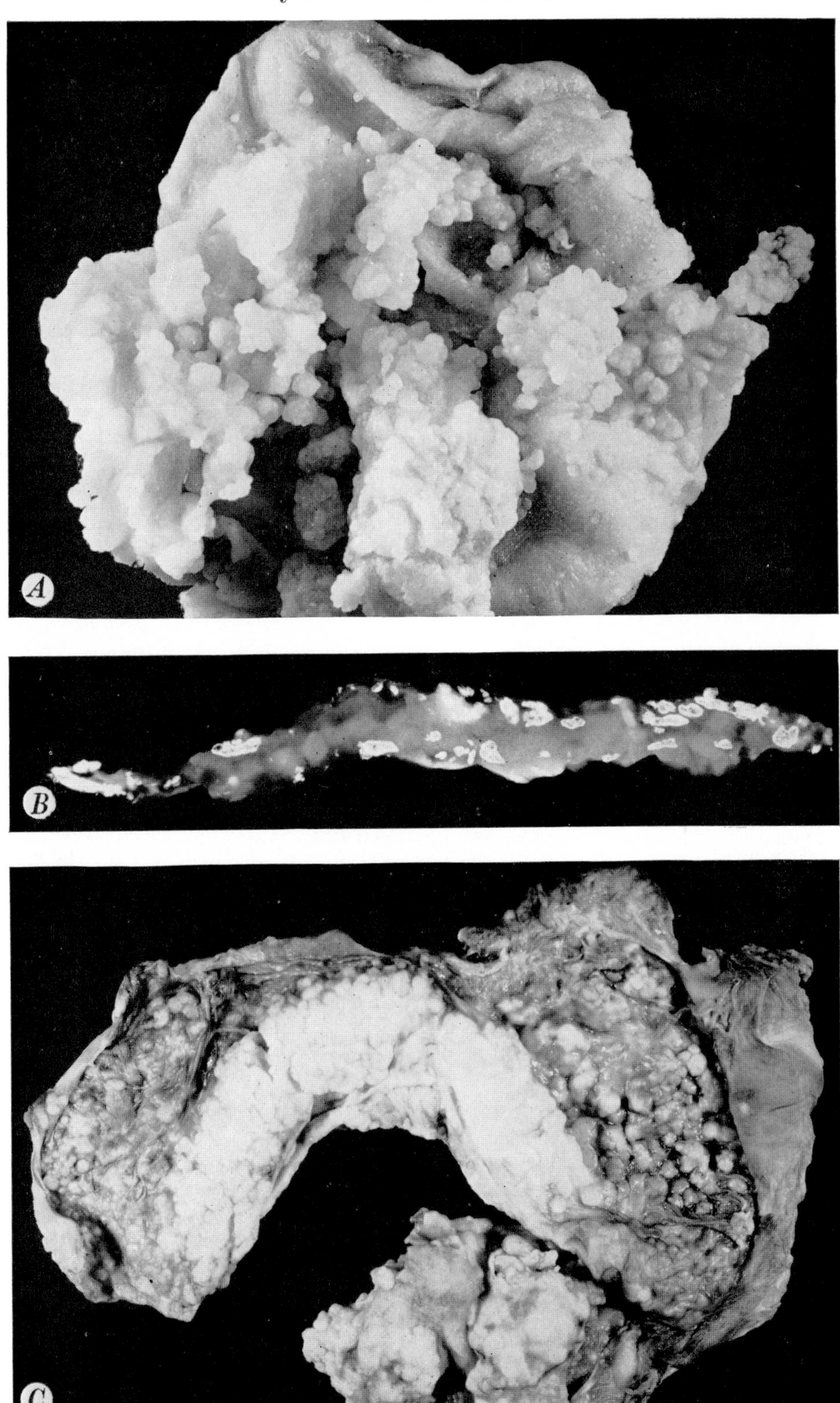


*Figure 177*

of the mesenchyme that gives rise to the bones (*i.e.*, the skeletogenic mesenchyme). Indeed, in some lower animal forms, the synovial membrane of the knee joint, for instance, contains considerable cartilage normally (see Lubosch). However, in cases of synovial chondromatosis, concrete histologic evidence of cartilaginous metaplasia of the synovial connective tissue usually has to be searched for, even when the specimen represents the condition in florid form. If one examines many sections prepared from different areas of such a lesion, one will encounter, here and there, a nest of connective-tissue cells which are swelling and apparently undergoing transformation into cartilage. Once cartilage formation has been initiated at a given site, increase in size of the cartilage focus results from multiplication of the cartilage cells and not from cartilage accretion by further metaplasia of the surrounding connective tissue.

The growing nodules of cartilage compress the neighboring connective tissue, so that they appear surrounded by fibrous capsules. Those cartilage nodules which have not as yet become calcified or ossified are often richly cellular. Also in line with the fact that such nodules represent actively growing foci of cartilage is the presence of a fair number of cartilage cells with double nuclei. Some of the nuclei may be plump, but cells with bizarre nuclei are not to be observed. Altogether, these findings in regard to the cell nuclei in synovial chondromatosis are not to be viewed as early stigmata of chondrosarcoma, as they might have to be if noted in relation to a central cartilaginous lesion of bone which has taken on a spurt of growth. That is, in connection with synovial chondromatosis it is well to remember that the presence of plumpish nuclei and of more than an occasional cell with a double nucleus indicates merely that the cartilage area in question is actively growing.

The cartilage foci which are undergoing calcification show more or less heavy incrustation of the cartilage matrix with granules of calcium. Heavy calcification of a focus of cartilage is usually a forerunner of ossification of the area in question. A prerequisite of ossification appears to be invasion of the calcified area by blood vessels. These apparently bring in osteoblasts on their walls, layers of lamellar bone are deposited, and bone is substituted for the calcified cartilage by the process of creeping replacement. In the interior of an ossific focus which has substantially replaced a focus of calcified cartilage, one may even find fatty marrow. (See Fig. 178.)

Mention has already been made of the fact that, in an area in which the cartilage is growing actively, many cells with plump nuclei and double nuclei are often to be observed. However, such findings should not lead to the conclusion that such an area is undergoing sarcomatous transformation. It is, of course, theoretically conceivable that a chondrosarcoma might evolve in a synovial membrane which is the

***Figure 178***

*A*, Photomicrograph (× 20) illustrating the histologic pattern presented by tissue from the specimen shown in Figure 177-*C*. Note the numerous discrete but closely set nodules of cartilage, some of which are still uncalcified while others are calcified and even being replaced by osseous tissue. Some of the cartilage foci show dark staining of their matrix with hematoxylin. This alteration in staining reflects a physicochemical change which precedes calcification of the matrix. The histologic details presented by the two nodules in the lower part of the picture, to the right of the center, are illustrated in *B*.

*B*, Photomicrograph (× 65) showing, above, a cartilage nodule which had become heavily encrusted with calcium and then invaded by blood vessels. One can see that osseous tissue is being laid down about the blood vessels and is replacing the calcified cartilage. Below this partly calcified and ossified nodule there is one which is still uncalcified. In that nodule the cartilage is rather cellular, and the nodule is surrounded by a layer of condensed connective tissue.

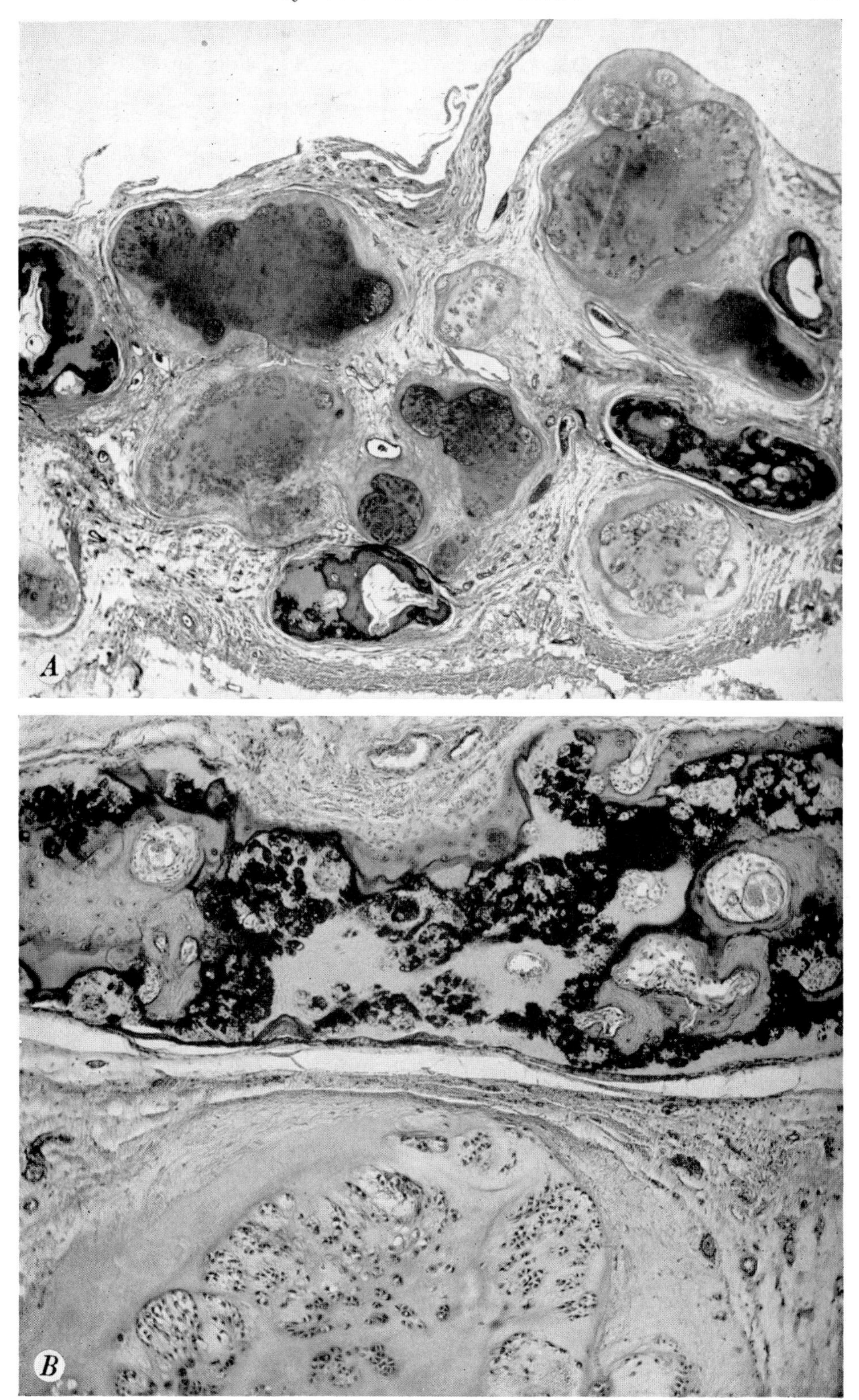


*Figure 178*

site of chondromatosis. However, the writer's personal experience includes no case in which this happened. Indeed, the only instances in which he has seen chondrosarcomatous involvement of the synovium at all were cases in which a chondrosarcoma had invaded the joint cavity and seeded itself in the synovium. One of these instances is represented by the large soft-tissue chondrosarcoma of the knee area which is illustrated in Figures 163-*C* and *D*.

### TREATMENT

The treatment consists in principle of clearing the joint of its free bodies and removing the affected synovium. In considering how much of the synovium should be excised, it should be borne in mind that any remaining synovium constitutes a possible source of new bodies, and the synovectomy should therefore be as nearly complete as possible. As to the free bodies, it is not unusual to find, from postoperative roentgenographs, that some still remain, although it had been thought that all had been removed. The remaining ones are such as had been concealed in some articular recess inaccessible through the surgical incision made. However, cases have been reported in which bodies not removed have decreased in size and even disappeared.

If, in a case suspected of representing synovial chondromatosis, the synovial membrane does not show any areas of cartilaginous or osteocartilaginous transformation, it will be sufficient to remove the bodies from the articular cavity unless the synovium is found abnormal in some other respect. As already indicated, such cases do not represent actual instances of synovial chondromatosis, and not infrequently the basis for the formation of the joint bodies remains obscure. On the other hand, the case may be one in which the joint bodies are ascribable to the presence of an osteoarthritis, associated with thickening and villous hypertrophy of the synovial membrane. In such an instance, the decision about the details of the surgical intervention has to be guided by that diagnosis.

## BURSAL AND TENOSYNOVIAL CHONDROMATOSIS

In analogy with articular chondromatosis, the terms *bursal* and *tenosynovial chondromatosis* are strictly applicable only to those cases in which the lining of the affected bursa or tendon sheath is itself the site of formation of cartilaginous or osteocartilaginous bodies. On this basis, instances of *exostosis bursata* with free cartilaginous or osteocartilaginous bodies in the bursal cavity should not be included in the category of bursal chondromatosis unless it can be established that the bodies had their origin in the bursal wall which had developed over an exostosis. Unquestionable instances of both tenosynovial and bursal chondromatosis (that is, cases meeting the indicated requirement as to pathogenesis) are certainly rare.

A clear-cut case of tenosynovial chondromatosis was described by Albertini. The site of the lesion was a tendon sheath on the back of a wrist. The sheath was hypertrophied and contained imbedded cartilage bodies, and many free cartilage bodies were also present in the space bordered by the sheath. The present writer, too, has observed a case in point. The site of the lesion was a tendon sheath compartment over the radiocarpal articulation. The lining of the sheath presented 3 cartilaginous bodies hanging from it by pedicles. An instance of chondromatosis involving a metacarpophalangeal joint is described by Lindén.

A case of bursal chondromatosis in which the lesion was in an ileopectineal bursa was described by Lehner. The affected bursal wall showed cartilaginous bodies, some of which had become ossified, and the bursal cavity contained many rice-sized cartilaginous bodies. An instance in which the lesion had developed in a popliteal bursa was described by Zadek, and the present writer had examined the lesional tissue in that case. The popliteal bursa in question did not communicate with the knee joint, and the synovial membrane and articular cavity of the knee showed nothing remarkable. A pertinent case again involving a popliteal bursa is reported by Hautkappe.

## INTRACAPSULAR AND PARA-ARTICULAR CHONDROMA

The connective tissue of the outer or fibrous coat of the capsule of a joint and/or the connective tissue in the vicinity of the capsule is occasionally the site of cartilaginous metaplasia. The resultant *intracapsular* or *para-articular chondromas* vary in size. Those which develop in the vicinity of small joints are usually not more than 1 or 2 cm. in their largest dimension. However, those which evolve in relation to a large joint (usually a knee joint) may measure as much as 5 cm. or more in their greatest dimension.

The subject is likely to be a young adult. More often than not, there is no history of trauma. The clinical complaints are generally of some months' or even of several years' standing and often amount only to awareness of a local tissue mass, some local discomfort, and perhaps some limitation of motion.

In one of several cases studied by the writer, there was a slowly enlarging mass in the knee area. At the surgical intervention the lesional tissue was found to be entirely extracapsular. It had displaced the patella but was not attached to the latter. The extirpated tumor mass measured 6 cm. in its greatest dimension and was surrounded by connective tissue which was thick and collagenous in some places. When cut open, it was found to be composed of foci of cartilage showing areas of ossification. On microscopic examination it could be noted that it was where the lesional cartilage had become vascularized that this ossification was taking place.

In another case in point, the extracapsular mass was located on the medial side of the patellar ligament. The extirpated specimen measured 7 cm. in its largest dimension, and it was also encapsulated by fibrous tissue. On gross section, the tumor mass was found to consist of rather closely set foci of cartilage. Some of these showed no evidences of ossification, while others had been largely replaced by osseous tissue through the process of endochondral ossification. (See Fig. 179.)

Whether located in or adjacent to the capsule, the lesional cartilage may become substantially or completely ossified in the course of time. The cases of capsular osteoma of the knee joint described by Kautz are apparently instances of this kind. A case in which a large osseous mass apparently representing a chondroma which had developed in the infrapatellar fat pad and had become ossified was described by Roth. The writer too has seen a relevant case.

## HEMANGIOMA OF JOINTS

Occasionally a joint is the site of a *hemangioma,* and it is nearly always a knee joint that is affected in such cases. The involvement may be limited to the synovial membrane, but often includes also the outer or fibroligamentous layer of the joint capsule, and may perhaps even be restricted to that part of the capsule. In cases in which the capsular apparatus as a whole is more or less affected, it is not unusual also to find hemangiomatous involvement of the regional soft tissues. Indeed, in such cases the regional bones, too, may be affected in one way or another.

## CLINICAL CONSIDERATIONS

Hemangioma involving articular capsules is by no means common. Indeed, the pertinent literature to 1958 seems to include only about 50 cases (see Bennett and Cobey, Jacobs and Lee, and Lewis *et al.*). Furthermore, as already implied, it is only rarely that an articular hemangioma appears elsewhere than in a knee joint. As to age incidence, many of the subjects are adolescents or young adults at the time when the condition is first diagnosed. However, in such subjects, a clinical history of difficulty dating back to early or middle childhood is often obtained. This early onset of the manifestations of articular hemangioma is in harmony with the idea that the most plausible basis for the condition is a local congenital vascular malformation. It is true that some of the patients give a history of antecedent and supposedly causal trauma. However, the latter probably only stimulates the evolution of a condition that was already present or merely calls attention to it.

A knee joint which is the site of a capsular hemangioma is more or less enlarged and may show some limitation of motion. The subject is likely to report that the affected joint is somewhat painful under ordinary use. In addition, one may elicit a history of intermittent attacks of sharp pain in the joint, accompanied by acute swelling. Not infrequently, such an attack is precipitated by an acute trauma to the joint. Palpation of an affected joint which is not acutely painful and swollen often reveals the presence of an elastic mass which tends to diminish in size if the extremity is elevated. Tenderness, usually limited to the region of the palpable mass, is also present. Puncture of the joint may release variable amounts of hemorrhagically discolored fluid.

*X*-ray examination of the affected knee is often not of much help in the establishment of the diagnosis. In particular, especially in a young subject, the contour of the bones entering into the formation of the joint is not likely to be found modified. On the positive side, the *x*-ray picture may reveal a vague soft-tissue shadow in the region of the affected joint, but this is an ambiguous finding unless the soft-tissue mass shows radiopacities representing phleboliths in the vascular channels of the lesional tissue. However, phleboliths are rarely encountered in connection with hemangiomas of articular capsules unless there is concomitant angiomatous involvement of the musculature and other soft parts overlying the joint in question. Indeed,

### *Figure 179*

*A*, Roentgenograph of a knee area showing a para-articular tumor which had developed outside of the fibrous capsule of the joint, just to the medial side of the patellar ligament. The lesional tissue was found to consist of a number of agglomerated foci of cartilage, many of which were in the process of ossification (see *B* and *C*). The patient was a woman 37 years of age whose chief complaint was pain in the knee, particularly after exercise. She dated the onset of her pain to an injury sustained 3 years previously, but stated that the knee had also been injured 6 years and 17 years before then. Since the complaints dated only from the most recent injury, it seems reasonable to doubt the importance of trauma in the causation of the condition. During the surgical removal of the lesion, the capsule of the joint was opened, and the synovial membrane and articular cartilages were inspected and found to present nothing remarkable.

*B*, Photograph (slightly enlarged) showing the appearance of the extirpated tumor mass after it had been cut open. It is composed of small and large clearly delimited foci of cartilage which are imbedded in edematous connective tissue.

*C*, Photomicrograph (× 4) illustrating the pattern of the lesional tissue. Some of the foci of cartilage are still uncalcified; others show calcified cores without ossification; and still others can be seen to have undergone almost complete replacement (proceeding centrifugally) by osseous tissue containing bone marrow.

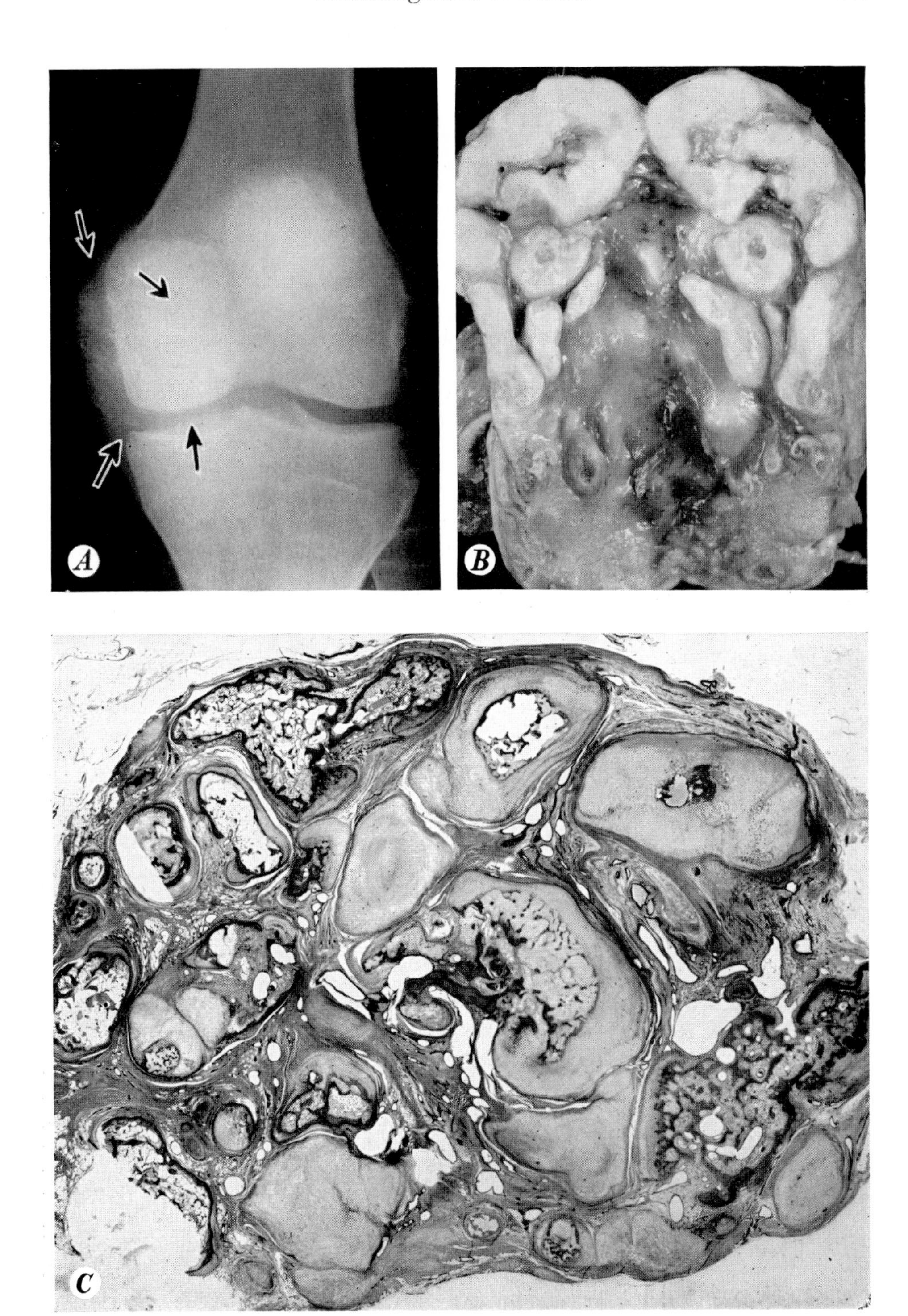


*Figure 179*

a capsular hemangioma may easily go unrecognized clinically unless a cue is offered through the detection of phleboliths or through the suggestive finding of angiomata in the skin, locally or elsewhere.

## PATHOLOGIC FINDINGS

Anatomically, hemangiomas of joints are of two types—circumscribed and diffuse. The circumscribed lesions may be stalked or sessile. A common site for them is the infrapatellar fat pad, although they may be located elsewhere. The pedunculated lesion described by Osgood was a reddish encapsulated tumor measuring $8 \times 3 \times 1\frac{1}{2}$ cm. and was attached to the infrapatellar fat pad. However, most of the stalked hemangiomas are smaller than this. The localized sessile hemangiomas are also usually of small size.

The lesions described as representing diffuse hemangiomatous involvement of the synovium sometimes raise problems of anatomic interpretation. Reichel and Nauwerck describe a lesion involving a knee joint in which the synovium showed brownish red discoloration and was studded by papillary polypoid projections. It may well be that this case and some of the other cases which have been placed in the category of diffuse hemangioma actually represent instances of diffuse pigmented villonodular synovitis (see p. 534). However, there are other cases in the literature which are so clear-cut that their interpretation as instances of articular hemangioma presents no problem. (See Fig. 180.) In one such case or another, the synovium of the joint is found more or less completely permeated by large masses of dark red vascular tissue presenting dilated intertwining blood channels. In other instances, not only the synovium but also the fibroligamentous part of the capsule, the muscles, and other soft parts in the region present this appearance (see Brodsky). In instances of such extensive involvement, the articular bone ends, too, may be affected (see Haas).

If the hemangioma is of the diffuse type, and particularly if it is associated with hemangiomatous involvement of the soft tissues about the joint, the *microscopic pattern* of the tissue removed from the joint is likely to be that of a so-called venous angioma. The prominent feature of this pattern is the presence of numerous dilated and tortuous vascular channels with moderately thick walls containing

### *Figure 180*

*A*, Roentgenograph showing the knee area of a child who was found to have diffuse hemangiomatous involvement of the capsule of the joint, associated with hemangiomatosis of the soft tissues of the extremity in question (see *B*). There is some suggestive swelling of the soft tissues in the region of the joint, but in view of the absence of phleboliths in the lesional tissue, the *x*-ray picture is not helpful in establishing the diagnosis. The patient was a boy 7 years of age who had had difficulty with the knee in question from the age of 3. In particular, there was a history of recurrent attacks of pain and swelling of the knee, usually ensuing upon mild trauma and relieved by some days of bed rest. Though the *x*-ray findings yielded no clue to the diagnosis, the latter was suggested by the fact that from very early childhood the skin on the outer aspect of the leg had presented blotchy bluish discoloration.

*B*, Photograph revealing the exposed joint area as it appeared in the course of the surgical intervention. Note the extensive hemangiomatous involvement of the synovial membrane, joint capsule, and local musculature.

*C*, Photomicrograph (× 65) showing the histologic appearance presented by the resected synovium. The pattern is that of a so-called venous hemangioma, being characterized by the presence of tortuous vascular channels with moderately thick walls. (The illustrative material in this case was supplied by Dr. Alexander E. Brodsky of Houston, Texas.)

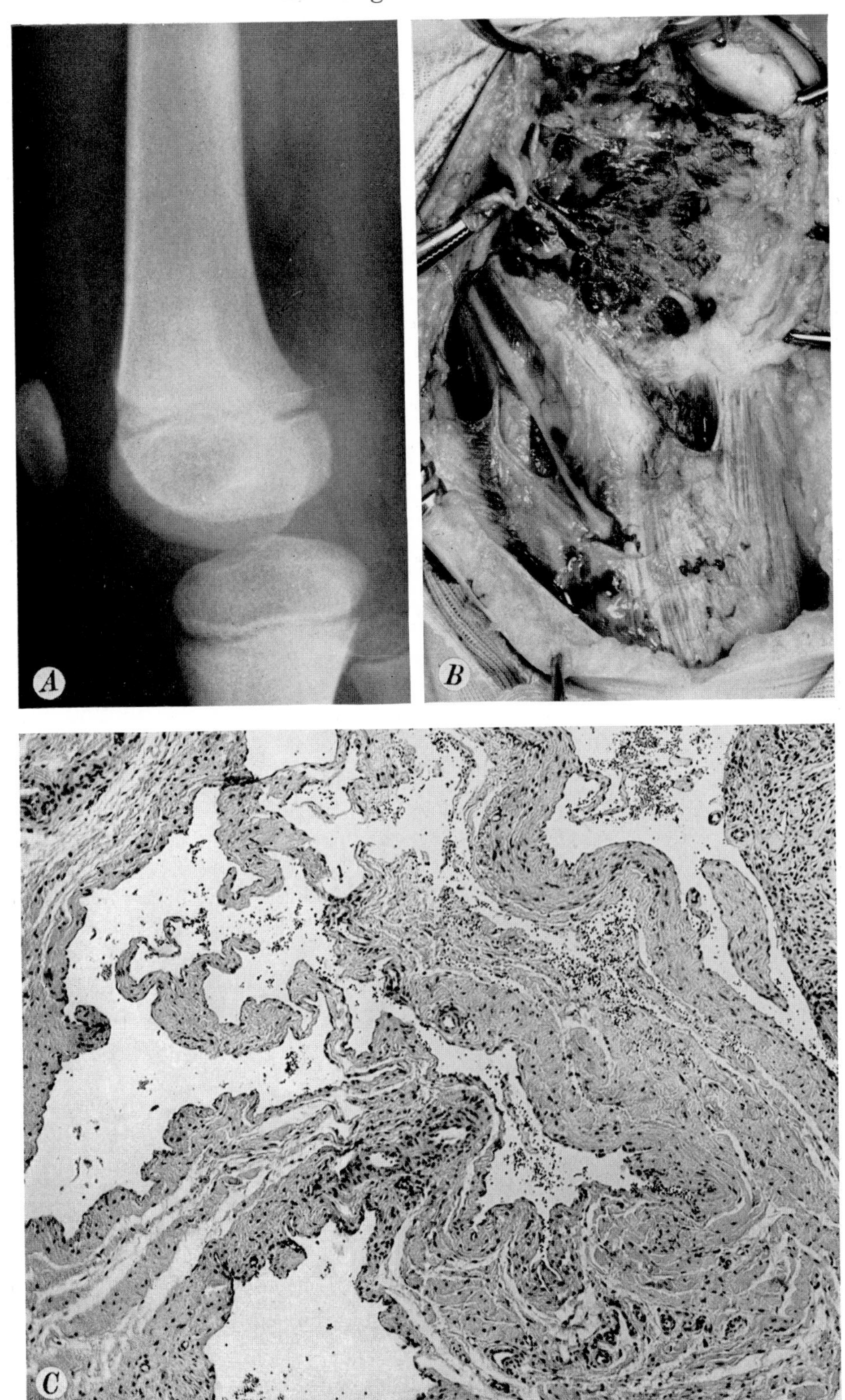

*Figure 180*

smooth muscle cells in variable amounts. On the other hand, if the lesion is of the circumscribed type, the histologic pattern is likely to be that of the so-called capillary and/or cavernous hemangioma. That is, the lesional tissue will be found composed of small, thin-walled capillaries distributed irregularly through the tissue (capillary hemangioma), or the thin-walled vascular channels may be widely dilated (cavernous hemangioma). Within a particular specimen, however, some of the capillaries may be small and others widely dilated.

### TREATMENT

If the surgeon enters the joint and finds a circumscribed (pedunculated or sessile) hemangioma, the procedure indicated is local excision of the lesion, giving it a wide berth. If this is carried out, there is little likelihood of recurrence. If the case is one of diffuse involvement, the difficulty of eradicating the lesional tissue completely favors recurrence of the lesion. If the regional soft tissues are involved in addition to the articular capsule, the likelihood of recurrence is, of course, increased. In cases in which complete excision of the lesional tissue has not been possible, recurrence may take place even if the surgical intervention has been supplemented by *x*-ray therapy. Finally, it is worth noting in connection with treatment and prognosis that there seems to be no recorded instance in which a capsular hemangioma has undergone spontaneous malignant transformation.

## HEMANGIOMA OF TENDON SHEATHS

Occasionally a tendon sheath is the site of a hemangioma. The lesion may be confined to the sheath, but sometimes involves the peritendinous fat and local muscles and may even implicate the tendon itself (see Burman and Milgram, and Harkins). The most common sites for tendon sheath hemangioma are the forearm (near the wrist) and the leg and foot (near the ankle). The subjects are likely to state that a trauma has either instigated the development of the lesion or accelerated its growth. The condition is rarely diagnosed clinically. However, reduction in size of the lesion when the limb is elevated is a highly suggestive finding, and the observation of phleboliths in the *x*-ray picture is strongly confirmative. If the lesion cannot be completely excised at the surgical intervention, *x*-ray treatment may shrink or obliterate such lesional tissue as remains. (See Fig. 181.)

***Figure 181***

*A*, Photograph showing a swelling on the dorsum of a hand and wrist, due to hemangiomatous involvement of the extensor tendon sheaths. The patient was a woman 36 years of age, and the local mass, which had been present for about a year, had gradually been increasing in size. Its presence was associated with some pain and limitation of motion. At the time when this picture was taken, the lesional area measured 4.5 cm. in diameter and about 2 cm. in thickness, and the mass was soft and somewhat fluctuant. At operation, the surgeon encountered a reddish vascular tumor which surrounded the local extensor tendons. The hemangioma was excised, and follow-up examination 2½ years later failed to reveal evidence of recurrence. (The clinical history and photograph in this case were supplied by Dr. Herbert Sandick of Pittsfield, Massachusetts.)

*B*, Photomicrograph (× 65) showing the histologic pattern of the lesional tissue from the case illustrated in *A*. The thickened tendon sheath is permeated by numerous dilated capillaries which are engorged with red blood cells, the pattern being that of a capillary hemangioma.

*C*, Photomicrograph (× 65) showing the pattern of a cavernous hemangioma presented by a tendon sheath hemangioma in another case. Note the extremely dilated, thin-walled, and engorged capillaries.

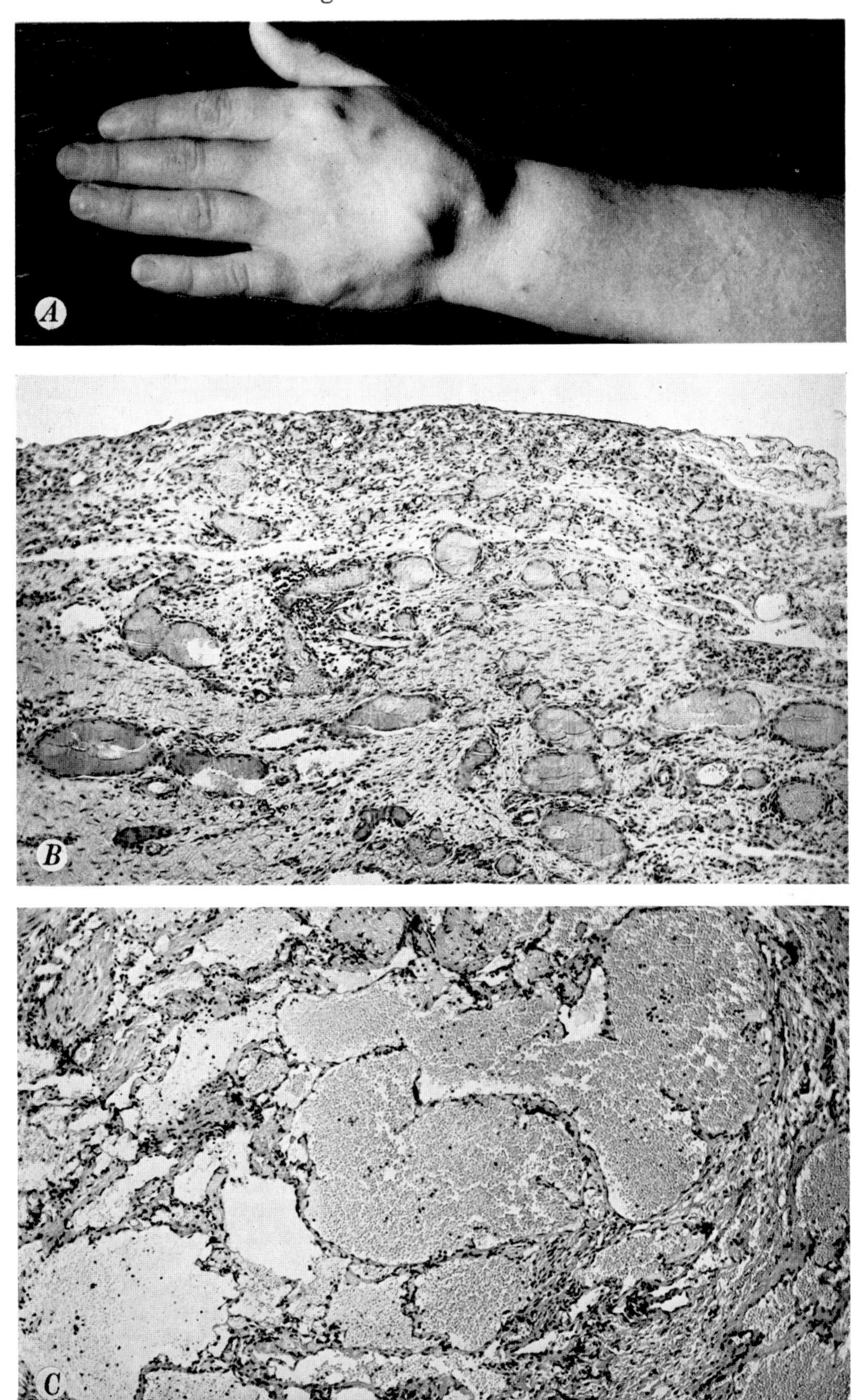


*Figure 181*

## LIPOMA AND FIBROMA OF ARTICULAR CAPSULES

**Lipoma.**—A lipoma—that is, a well circumscribed benign tumor composed of mature adipose tissue—is of rare occurrence as a primary lesion of an articular capsule. Of course, one must exclude from the category of articular lipoma the condition unfortunately named "lipoma arborescens" of the synovium. The latter represents merely a coarsely villous and/or polypoid synovial proliferation which may be circumscribed or diffuse and which appears in response to chronic irritation of the synovial membrane. Some cases of "lipoma arborescens" of tendon sheaths and even of bursae mucosae have also been described, but such lesions too represent merely inflammatory proliferations of the lining of the structures in question. Furthermore, the so-called Hoffa's disease, which has sometimes also been loosely interpreted as an expression of capsular lipoma, should likewise be excluded from that category. Hoffa himself defined that condition as a traumatic-inflammatory hypertrophy of the subsynovial fat normally present in the region of the patellar ligament. Confusion with primary capsular lipoma might also arise in a case in which a lipoma developing in the soft tissues about a large joint has extended through the capsule into the articular cavity (see Schwartz, and Metzler).

In almost all of the relatively few acceptable cases of capsular lipoma which have been reported, the lesion was in the knee joint. There the lipoma is likely to take its origin from the subsynovial fat on either side of the patellar ligament or on the anterior surface of the femur. The lesion is usually small (seldom exceeding the size of a hen's egg) and may even be stalked. A stalked lipoma may become strangulated through twisting of the pedicle (see Diamant-Berger). In a case of capsular lipoma seen by the present writer, the lesion was attached to the synovium in the region of the anterior horn of the medial meniscus, and it presented in the joint as a lobulated tumor mass measuring 6 × 4 × 2 cm. The patient was a woman 52 years of age who had been aware for a number of years that the knee was swollen, but who entered the hospital on account of acute pain and swelling apparently due to jamming of the lipoma between the articular bone ends. The nature of the condition was recognized only when the joint was explored, and this was also what happened in the other cases of capsular lipoma reported in the literature.

**Fibroma.**—As already indicated, the older literature contains some references to cases of fibroma of joints (see Robson, Sonntag, and also Kott). In the light of present knowledge, most of the cases reported as instances of synovial fibroma seem to be interpretable rather as localized expressions of pigmented villonodular synovitis (p. 545). The confusion is created by the fact that these nodular synovial lesions have undergone a certain amount of fibrous scarring in consequence of interference with their blood supply, through compression of the lesional tissue between the articular bone ends. Similarly, most of the cases reported under the heading of tenosynovial fibroma are not true examples of fibrous tumors of tendon sheaths. Undoubtedly they represent cases of localized nodular tenosynovitis (p. 549) in which the lesional tissue has become highly scarified and collagenized. Indeed, the ultimate form of such lesions is often that of a small, hard, fibrous nodule in which multinuclear giant cells and polyhedral stromal cells are no longer evident as they are in the earlier stages of development of the lesion in question.

### REFERENCES

von Albertini, A.: Demonstration eines seltenen Falles von Chondromatose der Sehnenscheide, Schweiz. med. Wchnschr., *66*, 82, 1936.

Beckman, T., and Ivarsson, G: Uber sogenannte Chondromatose der Gelenkkapsel, Acta chir. scandinav., *63*, 551, 1928.

Bennett, G. E., and Cobey, M. C.: Hemangioma of Joints, Arch. Surg., *38*, 487, 1939.
Brodsky, A. E.: Synovial Hemangioma of the Knee Joint, Bull. Hosp. Joint Dis., *17*, 58, 1956.
Burman, M. S., and Milgram, J. E.: Haemangioma of Tendon and Tendon Sheath, Surg., Gynec. & Obst., *50*, 397, 1930.
Diamant-Berger, L.: Un cas de volvulus d'un lipome pédiculé intra-articulaire du genou, Bull. et mém. Soc. nat. de chir., *56*, 744, 1930.
Fisher, A. G. T.: A Study of Loose Bodies composed of Cartilage or of Cartilage and Bone occurring in Joints. With Special Reference to their Pathology and Etiology, Brit. J. Surg., *8*, 493, 1920–21.
Freund, E.: Chondromatosis of the Joints, Arch. Surg., *34*, 670, 1937.
Haas, A.: Über Gefässtumoren der Kniegelenkkapsel, Deutsche Ztschr. f. Chir., *173*, 130, 1922.
Harkins, H. N.: Hemangioma of a Tendon or Tendon Sheath, Arch. Surg., *34*, 12, 1937.
Hautkappe, W.: Über die seltene Lokalisation einer Chondromatose in einem Kniegelenksganglion, Zentralbl. f. Chir., *77*, 379, 1952.
Henderson, M. S., and Jones, H. T.: Loose Bodies in Joints and Bursae Due to Synovial Osteochondromatosis, J. Bone & Joint Surg., *21*, 400, 1923.
Hoffa, A.: Zur Bedeutung des Fettgewebes für die Pathologie des Kniegelenks, Deutsche med. Wchnschr., *30*, 337, 388, 1904.
Jacobs, J. E., and Lee, F. W.: Hemangioma of the Knee Joint, J. Bone & Joint Surg., *31-A*, 831, 1949.
Janker, R.: Über Chondromatose der Gelenkkapsel, Deutsche Ztschr. f. Chir., *211*, 135, 1928.
Jones, H. T.: The Histogenesis of Cartilage as Shown in Chondromatosis of the Knee Joint, J. Bone & Joint Surg., *25*, 310, 1927.
Kautz, F. G.: Capsular Osteoma of the Knee Joint, Radiology, *45*, 162, 1945.
Kott, B.: Eine seltene Geschwulst des Semilunarknorpels, Deutsche Ztschr. f. Chir., *202*, 406, 1927.
Lehner, A.: Zur Schleimbeutel- und Gelenkosteochondromatose, Schweiz. med. Wchnschr., *67*, 634, 1937.
Lewis, R. C., Jr., Coventry, M. B., and Soule, E. H.: Hemangioma of the Synovium. Presented at the meeting of American Academy of Orthopaedic Surgeons, February 6, 1958.
Leydig, S. M., and Odell, R. T.: Synovial Osteochondromatosis, Surg., Gynec. & Obst., *89*, 457, 1949.
Lindén, O.: Case of Chondromatosis of a Metacarpo-Phalangeal Joint, Acta chir. scandinav., *75*, 181, 1934.
Lubosch, W.: *Bau und Entstehung der Wirbeltiergelenke*, Jena, G. Fischer, 1910.
Metzler, F.: Über einen Fall von Gelenkslipom, Deutsche Ztschr. f. Chir., *196*, 326, 1926.
Osgood, R. B.: Angioma of the Knee-joint, S. Clin. North America, *1*, 681, 1921.
Phemister, D. B.: The Causes of and Changes in Loose Bodies Arising from the Articular Surface of the Joint, J. Bone & Joint Surg., *22*, 278, 1924.
Reichel, and Nauwerck, C.: Eine echte Zottengeschwulst (Angiofibrom) des Kniegelenks, Arch. f. klin. Chir., *95*, 899, 1911.
Rixford, E.: Osteochondromatosis, Ann. Surg., *92*, 673, 1930.
Robson, A. W. M.: A Case of Polypoid Growths in the Knee Joint; Removal, Lancet, *1*, 934, 1891.
Rostock, P.: Die Gelenkchondromatose, Beitr. z. klin. Chir., *144*, 58, 1928.
Roth, P. B.: Ossifying Chondroma Replacing the Infrapatellar Pad of Fat, Proc. Roy. Soc. Med., *37*, 279, 1944.
Schiltenwolf, K.: Über einen seltenen Fall von Schultergelenkschondrom, Zentralbl. f. Chir., *77*, 1274, 1952.
Schwartz,: Énorme lipomatose péri et intra-articulaire du genou, Bull. et mém. Soc. de chir. de Paris, *30*, 207, 1904.
Sonntag, E.: Fibromatöse Wucherung in der fibrösen Kniegelenkkapsel, Zentralbl. f. Chir., *51*, 515, 1924.
Suermondt, W. F.: Tumours of the Joint Capsule, Arch. chir. neerl., *2*, 278, 1950.
Zadek, I.: Osteochondromatosis of a Popliteal Bursa, Bull. Hosp. Joint Dis., *5*, 12, 1944.

Chapter

# 32

# Synovial Sarcoma and Other Malignant Articular Tumors

In this chapter we are concerned almost solely with the so-called *synovial sarcoma* (*synovioma*). It is a curious fact that, except for this tumor (which itself only rarely develops within a joint), there are no primary malignant tumors which may be considered indigenous to articular capsules, bursae, or tendon sheaths. Theoretically, a sarcoma of almost any of the recognized types might develop in one of these structures. Practically, however, it appears that such tumors hardly ever arise in them, and this has certainly been the writer's own experience. The contrary impression conveyed by the older literature is probably to be accounted for, at least in part, by the fact that lesions which would now be called synovial sarcomas had been misinterpreted as fibrosarcomas, reticulum cell sarcomas, malignant endotheliomas, etc.

On the other hand, there can be no doubt that one or another primary malignant tumor in the articular end of a bone sometimes extends into the joint and seeds itself in the synovial membrane. This can occasionally also happen in connection with one or another of the soft-tissue sarcomas developing in the immediate vicinity of a joint. Indeed, the only chondrosarcomas which the writer has seen in relation to joints were those which had either broken into the latter from an affected articular bone end or reached the joint space after having developed in the soft tissues and penetrated the joint capsule.

Furthermore, none of the benign hyperplasias or tumorous conditions which may affect the synovial lining of a joint or the lining of a bursa or tendon sheath (notably pigmented villonodular synovitis, synovial chondromatosis, and synovial hemangiomatosis) ever undergo malignant transformation.

## SYNOVIAL SARCOMA (SYNOVIOMA)

The *synovial sarcoma* (*synovioma*) is a highly malignant tumor which is generally encountered in the vicinity of a joint (most often a large one). Though these names imply that the tumor starts its development in the synovial lining of a joint capsule, this is only infrequently the case, as has already been mentioned. Indeed, it usually starts in the para-articular soft parts just beyond the confines of the capsule, though it may eventually penetrate the latter and invade the synovial membrane. However, in a case in which the membrane is found involved, it may be difficult to decide whether the tumor actually began its development there or whether the membrane became involved secondarily.

Bursae and tendon sheaths, too, are only rarely the actual site of origin of a synovial sarcoma. When the tumor appears in connection with them, the findings again usually indicate that it had invaded, rather than started in, the lining of the structure in question. Finally, it should be pointed out that a so-called synovial sarcoma has been known to develop even at a considerable distance from a joint—

for instance, in an intermuscular space. In such a case, of course, the tumor cannot be related at all to a pre-existing synovial structure—that is, the lining of a joint capsule, bursa, or tendon sheath.

All this raises questions about the *nature* of the lesion and about the matter of *terminology* in relation to it. The tumor presents a highly distinctive histologic pattern which may be more strikingly developed in some lesions (or parts of a lesion) than in others. The histologic feature which gives the tumor its special character is the presence of clefts and tubular spaces lined by cells capable of secreting a mucin-like substance. It is this trait that suggests a relationship of the lesional tissue to synovial lining structures. Indeed, one can account for the clefts and spaces, along with some of the other cytologic features of the lesion, on the basis that the tumor is derived from specialized connective tissue having the same potentialities for differentiation as the specialized mesenchyme which, in the course of skeletogenesis, gives rise to the synovial linings of joints.

Currently, the term favored for the lesion is "synovioma"—the name suggested by Smith. The term "synovial sarcoma" is also often employed, and frequently the two terms are used interchangeably, even in the same discussion. There are also those who speak of "malignant synovioma" because they wish to point up a contrast between that lesion and what they call "benign giant-cell synovioma" (see Wright). These so-called benign giant-cell synoviomas represent the pigmented villonodular synovial, bursal and tenosynovial lesions which are discussed in Chapter 30. These lesions are not tumors in the strict sense of the word, but represent inflammatory-hyperplastic proliferations. This fact and the ominous implication of the term "synovioma" in general suggest that one ought to avoid the term "benign synovioma" in any connection.

## CLINICAL CONSIDERATIONS

**Incidence and Localization.**—In respect to general incidence, the synovioma is still to be regarded as a rather uncommon tumor. However, it is not so rare as it was thought to be when its histologic features were less familiar and the lesion was more often confused with various other sarcomas. Thus, Haagensen and Stout, evaluating the relevant literature to 1944, found only 95 cases which they held to be acceptable, and they supplement these with 9 of their own. Since then, numerous additional reports have appeared, and those who discuss relatively large series of cases collected from the files of their own institutions include Bennett, Tillotson *et al.*, Pack and Ariel, and Wright. The writer's experience with the lesion comprises 14 cases, of which 4 were previously reported (see Jaffe and Lichtenstein).

As to age incidence, it is clear that a definite majority of the subjects are young adults. The rest are mainly adolescents or middle-aged adults, and very few are young children or old people. As to sex incidence, if either sex is predilected at all, it is the female.

In respect to location, a synovioma is much more likely to be encountered in a lower than in an upper limb. Indeed, on the basis of the collected literature, it appears that the preponderance of lower limb over upper limb involvement is about 4 to 1. However, in the cases covering the writer's own total experience, there was no such difference, the two parts being involved with equal frequency. In any event, if the lesion is in a lower extremity, its most common location by far is in the region of the knee, and particularly in the popliteal area. In an upper extremity, the lesion is encountered not infrequently at the elbow, but apparently more often in the region of the hand or wrist. The foot and ankle are also not uncommon sites for the synovioma.

**Clinical Complaints and Findings.**—The duration of complaints by the time surgical intervention is undertaken may be only a few months but is often 2 or 3 years or longer. Many of the subjects state that the first difficulty noted was gradually increasing pain at the affected site. Others may have become aware of a "lump" even

***Figure 182***

*A*, Roentgenograph of a knee in which the anterior compartment of the joint is the site of a lesion established as a synovioma on the basis of microscopic examination of the lesional tissue. Note the numerous small radiopacities in the globular soft-tissue mass. These were found to represent areas in which the tumor tissue had undergone focal necrosis, and the necrotic areas had become the site of calcium deposition. While the radiopacities might lead one to suspect a synovioma, they also suggest various other conditions, such as synovial hemangioma with phleboliths, and synovial chondromatosis. Furthermore, the intra-articular location of the lesion favors a diagnosis of one of these other conditions rather than of synovioma, since the latter only rarely starts within a joint. The patient was a girl 10 years of age whose difficulties relating to the knee were of $1\frac{1}{2}$ years' standing. These consisted of slight swelling of the knee, local tenderness, and pain sufficient to make her favor the limb in question. Since a synovioma was not suspected on clinical grounds, the initial surgical intervention was mere excision of the tumor mass. The diagnosis having been established, the limb was promptly amputated through the upper third of the thigh, and this procedure was followed by extensive dissection of the regional lymph nodes. Nevertheless, the patient died of metastases within a few months.

*B*, Roentgenograph showing a soft-tissue mass between the proximal phalanges of the first and second toes of a foot. The lesional mass, which has separated the toes considerably, shows a good deal of radiopacity. Note that there is no bone destruction or involvement of the regional metatarsophalangeal joints. The patient was a woman 28 years of age who had been aware for 2 years of a small mass between the toes in question. The mass was sensitive to touch but had caused her no other inconvenience until about 1 month before this picture was taken. At that time she began to complain of pain on walking, and increase in size of the mass began to make it difficult for her to put on her shoe. The initial surgical intervention consisted of excision of the tumor, which shelled out in one piece with great ease. The diagnosis of synovioma was then established on the basis of microscopic examination of the tumor tissue. An amputation was then done at the level of the lower third of the leg, and this procedure was followed by removal of the inguinal lymph nodes. Examination of the patient $7\frac{1}{2}$ years after the amputation showed her to be in good health and apparently cured.

*C*, Roentgenograph showing a large soft-tissue mass representing a synovioma in the region of the elbow. The tumor shadow, which is of water-clear density, is not lobulated. Note that, in this case, radiopacities are not present. The patient was a man 35 years of age who became aware of the lesion only 7 months before he died. He first sought advice because he had noted a small painless lump on the flexor surface of the elbow. Within 3 months, the tumor had grown to the large size shown in the picture, but its presence was still not associated with pain or limitation of motion. At this time, pulmonary metastases were already present, though the surgeon was not aware of that fact when he carried out a local excision of the tumor. The patient died 4 months later from metastases, which were mainly in the lungs.

*D*, Roentgenograph showing a synovioma, again in the region of the elbow. However, in this tumor a good deal of spotty radiopacity is present. On the basis of the *x*-ray picture, one might even suspect that the lesion was a soft-tissue chondrosarcoma rather than a synovioma. The patient was a woman 41 years of age whose tumor was of at least 4 years' standing when this picture was taken. Originally, she complained of tenderness in the region of the elbow, and a barely perceptible local swelling could be detected on physical examination. The *x*-ray picture showed several radiopacities in the region of the head of the radius. At that time the patient was advised to have the mass biopsied, but did not take the advice. During the intervening 4 years the tumor grew slowly, without causing much pain or interfering seriously with functioning of the elbow. Finally, the lesion did come to biopsy, and the diagnosis of synovioma was made. However, no further information is available in this case.

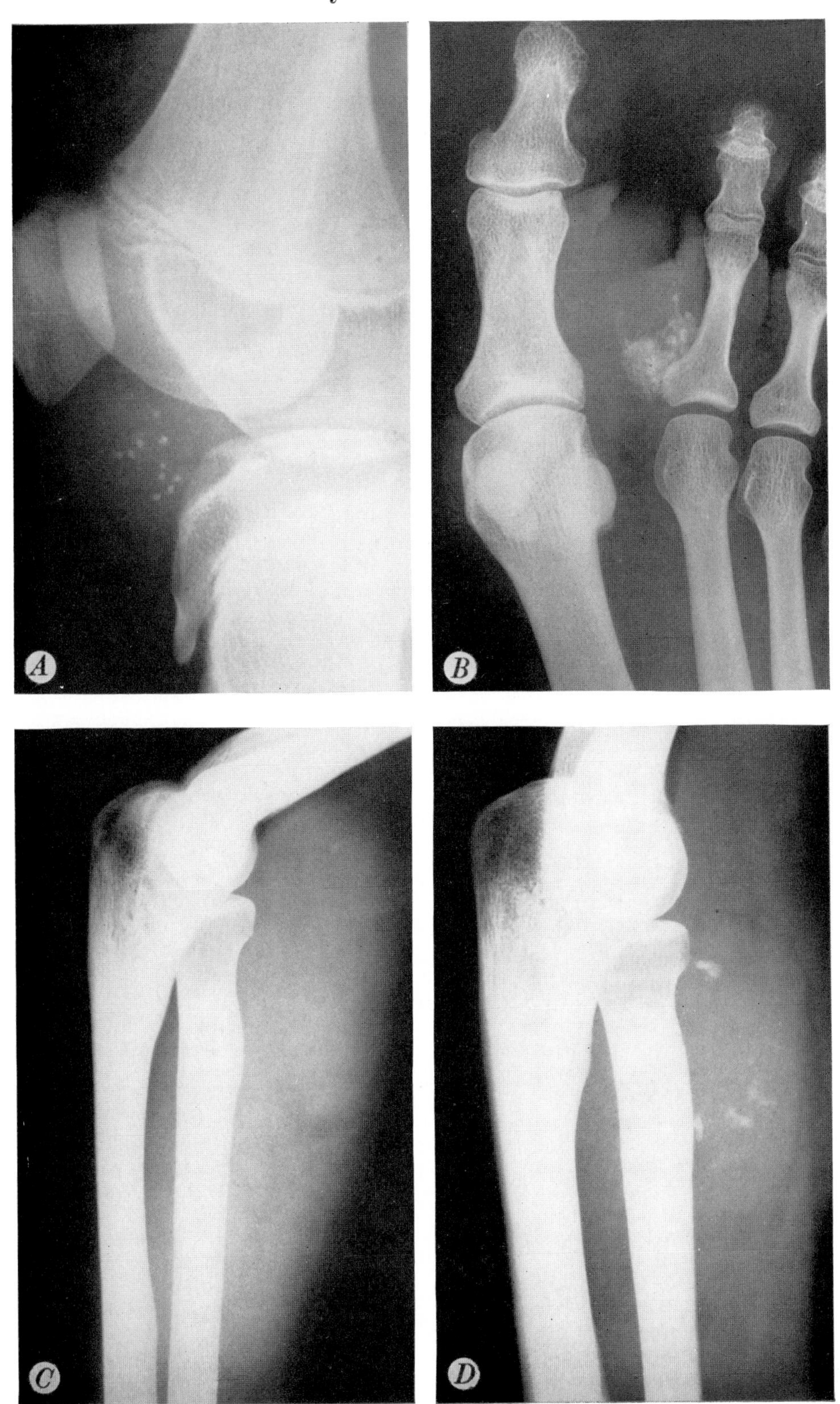


*Figure 182*

before the area became painful. The affected region is likely to be found somewhat enlarged and tender and to present a palpable mass. There may be some local heat and perhaps also some slight limitation of motion. Some of the patients give a history of antecedent trauma, but the proportion is so small that it is clear that trauma has no causal significance in relation to the lesion.

Only infrequently is the condition diagnosed before operation. However, the roentgenographic findings, properly evaluated in the light of the clinical history and notably the location of the lesion, may lead one to suspect the presence of a synovioma. The definitive diagnosis has to be based on microscopic examination of tissue from the lesion.

## ROENTGENOGRAPHIC FINDINGS

As has already been pointed out, a synovioma is usually found located in the vicinity of a joint but only rarely within a joint space proper. (See Fig. 182.) The para-articular orientation of the tumor is such that it generally makes contact with the joint capsule. The surface of contact of the tumor with the capsule stands out most clearly in relation to the knee joint, but is usually not extensive in any event. As to the joint itself, the *x*-ray picture is not likely to reveal any alteration in its bone contours or any fluid in the articular space. Indeed, a synovioma only rarely causes erosion of the bones in its vicinity or even periosteal new bone deposition (see Sherman and Chu).

The size of the soft-tissue mass representing the tumor may range from 2 or 3 cm. to 10 cm. or more in its greatest dimension. The mass is likely to be smaller if the tumor is in a foot or hand than if it is in a knee or elbow region. It is usually roundish or oval and is not likely to be lobulated. Its periphery may be distinguished from the neighboring soft tissues, but is not sharply outlined. The shadow cast by the tumor as a whole tends to be of water density and is often homogeneous. On the other hand, there are a good many cases in which the lesion shows spots of radiopacity here and there in its *x*-ray picture. Occasionally a lesion may even show a good deal of such spotty radiopacity. The latter represents focal calcification going on in the tumor tissue, as can be demonstrated on microscopic examination.

It was Lewis who stressed the presence of radiopacity in connection with the roentgenographic picture of synovioma. He emphasized it, particularly in relation to the knee, as a finding which was helpful in the differential diagnosis between

### *Figure 183*

*A*, Photomicrograph (× 125) showing the histologic pattern of a synovioma which was composed of spindle cells practically throughout. The winding clefts lined by cuboidal cells shown on the right were found only in a single small area of 1 of the 5 blocks of the lesional tissue taken for microscopic examination. If the field presenting this pattern had not come under observation, the lesion might have been misdiagnosed as a poorly differentiated fibrosarcoma. The tumor was in a foot of a man 30 years of age. The treatment consisted of local excision, followed by amputation through the leg when the nature of the lesion became apparent.

*B*, Photomicrograph (× 125) of tissue from a synovioma in which clefts and spaces lined by cuboidal ("pseudoepithelial") cells dominated the histologic pattern of the lesional tissue almost throughout. Many of the lined clefts and spaces reveal evidence of a mucoid substance. Note also the bits of dark-staining calcium. The lesion was located deep in the thigh and was adherent to the femur at a point lateral to the lesser trochanter. The patient was a girl 17 years of age, and the definitive treatment was disarticulation of the limb at the hip joint.

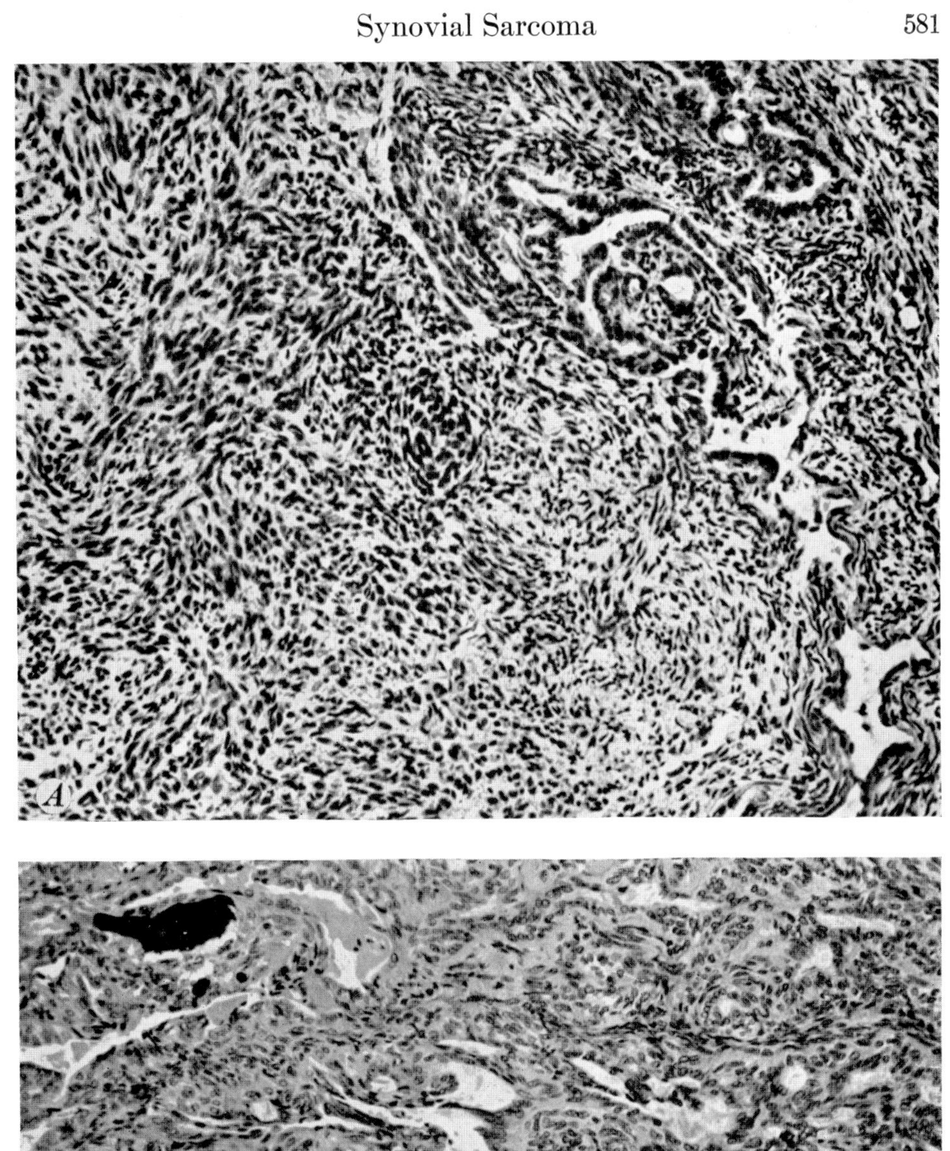

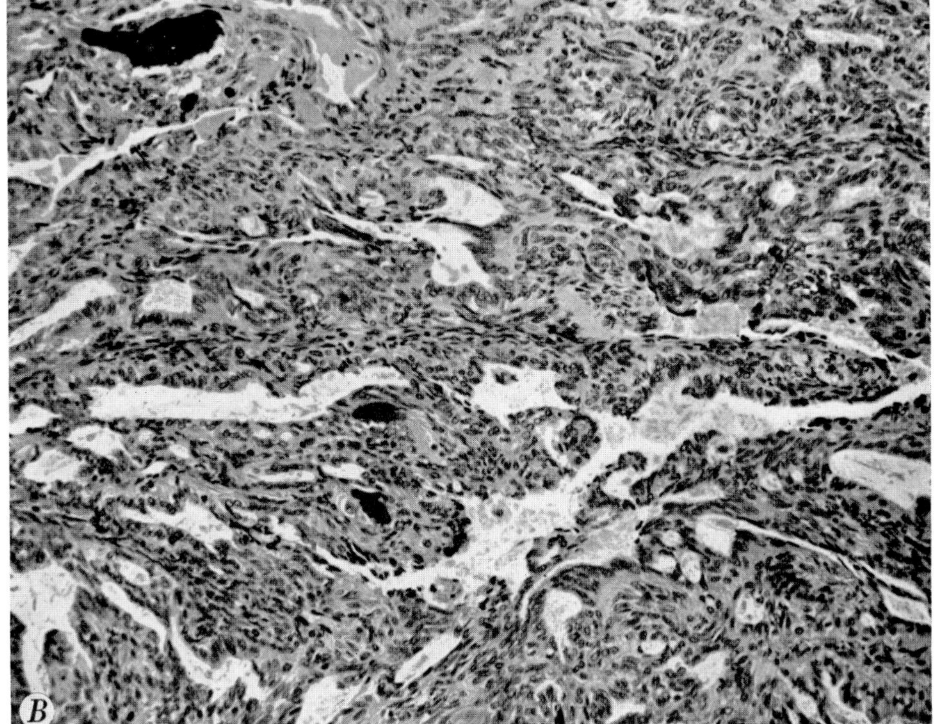

*Figure 183*

*synovioma* and *pigmented villonodular synovitis.* Specifically, pigmented villonodular synovitis does not show spotty radiopacity. Again in contrast to synovioma, the soft-tissue mass in that lesion is usually entirely intra-articular, is often lobulated and nodular, and is associated with the presence of fluid in the joint space.

It must be remembered, however, that lesions other than the synovioma, occurring in the vicinity of joints or even within them, may show spotty radiopacity. Thus a *soft-tissue chondrosarcoma* in the region of a joint (p. 520) usually presents at least some spots of radiopacity and might hence be mistaken for a synovioma if too much emphasis is placed upon the diagnostic significance of that finding. In a case of *synovial chondromatosis* (p. 561) the *x*-ray picture usually also shows spotty radiopacity in the affected joint (generally a knee). On the other hand, in the relatively rare instances in which a synovioma is found confined to a joint space (see Fig. 182-*A*), the presence of radiopacities in the lesional tissue might lead one to interpret the condition as synovial chondromatosis instead of synovioma. Furthermore, spotty radiopacities are observed in connection with *hemangiomas* appearing in the vicinity of joints or even within them. In these cases the radiopacities represent phleboliths and are usually clear-cut, roundish, and very dense (see Figs. 72-*C* and 166-*B*). Finally, even a *fibrosarcoma* developing in the vicinity of a joint may have to be differentiated from a synovioma if, as sometimes happens, it shows spotty radiopacity representing calcification of focal areas of necrosis.

## PATHOLOGIC FINDINGS

**Gross Pathology.**—When exposed at the surgical intervention, a synovioma is usually found adherent to the outer coat of the capsule of a joint. Exceptionally, it is found within the substance of the capsule and projects into the articular cavity. Whether small or large, the tumor is likely to be semi-firm, though occasionally it may feel quite firm. Except in those rare cases in which the lesion is intra-articular, the tumor mass is usually found well circumscribed and covered by a pseudocapsule composed of compressed adjacent tissue. When cut open, the tumor is likely to appear pinkish gray for the most part, but may also show yellow areas (where the tissue has undergone necrosis) and brown or red areas (where there has been recent hemorrhage into it). Here and there, the lesional tissue may be somewhat gritty, in consequence of the presence of calcium.

**Microscopic Pathology.**—The tissue pattern of a synovioma is given its character by two types of cells which are closely intermingled. In different lesions and even

### *Figure 184*

*A*, Photomicrograph (× 65) illustrating the histologic pattern presented by many areas of the synovioma shown in Figure 182-*C*. The numerous small spaces are bordered by thick collars of pale-staining roundish cells representing the so-called synovial cells. Under higher magnification it would be apparent that in some places the cells lining the spaces are cuboidal, while in others they are small and roundish and hardly different from the cells composing the collars about the spaces. (For further details, see Fig. 185-*A*.)

*B*, Photomicrograph (× 65) showing a different histologic pattern presented by many areas of another synovioma. In the lower part of the picture one can see long, drawn-out tubules which, under higher magnification, are found to be lined by flat cuboidal cells. In the upper half of the picture one notes wide, irregular spaces outlined by "pseudoepithelial" papillary proliferations almost suggesting the pattern of a papillary adenocarcinoma. The stroma between the tubules and spaces is composed of long, drawn-out spindle cells suggestive of fibrosarcoma. The tumor was in the region of the ankle, and the patient was a boy 18 years of age.

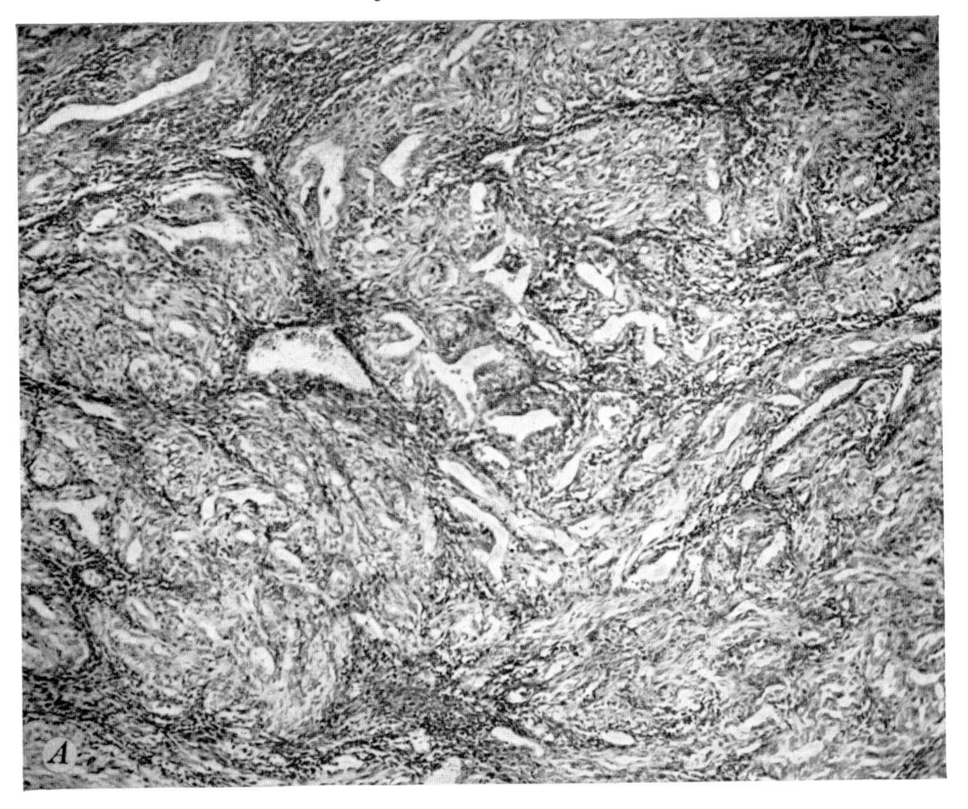


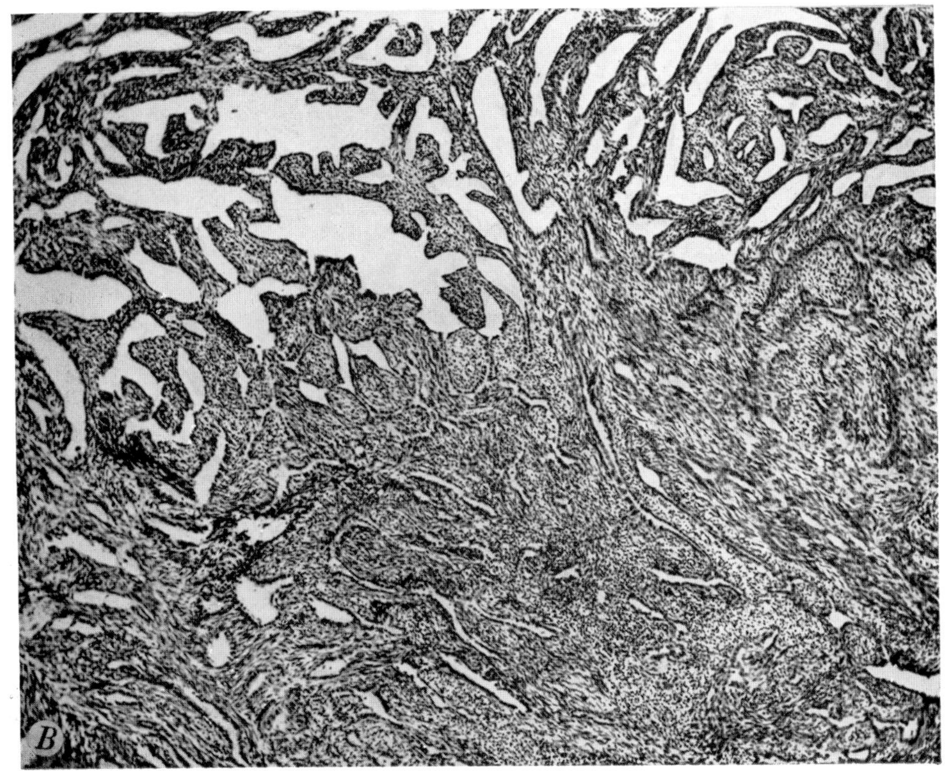


***Figure 184***

in different parts of the same lesion, they may be present in various proportions and various stages of differentiation. One of the cell types in question, which may be interpreted as the *fibrosarcomatous component* of the lesional tissue, is represented mainly by drawn-out spindle-shaped cells, associated with reticulin fibers and/or collagen. The other cellular constituent, which may be regarded as the *synovial component* of the lesional tissue, presents a good deal of variety in respect to the cytologic details of its cells and the pattern of their arrangement. These cells may be somewhat elongated and plump, or polygonal, and may be present in compact sheets, cords, or nests. They are also to be found lining slits and spaces, and in these sites they may be elongated, cuboidal, or even columnar. (See Figs. 183, 184 and 185.)

Whether the so-called fibrosarcomatous and synovial components of the tumor actually represent two generically distinct cell types is difficult to say. It may well be that they do not, and that the spindle cells represent the more primitive cell type, from which the synovial cells are derived by further differentiation. In any event, the form and arrangement of the synovial cells, the fact that they are capable of producing a mucin-like substance, and their behavior when cultivated *in vitro* seem to relate these cells in particular to the specialized mesenchymal tissue out of which the synovial linings of joints are formed (see Haagensen and Stout, Bennett, Murray *et al.*, and King).

In one lesion or another, the fibrosarcomatous tissue may so dominate the picture that one may have to examine many areas of the lesion to find synovial tissue elements and thus establish the lesion as a synovioma. Hence, one can understand why a synovioma whose histologic pattern is dominated by spindle cells might be misinterpreted as a fibrosarcoma. On the other hand, in a lesion or lesional area in which synovial elements dominate the histologic picture, the cytologic pattern as a whole may likewise not readily convey the nature of the lesion, unless the tissue sections also show that lined clefts and spaces have been formed. In the absence of clefts and spaces, the lesion might be thought to represent a sarcoma of undifferentiated type, or even an alveolar sarcoma or a reticulum cell sarcoma.

The lined spaces to be observed in the tumor tissue take many forms, such as mere slits, larger clefts, or structures suggesting acini, drawn-out tubules, and branching glandular formations. In a particular synovioma the spaces may be quite numerous and be manifest in all their variety if many areas from the specimen are studied. On the other hand, another synovioma may show relatively few of them, and these may even be mainly slits and clefts.

The cells lining the spaces may appear elongated and plump, but are usually cuboidal and sometimes even columnar, especially if the spaces take the form of pseudoglandular formations. In some places the lining cells may even be found projecting into the lumina as papillary formations. In any event, the cells lining the gland-like spaces are not delimited by a basement membrane.

### *Figure 185*

*A*, Photomicrograph (× 250) illustrating the appearance of a tissue field near the one shown in Figure 184-*A*. Lumina (spaces) have formed in the originally compact masses of roundish, so-called synovial cells. In some places the cells outlining the lumina are indistinguishable from the roundish cells in the compact cell masses. In other places, however, the lining cells have become cuboidal. Note also that the lining cells are not separated from the surrounding cells by a basement membrane.

*B*, Photomicrograph (× 250) illustrating the pattern observed in a synovioma in which lined spaces were present almost throughout the tumor. In some places the cells outlining the spaces are columnar. Mucoid secretion is present within the spaces.

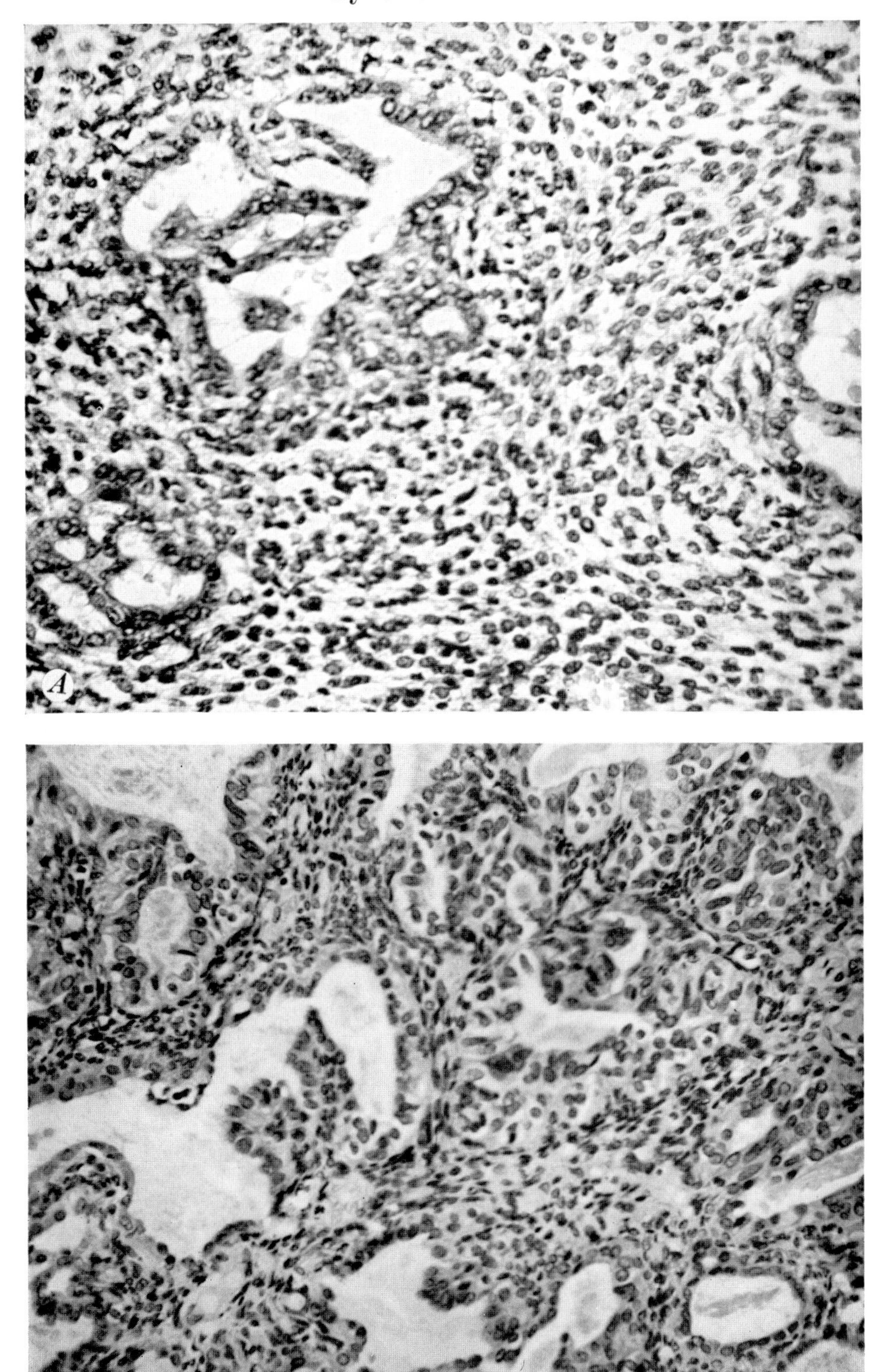


***Figure 185***

Many of the spaces may be found to contain secretion which, when stained with mucicarmine, reveals its mucoid nature. The glandular and tubular spaces lined by cuboidal and/or columnar cells may give the synovioma the imprint of an epithelial tumor. Hence, one can understand why the older pathologists, when they encountered such a lesion, often referred to it as a sarcocarcinoma. Calcification is also seen fairly often in synoviomas. Usually it takes the form of minute scattered spherical concretions (calcospherites), discernible only on histologic examination of the tissue. An occasional lesion also shows large areas of calcification at sites where the tumor tissue has undergone necrosis. It is these large areas that are likely to be reflected as radiopacities in the *x*-ray picture of the lesion.

As already indicated, there is the possibility of misinterpreting a diffuse pigmented villonodular synovial lesion as a synovial sarcoma. This confusion is usually due to incorrect evaluation of the microscopic findings, especially when the villonodular proliferations have become fused and compacted. Under these circumstances, a villonodular lesion is likely to show numerous lined clefts and spaces. However, the lining cells are generally small and often flattened (rather than plump, cuboidal or columnar) and usually contain a good deal of hemosiderin pigment. Furthermore, the cells between the spaces are, on the whole, round cells which possess phagocytic capacity, and many of them can be seen to have taken up hemosiderin and/or lipid. The cellular elements of a synovioma, on the other hand, do not show phagocytic capacity and do not contain hemosiderin and lipid. Finally, the pigmented villonodular lesion is likely to present small multinuclear giant cells, sometimes in great numbers, which a synovioma again does not do. (See Figs. 169, 170 and 171, illustrating the histopathology of diffuse pigmented villonodular synovitis.)

In connection with the roentgenographic aspects of synovioma, certain differences between that lesion and pigmented villonodular synovitis have also been pointed out. These center around the fact that the synovioma is nearly always outside the limits of the capsule, while the pigmented villonodular lesion has an intra-articular location. Also, the shadow cast by a large villonodular lesion, in contrast to that cast by a synovioma, is usually lobulated. Furthermore, it does not contain radiopacities reflecting calcification, as a synovioma shadow not infrequently does. In addition, of course, the gross appearance of the lesional tissue in the two conditions is quite different.

## PROGNOSIS AND TREATMENT

In view of the great frequency with which the synovioma metastasizes, the hope for cure resides mainly in early diagnosis and prompt radical surgical intervention. Unfortunately, the lesion may be present for months or even several years before it receives appropriate attention. This happens because the tumor often grows slowly, the local complaints associated with it are usually mild, and the true nature of the lesion is ordinarily not suspected on the basis of the clinical and roentgenographic findings. It is thus apparent why, in so many of the cases reported in the literature, the initial surgical intervention has consisted of enucleation of the tumor or mere excision, perhaps not even in one piece. Lack of awareness of the seriousness of the condition also explains why the initial surgical intervention is often not preceded by study of a biopsy specimen, which might have alerted the surgeon to the fact that he was dealing with a synovioma.

At any rate, a surgical intervention which merely removes the tumor without including the surrounding local tissue will almost certainly be followed by a recurrence within a few months or possibly a year or two. Furthermore, pulmonary metastases often develop even before the lesion recurs, indicating that the tumor had already metastasized before the excision or was disseminated in the course of it. If an amputation is done shortly after the excision, the patient is still quite likely to succumb to metastases sooner or later. This is an even stronger possibility if the amputation has been deferred until a recurrence has been noted.

All this taken together indicates that lowering of the hitherto extremely high general mortality rate for synovioma (at least 90 per cent) can be expected only to the extent to which a diagnosis is established early (through study of a small but adequate incisional biopsy specimen) and the affected limb is ablated at a level well beyond the site of the tumor. As to the site of amputation, the latter should be carried out (for instance) through the middle of the leg if the lesion is in the foot or ankle region and through the middle of the thigh if the lesion is in the region of the knee, and a hindquarter amputation should be done if the lesion is in the hip region. When metastases develop, they are mainly in the lungs, and the latter are frequently the only site of metastasis. However, in some cases the metastases may be quite generalized and even involve bones.

Despite the general desirability of amputation as the primary intervention, a cure is sometimes achieved by means of a radical local excision which gives the tumor a rather wide berth. It is sometimes also attained if an amputation is done as a secondary intervention soon after local excision or even after a recurrence which has followed such an excision. Not infrequently, metastases are found in the regional lymph nodes, if there has been a recurrence. Thus, at a subsequent intervention it is advisable to dissect out the lymph nodes immediately above the amputation site.

The writer has even studied material from a case in which a patient affected with a synovioma in the vicinity of a shoulder joint was still alive and well 6 years after local excision of the tumor, which was already a recurrent one. In that case the patient received 6,000 r of radiation to the lesional site after the recurrent tumor had merely been excised. The role of the radiation in this apparent cure cannot be evaluated. In general, however, radiation has not been found to be of benefit in connection with synovioma. In any event, an exceptional case such as this should not count very heavily against the principle of early and radical surgical treatment for synovioma.

## REFERENCES

Bennett, G. A.: Malignant Neoplasms Originating in Synovial Tissues (Synoviomata), J. Bone & Joint Surg., *29*, 259, 1947.

Berger, L.: Synovial Sarcomas in Serous Bursæ and Tendon Sheaths, Am. J. Cancer, *34*, 501, 1938.

Briggs, C. D.: Malignant Tumors of Synovial Origin, Ann. Surg., *115*, 413, 1942.

Craig, R. M., Pugh, D. G., and Soule, E. H.: The Roentgenologic Manifestations of Synovial Sarcoma, Radiology, *65*, 837, 1955.

Fisher, H. R.: Synovial Sarcomesothelioma (Sarcoendothelioma), Am. J. Path., *18*, 529, 1942.

Gold, A. M.: Synovial Sarcoma of the Shoulder Region, Bull. Hosp. Joint Dis., *15*, 79, 1954.

Haagensen, C. D., and Stout, A. P.: Synovial Sarcoma, Ann. Surg., *120*, 826, 1944.

Hartz, P. H.: Cancerous Synovial Tumors, Arch. Path., *40*, 88, 1945.

Jaffe, H. L., and Lichtenstein, L.: Synovial Sarcoma (Synovioma), Bull. Hosp. Joint Dis. *2*, 3, 1941.

Jönsson, G.: Malignant Tumors of the Skeletal Muscles, Fasciæ, Joint Capsules, Tendon Sheaths and Serous Bursæ, Acta radiol. (Suppl. 36), 1938.

King, E. S. J.: Tissue Differentiation in Malignant Synovial Tumours, J. Bone & Joint Surg., *34-B*, 97, 1952.

Knox, L. C.: Synovial Sarcoma, Am. J. Cancer, *28*, 461, 1936.

Lejars, and Rubens-Duval: Les sarcomes primitifs des synoviales articulaires, Rev. de chir. Paris, *41*, 751, 1910.

Lewis, R. W.: Roentgen Diagnosis of Pigmented Villonodular Synovitis and Synovial Sarcoma of the Knee Joint, Radiology, *49*, 26, 1947.

MORETZ, W. H.: Malignant Tumors Arising from the Synovial Membrane with Report of Four Cases, Surg., Gynec. & Obst., *79*, 125, 1944.

MURRAY, M. R., STOUT, A. P., and POGOGEFF, I. A.: Synovial Sarcoma and Normal Synovial Tissue Cultivated *in Vitro*, Ann. Surg., *120*, 843, 1944.

PACK, G. T., and ARIEL, I. M.: Synovial Sarcoma (Malignant Synovioma), Surgery, *28*, 1047, 1950.

SABRAZÈS, J., LOUBAT, E., DE GRAILLY, R., and MAGENDIE, J.: Synovialosarcomes, Gaz. hebd. d. sc. méd. de Bordeaux, *55*, 754, 1934.

DE SANTO, D. A., TENNANT, R., and ROSAHN, P. D.: Synovial Sarcomas in Joints, Bursæ, and Tendon Sheaths, Surg., Gynec. & Obst., *72*, 951, 1941.

SHERMAN, R. S., and CHU, F. C. H.: A Roentgenographic Study of Synovioma, Am. J. Roentgenol., *67*, 80, 1952.

SMITH, L. W.: Synoviomata, Am. J. Path., *3*, 355, 1927.

TILLOTSON, J. F., McDONALD, J. R., and JANES, J. M.: Synovial Sarcomata, J. Bone & Joint Surg., *33-A*, 459, 1951.

WRIGHT, C. J. E.: Malignant Synovioma, J. Path. & Bact., *64*, 585, 1952.

Chapter

# 33

# Tumors Metastatic to the Skeleton

In this chapter we are concerned mainly with the distribution and evolution of skeletal metastases, rather than with morphologic details relating to the metastases or to the primary tumors from which they were seeded. While both carcinomas and sarcomas metastasize to bones, the great majority of metastatic cancerous skeletal lesions represent metastases from carcinomas. It should be noted, furthermore, that the skeleton is one of the most common sites of cancer metastasis. Indeed, in cases of cancer which have run a protracted clinical course, the more thoroughly one investigates the bones at autopsy, the greater the probability that skeletal metastases will be found. The writer's own relevant experience indicates that they occur much more frequently than is generally supposed. In fact, he holds that skeletal involvement by metastases is probably just as common as pulmonary or hepatic involvement.

Very often, in a case of cancer, clinical difficulties arising from a metastatic bone lesion are the presenting complaints, the primary tumor being clinically silent. Not infrequently, in these cases it is too readily taken for granted that the skeletal lesion represents a primary bone tumor. Consequently, the general examination of the patient may be quite perfunctory and may fail to reveal the actual primary lesion, although the latter might rather easily have been detected. Furthermore, in a case in which one does suspect that the bone lesion represents a focus of metastatic cancer, clinical study of the patient directed toward discovery of the primary lesion is nevertheless often not immediately rewarding. Examination of a biopsy specimen from the presenting bone lesion in such a case frequently resolves the diagnostic dilemma. In addition to revealing that the lesion is a metastatic cancer, the pattern of the lesional tissue often allows one to deduce the site of the primary growth. On the other hand, this pattern may be ambiguous because the cancer cells are undifferentiated, so that the site of the primary lesion cannot be surmised. In the course of time, that lesion may give rise to clinical manifestations and its site be revealed in that way. Occasionally, however, the primary tumor is still clinically obscure even at the time of the patient's death, and in rare instances it may even be overlooked at autopsy.

Why the first site of metastasis from a cancer is so often one or another bone is an interesting question. Furthermore, one wonders why, in an occasional instance, much of the skeleton may eventually become heavily riddled by cancer while visceral metastases (and notably hepatic and pulmonary metastases) are entirely or almost entirely lacking. These questions are discussed in the section dealing with the routes by which cancer cell emboli are seeded in the bones.

In the section dealing with the roentgenographic *vs.* the anatomic findings relating to skeletal metastases, stress is laid on the fact that a focus of metastasis is not likely to become evident in the clinical roentgenographs unless a good deal of osteolysis or osteoplasia has taken place in the affected bone area or unless the contour of the affected bone part has been changed. In this connection, it is pointed out that a vertebral column removed at autopsy and containing metastatic lesions may not readily reveal them on roentgenographic study of the column.

In respect to certain of the clinical manifestations of cancer metastatic to the skeleton, the discussion centers around the question of the hypercalcemia that occasionally develops either as a result of widespread osteolysis or in consequence of the therapeutic use of hormones against the metastases.

The final section of the chapter deals with pulmonary hypertrophic osteoarthropathy. This subject is not, of course, directly pertinent to the matter of tumors metastatic to the skeleton. The section is an *addendum* to the chapter, included because the condition is sometimes encountered as a manifestation of pulmonary metastasis from a primary bone sarcoma or from a sarcoma primary in the soft tissues overlying a bone part. However, it is pointed out that there are also many other circumstances under which pulmonary hypertrophic osteoarthropathy appears.

## ROUTES OF METASTASIS TO THE SKELETON

The route by which cancer cell emboli ordinarily reach the skeleton is the blood stream (venous or arterial). The part played by the lymphatic system as a route by which cancer cell emboli are transported directly to bones is unimportant, in accordance with the apparent absence of lymph channels in the bone marrow. The direct invasion of a skeletal area by a cancerous growth in an adjacent organ or other soft part does not concern us here.

In relation to the development of secondary deposits of cancer in the skeleton, it is necessary to bear in mind that cancer cell emboli (from a carcinoma or a sarcoma) which have lodged in the marrow of a particular bone site at any one time do not necessarily survive. However, those which do remain viable tend to multiply and, sooner or later, completely crowd out the local marrow cells and fill the intertrabecular marrow spaces of the area. Further growth of the metastatic focus may lead to lysis of the regional osseous tissue and/or provoke the reactive deposition of new bone in the metastatic area. In consequence, the bone region in question may come to show changes detectable even roentgenographically, in the form of increased radiolucency and/or radiopacity.

As already indicated, a skeletal focus of cancer metastasis very often appears as the presenting lesion (for instance, in a vertebral body, in a pelvic bone, or in the upper end of a femur) and is frequently the only metastatic lesion demonstrable

***Figure 186***

*A*, Illustration of the anastomoses between the vertebral and caval venous systems in the lumbar and sacral regions of the rat. The upper part of the picture shows the anastomotic relationships as demonstrated by a vinylite-plastic corrosion preparation. The pelvic veins are on the right, and the form of the kidney is apparent in the center. The vertebral veins form the dense plexus extending along the top of the corrosion specimen. The large dark vessel below these veins is the inferior vena cava. The lower part of the picture is a diagrammatic representation of the anastomoses of the vertebral and caval systems and of the connections at each segmental level.

*B*, Illustration of the anastomoses between the vertebral and caval venous systems in the cephalic and thoracic regions of the rat. The anastomotic connections as demonstrated in a vinylite-plastic corrosion preparation are shown in the upper part of the picture. The lower part of the picture again illustrates the anastomoses in diagrammatic form. The network of veins above the azygos veins is extrathoracic in position and therefore not affected by changes in intrathoracic pressure. (This illustration is reproduced from the article by Coman and deLong 'Cancer, *4*, 610, 1951' with the kind permission of the authors and the editor of the journal.)

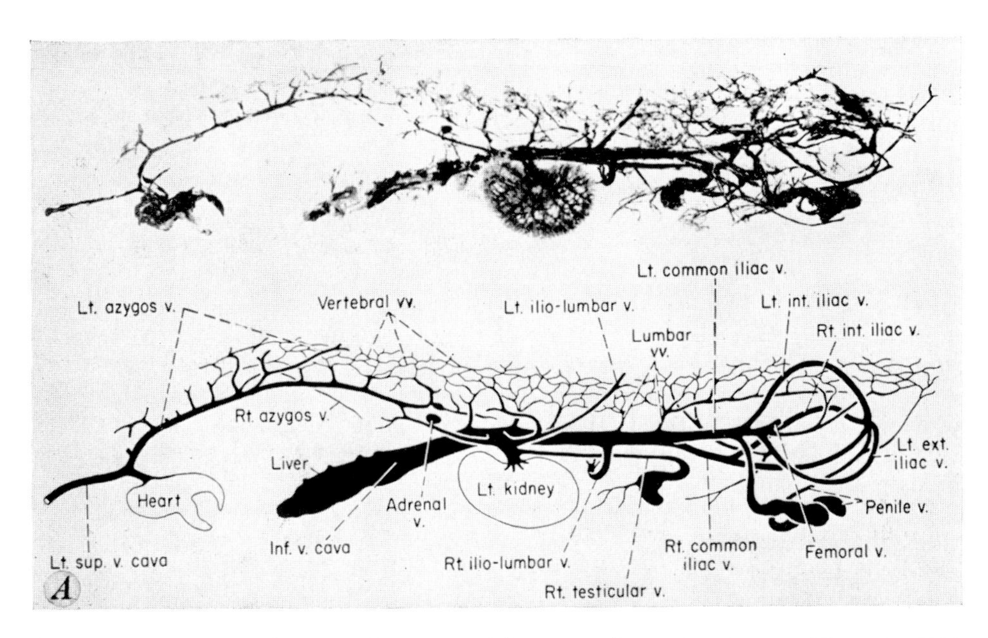
Lt. common iliac v.
Lt. azygos v.
Vertebral vv.
Lt. ilio-lumbar v.
Lt. int. iliac v.
Lumbar vv.
Rt. int. iliac v.
Rt. azygos v.
Lt. ext. iliac v.
Liver
Lt. kidney
Heart
Adrenal v.
Penile v.
Inf. v. cava
Rt. common iliac v.
Femoral v.
Lt. sup. v. cava
Rt. ilio-lumbar v.
A
Rt. testicular v.

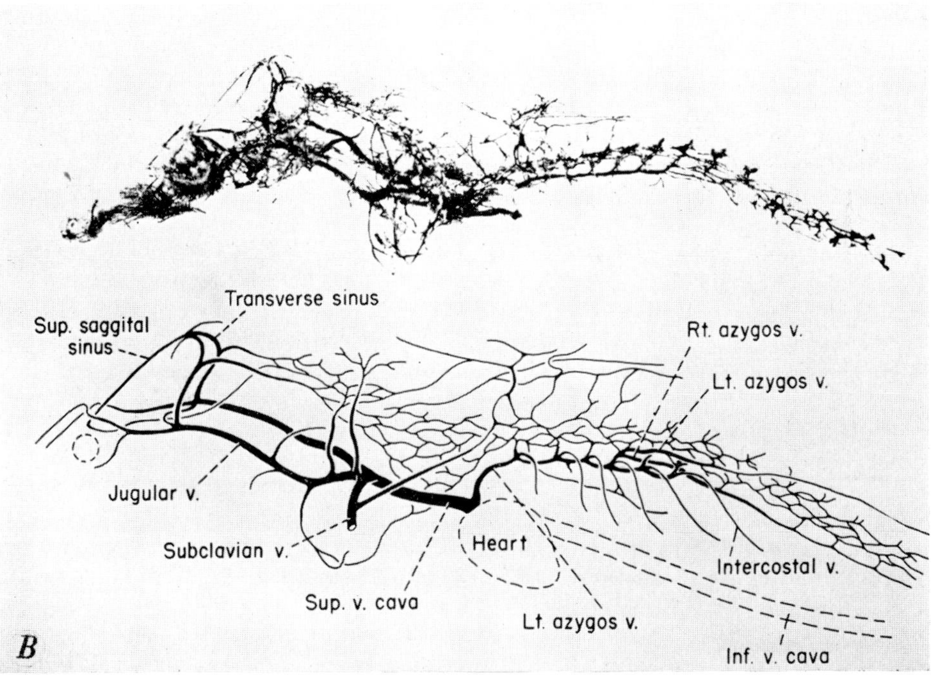
Transverse sinus
Sup. saggital sinus
Rt. azygos v.
Lt. azygos v.
Jugular v.
Subclavian v.
Heart
Intercostal v.
Sup. v. cava
Lt. azygos v.
B
Inf. v. cava

*Figure 186*

clinically and roentgenographically when the patient first comes under treatment. These facts are of particular interest in connection with the routes by which cancer metastasizes to the skeleton. So is the fact that the skeleton is sometimes found heavily riddled by metastases at autopsy, while the viscera are still entirely free of them. These findings are consistent with the idea that cancer cell emboli (from which the metastatic tumor growths develop) can reach the skeleton by way of the blood stream directly—that is, without first traveling to the lungs.

Anatomic studies undertaken by Batson to account for this seemingly "paradoxical" distribution of metastases resulted in his demonstration of the importance of the so-called "vertebral vein system" in this connection. Specifically, injection experiments led him to the conclusion that such metastases are to be explained on the basis of a network of valveless veins around the spinal dura mater and the vertebræ which also has cranial and body wall connections and even connections with the veins in the walls of the blood vessels of the extremities. He held this vertebral vein system to be an independent one existing in addition to the already recognized caval, portal, azygos, and pulmonary vein systems but connecting with these and providing bypasses for them. Because of the communications of the vertebral vein system with the superior and inferior vena cava, the two major caval veins are, in a sense, also linked without the intermediation of the lungs.

This so-called vertebral vein system is conceived as a venous pool, or lake, in which the flow is very sluggish and subject to arrest and even reversal. It provides a series of passageways by which cancer cell emboli can be seeded directly into the bones, bypassing the liver and lungs. In particular, Batson was able to show by injection experiments that the prostatic vein plexus can be made to drain into the vertebral vein plexus. The possibility of such a drainage path, leading to bypassing of the caval system, would explain the early and sometimes exclusive occurrence in the skeleton of metastases from cancer of the prostate. Also, injection of breast venules demonstrated the vertebral vein pattern by which cancer cell emboli from the breast can likewise, as they so often do, spread first to bones of the trunk and skull. Cancer cell emboli from a carcinoma of the thyroid or even of the stomach, for instance, may also drain into the vertebral vein system and thus metastasize directly to bones.

The anatomic findings of Batson relating to the vertebral vein system in man and the conclusions which he reached in regard to the possible role of this system in the spread of metastases have received confirmation in experimental studies on animals. In this connection, Coman and deLong injected suspensions of cancer cells into the femoral veins of rats, while applying moderate pressure to the abdomen. They found that under these conditions some of the tumor cells entering the pelvic veins reached the lumbar vertebræ directly by way of the vertebral vein system, although others continued on to the lungs by way of the caval system. Using injection-corrosion techniques, these investigators also worked out in detail the anatomic relationships of the vertebral venous system with the caval system of rats. The anastomotic connections between these two systems in the rat were found to correspond in general to those observed in regard to man. (See Fig. 186.)

As already indicated, the vertebral vein system is not the only vascular route by which cancer cells reach the bones. For instance, cancer cells from a focus of tumor (primary or metastatic) in the lung may enter the pulmonary vein, reach the arterial side of the circulation, and be carried to one or another bone site (among other sites) by the arterial blood stream. Such tumor cell emboli may lodge in a bone or bones not only of the axis and trunk, but also of the extremities. Furthermore, cancer cell emboli reaching the lungs by way of the caval circulation apparently sometimes even pass through the lungs instead of being arrested in them.

They would then likewise enter the arterial circulation, and some of them could make their way to a skeletal site, though of course they, too, could reach other sites also. In all probability, however, metastases become established in the skeleton much more often by cancer cell emboli which get to the bones through the vertebral vein system than by those which reach them through the arterial route.

In relation to the establishment of a focus of cancer metastasis in any site (whether in a bone or elsewhere), it is apparently of crucial importance that cancer cell emboli reach the site in adequate numbers, so that at least some of them will survive and multiply (see Coman *et al.*). How much importance should be attached to the role of a favorable tissue "soil" at the site of lodgment of the cancer cells for the development of metastases is not clear in the light of our present knowledge.

It is pertinent in this connection that carcinoma of the prostate comes to be associated with metastatic bone lesions in a very large proportion of the cases, while a carcinoma of the bladder, uterus, or ovary establishes bone metastases much less frequently. In relation to all these cancers, the venous drainage occurs by way of the pelvic veins, which not only drain into the caval system, but have communications with the vertebral venous system. Thus the possibility for skeletal lodgment of cancer cell emboli from all these various organs at least in the marrow of the vertebral column is potentially great. One may therefore infer that when cancer cells from a prostatic carcinoma reach and grow in the local capillary bed they are much more likely, for some reason or other, to separate off in large numbers and reach the bone marrow by way of the vertebral vein system than are cancer cells which have extended into the regional capillary bed from a tumor of the bladder, uterus, or ovary. If this is not the explanation for these differences, one has to fall back on the idea that the bone marrow does not constitute as favorable a "soil" for the survival of cancer cell emboli from these latter organs as from the prostate.

## A FOCUS OF SKELETAL METASTASIS AS THE PRESENTING LESION

As already indicated, many cases of cancer first attract clinical notice through complaints referable to a metastatic bone lesion, while the primary tumor (most often in the breast, prostate, lung, kidney, or thyroid) is still clinically silent or at least inconspicuous. The metastatic lesion is likely to be in the thoracic or lumbar part of the vertebral column, the upper part of a femur or humerus, a rib, or the iliac portion of an innominate bone. On the other hand, it is only exceptionally located in a bone distal to the knee joint, and hardly ever in a bone distal to the elbow joint. In many of the cases in question, a careful physical examination of the patient (along with the findings from pertinent roentgenographic and serum biochemical studies) will suffice to reveal the site of the primary tumor. In other cases, there may be difficulty in locating it, and, indeed, occasionally the primary lesion remains occult for a long time.

In a case in which the primary lesion is not readily found, biopsy of the bone lesion is indicated. Microscopic examination of the specimen will at least settle any doubts as to whether the bone lesion actually represents a malignant tumor and will nearly always indicate whether it is a primary or a metastatic cancer. In addition to confirming the suspected malignant character of the bone lesion, the cellular pattern of the tumor tissue may indicate the precise organ from which the tumor cells in the metastatic focus were derived. On the other hand, the pattern may only suggest one of several possible sites for the primary cancer, indicating the need for still further clinical investigation of the case. In some instances, however, the cellular pattern presented by the tumor tissue may be so lacking in differentiation that it offers practically no clue at all to the site of the primary lesion. Indeed, it may even mislead one into thinking that the bone lesion in question is a primary rather than a metastatic tumor. (See Figs. 187 and 188.)

In a case of *hypernephroma,* a focus of skeletal metastasis is not infrequently the presenting lesion, the existence of the renal tumor being unrecognized because it has not given rise to any clinical complaints. The skeletal lesion in question is commonly located in a long bone (though it may be in a flat bone) and is often of fairly large size. In the *x*-ray picture the affected bone area usually appears radiolucent, and if it has undergone expansion of its contour, the lesional area is also likely to appear "multiloculated." There is nothing diagnostically distinctive about this picture, and one might even interpret it as representing a focus of myeloma,

***Figure 187***

*A*, Roentgenograph showing erosion of the cortex of a femur from the periosteal side by a metastatic epidermoid carcinoma. This was the presenting lesion in the case in question, and the primary cancer was clinically occult. The patient was a man 80 years of age whose complaints referable to the limb in question were of 5 months' standing. In particular, he gave a history of local pain associated with the development of a palpable tumor mass. Clinically the lesion was interpreted as a sarcoma which had started in the soft tissues of the thigh and was invading the cortex. The nature of the lesion as a focus of metastatic epidermoid carcinoma was established by histologic examination of tissue from the lesional site. As noted, the primary site of the epidermoid carcinoma was not discovered in this case while the patient was hospitalized. However, it may be of interest in this connection that in 2 other cases observed by the writer in which the cortex of a femoral shaft was being eroded from the periosteal side by an epidermoid carcinoma the primary tumor was found to be in the lung.

*B*, Roentgenograph showing the upper end of a humerus which is the site of an osteoplastic metastasis from a carcinoma of the prostate. The tumor in the humerus was the presenting lesion in this case. This *x*-ray picture created diagnostic confusion on a clinical basis because it so strongly suggested a so-called sclerosing osteogenic sarcoma with "sunburst" periostitis. Indeed, on that account, no thought was given at first to the possibility that one might be dealing with a metastatic tumor. The patient was a man 48 years of age whose difficulties relating to the humerus (pain and local swelling) were of 5 months' standing. A biopsy established the carcinomatous nature of the lesion, and the primary tumor was then found to be in the prostate. Rather surprisingly, neither the pelvic bones nor the lumbar vertebræ yet showed any clear-cut roentgenographic evidences of metastasis.

*C*, Roentgenograph illustrating collapse of the first lumbar vertebra, resulting from involvement by a metastatic cancer and appearing as the presenting lesion. The patient was a man 55 years of age whose complaint was of increasing pain in the back of 10 months' standing. The history and physical examination gave no indication of the possible site of the primary tumor. Aside from the findings relating to the lumbar part of the column, clinical study of the patient showed that the right clavicle was thickened. *X*-ray examination revealed the presence of destructive and sclerotic changes in the clavicle, and a biopsy of that bone established the presence of metastatic cancer. However, the histologic pattern of the cancer, though it was clearly that of a carcinoma, was not such that one could be certain about the organ from which it came.

*D*, Roentgenograph showing an osteolytic lesion in an ilium, representing a focus of metastasis from a cancer of the breast. The patient was a man 65 years of age who entered the hospital because of pain radiating down the left thigh, pain in the hip, and increasing weakness of the extremity in question. The complaints were of 9 months' standing, and there were no complaints referable to the breast. The fact that a breast cancer was present was overlooked by the orthopaedic surgeon, since his attention was focused on the lesion in the ilium. The histologic appearance of the biopsy specimen from the ilium not only indicated that the lesion was a metastatic cancer, but suggested that the primary tumor was in the breast, where indeed it was found.

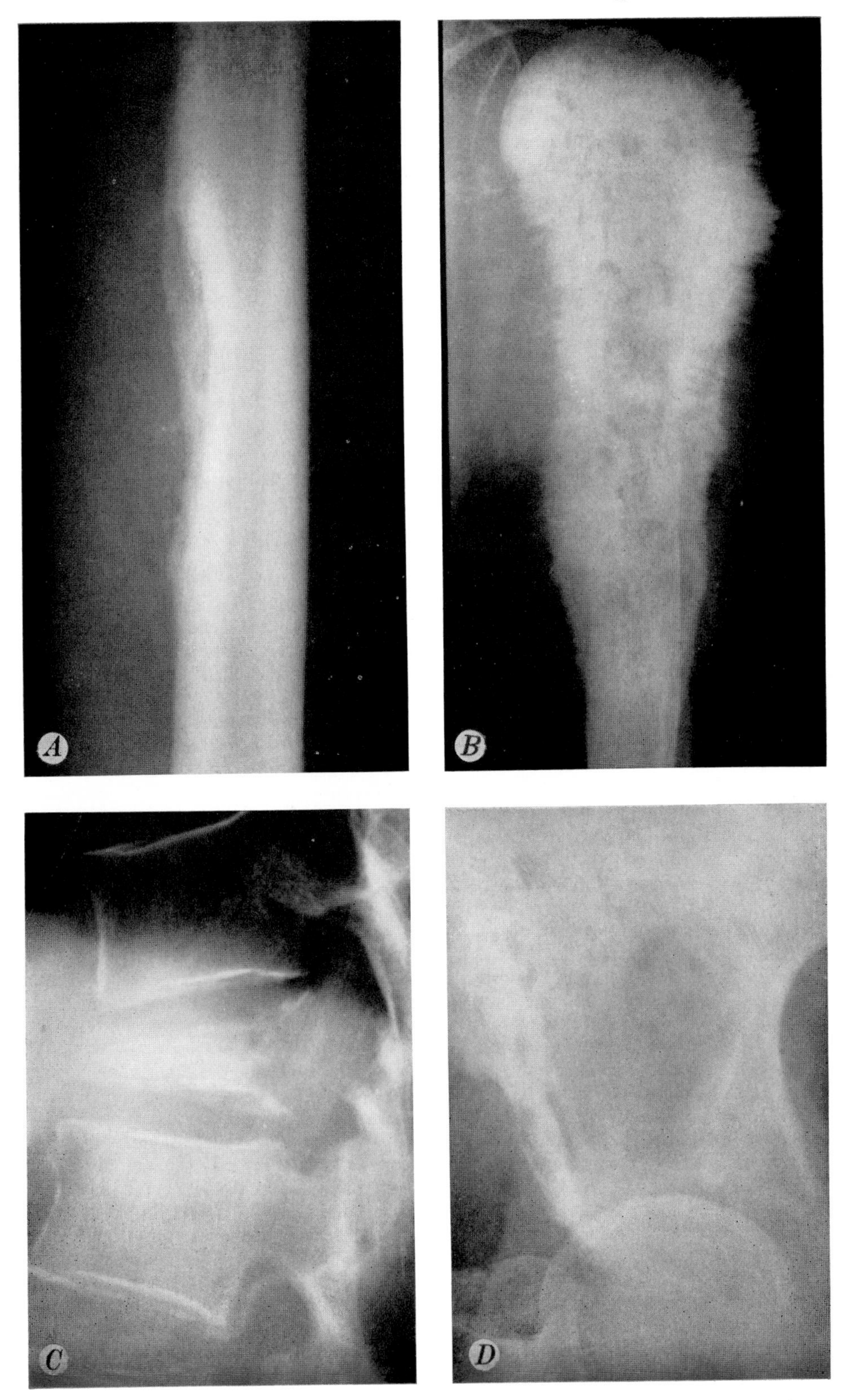


*Figure 187*

for instance. If the bone lesion is biopsied, however, the histologic pattern of the tumor tissue nearly always indicates that the primary lesion is a hypernephroma. Of special interest in connection with hypernephroma is the fact that a solitary focus of skeletal metastasis may be the only metastatic lesion present, at least for some time, insofar as one can judge from roentgenographic examination of the patient. It is on account of this fact that removal of the tumorously affected kidney and subsequent ablation of the affected bone part has sometimes been practiced. However, it is not likely that this procedure effects a permanent cure except in rare instances.

In a case of carcinoma of the *thyroid,* it is again not unusual for a focus of skeletal metastasis to be the source of the presenting complaints. The skeletal lesion ordinarily shows up in the *x*-ray picture as a focus of osteolysis which may be more or less uniformly radiolucent or appear loculated. The fact that the primary tumor is in the thyroid is often not recognized until tissue removed in the course of a biopsy on the skeletal lesion is examined histologically. The association is then a rather simple matter, since the cytologic pattern of the tissue from the metastatic focus nearly always clearly suggests a thyroid origin. Interestingly enough, despite the accessibility of the thyroid to physical examination, the fact that the gland is the site of a

***Figure 188***

*A*, Roentgenograph showing evidence of osteolytic destruction of parts of the 6th, 7th, and 8th thoracic vertebræ in a case of metastatic cancer in which involvement of these vertebræ constituted the presenting clinical lesion. The patient was a man 38 years of age who had been suffering from increasing pain (local and radiating) in the midthoracic region. A few days prior to admission to the hospital, he had developed difficulty in walking, associated with paresthesias of the lower abdomen and lower limbs. Physical examination revealed pronounced weakness of these limbs and other neurological signs pointing to compression of the cord at the level of the 7th and 8th thoracic vertebræ. A laminectomy was done as an emergency measure to avert the development of a complete transverse myelitis, and tissue obtained in the course of the intervention revealed the presence of an epidermoid carcinoma. During the 5 months preceding the patient's death, many clinical examinations were made in a search for the primary tumor, but with negative results. The autopsy, too, failed to reveal the site of the primary lesion. The latter was not in the lungs, and indeed the lungs were found completely free of tumor. There was a suspicion, on the basis of roentgenographic study of the skull during life, that the primary lesion might have been in the right antrum, but it was not possible to follow this clue at autopsy.

*B*, Photograph showing, in sagittal section, the affected part of the column in the case illustrated in *A*. The 6th, 7th, and 8th thoracic vertebræ are strikingly involved by tumor, the body of the 8th showing complete collapse. The contour of the spinal canal is deformed, and a large tumor mass is present at the site of the previous laminectomy. Histologic examination of the affected vertebral bodies showed that wherever the tumor tissue was present the original osseous tissue had been destroyed, and the osteolysis was not associated with any reactive osteoplasia.

*C*, Photograph showing, in sagittal section, a part of the cervicothoracic portion of a vertebral column which is the site of metastatic involvement by a mucous adenocarcinoma. Autopsy revealed that the primary site of the cancer was the first branch of the right bronchus. The patient was a man 69 years of age who entered the hospital because of pain in the cervical region of 3 months' duration, and because of weakness and paresthesias of the upper extremities. *X*-ray examinations done at the time of admission revealed collapse of the body of the 7th cervical vertebra and the presence of a tumor in the right lung. Thus, in this case, too, it was complaints arising from involvement of vertebræ that brought the patient to the hospital, while the primary lesion was clinically silent. The patient died 7 months after the onset of his complaints. Note the almost total collapse of the body of the 7th cervical vertebra and partial collapse of the body of the 1st thoracic vertebra. Observe also that bulging of these bodies posteriorly has narrowed the vertebral canal and compressed the cord.

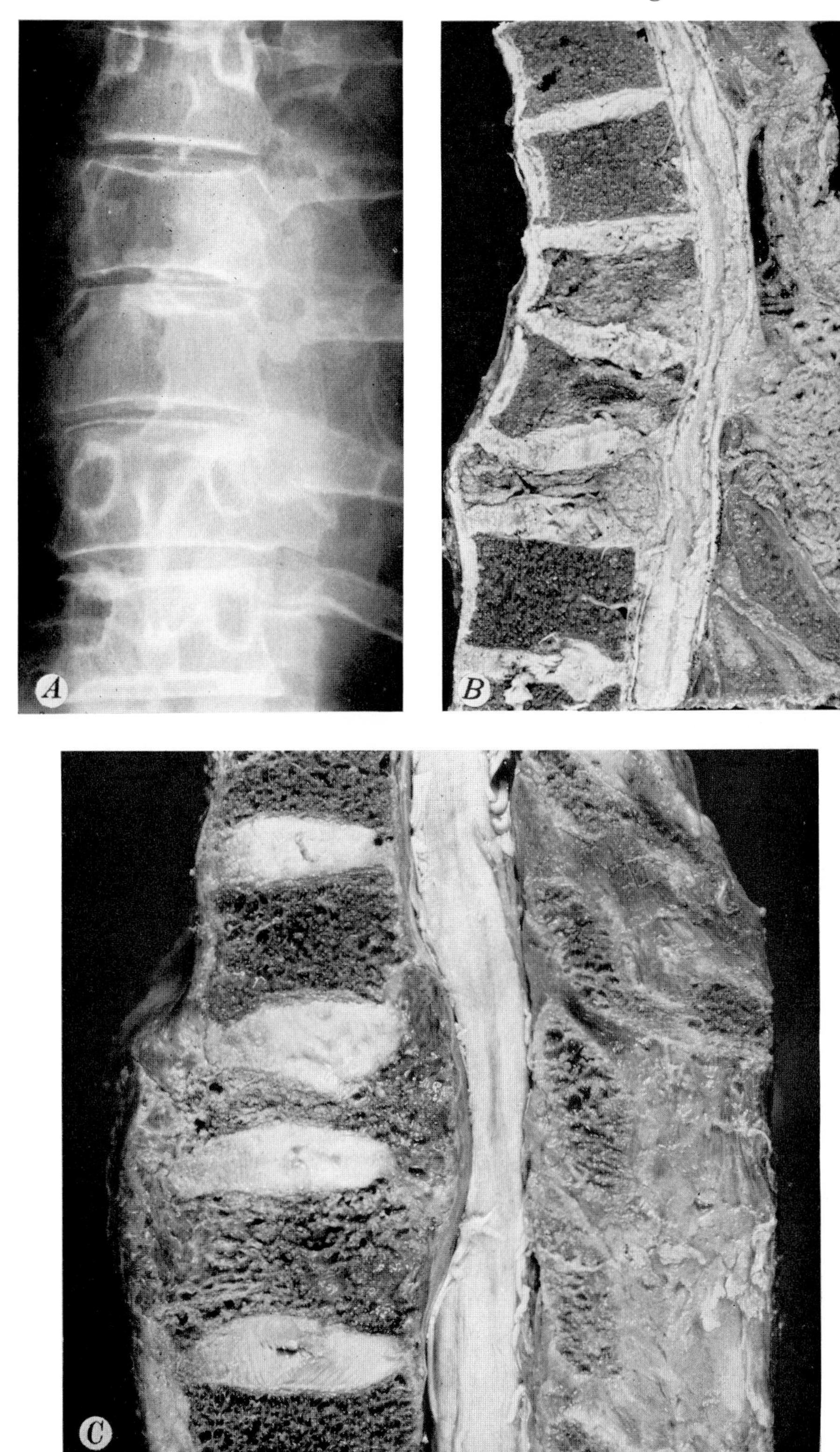


*Figure 188*

cancer is often overlooked clinically. Thus, not infrequently, the first recognition of that fact comes from study of the biopsy specimen from a focus of skeletal metastasis which it has produced.

In regard to cancer of the *prostate,* it is by no means unusual for the patient to seek medical attention merely on account of low back pain. In the majority of such cases, roentgenographic examination will show in particular that the lower part of the vertebral column and/or the pelvic bones are the site of extensive radiopacities representing osteoplastic metastases. Further study of the patient is very likely to reveal that the prostate is enlarged and is the site of one or more extremely firm nodular masses representing the carcinoma. Under these circumstances, the serum acid phosphatase value is usually found elevated. Indeed, the clinical diagnosis of prostatic carcinoma with skeletal metastases presents no problem in such a case when these various findings are considered together.

On the other hand, there are occasional cases of prostatic carcinoma in which it is complaints due to skeletal involvement that lead the patient to seek medical care, but in which the fact that he is affected with a carcinoma of the prostate is not revealed until some time later and perhaps only at autopsy. A case in point observed by the writer was that of a man 74 years of age who entered our hospital on account of swelling of the lower part of the right leg of about 6 months' duration. *X*-ray examination of the leg in question disclosed extensive tumorous involvement, osteoplastic in character, of much of the tibia and fibula. A skeletal survey revealed, furthermore, that osteoplastic metastases were also present in the scapula, ribs, vertebral column, and pelvic bones, though these were asymptomatic. The lungs revealed no evidence of involvement.

On clinical examination, the prostate was found to be small, nontender, and free of any firm nodular masses. Furthermore, the serum acid phosphatase value was found to be within normal limits. Thus, despite the fact that the skeletal changes visible in the *x*-ray pictures were highly suggestive of metastases from a carcinoma of the prostate, the clinical and biochemical findings did not sustain this impression. Biopsy of the affected fibula established the presence of metastatic cancer, but the cellular pattern of the tumor tissue was not such as to indicate definitively that the primary tumor was in the prostate. It was only at autopsy (about 6 weeks after the patient's admission to the hospital) that this fact was uncovered. Though the prostate was small, weighing only 20 gms., it was the site of a rather anaplastic carcinoma.

These few examples will suffice to point up the diagnostic problems which may arise when a focus of skeletal metastasis is the presenting lesion in a case of cancer. However, it should be noted that, in cases in which a cancer is known to be present in some organ and in which there are no complaints referable to the bones, roentgenographic examination of the skeleton may nevertheless reveal the presence of a suggestive or even clear-cut bone lesion. Under these circumstances, if the skeletal survey had not been made, the case might not be recognized as one in which metastases were already present early in the course of the disease. Furthermore, even if the clinical roentgenographs had not revealed findings suggestive of metastasis, one still cannot be certain that some bone part was not already affected. Indeed, unless the metastatic cancer has produced a good deal of alteration in the architecture of the osseous tissue at its site, the metastatic focus is not likely to be apparent in the clinical roentgenographs.

## INCIDENCE AND LOCALIZATION OF SKELETAL METASTASES

The fact that a focus of skeletal metastasis is frequently the presenting lesion in a case of cancer involving some organ, for instance, was discussed in the previous section. It was also pointed out there that one or more skeletal metastases may be present early in the course of a case of cancer without giving rise to clinical complaints. Furthermore, it was indicated that even if the roentgenographs fail to reveal skeletal metastases, these are sometimes already present. One must also recognize that in cases of cancerous disease of long standing, in which metastases are already present in the lungs and/or liver, clinical roentgenographs of the skeleton are likewise an unsatisfactory gauge of the presence and extent of metastases. Even if they do reveal a few metastatic lesions, the roentgenographs still give a very inadequate picture of the extent of the total skeletal involvement. Indeed, there may be widespread metastases to the bones which may not show up at all in roentgenographs taken even shortly before death.

**Incidence.**—In evaluating published reports on the incidence of skeletal metastasis, it is particularly important to take into account the circumstances under which the metastases came to attention. For instance, if a report is heavily weighted with cases in which a focus of skeletal metastasis was the presenting lesion, the reported figures on incidence must be interpreted with certain reservations. Notably, as implied, such figures give no indication of the extent to which skeletal metastases that are clinically silent or roentgenographically undetectable are present in the total series of the cases reported. If a report is heavily weighted with cases in which the patient continued to survive for years after treatment of the primary lesion but still died from the effects of cancer, the reported figures on the incidence of skeletal metastases must likewise be critically considered. In evaluating such reports, one must ask whether the figures on skeletal metastasis are based largely on antemortem roentgenographic study of the skeleton or on autopsy findings. If the estimate of incidence is based largely on roentgenographic findings, one must be aware that, as already noted, skeletal metastases may be present without being apparent in the *x*-ray pictures. Even if the estimate is based on autopsy findings, one may well ask whether the decision about the presence or absence of skeletal metastases was founded on adequate sampling of the skeleton.

In the final analysis, the actual ultimate incidence of skeletal metastases in connection with cancer can be ascertained only on the basis of anatomic study of many bones in cases which have run their full course. Obviously, a comprehensive investigation of the skeleton at autopsy involves certain practical difficulties. However, the bones of the trunk are so definitely predilected that their condition in respect to metastasis can be regarded as a criterion for the skeleton as a whole. Indeed, before maintaining that skeletal metastases are not present in a case of cancer which has come to autopsy, one should remove and examine at least a large segment of the vertebral column, many ribs, the sternum, and parts of both iliac bones.* If no metastases are found in any of these skeletal areas, it is not likely, though still possible, that some are present elsewhere in the skeleton. If the skeletal areas in question do show metastases, there is a strong likelihood that other bones (notably the calvarium, the upper ends of the femora, and/or the bones of the shoulder girdle) will also show them.

In the older literature, the over-all incidence of metastasis of cancer to the skeleton is reported to be about 13 per cent as calculated on the basis of large series of cases coming to autopsy (see Willis, and Walther). This figure relates to miscellaneous cases representing carcinomas and sarcomas of various kinds and of various degrees of known metastatic potential. In comparison with the current findings on the

*The procedure which we employ, as part of our routine autopsy technique, for removing a large segment of the vertebral column has been described by Selin *et al.* In the article in question, directions are also given for reconstructing the column into a unit which will remain firm under subsequent handling of the body. In addition, there are outlined briefly various ways of gross sectioning of the column, directed toward the demonstration of particular pathologic alterations.

incidence of skeletal metastasis in cases of cancer coming to autopsy, the value of 13 per cent is certainly very low.

The explanation for the discrepancy lies partly in the fact that improvements in the methods of prevention and in the management of surgical shock and postoperative infection have greatly reduced the proportion of cancer cases coming to autopsy in which the patient has died very shortly after surgery undertaken in connection with treatment of the primary lesion. Since skeletal metastases may not yet have developed in these instances, the inclusion of large numbers of such cases in any series would naturally reduce the over-all incidence of skeletal metastasis. Furthermore, improved medical management of cancer patients has tended to lengthen the period of survival, so that on this account, also, the time during which skeletal metastases might develop has been increased. Indeed, on the basis of his own experience in regard to fatal cases of cancer which have come to autopsy in recent years, and in which the bones have been adequately sampled, the writer rates the over-all incidence of skeletal metastasis at 70 per cent or more, rather than 13 per cent. If one considers only the most common carcinomas (notably those of the breast, lung, prostate, kidney, and thyroid), the incidence of skeletal metastasis in cases which have run their full clinical course is probably about 85 per cent.

**Localization.**—As to the sites of skeletal metastasis, the outstandingly frequent involvement of the vertebral column has already been noted. Indeed, if there are metastases in the skeleton at all, they will almost certainly be present in the vertebral column, whether other skeletal areas are also involved or not. Within the column, one, several, or many vertebræ (including those of the sacrum) may be affected. When vertebral metastases from all primary sites are considered together, it is the thoracic region of the column that is found to be most often and most heavily affected, and the lumbar area comes next in order. However, for cancer primary

***Figure 189***

*A*, Roentgenograph showing, in lateral projection, the lower 3 thoracic and the 1st lumba vertebral bodies of a column removed at autopsy in a case of mucinous adenocarcinoma primary in the colon. Despite the fact that all the overlying soft tissues have been cleared away, one cannot see any clear-cut evidence of metastatic involvement of the vertebral bodies in question. (This picture was taken on non-screen film with a conventional diagnostic *x*-ray unit.)

*B*, Photograph showing, in sagittal section, the 4 vertebræ illustrated in *A*. Note that the anterior upper portion of the 10th thoracic body and the posterior upper portion of the 1st lumbar body present foci of mucinous cancer which are just perceptible to the nakes eye.

*C*, Roentgenograph of a 6 mm. slice of the bodies shown in *B*. The picture was taken on non-screen film, also with a conventional diagnostic *x*-ray unit, but the exposure time was modified for the thinness of the tissue slice. Under these conditions, the involvement of the 10th thoracic and 1st lumbar bodies has become apparent through alteration in the details of the trabecular patterns. Observe also that the 12th vertebra, too, appears to be the site of the lodgment of tumor tissue, though this was not apparent in the gross specimen. Compare these affected vertebral bodies with the 11th vertebral body, whose trabecular architecture presents a fairly normal pattern.

*D*, Photomicrograph (× 5) showing the focus of metastatic cancer in the upper right-hand corner of the 10th thoracic vertebra illustrated in *B* and *C*. In this photomicrograph the postion of the focus of tumor is reversed, and it appears in the upper left-hand corner of the picture. However, it is clear that one is dealing with the same focus, since one can see the anterior ligament to the left of it. Note also that the tumor has not completely destroyed the original osseous tissue of the site, and that, on the other hand, there is no new bone deposition (osteoplastic reaction) either.

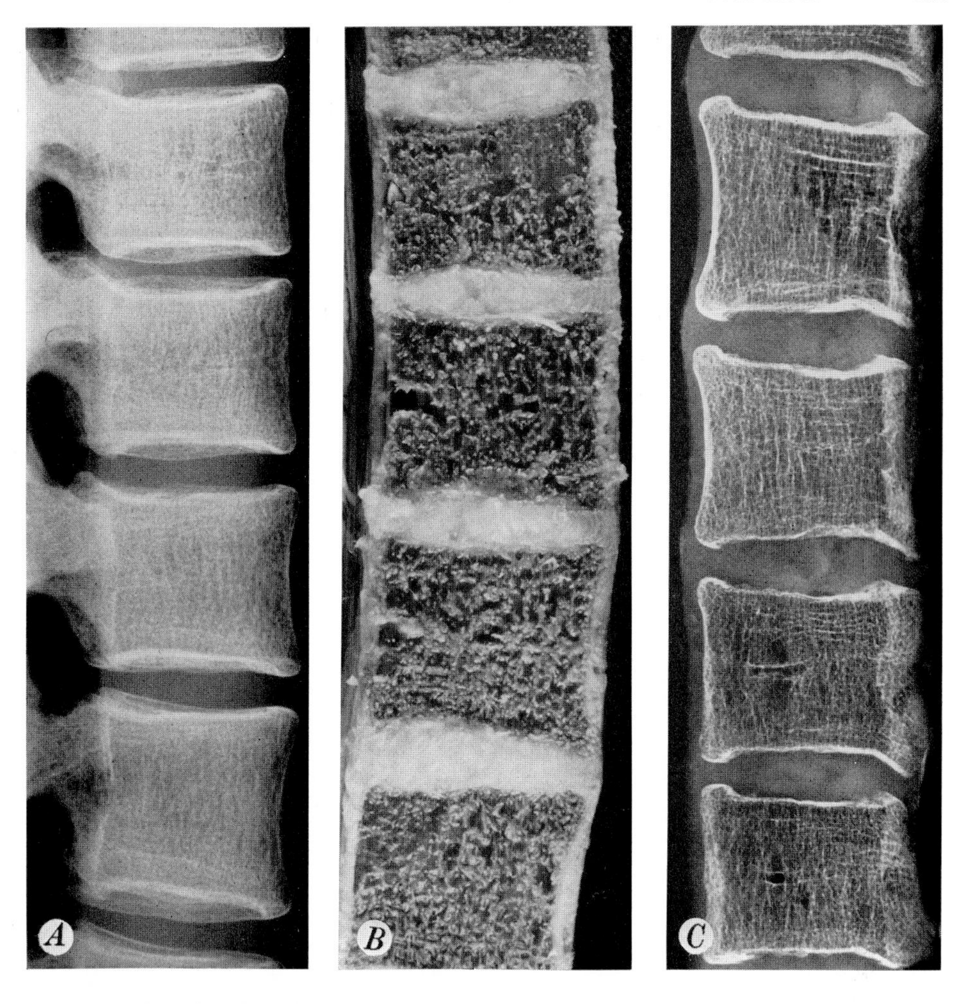


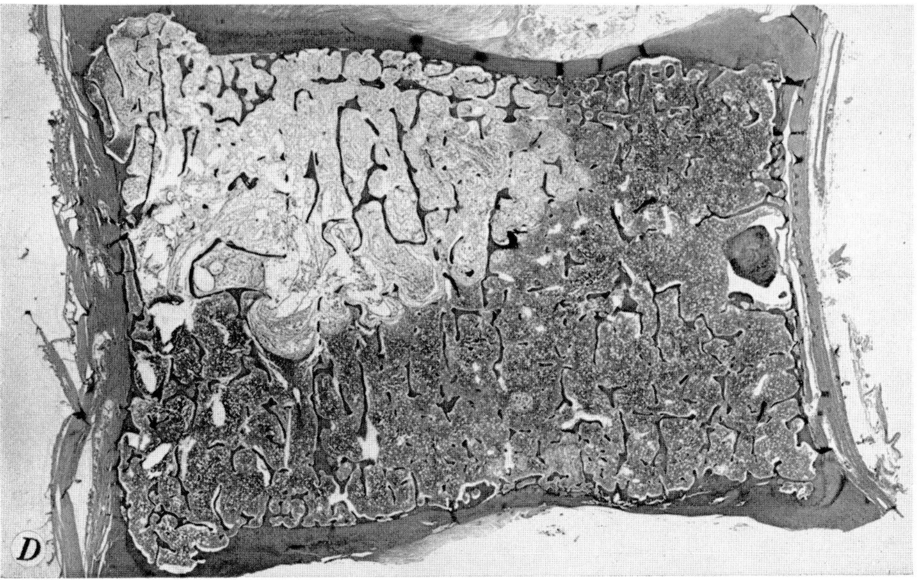


*Figure 189*

in the prostate in particular, the vertebral sites of predilection are the lumbar area and the sacrum.

The sternum and ribs and the upper part of the femur are also common sites of metastasis, though ranking definitely below the vertebral column. The three skeletal sites which seem to rank next in order of frequency of involvement are the innominate bone, the calvarium, and the humerus. However, in regard to these sites, too, certain primary cancers show special predilections. Thus the innominate bones are among the most frequent sites of skeletal involvement when the primary tumor is in the prostate, and the skull bones are almost always (and usually heavily) implicated when the primary lesion is a neuroblastoma, which usually arises in an adrenal gland.

Occasionally a metastatic lesion is found in a scapula or clavicle. Metastases to other skeletal sites, including jawbones, have been known to occur but are uncommon. In this connection it can be said in general that bones distal to the knee joint, and particularly those distal to the elbow joint, are very exceptional sites for metastasis.

## ROENTGENOGRAPHIC *VS.* ANATOMIC FINDINGS RELATING TO SKELETAL METASTASES

Comparative studies undertaken to elucidate the conditions under which skeletal metastases show up in the *x*-ray picture have dealt mainly with the vertebral column (see Borak, Young and Funk, and Bachman and Sproul). The clearest roentgenographic sign of metastatic involvement of a vertebral body, and the one least likely to be obscured by the intervening soft tissues, is alteration of its contour. In particular, part of the outline of the body may be blurred, the contour of the

***Figure 190***

*A*, Photograph showing, in sagittal section, the lower 4 lumbar vertebræ, which are the site of metastases from a cancer primary in the left breast. The patient was a woman 57 years of age who died 2½ years after mastectomy. Terminally, she presented toxic manifestations of hypercalcemia which were apparently induced (or at least aggravated) by the hormone therapy she received for several months before her death. (For the renal changes associated with the hypercalcemia in this case, see Figs. 193-*A* and *B*.)

*B*, Roentgenograph of a 6 mm. slice of the bodies shown in *A*. However, the picture is oriented so that the anterior surface of the column is on the right-hand side, instead of being on the left as it is in *A*. It is interesting to compare the alterations observed roentgenographically in each of the affected vertebral bodies with those shown in the corresponding gross picture. In some areas the changes do not stand out so well in the *x*-ray picture as they do in the photograph of the gross specimen, and vice versa. (Industrial type M film was used, and the picture was taken with a 50 kilovolt industrial *x*-ray unit adapted for roentgenographing tissues.)

*C*, Roentgenograph (somewhat enlarged) of a 1 mm. slice cut from the surface of the 2nd lumbar body shown in *B*. This picture, too, was taken with the industrial *x*-ray unit, and industrial type M film was again used. Certain details of the changes going on in the vertebral body are brought out in this picture which were not observed in the 6 mm. slice shown in *B*. For instance, the small, roundish radiolucent area apparent in the 1 mm. roentgenograph slice cannot be seen in the 6 mm. slice, though it can be seen in the photograph of the gross specimen.

*D*, Roentgenograph (somewhat enlarged) of a 1 mm. slice cut from the surface of the 4th lumbar vertebra shown in *B*, bringing out the details of the changes. The orientation is somewhat different, however, the anterior border of the body being on the left in this *x*-ray picture and on the right in *B*.

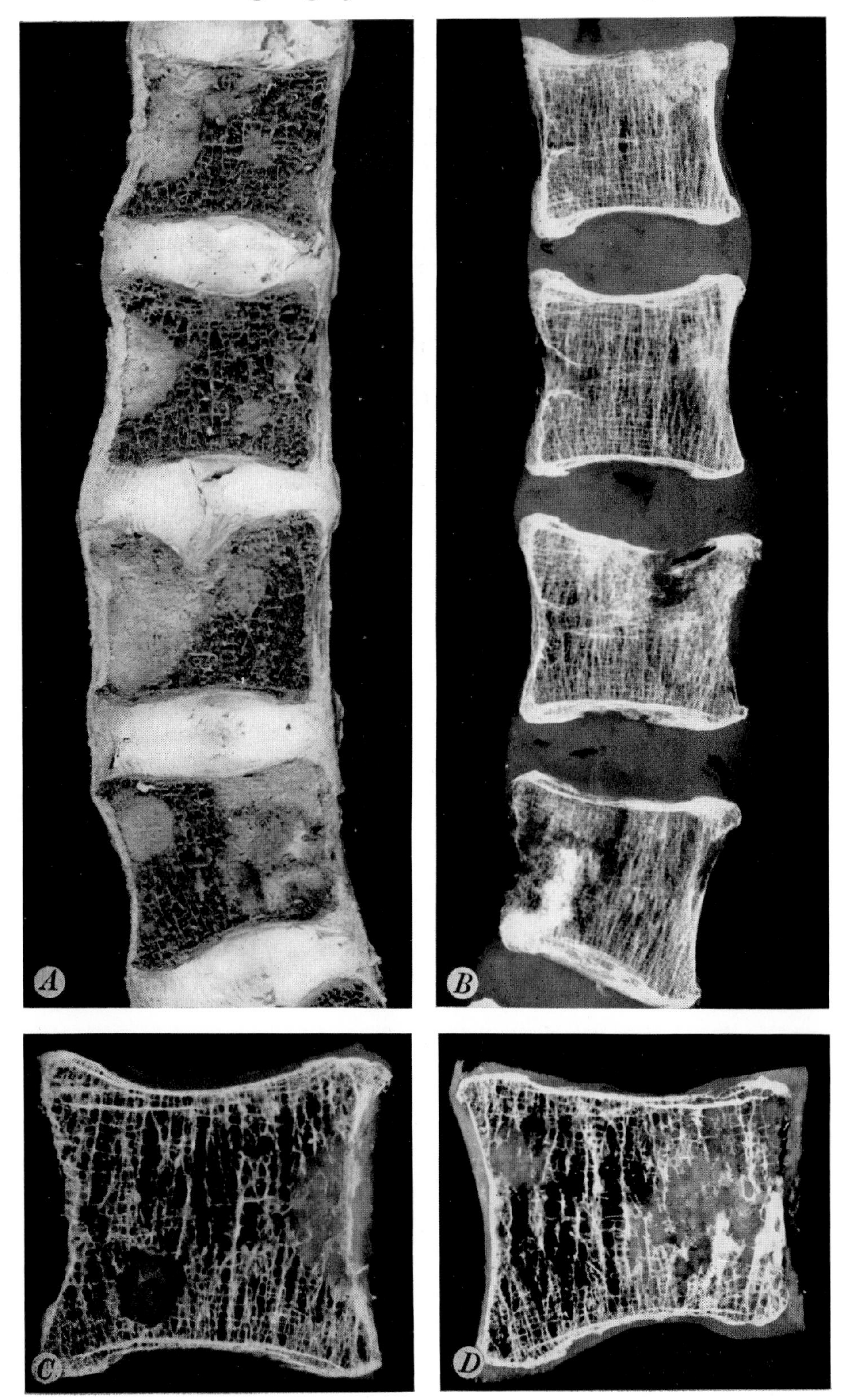


***Figure 190***

body may show some deformation, the body may have suffered partial compressional collapse, or it may even have undergone such radical change in contour as to appear wedged.

In the absence of alteration in contour, an affected vertebral body may still be substantially filled by tumor tissue, and yet the clinical roentgenographs may fail to reveal changes. If none are to be seen, it is because the presence of the tumor tissue is not associated with lytic destruction of large amounts of the spongy bone or with manifestations of an osteoplastic reaction—that is, the formation of new bone in the region of the tumor. Indeed, changes may not be apparent under these conditions even if the vertebral body in question has been removed at autopsy, hemisectioned, and then roentgenographed. Furthermore, even if affected vertebral bodies are the site of a certain amount of lytic destruction or osteoplastic reaction, the involvement may be prevented from showing up in clinical roentgenographs by excessive thickness of the intervening soft tissues. (See Figs. 189 and 190.)

Various workers have made studies comparing the roentgenographic with the gross and microscopic findings relating to segments of the vertebral column in cases of cancer coming to autopsy. Bachman and Sproul, in particular, correlated the anatomic findings not only with those from the last antemortem *x*-ray picture of the spine, but also with tomographs and conventional *x*-ray pictures of the spine made just before the autopsy. Among the 31 specimens in their series in which the presence of metastases was established by the anatomic findings, there were only 15 (48 per cent) in which metastases were visualized roentgenographically. Like others, these workers found that the size of a metastatic focus was of crucial significance insofar as the roentgenographic demonstrability of the lesion was concerned. However, even a lesion 1.5 cm. or more in diameter was often not demonstrable roentgenographically unless its presence was associated with a good deal of local osteolysis on the one hand or osteoplastic reaction on the other. It is worth noting also that anteroposterior tomography was not more successful than the conventional roentgenographs in revealing occult metastases.

The ribs, sternum, iliac bones, and the metaphysial ends of certain long bones may likewise contain considerable tumor tissue in the spongy marrow spaces without presenting roentgenographic evidence of this. Indeed, the tumor may even have induced a good deal of lytic destruction of the spongy trabeculæ, but here again this may not be demonstrable in the clinical *x*-ray pictures because the regional cortex has not been destroyed or otherwise modified. The patient may even have had pain localized to one of these sites, perhaps for weeks, before changes finally became apparent roentgenographically in the site in question. However, if a cancer patient complains of pain referable to a site where the cortical bone is thick (the calvarium or the midshaft of a long bone, for example), the great likelihood is that destructive changes will already be evident in the *x*-ray picture. On the other hand, these sites are often found to present evidence of considerable osteolysis in the absence of related clinical complaints.

## OSTEOLYTIC *VS.* OSTEOPLASTIC SKELETAL METASTASES

The terms "osteolytic" and "osteoplastic" metastases have traditionally been used to point up certain roentgenographic and anatomic contrasts among skeletal metastases. In a focus of osteolytic metastasis, the anatomic picture is dominated by dissolution and/or actual destruction of the original osseous tissue at the affected bone site. Consequently, if obliteration of the original osseous tissue is sufficiently extensive, the lesional area in question appears more or less radiolucent in the *x*-ray picture. In a focus of osteoplastic metastasis, the anatomic picture is one in which the deposition of new bone definitely predominates over any osteolysis that is or has been occurring. So much new bone may have formed that the area appears densely sclerotic even on gross examination. Such a lesional area tends to be manifest roentgenographically as a focus of more or less pronounced radiopacity. By and large, osteoplastic metastases are much more likely to show up roentgenographically at an early stage of their development in any site than are osteolytic metastases. Furthermore, even very extensive osteoplastic metastases are frequently demonstrable in the absence of clinical complaints referable to them.

In designating skeletal metastases from a particular primary growth as either predominantly osteolytic or predominantly osteoplastic, one is making a rough but serviceable distinction. However, no useful purpose seems to be served by attempting to establish gradations of osteolysis and osteoplasia within the two groups. Also, a decision as to whether the metastases from a cancer in a particular case are to be classed on the whole as osteolytic or osteoplastic should not be made on the basis of study of mere isolated areas of metastasis. For instance, in a case in which the metastases from a cancer are of the essentially osteolytic type, one or more affected vertebral bodies may show a good deal of sclerosis, due to compressional collapse. Thus, on the basis of the appearance of the collapsed vertebræ alone, the case might be interpreted as one showing osteoplastic metastases, despite the fact that the metastases elsewhere in the skeleton were predominantly osteolytic. Actually, the new bone seen within the compressed and collapsed vertebral bodies under these conditions represents mainly internal fracture callus formed in reaction to the collapse, and not new bone formed in response to the presence of the tumor tissue. Furthermore, skeletal metastases from certain primary cancers (notably carcinoma of the breast) often produce both osteolytic and osteoplastic metastases. In such a case, one would, of course, be overlooking the osteolytic metastases if one drew conclusions regarding the nature of the metastases from study of an osteoplastic area alone.

Be that as it may, there are certain cancers whose skeletal metastases tend strongly to be of the osteolytic type. (See Fig. 191.) These include hypernephroma, carcinoma of the thyroid, carcinomas of the lower bowel, and neuroblastoma (primary in the adrenal or elsewhere). A considerable proportion of metastases from cancers primary in the breast are likewise essentially of the osteolytic type. However, as already noted, there are a good many cases of breast cancer in which the metastases also show evidences of osteoplasia. Indeed, in such cases, osteolytic and osteoplastic areas may be found intermingled, as is usually best demonstrated in affected vertebral bodies.

In connection with bronchogenic carcinoma (and also, in the writer's experience, with signet cell carcinoma of the stomach), the skeletal metastases tend on the whole to be of the osteoplastic type. However, as is well known, it is cancer of the prostate that produces osteoplastic skeletal metastases most regularly and in the most pronounced form. Indeed, affected vertebræ may appear densely sclerotic throughout, though others may still show small areas which have not yet undergone this change. Other bones, too (the innominate bones, ribs, upper ends of the femora), when cut open, often reveal smaller or larger roundish, dense, osteoplastic areas. Also, in cases of skeletal metastasis from prostatic carcinoma, the cortices of affected bones may be found roughened by osteophytic deposits. These represent periosteal new bone that has formed in reaction to the presence of tumor cells which have penetrated the cortex and settled beneath the periosteum.

It seems appropriate to note here that there are certain conditions under which osteoplastic metastases may be simulated. For instance, on gross inspection, a sectioned vertebral column sometimes creates the illusion that it is the site of osteoplastic metastasis merely because the marrow spaces of the vertebral bodies are very tightly packed with cancer cells. In such a case, it is not until one studies histologic sections from the affected bones that the erroneous impression is corrected, because one fails to find evidence of new bone deposition and notes that the original osseous trabeculæ are also essentially unmodified. Another circumstance which may deceive one is observed sometimes in connection with metastatic foci of keratinizing epidermoid carcinoma from the lung, for instance. Grossly, such foci of bone metastasis may appear gritty, and roentgenographically they may cast radiopaque shadows. Histologic examination shows, however, that osseous tissue has not been laid down in these metastatic lesions and that the impression that this has happened is created merely by the fact that the keratinized epidermoid carcinoma metastases are the site of calcium deposition.

In the evolution of *osteolytic metastases,* growth pressure from the proliferating tumor tissue upon the regional osseous tissue seems to play the dominant role in the osteolysis. As the tumor cells come to fill the intertrabecular marrow spaces and abut against the osseous trabeculæ, the latter tend to become thinned and may even disappear in some places. Osteoclasts play little if any part in the resorption of the osseous tissue. Indeed, they are sparse on the whole and sometimes have to be searched for. As the focus of tumor grows larger, more of the trabeculæ undergo dissolution, and a particular area under observation may be found completely devoid of them.

However, what has just been said relates only to areas of osteolytic metastasis in which the tumor tissue is viable and proliferating. In areas in which the tumor tissue has become necrotic, any osseous tissue still present will likewise be found necrotic and even fragmented. If the necrotic area becomes revascularized, one may note some evidences of new bone deposition on the previously necrotic osseous trabeculæ, and the necrotic tumor tissue itself may have become scarified. Furthermore, if a vertebral body which has been the site of massive osteolytic metastasis has collapsed, considerable new bone formation (representing internal callus) may occur at the site. This is to be observed if the area has become revascularized and there has been a long interval between the occurrence of the collapse and the anatomic examination of the vertebra in question.

***Figure 191***

*A*, Roentgenograph of the lumbar area from a sagittally sectioned vertebral column showing extensive osteolysis produced by metastases from a carcinoma of the stomach. The patient was a woman 35 years of age who entered the hospital with a history of gastric complaints of only 10 weeks' standing and died 1 month later. No surgical intervention was undertaken, since it was apparent at the time of admission that widespread metastases were already present. Note the numerous large areas of striking radiolucency in the vertebral bodies and spinous processes and the generally rarefied status of these bones.

*B*, Photograph showing the appearance of the lower 4 lumbar vertebræ illustrated in *A*, after the specimen had been macerated to remove the overlying soft parts and the tumor tissue. The extensive lytic destruction which the metastatic tumor had induced in the vertebral bodies stands out very clearly.

*C*, Photomicrograph (× 10) showing part of a vertebral body which is the site of an osteolytic metastasis from a cancer primary in a breast. The anterior ligament can be seen at the upper border of the picture, and part of the intervertebral disk can be seen at the right. Almost nothing is left of the original osseous tissue at the site of the metastasis. (The osteolytic changes illustrated in this figure contrast strikingly with the osteoplastic changes shown in Fig. 192.)

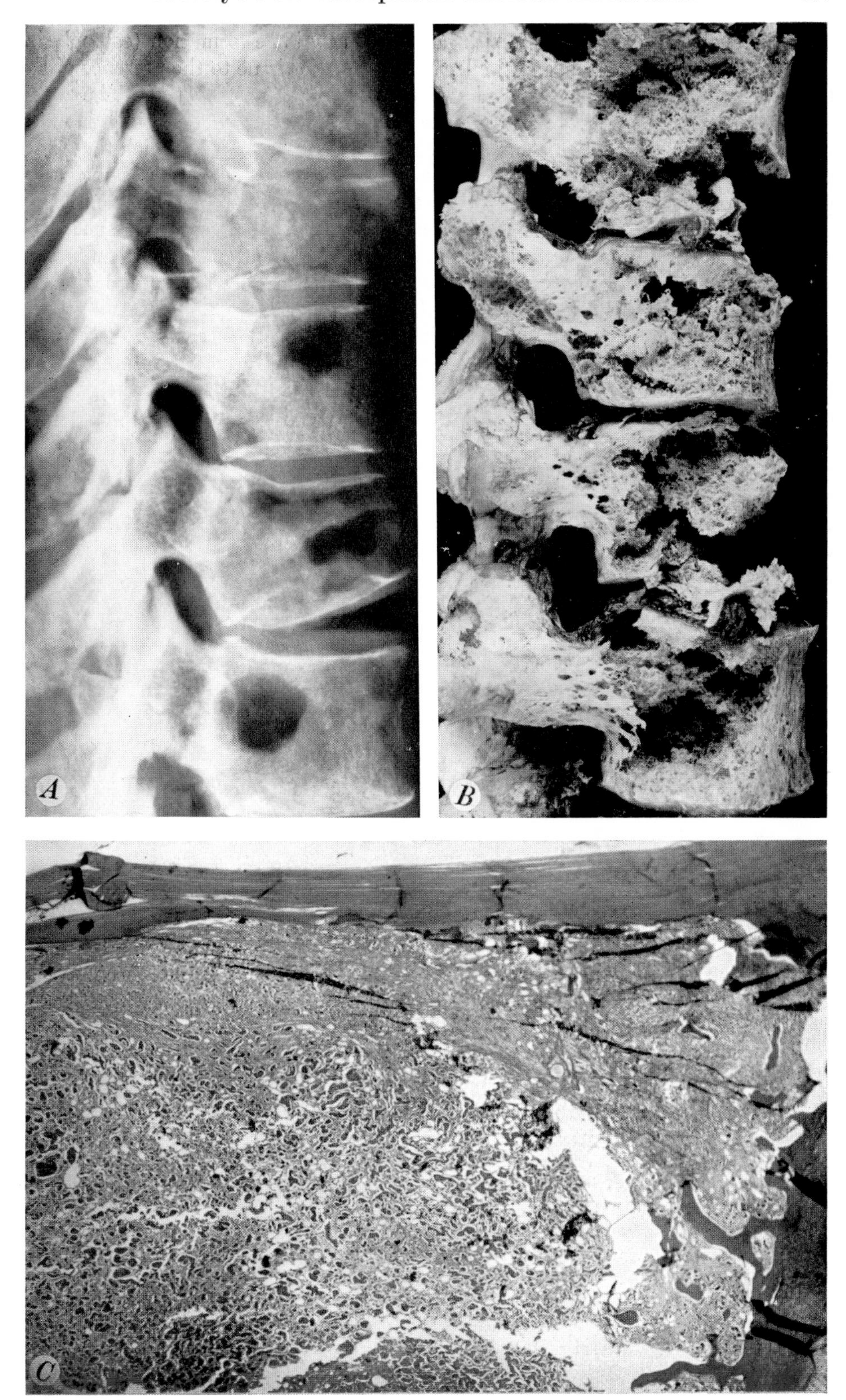


*Figure 191*

In the evolution of *osteoplastic metastases,* the new bone formation (osteoplasia) represents a reactive response of the local osteogenetic tissue to the presence of the tumor; the tumor cells apparently play no direct role in the osteogenesis. The extent of the osteoplasia observed in a particular area or in a given metastatic lesion as a whole may vary. One may encounter an osteoplastic metastasis in which the osteoplasia is associated with a good deal of osteolysis. On the other hand, in some osteo plastic foci, osteoplasia is so active that the concomitant osteolysis is completely submerged. Under these circumstances, much of the original osseous tissue at the site of the metastasis may even have been preserved. What one finds then is considerable new bone present between cancer cells in the marrow spaces and apposed on the original osseous tissue. (See Fig. 192.)

In regard to what instigates the osteoplasia, the writer does not wish to go beyond his statement that the occurrence of considerable new bone formation in a metastatic lesion represents a reactive response of the local osteogenetic tissue to the presence of the tumor. In particular, he does not wish to imply, as some have done, that a focus of metastasis at a given site is osteoplastic merely because the rate of bone repair is greater than the rate of bone destruction at that site. The interpretation of the osteoplastic response solely as a reparative reaction is appropriate only in connection with new bone formation representing callus repair at a site of metastatic cancer. A good many other theories have been advanced to account for the appearance of osteoplastic metastases. However, none of the explanations seem to be applicable to all the conditions under which such metastases appear.

## CERTAIN CLINICAL AND BIOCHEMICAL CONSIDERATIONS

The possible presence of a *hypercalcemia* must always be borne in mind in connection with cancer metastatic to the skeleton. In an adult, a definite hypercalcemia is represented by a serum calcium value of 11.5 mg. per 100 cc. or more—that is,

***Figure 192***

*A*, Roentgenograph of a longitudinally sliced segment of a vertebral column showing 4 vertebral bodies (11th and 12th thoracic and 1st and 2nd lumbar) altered by osteoplastic metastases from a carcinoma of the prostate. Note the wide variation in the degree of radiopacity presented by the different vertebral bodies. The patient was a man 68 years of age who entered the hospital on account of pain of 8 months' standing. The pain was centered in the lower part of the back and radiated to the buttocks and lower limbs. The patient died 2 days after admission, and the cause of death was massive pulmonary embolism. Although at the autopsy the vertebral column was found extensively involved by metastases, no metastases were found either in the lungs or in the liver.

*B*, Photograph illustrating the appearance of the uppermost vertebral body shown in *A*, after it had been macerated. Note the close compaction of the osseous tissue (new bone formed in reaction to the presence of the cancer) throughout most of the body. To the left, one sees a small area in which the architecture of the spongy bone is still relatively normal. There is striking correspondence in detail between the gross appearance of this macerated body and the *x*-ray appearance it presents.

*C*, Photograph showing the most intensely sclerotic body illustrated in *A*, after it had been macerated. Note that the compaction of the newly formed osseous tissue is so dense that the affected surface of the body looks almost like coarse pumice stone.

*D*, Photomicrograph (× 5) presenting a survey view of a histologic section prepared from the particularly sclerotic body shown in *C*. The reactively formed and condensed new bone has largely crowded out the tumor tissue.

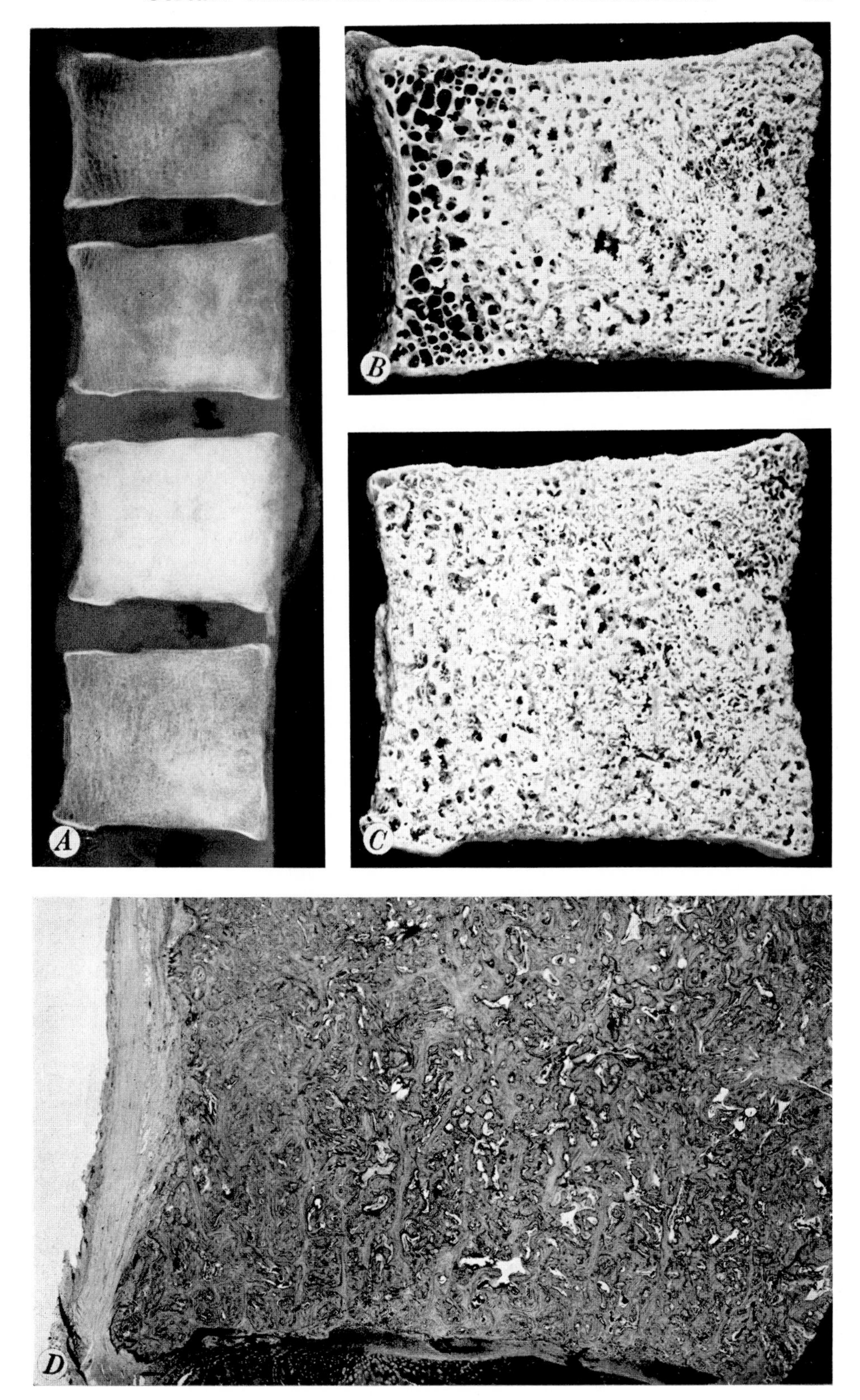


*Figure 192*

a value 1 mg. above the normal upper limit of the serum calcium value.* Values of 13 to 15 mg. represent a pronounced hypercalcemia, and values definitely above 15 indicate a hypercalcemia so extreme that it is almost certain to be associated with severe toxic effects (see Jaffe and Bodansky).

Clinically, the toxic manifestations of hypercalcemia include: (1) gastrointestinal disturbances (anorexia, nausea, vomiting leading to loss of water and electrolytes, and constipation); (2) neurological symptoms (apathy, weakness, drowsiness sometimes merging into disorientation and stupor or coma); (3) cardiac aberrations

*As determined in the morning after a fast of about 12 hours, practically all *normal calcium values* of human blood serum fall within the following limits: 9.5 to 10.5 mg. per 100 cc. for adults, 10.0 to 11.5 for children, and 10.5 to 12 for neonates and other infants. It should also be noted that, in a normal subject, these individual values remain practically the same from morning to morning. Indeed, through the balance maintained between the factors of calcium absorption, excretion, and storage in or release from the tissues, the serum calcium value readily restabilizes itself after any modification which food consumption, fasting, exercise, etc. may tend to introduce in the course of the day.

In evaluating a serum calcium finding, consideration must also be given to the findings in respect to the serum *inorganic phosphate* and the total serum protein. It is well known that an increase in the serum inorganic phosphate value (normal value 2.5 to 4.0 mg. per 100 cc. in adults) tends to be associated with a reduction in the calcium value, and vice versa. This reciprocal relation is one to be expected theoretically. It is observed clinically and experimentally under certain conditions, but under other circumstances it may be masked. In any event, in a cancer patient in whom the serum inorganic phosphate value is definitely elevated, the presence of a calcium value which even lies at or near the upper limits of the normal may be held to point in the direction of hypercalcemia.

In connection with the value of the total *serum proteins* (normal value 6.5 to 7.5 gm. per 100 cc.), it should be borne in mind that about 40 per cent of the serum calcium is combined with the albumin fraction of the serum protein. Hence, a decrease in the serum protein, due to a decrease in the albumin fraction, is reflected in a decrease in the serum calcium value. Thus, in a case of cancer in which the patient has skeletal metastases and a reduced serum protein value on account of cachexia, a serum calcium value even at the upper limit of the normal range could be held to represent at least a slight degree of hypercalcemia.

## *Figure 193*

*A*, Roentgenograph of a 3 mm. slice of part of a kidney from the case illustrated in Fig. 190, in which widespread skeletal metastases were associated with hormone-induced hypercalcemia. The serum calcium value was 18.3 mg. per cent the day before the patient died. Note the profuse delicate radiating streaks of radiopacity representing calcium in the collecting tubules.

*B*, Photomicrograph (× 12) presenting a survey view of a small area of the cortex of the kidney shown in *A*. The dark streaks represent the calcium in the renal tubules.

*C*, Photograph of a patient affected with a bronchogenic carcinoma and manifesting pulmonary hypertrophic osteoarthropathy. He was admitted to our hospital because of complaints relating to his joints, the pulmonary lesion being clinically occult. These complaints had been present for about 1 year. In particular, the finger joints, knees, ankles, shoulder joints, and wrist joints were swollen, painful, warm, and tender, and restricted in their motion. Indeed, the clinical picture at the time of admission suggested a rheumatoid polyarthritis, and the fact that the patient's complaints were to be related to a bronchogenic carcinoma was first suggested by the presence of widespread osteoperiostitis as revealed by a roentgenographic skeletal survey.

*D*, Photograph showing the clubbing of the ends of the fingers and the swelling of the wrist and finger joints of the left hand shown in *C*.

*E*, Roentgenograph of part of the hand of the patient shown in *C*. Note the periosteal new bone deposition on the proximal phalanges of the fingers and on the metacarpal bones. An osteoperiostitis was also present on the bones of the right hand, as well as on the long bones—particularly those of the legs and forearms. It was these findings that led to roentgenographic examination of the chest, which revealed the tumor in the right lung.

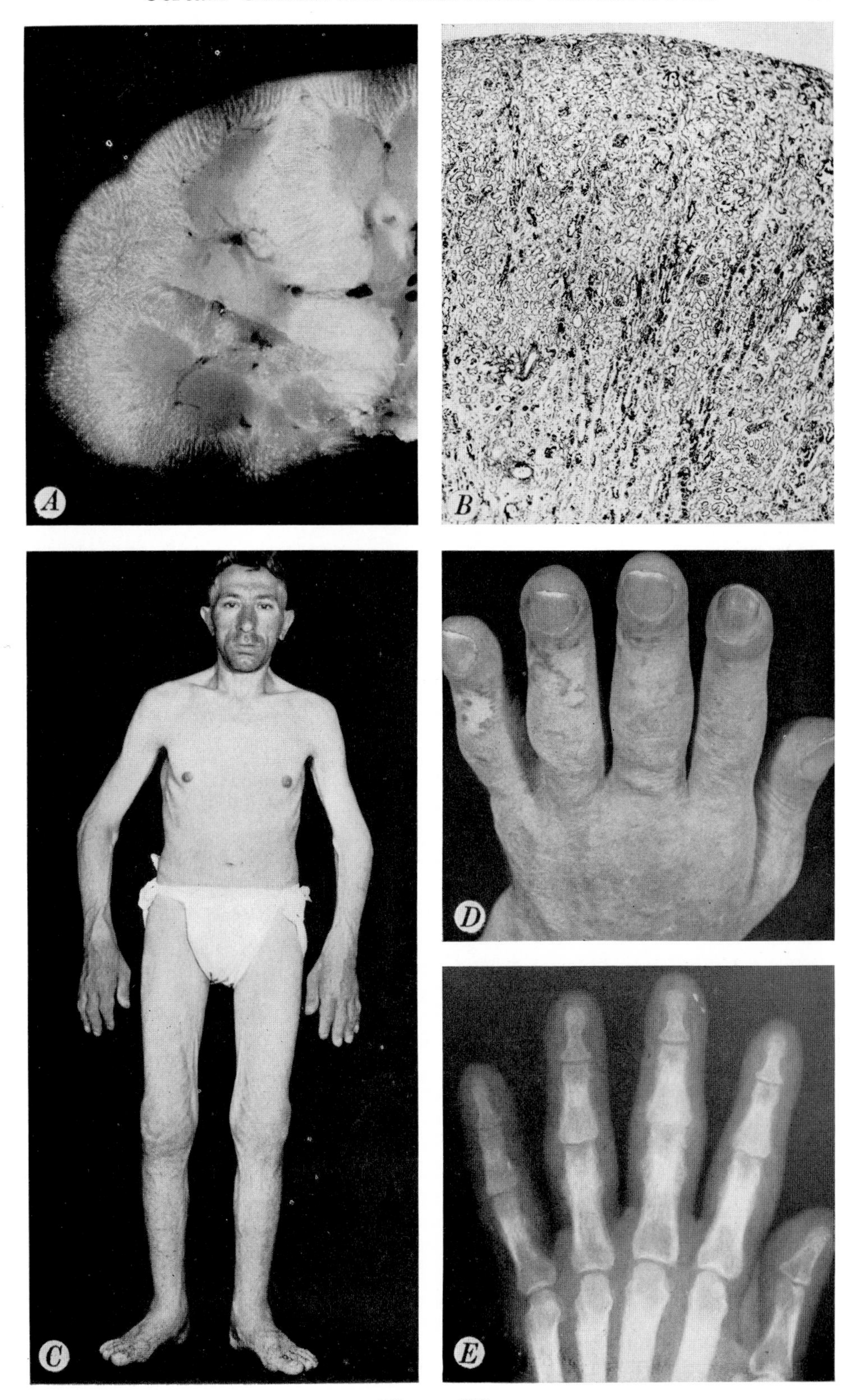


*Figure 193*

and even vascular collapse; and (4) renal disturbances (polyuria leading to further loss of water and electrolytes, and even eventual renal failure). Hypercalcemia is usually also associated with increased urinary excretion of calcium (hypercalciuria) and the deposition of calcium (metastatic calcification) in various organs and especially in the kidneys (see Fig. 193-*A* and *B*).

Of course, cancer metastatic to the skeleton is not the only condition which may give rise to hypercalcemia. Indeed, the clinicopathologic manifestations of the syndrome are more or less the same, whether it is caused by hyperparathyroidism, vitamin D poisoning, widespread osteolysis due to multiple myeloma, or cancer metastatic to the skeleton (see Jaffe, Kennedy *et al.*, and Myers).

Although it is certain that hypercalcemia occurs fairly frequently in cases of cancer metastatic to the skeleton, there are a number of factors which make it difficult to establish its true incidence. In many cases it is absent in the early phases of the metastatic spread of the cancer to the skeleton. Then again, the hypercalcemia is often transient and intermittent. Thus, it may actually have been present before the serum calcium determination had been made, be absent at the time of the determination, and reappear subsequently. In any event, the usual explanation for the occurrence of hypercalcemia in cases of cancer metastatic to the skeleton is lytic destruction of the osseous tissue at the sites of the metastases and release of calcium into the blood stream.

Interestingly enough, too, there are rare cases in which a patient affected with cancer of some organ is found to have a hypercalcemia even though skeletal metastases are not demonstrable roentgenographically or perhaps even at autopsy. Such patients have also been known to present mild clinical manifestations of hypercalcemia, and it is reported that the latter may disappear after surgical removal of the primary cancer. The pathogenetic mechanism underlying the hypercalcemia in such cases has not as yet been clarified (see Plimpton and Gellhorn).

Woodard has contributed data on the serum calcium value in a large series of patients (not under active therapy) who had metastases to the skeleton from cancers primary in various sites. She found that in 8 to 9 per cent of such patients there was evidence of hypercalcemia. However, the serum calcium value was seldom extremely high, usually lying between 11.5 and 12.5 mg. per 100 cc. and rarely being above 13. It is when the primary cancer is in the breast, lung, or kidney that *"spontaneous" hypercalcemia* is most likely to be present. As already indicated, the hypercalcemia is related to the occurrence of osteolysis at the sites of metastasis, and the metastases produced by these cancers are not infrequently of the osteolytic type. Occasionally, osteolytic metastases produce devastating destruction of the skeleton, and when this happens, the serum calcium value may be found to be as high as 18 mg. per 100 cc. or even higher. On the other hand, skeletal metastases from prostatic carcinoma are nearly always overwhelmingly osteoplastic, and in such cases, accordingly, hypercalcemia is seldom observed.

The introduction of steroid hormone therapy as a palliative procedure in the treatment of patients affected with advanced mammary cancer has created the problem of *"induced" hypercalcemia.* Though this complication is not very common, it does seem to be established that it is more likely to occur in connection with the use of androgenic hormones than of estrogenic hormones. Apparently it is to be observed only among those cases of mammary cancer in which skeletal metastases are present. Induced hypercalcemia represents a serious complication, since the serum calcium value may rise to extremely high levels and the patients may develop the toxic manifestations which characterize the hypercalcemia syndrome.

In a patient under hormone treatment who does not show roentgenographic evidence of skeletal involvement, the appearance of clinical evidence of hypercalcemia is a strong indication that such involvement is present nevertheless.

Furthermore, an elevation of the serum *alkaline phosphatase* value during hormone therapy (in the absence of detectable liver disease) is likewise presumptive evidence of the presence of skeletal metastases, even though these were not apparent roentgenographically (see Kennedy *et al.*).

If hypercalcemia becomes manifest in the course of the treatment, hormone therapy should be discontinued, at least temporarily. The administration of parenteral fluid to prevent severe dehydration should be begun immediately, and measures should be undertaken to combat electrolyte imbalance. The calcium intake should be kept at a low level. Some patients have been benefited by the administration of cortisone. If not corrected, the toxic effects of a pronounced hypercalcemia may rapidly lead to death of the patient.

## PULMONARY HYPERTROPHIC OSTEOARTHROPATHY

As was already indicated in the introductory section of this chapter, the subject of so-called *pulmonary hypertrophic osteoarthropathy* is not directly germane to the question of tumors metastatic to the skeleton. It is being discussed nevertheless because it not infrequently evolves in a patient presenting pulmonary metastases from a primary bone sarcoma (most often an osteogenic sarcoma). When the underlying pulmonary lesion is not a sarcoma metastatic from a bone, it may be a sarcoma metastatic from the soft tissues, or a pulmonary carcinoma (either primary or metastatic). Furthermore, the pulmonary disease provoking a hypertrophic osteoarthropathy may even have its basis in an infection, appearing, for instance, in connection with a tuberculous or nontuberculous lung abscess or a chronic bronchiectasis.

The principal components of the clinicopathologic complex represented by pulmonary hypertrophic osteoarthropathy are: (1) pulmonary disease of one type or another; (2) clubbing (drumstick enlargement) of the ends of the fingers and toes, due mainly or entirely to thickening of the subungual soft tissues; (3) periosteal new bone deposition (osteophytosis) found particularly on the tubular bones of the extremities; and (4) painful swelling of joints, apparently initiated by inflammatory changes in the synovial membrane. However, in some cases the extrapulmonary findings consist of drumstick fingers alone, or rather widespread osteoperiostitis (osteophytosis) alone, or of both of these features with or without articular changes.*

### CLINICAL CONSIDERATIONS

In a young patient presenting pulmonary metastases from an osteogenic sarcoma of bone, manifestations of pulmonary hypertrophic osteoarthropathy may easily

*Clubbing of the fingers and toes may, of course, be observed with conditions other than pulmonary disease—notably with cardiac disease. Osteophytosis (with or without the clubbing) is occasionally also found in connection with disease of the heart, liver (including biliary passages) and intestinal tract (see Locke). Clubbing of the fingers and toes and widespread osteophytosis have even been noted in connection with hypothyroidism developing after thyroidectomy for Graves' disease (see Thomas). Furthermore, clubbing and rather widespread periosteal new bone deposition have been reported as occurring without disease of the lungs or heart, or indeed of any other organ. Such cases are rare and should be held apart from cases of pulmonary hypertrophic osteoarthropathy. The condition they represent is denoted as "idiopathic familial generalized hyperostosis" or "generalized hyperostosis with pachydermia." The disease usually sets in around puberty, progresses for a number of years, and comes to a standstill spontaneously. Its initial manifestations are extensive osteophytosis, and pachydermia of the forearms and legs and sometimes of the scalp and forehead. These changes are followed by ossification of ligaments and bony ankylosis of many of the joints. Finally, the patient may present neurological manifestations due to pressure from vertebral osteophytes upon the spinal cord and nerve roots (see Uehlinger).

fail to arouse much interest because of the gravity of the subject's general condition. This may also be the case in the terminal stages of illness when an older patient is suffering from metastases to the lungs—for instance, from a soft-tissue sarcoma or from a carcinoma. In either case, it may be the casual finding of periosteal new bone deposition in the course of a roentgenographic skeletal survey that first calls attention to the presence of the condition.

On the other hand, in an occasional instance, it is the manifestations of pulmonary hypertrophic osteoarthropathy that occupy the foreground of the clinical picture. This happens especially in connection with cases of primary bronchogenic carcinoma, and sometimes the pulmonary tumor is even clinically occult. Indeed, in 2 cases observed by the writer, the knee joints and the small joints of the hands and feet were so painful and swollen that, if the skeletal roentgenographs had not disclosed widespread osteophytosis, the presenting articular complaints and findings could have been misinterpreted as those of rheumatoid arthritis. In both of these cases, it was only after discovery of the osteoperiostitis that roentgenographs of the lungs were taken and the presence of a bronchogenic carcinoma was discovered. (See Fig. 193-*C*, *D*, and *E*.)

In an adult in whom the hypertrophic osteoarthropathy is present in very pronounced form, there may be striking enlargement of the hands and feet. On this account, there is the possibility that at first sight the patient in question might be regarded as an acromegalic. In fact, it was this confusion that led Marie to delimit the concept of "pulmonary hypertrophic osteoarthropathy" and to distinguish the hand and foot changes associated with it from those of acromegaly, of which he likewise gave the classic description. Despite the impression of acromegaly which may be created by the appearance of a patient affected with hypertrophic pulmonary osteoarthropathy, anatomic examination of the pituitary fails to reveal the changes characteristically associated with acromegaly.

As Marie pointed out, in pulmonary hypertrophic osteoarthropathy, in contrast, to acromegaly, the ends of the fingers have a drumstick shape, the nails are curved.

### *Figure 194*

*A*, Roentgenograph showing periosteal new bone deposition on the *left* tibia and fibula in the case of a child presenting pulmonary metastases from an osteogenic sarcoma. The primary site of the sarcoma was the *right* tibia, and that leg had been amputated 22 months before this roentgenograph was taken. At this second admission, a skeletal survey also showed the presence of osteophytosis on both radii and ulnæ and on practically all the metacarpal and metatarsal bones. The patient died 2½ years after the amputation, and autopsy revealed not only pulmonary metastases, but a number of skeletal metastases.

*B*, Photograph of the tibia and fibula shown in *A*, after they had been removed at autopsy and sectioned in the longitudinal plane. Note the layers of new bone on their cortices and the normal architecture of their spongiosa.

*C*, Photograph of a transverse slice through the shaft of the tibia shown in *B*, before that bone had been cut in the long axis. Observe that the osteophytic deposit extends around the entire circumference of the bone, but is not of uniform thickness. The original cortex stands out most clearly below and to the right. On the left, it is more obscure, because it is undergoing resorption (see *D*).

*D*, Roentgenograph of the slice of thickened cortex shown in *C*. Note the circumferential layering of the periosteal new bone and the small roundish radiolucencies on the left in the original cortical bone where the latter is undergoing resorption.

*E*, Photomicrograph (× 6) illustrating the pattern of the cortical bone and of the periosteal deposit present on the left in *C* and *D*. The subperiosteal new bone has been deposited in ring-like layers. In the central portion of the picture, the original cortex is undergoing porotification, while on the left and below, it is still compact.

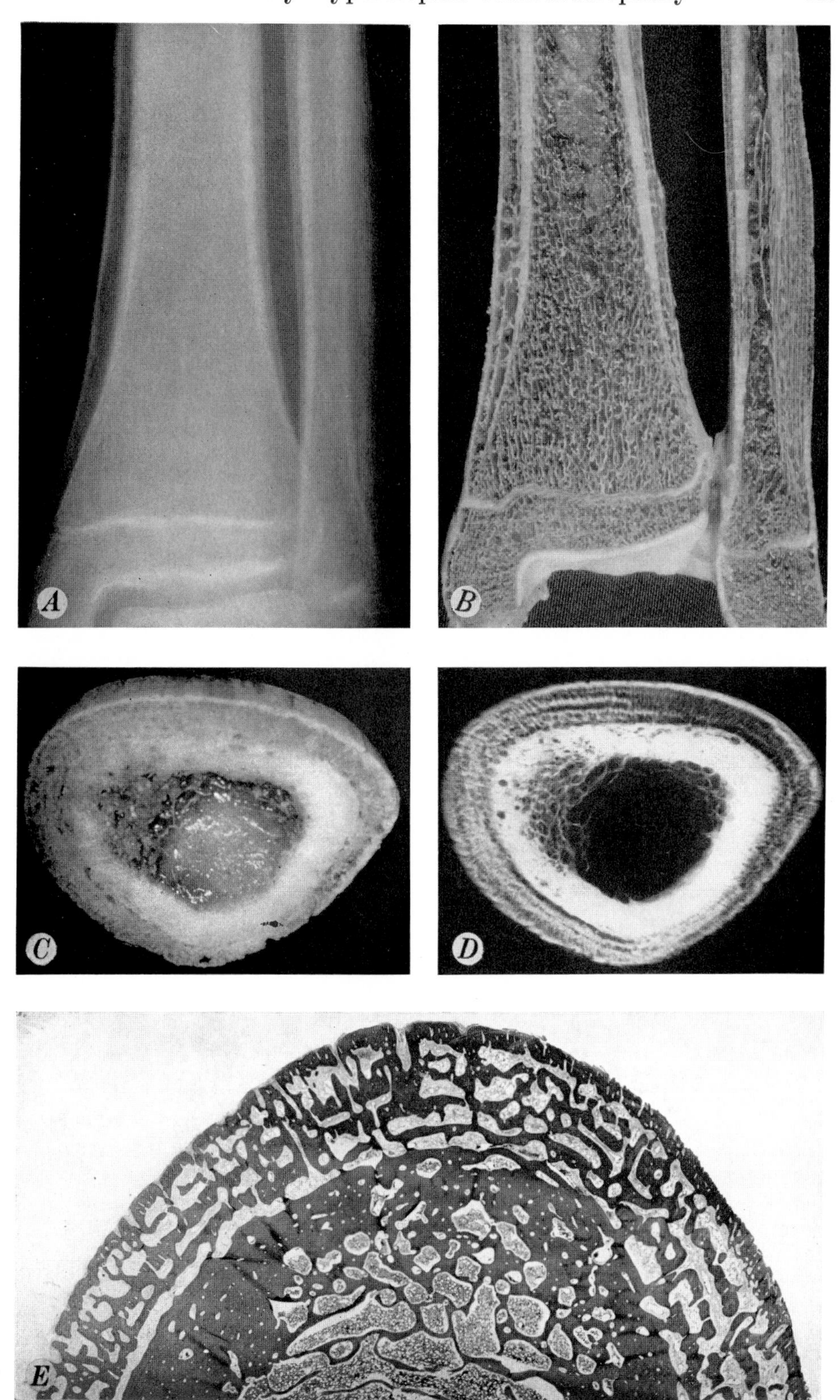


*Figure 194*

and the acral enlargement extends somewhat above the wrists and ankles. As an additional point of differentiation, he stressed the absence of the enlargement of the lower jaw which is regularly found in acromegaly. Historically, it is of interest that Bamberger independently antedated Marie's description of the skeletal changes associated with pulmonary disease, so that the clinicopathologic complex in question is sometimes also denoted as Bamberger-Marie's disease.

## PATHOLOGY OF THE SKELETAL ALTERATIONS

As already indicated, it is the tubular bones of the extremities that show the periosteal new bone apposition and resultant cortical thickening most regularly and prominently (see Crump, and Gall *et al.*). Furthermore, within a given tubular bone, the involvement is usually most intense about the middle of the shaft, becoming gradually less so toward the ends of the bone. The epicondyles and the sites of insertion of tendons usually do not become excessively prominent. Among the long tubular bones, the radius and ulna and the tibia and fibula are usually more severely affected than the humerus and femur. (See Fig. 194.) Of the short tubular bones, the metacarpals and metatarsals are more heavily involved than the phalanges. Indeed, the terminal phalanges often escape completely, though they sometimes show tufting at their distal ends.

The bones of the trunk are relatively little affected and seem often to be spared altogether. However, one may find some osteophytic deposition upon the cortices of the clavicles. The cortices of the ribs are modified only slightly if at all. The same statement applies to periosteal new bone apposition on the vertebral bodies. Osteophytic thickening of the iliac crests is not exactly uncommon, but new bone deposition upon the flat surfaces of the iliac bones is distinctly unusual. The skull bones are usually completely spared. However, in rare instances, periosteal new bone has been noted on the inner surface of the calvarium and on the nasal bones.

As revealed microscopically, notably in the study by Crump, the osteoperiostitic deposit is at first sharply demarcated from the original cortex and is composed of meshy trabeculæ of primitive bone. As the deposit, which does not appear as an even cuff, becomes thicker, much of the deeper part of it undergoes lamellar reconstruction and becomes denser, though never as compact as the original cortex was. On the other hand, the latter undergoes a certain amount of porotification (as do also the deeper layers of the periosteal new bone), so that the once sharp line of demarcation between the old and new cortical bone gradually becomes obliterated. Indeed, in some bones, especially the short tubular ones, the new and what remains of the old cortex become practically uniform in structure throughout their whole depth, if the patient survives for a long time. Finally, it should be noted that there is no endosteal deposition of bone. In fact, the subcortical and subchondral spongy trabeculæ tend to undergo some resorption, and where this occurs the intertrabecular marrow becomes slightly fibrosed.

As to the status of the joints, it should be noted first that the enlargement of articular regions and the limitations of motion so often observed clinically are sometimes dependent upon thickening of the bone ends from the periosteal deposits and are not necessarily associated with any alterations in the articular tissues themselves. Nevertheless, in some cases, the latter, too, are affected. When the joints are involved, postmortem examination will reveal inflammatory changes in the synovial membrane, with thickening of the membrane and sometimes also intra-articular effusion. In addition, the articular cartilages may be found modified by connective tissue pannus extending out from the inflamed membrane and by subchondral vascularization. These articular changes are especially likely to be encountered in adults whose pulmonary osteoarthropathy is of long standing.

The pathogenetic mechanism underlying pulmonary hypertrophic osteoarthropathy has not yet been adequately explained. Among the various hypotheses proposed are those which would base the condition on irritation by circulating toxic products from the pulmonary lesion, changes in blood supply induced by the underlying disease, or even endocrine imbalance. However, no hypothesis has yet been offered which seems to account for the condition under all the circumstances of its occurrence or to explain all the facets of its manifestations (see Mendlowitz).

## REFERENCES


Bachman, A. L., and Sproul, E. E.: Correlation of Radiographic and Autopsy Findings in Suspected Metastases in the Spine, Bull. New York Acad. Med., *31*, 146, 1955.

Baker, W. H.: Abnormalities in Calcium Metabolism in Malignancy; Effects of Hormone Therapy, Am. J. Med., *21*, 714, 1956.

Bamberger, E.: Ueber Knochenveränderungen bei chronischen Lungen- und Herzkrankheiten, Ztschr. f. klin. Med., *18*, 193, 1891.

————: Case Report, Wien. klin. Wchnschr., *2*, 226, 1889.

Baserga, R., and Saffiotti, U.: Experimental Studies on Histogenesis of Blood-Borne Metastases, Arch. Path., *59*, 26, 1955.

Batson, O. V.: The Function of the Vertebral Veins and Their Role in the Spread of Metastases, Ann. Surg., *112*, 138, 1940.

————: The Vertebral Vein System as a Mechanism for the Spread of Metastases, Am. J. Roentgenol., *48*, 715, 1942.

Bigler, F. C.: The Morphology of Clubbing, Am. J. Path., *34*, 237, 1958.

Borak, J.: Relationship Between the Clinical and Roentgenological Findings in Bone Metastases, Surg., Gynec. & Obst., *75*, 599, 1942.

Coman, D. R.: Mechanisms Responsible for the Origin and Distribution of Blood-borne Tumor Metastases, Cancer Research, *13*, 397, 1953.

Coman, D. R., and deLong, R. P.: The Role of the Vertebral Venous System in the Metastasis of Cancer to the Spinal Column. Experiments with Tumor-Cell Suspensions in Rats and Rabbits, Cancer, *4*, 610, 1951.

Coman, D. R., deLong, R. P., and McCutcheon, M.: Studies on the Mechanisms of Metastasis. The Distribution of Tumors in Various Organs in Relation to the Distribution of Arterial Emboli, Cancer Research, *11*, 648, 1951.

Crump, C.: Histologie der allgemeinen Osteophytose. (Ostéoarthropathie hypertrophiante pneumique.) Virchows Arch. f. path. Anat., *271*, 467, 1929.

Forschbach, G.: Die Ostéoarthropathie hypertrophiante pneumique. (Zur Fernwirkung intrathorakaler Tumoren.) Arch. klin. Chir., *281*, 18, 1955.

Fried, B. M.: Chronic Pulmonary Osteoarthropathy: Dyspituitarism as a Probable Cause, Arch. Int. Med., *72*, 565, 1943.

Gall, E. A., Bennett, G. A., and Bauer, W.: Generalized Hypertrophic Osteoarthropathy, Am. J. Path., *27*, 349, 1951.

Griboff, S. I., Herrmann, J. B., Smelin, A., and Moss, J.: Hypercalcemia Secondary to Bone Metastases from Carcinoma of the Breast. I. Relationship Between Serum Calcium and Alkaline Phosphatase Values, J. Clin. Endocrinol., *14*, 378, 1954.

Gutman, A. B.: Tumors of the Skeletal System: Medical Aspects, Bull. New York Acad. Med., *23*, 512, 1947.

Jaffe, H. L.: Hyperparathyroidism (Recklinghausen's Disease of Bone), Arch. Path., *16*, 63 and 236, 1933.

Jaffe, H. L., and Bodansky, A.: Serum Calcium: Clinical and Biochemical Considerations, J. Mt. Sinai Hosp., *9*, 901, 1943.

————: Diagnostic Significance of Serum Alkaline and Acid Phosphatase Values in Relation to Bone Disease, Bull. New York Acad. Med., *19*, 831, 1943.

Kennedy, B. J., Tibbetts, D. M., Nathanson, I. T., and Aub, J. C.: Hypercalcemia, a Complication of Hormone Therapy of Advanced Breast Cancer, Cancer Research, *13*, 445, 1953.

Locke, E. A.: Secondary Hypertrophic Osteo-Arthropathy and Its Relation to Simple Club-Fingers, Arch. Int. Med., *15*, 659, 1915.

Makrycostas, K.: Zur Histologie der Osteomalacia carcinomatosa, Frankfurt. Ztschr. Path., *40*, 501, 1930.

Marie, P.: De l'ostéo-arthropathie hypertrophiante pneumique, Rev. de méd., *10*, 1, 1890.

Mendlowitz, M.: Clubbing and Hypertrophic Osteoarthropathy, Medicine, *21*, 269, 1942.

Milch, R. A., and Changus, G. W.: Response of Bone to Tumor Invasion, Cancer, *9*, 340, 1956.

Myers, W. P. L.: Hypercalcemia in Neoplastic Disease, Cancer, *9*, 1135, 1956.

———: Cortisone in the Treatment of Hypercalcemia in Neoplastic Disease, Cancer, *11*, 83, 1958.

Odell, R. T., and Key, J. A.: Lumbar Disk Syndrome Caused by Malignant Tumors of Bone, J.A.M.A., *157*, 213, 1955.

Plimpton, C. H., and Gellhorn, A.: Hypercalcemia in Malignant Disease without Evidence of Bone Destruction, Am. J. Med., *21*, 750, 1956.

Rothendler, H. H.: Pulmonary Hypertrophic Osteoarthropathy, Bull. Hosp. Joint Dis., *7*, 43, 1946.

Selin, G., Schlyen, S., and Jaffe, H. L.: Vertebral Column. Methods for Removal, Reconstruction, and Gross Sectioning, Arch. Path., *55*, 245, 1953.

Shapiro, S.: Ossifying Periostitis of Bamberger-Marie (Secondary Hypertrophic Pulmonary Osteoarthropathy), Bull. Hosp. Joint Dis., *2*, 77, 1941.

Thomas, H. M., Jr.: Acropachy, Arch. Int. Med., *51*, 571, 1933.

Uehlinger, E.: Hyperostosis generalisata mit Pachydermie. (Idiopathische familiäre generalisierte Osteophytose Friedreich-Erb-Arnold.) Virchows Arch. f. path. Anat., *308*, 396, 1941.

Walther, H. E.: *Krebsmetastasen*, Basel, Benno Schwabe & Co., 1948.

Warren, S., Harris, P. N., and Graves, R. C.: Osseous Metastasis of Carcinoma of the Prostate, Arch. Path., *22*, 139, 1936.

Willis, R. A.: A Review of Five Hundred Consecutive Cancer Autopsies, M. J. Australia, *28*, 258, 1941.

Woodard, H. Q.: Changes in Blood Chemistry Associated with Carcinoma Metastatic to Bone, Cancer, *6*, 1219, 1953.

Young, J. M.: The Thoracic Duct in Malignant Disease, Am. J. Path., *32*, 253, 1956.

Young, J. M., and Funk, F. J., Jr.: Incidence of Tumor Metastasis to the Lumbar Spine. A Comparative Study of Roentgenographic Changes and Gross Lesions, J. Bone & Joint Surg., *35-A*, 55, 1953.

Zeidman, I.: Metastasis: A Review of Recent Advances, Cancer Research, *17*, 157, 1957.

Zeidman, I., Copeland, B. E., and Warren, S.: Experimental Studies on the Spread of Cancer in the Lymphatic System. II. Absence of a Lymphatic Supply in Carcinoma, Cancer, *8*, 123, 1955.

Zemgulys, J.: Krebsmetastasen im Knochensystem mit besonderer Berücksichtigung der Wirbelsäule und der Osteophytosis carcinomatosa, Ztschr. f. Krebsforsch., *34*, 266, 1931.

# Index


A

ACHONDROPLASIA, 152
Adamantinoma of jawbones, 425 (*see also* Ameloblastoma)
Adamantinoma of limb bones, 213–223
clinical considerations, 213
clinical complaints, 213
incidence, 213
localization, 213
differential diagnosis, 222
metastasis of, 220
nature and genesis, 220
epithelial nature of lesion, 221
mesodermal nature of lesion, 221
pathologic findings, 216
roentgenographic findings, 214
trauma, role of, 214
treatment, 222
Adipose tissue tumors, 507
lipoma, 507
liposarcoma, 507
Albright's disease (*see* Fibrous dysplasia)
Ameloblastic fibroma, 448
Ameloblastoma of jawbones, 213, 216, 218, 220, 221, 429, 430, 435, 442–448
Amyloid deposition in myeloma, 390
Anatomic *vs.* roentgenographic findings relating to skeletal metastases, 602–604
Aneurysm, benign bone, 54
malignant bone, 260
Aneurysmal bone cyst, 22, 39, 40, 54–62, 74, 230
clinical considerations, 56
clinical complaints, 56
incidence, 56
localization, 56
differential diagnosis, 60
aneurysmal giant-cell tumor, 61
atypical giant-cell tumor, 61
hemangioma of bone, 61
osteogenic sarcoma, 60
pulsating giant-cell tumor, 61
subperiosteal giant-cell tumor, 61
nature and genesis, 60
nomenclature, 54
pathologic findings, 58
roentgenographic findings, 58
trauma as a factor in, 56
treatment, 61
Angioblastoma of bone, 222
Angioblastoma of bone, malignant, 213, 220, 222
Angioendothelioma of bone, 346
Angioma, vertebral, 228 (*see also* Hemangioma of bone)
Angiosarcoma of bone (*see* Malignant vascular tumors)
Articular tumors, benign, 558–575
Articular tumors, malignant, 576–588

B

BATSON's vertebral vein system, 592
Bence Jones proteins in myeloma, 378
Benign articular tumors, 558–575
Benign chondroblastoma, 40, 44–53, 182, 210, 211
clinical considerations, 44
clinical complaints, 45
incidence, 44
localization, 44
differential diagnosis, 52
chondrosarcoma, 46, 52
enchondroma, 46, 52, 53
giant-cell tumor, 46, 52
nomenclature, 44
pathologic findings, 46
gross, 46
microscopic, 48
roentgenographic findings, 45
treatment, 53
postirradiation chondrosarcoma, 53, 497
Benign chordoma, 452
Benign giant-cell synovioma, 533, 544, 577
Benign metastasizing hemangioma, 238, 341
Benign osteoblastoma, 94, 107–116
clinical considerations, 108
clinical complaints and findings, 108
incidence, 108
localization, 108
differential diagnosis, 112
giant-cell tumor, 116
osteogenic sarcoma, 114
osteoid-osteoma, 112
nomenclature, 107
giant osteoid-osteoma, 107, 114
osteogenic fibroma, 107
pathologic findings, 110
gross, 110
microscopic, 112
roentgenographic findings, 110
treatment, 116
Benign vascular tumors of bone, 224–239
Biopsy as a diagnostic procedure, 14
needle (closed), 15
surgical (open), 16
frozen *vs.* paraffin section, 16
Bone abscess, intracortical, 90, 104
Bone abscess, solitary, 98, 104
Bone cyst, aneurysmal (*see* Aneurysmal bone cyst)

Bone cyst, hemangiomatous, 54
Bone cyst, solitary (*see* Solitary bone cyst)
Bone cyst, unicameral (*see* Solitary bone cyst)
Bone growth retardation following radiation, 490
Bone invasion by tumors of overlying soft parts, 502–531
Bone lesions associated with neural tumors, 240–255
Bone sarcoma following external radiation, 479, 491–497
Bone sarcoma following internal radiation, 479–482, 497–501
Bronchogenic carcinoma, skeletal metastasis from, 605
"Brown tumor" of hyperparathyroidism, 19, 34, 38, 426, 449
Bursal chondromatosis, 566
Bursitis, pigmented villonodular, 532, 548

C

CALVARIAL hemangioma (*see* Hemangioma of bone)
Cancer metastatic to the skeleton (*see* Metastasis of tumors to skeleton)
Carcinoma complicating osteomyelitis, 474
Cartilage tumors invading bone, 518
juxtacortical chondroma, 196, 518
juxtacortical chondrosarcoma, 518
soft-tissue chondrosarcoma, 520
Cementoblastoma, 436
Cementoma, 435, 436
fibrocementoma, 438
sclerosing, 438, 440
Central chondrosarcoma of bone (*see* Chondrosarcoma of bone, central)
Chondroblastoma, benign (*see* Benign chondroblastoma)
Chondrodysplasia, hereditary deforming, 150
Chondroma, eccentric (*see* Juxtacortical chondroma)
Chondroma, intracapsular, 567
Chondroma, juxtacortical (*see* Juxtacortical chondroma)
Chondroma, malignant, 164, 166
Chondroma, para-articular, 198, 567
Chondroma, periosteal (*see* Juxtacortical chondroma)
Chondroma of soft tissues, 520
Chondroma, solitary central (*see* Solitary enchondroma)
Chondromatosis, bursal, 566
Chondromatosis, synovial (*see* Synovial chondromatosis)
Chondromatosis, tenosynovial, 566
Chondromyxoid fibroma, 50, 52 203–212, 222, 299, 302, 330, 436
clinical considerations, 203
clinical complaints, 204
incidence, 203
localization, 203
Chondromyxoid fibroma, differential diagnosis, 210
benign chondroblastoma, 210, 211
chondrosarcoma of bone, 203, 210, 211
enchondroma, 211
myxoma of bone, 211
myxosarcoma of bone, 211
solitary bone cyst, 211
pathologic findings, 208
recurrence and malignant transformation, 210
roentgenographic findings, 206
treatment, 211
Chondromyxosarcoma, 203, 211
Chondro-osteosarcoma, 164, 274, 315
Chondrosarcoma as a complication of multiple enchondromatosis, 194, 320
Chondrosarcoma as a complication of multiple exostosis, 164
Chondrosarcoma as a complication of solitary enchondroma, 177, 180, 326
Chondrosarcoma as a complication of solitary exostosis, 150
Chondrosarcoma of bone, 46, 52, 134, 150, 164, 203, 210, 211, 256, 274, 314–340, 426, 460
nomenclature, 314, 315
primary, 314
secondary, 314
Chondrosarcoma of bone, central, 46, 52, 315–332
clinical considerations, 316
clinical complaints and findings, 316
incidence, 316
localization, 316
differential diagnosis, 318, 330
chondromyxoid fibroma, 330
infarct, bone, 318
osteogenic sarcoma, 318, 331
evolution of, 314, 315, 326
extension and metastasis, 330
pathologic findings, 320
gross, 320
microscopic, 326
roentgenographic findings, 317
trauma as a factor in, 317
treatment, 331
Chondrosarcoma of bone, peripheral, 332-340
clinical considerations, 332
clinical complaints and findings, 333
incidence, 332
localization, 332
differential diagnosis, 333, 334
juxtacortical osteogenic sarcoma, 334
osteocartilaginous exostosis, 333
evolution of, 332, 333
pathologic findings, 333
gross, 334
microscopic, 336
roentgenographic findings, 333
trauma as a factor in, 333
treatment, 338
Chondrosarcoma of soft tissues, 561, 582
Chondrosarcoma of soft tissues invading bone, 520–521

Chondrosarcoma of soft tissues invading bone,
clinical considerations, 520
pathologic findings, 521
treatment, 521
Chordoma, 451–462
clinical considerations, 452
clinical complaints and findings, 453
incidence, 452
localization, 452
ecchordosis physaliphora spheno-occipitalis, 452, 456
metastasis of, 461
nomenclature, 451, 452
pathologic findings, 456
gross, 458
microscopic, 460
*vs.* chondrosarcoma, 460
roentgenographic findings, 454
trauma as a factor in, 453
treatment, 461
Classification of skeletal tumors, 9
evaluation of methods of, 9–12
general orienting system of, 9
Phemister's, 10
Registry of Bone Sarcoma, 10
Codman tumor, 40, 44
Cortical fibrous defect (*see* Fibrous cortical defect)
Cranial hemihypertrophy, 139
Cranial hyperostosis, unilateral, 138
Cystlike bone lesions, multiple, 249
Cysts of jawbones (*see* Jawbone cysts)

D

Dentigerous cysts, 429
Dentinoma, 435
Desmoplastic fibroma of bone, 298–303, 426
clinical considerations, 299
clinical complaints, 299
incidence, 299
location, 299
differential diagnosis, 300
chondromyxoid fibroma, 299, 302
fibrosarcoma, well differentiated, 300
fibrous dysplasia, 302
non-ossifying fibroma, 299, 302
nomenclature, 298
pathologic findings, 299
gross, 299
microscopic, 300
roentgenographic findings, 299
treatment, 302
Diagnostic approach to skeletal tumors, 12
correlation of clinical, *x*-ray and pathologic findings, 12–14
Diaphysial aclasis, 150, 165
Diffuse pigmented villonodular synovitis (*see* Synovitis, diffuse pigmented villonodular)
Disappearing multilocular cystlike lesions, 249
Distribution of cancer metastases to skeleton, 598, 600

E

Ecchondrosis, 156, 165
Ecchordosis physaliphora spheno-occipitalis, 452, 456
Embryonal rhabdomyosarcoma, 514
Enameloma, 435
Enchondroma, solitary (*see* Solitary enchondroma)
Enchondromatosis (*see* Multiple enchondromatosis)
Endothelial myeloma of bone (*see* Ewing's sarcoma)
Endothelioma, diffuse (*see* Ewing's sarcoma)
Enostosis, solitary, 96, 104
Eosinophilic granuloma, 73, 90
*vs.* Ewing's sarcoma, 354, 363
*vs.* Hodgkin's disease, 410
Epulis, giant-cell, 426
Ewing's sarcoma, 310, 350–368, 426
clinical considerations, 351
clinical complaints and findings, 351
incidence, 351
localization, 351
differential diagnosis, 354, 356, 363
eosinophilic granuloma, 354, 363
metastatic carcinoma, undifferentiated, 366
neuroblastoma, 350, 351, 363
osteogenic sarcoma, 363
osteomyelitis, 354
primary reticulum cell sarcoma, 366, 420
nomenclature, 350
pathologic findings, 357
gross, 357
microscopic, 360
prognosis, 367
roentgenographic findings, 354
treatment, 367
*vs.* primary reticulum cell sarcoma, 420
Exostosis bursata, 148, 158, 566
Exostosis, ivory, 143
Exostosis, multiple osteocartilaginous (*see* Multiple osteocartilaginous exostosis)
Exostosis, solitary osteocartilaginous (*see* Solitary osteocartilaginous exostosis)
Exostosis, subungual, 143
Extraskeletal osteogenic sarcoma, 296

F

Fibrocementoma, 436, 438
Fibrocystic disease of bone, 70, 118
Fibroma, ameloblastic, 448
Fibroma, articular capsules, 574
Fibroma, chondromyxoid (*see* Chondromyxoid fibroma)
Fibroma, desmoplastic, of bone (*see* Desmoplastic fibroma of bone)
Fibroma, non-ossifying (*see* Non-ossifying fibroma)
Fibroma, odontogenic, 436
Fibro-osseous dysplasia (*see* Fibrous dysplasia)

Fibrosarcoma of bone, 23, 28, 75, 134, 256, 274, 298–313, 426
clinical considerations, 306
clinical complaints, 306
clinical course, 308, 312
incidence, 306
location, 306
nomenclature, 304
pathologic findings, 310
poorly differentiated, 312
well differentiated, 310
roentgenographic findings, 308
differential diagnosis, 300, 310
trauma as a factor in, 306
treatment, 312
Fibrosarcoma of soft tissues invading bone, 503–507
clinical considerations, 503
pathologic findings, 504
poorly differentiated, 506
well differentiated, 506
roentgenographic findings, 503
treatment, 506
recurrence and metastasis, 506
Fibrous cortical defect, 76–91, 200, 248
clinical considerations, 78
clinical complaints, 80
incidence, 78
localization, 78
differential diagnosis, 88
intracortical bone abscess, 90
osteoid-osteoma, 90
pathogenesis, 82
evolution, 78, 82
spontaneous regression, 82
transition to non-ossifying fibroma, 76, 82
pathologic findings, 80
roentgenographic findings, 80
multiple involvement, 78, 84
trauma in relation to, 80, 84
treatment, 83
Fibrous dysplasia, 70, 73, 117–142, 186, 249, 275, 302, 425, 426
biochemical findings, 124
clinical considerations, 118
clinical complaints, 119
distribution of skeletal involvement, 118, 136, 425, 426
incidence, 118
pigmentation, abnormal cutaneous, 120
precocity, growth and sex, 122
various other aberrations, 117, 124
course of disease in skeleton, 130
differential diagnosis, 134
bone cyst, solitary, 134
cranial hyperostosis, 138
enchondroma, solitary, 136
enchondromatosis, 130, 139
fibrous osteoma, jawbones, 136, 138
Hand-Schüller-Christian disease, 139
hyperparathyroidism, 139
leontiasis ossea, 138
lipid granulomatosis, 126, 139
Fibrous dysplasia, differential diagnosis, neurofibromatosis, 140
non-ossifying fibroma, 136
ossifying fibroma, jawbones, 136
monostotic and polyostotic, 118
nature and genesis, 117
nomenclature, 118
pathologic findings, 124
gross, 124
microscopic, 126
roentgenographic findings, 128
sarcoma as a complication of, 134
solitary focus of, 173, 182
stabilization of skeletal changes, 130
treatment, 140
postirradiation sarcoma, 497
Fibrous osteoma of jawbones, 118, 136, 138, 426
Fissural cyst of jawbones, 432
Follicular cysts of jawbones, 426, 429
Fracture complicating radiation osteitis, 491

G

Ganglioneuroma of bone, 240
Generalized hyperostosis with pachydermia, 613
Generalized malignant lymphoma (*see* Lymphoma, generalized)
Giant-cell epulis, 426
Giant-cell reparative granuloma of jawbones, 20, 36, 426, 449
Giant-cell reparative granuloma, peripheral, 426
Giant-cell sarcoma, 18
Giant-cell synovioma, benign, 533, 544, 577
Giant-cell tumor of bone, 18–43, 44, 46, 50, 52, 61, 70, 73, 83, 88, 90, 116, 173, 177, 182, 310
aneurysmal, 61
"atypical" or "subperiosteal," 39, 54, 61
calcifying, 44
clinical considerations, 18
clinical complaints and findings, 22
incidence, 18
localization, 19
differential diagnosis, 23, 32
aneurysmal bone cyst, 39
benign chondroblastoma, 40
"brown tumor" of hyperparathyroidism, 34, 38
Codman tumor, 40
enchondroma, solitary, 23
fibrosarcoma, 23
multiple myeloma, 23
non-ossifying fibroma, 40
reparative granuloma of jawbones, 36
solitary bone cyst, 23, 40
epiphyseal chondromatous, 44
histologic pattern *vs.* clinical behavior, 30
grading of giant-cell tumor, 30
jawbone involvement by, 448
malignant, 26, 28, 30
metastasis of, 28, 31

Giant-cell tumor of bone,multiple lesions, 22
nature and genesis, 28
nomenclature, 18, 28
Paget's disease complicated by, 20, 470
pathogenesis, 23
pathologic findings, 23
gross, 23
microscopic, 26, 30
grading of pattern, 30
recurrence and metastasis, 24, 26, 28, 31
postirradiation sarcoma, 42, 494
pulsating, 61
recurrence, 24, 26, 31
roentgenographic findings, 22
serum biochemical findings, 22, 36
trauma, role of, 22, 30
treatment, 41
Giant-cell tumor of bursa, 533, 548
Giant-cell tumor of synovium, 533, 534, 549
Giant-cell tumor of tendon sheath, 533, 549
Giant follicle lymphoma, 414
Giant osteoid-osteoma, 94, 107, 114
Globulomaxillary cyst, 432
Glomangioma, 254
Glomus tumor of bone, 240, 254, 530
Granular cell myoblastoma (malignant) invading bone, 512

H

HAND-SCHÜLLER-CHRISTIAN disease, 139
Hemangioendothelioma of bone, malignant (*see* Malignant vascular tumors)
Hemangioma, benign metastasizing, 238, 341
Hemangioma of bone, 54, 61, 224-237
calvarial, 230
clinical considerations, 232
differential diagnosis, 232
pathologic findings, 234
roentgenographic findings, 232
treatment, 236
rare skeletal sites, 236
primary involvement, 236
secondary involvement, 237
vertebral, 224
clinical complaints, 225
incidence, 224
differential diagnosis, 228
aneurysmal bone cyst, 230
pathologic findings, 226
gross, 226
microscopic, 228
roentgenographic findings, 225
treatment, 230
Hemangioma of joints, 567–572, 582
clinical considerations, 568
pathologic findings, 570
roentgenographic findings, 568
treatment, 572
Hemangioma of musculature, 228, 237
Hemangioma of soft tissues invading bone, 527–530
clinical considerations, 528
diffuse, 527
localized, 527
pathologic findings, 530
roentgenographic findings, 528
Hemangioma of tendon sheaths, 572
Hemangiomatosis of bone, 237
Hemangiomatosis of soft tissues, 237
Hemangiomatosis of soft tissues invading bone, 527
Hemangiomatous bone cyst, 54
Hemangiopericytoma, 254, 341
Hemangiosarcoma of bone (*see* Malignant vascular tumors)
Hemorrhagic extravasation cyst, mandible, 434
Hereditary multiple exostosis (*see* Multiple osteocartilaginous exostosis)
Hodgkin's disease, 407, 410
Hodgkin's sarcoma, 408
Hypercalcemia due to skeletal metastases, 608, 612
Hypercalcemic syndrome, 610
treatment, 613
Hypernephroma, skeletal metastasis from, 594
Hyperostosis, familial idiopathic, 613
Hyperparathyroidism, 22, 38
biochemical findings in, 36
"brown tumor" of, 19, 34, 38, 426, 449
*vs.* fibrous dysplasia, 139
Hypertrophic pulmonary osteoarthropathy (*see* Pulmonary hypertrophic osteoarthropathy)

I

IDIOPATHIC familial generalized hyperostosis, 613
Inclusion cyst, epithelial, 173, 430
Infarct of bone, 182, 318
Intracapsular chondroma, 567
Intracortical bone abscess, 90, 104
Intramedullary lesions in neurofibromatosis, 248
Invasion of bone by tumors of overlying soft parts, 502–531
chondrosarcoma, 518, 520
fibrosarcoma, 503
glomus tumor, 254, 530
granular cell myoblastoma, 512
hemangioma, localized, 527
hemangiomatosis, 527
leiomyosarcoma, 512
liposarcoma, 507
osteogenic sarcoma, 521
rhabdomyosarcoma, 513
Ionizing radiation, injury from, 397, 479
Ivory exostosis, 143

J

JAWBONE cysts, 426–435
nonodontogenic (epithelialized), 430–434
fissural and vestigial, 432–434
globulomaxillary, 432
median, 432
naso-alveolar, 434
nasopalatine, 434

Jawbone cysts, nonodontogenic (nonepithelialized), 434–435
solitary hemorrhagic, 434
traumatic, 434
odontogenic, 426–430
follicular, 426, 429
dentigerous, 429
primordial, 430
periodontal, 428
radicular, 428
Jawbone tumors, 435–450
ameloblastoma, 429, 430, 435, 442
cementoma, 435, 436
fibrocementoma, 438
sclerosing, 438, 440
dentinoma, 435
enameloma, 435
myxoma, 435
odontoma, 425, 435, 448
other lesions, 425–426, 448–450
"brown tumor" of hyperparathyroidism, 426, 449
fibrous dysplasia, 425, 426
giant-cell reparative granuloma, 426, 449
osteofibroma, 426
peripheral giant-cell reparative granuloma, 426
Joints, fibroma of, 574
Joints, hemangioma of (*see* Hemangioma of joints)
Joints, lipoma of, 574
Juxtacortical chondroma, 196–202, 248, 518
clinical considerations, 196
clinical complaints and findings, 196
incidence, 196
localization, 196
differential diagnosis, 200
fibrous cortical defect, 200
tenosynovitis, pigmented villonodular, 200
various other conditions, 202
pathologic findings, 197
roentgenographic findings, 197
treatment, 202
Juxtacortical chondrosarcoma, 518
Juxtacortical osteogenic sarcoma, 256, 262, 274, 279–297, 334, 518
clinical considerations, 280
clinical complaints and findings, 280
clinical course, 282
incidence, 280
location, 280
differential diagnosis, 290
myositis ossificans, 286, 290
osteochondroma, atypical, 279, 288, 294
osteogenic sarcoma, extraskeletal, 296
periostitis, post-traumatic, 286, 292
nomenclature, 279
pathologic findings, 286
gross, 286
microscopic, 288
Juxtacortical osteogenic sarcoma, roentgenographic findings, 286
treatment, 296
recurrence and metastasis, 282, 284

K

KAPOSI's sarcoma, 341

L

LATERAL cyst of jawbone, 428
Leiomyosarcoma invading bone, 512
Leontiasis ossea, 138
Lesions of jawbones, 425–450
Leukemia, 396–406, 480
acute, 397
chronic, 398
cytologic types, 397
incidence, 396
ionizing radiation and, 397
skeletal manifestations of, 398
in adults, 402
in children, 398
treatment, 399, 406
Lipid granulomatosis, 126, 139
Lipoma of articular capsules, 574
Lipoma of bone, 228, 230
Lipoma of soft tissues, 507
Liposarcoma of bone, 507
Liposarcoma of soft parts invading bone, 507–510
general considerations, 507
pathologic findings, 508
poorly differentiated, 508
well differentiated, 508
roentgenographic findings, 507
treatment, 510
Localized nodular synovitis (*see* Synovitis, localized nodular)
Localized nodular tenosynovitis (*see* Tenosynovitis, localized nodular)
Lymphangioma of bone, 238
Lymphangiosarcoma of bone (*see* Malignant vascular tumors)
Lymphoma, generalized, 406–415
general considerations, 406
skeletal changes, 407
in giant follicle lymphoma, 414
in Hodgkin's disease, 407
in lymphosarcoma, 410
in reticulum cell sarcoma, 414
treatment, 414
Lymphoma primary in bone, 396, 415–424
general considerations, 415
primary reticulum cell sarcoma of bone, 416–423
clinical considerations, 418
course, 422
differential diagnosis, 419
Ewing's sarcoma *vs.*, 420
pathologic findings, 419
roentgenographic findings, 418
treatment, 423
Lymphosarcoma, 410

M

MAFFUCCI's syndrome, 185, 186
Malignant articular tumors, 576–588
Malignant bone aneurysm, 260
Malignant granular cell myoblastoma invading bone, 512
Malignant hemangioendothelioma of bone (*see* Malignant vascular tumors)
Malignant lymphoma (*see* Lymphoma)
Malignant synovioma (*see* Synovial sarcoma)
Malignant vascular tumors of bone, 341–349
clinical considerations, 341
differential diagnosis, 346
pathologic findings, 342
gross, 342
microscopic, 344
roentgenographic findings, 342
treatment, 348
Marble bone disease, 399
Median cysts of jawbones, 432
Meningioma, hyperostosis from, 234
Mesenchymoma, 502
Mesodermal tumors invading bone, 502
Mesothorium, damaging effects of, 479–501
Metaphysial fibrous defect (*see* Fibrous cortical defect and non-ossifying fibroma)
Metastasis of tumors to skeleton, 589–613
biochemical and clinical considerations, 608
alkaline phosphatase, 613
calcification, metastatic, 612
hypercalcemia, hormone-induced, 612
hypercalcemia, spontaneous, 608, 612
hypercalcemic syndrome, 610
hypercalciuria, 612
focus of metastasis as presenting lesion, 593
bronchogenic cancer, 605
hypernephroma, 594
prostatic cancer, 598, 605
thyroid cancer, 596
incidence of metastases, 598
localization of metastases, 598, 600
osteolytic *vs.* osteoplastic metastases, 604
evolution of osteolytic, 606
evolution of osteoplastic, 608
general considerations, 604
roentgenographic *vs.* anatomic findings relating to, 602
routes of metastasis, 590
arterial blood stream, 592
caval vein system, 592
lymphatic system, 590
vertebral vein system, 592
sites of predilection, 600
Metastatic skeletal focus as presenting lesion, 593–598
Monostotic fibrous dysplasia, 118
Multicentric osteogenic sarcoma of bone, 266
Multiple cystlike bone lesions, 249
Multiple enchondromatosis, 118, 119, 130, 139, 151, 166, 169–195, 314, 316, 326
chondrosarcoma as a complication, 194, 320
clinical considerations, 185
clinical emergence of disorder, 185
course of disorder, 185
distribution of bone lesions, 185
nonskeletal manifestations, 186
nomenclature, 184
pathogenesis, 192
pathologic findings, 188
gross, 188
microscopic, 192
roentgenographic findings, 188
treatment, 194
Multiple myeloma (*see* Myelomatosis)
Multiple osteocartilaginous exostosis, 143–168, 192, 314, 333
chondrosarcoma as a complication, 164
clinical considerations, 151
clinical emergence of disorder, 151
clinical features, 151
forearm deformity, 154, 185
distribution of lesions, 155–158
incidence, 151
differential diagnosis, 166
enchondromatosis, 166
inheritance of, 154
nomenclature, 150
pathogenesis, 164
pathologic findings, 155
gross, 155
microscopic, 160
roentgenographic findings, 155
treatment, 167
Muscle tumors invading bone, 510–516
granular cell myoblastoma, malignant, 512
leiomyosarcoma, 512
rhabdomyosarcoma, 513
Myeloid sarcoma, 18
Myeloid tumor, 18
Myeloma of bone, solitary, 370, 379
Myeloma kidney, 389
Myeloma, multiple (*see* Myelomatosis)
Myeloma, plasma cell, 369, 386
Myelomatosis, 22, 23, 36, 369–395
biochemical findings, 375
Bence Jones proteinuria, 378
serum alkaline phosphatase, 376
serum calcium, 376
serum inorganic phosphate, 376
serum proteins, 378
bone marrow smears, 375, 393
other hematologic findings, 372, 375
clinical considerations, 372
clinical complaints, 372
clinical course, 372
incidence, 372
differential diagnosis, 384, 388, 392
pathologic extraskeletal findings, 389
amyloid deposits, 390
calcification, metastatic, 390
myeloma kidney, 389

Myelomatosis, pathologic extraskeletal findings, visceral involvement, 389
pathologic skeletal findings, gross, 379
diffuse myeloma, 382
multiple myeloma, 382
solitary myeloma, 379
pathologic skeletal findings, microscopic, 386
amyloid deposition, 390
roentgenographic findings, skeletal, 379
treatment, 393
Myelosclerotic anemia, 406
Myoblastoma, malignant granular cell, invading bone, 512
Myositis ossificans, 286, 290, 527
Myxochondrosarcoma of bone, 315, 330
Myxoma of jawbone, 211, 435
Myxosarcoma of bone, 211

N

Naso-alveolar cyst, 434
Nasopalatine cyst, 434
Neural tumors and associated bone lesions, 240–255
Neurilemmoma of bone, 240
Neuroblastoma, metastasis from, 350, 351, 363, 399, 602
Neurofibroma of bone, solitary, 240
Neurofibromatosis, 140, 202, 242-254
bone involvement in, 242
clinical considerations, 242
erosive lesions of bone cortex, 246
intramedullary bone lesions, 248
pseudarthrosis, 250
scoliosis, 250
Neuromyo-arterial glomus, 254
Nonodontogenic cysts of jawbones, 430–435
Nonossifying fibroma, 18, 40, 76–91, 136, 222, 248, 299, 302
clinical considerations, 83
clinical findings, 84
incidence, 83
localization, 83
differential diagnosis, 88
giant-cell tumor, 88, 90
xanthogranuloma, 90
nomenclature, 83
pathologic findings, 86
roentgenographic findings, 84
multiple involvement, 84, 249
treatment, 90
Nonosteogenic fibroma (*see* Nonossifying fibroma)
Notochord, 451

O

Odontoblastoma, 448
Odontogenic cysts, 426–430
Odontogenic fibroma, 436
Odontogenic tumors, 435–448
Odontoma, 425, 435, 448
Ollier's disease, 119, 130, 139, 184
Ossifying fibroma of jawbones, 118, 136
Osteitis fibrosa, 70, 118
Osteitis, radiation (*see* Radiation osteitis)
Osteoarthropathy, hypertrophic pulmonary (*see* Pulmonary hypertrophic osteoarthropathy)
Osteoblastoma, benign (*see* Benign osteoblastoma)
Osteocartilaginous exostosis, multiple (*see* Multiple osteocartilaginous exostosis)
Osteocartilaginous exostosis, solitary (*see* Solitary osteocartilaginous exostosis)
Osteochondritis dissecans, 96
Osteochondroma, 173
Osteochondroma, atypical, 279, 288, 294
Osteochondroma, solitary (*see* Solitary osteocartilaginous exostosis)
Osteochondromatosis, synovial, 558
Osteochondrosarcoma of bone, 164, 274, 315
Osteoclastoma of bone, 18
Osteofibroma of jawbones, 136, 426
Osteogenic disease, 151, 166
Osteogenic fibroma of bone, 107
Osteogenic sarcoma, juxtacortical (*see* Juxtacortical osteogenic sarcoma)
Osteogenic sarcoma of bone, 46, 60, 100, 104, 107, 110, 114, 134, 164, 232, 256–278, 286, 304, 310, 314, 318, 331, 363, 426
clinical considerations, 257
clinical complaints and findings, 257
incidence, 257
localization, 257
multicentric primary, 266
serum alkaline phosphatase, 258
differential diagnosis, 272
chondrosarcoma, 274
fibrosarcoma, 274
fibrous dysplasia, 275
juxtacortical osteogenic sarcoma, 274
other lesions, 275
metastasis of, 266, 277
nomenclature, 256
osteolytic and sclerosing, 28, 60, 260, 267
pathologic findings, 260
gross, 262
microscopic, 268
phosphatase in tumor tissue, 272
terminology in relation to pathologic features, 260
primary multicentric, 266
prognosis, 276
roentgenographic findings, 267
trauma as a factor in, 258
treatment, 276
Osteogenic sarcoma of soft parts invading bone, 521–527
clinical considerations, 521
differential diagnosis. 526
post-traumatic myositis ossificans, 527
pseudomalignant osseous tumor of soft tissues, 526
pathologic findings, 524
roentgenographic findings, 522
Osteoid-osteoma, 90, 92–106, 112, 275
clinical considerations, 94

Osteoid-osteoma, clinical considerations, clinical complaints and findings, 94
aspirin as palliative for pain, 95
sympathetic synovitis, 95
incidence, 94
localization, 94
delimitation of concept, 92
differential diagnosis, 96, 104
bone abscess, 98, 104
enostosis, solitary, 96, 104
osteochondritis dissecans, 96
osteogenic sarcoma, 100, 104
nature and genesis, 102
nomenclature, 94
giant osteoid-osteoma, 94, 107, 114
pathologic findings, 98
recurrence, 105
roentgenographic findings, 95
trauma as a factor in, 95
treatment, 105
Osteolytic *vs.* osteoplastic cancer metastases, 604
Osteoma, fibrous, of jawbones, 118, 136, 138, 426
Osteoma of skull bones, 138
Osteomyelitis complicated by sarcoma, 476
Osteomyelitis complicated by squamous cell carcinoma, 474
Osteomyelitis complicating radiation osteitis, 490
Osteomyelitis, hemorrhagic, 18
Osteopetrosis, 399
Osteoplastic *vs.* osteolytic cancer metastases, 604
Osteosarcoma of bone (*see* Osteogenic sarcoma)
Osteosclerosis, 399, 404

P

PAGET's disease of bone, 20, 128, 257, 266, 463–472
giant-cell tumor complicating, 20, 470
sarcoma complicating, 463
clinical emergence of the, 466
clinical findings, 468
incidence, 464
pathologic findings, 469
roentgenographic findings, 468, 469
serum alkaline phosphatase, 469
treatment and prognosis, 470
Para-articular chondroma, 198, 520, 558, 567
Parosteal osteogenic sarcoma (*see* Juxtacortical osteogenic sarcoma)
Parosteal osteoma (*see* Juxtacortical osteogenic sarcoma)
Periapical cyst of jawbones, 428
Periodontal (radicular) cysts, 428
Periosteal chondroma (*see* Juxtacortical chondroma)
Periosteal desmoid, 82
Periostitis, post-traumatic, 286, 292
Peripheral chondrosarcoma of bone (*see* Chondrosarcoma of bone, peripheral)
Peripheral giant-cell reparative granuloma, 426
Phemister's classification of primary bone tumors, 10
Phosphatase, serum alkaline, in fibrous dysplasia, 124, 139
in myeloma, 376
in osteogenic sarcoma of bone, 258, 272
in Paget's disease, 469
with skeletal metastases, 613
Pigmentation, cutaneous, in fibrous dysplasia, 120
in neurofibromatosis, 242
Pigmented synovitis, diffuse villonodular (*see* Synovitis, diffuse pigmented villonodular)
Pigmented synovitis, localized nodular (*see* Synovitis, localized nodular)
Pigmented tenosynovitis, diffuse villonodular, 554–556
Pigmented tenosynovitis, localized nodular (*see* Tenosynovitis, localized nodular)
Pigmented villonodular bursitis, 532, 548
Plasma cell leukemia, 372, 375
Plasma cell myeloma (*see* Myelomatosis)
Plasmacytoma of bone, solitary, 370, 379
Polyostotic fibrous dysplasia, 118
Postradiation injury, 479–491
general considerations, 479
genetic effects, 482
leukemia, 480
radiation osteitis, 482
fracture complicating, 491
osteomyelitis complicating, 490
retardation of bone growth, 490
Postradiation sarcoma (*see* Radiation-provoked bone sarcoma)
Post-traumatic myositis ossificans, 286, 290, 527
Post-traumatic periostitis, 286, 292
Primary chondrosarcoma of bone, 314
Primary lymphoma of bone (*see* Lymphoma primary in bone)
Primary multicentric osteogenic sarcoma of bone, 266
Primary reticulum cell sarcoma of bone, 275, 366, 416 (*see also* Lymphoma primary in bone)
Primordial cyst of jawbones, 430
Prostatic cancer, skeletal metastasis from, 598, 605
Pseudarthrosis in neurofibromatosis, 250
Pseudomalignant osseous tumor of soft tissues, 526
Pulmonary hypertrophic osteoarthropathy, 613–617
clinical considerations, 613
pathologic findings, 616

R

RADIATION osteitis, 479, 482–500
bone growth, retardation of, 390
damaging effects of external radiation, 484
damaging effects of internal radiation, 484, 497
fracture complicating, 491
osteomyelitis complicating, 490

Radiation osteitis, pathologic findings, 488
roentgenographic findings, 486
Radiation-provoked bone sarcoma, 479, 491–501
following external radiation, 491–497
of benign chondroblastoma, 44, 497
of fibrous dysplasia, 497
of giant-cell tumor, 42, 494
of solitary bone cyst, 74, 496
following internal radiation, 479–482, 497–501
for therapeutic purposes, 498
in watch dial workers, 498
Radicular (periodontal) cysts, 428
Radioactive isotopes, damaging effects of, 479–501
Radium, damaging effects of, 479–501
Recklinghausen's disease of bone, 118
Registry of Bone Sarcoma classification, 9, 10, 256, 279
Residual cyst of jawbones, 428
Retardation of bone growth following radiation, 490
Reticulosarcoma of bone marrow (*see* Ewing's sarcoma)
Reticulum cell sarcoma, 414, 419, 584
Reticulum cell sarcoma, primary, of bone, 275, 366, 416 (*see also* Lymphoma primary in bone)
Rhabdomyosarcoma invading bone, 513–516
alveolar, 514
botryoid, 514
embryonal, 514
pleomorphic, 513
Roentgenographic *vs.* anatomic findings relating to skeletal metastases, 602–604
Round cell sarcoma of bone (*see* Ewing's sarcoma)
Routes of cancer metastasis to skeleton, 590–593

S

SARCOCARCINOMA, 586
Sarcoma complicating enchondroma, solitary, 180, 326, 463
enchondromatosis, 194, 320, 463
exostosis, multiple, 164, 463
exostosis, solitary, 150, 463
fibrous dysplasia, 134
giant-cell tumor, 42, 494
osteomyelitis, 476
Paget's disease, 463
Sarcoma of bone following irradiation, 491–501
of benign chondroblastoma, 53, 497
of fibrous dysplasia, 497
of giant-cell tumor, 42, 494
of solitary bone cyst, 74, 496
Sarcoma, synovial (*see* Synovial sarcoma)
Scoliosis in neurofibromatosis, 250
Secondary chondrosarcoma of bone, 314
Serum calcium, in metastatic cancer, 608, 610, 612
in myeloma, 376
Serum proteins in myeloma, 378
Bence Jones, 378, 379
hyperglobulinemia, 379
Skeletal changes in leukemia, 396–406
Skeletal changes in lymphoma, 407–424
Skeletal hemangiomatosis, 237
Solitary bone cyst, 23, 40, 54, 58, 60, 63–75, 134, 173, 182, 211, 241, 310
active and latent, 72, 74
clinical considerations, 63
clinical complaints, 64
fracture healing, 64
incidence, 63
localization, 63
differential diagnosis, 72
aneurysmal bone cyst, 74
enchondroma, 73
eosinophilic granuloma, 73
fibrous dysplasia (solitary), 73
giant-cell tumor, 73
natural course of, 72
pathogenesis, 70
traumatic factor in, 64, 70
pathologic findings, 68
roentgenographic findings, 64
sarcoma following radiation of, 74, 496
treatment, 74
recurrence, 74
Solitary enchondroma, 23, 46, 52, 53, 73, 136, 169–195, 198, 211, 314, 318, 326, 426
clinical considerations, 169
age and sex incidence, 169
clinical complaints and findings, 172
localization, 169
differential diagnosis, 182
benign chondroblastoma, 182
bone infarct, 182
epithelial inclusion cyst, 173
fibrous dysplasia, solitary focus of, 173, 182
giant-cell tumor, 173, 177, 182
osteochondroma, 173
solitary bone cyst, 173, 182
pathogenesis, 174
pathologic findings, 176
gross, 176
microscopic, 177
evaluation of benignity, 178
roentgenographic findings, 172
sarcomatous transformation, 180
treatment and prognosis, 182
Solitary osteocartilaginous exostosis, 143–168. 314
clinical considerations, 143
clinical complaints, 144
incidence, 143
localization, 144
pathologic findings, 146
roentgenographic findings, 148
sarcoma as a complication, 150
treatment, 150
Strontium-90, damaging effects of, 479–501
Subungual exostosis, 143
Sympathicoblastoma, 363
Synovial chondromatosis, 198, 558–566, 582
clinical considerations, 558
differential diagnosis, 564
pathologic findings, 560

Synovial chondromatosis, pathologic findings,
gross, 560
microscopic, 562
roentgenographic findings, 559
treatment, 566
Synovial hemangioma (*see* Hemangioma of joints)
Synovial sarcoma (synovioma), 213, 216, 220, 221, 222, 576–588
clinical considerations, 577
clinical complaints and findings, 578
incidence, 577
localization, 577
differential diagnosis, 582, 586
chondromatosis, synovial, 582
chondrosarcoma, soft-tissue, 582
fibrosarcoma, soft-tissue, 582, 584
hemangioma, 582
pigmented villonodular synovitis, 582, 586
reticulum cell sarcoma, 584
sarcoma, undifferentiated, 584
nomenclature, 577
pathologic findings, 582
prognosis, 586
roentgenographic findings, 580
treatment, 586
Synovioma, benign giant-cell, 533, 544, 577
Synovitis, diffuse pigmented villonodular, 532, 534–545, 582, 586
clinical considerations, 534
nomenclature, 532, 533
pathogenesis, 542
pathologic findings, 538
gross, 538
microscopic, 540
roentgenographic findings, 538
bone erosion, 533, 538
treatment, 545
Synovitis, localized nodular, 532, 545–548
clinical considerations, 545
nomenclature, 532, 533
pathologic findings, 546
gross, 546
microscopic, 548
Synovitis, sympathetic, in osteoid-osteoma, 95

T

Tenosynovial chondromatosis, 566
Tenosynovial hemangioma, 572
Tenosynovitis, diffuse pigmented villonodular, 554–556
Tenosynovitis, localized nodular, 200, 549–554
clinical considerations, 549
nomenclature, 532, 533
Tenosynovitis, localized nodular, pathologic findings, 549
gross, 549
microscopic, 552
treatment, 554
Thyroid cancer, skeletal metastasis from, 596
Traumatic cyst of mandible, 434
Tuberous sclerosis, 246
Tumeur à myéloplaxes, 18
Tumors developing at sites of osteomyelitis, 472–478
Tumors developing at sites of Paget's disease, 463–472
Tumors invading bone from overlying soft parts, 502–531
Tumors metastatic to the skeleton (*see* Metastasis of tumors to skeleton)

U

Unicameral bone cyst (*see* Solitary bone cyst)

V

Vascular tumors of bone, benign, 224–239
Vascular tumors of bone, malignant, 341–349
Vascular tumors of soft tissues invading bone, 527–530
glomus tumor, 530
hemangioma, localized, 527
hemangiomatosis, 527
Vertebral hemangioma (*see* Hemangioma of bone)
Vertebral lipoma, 228
Vertebral vein system, 592
anatomic connections, 592
metastasis via, 592
Vestigial cysts of jawbones, 434
Villonodular bursitis, pigmented, 532, 548
Villonodular synovitis, localized (*see* Synovitis, localized nodular)
Villonodular synovitis, pigmented (*see* Synovitis, diffuse pigmented villonodular)
Villonodular tenosynovitis, localized (*see* Tenosynovitis, localized nodular)
Villonodular tenosynovitis, pigmented diffuse, 554–556

X

Xanthofibroma of bone, 90
Xanthogranuloma of bone, 83, 90
Xanthogranuloma of tendon sheath, 533
Xanthoma of bone, 83, 90
Xanthoma of tendon sheath, 533
Xanthoma tuberosum multiplex, 549
*X*-rays, damaging effects of, 479–501